BIOMEDICAL ETHICS

SIXTH EDITION

BIOMEDICAL ETHICS

THOMAS A. MAPPES
Frostburg State University

DAVID DEGRAZIA
George Washington University

Boston   Burr Ridge, IL   Dubuque, IA   Madison, WI   New York   San Francisco   St. Louis
Bangkok   Bogotá   Caracas   Lisbon   London   Madrid
Mexico City   Milan   New Delhi   Seoul   Singapore   Sydney   Taipei   Toronto

McGraw-Hill Higher Education

A Division of The **McGraw·Hill** *Companies*

BIOMEDICAL ETHICS, SIXTH EDITION

Published by McGraw-Hill Higher Education, an imprint of The McGraw-Hill Companies, Inc., 1221 Avenue of the Americas, New York, NY 10020. Copyright © 2006, 2001, 1996, 1991, 1986, 1981 by The McGraw-Hill Companies, Inc. All rights reserved. No part of this publication may be reproduced or distributed in any form or by any means, or stored in a database or retrieval system, without the prior written consent of The McGraw-Hill Companies, Inc., including, but not limited to, in any network or other electronic storage or transmission, or broadcast for distance learning.

Some ancillaries, including electronic and print components, may not be available to customers outside the United States.

This book is printed on acid-free paper.

3 4 5 6 7 8 9 0 QPF/QPF 0 9 8 7 6

ISBN 978-0-07-297644-1
MHID 0-07-297644-6

Editor-in-chief: *Emily J. Barrosse*
Publisher: *Lyn Uhl*
Senior sponsoring editor: *Jon-David Hague*
Editorial coordinator: *Allison Rona*
Marketing manager: *Zina Craft*
Project manager: *Judy Ludowitz/Carlisle Publishers Services*
Production supervisor: *Tandra Jorgensen*
Design manager: *Preston Thomas*

This book was set in 10/12 Times Roman by Carlisle Communications and printed on 45# New Era Matte by Quebecor World, Fairfield.

Library of Congress Cataloging-in-Publication Data

Biomedical ethics / [edited by] Thomas A. Mappes, David DeGrazia.
  -- 6th ed.
    p. ; cm.
  Includes bibliographical references.
  ISBN 0-07-297644-6
  1. Medical ethics. 2. Bioethics.   I. Mappes, Thomas A.
 II. DeGrazia, David.
  [DNLM: 1. Bioethics. 2. Ethics, Medical.   W 50 B6153 2005]
 R724.B49 2005
 174.2--dc22
                          2005017337

ABOUT THE AUTHORS

THOMAS A. MAPPES holds a B.S. in chemistry from the University of Dayton and a Ph.D. in philosophy from Georgetown University. He is professor of philosophy at Frostburg State University, where he has taught since 1973. He is the coeditor (with Jane S. Zembaty) of *Social Ethics: Morality and Social Policy* (McGraw-Hill, 6th ed., 2002) and his published work appears in journals such as *American Philosophical Quarterly* and *Kennedy Institute of Ethics Journal.*

DAVID DeGRAZIA earned a B.A. from the University of Chicago, an M.St. from Oxford University, and a Ph.D. from Georgetown University, each in philosophy. He is professor of philosophy at George Washington University, where he has taught since 1989. His publications include *Taking Animals Seriously* (Cambridge University Press, 1996), *Human Identity and Bioethics* (Cambridge University Press, 2005), and articles in such journals as *Philosophy and Public Affairs, The Philosophical Forum, The Hastings Center Report,* and *History of Philosophy Quarterly.*

In memory of Albin J. Mappes (1919-2003)

CONTENTS

Preface   *xvii*

CHAPTER 1   GENERAL INTRODUCTION   1

THE NATURE OF BIOMEDICAL ETHICS   1

RECENTLY DOMINANT ETHICAL THEORIES   4
The Critical Assessment of Competing Ethical Theories   5
Teleological Versus Deontological Theories   6
Act-Utilitarianism   7
Rule-Utilitarianism   13
Kantian Deontology   17
W. D. Ross's Theory of Prima Facie Duties   23

THE PRINCIPLES OF BIOMEDICAL ETHICS   26

ALTERNATIVE DIRECTIONS AND METHODS   27
Virtue Ethics   28
The Ethics of Care and Feminist Ethics   30
Casuistry: Case-Based Reasoning In Historical Context   33
Reflective Equilibrium and Appeals to Coherence   36

CONFRONTING ETHICAL RELATIVISM   38

FUNDAMENTAL CONCEPTS AND PRINCIPLES   40
Autonomy   40
Liberty-Limiting Principles   46
Paternalism   48

NOTES   53

ANNOTATED BIBLIOGRAPHY   55

APPENDIX: SELECTED REFERENCE SOURCES IN BIOMEDICAL
     ETHICS   57
Print Resources   57
Web Resources   57

CHAPTER 2   THE PHYSICIAN-PATIENT RELATIONSHIP   59

INTRODUCTION   59
Physicians' Obligations and Virtues   59
Paternalism and Respect for Patient Autonomy   60
Truth Telling   62
Informed Consent   64
The Practice of Medicine in a Multicultural Society   67
Contested Therapies Within the Physician-Patient Relationship   67
Conflicts of Interest, Problems of Conscience, and Managed Care   69
Notes   70

PHYSICIANS' OBLIGATIONS AND VIRTUES   70
The Hippocratic Oath   70
Council on Ethical and Judicial Affairs, American Medical Association,
    Fundamental Elements of the Patient-Physician Relationship   71
Edmund D. Pellegrino, *The Virtuous Physician and the
    Ethics of Medicine*   72

PHYSICIAN-PATIENT MODELS AND PATIENT AUTONOMY   76
James F. Childress and Mark Siegler, *Metaphors and Models
    of Doctor-Patient Relationships: Their Implications for Autonomy*   76
Terrence F. Ackerman, *Why Doctors Should Intervene*   85

TRUTH TELLING   90
Roger Higgs, *On Telling Patients the Truth*   90
Benjamin Freedman, *Offering Truth: One Ethical Approach to the Uninformed
    Cancer Patient*   95

INFORMED CONSENT   102
Judge Spotswood W. Robinson III, *Opinion in* Canterbury v. Spence   102
President's Commission for the Study of Ethical Problems
    in Medicine and Biomedical and Behavioral Research,
    The Values Underlying Informed Consent   106
Howard Brody, *Transparency: Informed Consent in Primary Care*   112

THE PRACTICE OF MEDICINE IN A MULTICULTURAL SOCIETY   118
Ruth Macklin, *Ethical Relativism in a Multicultural Society*   118
Kenneth Kipnis, *Quality Care and the Wounds of Diversity*   127

CONTESTED THERAPIES WITHIN THE PHYSICIAN-PATIENT
RELATIONSHIP   131
Franklin G. Miller, Howard Brody, and Kevin C. Chung,
    Cosmetic Surgery and the Internal Morality of Medicine   131
Claudia Mills, *One Pill Makes You Smarter: An Ethical
    Appraisal of the Rise of Ritalin*   140

CONFLICTS OF INTEREST, PROBLEMS OF CONSCIENCE, AND
MANAGED CARE   144
Marcia Angell, *The Doctor as Double Agent*   144
Daniel Callahan, *Managed Care and the Goals of Medicine*   149
James F. Childress, *Conscience and Conscientious Actions in the
    Context of MCOs*   154

ANNOTATED BIBLIOGRAPHY   159

CHAPTER 3   **HOSPITALS, NURSES, FAMILIES, AND MEDICAL CONFIDENTIALITY   162**

INTRODUCTION   162
Professional Statements Regarding Patients' Rights and Professionals'
    Obligations   162
The Role and Responsibilities of Nurses   163
Families and Medical Decision Making   164
Confidentiality and Conflicting Obligations   168
Notes   169

PROFESSIONAL STATEMENTS   170
American Hospital Association, *The Patient Care Partnership: Understanding*
    Expectations, Rights and Responsibilities   170
American Nurses Association, *Code of Ethics for Nurses*   172

THE ROLE AND RESPONSIBILITIES OF NURSES   173
Lisa H. Newton, *In Defense of the Traditional Nurse*   173
Helga Kuhse, *Advocacy or Subservience for the Sake of Patients?*   180
Amy M. Haddad, *The Nurse/Physician Relationship and Ethical*
    Decision Making   188

FAMILIES AND MEDICAL DECISION MAKING   192
Thomas A. Mappes and Jane S. Zembaty, *Patient Choices, Family Interests,*
    and Physician Obligations   192
Bonnie Poitras Tucker, *Deaf Culture, Cochlear Implants, and*
    Elective Disability   201
Sherri A. Groveman, *The Hanukkah Bush: Ethical Implications in the*
    Clinical Management of Intersex   207

CONFIDENTIALITY   211
Justice Mathew O. Tobriner, *Majority Opinion in* Tarasoff v. Regents
    of the University of California   211
Justice William P. Clark, *Dissenting Opinion in* Tarasoff v. Regents
    of the University of California   215
Please Don't Tell!: A Case About HIV and Confidentiality (with commentaries
    by Leonard Fleck and Marcia Angell)   218

ANNOTATED BIBLIOGRAPHY   222

CHAPTER 4   **HUMAN AND ANIMAL RESEARCH   224**

INTRODUCTION   224
Conceptual Issues   224
The Justification of Research Using Human Subjects   225
The Informed-Consent Requirement   227
Proxy Consent for Research Subjects Incapable of Informed
    Consent   228
Experimental Design and Research in Developing Nations   230
Animal Research   232
Notes   233

ETHICAL CODES   234
The Nuremberg Code   234
World Medical Association, *Declaration of Helsinki*   235

Council for International Organizations of Medical Sciences, *International Guiding Principles for Biomedical Research Involving Animals*   239

RESEARCH INVOLVING "VULNERABLE" POPULATIONS   240
Barry F. Brown, *Proxy Consent for Research on the Incompetent Elderly*   240
Patricia A. King, *The Dangers of Difference*   247
Alexander Morgan Capron, *Ethical and Human-Rights Issues in Research on Mental Disorders that May Affect Decision-Making Capacity*   251

EXPERIMENTAL DESIGN AND RANDOMIZED CLINICAL TRIALS   257
Samuel Hellman and Deborah S. Hellman, *Of Mice but Not Men: Problems of the Randomized Clinical Trial*   257
Don Marquis, *How to Resolve an Ethical Dilemma Concerning Randomized Clinical Trials*   262

CLINICAL TRIALS IN DEVELOPING COUNTRIES   266
Leonard H. Glantz, George J. Annas, Michael A. Grodin, and Wendy K. Mariner, *Research in Developing Countries: Taking Benefit Seriously*   266
Baruch Brody, *Ethical Issues in Clinical Trials in Developing Countries*   272

ANIMAL RESEARCH   276
Carl Cohen, *The Case for the Use of Animals in Biomedical Research*   276
Edwin Converse Hettinger, *The Responsible Use of Animals in Biomedical Research*   283
David DeGrazia, *The Ethics of Animal Research: What Are the Prospects for Agreement?*   289

ANNOTATED BIBLIOGRAPHY   299

CHAPTER 5   DEATH AND DECISIONS REGARDING LIFE-SUSTAINING TREATMENT   302

INTRODUCTION   302
The Definition and Determination of Death   302
Competent Adults and the Refusal of Life-Sustaining Treatment   304
DNR Orders and Medical Futility   305
Advance Directives and Treatment Decisions for Incompetent Adults   306
The Treatment of Impaired Infants   307
Notes   308

THE DEFINITION AND DETERMINATION OF DEATH   309
President's Commission for the Study of Ethical Problems in Medicine and Biomedical and Behavioral Research, *Why "Update" Death?*   309
Charles M. Culver and Bernard Gert, *The Definition and Criterion of Death*   312
Martin Benjamin, *Pragmatism and the Determination of Death*   319

**COMPETENT ADULTS AND THE REFUSAL OF LIFE-SUSTAINING
TREATMENT   327**

Council on Ethical and Judicial Affairs, American Medical Association,
    Withholding and Withdrawing Life-Sustaining Treatment   327

Tia Powell and Bruce Lowenstein, *Refusing Life-Sustaining Treatment After
    Catastrophic Injury: Ethical Implications*   330

Vicki Michel, *Suicide by Persons with Disabilities Disguised as the Refusal of
    Life-Sustaining Treatment*   335

DNR ORDERS AND MEDICAL FUTILITY   340

Tom Tomlinson and Howard Brody, *Ethics and Communication in Do-Not-
    Resuscitate Orders*   340

Mark R. Wicclair, *Medical Futility: A Conceptual and Ethical
    Analysis*   345

**ADVANCE DIRECTIVES AND TREATMENT DECISIONS FOR
INCOMPETENT ADULTS   350**

Thomas A. Mappes, *Some Reflections on Advance Directives*   350

Norman L. Cantor, *My Annotated Living Will*   357

Rebecca Dresser, *The Conscious Incompetent Patient*   363

THE TREATMENT OF IMPAIRED INFANTS   365

John A. Robertson, *Involuntary Euthanasia of Defective Newborns*   365

Members of The Hastings Center Research Project on the Care of Imperiled
    Newborns, *Standards of Judgment for Treatment of Imperiled
    Newborns*   371

ANNOTATED BIBLIOGRAPHY   375

**CHAPTER 6   SUICIDE, PHYSICIAN-ASSISTED SUICIDE, AND ACTIVE
EUTHANASIA   377**

INTRODUCTION   377

What Is Suicide?   377

The Morality of Suicide   379

The Morality of Active Euthanasia   379

Physician-Assisted Suicide   381

Physician-Assisted Suicide, Active Euthanasia, and Social Policy   382

Notes   384

THE MORALITY OF SUICIDE   384

Immanuel Kant, *Suicide*   384

R. B. Brandt, *The Morality and Rationality of Suicide*   388

THE MORALITY OF ACTIVE EUTHANASIA   395

James Rachels, *Active and Passive Euthanasia*   395

Daniel Callahan, *Killing and Allowing to Die*   399

Dan W. Brock, *Voluntary Active Euthanasia*   401

**THE SUPREME COURT, PHYSICIAN-ASSISTED SUICIDE, AND
TERMINAL SEDATION   404**

Chief Justice William H. Rehnquist, *Opinion of the Court in
    Washington v. Glucksberg*   404

Chief Justice William H. Rehnquist, *Opinion of the Court in
    Vacco v. Quill*   409

Justice Sandra Day O'Connor, *Concurring Opinion in* Washington v. Glucksberg *and* Vacco v. Quill   413

David Orentlicher, *The Supreme Court and Physician-Assisted Suicide: Rejecting Assisted Suicide But Embracing Euthanasia*   414

PHYSICIAN-ASSISTED SUICIDE, ACTIVE EUTHANASIA, AND SOCIAL POLICY   417

Timothy E. Quill, Christine K. Cassel, and Diane E. Meier, *Care of the Hopelessly Ill: Proposed Clinical Criteria for Physician-Assisted Suicide*   417

The Oregon Death with Dignity Act   420

Franklin G. Miller, Timothy E. Quill, Howard Brody, John C. Fletcher, Lawrence O. Gostin, and Diane E. Meier, *Regulating Physician-Assisted Death*   426

John D. Arras, *On the Slippery Slope in the Empire State: The New York State Task Force on Physician-Assisted Death*   431

James L. Bernat, Bernard Gert, and R. Peter Mogielnicki, *Patient Refusal of Hydration and Nutrition: An Alternative to Physician-Assisted Suicide or Voluntary Active Euthanasia*   438

ANNOTATED BIBLIOGRAPHY   445

CHAPTER 7   ABORTION AND RESEARCH ON EMBRYONIC STEM CELLS   448

INTRODUCTION   448

Abortion: The Ethical Issue   448

The Conservative View and the Liberal View   450

Moderate Views   451

Abortion and Social Policy   453

Research on Embryonic Stem Cells   455

Notes   456

THE MORALITY OF ABORTION   457

Pope John Paul II, *The Unspeakable Crime of Abortion*   457

Mary Anne Warren, *On the Moral and Legal Status of Abortion*   459

Don Marquis, *Why Abortion is Immoral*   466

Judith Jarvis Thomson, *A Defense of Abortion*   471

Margaret Olivia Little, *The Morality of Abortion*   479

ABORTION AND SOCIAL POLICY   483

Justice Harry Blackmun, *Majority Opinion in* Roe v. Wade   483

George J. Annas, *"Partial-Birth Abortion" and the Supreme Court*   488

RESEARCH ON EMBRYONIC STEM CELLS   493

National Institutes of Health, *Stem Cells: A Primer*   493

Bonnie Steinbock, *What Does "Respect for Embryos" Mean in the Context of Stem Cell Research?*   498

President's Council on Bioethics, *The Moral Case Against Cloning-for-Biomedical-Research*   501

ANNOTATED BIBLIOGRAPHY   508

CHAPTER 8   GENETICS AND HUMAN REPRODUCTION   511

INTRODUCTION   511
Genetic Disease and the Language of Genetics   511
Prenatal Diagnosis and Selective Abortion   513
Morality and Reproductive Risk   514
Reproductive Technologies and the Treatment of Infertility   514
Reproductive Technologies: Ethical Concerns   516
Human Cloning   517
Preimplantation Genetic Diagnosis   519
Genetic Engineering, Gene Therapy, and Enhancement   519
Notes   520

REPRODUCTIVE RISK, PRENATAL DIAGNOSIS, AND SELECTIVE ABORTION   521
Leon R. Kass, *Implications of Prenatal Diagnosis for the Human Right to Life*   521
Laura M. Purdy, *Genetics and Reproductive Risk: Can Having Children be Immoral?*   526

REPRODUCTIVE TECHNOLOGIES   532
Peter Singer, *IVF: The Simple Case*   532
Susan Sherwin, *Feminist Ethics and In Vitro Fertilization*   536
The New York State Task Force on Life and the Law, *Ethical Debates about Infertility and its Treatment*   541
President's Council on Bioethics, *Assisted Reproduction*   548

GAMETE DONATION AND SURROGACY   553
Thomas H. Murray, *Families, the Marketplace, and Values: New Ways of Making Babies*   553
Bonnie Steinbock, *Surrogate Motherhood as Prenatal Adoption*   561

HUMAN CLONING   565
Leon R. Kass, *Cloning of Human Beings*   565
Thomas H. Murray, *Even If It Worked, Cloning Wouldn't Bring Her Back*   568
Robert Wachbroit, *Genetic Encores: The Ethics of Human Cloning*   571

PREIMPLANTATION GENETIC DIAGNOSIS   577
John A. Robertson, *Extending Preimplantation Genetic Diagnosis: Medical and Non-Medical Uses*   577
President's Council on Bioethics, *Selecting Embryos for Desired Traits*   583

GENE THERAPY   586
Sophia Kolehmainen, *The Dangerous Promise of Gene Therapy*   586
Marina Cavazzana-Calvo, Adrian Thrasher, and Fulvio Mavilio, *The Future of Gene Therapy: Balancing the Risks and the Benefits of Clinical Trials*   590
LeRoy Walters and Julie Gage Palmer, *Germ-Line Gene Therapy*   594

GENETIC ENHANCEMENT   601
Walter Glannon, *Genetic Enhancement*   601
Dan W. Brock, *Genetic Engineering*   606

ANNOTATED BIBLIOGRAPHY   612

CHAPTER 9   SOCIAL JUSTICE AND HEALTH-CARE POLICY   615

INTRODUCTION   615
Justice, Rights, and Societal Obligations   617
Rationing, Managed Care, and Health-Care Reform
   in the United States   620
Systems of Health-Care Delivery and Finance: Four International
   Perspectives   624
Notes   627

JUSTICE, RIGHTS, AND SOCIETAL OBLIGATIONS   628
Allen Buchanan, *Justice: A Philosophical Review*   628
Kai Nielsen, *Autonomy, Equality and a Just Health Care System*   639

**RATIONING, MANAGED CARE, AND HEALTH-CARE REFORM IN THE
UNITED STATES   645**
Norman Daniels, *Is the Oregon Rationing Plan Fair?*   645
Allen Buchanan, *Managed Care: Rationing Without Justice, but not
   Unjustly*   652
Leonard M. Fleck, *Rationing: Don't Give Up*   660
Norman Daniels and James Sabin, *Closure, Fair Procedures, and Setting Limits
   Within Managed Care Organizations*   663
Ezekiel Emanuel, *Health Care Reform: Still Possible*   669

INTERNATIONAL MODELS AND PERSPECTIVES   672
Pat Armstrong, *Managing Care the Canadian Way*   672
John K. Iglehart, *Restoring the Status of an Icon: A Talk with Canada's
   Minister of Health*   674
Gerd Richter, *The German Health Care System*   681
Nicholas Mays and Justin Keen, *Will the Fudge on Equity Sustain the
   NHS into the Next Millennium?*   684
Giovanna Ruberto, *Ethics, Politics, and Priorities in the Italian
   Health-Care System*   689

ANNOTATED BIBLIOGRAPHY   694

Appendix: Case Studies   697
About the Contributors   719

PREFACE

This sixth edition of *Biomedical Ethics,* like its predecessors, is designed to provide an effective teaching instrument for courses in biomedical ethics. Although the basic character of the book remains unchanged, it has been substantially revised and updated. About one third of the book's readings are new to the sixth edition, and several new chapter sections have been developed. For example, there are now sections on contested therapies in the physician-patient relationship (Chapter 2), research on embryonic stem cells (Chapter 7), and preimplantation genetic diagnosis (Chapter 8). Other notable changes include the addition of a new pair of articles in Chapter 3—one article on cochlear implants, the other on the clinical management of intersex—dealing with difficult decisions that parents must sometimes make for their children, the inclusion in Chapter 4 of several new articles on the ethics of experimentation, the addition of an article in Chapter 5 that presents a disability-rights perspective on the refusal of life-sustaining treatment, the inclusion in Chapter 6 of the Oregon Death with Dignity Act, and an expanded treatment of gene therapy and genetic enhancement in Chapter 8. In Chapter 9, the reorganization of chapter material and the incorporation of three new articles has resulted in the formation of a section entitled "Rationing, Managed Care, and Health-Care Reform in the United States," and the section on international models and perspectives has been expanded to include two articles on the Canadian health-care system and one each on the German, English, and Italian systems. Also noteworthy, a discussion of ethical relativism has been added to the General Introduction (Chapter 1), and that chapter's appendix of reference sources in biomedical ethics has been expanded.

In this sixth edition we have retained the various structural features that made earlier editions of the book effective teaching instruments. We have maintained the comprehensive character of the text, have once again organized the subject matter so that it unfolds in an effective and natural fashion, and have retained helpful editorial features such as the argument sketches that precede each selection and the annotated bibliographies at the end of each chapter. We have also retained and updated the appendix of case studies. Finally, inasmuch as the value of any textbook anthology is largely dependent upon the quality of its readings, we have once again assembled a set of readings characterized by high-quality analysis and, to the greatest extent possible, clarity of writing style. As in the past, we have also taken care to choose readings that reflect diverse viewpoints with regard to the leading issues in biomedical ethics.

The introductions to each chapter of this book provide one of its most important editorial features. In the introductions we explicitly identify the central issues in each chapter and scan the various positions on these issues together with their supporting argumentation.

Whenever possible, we draw out the relationship between the arguments that appear in a certain chapter and the ethical concepts and approaches discussed in the General Introduction. Whenever necessary, we also provide background conceptual clarification and factual information. In this vein, as a matter of course, we explicate the meaning of technical biomedical terms and introduce relevant biomedical information. The purpose of the chapter introductions is to enhance the effectiveness of the book as a teaching instrument. This same central purpose is shared by the book's other editorial features, which include the argument sketches preceding each selection and the annotated bibliographies at the end of each chapter. The annotated bibliographies provide substantial guidance for further reading and research. The various entries in the bibliographies, like the various readings in each chapter, reflect diverse viewpoints.

The first three editions of *Biomedical Ethics* were developed through the joint efforts of Thomas A. Mappes and Jane S. Zembaty. This sixth edition, as well as the fourth and fifth, was developed through the joint efforts of Thomas A. Mappes and David DeGrazia. One of the present editors (T.A.M.) would like to express his gratitude to Jane Zembaty for three decades of friendship and professional collaboration (which is ongoing in connection with other projects). Both of the present editors (T.A.M. and D.D.) want to acknowledge their extensive indebtedness to her for numerous passages, analyses, organizational structures, and insights originally embodied in earlier editions and carried over to the sixth.

We wish to thank George Washington University and Frostburg State University for their support of this project. We are indebted to the Kennedy Institute, Georgetown University, whose bioethics library has been a significant ally in our research efforts. We greatly appreciate the helpful assistance of all the library staff, especially Martina Darragh and Mary Ruof. We are also indebted to the reference librarians at Frostburg State University and to the following professors who provided McGraw-Hill with useful review information: Jay Ciaffa, Xavier University of Louisiana; Gerald Dworkin, University of California, Davis; Karen L. Hornsby, North Carolina A & T State University; Christopher Williams, University of Nevada, Reno; and David Yount, Mesa Community College. We are especially grateful to Jon-David Hague and Allison Rona at McGraw-Hill, for their consistent responsiveness to our needs and concerns, and to Joy Kroeger-Mappes, Frostburg State University, for her valuable suggestions and advice through all the editions of this book. Finally, we must express our thanks to Shelley Drees for her valuable help with manuscript preparation, and to Vera Mappes and Brandy Ritchie for their assistance in proofreading.

Thomas A. Mappes
David DeGrazia

BIOMEDICAL
ETHICS

CHAPTER 1

GENERAL
INTRODUCTION

A number of ethical issues can be identified as associated with the practice of medicine, the pursuit of biomedical research, or both. This set of ethical issues constitutes the subject matter of biomedical ethics. The proper task of biomedical ethics is to advance reasoned analysis in an effort to clarify and resolve such issues. What we term "biomedical ethics" is also commonly termed "bioethics." Although both terms are very well established and can be used interchangeably, *biomedical ethics* has the virtue of making more explicit the concern with issues associated with the practice of medicine. In any case, it is necessary in this context to understand *the practice of medicine* in an inclusive way, as referring not only to the professional activities of physicians but also to the distinctive activities of other health-care professionals.

THE NATURE OF BIOMEDICAL ETHICS

In order to situate biomedical ethics properly as a subdiscipline within the more general discipline of ethics, it is necessary to consider the nature of ethics as a philosophical discipline. *Ethics,* understood as a philosophical discipline, can be conveniently defined as the "*philosophical* study of morality." As such, it must be immediately distinguished from the *scientific* study of morality, often called "descriptive ethics." The goal of descriptive ethics is to attain empirical knowledge about morality. The practitioner of descriptive ethics is dedicated to describing existing moral views and, subsequently, explaining such views by advancing an account of their causal origin. Moral views, no less than other aspects of human experience, provide behavioral and social scientists a range of phenomena that stand in need of explanation. For example, why does a certain individual have such a Victorian view of sexual morality? A Freudian psychologist might attempt an explanation in terms of basic Freudian categories and early childhood experience. Why does a particular group of people manifest such a high incidence of moral advocacy for physician-assisted suicide? A sociologist might study the group in question and ultimately suggest an explanation based on factors such as the following: Many members of the group have seen loved ones die only after extensive suffering. Many members of the group identify themselves as nonreligious.

Ethics as a philosophical discipline stands in contrast to descriptive ethics. (Hereafter, the expression *ethics* is used to designate the philosophical discipline, as distinct from descriptive ethics.) Philosophers commonly subdivide ethics into (1) normative ethics and (2) metaethics, although the precise relationship of these two branches is a matter of some dispute. In normative ethics, philosophers attempt to determine what is morally right and what is morally wrong with regard to human action.[1] In metaethics, philosophers are concerned with tasks such as analyzing the nature of moral judgments and specifying appropriate methods for the justification of particular moral judgments and theoretical systems. It seems plausible to maintain that deliberations in normative ethics are to some extent dependent upon and cannot be completely detached from metaethical considerations. Whatever the precise relationship between normative ethics and metaethics, it is important to see that *normative ethics* is logically distinct from *descriptive ethics.* Whereas descriptive ethics attempts to describe (and explain) those moral views that in fact *are accepted,* normative ethics attempts to establish which moral views are *justifiable* and thus *ought to be accepted.* In *general* normative ethics, the task is to advance and provide a reasoned justification of an overall theory of moral obligation, thereby establishing an ethical theory that provides a general answer to the question, "What is morally right and what is morally wrong?" In *applied* normative ethics, as opposed to general normative ethics, the task is to resolve particular moral problems—for example, the issue of whether abortion can be morally justified, and, if so, under what conditions.

In light of the distinctions just made, it is now possible to identify biomedical ethics as one branch of applied (normative) ethics.[2] The task of biomedical ethics is to resolve ethical problems associated with the practice of medicine and/or the pursuit of biomedical research. Clearly, since there are ethical problems associated with other aspects of life, there are other branches of applied ethics. Business ethics, for example, is concerned with the ethical problems associated with the transaction of business. Importantly, in all branches of applied ethics, the particular issues under discussion are *normative* in character. Is this particular practice right or wrong? Is it morally justifiable? In applied ethics, the concern is not to establish which moral views people do, in fact, have. That is a descriptive matter. The concern in applied ethics, as in general normative ethics, is to establish which moral views are justifiable.

Questions such as the following are raised in biomedical ethics: Is a physician morally obligated to tell a terminally ill patient that he or she is dying? Are breaches of medical confidentiality ever morally defensible? Can euthanasia be morally justified? Is surrogate motherhood morally justified? Normative ethical questions such as these are concerned with the morality of certain acts and practices. Other questions in biomedical ethics focus on the ethical justifiability of laws. For example, is society justified in having laws that restrict the availability of abortion? Should we have laws that prohibit physician-assisted suicide? Should we have laws that prohibit research on human cloning or embryonic stem cells? The appearance of questions of this latter type shows that deliberations in biomedical ethics are intertwined not only with deliberations in general normative ethics but also with deliberations in social-political philosophy and the philosophy of law. In these latter disciplines, a central theoretical question concerns the justifiable limits of law. Strictly speaking, if biomedical ethics is a type of applied ethics, ethics must be broadly understood as overlapping with social-political philosophy and the philosophy of law.

Although many of the ethical issues falling within the scope of biomedical ethics have historical roots, especially insofar as they are related to various codes of medical ethics, biomedical ethics did not crystallize into a full-fledged discipline until somewhat recently. Only since about 1970 have the various trappings of a relatively autonomous discipline become manifest. Numerous centers for research in biomedical ethics now exist. Three of the most prominent are the Hastings Center (now located in Garrison, New York), the Joseph and Rose Kennedy Institute of Ethics, Georgetown University (Washington, D.C.), and the Center for Bioethics, University of Pennsylvania (Philadelphia). New journals continue to appear, conferences abound, and the field has its own encyclopedia, *The Encyclopedia of Bioethics,* first published in 1978. An increasing number of philosophers, theologians, lawyers, and other professionals now identify biomedical ethics as an area of specialization.

If, as is clear, many of the ethical issues falling within the scope of biomedical ethics have historical precedents, why has the field emerged as a vigorous and highly visible discipline only somewhat recently? Two cultural developments are at the root of the contemporary prominence of biomedical ethics: (1) the awesome advance of biomedical research as attended by the resultant development of biomedical technology and (2) the practice of medicine in an increasingly complicated institutional setting.

Consider first the impact of recent biomedical research. It has been responsible not only for creating historically unprecedented ethical problems but also for adding new dimensions to old problems and making the resolution of those old problems a matter of greater urgency. Some developments—for example, those associated with reproductive technologies such as in vitro fertilization and, more recently, cloning—seem to present us with ethical problems that are genuinely unprecedented. More commonly, however, the advance of biomedical research has simply added complexity to old problems and created a sense of urgency with regard to their solution. Euthanasia is not a new problem; however, our ability to save the lives of severely impaired newborns who would have died in the past and our ability to sustain the biological processes of permanently unconscious patients have added new dimensions and, surely, a new urgency. Abortion is not a new problem, but the development of various techniques of prenatal diagnosis has created the new possibility of abortion based on genetic information. Indeed, the many successes of biomedical research in our own time, as manifested in the associated technological developments, call attention to the value of systematic biomedical research on human subjects and thus occasion reexamination of ethical constraints with regard to human experimentation.

The practice of medicine in an increasingly complicated institutional setting is, along with the advance of biomedical research, largely responsible for the contemporary prominence of biomedical ethics. In the past, the practice of medicine was largely confined within the bounds of the physician-patient relationship. Now, however, hospitals and other health-care institutions are intimately intertwined with physicians and allied personnel in the delivery of medical care. We have also witnessed an extension of the consumer rights movement into the health-care arena, a heightened emphasis on the legal requirements of informed consent, and an accompanying escalation of concern within the health-care community about legal liability. As a result, health-care professionals and institutions now find it necessary to pay closer attention to the interplay among medical, legal, and ethical considerations. Moreover, as a society we have become increasingly conscious of possible tensions between social justice and economic constraints—tensions that are acutely felt in confronting the general question of whether there is a right to health care, as well as specific problems of allocation such as those associated with managed care.

It is frequently said that biomedical ethics is an interdisciplinary field, and some explication of its interdisciplinary character might prove helpful. First, biomedical ethics is interdisciplinary within philosophy itself, inasmuch as deliberations in biomedical ethics are intertwined not only with deliberations in general normative ethics but also with deliberations in social-political philosophy and the philosophy of law. Second, biomedical ethics is interdisciplinary precisely because the issues under discussion are frequently approached not only from the vantage point of moral philosophy (the principal vantage point in the collection of readings in this text) but also from the vantage point of moral theology. Whereas philosophical arguments are constructed without presupposing the truth of any religious claims, that is, without reliance on religious *faith,* theological arguments are generally constructed within a faith framework. There is yet a third—and most significant—way in which biomedical ethics is interdisciplinary, and that is by reference to the disciplines of medicine and biology. Medical judgments and the findings of biology often play a crucial role in ethical deliberations. (The findings of the social sciences can be relevant as well.) It is also important to recognize that the *experience* of health-care professionals and biomedical researchers is often essential to ensure that ethical discussions retain firm contact with the concrete realities that permeate the practice of medicine and the pursuit of biomedical research.

Although the issues of biomedical ethics are essentially normative, they are intertwined with both conceptual issues and factual (i.e., empirical) issues. For example, suppose we are concerned with the ethical acceptability of intervention for the sake of preventing a person from committing suicide. Our basic concern is with a normative question; however, we must face the problem of clarifying the nature of suicide, a conceptual issue. For example, if a Jehovah's Witness, on the basis of religious principle, refuses a life-saving blood transfusion, is the resultant death to be classified as a suicide? In addition to facing conceptual perplexities, we are also faced with an important factual question: Do those who typically attempt suicide really want to die? Presumably psychologists have important things to tell us on this score. In the end, of course, we want to reach an ethical conclusion. However, ethical deliberations must proceed in the light of conceptual structures and factual beliefs. In the case of some issues in biomedical ethics, underlying factual issues are especially prominent. For example, in addressing the normative question of whether it is ever morally permissible to use children as research subjects, it is important to consider a factual question: To what extent can therapeutic techniques be developed for children in the absence of research employing children as research subjects? In the case of other issues in biomedical ethics, associated conceptual issues command special attention. For example, one could hardly discuss the normative issue of whether it is appropriate to transplant vital organs from brain-dead patients without closely examining the concept of death.

It is helpful to approach the literature of biomedical ethics with an eye toward distinguishing conceptual, factual, and normative issues. Furthermore, with regard to normative issues, which are the central issues of biomedical ethics, one cannot hope to situate argumentation in biomedical ethics properly without some awareness of the various types of ethical theory developed in general normative ethics. Such theories provide the frameworks within which many of the arguments in biomedical ethics are formulated.

RECENTLY DOMINANT ETHICAL THEORIES

An ethical theory provides a framework that can be used to determine what is morally right and morally wrong regarding human action in general, or what is morally good and morally bad regarding human character in general. The discussion of ethical theories in this section is restricted in two ways. First, consideration is limited to theories of right and wrong action, as opposed to theories of good and bad character (which fall naturally under the heading of virtue ethics, an approach that is explicated in a later section of this chapter). Second, consideration is limited to those theories of right and wrong action that commanded the most attention in the twentieth century. These recently dominant theories are frequently reflected in arguments advanced in biomedical ethics.

An ethical theory—as discussed in this section—provides an ordered set of moral standards (in some cases, simply one ultimate moral principle) that is to be used in assessing what is morally right and what is morally wrong regarding human action in general. A proponent of any such theory puts it forth as a framework with which a person can correctly determine, on any given occasion, what he or she (morally) ought to do.

THE CRITICAL ASSESSMENT OF COMPETING ETHICAL THEORIES

Since a number of competing ethical theories may be identified, the question that immediately arises is what criteria are relevant to an assessment of these competing theories. There is no easy way to answer this very fundamental and very controversial question, but let us start with those considerations whose relevance is unlikely to be disputed. Any theory in any field is rightly expected to be internally consistent. Thus, a theory can be faulted on the basis of inconsistency. In a similar vein, any theory is surely flawed to the extent that it is either unclear or incomplete. In addition, a theory should be as simple as it can be without entailing a failure to satisfy other relevant criteria, such as clarity and completeness.

If the above considerations are relevant to a critical assessment of theories in any field, we must yet identify considerations relevant to our particular concern, the critical assessment of (normative) ethical theories. Responsive to this task, it is suggested that the following criteria embody the two most important considerations. (1) The implications of an ethical theory must be largely reconcilable with our experience of the moral life. (2) An ethical theory must provide effective guidance where it is most needed, that is, in those situations where substantial moral considerations can be advanced on both sides of an issue. In embracing the priority of criteria 1 and 2 we are saying that an adequate ethical theory must achieve two major goals. An adequate ethical theory must accord with the moral life as we experience it, and it must function heuristically by guiding us when we are confronted with moral perplexity. An ethical theory should, on the one hand, make sense out of the moral life by exhibiting the basic features of our ordinary moral thinking. On the other hand, it should illuminate our moral judgment precisely where it is experienced to falter—in the face of moral dilemmas.

There is certainly no suggestion here that the standards embodied in criteria 1 and 2 can be applied in some mechanical fashion to assess the relative adequacy of a proposed ethical theory. Intellectual judgments on these matters are necessarily complex and subtle. In saying, for example, that an adequate ethical theory must accord with our experience of the moral life, we certainly do not want to insist that each and every divergence from the verdict of "commonsense morality" must be interpreted as counting against an ethical theory. Perhaps we would be better advised to revise our moral judgment in light of the theory. (In empirical science, fact-theory mismatches are sometimes resolved not by modifying the theory but by reinterpreting the facts in the light of the theory.) In embracing criterion 1 we undoubtedly commit ourselves to a point of view incompatible with the acceptance of an ethical theory that is revisionary in some wholesale sense, but we do not commit ourselves to the view that "commonsense morality" is sacrosanct. If an ethical theory successfully captures the basic features of our ordinary moral thinking, it will, of course, be true that its implications in large measure accord with our ordinary moral thinking. If the theory, however, cannot be reconciled with a relatively smaller range of our ordinary moral judgments, we may decide to interpret this disharmony as the product of some inadequacy in "commonsense morality" rather than as an inadequacy in the proposed theory.

TELEOLOGICAL VERSUS DEONTOLOGICAL THEORIES

With the introduction of criteria 1 and 2, we are now prepared to undertake a survey of alternative ethical theories. Our immediate concern is the identification, articulation, and critical consideration of those ethical theories that are the most prominent theories in general normative ethics—commanding the most attention in the twentieth century—and frequently reflected in argumentation advanced in biomedical ethics. In a later section, under the heading of "Alternative Directions and Methods," some additional theoretical perspectives that are important in biomedical ethics are presented.

In contemporary discussions, ethical theories are often grouped into two basic, and mutually exclusive, classes—*teleological* and *deontological*. Any ethical theory that claims the rightness and wrongness of human action is *exclusively* a function of the goodness and badness of the consequences resulting directly or indirectly from that action is a teleological theory. Consequences are all-important here. A deontological theory maintains, in contrast, that the rightness and wrongness of human action is *not exclusively* (in the extreme case, not at all) a function of the goodness and badness of consequences. Accordingly, a theory is deontological (rather than teleological) if it places limits on the relevance of teleological considerations. Thus, an ethical theory in which the moral rightness and wrongness of human action is construed as totally independent of the goodness and badness of consequences would be only one kind, albeit the strongest or most extreme kind, of deontological theory.

The most prominent teleological ethical theory is the theory known as "utilitarianism." The adequacy of utilitarianism and the issue of its proper explication continue to be significant concerns in contemporary discussions of ethical theory. For this reason, and especially because much argumentation in biomedical ethics is based on utilitarian reasoning, utilitarianism warrants our detailed attention. However, it should first be noted that utilitarianism is not the only ethical theory that is correctly categorized as teleological. One other notable teleological theory is the theory known as "ethical egoism." The basic principle of ethical egoism can be phrased as follows: *A person ought to act so as to promote his or her own self-interest.* An action is morally right if, when compared with possible alternatives, its consequences are such as to generate the greatest balance of good over evil *for the agent.* (The impact of action on other people is irrelevant except as it may indirectly affect the agent.) Ethical egoism is a teleological theory precisely because, by the terms of the theory, the rightness and wrongness of human action is exclusively a function of the goodness and badness of consequences.

Ethical egoism is an enormously problematic theory, one whose implications seem to be intensely at odds with our ordinary moral thinking. Under certain conditions, ethical egoism leads us to the conclusion that it is a person's moral obligation to perform an action that is flagrantly antisocial in nature. Consider this example. Mr. A loves to set buildings on fire; nothing makes him happier than watching a building burn. He recognizes that arson destroys property and subjects human life to serious risk, but he happens to be a thoroughly unsympathetic person, one whose well-being is not negatively affected by the misfortune

of others. Of course, it is not in A's self-interest (and thus would not be A's moral obligation) to burn down a building if there is a good chance that he will be caught. (The punishment for arson is severe.) However, if A is very clever and if it is virtually certain that he
will not be caught, ethical egoism seems to imply that arson is the morally right thing for
him to do.

Another problematic feature of ethical egoism is that it cannot be publicly advocated
without inconsistency. Suppose that Ms. B embraces ethical egoism. Accordingly, she considers it her moral obligation always to act in such a way as to promote her individual self-
interest. Should she now publicly advocate ethical egoism, that is, encourage others to
adopt the view that each person's moral obligation is to act in such a way as to promote his
or her individual self-interest? No. Since it is to *her* advantage that others *not* act egoisti-
cally, it follows that it would be immoral for her to publicly advocate ethical egoism.

In reducing morality to considerations of personal prudence, it can be argued, ethical
egoism destroys the very sense behind morality. Morality, it would seem, functions (at least
in part) to restrict the pursuit of personal self-interest. It is not that morality prohibits the
pursuit of personal self-interest; rather, it places limits on this pursuit. In "collapsing"
morality into prudence, ethical egoism does not accord with a commonly experienced phenomenon of the moral life, the tension between self-interest and morality, between "what
would be best for me" and "what is the morally right thing."

In fairness to ethical egoism, it must be noted that its proponents have sometimes devised ingenious arguments in an attempt to minimize the sort of difficulties just discussed.
However, ethical egoism is not widely defended in contemporary discussions of ethical theory, and it surely plays an insignificant role in discussions of biomedical ethics. It has been
introduced primarily as a notable instance of a teleological yet nonutilitarian theory. Attention will now be focused on utilitarianism.

In its classical formulation, utilitarianism is found most prominently in the works of two
English philosophers, Jeremy Bentham (1748–1832) and John Stuart Mill (1806–1873). In
contemporary discussions, a distinction is made between two kinds of utilitarianism—
act-utilitarianism and *rule-utilitarianism.* Although it is somewhat controversial whether a
significant distinction can be maintained between these two versions of utilitarianism, it is
presumed for the sake of exposition that two distinct utilitarian ethical theories can indeed
be articulated.[3]

ACT-UTILITARIANISM

Human action typically takes place within the fabric of our social existence. Thus, an action performed by one person often affects not only the agent but also the lives of many others. Consider a man who refuses to stop smoking even though he suffers from emphysema.
He will not be the only one to suffer the consequences; certainly those who care about him
will also. His refusal to give up smoking, since it has the effect of further damaging his
health, also produces a higher level of anxiety among the members of his family. Among
the other detrimental consequences of his continuing to smoke is the negative impact on
any nonsmokers in the vicinity when he smokes: annoyance, displeasure, and the like.
However, the various consequences of a single action are seldom uniformly good or uniformly bad. In addition to the bad consequences already indicated, there are also a number
of good consequences that result from the refusal to stop smoking. Most notably, the emphysema patient continues to derive the satisfaction associated with cigarette smoking. In

addition, it is likely that his continuing to smoke will make him less irritable around others. When the various consequences of a single action are fully analyzed, more often than not we find ourselves confronted with a mixture of good and bad. For example, if a person throws a late-night party, it is true that those in attendance may have a very good time, but it is also true that the neighbors may lose out on some much needed sleep.

The basic principle of act-utilitarianism can be stated as follows: *A person ought to act so as to produce the greatest balance of good over evil, everyone considered.* Act-utilitarianism stands in vivid contrast to ethical egoism, which directs a person always to act so as to produce the greatest balance of good over evil *for oneself* (i.e., the agent). The act-utilitarian is committed to the proposition that the interests of everyone affected by an action are to be weighed in the balance along with the interests of the agent. Everyone's interests are entitled to an impartial consideration. According to the act-utilitarian, an action is morally right if, when compared with possible alternatives, its likely consequences are such as to generate the greatest balance of good over evil, everyone considered. If we refer to the net balance of good over evil (everyone considered) that is likely to be produced by a certain action as its (overall) *utility,* then we can say that act-utilitarianism directs a person always to choose that alternative that has the greatest utility. Thus, we can express the basic principle of act-utilitarianism as follows: A person ought to act so as to maximize utility.

For the act-utilitarian, calculation is a paramount element in the moral assessment of action. The question is always this: What is the utility of each of my alternatives in this particular set of circumstances? However, any system of utilitarian calculation must ultimately be anchored in some conception of intrinsic value (i.e., that which is good or desirable in and of itself). The act that will maximize utility (by our definition) is the act that is likely to produce the greatest balance of good over evil, everyone considered. However, what is to count as "good" and what as "evil" in our calculations? The answers provided within the framework of classical utilitarianism reflect a so-called hedonistic theory of intrinsic value. According to Bentham, only pleasure (understood broadly to include any type of satisfaction or enjoyment) has intrinsic value; only pain (understood broadly to include any dissatisfaction, frustration, or displeasure) has intrinsic disvalue. According to Mill, only happiness has intrinsic value; only unhappiness has intrinsic disvalue. To what extent there is substantive disagreement between Bentham and Mill on this matter is a complex question that cannot be dealt with here. It should be mentioned, however, that many contemporary utilitarian thinkers have embraced more elaborate and nonhedonistic theories of intrinsic value.[4] Nevertheless, for the sake of exposition, we shall presume that a hedonistic theory of intrinsic value, in the spirit of Bentham and Mill, underlies utilitarian calculation.

In the spirit of act-utilitarianism, in order to determine what I should do in a certain situation, I must first attempt to delineate alternative paths of action. Next, I attempt to foresee the consequences (sometimes numerous and far-reaching) of each alternative action. Then I attempt, in each case, to evaluate the consequences and to weigh the good against the bad, considering the impact of my action on everyone whom it is likely to affect. Such a reckoning will reveal the act that is likely to produce the greatest balance of good over evil, and this act is the morally right act for me in my particular circumstances. (If it appears likely that two competing actions would produce the same balance of good over evil, then either action will qualify as morally correct.) In some situations, it is true that no matter what I do, more evil (pain or unhappiness) will come into the world than good (pleasure or happiness). In such unfortunate situations, according to the act-utilitarian, the morally right act is the one that will bring the least unfavorable balance of evil and good into the world.

Act-utilitarianism can rightly be understood as a form of "situation ethics." The act-utilitarian has no sympathy for the notion that certain kinds of actions are intrinsically wrong, that is, wrong by their very nature. Rather, a certain kind of action (e.g., lying) may be wrong in one set of circumstances yet right in another. The circumstances in which an action is to be performed are relevant to its morality (i.e., its rightness or wrongness) because the consequences of the action will vary depending upon the circumstances. Thus, the morality of action is a function of the situation confronting the agent—"situation ethics."

The situational character of act-utilitarianism is reflected in the act-utilitarian attitude toward moral rules. Among the "commonsense rules of morality" are the following: "do not kill," "do not injure," "do not steal," "do not lie," "do not break promises." According to the act-utilitarian, these rules are to be understood merely as rules of thumb. They are, for the most part, reliable guides for human action, especially relevant when time constraints undermine the possibility of careful calculation. In most circumstances, acting in accordance with a moral rule is the way to maximize utility, but in some cases this is not so. In these latter cases, whenever there is good reason to believe that breaking a moral rule will produce a greater balance of good over evil (everyone considered), the right thing to do is to break it. In such a case, it would be wrong to follow the rule. Lying is usually wrong, breaking promises is usually wrong, killing is usually wrong; however, whenever circumstances are such that there is good reason to believe that breaking a certain moral rule will maximize utility, the rule should be broken. Of course, the act-utilitarian insists, one must be cautious in concluding that any given exception to a moral rule is indeed justified. One must be wary of rationalization and not allow one's own interests to weigh more heavily than the interests of others in the utilitarian calculation. Most importantly, one must not be simpleminded in a consideration of the likely consequences of breaking a moral rule. Indirect and long-term consequences must be considered as well as direct and short-term consequences. Lying on a certain occasion may seem to promote most effectively the interests of those immediately involved, but perhaps the lie will provide a bad example for less reflective people, or perhaps it will contribute to a general breakdown of trust among human beings. In this same vein, one prominent contemporary act-utilitarian emphasizes the significance of the long-term, indirect consequences of promise breaking, while at the same time exhibiting the underlying act-utilitarian attitude toward moral rules:

> The rightness or wrongness of keeping a promise on a particular occasion depends only on the goodness or badness of the consequences of keeping or of breaking the promise on that particular occasion. Of course part of the consequences of breaking the promise, and a part to which we will normally ascribe decisive importance, will be the weakening of faith in the institution of promising. However, if the goodness of the consequences of breaking the rule is *in toto* greater than the goodness of the consequences of keeping it, then we must break the rule. . . .[5]

Act-utilitarianism has often been criticized on the grounds that, due to the extensive sort of calculations it seems to demand, it cannot function as a useful guide for human action. In the spirit of this criticism, the following questions are asked: How can I possibly predict all the consequences of my actions? How am I to assign weights to the various kinds of human satisfactions—for example, the pleasure of eating a candy bar versus the aesthetic enjoyment of the ballet? How am I to weigh the anxiety of one person against the inconvenience of another? Besides, how am I supposed to have time to do these extensive calculations? Act-utilitarians, in response to such questions, usually appeal rather directly to "common sense." They say, typically, that there is no escape from a consideration of probabilities in rational decision making; predict as best you can and weigh as best you can, considering the time you have available for deliberation. All that can be expected is that you come to grips with the likely consequences of your alternatives in a serious-minded, sensible way and then act accordingly.

Examples of Act-Utilitarian Reasoning in a Biomedical Context   The following examples are provided in an effort to exhibit act-utilitarian reasoning as it might arise in a biomedical context. It is not claimed that an act-utilitarian must necessarily reach the conclusion suggested in each case. It is claimed only that an act-utilitarian might plausibly reach the stated conclusion.

(1) A severely impaired newborn, believed to have no realistic chance of surviving more than a few weeks, has contracted pneumonia. (The treatment of impaired newborns is discussed in Chapter 5.) A physician, in conjunction with the parents of the infant, must decide whether to fight off the pneumonia with antibiotics, thereby prolonging the life of the infant. The alternative is simply to allow the infant to die. It seems clear that the interests of all those immediately involved are best served by deciding not to treat the pneumonia. Surely the infant has nothing to gain, and something to lose, by a slight extension of a pain-filled life. The parents, whose suffering cannot be eradicated whatever action is taken, nevertheless will find some relief knowing that their child's suffering has ended. In addition, hospital resources can be better utilized than to prolong the dying process of an infant who cannot benefit from further treatment. However, there may be decisive consequences of allowing death to occur that are indirect and long-term. Perhaps allowing this infant to die will contribute to a breakdown of protective attitudes toward infants in general. No, the risk of this untoward consequence seems minimal. Withholding antibiotics, thereby allowing the infant to die, is the right thing to do in this case.

(2) A biomedical researcher, on the basis of animal studies she has conducted, believes that a certain drug therapy has great promise for the treatment of a particular kind of cancer in human beings. (The use of animals in research is discussed in Chapter 4.) At present, however, her primary concern is to establish an appropriate dosage level for human beings; there have been several troublesome side effects exhibited by the animals who received large doses of the drug. Over the years, the researcher has found that students at her university are very willing to volunteer as research subjects in experiments that can be identified as presenting only minimal risks to themselves. They are, however, understandably reluctant to volunteer for experiments that seem to present more substantial risks. The researcher in this case cannot honestly say that there are no substantial risks for research subjects. She expects, in particular, that perhaps 30 to 40 percent of the research subjects will have to contend with very prolonged nausea. However, if she is honest in conveying this information to potential research subjects, it is unlikely that they will volunteer in sufficient numbers. (The ethics of experimentation on human subjects is discussed in Chapter 4.) Perhaps, she reasons, it is justifiable in this case to withhold information about the risk of very prolonged nausea. After all, it is very likely that numerous people will eventually derive great benefit from the therapeutic technique under study. Surely this likely benefit far outweighs the short-term discomfort of a much smaller number. But consider the very real possibility that the deception would come to light. If those who routinely volunteer as research subjects are given a reason to distrust those conducting the experiments, the overall research effort on campus will be negatively affected. Moreover, publicity about the decep-

tion would create a major public relations scandal for the university, forcing it to devote valuable time, energy, and money to repairing its reputation. These seem to be decisive considerations. In this case, then, deception would be wrong. (If there were no realistic chance of the deception's being discovered, it seems that the conclusion would be different.)

(3) The setting is in the 1960s, when kidney dialysis machines are scarce, and it is not possible for all who need them to be given access. A hospital administrator or perhaps a committee has been charged with the responsibility of deciding, in essence, whose lives will be saved. (Such decisions are often referred to as "microallocation decisions.") On a particular occasion, when there is room for one more patient, there are two candidates in great need. One of the candidates, a civic-minded woman of 40, is married and the mother of four children. The other candidate, an unmarried man of the same age, is known to be a drifter and an alcoholic. It seems clear, at first glance, that the consequences of saving the woman's life are far superior to those of saving the man's life. Her husband, her children, and the community in general would be negatively affected in very substantial ways by her death. However, is it not problematic to accord a person access to a scarce medical resource on the basis of his or her social role? If a precedent of this sort is set, will not those whose lives are less "socially useful" become somewhat anxious and fearful? On the other hand, perhaps this negative consequence will be balanced by a positive consequence; that is, people will be more inclined to become "socially useful." It still seems clear that the woman in this case should have priority over the man.

Critical Assessment of Act-Utilitarianism Act-utilitarianism arguably fares poorly when measured against a previously identified standard: The implications of an ethical theory must be largely reconcilable with our experience of the moral life. In a number of ways, it can be argued, act-utilitarianism clashes with our experience of the moral life. This perceived failure to accord with our ordinary moral thinking is reflected in the following well-known objections to act-utilitarianism.

(1) Act-Utilitarianism Confronts Individuals with an Overly Demanding Moral Standard. We are accustomed to thinking that at least some of our decisions are matters of "mere prudence," rightly decided on the basis of "what is best for me." Which major a college student should choose is a good example of a choice that we are inclined to consider essentially a nonmoral matter, a matter of "mere prudence." According to the act-utilitarian, however, a person is continually under a moral obligation to produce the greatest balance of good over evil, everyone considered. Whereas ethical egoism seems to wrongly "collapse" morality into prudence, it would seem that act-utilitarianism "expands" morality so as to destroy the realm of prudence. No aspect of a person's life can be considered merely a matter of prudence. Every decision is a moral decision, to be made on the basis of utilitarian calculation. However, no matter how noble it might be for a college student to decide his or her major on the basis of a utilitarian calculation, it would seem that one is certainly not under an obligation to proceed in this manner. Doing so, we would ordinarily say, is not one's duty but, rather, is something "above and beyond the call of duty." Act-utilitarianism, in directing a person always to act so as to maximize utility, seems problematically to imply that it is one's duty to act in a way that we ordinarily consider "above and beyond the call of duty."

(2) Act-Utilitarianism Does Not Accord with Our Experience of Particular, Morally Significant Relationships. In our experience of the moral life, we are continually aware of highly particular, morally significant relationships that exist between ourselves and others.

We are related to particular individuals in a host of morally significant ways, such as spouse to spouse, parent to child, creditor to debtor, promisor to promisee, employer to employee, teacher to student, physician or nurse to patient. In view of such relationships, it is ordinarily thought, we have special obligations—obligations that restrict the effort to maximize utility. Parents, we are strongly inclined to say, are obligated to care for their children even if there is good reason to think that the time and energy necessary for this task would maximize utility if redirected to some other task. In the same way, by virtue of the special relationship that exists between a physician and a patient, would it not be wrong for a physician to make decisions regarding a patient's treatment in the manner of an act-utilitarian? For a physician to compromise the interests of an individual patient in an effort to maximize utility surely seems wrong. W. D. Ross, who has vigorously pressed this overall line of criticism against act-utilitarianism, asserts that the "essential defect of the . . . theory is that it ignores, or at least does not do full justice to, the highly personal character of duty."[6]

(3) Act-Utilitarianism Does Not Accord with Our Conviction That Individuals Have Rights. The notion of rights plays an important part in our ordinary moral thinking, but act-utilitarianism seems incapable of accommodating this notion. Moreover, in certain circumstances, the action that would maximize utility (and thus the right action, according to the act-utilitarian) is one that we are inclined to consider seriously immoral precisely because it entails the violation of some person's right. For example, it seems that act-utilitarianism would allow an innocent person to be unjustly punished, as long as circumstances were such as to make this line of action the one that would generate the greatest balance of good over evil. Suppose extreme social unrest has been created by a wave of unsolved crimes. The enraged crowd will violently erupt, bringing massive evil into the world, unless the authorities punish someone (anyone) in an effort to appease the appetite for vengeance. So act-utilitarianism seems to allow the unjust treatment of a person as a scapegoat, as a mere means to a social end. But surely an innocent person has a right not to be punished, and it is by reference to this right that the wrongness of scapegoating is most naturally understood. Similarly, "the common moral opinion that painless undetected murders of old unhappy people are wicked, no matter what benefits result"[7] can be thought to rest on the contention that people, however old and unhappy, nevertheless have a *right* to life. It is often asserted against act-utilitarianism that it is a defective theory because it allows "the end to justify the means." At least part of the sense behind this charge can be made out in reference to the notion of rights. Certain means of achieving a desirable social end are simply wrong because they entail the violation of a person's right. Contrary to act-utilitarianism, such means cannot be justified by the end.

Act-utilitarians have responded in two ways to the overall claim that the theory cannot be reconciled with our ordinary moral thinking. Some say, in essence, "so much the worse for our ordinary moral thinking." In their view, we must simply overhaul our collective moral consciousness and embrace the mind-set of the act-utilitarian. Most act-utilitarians, however, do not adopt this revisionary stance. Rather, they seek to demonstrate that the clash between act-utilitarianism and our ordinary moral thinking is not nearly so severe as the above criticisms suggest. They argue that, when act-utilitarianism is properly applied, when all the significant long-term, indirect consequences are taken into account, the theory does not give rise to conclusions that seem so patently objectionable. It is very doubtful, however, that this strategy of argument can completely rescue act-utilitarianism from its difficulties.

Perhaps act-utilitarianism fares better when measured against the second of our previously identified standards: An ethical theory must provide effective guidance where it is most needed. At the very least, it must be said in favor of act-utilitarianism that it provides a reasonably clear decision procedure, a sense of direction, for the resolution of moral dilemmas. In the face of moral considerations that incline our judgment in conflicting ways, act-utilitarianism counsels us to analyze the likely consequences of alternative actions in order to determine the alternative that will maximize utility. Still, however well act-utilitarianism might be thought to fare with regard to our second standard—and even that is debatable—it seems to encounter significant problems when measured against our first standard. Indeed, in contemporary times, most utilitarian thinkers have rejected act-utilitarianism in favor of a theory known as rule-utilitarianism.[8]

RULE-UTILITARIANISM

The basic principle of act-utilitarianism has previously been formulated as follows: A person ought to act so as to produce the greatest balance of good over evil, everyone considered. In contrast, the basic principle of rule-utilitarianism can be formulated as follows: *A person ought to act in accordance with the rule that, if generally followed, would produce the greatest balance of good over evil, everyone considered.* If the demand to produce the greatest balance of good over evil, everyone considered, is referred to as the principle (standard) of utility, then the principle of utility is the basic ethical principle in both the act-utilitarian and the rule-utilitarian systems. However, in the act-utilitarian system, determining the morally correct action is a matter of assessing alternative actions directly against the standard of utility, whereas in the rule-utilitarian system determining the morally correct action involves an *indirect* appeal to the principle of utility. In the spirit of rule-utilitarianism, a moral code is first established by reference to the principle of utility. That is, a set of valid moral rules is established by determining which rules (as opposed to conceivable alternatives), if generally followed, would produce the greatest balance of good over evil. In rule-utilitarianism, individual actions are morally right if they are in accord with those rules.

The difference between act-utilitarian reasoning and rule-utilitarian reasoning can be represented schematically as follows:

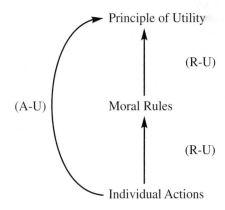

Act-utilitarian reasoning embodies a single-stage procedure; rule-utilitarian reasoning, a two-stage procedure. Because the act-utilitarian is committed to assessing individual actions strictly on the basis of utilitarian considerations, act-utilitarianism is often referred to as "extreme" or "unrestricted" utilitarianism. Because the rule-utilitarian is committed to developing a moral code (a set of moral rules) on the basis of utilitarian considerations and then assessing individual actions, not on the basis of utilitarian considerations but on the basis of accordance with the moral rules that have been established, rule-utilitarianism is often referred to as "restricted" utilitarianism.

For the act-utilitarian, moral rules have a very subordinate status. They are merely "rules of thumb," providing some measure of practical guidance. For the rule-utilitarian, moral rules assume a much more fundamental status, indeed a theoretical primacy. Only in reference to established moral rules can the moral assessment of individual actions be carried out. Thus, the first and most crucial step for the rule-utilitarian is the articulation of a set of moral rules, themselves justified on the basis of utilitarian considerations. Underlying this task is the question of which rules (as opposed to conceivable alternatives), if generally followed, would produce the greatest balance of good over evil, everyone considered. That is, which rules, if adopted or recognized in our moral code, would maximize utility?

As a first approximation of a set of moral rules that could be justified on the basis of utilitarian considerations, consider the "commonsense rules of morality," such as "do not kill," "do not steal," "do not lie," "do not break promises." It is not difficult to think of such rules as resting upon a utilitarian foundation. Surely the consequences of the adoption of the rule "do not kill" are dramatically better than the consequences of the adoption of the rule "kill whenever you want." If the latter rule were generally followed, society would give way to anarchy. Similarly, the consequences of the adoption of the rule "do not steal" are dramatically better than the consequences of the adoption of the rule "steal whenever you want." If the former rule is generally followed, individuals will enjoy an important measure of personal security. If the latter rule were adopted by a society, anxiety and tension would dominate social existence. As for lying and promise breaking, if people felt free to engage in such behavior, the numerous advantages that derive from human trust and cooperation would evaporate. However, the rules thus far exhibited as having a utilitarian foundation are essentially prohibitions. Are there not also rules of a more positive sort that could also be justified on the basis of utilitarian considerations? It would seem so. Consider rules such as "come to the aid of people in distress" and "prevent innocent people from being harmed." It surely seems that human welfare would be enhanced by the adoption of such rules as part of the overall fabric of our moral code.

According to the rule-utilitarian, an individual action is morally right when it accords with the rules or moral code established on a utilitarian basis. However, the account of moral rules thus far presented is too simplistic. In order to be plausible, the rules that constitute the moral code must be understood as incorporating certain exceptions. The need to recognize justified exceptions is perhaps most apparent when we remember that moral rules, if stated unconditionally, can easily come into conflict with each other. When an obviously agitated person waves a gun and inquires as to the whereabouts of a third party, it may not be possible to act in accordance with both the rule "do not lie" and the rule "prevent innocent people from being harmed." Indeed, it is precisely this sort of situation that inclines us to consider incorporating an exception into our rule against lying. Suppose we say, "Do not lie *except* when necessary to prevent an innocent person from being seriously harmed." When the possibility of a justified exception is raised, the rule-utilitarian employs the following decision procedure. The question is posed, "Would the adoption of the rule with the exception have better consequences than the adoption of the rule without the exception?" If so, the exception is a justified one; the rule incorporating the exception has greater utility than the rule without the exception. In the face of our proposed exception to the rule against lying, the rule-utilitarian would probably conclude that it does constitute a justified exception. The adoption of the rule "do not lie *except* when necessary to protect an innocent person from being seriously harmed" would seem to preserve essentially all the social benefits provided by the adoption of the rule "do not lie," while bringing about an additional social benefit, an increased measure of personal security for potential victims of assault.

Examples of Rule-Utilitarian Reasoning in a Biomedical Context (1) A substantial problem in biomedical ethics (discussed in Chapter 2) is whether it is ever right for a physician to lie to a patient, saying that the patient's illness is not terminal when it is believed to be so. The rule-utilitarian would conceptualize this issue as raising the possibility of a justified exception to the rule against lying. (Notice that an act-utilitarian, in contrast, would insist on assessing every individual case on its own utilitarian merits.) Suppose we consider incorporating into the rule against lying an exception to this effect: "*except* when in the judgment of a physician it would be better for a patient not to know that his or her illness is believed to be terminal." Would the adoption of the rule incorporating this exception have better consequences than the adoption of the rule without the exception? The correct answer to this question is perhaps arguable, but it would seem that the rule-utilitarian would conclude that the proposed exception is an unjustified one. It is perhaps true that adoption of a rule incorporating the proposed exception would result in many patients' being spared (at least temporarily) the distress that accompanies knowledge of one's impending death. On the other hand, it seems that this gain would be dwarfed by the distress and anxiety that would emerge from the erosion of trust within the confines of the physician-patient relationship. Whether a more limited exception could be formulated to a rule-utilitarian's satisfaction remains an open question.

(2) Another substantial problem in biomedical ethics (discussed in Chapter 6) has to do with the morality of mercy killing. Suppose a terminally ill patient, in great pain, requests that a physician terminate his or her life by administering a lethal dose of a drug. Such a case raises the issue of voluntary (active) euthanasia. The rule-utilitarian would conceptualize this issue (and other issues, such as suicide and abortion) as raising the possibility of a justified exception to our rule against killing. Notice that at least one exception to our rule against killing is relatively uncontroversial. Killing in self-defense is justifiable, according to the rule-utilitarian, because although the adoption of the rule "do not kill" has dramatically better consequences than the adoption of the rule "kill whenever you want," adoption of the rule "do not kill *except* in self-defense" has still better consequences. As for voluntary (active) euthanasia, perhaps we should say that strong rule-utilitarian arguments can be advanced on both sides of the issue. Rule-utilitarian proponents of voluntary (active) euthanasia emphasize that social acceptance of this practice would result in great benefits— the primary one being that many dying people would be able to escape an extension of an anguished dying process. On the other side of the issue, however, we find, among a number of important concerns, insistence that availability of the lethal dose would create a climate of fear and anxiety among the elderly. Will dying people not come to feel that their families, to whom they have become a burden, expect them to ask for the lethal dose?

(3) A final illustration of rule-utilitarian reasoning in a biomedical context can be presented in reference to the principle of medical confidentiality (discussed in Chapter 3). This principle, which has an obvious basis in a rule-utilitarian structure, demands that information revealed within the context of a therapeutic relationship be held confidential. If patients could not rely on this expectation, they would be reluctant to communicate information that is essential to their proper treatment. Still, are there not justifiable exceptions to the principle of medical confidentiality? Suppose, for example, a patient reveals to his or her therapist an intention to kill or injure a third party. Is it not incumbent upon the therapist to break medical confidentiality in an effort to ensure protection for the third party? The situation just described is the basis of the *Tarasoff* case considered in Chapter 3, and rule-utilitarian arguments on both sides of the issue can be found in the judicial opinions presented. There is an obvious benefit associated with the recognition of an exception to medical confidentiality based on the interests of innocent third parties; namely, threatened people will sometimes be saved from injury and death. On the other hand, it is argued, emotionally disturbed patients are likely to become more inhibited in communicating with therapists; thus, their treatment will be inhibited, and a greater incidence of violence against innocent people will result.

Critical Assessment of Rule-Utilitarianism Rule-utilitarianism, it would seem, goes some distance toward alleviating the perceived difficulties of act-utilitarianism. Although act-utilitarians have charged rule-utilitarians with "superstitious rule-worship,"[9] it is act-utilitarianism rather than rule-utilitarianism that seems to clash with our ordinary moral thinking on this score. Rule-utilitarianism seems to fare at least somewhat better than act-utilitarianism when measured against the standard that the implications of an ethical theory must be largely reconcilable with our experience of the moral life.

Whereas act-utilitarianism seems to confront individuals with an overly demanding moral standard, placing each of us under a continuing obligation to maximize utility with each of our actions, rule-utilitarianism may prove to be far less demanding of individuals. It requires only that individuals conform their actions to the rules that constitute a utilitarian-based moral code, which may not include any rules that prove overly demanding. Rule-utilitarianism also seems to accord reasonably well with our experience of particular, morally significant relationships. We commonly perceive ourselves as having special obligations arising out of our various morally significant relationships, and we think of these obligations as incompatible with functioning in the manner of an act-utilitarian. For example, parents have a special obligation to care for their children, physicians have a special obligation to act in the interests of their patients, and so forth. Such special obligations can be understood as having a rule-utilitarian foundation, as deriving from rules that, if generally followed, would maximize utility. Thus, rule-utilitarianism seems to remedy another perceived difficulty of act-utilitarianism.

It is less clear that rule-utilitarianism is capable of providing a complete remedy for another perceived difficulty of act-utilitarianism, that is, its inability to provide an adequate theoretical foundation for individual rights. Surely rule-utilitarianism does not lead us as easily as does act-utilitarianism to conclusions that are incompatible with our ordinary moral thinking about the rights of individuals. For example, in suggesting that the painless murder of an old, unhappy (but not suicidal) person is the right thing as long as it can be done in complete secrecy, act-utilitarianism seems to clash violently with our conviction that such an action is patently objectionable, inasmuch as it constitutes a violation of a person's right to life. Rule-utilitarianism, in contrast, would never lead us to the conclusion that this sort of killing is morally legitimate. Surely the consequences of adopting the rule "do not kill *except* in the case of old, unhappy people who can be killed in complete secrecy" are dramatically worse than the consequences of adopting the rule without such an exception. If the rule with the exception were adopted, the lives of elderly people would be filled with anxiety and fear; moreover, people attempting to follow such a rule would no doubt sometimes kill old, *happy* people, mistakenly believing them to be unhappy. In addition to rescuing utilitarian thinking from such obvious clashes with our ordinary moral thinking, rule-utilitarianism suggests a way of accommodating the notion of individual rights. Just as our special obligations can be understood as deriving from rules in a utilitarian-based moral code, so, too, can an individual's rights be understood in this fashion. A person's right to life, for example, can be understood as a correlate of our utilitarian-based rule against killing. Of course, whatever exceptions are properly incorporated into our rule against killing will factor out as limitations on a person's right to life. Whether rule-utilitarianism in this manner can provide an adequate theoretical foundation for individual rights is a very controversial matter. Its critics charge that it cannot.

Closely related to the claim that rule-utilitarianism does not provide an adequate theoretical foundation for individual rights is the somewhat broader claim that rule-utilitarianism fails to provide an adequate theoretical grounding for what we take to be the obligations of justice. This broader criticism, which is also vigorously advanced against act-utilitarianism, is perhaps the principal residual difficulty confronting rule-utilitarianism. Critics of rule-utilitarianism allege, for example, that the theory is compatible with the blatant injustice of enslaving one segment of a society's population or at least discriminating against this segment. The idea is that social rules discriminating against an explicitly identified minority group might maximize utility by bringing about more happiness in the advantaged majority than unhappiness in the disadvantaged minority. Rule-utilitarians are inclined to argue in response to this line of criticism that, when the consequences of adopting "unjust rules" are completely analyzed, it is never true that their adoption can be justified on utilitarian grounds. Rather, the rule-utilitarian contends, "the rules of justice" rest on a secure utilitarian foundation. Whether rule-utilitarianism, in this manner, can adequately be reconciled with the perceived obligations of justice is a matter of contemporary debate.

Rule-utilitarianism also seems to fare reasonably well when measured against the second of our suggested standards: An ethical theory must provide effective guidance where it is most needed. In a dilemma, where one moral rule, or principle, inclines us one way and another moral rule, or principle, inclines us another way, the rule-utilitarian instructs us to establish relative priority by considering the consequences of incorporating appropriate exceptions into the rules that are in conflict. The dilemma is to be resolved by adoption of a rule that will maximize utility. Although this decision procedure sometimes entails very complex factual analysis and deliberation, it does seem to provide us a substantial measure of explicit guidance. Since rule-utilitarianism also seems to be reasonably harmonious with our ordinary moral thinking, it is an ethical theory that cannot easily be dismissed.

KANTIAN DEONTOLOGY

The most prominent of the classical deontological theories is that developed by German philosopher Immanuel Kant (1724–1804). Kantian deontology continues to command substantial attention in contemporary discussions of ethical theory and, importantly, is the underlying framework of much argumentation in biomedical ethics. In both of these respects, Kantian deontology is similar to utilitarianism and, like utilitarianism, warrants our detailed attention.

Kant sees utilitarianism as embodying a radically wrong approach in ethical theory. He emphasizes the need to avoid the "serpent-windings" of utilitarian thinking and refers to the principle of utility as "a wavering and uncertain standard." There is indeed a single, fundamental principle that is the basis of all moral obligation, but this fundamental principle is *not* the principle of utility. The supreme principle of morality, the principle from which all of our various duties derive, Kant calls the "categorical imperative."

Although our present objective is an exposition of Kantian deontology, the enormous complexity of Kant's moral philosophy is a formidable obstacle to any concise exposition of the structure of Kant's ethical system. In particular, we are faced with the problem that Kant formulated the basic principle of his system, the categorical imperative, in a number of different ways. Although Kant insists that his various formulations are all equivalent, this contention is explicitly denied by many of his expositors and critics. Thus, if we are to provide a coherent account of Kantian deontology, mindful of the need to provide an account that is especially useful in dealing with issues in biomedical ethics, it seems advisable to settle on a favored formulation of the categorical imperative. Since two of Kant's formulations of the categorical imperative are especially prominent, it will suffice for our purposes to choose a favored formulation from these two.

According to what we will call the "first formulation," the categorical imperative tells us: "Act only on that maxim through which you can at the same time will that it should become a universal law."[10] According to what we will call the "second formulation," the categorical imperative tells us: "Act in such a way that you always treat humanity, whether in your own person or in the person of any other, never simply as a means, but always at the same time as an end."[11] The first formulation of the categorical imperative has often been compared to the Golden Rule ("Do unto others as you would have them do unto you"), and it may be true that these principles, when suitably interpreted, have roughly the same implications. At any rate, Kant apparently considered the first formulation to be the most basic of all his formulations, yet despite this fact, and despite the fact that ethical theorists have tended to pay more attention to the first formulation than the second, it is the second formulation that we take to have greater promise for the task at hand. Two major reasons can be advanced for choosing to exhibit the structure of Kant's ethical system in reference to the second formulation of the categorical imperative. First, the second formulation embodies a central notion—respect for persons—that is somewhat easier to grasp and apply than the more formalistic notion of universalizability, which is the core element of the first formulation. Second, when argumentation in biomedical ethics reflects a Kantian viewpoint, it is almost always couched in terms of the second formulation rather than the first.

Kantian deontology is an ethics of respect for persons. In Kant's view, every person, by virtue of his or her humanity (i.e., rational nature) has an inherent dignity. All persons, as rational creatures, are entitled to respect, not only from others but from themselves as well. Thus, the categorical imperative directs each of us to "act in such a way that you always treat humanity, whether in your own person or in the person of any other, never simply as a means, but always at the same time as an end." From this fundamental principle, according to Kant, a host of particular duties can be derived. The resultant system of duties includes duties to self as well as duties to others. In each of these cases, "perfect duties" must be distinguished from "imperfect duties," thus generating a fourfold classification of duties: (1) perfect duties to self, (2) imperfect duties to self, (3) perfect duties to others, and

(4) imperfect duties to others. Although the distinction between perfect and imperfect duties is not a transparent one, its structural importance in the Kantian system is hard to overemphasize. Perfect duties require that we do or abstain from certain acts. *There are no legitimate exceptions to a perfect duty.* Such duties are binding in all circumstances, because certain kinds of action are simply incompatible with respect for persons, hence strictly impermissible. Imperfect duties, by contrast, require us to pursue or promote certain goals (e.g., the welfare of others). However, action in the name of these goals must never be at the expense of a perfect duty. One of Kant's most prominent commentators relates the distinction between perfect and imperfect duties to the categorical imperative in the following way: "We transgress perfect duties by treating any person *merely* as a means. We transgress imperfect duties by failing to treat a person as an end, even though we do not actively treat him as a means."[12]

Our discussion of Kant's fourfold classification of duties begins with a consideration of perfect duties to others. A transgression in this category of duty occurs whenever one person treats another person merely as a means. It is strictly impermissible for person A to treat person B merely as a means because such treatment is incompatible with respect for B as a person. Notice that Kant does not claim that it is morally wrong for one to use another as a means. His claim is that it is morally wrong for one person to use another *merely* as a means. In the ordinary course of life, it is surely unavoidable (and morally unproblematic) that each of us in numerous ways uses others as means to achieve our various ends. A college teacher uses students as a means to achieve his or her livelihood. A college student uses instructors as a means of gaining knowledge and skills. Such human interactions, presumably based on the voluntary participation of the respective parties, are quite compatible with a principle of respect for persons. However, respect for persons entails that each of us recognizes the rightful authority of other persons (as rational beings) to conduct their individual lives as they see fit. We may legitimately recruit others to participate in the satisfaction of our personal ends, but they are used merely as a means whenever we undermine the voluntary or informed character of their consent to interact with us in some desired way. Person A coerces person B at knifepoint to hand over $200. A uses B merely as a means. If A had requested of B a gift of $200, leaving B free to determine whether or not to make the gift, A would have proceeded in a manner compatible with respect for B as a person. Person C deceptively rolls back the odometer of a car and thereby manipulates person D's decision to buy the car. C uses D merely as a means. C has acted in a way that is strictly incompatible with respect for D as a person.

In the Kantian system, among the most notable of our perfect duties to others are (1) the duty not to kill an innocent person, (2) the duty not to lie, and (3) the duty to keep promises. Murder (the killing of an innocent person), lying, and promise breaking are actions that are intrinsically wrong. However beneficial the consequences of such an action might be in a given circumstance, the action is strictly impermissible. (Notice the anti-utilitarian character of Kant's thinking.) The murderer exhibits obvious disrespect for the person of the victim. The liar, in misinforming another person, violates the respect due to that person as a rational creature with a fundamental interest in the truth. A person who makes a promise issues a guarantee upon which the recipient of the promise is entitled to rely in his or her future planning. The person who breaks a promise shows disrespect for another by undermining the effort to conduct the affairs of one's life. By murdering, lying, or breaking a promise, an agent uses another person merely as a means to the agent's own ends.

According to Kant, each person has not only perfect duties to others but also perfect duties to self. The categorical imperative demands that no person (including oneself) be treated merely as a means. It is no more permissible to manifest disrespect for one's own person than to do so for the person of another. Kant insists, for example, that each person has a perfect duty to self to avoid drunkenness. Since drunkenness undermines a person's rational capacities, it is incompatible with respect for oneself as a rational creature. Kant believes that individuals debase themselves in the effort to achieve pleasure via inebriation. Inebriates treat themselves merely as a means (to the end of pleasure). But surely the foremost example of a perfect duty to self in the Kantian system is the duty not to commit suicide. To terminate one's own life, Kant insists, is strictly incompatible with respect for oneself as a person. In eradicating one's very existence as a rational creature, a person treats oneself merely as a means (ordinarily to the end of avoiding discomfort or distress). Suicide is an action that is intrinsically wrong, and there are no circumstances in which it is morally permissible.

In addition to the notion of perfect duties (both to self and others), the Kantian system also incorporates the notion of imperfect duties. Whereas perfect duties require, in essence, strict abstention from those actions that involve using a person merely as a means, imperfect duties have a very different underlying sense. Imperfect duties require the promotion of certain goals. In broad terms, there are two such goals—an agent's personal perfection (i.e., development) and the happiness or welfare of others. Respect for oneself as a person requires commitment to the development of one's capacities as a rational being. Thus Kant spoke of an imperfect duty to self to develop one's talents. The sense of this duty is that, by and large, it is up to each individual to decide which talents to cultivate and which to deemphasize. But a person is not free to abandon the goal of personal development. Although the duty to develop one's talents requires no *specific* actions, it does require each individual to formulate a plan of life that embodies a commitment to the goal of personal development.

Before discussing Kant's final category of duty, imperfect duty to others, it will prove helpful to introduce the notion of *beneficence*.[13] If one acts in such a way as to further the happiness or welfare of another, then one acts beneficently. (A benevolent person is one who is inclined to act beneficently.) Beneficence may be contrasted with *nonmaleficence,* which is ordinarily understood as the noninfliction of harm on others. One who harms ("does evil" to) another acts in a maleficent fashion. One who *refrains* from harming others acts in a nonmaleficent fashion. One who acts, in a more positive way, to contribute to the welfare of others acts in a beneficent fashion. Beneficence is a generic notion that can best be understood as including the following types of activity: (1) preventing evil or harm from befalling someone, (2) removing an evil that is presently afflicting someone, and (3) providing benefits ("doing good") for someone. Although it is sometimes difficult to decide which of these categories is the most appropriate classification for a particular beneficent action, the following examples seem relatively straightforward. Pushing someone out of the path of an oncoming car is an example of the first type of activity. Curing a patient's disease is an example of the second. Giving someone a $100 gift is an example of the third.

According to Kant, respect for other persons requires not only that we avoid using them merely as a means (by the observance of our perfect duties to others) but also that we commit ourselves in some general way to furthering their happiness or welfare. Thus, Kant considers what we will call the "duty of beneficence" to be an imperfect duty to others. As with the duty to develop our talents, an imperfect duty to self, the duty of beneficence requires no *specific* actions. One does not violate the duty of beneficence by refusing to act beneficently in any individual case where the opportunity arises. What is required instead of specific actions is that each person incorporate into his or her lifeplan a commitment to promote the well-being of others. Individuals are free to choose the sorts of actions they will embrace in an effort to further the well-being of others (e.g., contributing to the relief of famine victims); they are not free to abandon the general goal of furthering the well-being of others.

Since the duty of beneficence is an imperfect duty in the Kantian system, action in the name of beneficence must never be taken at the expense of a perfect duty. For example, it is impermissible to lie or break a promise in an effort to save a third party from harm. The same is true with regard to the imperfect duty to develop one's talents. For example, if one has resolved (quite properly) to develop one's creative powers, it is nevertheless impermissible to do so by "creatively" defrauding others.

The Kantian Framework in a Biomedical Context With our exposition of Kantian deontology now complete, we are in a position to exhibit some of the more important implications of this ethical theory in the realm of biomedical ethics. To begin with, the theory has an obvious relevance to the much discussed problem of whether or not a physician may justifiably lie to a patient (an issue discussed in Chapter 2). Since every person has a perfect duty to others not to lie, a straightforward implication of Kantian deontology is that a physician may *never* lie to a patient. If a patient diagnosed as terminally ill by a physician inquires about his or her prognosis, the physician may be much inclined to lie, motivated by a desire to protect the patient from the psychological turmoil that would accompany knowledge of his or her true condition; but action in the name of beneficence (an imperfect duty) may never be at the expense of a perfect duty. This same analysis is relevant to the use of placebos by physicians. Sometimes a patient becomes psychologically dependent on a certain medication. When the medication is discontinued, because the physician is convinced it is no longer needed and because its continued use represents a threat to health, the patient complains of the reemergence of symptoms. If such a patient is given a placebo, that is, a therapeutically inert but harmless substance, misrepresented as a medication, the patient may feel fine. Nevertheless, despite the fact that placebos may be capable of enhancing patient welfare, their use is morally impermissible, at least in cases involving an explicit lie.

Kantian deontology has some very important and very direct implications for the ethics of experimentation with human subjects (a topic discussed in Chapter 4). Since it is morally wrong for any person to use any other person merely as a means, it follows that it is morally wrong for a biomedical researcher to use a human research subject merely as a means. From this consideration it is but a short step to the requirement of voluntary informed consent as a basic principle of research ethics. If a researcher is engaged in a study that involves human subjects, we may presume that the immediate "end" being sought by the researcher is the successful completion of the study. But notice that the researcher may desire this particular end for any number of reasons: the speculative understanding it will provide; the technology it will make possible; the eventual benefit to humankind; personal recognition in the eyes of the scientific community; a raise in pay; and so forth. This mixture of self-centered and benevolent motivations may be considered the researcher's less immediate ends. If researchers are to avoid using their research subjects merely as means (to the ends of the researchers), surely they must refrain from coercing the participation of their subjects and provide information about the research project (most notably, risks to the subjects) sufficient for the subjects to make a rational decision with regard to their personal participation. Thus, respect for persons demands that researchers honor the requirement of voluntary informed consent.

Suppose a researcher explains to a potential research subject how important it is that he or she consent to participate. There is no question but that the research project at issue, if brought to a successful conclusion, will provide substantial benefit to humankind. Does the potential subject have a moral obligation to participate? Surely not. Within the framework of Kantian deontology, the duty of beneficence is an imperfect duty. A person must on occasion act beneficently, but there is no obligation to perform any *specific* beneficent action.

Critical Assessment of Kantian Deontology Are the implications of Kantian deontology largely reconcilable with our experience of the moral life? Can this theory provide effective guidance in the face of perceived moral dilemmas? These two questions reflect the criteria suggested earlier as most central to the assessment of the relative adequacy of an ethical theory.

Before indicating some of the ways in which Kantian deontology can be thought to be at odds with our ordinary moral thinking, it is important to emphasize that the theory does successfully account for crucial aspects of our experience of the moral life. To begin with, Kantian deontology provides an obvious foundation for the "commonsense rules of morality." The wrongfulness of actions that fly in the face of these rules—actions such as killing, injuring, stealing, lying, breaking promises—can very plausibly be understood as flowing from the categorical imperative. The Kantian deontologist maintains that these actions are wrong because they involve treating another person merely as a means, and there is something very compelling about the notion of respect for persons as the core notion of morality.

Kantian deontology also seems to provide a secure foundation for the notion of individual rights, a notion that is very prominent in our ordinary moral thinking. Individual rights, in the Kantian system, are to be understood as the correlates of our perfect duties to others. (Imperfect duties, in contrast, do not generate rights.) For example, each of us has a perfect *duty* not to kill an innocent person; thus, every innocent person has a *right* not to be killed. More generally, every person has a right not to be used by another merely as a means. An innocent person has a right not to be punished, no matter how socially desirable the consequences might be in a certain set of circumstances. A potential research subject has a right not to be coerced or deceived into participation, even if the satisfactory completion of the study promises great benefit for humankind. In its insistence that individual rights cannot be overridden by "utilitarian" considerations, Kantian deontology achieves accord with our firmly entrenched (if somewhat vague) conviction that the end does not justify the means.

However, there are aspects of Kantian deontology that cannot be easily reconciled with our experience of the moral life. One very prominent difficulty has to do with the Kantian contention that keeping promises and not lying are both duties of perfect obligation. We are quite at home, in our ordinary moral thinking, with both a duty to keep promises and a duty not to lie, but it is the exceptionless character of these duties in the Kantian system that we find troublesome. Surely in extreme cases, we are inclined to say, these duties must yield to more weighty moral considerations. For example, if a person breaks a rather trivial promise (say, to return a book at a certain time) in order to respond to the needs of a person in serious distress, surely he or she has not acted immorally. Or again, if a person lies to a would-be murderer about the whereabouts of the intended victim, surely the liar has not (all things considered) acted immorally. The Kantian deontologist sees in such examples a clash between a perfect duty and the imperfect duty of beneficence, and the Kantian teaching is that the former may never yield to the latter. But it would seem that a theory with such implausible implications stands in need of revision. Perhaps the problem is not only that Kantian deontology overstates the significance of certain "perfect" duties but also that it understates the significance of the duty of beneficence, at least that aspect of beneficence that has to do with preventing serious harm from befalling another or alleviating the serious distress of another.

In our everyday existence as moral agents, we are accustomed to the idea that we have a number of important duties to others. It is less clear that the Kantian notion of duties to self can be satisfactorily reconciled with our experience of the moral life. This is difficult territory. For one thing, the issue of suicide (discussed in Chapter 6) seems to confound our moral "common sense" in a way that blatant wrongs such as murder, rape, and slavery do not. Still, despite significant disagreement, suicide is considered by many to be morally wrong. But the issue is this: Do those who consider suicide morally wrong experience the duty not to commit suicide as a duty to self? It seems more likely that this duty is experienced as a duty to others (who may be negatively affected by one's suicide) or, in the case of religious believers, as a duty to God. (Whether a similar argument would be persuasive with regard to the imperfect duty to develop one's talents is unclear.)

It cannot be denied that Kantian deontology, to a substantial degree, is reconcilable with our experience of the moral life. On the other hand, it appears that the theory is attended with some significant and unresolved difficulties. How does Kantian deontology fare when measured against the second of our standards, the requirement that an ethical theory provide effective guidance in the face of moral dilemmas? Once again, it seems, the verdict is somewhat mixed.

It might be argued that Kantian deontology, by sorting our various duties into the categories of perfect and imperfect and assigning priority to perfect duties, provides us with a structure in terms of which moral dilemmas can be resolved. This is perhaps true to the extent that our perplexity can be analyzed in terms of perfect duties marshaled against imperfect duties, but even here it is difficult to overlook the fact that the priority of perfect over imperfect duties is itself a somewhat problematic feature of Kantian deontology. One is tempted to say that, even if the theory provides reasonably *clear* guidance, it sometimes fails to provide *correct* guidance.

W. D. ROSS'S THEORY OF PRIMA FACIE DUTIES

In a book entitled *The Right and the Good* (1930), English philosopher W. D. Ross proposed a deontological theory that has received considerable attention among ethical theorists. The point of departure for the development of Ross's theory is his concern to provide a defensible account of "cases of conscience," that is, situations that confront us with a conflict of duties. One perceived line of obligation pulls us in one direction; another perceived line of obligation pulls us in a contrary direction. We find ourselves unsettled and uncertain but cannot avoid a choice. Which duty takes precedence over the other? The parent of a young child has promised to attend a community meeting, but the child seems to need special attention. Since our social existence is complex, conflict-of-duty situations are a recurrent feature of our daily life. In the biomedical context, such situations are pervasive.

For understandable reasons, Ross maintains that neither the Kantian nor the utilitarian can provide an account of conflict-of-duty situations that harmonizes with what he calls "ordinary moral consciousness." We have just considered the relevant deficiency in the Kantian approach. It is implausible to maintain that the duty of beneficence can never take precedence over the duty to keep promises or the duty not to lie. As for the utilitarian approach (and here it is clear that Ross has act-utilitarianism in mind), this theory's insistence that in reality we have only the one duty of maximizing utility clashes with our conviction that we have distinct lines of obligation to distinct people. In order to provide an adequate account of conflict-of-duty situations, Ross maintains, it is essential to introduce the notion of "prima facie duty." The Latin phrase *prima facie,* now commonplace in moral philosophy, literally means "at first glance." But the word *conditional* best expresses the sense of the phrase as Ross intends it. A prima facie duty is a conditional duty. A prima facie duty (as opposed to an absolute duty) can be overridden by another prima facie duty that in a particular set of circumstances is more stringent.

According to Ross, there are no absolute, or unconditional, duties (such as "Never lie"), only prima facie duties. But what is the basis of our prima facie duties? Both the utilitarian and the Kantian assert that our various duties have a unitary basis in a fundamental principle of morality. The utilitarian believes that our various duties can be derived from the principle of utility. The Kantian believes that our various duties can be derived from the categorical imperative. Ross, in vivid contrast, maintains that our various prima facie duties have no unitary basis. Rather, they emerge out of our numerous "morally significant relations," relations such as promisee to promiser, creditor to debtor, spouse to spouse, child to parent, friend to friend, citizen to the state, fellow human being to fellow human being. "Each of these relations is the foundation of a *prima facie* duty, which is more or less incumbent on me according to the circumstances of the case."[14]

In unproblematic circumstances, where we are bound by only one prima facie duty, this particular prima facie duty is our *actual* duty. In conflict-of-duty situations, where two (or more) prima facie duties compete for priority, only one of these duties, the more stringent one in the circumstances, can be our actual duty. We have, for example, both a prima facie duty to keep promises and a prima facie duty to assist those who are in need. According to Ross, when these two duties come into conflict, it is clear (in terms of our "ordinary moral consciousness") that the duty to keep promises is usually more incumbent upon us than the duty to assist those who are in need. However, if the promise is relatively trivial and the need of another is compelling—a matter of serious distress—then it is equally clear that the priority is reversed. In the difficult cases, Ross maintains, there is in principle no hard-and-fast rule to apply. In his view, the best anyone can do is to make a reflective, "considered decision" as to which of the competing prima facie duties has the priority in any given situation.

According to Ross, "there is nothing arbitrary about [our] *prima facie* duties. Each rests on a definite circumstance which cannot seriously be held to be without moral significance."[15] Accordingly, he proposes the following division of our prima facie duties.

(1) *Duties of fidelity* include keeping promises, honoring contracts and agreements, and telling the truth. Duties in this class rest on a person's previous acts. In giving one's word to do something, a person creates the duty to do so. (Ross thinks that by entering a conversation, a person implicitly agrees to tell the truth.) Notice that a person's so-called role responsibilities can be identified as an important subclass of duties of fidelity. For example, a teacher has certain responsibilities as a teacher, a physician certain responsibilities as a physician, and a nurse certain responsibilities as a nurse. In taking on a certain social role, a person brings into existence various duties of fidelity. In addition, further duties of fidelity arise out of agreements (both explicit and implicit) that a person enters into while functioning in a professional capacity.

(2) *Duties of reparation* also rest on a person's previous acts. Any person, by wrongfully treating someone else, creates the duty to rectify the wrong that has been perpetrated. For example, if A steals a certain amount of money from B, A thereby brings into existence the duty to repay this amount. (3) *Duties of gratitude* rest upon previous acts of other persons, namely, beneficial services provided by them. If A has provided a good service for B when B was in need, B thereby stands under a duty to provide a good service for A when A is in need.

(4) *Duties of beneficence* "rest on the mere fact that there are other beings in the world whose condition we can make better."[16] (5) *Duties of nonmaleficence* rest on the complementary fact that we can also make the condition of other beings worse. The duties in this category, which Ross recognizes as especially stringent, can be summed up under the heading of "not injuring others." The duty not to kill is an obvious example.

(6) *Duties of justice* "rest on the fact or possibility of a distribution of pleasure or happiness (or of the means thereto) which is not in accordance with the merit of the persons concerned."[17] Benefits are to be distributed in accordance with personal merit, and existing unjust patterns of distribution are to be rectified. (7) *Duties of self-improvement* "rest on the fact that we can improve our own condition."[18]

Prima Facie Duties in a Biomedical Context Ross's framework of prima facie duties is helpful for conceptualizing many of the moral dilemmas that arise in a biomedical context. In analyzing such dilemmas as they arise from the point of view of health-care professionals, the category of duties of fidelity is especially important. Consider, for example, the physician-patient relationship (a topic discussed in Chapter 2). The social understanding or implicit agreement that underlies this relationship undoubtedly includes a number of important provisions. Among these are the provision that the physician is to act in the best medical interest of the patient and the provision that the physician is to keep confidential any personal information that comes to light within the context of the physician-patient relationship. In the very act of accepting a patient for treatment, a physician thereby incurs a number of important prima facie duties of fidelity.

Suppose a physician is convinced that lying to a patient is in the best medical interest of the patient. In Ross's scheme, the prima facie duty not to lie, itself a duty of fidelity, comes into conflict with another duty of fidelity, the prima facie duty to act in the best medical interest of the patient. Since neither duty is unconditional, in one case the duty not to lie might be more incumbent upon the physician, whereas in another case the duty to act in the best interest of the patient might be the more stringent duty. Suppose, in a different case, a physician is treating a patient suffering from a condition that renders the patient in his or her occupation a danger to others. In addition, suppose that the patient is a bus driver subject to blackouts. The patient is desperate to keep his or her job and refuses to divulge the problem to his or her employer. Should the physician break medical confidentiality and notify the patient's employer in an effort to ensure the public safety? In this case, the prima facie duty of beneficence comes into conflict with a duty of fidelity, the prima facie duty to keep medical confidentiality. (Justifiable exceptions to the duty to keep medical confidentiality are discussed in Chapter 3.)

Among the explicit role responsibilities of a typical hospital nurse is the obligation to follow a physician's orders in the treatment of patients. By the simple act of accepting employment in the hospital setting, a nurse thereby incurs, among other numerous duties of fidelity, the prima facie duty to obey a physician's orders. An important moral dilemma for the hospital nurse arises when, in the judgment of the nurse, following a physician's order would be detrimental to the patient. (This dilemma is discussed in Chapter 3.) Thinking in terms of Ross's theory, we can structure the dilemma as follows. The prima facie duty to follow a physician's orders comes into conflict with two other prima facie duties. First, there is a relevant duty of nonmaleficence. A nurse should not act in a way that would, in effect, injure another person. Second, there is another relevant duty of fidelity, deriving from the fact that a nurse has an implicit contract or agreement with the patient to act in his or her best medical interest. Is the collective force of these two prima facie duties more incumbent upon the nurse than the prima facie duty to follow a physician's orders? Since the duty of nonmaleficence is recognized by Ross (and "ordinary moral consciousness") as especially stringent, it seems that, in most cases, at least where the potential harm to patients is significant, the nurse must conclude that it would be wrong to follow the physician's order.

Abstracting from any relevant role responsibilities on the part of health-care professionals, the issue of the moral justifiability of active euthanasia (discussed in Chapter 6) might be conceptualized, in accordance with Ross's scheme, as a moral dilemma involving the conflict between a duty of beneficence and a duty of nonmaleficence. A terminally ill person suffering unbearable pain could be understood to benefit from an immediate and painless death. Thus, we have on one hand a duty of beneficence—the prima facie duty to come to the assistance of a person in serious distress—and on the other hand a duty of nonmaleficence—the prima facie duty not to kill.

Critical Assessment of Ross's Theory Since Ross developed his theory of prima facie duties explicitly in reference to the promptings of "ordinary moral consciousness," it would be surprising if his theory could not be reconciled with our experience of the moral life. Indeed, let us put aside whatever worries might be expressed on this score, for there is a much more obvious deficiency in Ross's theory. Recall that we have asked not only that an ethical theory be largely reconcilable with our experience of the moral life but also that it provide us with effective guidance where it is most needed, in the face of moral dilemmas. And despite the fact that Ross's theory provides us with a helpful framework for conceptualizing our moral dilemmas, it provides us with virtually no substantive guidance for resolving them.

In the difficult cases, where two prima facie duties come into strong conflict, Ross holds that there are no principles we can appeal to in an effort to make an appropriate decision. The most we can do, in his view, is render a "considered decision" as to which duty is more incumbent upon us in a certain situation. Although it is fine to be told to make a considered decision, what exactly is worthy of consideration in reaching a decision? At this point, there is a strong argument for moving beyond Ross's theory. One plausible approach would identify *considerations of coherence* (within our overall system of moral convictions) as the relevant standard. (See the discussion "Reflective Equilibrium and Appeals to Coherence" later in this chapter.) If Ross's theory were supplemented with a coherence-based decision procedure, the advantages of thinking in terms of prima facie duties could be combined with a plausible methodology for mediating among conflicting duties.

THE PRINCIPLES OF BIOMEDICAL ETHICS

One prominent approach to problems in biomedical ethics has been articulated by Tom Beauchamp and James Childress in *Principles of Biomedical Ethics,* originally published in 1979. The basic idea is that problems can be appropriately identified, analyzed, and resolved by reference to a set of four principles, each of which corresponds to a prima facie (i.e., conditional) obligation. The four principles, tailored specifically to be relevant in the field of biomedical ethics, are as follows: the principle of respect for autonomy, the principle of nonmaleficence, the principle of beneficence, and the principle of justice.

This distinctive principle-based approach has much in common with W. D. Ross's theory of prima facie duties, which can also be understood as a principle-based approach. In each case, we are dealing with several prima facie principles of obligation. So in each case, it is common for the principles of the system to conflict, thus requiring a judgment as to which principle has overriding weight or significance in any particular set of circumstances.[19]

Frequent references to "the principles of biomedical ethics," both individually and collectively, can be found in the literature of biomedical ethics (including the readings collected in this textbook). As presented by Beauchamp and Childress, each of the principles must ultimately be understood by reference to numerous distinctions and clarifications. For our purposes, however, it is useful to identify a central (if less than complete) meaning for each principle. The *principle of respect for autonomy* requires that health-care professionals not interfere with the effective exercise of patient autonomy. (A suggested analysis of the concept of autonomy is presented in a later section of this chapter.) The *principle of nonmaleficence* requires that health-care professionals not act in ways that entail harm or injury to patients. The *principle of beneficence* requires that health-care professionals act in ways that promote patient welfare. (The closely related concepts of beneficence and nonmaleficence are briefly explicated in our earlier discussion of Kantian deontology.) The *principle of justice* requires that social benefits (e.g., health-care services) and social burdens (e.g., taxes) be distributed in accordance with the demands of justice. Although this articulation of the principle of justice is somewhat uninformative, it is impossible to give the principle any clearer content without considering questions that are at issue in competing theories of distributive justice. These theories are discussed in the introduction to Chapter 9.

ALTERNATIVE DIRECTIONS AND METHODS

By the 1990s a challenge was well underway both to recently dominant ethical theories (that is, those theories—discussed earlier—that commanded the most attention in the twentieth century) and to the idea that these theories can simply be *applied* to generate satisfactory solutions to concrete problems. In biomedical ethics, criticisms have increasingly been directed at two broad approaches to ethical reasoning. These approaches are known as *deductivism* and *principle-based ethics* (also called "principlism"). A deductivist theory, such as utilitarianism or Kantianism, features a single foundational principle that supposedly provides a basis for all ethical justification.[20] According to this approach, correct ethical judgments can, in principle, be derived from the foundation, given relevant factual information (e.g., concerning the consequences of possible actions, in utilitarianism). As we saw in the previous section, principle-based ethics features a framework of several principles, rules, or duties, none of which takes absolute priority over any other. In principle-based ethics, as it is commonly understood,[21] one considers whatever principles, rules, or duties are relevant in the circumstances, settling conflicts by determining which seems more weighty.[22] Specific criticisms of deductivism and principle-based ethics will emerge in the discussions of leading alternative approaches.

VIRTUE ETHICS

An emphasis on the moral evaluation of *actions* is common both to deductivist theories and to principle-based ethics. These approaches offer principles or rules of conduct as their main source of moral guidance. One is directed to maximize utility, never to treat persons as mere means to one's ends, or the like. Sometimes principles or rules are expressed in the language of rights and duties. For example, it is said that competent adults have a right to refuse medical treatment and health-care professionals have a duty to respect the decision making of competent adults. In contrast, virtue ethics, the tradition of Plato and Aristotle, gives *virtuous character* a preeminent place. For our purposes, virtues may be understood as character traits that are morally valued, such as truthfulness, courage, compassion, and sincerity. In virtue ethics, agents—those performing the actions—are the focus. Whereas the principal concern in an action-based approach to ethics is with the right thing to do, the principal concern in a virtue-based approach is with what kind of person to be.

In recent years there has been a significant revival of virtue ethics, a development affecting bioethics. Some theorists have argued that mainstream theories have overemphasized action-guides to the neglect of issues of character. What is needed, they maintain, is a *supplementation* of action-based ethics with virtue ethics. Other theorists have defended the more radical thesis that the neglect of virtue has caused action-based ethical theories to be *importantly misconceived* (so that merely supplementing them is insufficient). Among these theorists, some have argued for a robust *integration* of action-based ethics and virtue ethics (without giving priority to either), while others have gone further, calling for the *replacement* of action-based ethics by virtue ethics.

What arguments can be advanced in favor of virtue ethics? One difficulty with theories that are solely action-based is that they seem to neglect the fact that we often morally judge people's motivations and character, not just their actions. For example, in praising someone's kindness or criticizing a person's meanness, our evaluation makes no explicit reference to actions. Sometimes we even fault a person who acts rightly but with questionable motivation or attitude. For example, consider a person who gives to charities only when seeking public office, or a surgeon who only begrudgingly solicits a patient's informed consent to surgery. Conversely, sometimes we temper our blame of a person who has acted wrongly if, in doing so, admirable motives and character traits were displayed. For example, we might moderate our criticism of someone who lied to assuage another's feelings, even if we think lying was the wrong choice.

Another argument addresses what is most useful in guiding moral choice. It is claimed that principles, rules, and codes are of little use in actual decision making (e.g., in biomedical contexts). Such action-guides are too abstract to provide practical guidance. Moreover, they often conflict. (The suggestion that conflicts can be effectively resolved by appeal to an ethical theory immediately confronts the problem that there is such extensive disagreement on which theory is most adequate.) A more effective approach, according to this argument, is to cultivate enduring traits (such as competence, attentiveness, honesty, compassion, and loyalty) through education, the influence of role models, and habitual exercise of those traits. Such virtues, it is claimed, are a more reliable basis, in practice, for morally correct action than is knowledge of principles, rules, or codes.

The arguments surveyed so far are compatible with the program of supplementing action-based theories with virtue ethics. Even the idea that virtues are more useful in practice is consistent with these claims: (1) Ethics is more centrally concerned with what people should do (virtues being generally reliable means for doing the right thing); (2) right action, in principle, can be characterized without reference to virtue. However, the following arguments are more radical. They suggest that virtue is often at least as morally important or fundamental as right action and that sometimes the latter cannot even be characterized independently of virtue.

First, several philosophers have argued that in many cases right action cannot be described in an illuminating way without referring to virtue. Consider the idea that we should help those who are suffering. (This idea expresses a principle of action.) Truly helping someone often requires keen attention to the subtleties of the situation at hand to determine whether, and what sort of, intervention is called for. Would calling a particular student aside, telling him or her an anecdote, and offering advice be helpful, or would it be intrusive and condescending? One cannot reliably perform acts that are helpful (as opposed to intrusive or condescending) without exercising a capacity for discernment, which involves such virtues as emotional attunement and sympathetic insightfulness.[23] Since being helpful in such circumstances involves being virtuous, the proper conclusion is that virtue partly constitutes right action.

Second, the manner in which we act—what we express in our action—can matter as much as, or more than, what we do. (We might even say that our manner of acting is part of what we do.) Suppose Earl borrows money from his brother, Jake, and promises to repay him within a month. Four weeks later Jake gently reminds Earl of his promise. If Earl later storms into his brother's house, slams down the money, and marches off in resentment and anger, he has fulfilled his duty to keep a promise, but he has not acted well. A full account of how Earl should have conducted himself would include a description of the manner in which he should have acted (perhaps courteously). Here, again, the conclusion is that virtue partly constitutes right action.

Moreover, sometimes emotional responses, which can reveal a person's character, are of paramount moral importance (a point suggested in the last example). This is especially evident in situations in which no particular action is morally called for. For example, a social worker might be deeply affected by another social worker's detailed account of a patient who lost his job and committed suicide. If the two work at different hospitals, there is probably nothing the first social worker can do about the tragedy. However, her pain at a stranger's plight reveals virtue; complete indifference arguably would reveal a moral deficiency.[24]

While the previous arguments probably succeed in showing the need to integrate virtue ethics and action-based ethics, there are compelling reasons to resist the stronger thesis that virtue ethics should *replace* action-based approaches. First, while action-guides such as principles and rules are not exhaustive of what is important in the moral life, neither is virtue. One can be well motivated and have a good character yet act wrongly; conversely, acting without virtue does not *always* mean doing the wrong thing. (This is consistent with the view that virtue sometimes partly constitutes right action.) Morally, we are concerned with both action and character, doing and being.

Second, the specificity of such action-guides as rules, codes, and rights-claims often provides an attractive form of bottom-line moral protection. Rules such as those requiring informed consent for medical interventions and prohibiting psychotherapists from having sexual relations with psychiatric patients provide an important bedrock of action requirements. In fact, such rules can often help professionals establish relationships with patients in which certain virtues can be exercised more naturally.

Similarly, it seems unlikely that any specification of virtues would be sufficient to guide conduct. In bioethics we are interested in such questions as "Is it ever right for a psychotherapist to violate patient confidentiality, and, if so, when?" Such a question probably cannot be answered by appeal to virtue alone. In conclusion, it would seem that an adequate portrait of the moral life would include action-guides such as principles, rules, and rights-claims—not just virtues. The question we are left with, then, is not whether both virtues and action-guides have important places in ethical theory and bioethics but, rather, how to understand in greater detail their roles and relationship to one another.

How might virtues play a role in biomedical ethics? Here is one example. A physician has just received test results strongly suggesting that her 30-year-old patient has inoperable ovarian cancer. Neither of them expected such a calamity. The physician knows that she has an obligation to inform her patient of the results. However, in reflecting on how to broach and discuss this matter with her, the physician finds such principles as beneficence and nonmaleficence too general to be useful; no helpful rules of conduct come to mind, either. The physician keeps coming back to such ideas as *compassion, sensitivity,* and *honesty.* Although these words describe virtues, we could say that "Be compassionate," "Be sensitive," and "Be honest" are rules of action. Nevertheless, such instructions do not really tell the physician how to handle her delicate predicament. To handle it well, she will have to *be* compassionate, sensitive, and honest, and no set of rules can explain how to be that way. The physician, in other words, will have to manifest virtue. She might find it useful to model her behavior on that of a mentor or colleague whom she identifies as having the desired qualities.

THE ETHICS OF CARE AND FEMINIST ETHICS

The ethics of care and feminist ethics represent further challenges to recently dominant ethical theories, to deductivism, and to principle-based ethics. While the ethics of care and feminist ethics both stem importantly from the moral experience of women, they represent overlapping—but certainly not identical—sets of concerns.

Like virtue ethics, the ethics of care pays considerable attention to affective components of the moral life, but with special emphasis on empathy and concern for the needs of others, that is, on caring. Like casuistry (an approach discussed in the next section), the ethics of care emphasizes the particularities and context of moral judgment. It also underscores the moral importance of relationships and the responsibilities to which they give rise.

Perhaps more than any other work, Carol Gilligan's study of gender differences in ethical thinking has brought the ethics of care into the mainstream of philosophical discussion.[25] In a study of responses to moral conflicts, Gilligan finds that females often focus on details about the relationships among the persons involved and to seek innovative solutions that protect everyone's interests. In contrast, males typically try to identify and apply a relevant principle or rule (which they take to be universal or valid from an impartial perspective), even if doing so means sacrificing someone's interests. Gilligan calls the former approach an *ethic of care* (or responsibility) and the latter (which includes recently dominant ethical theories) an *ethic of justice.* She notes in her study that the empirical correlations are far from perfect; males sometimes work from the care perspective and women fairly often use the justice approach. In any event, the tendencies she notes are striking, for they suggest that traditional approaches to ethics have been more responsive to the moral experience of males than to that of females. Gilligan concludes that there is no reason to consider the care perspective inferior and that an ideal ethics would incorporate both approaches.

As originally characterized by Gilligan and now generally understood, the ethics of care downplays rights and allegedly universal principles and rules in favor of an emphasis on caring, interpersonal relationships, and context. Numerous specific criticisms of recently dominant ethical theories have been developed in the ethics of care literature. A summary of several critical arguments follows.

To begin with, there is a problematic presumption underlying theories such as utilitarianism and Kantianism. The presumption is that impartiality is a fundamental aspect of moral thinking. In reality, impartiality is a demand reflective of male thinking; the partiality that comes with caring relationships is no less legitimate. Indeed, certain relationships merit special weight. For example, in many contexts, a father should favor his own children's interests over those of other children. Moreover, the abstract principles of traditional theories have very limited practical use; contextualization and attention to detail are needed for problem solving in ethics. In many complex situations involving ethical conflicts, such principles as "Respect all persons as ends in themselves" and "Maximize utility" simply provide inadequate guidance.

Furthermore, ethical theories featuring abstract principles tend to neglect affective components of the moral life. Caring responsiveness to others' needs is often morally preferable to detached, dispassionate moral evaluation. For example, the ethics of care would strongly affirm a health-care professional's heartfelt dedication to a patient, without conditioning its value on good consequences or respect for persons. The abstract nature of recently dominant theories also tends to cover up certain morally salient experiences—such as being a woman, a parent, a minority, or a professional who has particular working relationships with other professionals.

A health-care professional working within the spirit of the ethics of care would bear in mind (or internalize) considerations such as these: (1) the individualized needs, both physical and psychological, of the patient; (2) how to respond in a caring, personalized manner to those needs; (3) the likely impact of various options on the quality of the relationships among the involved persons, including the patient and professional, but also other members of the health-care team and any involved family members; and (4) how to attain or maintain the best possible relationships among those persons. Suppose a nurse faces a conflict between loyalty to a patient and loyalty to the attending physician, who refuses to disclose certain medical options to the patient. The "justice" approach might view the dilemma in terms of overall utility, conflicting rights, or the like. In contrast, the ethics of care would emphasize the lived relationships and the responsibilities inherent in them, the impact of possible responses on those relationships, and the prospects for conflict resolution.

The relationship between *feminist ethics* and the ethics of care is a complex one, and this complexity is reflected in the different ways that various feminists have responded to the emergence and widespread discussion of the ethics of care. Some feminists have celebrated the reception accorded the ethics of care and feel validated by the recognition of a distinctly female moral perspective. Others, however, have reacted negatively to at least certain aspects of the ethics of care.

Feminist ethics can be initially characterized in the following ways. (1) As with the ethics of care, it is firmly committed to the view that the moral experience of women must be taken seriously (but often with a critical eye to the role that the subordination of women may play in shaping that experience). (2) It is deeply committed to the overriding moral importance of ending oppression—with special emphasis on the subordination of women.

These features of feminist ethics together motivate a redirection of focus to women (and, to an important extent, minorities and other historically disadvantaged groups). This focus includes both an emphasis on the importance of women's interests and special attention to issues that especially concern or affect women. Thus, in bioethics, feminist ethics urges careful examination of the interests of women in matters of reproduction and as the almost exclusive participants in the profession of nursing. Special attention is also given, for example, to the distinctive needs of women in the area of medical research, to the moral complexities of surrogate motherhood, and to arguably sexist undercurrents in the promotion of in vitro fertilization and in various medical practices surrounding childbirth.

In feminist ethics, a critical eye is turned toward practices and institutions that may perpetuate and legitimate forms of oppression. Some of these practices and institutions, feminists argue, are so deeply embedded in our culture that they go unnoticed. Accordingly, some feminists have charged proponents of the ethics of care with naïveté for accepting women's moral experiences at face value—without questioning the oppressive practices and attitudes that may have helped make certain experiences and ways of thinking typical for women. Perhaps women's proficiency at caring is related to their subordinate status.[26] In fact, nurturing, caring, and the disposition to preserve relationships at almost any cost may simply be the survival skills of an oppressed group; it has been noted that such dispositions are also found among persons of both genders who are members of groups that have been subjected to slavery or colonization.[27] Some feminists also argue that the value of mothering, so affirmed in the ethics of care, may be tied to the norm of the nuclear family— a norm that can be seen as discounting the perspectives of homosexuals, persons in single-parent families, and others who remain legally unmarried. They point out that caring has led some women to direct nearly all of their energies to others' needs, without adequately attending to their own. While caring is an admirable trait in many circumstances, these feminists maintain, it is sometimes better withheld when a focus on rights and autonomy is necessary. In general, they conclude, we must not valorize the traits that tend to perpetuate women's subordinate status.[28]

How might we assess the ethics of care and feminist ethics as alternatives to recently dominant theories and to the idea that these theories can simply be applied in order to resolve concrete problems? The care perspective's emphasis on relationships and the affective components of the moral life merits careful attention; arguably, the traditional theories greatly understate their significance. (Ross's theory, which highlights morally significant relationships, is a partial exception.) The critical-minded attention of feminist ethics to oppression, inequalities, and issues pertaining to women and other disadvantaged groups is surely valuable. In addition, the feminist caution about gender stereotyping is well taken. Uncritical acceptance of traditionally feminine and masculine qualities may lead too easily to the assignment of people to "appropriate" roles (such as women to midnight infant feedings and men to aggressive professional pursuits).

However, the distance between the perspectives presently under discussion, on the one hand, and recently dominant theories, on the other, can easily be overdrawn. Utilitarians, for example, should be firmly dedicated to the eradication of oppression (given all of its bad consequences). Kantian respect for persons, while perhaps vague and abstract, is at least compatible with caring and special relationships (the validity of which could be impartially recognized). Caring attention to particularities might even provide a useful way of specifying or supplementing abstract but worthy principles.

In the end, Gilligan argues that "care" and "justice" are both only parts of a broader ethics, and few proponents of the care perspective propose that it monopolize ethics. In a pluralistic spirit, one might adopt a similar attitude toward feminist ethics, concentrating on whatever insight and illumination this perspective brings to ethics. Following is a concluding suggestion from feminist philosopher Susan Sherwin:

> I do not envision feminist ethics to be a comprehensive . . . theory that can be expected to resolve every moral question with which it is confronted. It is a theoretical perspective that must be combined with other considerations to address the multitude of moral dilemmas that confront human beings. . . . Although very little of the literature in ethics addresses the issue of sexism or any other form of systematic oppression, surely the responsibility to do so in one's moral evaluations is implicit. Feminist ethics has assumed leadership in pursuing such analysis.[29]

CASUISTRY: CASE-BASED REASONING IN HISTORICAL CONTEXT

Casuistry, which has received a great deal of attention in recent years, is a method of moral reasoning that was reawakened from three centuries of slumber with the publication of *The Abuse of Casuistry,* by Albert Jonsen and Stephen Toulmin.[30] Following Aristotle and other philosophers as well as theologians throughout the ages, the authors contend that the "top-down" reasoning inherent in deductivism and principle-based ethics (as they understand it) is entirely inadequate for the resolution of concrete problems, such as those that arise in bioethics. (Jonsen and Toulmin never clearly distinguish deductivism and principle-based ethics. While some of their criticisms concern both approaches, others concern only deductivism.)

First, according to the casuists, no simple, unified ethical theory can capture the great diversity of our moral ideas, a consideration that helps to account for the fact that there is such extensive disagreement about ethical theories. Second, our actual moral thinking does not typically consist of straightforward deductive reasoning (deriving an ethical judgment from a supreme principle). *Practical wisdom* is required to determine which of various norms (principles or rules) applies in a complicated or ambiguous case. For example, if a patient awaiting admission to a fully occupied intensive care unit better fulfills admission criteria than someone already admitted, would it ever be right to admit the waiting patient if doing so would be detrimental to the one who would be displaced? Casuists doubt that the answers to such questions can be derived from a traditional ethical theory, such as utilitarianism or Kantianism, or from a set of abstract principles. Third, such approaches miss the fact that moral certainty, where it exists, concerns particular cases. For example, that a particular person acts wrongly in torturing for sadistic pleasure is far more certain than any full-blown ethical theory could be.

The alternative of casuistry is a form of case-based reasoning. It begins with clear "paradigm" cases in which some *maxim* (a relatively specific principle or rule) is clearly relevant and indicates the right action or judgment. For example, if we learn that a man stole a car just for a thrill, we know he acted wrongly. From this and similar cases we can extract a maxim, "Stealing is wrong," which holds in the absence of unusual circumstances. The paradigm cases illuminate other cases by way of analogy. Maxims are refined as new cases are confronted in which the norms apply ambiguously (for example, if someone finds an expensive watch in a classroom and does not attempt to locate its owner) or in conflict (for example, if someone believes that temporarily appropriating a bicycle is the only way to save an innocent person's life). Often, the refinements involve stating exceptions.

In order to reach a defensible moral judgment in any particular case, we must first determine which paradigms are relevant. Difficulties arise, of course, when paradigms fit only ambiguously or when two or more paradigms fit in conflicting ways. Jonsen and Toulmin see the history of moral practice as revealing an ongoing clarification of the use of paradigms and of admitted exceptions. This brings us to an important point.

Moral reasoning about cases cannot proceed without reference to actual moral traditions. Casuists assert the priority of *practice* over theory. Moral norms are to be found in practice; practice is not to be justified (or condemned) by absolute moral principles, because there are none. In rejecting the idea of a timeless, rationally required ethical theory, the casuists have important allies in such American pragmatists as William James (1842–1910) and John Dewey (1859–1952). But the emphasis on practice is not simply a broad historicism, grounding our understanding of morality in the developing Western moral tradition. Also crucial are the specific institutions and practices (such as those of American medicine) that provide the context for any set of ethical problems. To illustrate their method, casuists point to case law—including, in bioethics, classic cases such as *Quinlan, Conroy,* and *Cruzan,* which have greatly illuminated the ethics of terminating life-sustaining treatment.[31]

For an example of casuistry in action, consider the question of whether Jehovah's Witness parents have the right to refuse a blood transfusion for their young child who will die without one. Rather than appealing to an ethical theory or to general principles such as beneficence or respect for autonomy, a casuist would try to reason by analogy from cases about which we have relatively settled opinions. The casuist would cite various cases that support (1) the right of competent adults to refuse medical treatment for themselves and (2) the right of parents to make decisions for their children. Regarding the second right, we let parents send their children to private religious schools, for example. On the other hand, society tends to limit parental discretion if choices amount to serious neglect. Thus, while parents have much discretion over where to send their children to school, they may not keep them out of school (using the term broadly to include home schooling). The choice to keep them out of school is regarded as seriously detrimental to children's well-being. Similarly, a casuist might argue that because refusing a blood transfusion would ensure the child's death, such a choice would be seriously neglectful and therefore beyond the bounds of parental discretion. Unlike the parents, the child has not autonomously chosen to be a Jehovah's Witness. If and when the child becomes an adult, he or she may choose or reject this value system and make medical and other decisions accordingly.

How viable is casuistry as an alternative to recently dominant theories and top-down methods of ethical reasoning? It certainly avoids the remoteness from concrete problems that arguably plagues utilitarianism and Kantianism. Indeed, it seems to capture the way much of our ethical reasoning actually proceeds. Moreover, casuistry is capable of producing consensus even when people disagree about ethical theories. Furthermore, the casuists are surely right that at least some specific moral judgments are more certain than any ethical theory.

At the same time, a number of problems confront casuistry. Some concern the work of its currently leading proponents, Jonsen and Toulmin. For example, while they identify casuistry as an alternative to top-down approaches represented in the theories already described, they never clearly distinguish their primary targets: deductivism and principle-based ethics. This omission is significant, because some of their criticisms can be validly made against at most one of these approaches. For instance, while some specific moral judgments are more certain than any *complete ethical theory,* it is far from clear that such judgments are more certain than any *principle.* Since principle-based ethics involves the use of principles (as opposed to the use of a complete ethical theory), the casuists' point about the locus of ethical certainty may only constitute an advantage over deductivism.

One might therefore wonder whether casuistry is so different from principle-based ethics. Casuists claim that moral certainty is to be found in particular cases. However, giving priority to the particular over the general may be undermined by the following possibility: *Grasping the ethical significance of a case is indistinguishable from grasping a prima facie principle or rule that applies to that case.* We can grasp that a man beating a child is wrong. However, in order to make this judgment, we must also grasp the prima facie wrongness of some kind of action, such as harming the innocent or hurting children, for it is something about the man's action that is understood to make it wrong. There seems to be no reason to claim that judgments about particular cases are more certain than judgments about prima facie principles or rules relevant to such cases. Indeed, it is not clear that the two kinds of judgments can be completely separated.

Another possible charge against casuistry is that it is overly "intuitionistic" in resolving difficult cases. Suppose we start with the established view that a competent adult patient may refuse medical treatment. May such a patient also refuse all nutrition and hydration? If so, what makes this second kind of case *relevantly similar* to the first, such that the maxim guiding the first (respecting competent adult patients' refusals) applies also to the second? Where matters are debatable, how does one *justify* particular judgments? At this point, the casuist is likely to vest decision-making authority in community judgment. Such a judgment becomes incorporated into the community's evolving traditions and practices. For example, our society has judged that food and water can be thought of, in medical settings, as similar to medical care, so a competent adult patient may refuse them.

While casuistry can respond to the charge of being overly intuitionistic by appealing to traditions and practices, it must then confront the charge of being too *accepting* of the latter. Why take at face value the ethical convictions woven into our cultural traditions and professional practices? American medical practice, for instance, may embody a vision of the physician-nurse relationship that is elitist and sexist. Therefore, is it not unsound, as contemporary feminists would insist, to appeal to established medical practice in considering issues concerning the interactions of physicians and nurses? To take another example, arguably neither broad cultural traditions nor the professional practice of researchers has sufficient critical "edge" to confront squarely the question of whether animals should be used in biomedical research and, if so, with what restrictions.

Finally, by focusing so exclusively on cases, casuistry risks (1) being unable to make progress with especially controversial issues and (2) missing very general and fundamental issues, the resolution of which may be relevant to specific cases. As an example of problem (1), case analysis is almost certainly insufficient to illuminate the moral status of animals. In our society today there is fundamental disagreement about animals' moral status, so people are likely to have widely varying responses to individual cases. Regarding (2), fundamental issues can be missed because of excessive faith in precedents (judgments about previous cases). How do we know our precedents are right? For example, the fact that Medicare covers renal dialysis and kidney transplants, open-heart surgery, and certain other treatments may seem to weigh in favor of funding heart transplants. But perhaps we never should have funded those other treatments in the first place.[32]

In conclusion, while casuistry embodies important insights about ethical reasoning, it faces significant challenges. Contrary to the claims of recent defenders, casuistry may be compatible with principle-based ethics. Further reflection on its strengths and weaknesses may suggest that casuistry is best regarded as part of a more comprehensive model of ethical reasoning.

REFLECTIVE EQUILIBRIUM AND APPEALS TO COHERENCE

Recently dominant approaches (whether deductivist or principle-based) are sometimes criticized for viewing ethical justification as essentially "downward"; that is, *theories or principles,* assumed to be firmly established, are thought to justify our judgments about particular cases. On the other hand, casuistry may oversimplify the nature of ethical reasoning in the opposite direction. Casuists claim that ethical certainty lies in *cases,* the study of which allows us to identify maxims to be used and revised in exploring new cases. Arguably, each of these models is excessively rigid in giving priority to one level of ethical conviction: general norms (theories or principles) or particular cases. Perhaps our ethical insights and reasoning lack any such exclusive foundation.

According to the model of *reflective equilibrium,* formulated by John Rawls, no level of ethical conviction deserves such priority.[33] Justification occurs at all levels of generality: (1) theories, (2) principles and rules of differing degrees of specificity, and (3) judgments about cases. Judgments that seem especially compelling at any level can be used to revise less certain judgments at any other level.

The reflective-equilibrium model directs us to start with *considered judgments,* that is, those judgments about which we have a high degree of confidence after careful and extensive consideration. These judgments differ in some ways from the paradigm case judgments of casuistry. First, considered judgments may be of any level of generality. Some may be specific case judgments (as in casuistry); others may be rules such as a prohibition of rape; still others may be principles such as the principle of respect for autonomy. Second, a judgment counts as a considered judgment only if it is reasonably believed not to have resulted from bias. (Casuistry, again, ties its paradigm case judgments so closely to accepted practices that many such judgments may be suspected of bias.) Considered judgments serve as a basis for revising other ethical beliefs or judgments that one may hold, in an effort to achieve a more coherent overall set of beliefs. (What coherence involves is described later in this section.)

For example, one might initially believe it appropriate to deceive prospective participants in an important biomedical study if deception seems necessary to attract a sufficient number of participants. But Kant's principle that we should not treat persons merely as means casts doubt on this initial judgment. Prospective participants are not treated as ends in themselves unless they are given full information about what their participation would involve. This revision of judgments moves "downward" (from principle to case), but in the present model one may also revise "upward." For example, in consideration of a case in which a psychiatric patient threatens to kill an identified third party, we might revise a principle of patient confidentiality to allow exceptions in this sort of case.

One point stressed by defenders of the reflective-equilibrium model is that revisions are never considered final; we must always admit the possibility that our ethical convictions (sometimes even considered judgments) will require modification in light of further considerations. Thus, while we strive, through continual reflection, for a state of equilibrium in our total set of ethical convictions (hence the model's name), we are never finished with moral inquiry. New problems arise, and fresh information and novel insights make us question old judgments. As in casuistry, moral reasoning is viewed as dynamic and is not expected to produce a final, rationally necessary theory.

But how do we know which judgments or norms should get revised when there is a conflict? In the cases previously mentioned, why not (1) reject or revise the prohibition against treating persons merely as means or (2) retain confidentiality as an exceptionless principle, instead of the other way around in each case? How can we *justify* any particular resolution of conflicts? In brief, conflicts are to be settled by making revisions that seem to produce the greatest *coherence* in our overall system of ethical convictions.

Appeals to coherence may be understood, more specifically, to include requirements of logical consistency, argumentative support, and plausibility (reconcilability with our moral experience).[34] *Logical consistency* is simply the avoidance of outright contradiction. For example, it is logically inconsistent to hold that killing an innocent person is always wrong, yet hold that it would be right to grant this person's request to be killed on grounds of mercy. *Argumentative support* is the giving of reasons that back up one's ethical views (reasons that, of course, must be consistent with one's reasoning about other ethical issues). Thus, if one favors paternalistically prohibiting the use of certain drugs but opposes paternalistic seat belt laws, one must provide a reason that supports the claim that paternalism is justified in one case but not in the other. (Paternalism will be discussed in detail later in this chapter.) Wherever there is ethical controversy, lack of argumentative support for a particular position suggests dogmatism and invites reasonable doubts that the position is really justified. The third requirement for selecting from among alternative viewpoints is *plausibility*. Suppose someone argues that no actions are ethically right or wrong (a logically consistent position) and gives as a reason (argumentative support) for this view the fact that ethical judgments are subject to seemingly endless dispute. This view is utterly implausible. It implies that it is not wrong to commit genocide out of sheer racial hatred. Thus, in the present model one seeks logically consistent judgments, supported by ethical reasons or arguments, that are largely plausible upon reflection.[35]

The reflective-equilibrium model, involving appeals to coherence, appears to be gaining support as more theorists and professionals question the adequacy of more traditional approaches. The model is especially favored by those contemporary philosophers who identify with the spirit of the early American pragmatists (who saw ethical reasoning as dynamic and rejected claims of an absolute foundation for morality). The model incorporates the case-based reasoning of casuistry, as well as the downward argumentation associated with principle-based ethics.[36] It concedes to deductivism that sometimes theoretical thinking is needed to check our particular judgments. Depending upon how it is developed, the model can also include many insights and elements of virtue theory as well as the ethics of care and feminist ethics. Overall, it may seem to offer a flexible and balanced approach to moral reasoning.

Nevertheless, the model of reflective equilibrium has its difficulties. Arguably, it buys flexibility and freedom from dogmatism at the cost of vagueness and lack of structure. By contrast, deductivism, which identifies a single principle as a basis for ethical justification, provides a framework or method that may be easier to conceptualize. And casuistry, by focusing on concrete cases, may provide a clearer method for approaching some issues. A critic could argue that, in the reflective-equilibrium model, one might not know where to start or how to proceed. A defender of the model might respond as follows. Theoretically, we start with considered judgments; in practice, we often simply start wherever we have ethical concern, and we use various tools of reasoning as we work toward more coherent positions. While this model is receiving increasing attention in bioethics and appears to have many strengths, it may be premature to judge its overall adequacy as an alternative to casuistry and recently dominant approaches.

CONFRONTING ETHICAL RELATIVISM

In critically examining various ethical theories and methodologies in this introduction, we have implicitly assumed that there can be right and wrong answers to moral questions, reasonable and unreasonable moral positions, better and worse ways of addressing ethical issues. Naturally, this assumption underlies the theories and methodologies themselves, as each represents an effort to provide the most adequate approach to addressing moral questions. Moreover, the articles reprinted in this volume also seem to rely on this assumption in defending particular positions on issues in biomedical ethics. Indeed, the assumption that there can be right and wrong answers to moral questions is so fundamental that it is implicit in the very act of making a moral judgment. To judge, for example, that genocide is wrong is equivalent to believing that this judgment is *correct* and that someone who denies that genocide is wrong is *mistaken.* Unless we believe that moral judgments can be correct or incorrect, reasonable or unreasonable, there seems to be little point in discussing and debating ethical issues: If all moral judgments are *equally* correct or reasonable, why bother trying to persuade anyone of your position on some ethical issue? Our everyday practices of moral discussion assume that some moral answers are more adequate and defensible than others.

Nevertheless, many people wonder whether there are any *universal* moral judgments— that is, any moral judgments whose legitimacy or authority extends *across cultural boundaries.* Perhaps, as *ethical relativism* claims, moral judgments are justified only relative to one's culture and upbringing. Today ethical relativism is casually asserted by many students, faculty members, and other individuals in our culture (although by very few ethicists and moral philosophers). Why is ethical relativism so commonly asserted? The following considerations may provide part of the answer.

We are encouraged today to become better informed about cultures in other countries— as well as distinct cultures within our own (e.g., those of different ethnic groups)—and to be respectful of their traditions values, and beliefs. When one adopts such a multicultural attitude and appreciates differences among cultures in their moral practices and traditions, one might find it natural to think that no moral values are common to all human cultures. Moreover, since it is obvious that an individual's upbringing (e.g., one's religious education and the political values espoused by one's parents) and broader culture (e.g., secular, Western, democratic values) profoundly affect his or her moral outlook, one might infer that a person's moral judgments make sense only within this framework of values. For these and other reasons, increasingly many people appear to be attracted to ethical relativism.

Nevertheless, we believe that ethical relativism is not a viable option. Before outlining our reasons for rejecting this view, we must clarify that we are not rejecting certain important ideas that are sometimes associated with ethical relativism. First, we are not claiming that whenever two cultures approach a moral issue differently, one culture must be wrong. For example, in balancing the values of (1) individual autonomy and (2) familial closeness and solidarity, in cases where the two seem to conflict, one culture may tend to give greater weight to the first value while another culture places greater importance on the second— without either culture's priorities being unreasonable or even less reasonable than the other. How to set priorities among conflicting values is often a matter of reasonable disagreement. On the other hand, it might be unreasonable to place *no* value on individual autonomy or *no* value on familial closeness.

Second, in rejecting ethical relativism, we are not claiming that moral principles and rules are *absolute* in the sense of never having exceptions and never being justifiably overridden by other principles or rules. Our discussion of recently dominant ethical theories suggested that general principles and most rules must sometimes be overridden by other principles or rules and sometimes admit of exceptions. Rather than implying that moral principles and rules are absolute, the rejection of relativism implies that some of these norms are binding across cultures. For example, all persons, regardless of culture, have prima facie obligations to respect other people, to communicate truthfully and keep promises, and to refrain from harming others.

Third, in rejecting ethical relativism in favor of some universal norms, we are not claiming that *our* society's prevailing values are always correct. On the contrary, we are convinced that they are not always correct. For example, we believe that in the United States the "right" of individual citizens to own guns is prized too highly.

Interestingly, one consideration that is sometimes thought to support ethical relativism proves, upon close examination, to undermine it. Lately increasing emphasis has been placed on the importance of *tolerance,* the attitude that we should not be too quick to judge negatively those who have beliefs, traditions, and values that differ from our own. Thus, for example, people who are comfortable in mainstream twenty-first century American or Canadian society should not dismiss the value systems and ways of life that have characterized Native American societies. Note that this is an ethical judgment, which implies that it would be wrong or inappropriate to dismiss these alternative cultural practices out of hand. But tolerance, which is a component of respecting persons more generally, is presumably a value that all persons ought to recognize. One who urges tolerance is very unlikely to think rabid intolerance is just fine as long as one's own culture and upbringing favor intolerance. One is likely to think, rather, that a society that executes people for having particular religious beliefs is profoundly wrong to do so.

This example suggests another important point: While tolerance seems to set appropriate standards for behavior across cultures, it also has limits insofar as we need not tolerate or accept *all* differences among people and cultures. The imagined society's violent intolerance of particular religious beliefs is beyond the pale of reasonable differences—and in that sense intolerable. Similarly, we are hardly obligated to tolerate rape, slavery, genocide, racism, or any other flagrant abuse of human beings (or animals) anywhere. What we should tolerate, generally, are cultural differences that do not involve extensive and unambiguous harm or violation of human rights. This principle of tolerance, it seems, is valid across cultures, providing our first argument against ethical relativism.

Another reason to reject ethical relativism is the sheer implausibility of some of its implications. Suppose a society's values are such that the systematic rape, torture, and killing of a despised minority are judged by the overwhelming majority to be appropriate. If ethical relativism were correct, then we would have no basis for claiming that the majority's brutality toward the minority is wrong. Yet we do not think, "Well, we have our liberal, more gentle ways of treating minorities, they have their way of treating minorities, and neither approach is morally better or worse." Instead, we condemn the brutality. In doing so, and in making similar cross-cultural moral judgments (e.g., condemning slavery or apartheid), we reveal our deep conviction that some moral standards ought to be recognized as binding on everyone.

Now consider the fact that, when a particular culture changes morally, the change often impresses people within that culture as being an improvement. For example, it is widely believed today that greater equality among the races and sexes over the years represents *moral progress,* as does growing tolerance of and respect for gay people. But, if ethical relativism were true, there could be no such thing as moral progress. On this view, we lack any basis for saying that when most Americans accepted slavery, this was unenlightened or unjustified; the only values by which their practice could be appropriately judged are their own (racist) values of the time, and by these values slavery was justified. Those who believe moral progress is a meaningful concept should reject ethical relativism.

Finally, consider individuals who challenge currently prevailing values within their culture. Abolitionists did so during the time of slavery; today's animal rights activists furnish another example. If ethical relativism were correct, then the moral position of these reformers—their conviction that some current practice is unjustified—would often be hard to understand. According to ethical relativism, moral judgments are justified only relative to a culture. That means the reformers would be claiming, in effect, that their culture's practice (which they are criticizing) is inconsistent with the culture's values (the only possible basis for criticism). But frequently moral reformers are advancing a more fundamental criticism that targets some of their culture's basic values, such as unequal regard for different races or unequal consideration for different species. In such cases, reformers contend that some of their culture's prevailing values are wrong—a claim that would make no sense if relativism were true. One need not agree with the reformer's moral agenda to appreciate this argument against relativism; one need only grant that the reformer's moral claim is intelligible.

For all of these reasons, then, we do not believe that ethical relativism is a visible option. At the same time, we applaud the growth of *multiculturalism.* We understand multiculturalism, roughly, as an appreciation of the often differing values and traditions of different cultures, an openness to learning important practical lessons from other cultures, and a rejection of the assumption that our own culture's values are always superior and deserving of emulation by other cultures. Multiculturalism does not imply ethical relativism. Indeed, the recognition that our culture is not beyond reproach and that we may learn valuable moral lessons from other cultures implies that some moral standards are so reasonable they deserve to be embraced by all persons across cultures.

FUNDAMENTAL CONCEPTS AND PRINCIPLES

The concepts of autonomy and paternalism are of fundamental importance in biomedical ethics. Closely associated with these concepts is a set of principles called "liberty-limiting principles," which are often invoked in order to justify limitations on individual liberty. This section provides an examination of these concepts and principles.

AUTONOMY

Many discussions in biomedical ethics presume the importance of individual autonomy, stressing the right of autonomous decision makers to determine for themselves what will be done to their bodies. This "right of self-determination" is said to limit what physicians, nurses, and other health-care professionals can justifiably do to patients. In fact, this right is often taken so seriously that professionals who act against their patients' wishes, even to save their patients' lives, are condemned as morally blameworthy and leave themselves open to charges of battery. In view of all this, it is useful to discuss the following questions, the first a conceptual question and the second an ethical one. (1) What sense of autonomy is operative in the widespread presumption that individual autonomy is an important value? (2) What is the ethical basis for the value accorded to individual autonomy?

The Concept of Autonomy Autonomy is typically defined as self-governance or self-determination. Individuals are said to act autonomously when they, and not others, make the decisions that affect their lives and act on the basis of these decisions. This general characterization needs to be explicated, however, because autonomy is a complex notion. In fact, different ways of conceptualizing autonomy may be appropriate in different contexts. In this section we attempt to elucidate the sense of autonomy or self-determination that is most prominent in biomedical ethics, one that squares with our ethical ideas about respect for autonomy. Although one may meaningfully talk about individuals' lives and political states as autonomous, we will focus on the nature of *autonomous action* (including *autonomous choice,* choice being a kind of action), because whether a certain action is autonomous is often a central question in biomedical ethics; secondarily, we will also refer to autonomous *agents.* It is widely agreed that for an action to qualify as autonomous, it must be (1) intentional, (2) based on sufficient understanding, (3) sufficiently free of external constraints, and (4) sufficiently free of internal constraints.[37] A brief elaboration of these conditions should both clarify the concept of autonomous action and illustrate various ways in which action can be less than fully autonomous.

Intentionality Imagine a patient, Mark, who has just been admitted to the psychiatric unit of a hospital to receive treatment for depression. The day after his admission, a staff psychiatrist talks to him for an extended period of time, during which Mark is highly distracted. The psychiatrist then requests Mark's signature, which Mark provides, believing that he is consenting to remain in the hospital for several days. Suppose, however, that the paper Mark signs has nothing to do with remaining in the hospital. As the psychiatrist had attempted to explain, the paper is a consent form authorizing Mark's participation in a study of patients with a particular form of depression.

In this scenario, Mark intentionally signs a piece of paper and, in doing so, formally consents to participate in a study. But Mark does not *intentionally consent to participate;* his intention is to authorize an extended stay in the hospital. Clearly, Mark's consenting to participate is not an autonomous action. To perform an action autonomously, one must, as a first condition, intentionally perform that action. But one must also satisfy other conditions.

Understanding Imagine a second depressed patient, Judy, who is also approached about possible participation in a biomedical study. Suppose that Judy, unlike Mark, does intentionally consent to participate in the study described to her. But despite the psychiatrist's best efforts to explain clearly what the study would entail, Judy is confused by the long presentation of details. She very much hopes to receive the promising new medication whose effectiveness the study is designed to determine. Due to a number of factors—this hope, her belief that researchers would not ask her to participate in a study that could be contrary to her interests, and her difficulty absorbing large amounts of information in a single presentation—Judy misses one very salient detail: There is a 50 percent chance that she will be one of a group of patients who will receive an established medication with which Judy has had very unpleasant experiences in the past. Indeed, if she were to grasp that she might receive this medication, she would refuse to participate in the study.

In this example, Judy intentionally consents to participate in a study, but since she does so with *insufficient understanding* of what participation entails, her decision cannot count as autonomous. Sometimes insufficient understanding results from blameworthy actions of others. For example, if a physician lies, misleads, or presents significantly incomplete information to a patient, the patient's understanding of his or her options may be insufficient for an autonomous decision. In other cases, insufficient understanding is the result of a person's lacking the mental capacities needed for understanding. Although there are exceptions to the following generalization, children are ordinarily presumed to lack the mental capacities required for a sufficient understanding of the options involved in medical decision making. If we define *autonomous agents* as individuals who are generally capable of acting autonomously, we may restate the point by saying that children are ordinarily presumed to be *nonautonomous* agents.

It is important to recognize that understanding, however it comes about, is a matter of degree. Rarely, if ever, does one *perfectly* understand the implications and likely consequences of one's various options when confronted with an important decision. Because understanding is a matter of degree, autonomous action may also be conceptualized as being a matter of degree. Thus, on this way of thinking about autonomy, one may act more or less autonomously, making it sensible to say that adolescents and even children can act autonomously to some degree.

At the same time, certain purposes favor thinking of autonomy in terms of a threshold— or cut-off point—so that a given action either qualifies as autonomous or does not. Thinking of autonomy in this way requires that its conditions have cut-off points. Thus, we identify *sufficient* understanding as a condition for autonomous action (although we recognize that in practice it will sometimes be difficult to determine whether this somewhat vaguely stated threshold has been met). One purpose that favors a threshold conception of autonomous action is the need to determine whether a patient's consent to receive medical treatment qualifies as "informed consent"—which implies that the patient's act of decision making has been autonomous. If the patient's consent counts as informed consent, it is ordinarily respected; if it does not qualify as informed consent, the decision is viewed as problematic, and a proxy decision maker may need to be involved in the decision-making process. In this practical context, there is little or no room for thinking of consent as a matter of degree. Thus, there are pragmatic reasons, in some contexts, to conceptualize autonomous action as a threshold concept and not as a matter of degree. Accordingly, we identify sufficient understanding of what is at stake—of the implications and likely consequences of one's action, and those of available alternatives—as a condition of autonomous action.

Freedom from External Constraints Think of Rhee, a medical student, who is attending a concert the night before her final exam in anatomy class. She is free to leave anytime she chooses. Her actions result from her conscious intention to listen to a concert, and she clearly understands what she is doing and the implications of her choice—including the risk of doing substandard work on the final. Importantly, Rhee's choice to remain at the concert is also voluntary in the sense that it is free from external constraints.

External constraints may be understood as including physical barriers deliberately imposed by other individuals and different forms of coercion. (Although in a sense a person is "constrained" by the laws of physics from highjumping to the moon, such impersonal constraints are not relevant to the present conception of autonomy.) Prisoners are constrained by the physical barriers of locked doors and prison walls. If they attempt to escape from prison and are detected in the process, they are likely to encounter coercion from prison guards. Coercion involves the deliberate use of force or the threat of harm. The coercer's purpose is to get the person being coerced to do something that he or she would not otherwise be willing to do (in the present case, submit to continued incarceration). "Occurrent" coercion involves the use of physical force. "Dispositional" coercion involves the threat of harm.[38] An unscrupulous medical researcher, for example, might literally force individuals to participate as research subjects, as was done in Nazi Germany. This is occurrent coercion. The researcher might also bring about the desired participation by threatening reluctant patients with some harm, such as the withdrawal of care essential for their recovery. This is dispositional coercion. Moreover, regarding the threat of harm, individuals can coerce others either directly or by enacting laws that threaten them with harm. Laws as well as individuals can be coercive. For example, a physician is constrained from actively killing patients by laws that threaten harm (in the form of punishment) to those who do so.

Let us revise the story of Rhee the concert-goer in a way that makes the voluntariness of her actions more questionable. Suppose that her decision regarding what to do that evening is based mainly on strong pressure from her family members, who want Rhee to watch her father perform in the concert. Rhee, as it happens, comes from a culture in which family loyalty is prized very highly and paternal authority is generally respected. While it would seem exaggerated to say that Rhee is coerced into attending the concert, she clearly faces some external pressure. (There may be a point at which external pressure shades into coercion.) This suggests that freedom from external constraints is really a matter of degree— reinforcing the idea, suggested earlier in our discussion of understanding, that autonomy itself may be thought of as something that comes in degrees. In the present scenario, Rhee's decision to attend the concert might be considered less than fully autonomous but more autonomous than some actions (such as when coercion or physical barriers deliberately imposed by others constrain one's options).

In contexts where there is good reason to think of autonomy as a threshold concept, such that one's action either is autonomous or is not, the present condition may be stated this way: An autonomous action must be *sufficiently free of external constraints*. If an adult patient's choice to undergo surgery is largely her own choice, it can be considered sufficiently free of external constraints for her decision to count as autonomous, even if she feels slight pressure from her family or physician to consent.[39]

Freedom from Internal Constraints Imagine now a classmate of Rhee's, Salvator, who on the night before the final exam is imbibing beer at a fast pace in a pub near campus. Having had several beers, Salvator faces a choice: He can go home and open his anatomy textbook or he can stay at the pub and order another beer. He decides on the latter course. His decision is intentional, and he fully understands his options and their likely consequences. Furthermore, no one is coercing him to stay and party. Nor are there physical barriers, such as locked doors, that prevent him from leaving the pub. Is his choice to stay and have another beer autonomous? That depends on further detail.

Suppose Salvator has a severe case of alcoholism. Once he begins to drink, he feels an uncontrollable urge to keep drinking—*even though he thinks doing so is contrary to his best interests*—and this urge typically continues to exert its force until he passes out. Perhaps Salvator's going to the pub, ordering a drink, and beginning to imbibe were autonomous actions. (People might reasonably disagree about this, even if all the details of the case are provided.) But surely the uncontrollable urge to continue drinking, once drinking commences, that characterizes severe alcoholism creates an *internal constraint* that substantially reduces the autonomy of one's subsequent actions. A person who is driven by such an urge is, in an important sense, "out of control" and no longer self-determining.

As an alternative, suppose that Salvator is not an alcoholic but is a schizophrenic. (Schizophrenia is a mental illness characterized by disorganized and delusional thinking and, very frequently, auditory and visual hallucinations.) He generally functions well when he takes antipsychotic medications—indeed, well enough to attend medical school—but for some reason he stopped taking them several days ago. Now, the night before the final, he hears "voices" ("command" auditory hallucinations) telling him that he must go to the pub and drink heavily. He is terrified of these "voices" and unwilling to disobey them. He goes to the pub, orders a drink, and begins imbibing. He is thinking clearly enough to understand that this course of action is likely to lead to inebriation and places him at risk of doing poorly on the final.[40] No external constraints control his actions, but internal constraints—the "voices" and his terror at the thought of disobeying them—do control his actions. Salvator's actions are substantially nonautonomous.

While the unleashed urges of severe alcoholism and the power of "command" hallucinations are dramatic examples of internal constraints on action, there are also more common internal phenomena that, to some degree, constrain our actions and choices. Intense fears, acute pain or persistent discomfort, and strong emotions such as rage and grief sometimes influence us to make choices that represent departures from our stable values and usual priorities; that is, these phenomena sometimes cause us to act out of character with the result that we later feel that we were "not ourselves" in doing what we did.[41] Sometimes, however, these internal phenomena simply make it more difficult to behave as one normally would. Clearly, then, one can be *more or less* free of internal constraints. In contexts where it is helpful to think of autonomy as involving a threshold, this final condition may be stated as follows: One acts autonomously only if one's action is *sufficiently free of internal constraints.*

Let us bring together the conditions we have discussed. First, autonomy may be conceived of in terms of a threshold: One acts autonomously only if one acts intentionally, with sufficient understanding of what is at stake, and one's action is sufficiently free of external and internal constraints. Second, conceptualizing autonomous action as a matter of degree, we may say that one acts autonomously *to the extent* that one acts intentionally, with understanding, and freely of external and internal constraints.

Another, somewhat intuitive, way of conceptualizing autonomy is to say that one acts autonomously when one effectively deliberates about one's options, chooses the option that best realizes one's values and priorities, and acts accordingly. Effective deliberation involves that careful, thorough, clearheaded assessment of options that makes it possible to identify the option most in accord with one's values and priorities. Being neither careless, uninformed, nor distorted in any significant way, effective deliberation permits the agent to make decisions that are faithful to his or her sense of what is most important or most worth pursuing.

We may relate the aforementioned four conditions of autonomous action to the present, somewhat intuitive, conception in the following way. First, intentional action is implicit in the idea of the agent acting in accordance with his or her values and priorities following effective deliberation; if one acts other than as one intends (e.g., consenting to participate in a placebo-controlled clinical trial rather than consenting to receive treatment tailored to one's needs), one hardly acts as one chooses, much less in a way that promotes one's values and priorities. Second, sufficient understanding is required for effective deliberation insofar as significant misunderstandings threaten one's ability to make the choice that is most in tune with one's values and priorities. Third, an agent needs sufficient freedom from external constraints in order to act in accordance with the decision following effective deliberation; coercion or undue social pressure can prevent one from implementing one's decision. Fourth, freedom from internal constraints is necessary both for effective deliberation and for acting in accordance with one's considered decision. Sometimes internal constraints can distort one's perception of available options, resulting in insufficient understanding. For example, temporary depression might cause a person to view *no* option as worthwhile—all effort seeming hopeless—even though, in his or her normal, nondepressed mental condition, the agent would view one of the options as the best realization of his or her values and priorities. In other cases, internal constraints can, like external constraints, prevent one from carrying out the decision that reasoned deliberation identified as best. For example, a student may have deliberated effectively and decided that the best thing for her to do is to remain enrolled in a class and take the midterm, but the recent onset of major anxiety or a specific phobia may make her quite unable (at least without professional help) to walk to and enter the classroom where the midterm will be given. In this way, the four conditions stated in our analysis are necessary conditions for autonomous action even when the latter is understood in terms of effective deliberation, choice, and action—suggesting the coherence of our analysis with an alternative, intuitively plausible, conception.

Both in biomedical contexts and in social life generally, it is an especially important fact that, even when people are capable of acting autonomously, the actions of others often prevent them from doing so. A person's autonomy can be infringed upon, limited, or usurped by others in many ways. For example, lying, practicing other forms of deception, and failing to supply needed information all can undermine another person's understanding of his or her options, thereby preventing that person from *effectively deliberating* about those options. By contrast, coercion and the deliberate imposition of physical barriers can undermine a person's autonomy by constraining his or her *liberty of action*.[42] In each of these ways of undermining autonomy, one individual interferes in some way with the effective exercise of another's capacity to act autonomously, and this is incompatible with the ethical principle of respect for autonomy.

The Value of Autonomy What is the basis for the moral value accorded to individual autonomy? The strongest claims regarding its moral primacy come from Kant and from certain other deontologists. In Kant's view, persons, unlike things, must always be accorded respect as self-determining subjects. They must be treated as ends in themselves and never merely as objects. For Kant, the fundamental principle of morality, respect for persons as moral agents, entails respect for personal autonomy. Such respect is due them as a right—autonomous agents are entitled to respect. If persons were not taken to be autonomous agents, there would be no basis for the moral responsibility we have toward other human beings, which precludes our using them—as we do cattle, chickens, rocks, land, and trees—simply to serve our own ends. But how does Kant understand autonomy?

Kant's primary focus is on the autonomy of the will. For Kant, "Autonomy of the will is the property the will has of being a law to itself."[43] What Kant calls the "dignity of man as a rational creature" is based on human beings possessing just that property that enables them to govern their own actions in accordance with rules of their own choosing. Putting aside many complexities in Kant's own thinking, a Kantian position central in biomedical ethics describes autonomy in terms of self-control, self-direction, or self-governance. The individual capable of acting on the basis of effective deliberation, guided by reason, and neither driven by emotions or compulsions nor manipulated or coerced by others, is, on a Kantian position, the model of autonomy.

For utilitarians, autonomy is an important value. John Stuart Mill, who speaks of individuality rather than autonomy, argues, for example, that liberty of action and thought is essential in developing both the intellectual and character traits necessary for truly human happiness:

> The human faculties of perception, judgment, discriminative feeling, mental activity, and even moral preference, are exercised only in making a choice. He who does anything because it is the custom makes no choice. He gains no practice either in discerning or in desiring what is best. The mental and moral, like the muscular powers, are improved by being used. . . .
>
> He who lets the world, or his own portion of it, choose his plan of life for him, has no need of any other faculty than the ape-like one of imitation. He who chooses his plan for himself employs all his faculties. He must use observation to see, reasoning and judgment to foresee, activity to gather materials for decision, discrimination to decide, and when he has decided, firmness and self-control to hold to his deliberate decision. . . .
>
> Where, not the person's own character, but the traditions or customs of other people are the rule of conduct, there is wanting one of the principal ingredients of human happiness.[44]

For Mill, persons possessing "individuality" are autonomous in a very strong sense, reflectively choosing their own plans of life, making their own decisions without coercion or manipulation by others, and exercising firmness and self-control in acting on their decisions.

Despite the high value placed on autonomy by utilitarians, their interest in autonomy differs from the Kantian one. On a Kantian view, respect for the autonomy of rational agents is entailed by the fundamental principle of morality, which serves as a limiting criterion for all moral conduct. That is, it places limits on what one individual can do to another without acting immorally. As noted earlier, one person can never use another as a subject in a medical experiment without his or her consent, no matter what potential good consequences for society as a whole might result. For a utilitarian such as Mill, respect for individual autonomy has utility value. A society that fosters respect for persons as autonomous agents will be a more progressive and, on balance, a happier society because its citizens will have the opportunities to develop their capacities to act as rational, responsible moral agents. If it could be shown that respect for individual autonomy does not have sufficient utility value, the utilitarian might have no good grounds for objecting to practices that infringe upon that autonomy.

LIBERTY-LIMITING PRINCIPLES

Since autonomy is accorded such great moral value, a moral justification must be given for any infringement upon or limitation or usurpation of autonomy. Many discussions in biomedical ethics explore such *proposed* justifications. The following exposition centers on the most general kinds of reasons advanced in these discussions.

Six suggested general reasons, most frequently considered when limitations of liberty are at issue, are embodied in the following six principles, often called "liberty-limiting principles."[45] (Liberty, or freedom from external constraints, is one aspect or component of autonomy.) It is important to note at the outset that while some writers advance these principles as legitimate liberty-limiting principles, others argue against the legitimacy of many, or even most, of them.

1. A person's liberty is justifiably restricted to prevent that person from harming others (the harm principle).

2. A person's liberty is justifiably restricted to prevent that person from offending others (the offense principle).

3. A person's liberty is justifiably restricted to prevent that person from harming himself or herself (the principle of paternalism).

4. A person's liberty is justifiably restricted to benefit that person (the principle of extreme paternalism).

5. A person's liberty is justifiably restricted to prevent that person from acting immorally (the principle of legal moralism).

6. A person's liberty is justifiably restricted to benefit others (the social welfare principle).

These liberty-limiting principles are most frequently discussed when questions arise about the justification of coercive laws, such as laws limiting access to hallucinogenic drugs. But the considerations they embody are also pertinent when applied to individual acts and practices that infringe upon or limit others' autonomy. It should also be noted that more than one of these principles might be advanced to justify a proposed limitation or infringement.

The harm principle is the most widely accepted liberty-limiting principle. Few will dispute that the law is within its proper bounds when it constrains individuals from performing acts that will seriously harm other persons or will seriously impair important institutional practices. Laws that threaten thieves, murderers, and the like with punishment, for example, are usually perceived as a necessary part of any social system. Individual acts of coercion whose intent is to prevent individuals from harming others are also usually considered morally permissible. A bystander, for example, who prevents a terrorist from killing or wounding someone is praised and not blamed for interfering with the terrorist's action. Aside from the harm principle, however, the moral legitimacy of the liberty-limiting principles under discussion here is a matter of dispute.

According to the offense principle, the law may justifiably be invoked to prevent offensive behavior in public. "Offensive" behavior may be understood as behavior that causes shame, embarrassment, or discomfort to onlookers. In an example of the relevance of the offense principle to biomedical ethics, individuals who behaved offensively in public were sometimes, in the past, involuntarily committed to psychiatric hospitals, even though their behavior did not pose a serious threat of harm to themselves or others. Committing individuals to psychiatric hospitals simply because their behavior was considered offensively eccentric involved at least an implicit appeal to the offense principle. Attacks on the use of such grounds to deprive individuals of much of their liberty are attacks on the legitimacy of the offense principle.

According to the principle of legal moralism, liberty may justifiably be limited to prevent immoral behavior or, as it is often expressed, to "enforce morals." Acts such as kidnapping, murder, and fraud are undoubtedly immoral, but the principle of legal moralism does not have to be invoked to justify laws against them. An appeal to the harm principle already provides a widely accepted independent justification. The principle of legal moralism usually comes to the fore only when so-called victimless crimes are at issue. Is it justifiable to legislate against homosexual acts, gambling, or prostitution simply on the grounds that such activities are thought by some to be morally unacceptable? In biomedical ethics, the principle of legal moralism is sometimes invoked, at least implicitly, when it is argued that suicide is an immoral act and that, therefore, it is justifiable to act to prevent suicide, even if the decision to take one's own life is the result of careful deliberation. Many do not accept the principle of legal moralism as a legitimate liberty-limiting principle, however. Mill holds, for example, that to accept the principle is tantamount to permitting a "tyranny of the majority."

The social welfare principle also has some relevance in biomedical ethics. According to this principle, individual liberty can justifiably be restricted to benefit others. Such justifications are sometimes attempted in discussions of funding for certain public health-care programs, such as Medicaid in the United States. These programs are funded by tax revenues. Since individual taxpayers are not given the option not to pay that amount of their taxes that is directed toward these programs—which benefit others—the liberty of taxpayers is restricted in a way that might be justified by appeal to the social welfare principle.

The liberty-limiting principles that are most prominent in the literature of biomedical ethics are the paternalistic principles. Disagreements about the legitimacy of paternalistic justifications affect the resolution of a number of important issues in biomedical ethics. Physicians or nurses, for example, who lie to patients in order to spare them pain are often accused of acting paternalistically and therefore wrongly. The paternalistic justifications offered for certain laws that are of special concern in biomedical ethics are also frequently attacked. Among such laws are those that allow courts to commit individuals to psychiatric hospitals either in order to keep them from harming themselves or in order to force them to receive beneficial treatment. Because of the centrality of paternalism in biomedical ethics, it is essential to examine the concept of paternalism as well as some of the arguments offered both for and against paternalistic actions and practices.

PATERNALISM

The definition of *paternalism* that is perhaps most widely cited is Gerald Dworkin's: "[Paternalism is] the interference with a person's liberty of action justified by reasons referring exclusively to the welfare, good, happiness, needs, interests, or values of the person being coerced."[46] When paternalism in the legal system is at issue, this definition is acceptable, since laws, backed by force or the threat of harm, are by nature coercive and therefore restrictive of liberty. However, many of the actions considered paternalistic in biomedical ethics do not fit this definition. Consider the following examples:

(1) A patient has frequently asserted that he would immediately commit suicide if he were ever diagnosed with Alzheimer's disease, and his physician believes he is serious. The patient says that Alzheimer's disease is antithetical to everything he values in life. The physician has now arrived at a diagnosis of Alzheimer's disease, but she lies to the patient about the diagnosis She does so because she believes that a premature death is incompatible with the patient's best interests.

(2) A physician believes that surgery is the best available treatment for a patient's cancer. The physician does not disclose significant information about nonsurgical alternatives because he believes that the patient would be inclined to choose one of these alternatives, and he wants to ensure that the patient consents to the treatment that the physician believes to be in the patient's best interests.

Note that neither of these cases involves coercion or interference with a person's liberty of action, yet both can be correctly described as involving paternalism. In both cases, the physicians have infringed upon or limited the patients' autonomy. In both, the physicians have denied the patients information vital to effective deliberation and have done so for the patients' own good. The physicians have treated the patients as individuals incapable of making the correct judgments about their own best interests. In doing so, each physician has effectively usurped a patient's decision-making power, substituting his or her judgment for the patient's. While it is difficult to capture this sense of paternalism in a precise definition, a rough definition can be given as follows: *Paternalism* is the interference with, limitation of, or usurpation of individual autonomy justified by reasons referring exclusively to the welfare or needs of the person whose autonomy is being interefered with, limited, or usurped. (The sense of autonomy employed in this definition is autonomy as a matter of degree. Thus, our definition will cover both cases of strong paternalism and cases of weak paternalism, a distinction explained later in this discussion.)

Is such paternalistic behavior ever morally justified? If the answer is yes, under what conditions do paternalistic grounds constitute good reasons, either for using coercion or for effectively taking decisions out of individuals' hands for their own good? In considering the justifiability of paternalistic actions, it may be helpful to keep in mind the difference between the principle of paternalism and the principle of extreme paternalism. The latter applies to paternalistic actions whose intent is to benefit individuals, whereas the former applies to paternalistic actions whose intent is to keep individuals from harm.

In the framework of Kantian ethical theory, the moral centrality of individual autonomy seems to prohibit any paternalistic actions when the individuals affected are capable of self-governance or self-determination. It would always be morally wrong, for example, for physicians to withhold information about surgical procedures from patients simply because the physicians believed that their patients would refuse to undergo potentially beneficial procedures if informed of all the risks. Charles Fried, an ethicist (and former solicitor general) who adopts a Kantian approach to paternalism in the medical context, maintains that patients must never be denied relevant information. By withholding it, physicians treat patients as mere means to the end of improving their own health. In Fried's view, patients may never be treated simply as means to ends, even when the ends in question are their own ends (e.g., their restored health).[47]

John Stuart Mill provides the classic utilitarian statement on the illegitimacy of paternalistic actions. This statement is sometimes cited in court opinions concerning the right of self-determination in medical matters. Mill argues:

> [O]ne very simple principle [is] entitled to govern absolutely the dealings of society with the individual in the way of compulsion and control, whether the means used be physical force in the form of legal penalties, or the moral coercion of public opinion. That principle is, that the sole end for which mankind are warranted, individually or collectively, in interfering with the liberty of action of any of their number, is self-protection. That the only purpose for which power can be rightfully exercised over any member of a civilized community, against his will, is to prevent harm to others. His own good, either physical or moral, is not sufficient warrant. He cannot rightfully be compelled to do or forbear because it will be better for him to do so, because it will make him happier, because, in the opinion of other, to do so would be wise, or even right.[48]

In this statement, Mill asserts that while prevention of harm to others is sometimes sufficient justification for interfering with another's autonomy, the individual's own good never is. Mill rejects paternalistic interventions because of the high utility value that he assigns to individual autonomy. In assigning it this value, he assumes that individuals are, on the whole, better judges of their own interests than anyone else, so that minimizing paternalistic interventions will maximize human happiness. However, Mill himself qualifies his rejection of paternalism in the following way:

> [T]his doctrine is meant to apply only to human beings in the maturity of their faculties. We are not speaking of children, or of young persons below the age which the law may fix as that of manhood or womanhood. Those who are still in a state to require being taken care of by others, must be protected against their own actions as well as external injury.[49]

In the kinds of cases he cites, Mill assumes that people are justified in acting paternalistically because they are better judges of an individual's interest than the individual himself or herself. Arguing in this way, Mill seems to open the door for the justification of paternalism in the case of individuals who may not be able to identify and advance their own interests correctly because they lack the required level of ability for effective deliberation—and in particular for sufficiently understanding their options and the likely consequences of specific choices. Such individuals, often described as having diminished autonomy insofar as they lack the necessary abilities or capacities for self-determination, include young children and the severely mentally retarded. It is important to see that the paternalistic restrictions Mill would allow in this regard do typically amount to restrictions on individual autonomy— at least in a certain sense. To the extent that an individual is subject to coercion, individual liberty of action is restricted, and liberty of action may be understood as one aspect of individual autonomy. However, the paternalistic restrictions at issue here do not limit autonomy in the sense central to Mill's, as well as Kant's, moral position, since those whose liberty would be limited are substantially lacking in autonomy to begin with. (They are nonautonomous where autonomy is thought of as having a threshold.)

Many contemporary attempts to justify *some* paternalistic actions adopt an approach similar to Mill's, stressing the apparently diminished autonomy of those who are treated paternalistically. If their autonomy were not so compromised, the argument runs, they would want the benefits involved and would want to avoid harm. Those who argue in this way must deal with an underlying conceptual issue. They must identify the criteria that should be used in determining whether a person's autonomy is sufficiently diminished to justify paternalism. In light of our earlier discussion of autonomy, it seems plausible to hold the following view regarding diminished autonomy. When a person's ability to act autonomously is significantly constrained by intellectual deficits (e.g., lack of reasoning ability or ignorance of relevant facts) and cannot be easily augmented (e.g., by providing needed information), it is sufficiently impaired to justify paternalistic acts, especially when necessary to prevent serious, irrevocable harm. Two examples may be helpful here. People under the influence of hallucinogenic drugs who decide to leap from twentieth-floor windows in order to get home more quickly, believing that they (like Superman) can fly, are hardly acting in an autonomous manner. Their decisions are grossly inconsistent with available inductive evidence regarding what happens to human beings who leap out of windows and are therefore *irrational* in a familiar sense of the term. Severely retarded individuals who decide to go out alone in a busy city but are incapable of understanding traffic signals would also seem to be acting in a significantly nonautonomous way. They are unaware of the kind of risk they would be running by going out alone. In both cases, there is good reason to assume that the individuals are incapable, whether temporarily or permanently, of the level of understanding required for sufficiently autonomous decision making. Thus, paternalistic interventions seem to be justified.

Does the fact that a decision will result in death or some other serious, irrevocable harm *always* provide sufficient grounds for the claim that autonomy is so severely diminished that paternalism is justified? Some especially problematic cases involve decisions to attempt suicide. Many suicide attempts are the result of temporary disorientation associated with drugs, alcohol, or extreme, but reversible, depression. Decisions to attempt suicide in these cases are apparently due to insufficient understanding of one's situation and options— or perhaps internal constraints that impede effective deliberation—and can therefore be considered nonautonomous. Indeed, cases involving individuals who are so constrained in their reasoning that they are temporarily or permanently incapable of identifying the probable (severely harmful) consequences of their acts would seem to provide clear instances of autonomy that is sufficiently diminished to justify paternalism. However, some decisions to end or risk life may be based on carefully thought-out reasons and may be consistent with the person's own long-held conception of a satisfying or meaningful life or the result of a new but reflective reassessment of ultimate values and priorities. It would beg the question to assume—in an effort to justify paternalistic interventions—that all decisions to end or risk life are irrational (due to being based on insufficient understanding and/or insufficient freedom from internal constraints) and therefore nonautonomous. But perhaps in the case of those outcomes that are usually considered highly undersirable (e.g., death or severe injury) it should be presumed that the individual's choice is irrational and therefore nonautonomous. This presumption would justify, at best, temporarily constraining someone from certain acts in order to establish the rationality or irrationality of the choice.

In summary, it can plausibly be maintained that paternalistic interventions can be justified either (1) when intervention is responsive to the welfare of an individual whose autonomy is significantly diminished or (2) when temporary constraint is necessary to prevent a person from acting in a self-harming and *presumably* nonautonomous manner until it can be determined whether the individual is, in fact, acting autonomously. Paternalism in accordance with these two conditions is often called "weak paternalism," and it is entirely consistent with Mill's criticism of paternalism (which is essentially a rejection of so-called "strong paternalism"). The interventions that are characteristic of weak paternalism do not show a lack of respect for individual autonomy. In the first case, an individual is simply incapable of acting in a significantly autonomous manner. In the second, the point of the intervention is to ensure that an individual will not harm himself or herself while acting nonautonomously. Thus, the legitimacy of weak paternalism is widely accepted. In contrast, the legitimacy of strong paternalism is a hotly disputed issue. Strong paternalism is characterized by interventions that go beyond the limits set by conditions 1 and 2. Advocates of strong paternalism maintain that paternalistic interference with autonomous actions and choice can sometimes be justified.

Note that the distinction between weak and strong paternalism is not the same as the distinction between paternalism and extreme paternalism (as reflected in the statement of liberty-limiting principles). Discussions of the distinction between weak and strong paternalism often focus on actions and practices whose intention is to prevent harm and, thus, on the principle of paternalism rather than the principle of extreme paternalism. However, a similar distinction can be made in regard to extreme paternalism. A weak form of extreme paternalism would allow paternalistic interferences intended to benefit those whose autonomy is significantly diminished. This would stand in contrast to a strong form of extreme paternalism, which would allow beneficial paternalistic interferences even in the case of persons whose autonomy is not significantly diminished.

The mildly mentally retarded may pose special problems when questions of justified paternalism are raised, precisely because they *may* lack the cognitive abilities necessary for substantially autonomous action. Whether the mildly retarded lack such abilities is a matter of dispute, however. Many people classified as mildly mentally retarded are capable of substantially autonomous action if they are given appropriate training and information. In the case of mentally retarded individuals who are capable of substantially autonomous action, paternalistic treatment seems to be justified only if strong paternalism is justified. If strong paternalism is not justified in the case of those who are not mentally retarded, then it is hard to see why it would be justified in the case of mildly mentally retarded individuals capable of substantially autonomous action. On the other hand, in the case of mentally retarded individuals whose cognitive abilities are diminished to the point that paternalistic interferences in their lives would be instances of weak paternalism, paternalistic actions whose intent is to benefit these individuals could be as justifiable as those whose intent is to keep them from harm.

Is strong paternalism ever justified? One defense of strong paternalism rests on a prudential argument that itself appeals to the importance of autonomy. We are aware that we are often tempted to act in ways that are likely to frustrate our long-term interests. Indeed, we may do ourselves serious irreversible harm of a sort that would severely diminish our autonomy. We should be willing, therefore, to accept those paternalistic acts, laws, and practices whose intent is to protect individual autonomy from being severely diminished. This argument is advanced in order to justify both (1) laws, such as those against the sale of seriously mind-altering drugs, that protect us against our own weakness of will and (2) laws that allow courts and psychiatrists to commit the mentally ill to institutions against their will in order to keep them from the kind of self-harm that might reduce their autonomy. The same sort of prudential argument is sometimes invoked to justify paternalistic acts by physicians when these acts are performed to prevent serious deterioration of the patient's autonomy. However, some of the constraining interventions that seem to be justified by this line of argument are very problematic. Some individuals, for example, might prefer to give in to temptations, weighing the pleasures of using seriously mind-altering drugs more highly than its risks (including that of diminished autonomy). The appropriateness of involuntary civil commitment of the mentally ill is, of course, also quite disputable in cases involving strong paternalism (i.e., in cases in which the mental illness in question has not destroyed the person's capacity to make autonomous decisions).

In a different vein, indirect support for antipaternalism comes from certain sociologists, psychologists, and other social theorists who offer various analyses to explain the recent emphasis on antipaternalism in American society. They attribute much of this recent emphasis to a growing awareness of both the class differences in our society and the fact that those who perform paternalistic acts (e.g., psychiatrists, other physicians, judges) are usually members of the upper middle class, while those who are treated paternalistically are usually members of the poorer, less privileged classes. An awareness of this class difference, and of related differences in interests and values, raises serious doubts about the ability and willingness of those wielding paternalistic authority to act in the interests of those whom they typically constrain. On this analysis, it is not the moral legitimacy of the principle of paternalism that is really at issue when paternalistic acts and practices are increasingly rejected. Rather, at issue are the abuses resulting from so-called paternalistic acts that do not, in fact, benefit (or keep from harm) the individuals constrained but, rather, serve the ends of the members of the professions wielding paternalistic authority. This line of argument is intended to point out that the current antipaternalistic stress is probably not the result of conscious deliberation about the legitimacy of central ethical principles but a rejection of what passes as justified paternalism in a class society in which the "constrainers" are neither knowledgeable nor altruistic enough to perceive correctly the interests of those they constrain. However, these factual claims, if correct, tend to support a Mill-like thesis that, unless the interests and values of constrainers and constrainees coincide, individual well-being is better served in the long run if paternalism is rejected.

T.A.M. and D.D.

NOTES

1 Efforts to determine what is morally good and what is morally bad with regard to human character also fall under the heading of normative ethics. This aspect of normative ethics is of central importance in a school of thought known as *virtue ethics.* A discussion of virtue ethics is presented later in Chapter 1.

2 Some scholars prefer to identify biomedical ethics as a type of *practical ethics,* rather than *applied* ethics. Their underlying concern is to avoid any suggestion that particular moral problems can be effectively resolved simply by "applying" ethical theories or principles. We continue to employ the commonly used category of applied ethics, but in no way do we mean to imply the appropriateness of any mechanical "application" model. (See the section "Alternative Directions and Methods.")

3 In what follows, the two versions of utilitarianism are articulated in ways intended to emphasize a contrast between them. There are alternative ways of articulating both act-utilitarianism and rule-utilitarianism, and some of these articulations bring the two versions of utilitarianism much closer than our account suggests.

4 Probably a majority of contemporary utilitarians take the satisfaction of preferences to constitute intrinsic value. See, for example, Jonathan Glover, ed., *Utilitarianism and Its Critics* (New York: Macmillan, 1990), Part 2.

5 J. J. C. Smart, "Extreme and Restricted Utilitarianism," in Michael D. Bayles, ed., *Contemporary Utilitarianism* (New York: Doubleday, 1968), p. 100.

6 W. D. Ross, *The Right and the Good* (Oxford: Clarendon Press, 1930), p. 22.

7 Alan Donagan, "Is There a Credible Form of Utilitarianism?" in *Contemporary Utilitarianism,* p. 189. Donagan's point is that act-utilitarianism is "monstrous" and "incredible" because it seems to recommend such murders.

8 The distinction between act-utilitarianism and rule-utilitarianism is a distinction that has become prominent only in contemporary times. Accordingly, the writings of Bentham and Mill are somewhat ambiguous with regard to these categories. Although Bentham is probably rightly understood as an act-utilitarian, a very strong case can be made for interpreting Mill as a rule-utilitarian. See, for example, J. O. Urmson, "The Interpretation of the Moral Philosophy of J. S. Mill," in *Contemporary Utilitarianism,* pp. 13–24.

9 Smart, "Extreme and Restricted Utilitarianism," p. 107.

10 Immanuel Kant, *Groundwork of the Metaphysic of Morals,* trans. H. J. Paton (New York: Harper & Row, 1964), p. 88.

11 *Ibid.,* p. 96.

12 H. J. Paton, *The Categorical Imperative: A Study in Kant's Moral Philosophy* (Chicago: University of Chicago Press, 1948), p. 172.

13 The account of beneficience suggested here reflects an analysis originally presented by Tom L. Beauchamp and James F. Childress in Chapters 4 and 5 of *Principles of Biomedical Ethics* (New York: Oxford University Press, 1979).

14 Ross, *The Right and the Good,* p. 19.

15 *Ibid.,* p. 20.

16 *Ibid.,* p. 21.

17 *Ibid.*

18 *Ibid.*

19 Beauchamp and Childress, *Principles of Biomedical Ethics,* 5th ed. (2001), Chapter 1.

20 Such a foundational principle might have a complex structure (unlike that of utilitarianism or Kantianism). For example, a foundational principle might consist of two or more simpler principles arranged in a strict hierarchy.

21 But see the section "Reflective Equilibrium and Appeals to Coherence" later in the chapter.

22 We have noted that Beauchamp and Childress, *Principles of Biomedical Ethics,* is an influential work of principle-based ethics in biomedical ethics. Another is National Commission for the Protection of Human Subjects of Biomedical and Behavioral Research, *The Belmont Report: Ethical Principles and Guidelines for Research Involving Human Subjects* (Washington, DC: Government Printing Office, 1979).

23 Arguments of this sort can be found in, for example, Iris Murdoch, *The Sovereignty of Good* (London: Routledge and Kegan Paul, 1970); and Martha Nussbaum, *Love's Knowledge* (New York: Oxford University Press, 1990).

24 The last three paragraphs have benefited from ideas in Alisa L. Carse, "Rules of Conduct and the Uncodifiability of Virtue" (unpublished manuscript).

25 Carol Gilligan, *In a Different Voice: Psychological Theory and Women's Moral Development* (Cambridge, MA: Harvard University Press, 1982).

26 Susan Sherwin, *No Longer Patient: Feminist Ethics and Health Care* (Philadelphia: Temple University Press, 1992), p. 50.

27 See, e.g., Allison M. Jaggar, "Feminist Ethics: Projects, Problems, Prospects," in Claudia Card, ed., *Feminist Ethics* (Lawrence: University of Kansas Press, 1991), p. 89.

28 See Sherwin, *No Longer Patient,* pp. 49–51. Cf. Sara Ruddick, "Remarks on the Sexual Politics of Reason," in Eva Feder Kittay and Diana T. Meyers, eds., *Women and Moral Theory* (Savage, MD: Rowman & Littlefield, 1987), p. 246; John M. Broughton, "Women's Rationality and Men's Virtues: A Critique of Gender Dualism in Gilligan's Theory of Moral Development," in Mary Jeanne Larrabee, ed., *An Ethic of Care: Feminist and Interdisciplinary Perspectives* (New York: Routledge, 1993), p. 134; and Zella Luria, "A Methodological Critique," in Larrabee, *An Ethic of Care,* pp. 202–203.

29 Sherwin, *No Longer Patient,* p. 57.

30 Albert R. Jonsen and Stephen Toulmin, *The Abuse of Casuistry: A History of Moral Reasoning* (Berkeley: University of California Press, 1988). For a distinct version of casuistry, see Baruch Brody, *Taking Issue: Pluralism and Casuistry in Bioethics.* (Washington, DC: Georgetown University Press, 2003).

31 See *In re Quinlan,* 70 N.J. 10 (1976); *In re Conroy,* 486 A. 2d 1209 (N.J. 1985); and *Cruzan v. Director,* 110 S. Ct. 2841 (1990).

32 John D. Arras, "Getting Down to Cases: The Revival of Casuistry in Bioethics," *Journal of Medicine and Philosophy* 16 (1991), p. 46.

33 See "Outline for a Decision Procedure for Ethics," *Philosophical Review* 60 (1951), pp. 177–197; and *A Theory of Justice* (Cambridge, MA: Harvard University Press, 1971).

34 Strictly speaking, coherence involves other theoretical virtues as well, such as simplicity and clarity. Moreover, any proponent of this model—in fact, of any model or theory—must seek not only coherence among ethical beliefs but also coherence between ethical beliefs and empirical beliefs. Thus, the claim that surgery without anesthesia on dogs is morally appropriate because dogs are incapable of suffering is undermined by evidence showing that dogs, in fact, can suffer.

35 A commonly cited distinction pertaining to the present model is that between "narrow" and "wide" reflective equilibrium. See, for example, Norman Daniels, "Wide Reflective Equilibrium and Theory Acceptance in Ethics," *Journal of Philosophy* 76 (1979), pp. 256–282; and Margaret Holmgren, "The Wide and Narrow of Reflective Equilibrium," *Canadian Journal of Philosophy* 19 (1989), pp. 43–60.

36 Indeed, contrary to its reputation as an exclusively top-down form of reasoning, principle-based ethics may be best understood as a version of reflective equilibrium that emphasizes principles. See David DeGrazia, "Moving Forward in Bioethical Theory: Theories, Cases, and Specified Principlism," *Journal of Medicine and Philosophy* 17 (1992), pp. 511–539.

37 Authors writing on the nature of autonomous action present analyses that differ at the level of details, but leading contributions seem to agree that the conditions just stated are at least necessary for autonomous action. For example, the analysis of Beauchamp and Childress (*Principles of Biomedical Ethics,* 4th ed. [1994], p. 123) is close to the present analysis (and, in fact, significantly influenced it). Some authors, however, suggest—controversially—that the four conditions just stated are insufficient for autonomous action. According to these authors, autonomous action involves the exercise of the capacity to form higher-order values or desires about the desires (to do certain things) that are involved in intentional action. See,

e.g., Harry G. Frankfurt, "Freedom of the Will and the Concept of a Person," *Journal of Philosophy* 68 (1971), pp. 5–20; Gerald Dworkin, *The Theory and Practice of Autonomy* (Cambridge: Cambridge University Press, 1988), Chapter 1; and David DeGrazia, "Autonomous Action and Autonomy-Subverting Psychiatric Conditions," *Journal of Medicine and Philosophy* 19 (1994), pp. 279–297.

38 The distinction between occurrent and dispositional coercion is made by Michael D. Bayles in "A Concept of Coercion," in J. Roland Pennock and John D. Chapman, eds., *Coercion: Nomos XIV* (Chicago: Aldine-Atherton, 1972), pp. 16–29.

39 Some may find it plausible to understand freedom from external constraints as including *freedom of choice,* which is constrained by actions and policies that narrow the range of options that one can reasonably expect to be available to one. This understanding of freedom from external constraints is very broad (and controversial) because it implies that the *nonprovision* of certain goods or services can count as an external constraint, as well as disrespectful of autonomy. For example, excluding Medicaid coverage for a procedure that was previously funded—and that the poor can reasonably expect to be covered—would narrow some indigent persons' range of medical options and would therefore count as disrespectful of their autonomy.

40 Perhaps he does not sufficiently understand the alternative of studying; perhaps he thinks studying puts him in some kind of danger. In any case, his capacity to act autonomously is clearly compromised by the constraint described in the case.

41 Because nonautonomous action is often inconsistent with one's usual values and priorities—and is, therefore, in a sense less authentically "one's own"—autonomy is sometimes conceptualized as involving *authenticity.*

42 There are some situations in which constraining someone's liberty is compatible with respecting his or her autonomy. For example, suppose Salvator asks Danny to take away Salvator's car keys if the latter drinks too much at a party; Salvator does not trust himself to exercise good judgment while drunk. If, hours later, Salvator has imbibed excessively, Danny would not show disrespect for Salvator's autonomy by snatching away his car keys, thereby restricting his liberty at that moment. Or, to cite a famous example, if you see a man who is about to walk onto a seriously faulty bridge, you might grab him—much to his annoyance—and prevent his walking farther until you are sure that he knows the risks. Since not knowing the risks undermines the man's understanding of his options, this minor interference with his liberty is consistent with respecting his autonomy.

43 Kant, *Groundwork,* p. 108.

44 John Stuart Mill, *Utilitarianism, On Liberty, Essay on Bentham,* ed. Mary Warnock (New York: New American Library, 1962), pp. 185, 187. All quotations in this chapter are from this edition of *On Liberty.*

45 Joel Feinberg's discussion of such principles served as a guide for the formulations adopted here. See Joel Feinberg, *Social Philosophy* (Englewood Cliffs, NJ: Prentice-Hall, 1973), Chapter 2.

46 Gerald Dworkin, "Paternalism," *The Monist* 56 (1972), p. 65.

47 Charles Fried, *Medical Experimentation: Personal Integrity and Social Policy* (New York: American Elsevier, 1974), p. 101.

48 Mill, *On Liberty,* p. 135.

49 *Ibid.*

ANNOTATED BIBLIOGRAPHY

Beauchamp, Tom L., and James F. Childress: *Principles of Biomedical Ethics,* 5th ed. (New York: Oxford University Press, 2001). The authors defend and deploy a principle-based approach in biomedical ethics. An appendix presents detailed accounts of ten important cases.

Blustein, Jeffrey: *Care and Commitment: Taking the Personal Point of View* (New York: Oxford University Press, 1991). Blustein argues for a synthesis of insights from recently dominant ethical theories, the ethics of care, and recent philosophical work on personal integrity into a unified moral outlook.

Brody, Baruch: *Taking Issue: Pluralism and Casuistry in Bioethics* (Washington, DC: Georgetown University Press, 2003). Brody defends a unique variant of casuistry before employing it in exploring various issues in biomedical ethics.

Carse, Alisa L., and Hilde Lindemann Nelson: "Rehabilitating Care," *Kennedy Institute of Ethics Journal* 6 (March 1996), pp. 19–35. The authors identify four major criticisms that are commonly directed against the ethics of care, and they argue that the ethics of care can respond adequately to those criticisms.

Childress, James F.: *Who Should Decide? Paternalism in Health Care* (New York: Oxford University Press, 1982). In this extended discussion of paternalism, Childress examines the metaphors and principles underlying the disputes about professional paternalism in health care.

Christman, John, ed.: *The Inner Citadel: Essays on Individual Autonomy* (New York: Oxford University Press, 1989). This anthology provides a collection of articles on the nature and value of individual autonomy.

DeGrazia, David: "Moving Forward in Bioethical Theory: Theories, Cases, and Specified Principlism," *Journal of Medicine and Philosophy* 17 (October 1992), pp. 511–539. After challenging several leading methodologies in ethics, DeGrazia defends a "specified" principlism.

Dworkin, Gerald: *The Theory and Practice of Autonomy* (Cambridge: Cambridge University Press, 1988). In Part 1, Dworkin examines the nature and value of autonomy. In Part 2, he applies the general framework developed in Part 1 to various moral questions.

Foot, Philippa: *Virtues and Vices* (Oxford: Blackwell, 1978). Foot argues that virtue is more central, morally, than obligation; the paradigm moral person is one who is disposed by character to be rightly motivated.

Glover, Jonathan, ed.: *Utilitarianism and Its Critics* (New York: Macmillan, 1990). The various selections in this anthology incorporate both objections to utilitarianism and attempts to defend utilitarianism against the objections.

Holmes, Helen Bequaert, and Laura M. Purdy, eds.: *Feminist Perspectives in Medical Ethics* (Bloomington: Indiana University Press, 1992). The aim of this anthology is to show how feminist ethics and the ethics of care can advance medical ethics. Most of the contributors focus on specific issues in medical ethics that especially affect the interests of women.

Jonsen, Albert R., and Stephen Toulmin: *The Abuse of Casuistry: A History of Moral Reasoning* (Berkeley: University of California Press, 1988). After examining the history of casuistry and the criticism it has received, the authors argue for its revival.

Journal of Medicine and Philosophy 15 (April 1990). The articles included in this issue appear under the heading of "Philosophical Critique of Bioethics." Various methodological issues are considered, and several of the articles develop criticisms of the principle-based approach associated with Beauchamp and Childress in *Principles of Biomedical Ethics.*

Kant, Immanuel: *Groundwork of the Metaphysic of Morals,* translated and analyzed by H. J. Paton (New York: Harper & Row, 1964). In this work, a basic reference point, Kant offers an overall statement and defense of his ethical theory.

Korsgaard, Christine M.: *Creating the Kingdom of Ends* (Cambridge: Cambridge University Press, 1996). This collection of the author's essays represents a leading attempt to defend, refine, and engage Kant's moral philosophy.

Larrabee, Mary Jeanne, ed.: *An Ethic of Care: Feminist and Interdisciplinary Perspectives* (New York: Routledge, 1993). This anthology focuses on Carol Gilligan's work and its implications. Special attention is given to debates in moral philosophy, empirical claims in psychology about alleged gender differences in moral reasoning, and challenges to Gilligan's work that claim it excludes African American and other cultures.

Lindley, Richard: *Autonomy* (Atlantic Highlands, NJ: Humanities Press, 1986). After examining various conceptions of autonomy and some related principles, Lindley discusses several specific practical problems regarding autonomy, including social practices in regard to those who are mentally handicapped or mentally ill.

MacIntyre, Alasdair: *After Virtue: A Study in Moral Theory,* 2nd ed. (Notre Dame, IN: University of Notre Dame Press, 1984). Advancing the disquieting thesis that contemporary moral language consists of the fragmented remnants of a worldview no longer accepted in the secular West, MacIntyre advocates a return to Aristotelean virtue ethics.

Mill, John Stuart: *Utilitarianism, On Liberty, Essay on Bentham,* edited by Mary Warnock (New York: New American Library, 1962). In his famous essay "Utilitarianism," Mill offers a classic statement of the utilitarian position. In his equally well-known essay "On Liberty," he defends the classic liberal view regarding the limitation of individual liberty.

Rawls, John: *A Theory of Justice* (Cambridge, MA: Harvard University Press, 1971). In this classic work, Rawls presents and defends his theory of justice as an alternative to utilitarian theory. In doing so, he also argues for and uses the method of reflective equilibrium.

Sartorius, Rolf, ed.: *Paternalism* (Minneapolis: University of Minnesota Press, 1983). The various articles in this collection deal with the nature and justifiability of paternalism.

Sumner, L. W.: *Welfare, Happiness, and Ethics* (Oxford: Clarendon, 1996). Sumner defends an updated version of the theory that happiness constitutes an individual's good or well-being and argues that utilitarianism is the most promising approach to ethical and political theory.

Tong, Rosemarie: *Feminist Approaches to Bioethics: Theoretical Reflections and Practical Applications* (Boulder, CO: Westview, 1997). Tong articulates feminist and nonfeminist approaches to bioethics, defends the former, and explores implications for medical issues related to procreation.

Wolf, Susan, ed.: *Feminism & Bioethics: Beyond Reproduction* (New York: Oxford University Press, 1996). This anthology takes feminist theory beyond reproductive issues, tackling such problems as euthanasia, AIDS, the physician-patient relationship, and health-care reform.

APPENDIX: SELECTED REFERENCE SOURCES IN BIOMEDICAL ETHICS

PRINT RESOURCES

Craig, Edward, ed.: *The Routledge Encyclopedia of Philosophy* (New York: Routledge, 1998). This ten-volume resource contains articles on all major topics in philosophy including many in ethics.

Kennedy Institute of Ethics, Georgetown University: Scope Note series. This series provides extensive annotated bibliographies on a wide variety of issues in biomedical ethics. Currently Scope Notes are available on more than forty topics. They can be ordered toll-free by telephone at 800-MED-ETHX or by e-mail at bioethics@georgetown.edu.

Lineback, Richard H., ed.: *The Philosopher's Index* (Bowling Green, OH: Philosophers' Information Center). This reference source, updated quarterly, is "a current, comprehensive and easy-to-use subject and author index" to philosophical articles, books, anthologies, and contributions to anthologies. The subject index identifies useful material on virtually all major topics in biomedical ethics. A bibliography follows each article, and article abstracts are usually available.

Post, Stephen G., ed. in chief: *Encyclopedia of Bioethics,* 3rd ed. (New York: Macmillan, 2003). This five-volume set is a basic reference source in biomedical ethics, containing entries on virtually all major topics in biomedical ethics. Each article is followed by a selected bibliography.

Walters, LeRoy, and Tamar Joy Kahn, eds.: *Bibliography of Bioethics* (Washington, DC: Kennedy Institute of Ethics, Georgetown University). With volumes listed annually, this bibliography is exceptionally comprehensive.

WEB RESOURCES

Bioethics net (http://ajobonline.com). This resource is provided by the Center for Bioethics, University of Pennsylvania. It contains links to journals in biomedical ethics, updates and editorials on current issues, and a listing of jobs in the field. The center's online *American Journal of Bioethics* is accessible by subscription.

ETHX on the Web (www.georgetown.edu/research/nrcbl/). Sponsored by the Kennedy Institute of Ethics, Georgetown University, this source permits visitors to search for journal articles, book chapters, bills, laws, court decisions, books, and news articles pertaining to biomedical ethics and other types of professional ethics.

Locator Plus (http://locatorplus.gov). Sponsored by the National Library of Medicine, this resource allows visitors to search for books, journals, and audiovisuals, including many in biomedical ethics, in the National Library of Medicine collection.

PubMed (www.ncbi.nlm.nih.gov/entrez/query.fcgi). A service of the National Library of Medicine, PubMed includes more than 14 millions citations for articles in medicine and the life sciences, including articles in biomedical ethics. This resource also provides links to sites that provide full text articles.

THE PHYSICIAN-PATIENT RELATIONSHIP

INTRODUCTION

What moral rules should physicians observe in dealing with patients? What qualities of character will a virtuous physician exhibit? Are physicians ever morally justified in acting paternalistically toward their patients? Are they ever morally justified in withholding information from their patients, lying to them, or treating them without their consent? And what does morally valid consent involve? How should physicians negotiate the complexities of a multicultural environment, in which patients sometimes embrace values that differ significantly from those of the physician and his or her culture? Among the therapies and services that physicians are capable of providing, and legally permitted to provide, are there some that nevertheless distort the practice of medicine or the physician-patient relationship? Finally, with managed care dominating health-care delivery and finance, what sorts of conflicts of interest and problems of conscience do physicians face? Can the ethical practice of medicine and the integrity of individual practitioners survive the challenges posed by these conflicts and problems? This chapter confronts these and other fundamental moral issues associated with the physician-patient relationship and, therefore, with many of the other issues taken up in this book.

PHYSICIANS' OBLIGATIONS AND VIRTUES

The Hippocratic Oath, reprinted in this chapter, reflects the traditional paternalism of the medical profession. The oath requires physicians to act so as to benefit the sick and "keep them from harm," but says nothing about patients' rights. Until fairly recently, the codes of ethics developed by the American Medical Association revealed a similar approach. They articulated rules and virtues that should guide physicians in their professional relationships with patients and others but remained silent on patients' rights. For example, physicians were expected to promote their patients' well-being, but nothing was said about a patient's right to define his or her own "well-being"—or to participate in decisions affecting it. By contrast, the discussions that have taken place over the past three decades in biomedical ethics have frequently emphasized patients' rights, especially their right of self-determination. This emphasis reflects, among other factors, a growing change in lay attitudes toward physicians.

For a long time physicians were viewed as selfless individuals who could be expected to do everything in their power to benefit their patients. Patients, by contrast, were viewed as dependent individuals with an obligation to trust their physicians. It was often taken for granted that doctors—because of their presumed wisdom, objectivity, skill, and benevolence—were best positioned to decide what was in their patients' best interests. Professional codes of medical ethics reflected this view of the physician-patient relationship, affirming that physicians would act to benefit, and not exploit, the often vulnerable patients over whom they frequently held great influence and power.

Current attitudes toward physicians are somewhat different due to many factors. First among them, the physician-patient relationship has become increasingly impersonal as the growth of medical knowledge and technology has made medicine more complex. Growing complexity has led to increased specialization and the growth of large, depersonalized medical institutions. Second, the rise of "iatrogenic harm," illnesses and injuries resulting from medical interventions, has sometimes raised doubts about the skills and judgment of physicians. Third, it is commonly thought that many physicians engage in practices that compromise patients' interests either for the sake of physicians' financial gain or to protect the financial interests of an insurance company or program. In an article reprinted in this chapter, Edmund D. Pellegrino argues that physician virtue is of paramount importance in situations in which altruism and self-interest appear to conflict.

In keeping with such changing attitudes toward physicians, many recent discussions of medical ethics have attempted to expose and criticize the extensive paternalism embodied in traditional codes of medical ethics. Numerous authors have criticized professional codes that sanction paternalistic justifications for medical practices—such as lying for a patient's "own good"—that violate a patient's right to self-determination. But in several recent statements, including "Fundamental Elements of the Patient-Physician Relationship" (reprinted in this chapter), the American Medical Association acknowledges numerous patient rights, including the right to receive information relevant to one's medical care.

PATERNALISM AND RESPECT FOR PATIENT AUTONOMY

Is fostering a patient's well-being, in accordance with the traditional commitment, always compatible with respecting patient autonomy? In their analysis of several models—or metaphors—of the physician-patient relationship, James F. Childress and Mark Siegler suggest in this chapter that these two goals are not always compatible. The paternalism model, which emphasizes the traditional commitment to serve patient well-being, is usually inadequate in today's world, according to the authors. Physicians and patients may disagree in their health-related values (for example, if only the physician considers addiction to cigarettes a disease); or they may disagree about the relative value of health in comparison with other values (as when a Jehovah's Witness refuses a blood transfusion, knowing that death will inevitably result, while the patient's physician considers the transfusion necessary). As the authors put it, paternalism "tends to concentrate on care rather than respect, patients' needs rather than their rights, and physicians' discretion rather than patients' autonomy or self-determination."

That is not to say that paternalism is never justified, however. Childress and Siegler defend the commonly accepted form of paternalism (identified in Chapter 1 as *weak* paternalism) in which a patient is incompetent, or substantially lacking in decision-making capacity, and at risk of harm. Moreover, the authors ultimately recommend, for many physician-patient interactions in which the patient is competent, the metaphor of *negotiation*. This metaphor illuminates two important aspects of medical relationships: (1) the autonomy of both parties (where autonomy is construed not as a goal that in some cases might be imposed on a patient, but as a constraint on permissible interactions between autonomous persons), and (2) the ongoing nature of the relationship. The metaphor of negotiation invites both patient and physician to determine what they consider acceptable terms for continuing the relationship. Those terms may involve one or more of the models Childress and Siegler discuss—even paternalism, for a patient might autonomously decide to turn the medical decision-making reins over to a physician willing to take them.

As presented in Chapter 1, paternalism is the interference with, limitation of, or usurpation of individual autonomy justified by reasons referring exclusively to the welfare or needs of the person whose autonomy is being interfered with, limited, or usurped. In acting paternalistically, physicians in effect act as if they, and not their patients, can best identify what is in their patients' best interests as well as the best means to advance those interests. Many commentators contend that paternalism and respect for patient autonomy are incompatible. But Terrence F. Ackerman argues in this chapter that genuine respect for autonomy may require physicians to override patients' treatment-related preferences (suggesting at least weak paternalism) in order to help them regain some of the autonomy lost due to the constraining effects of illness. While affirming the importance of honesty and respect for patients' rights, Ackerman criticizes the interpretation of respect for autonomy that takes it to be essentially a principle of *noninterference*. To understand his concern, it is helpful to discuss two kinds of cases in which the values perceived as fundamental in physician-patient interactions—promotion of patient well-being and respect for patient autonomy—appear to conflict.

First, a patient's abilities to reason and deliberate may be so severely constrained by illness (e.g., high fever, delirium) that autonomous decisions are virtually impossible and apparent decisions may be inconsistent with the patient's history of decisions and values. In such cases, the promotion of a patient's well-being may require acting against his or her wishes as currently expressed. This would appear to violate the principle of respect for autonomy. But the conflict between the two values may be illusory. If the patient's autonomy is severely diminished and the desires expressed are inconsistent with the patient's history and values, the principle of respect for autonomy would not even seem to apply. When there are compelling reasons to believe that a patient's decisions are not autonomous and that as a result the patient cannot exercise the right of self-determination, no paternalistic violation of that right—no *strong* paternalism—is involved when a physician makes decisions for the patient.

Second, a patient and physician may disagree about just what constitutes the patient's well-being (a point noted by Childress and Siegler). A physician, for example, might insist on continuing aggressive treatment for a cancer patient, even though past treatment has brought no positive results. The patient might have a strong desire to discontinue the recommended therapy and die without the additional discomforts caused by the therapy. To foster the patient's well-being, then, the physician might think it necessary to override the patient's decision paternalistically. Here the physician may see a conflict between two obligations: an obligation to promote the patient's well-being, as understood from an objective medical standpoint, and an obligation to respect the patient's right of self-determination. The physician may believe that virtually any chance of prolonging life justifies continuing treatment. But while the prolongation of life is generally regarded as a good, and premature death a harm, the paternalistic model itself does not commit one to the prolongation of life irrespective of the harms the patient might incur. Thus, the physician's belief that this life must be prolonged, whatever the discomfort to the patient and no matter how brief the extension of life, is apparently due to the physician's own values rather than to some indisputably objective medical values. The patient, meanwhile, may believe that a few extra days or weeks of uncomfortable in-hospital life, with an extremely small chance of further prolonging life, are not worth the price. If the patient's decision is the result of reflection and is in keeping with his or her history of decisions and values, respect for autonomy would seem to require acting in accord with the *patient's* conception of his or her well-being. If the patient's decision is not in accord with his or her history of decisions and values but is the result of a careful, reflective revision of those values, respect for autonomy would again seem to require acting in accord with the patient's choices. The conflict here is not between an obligation to respect autonomy and an obligation to promote patient well-being, but between two different conceptions of "well-being." The conflict arises because what constitutes a person's well-being is, at least to some extent, a subjective or personal judgment.

The problematic cases that concern Ackerman arise because of the constraining effects illness has on autonomy. In relation to the first kind of case, for example, it is sometimes difficult to judge to what extent a patient's capacity for clear-headed deliberation is undermined. In the face of such uncertainty, does the physician's obligation to promote the patient's well-being entail an obligation to act so as to "restore the patient's autonomy" to the greatest extent possible, even if this involves some measure of paternalism? Ackerman holds that the physician's obligation is to act to restore autonomy—suggesting (in Childress and Siegler's terms) that autonomy is a goal to be sought when it is absent or diminished, not just a constraint on physician-patient interactions when the patient is already considered autonomous. Ackerman gives examples intended to show how psychological states, such as depression, or social factors, such as family influence, can constrain a patient's decision making. He argues that physicians have an obligation to act in ways that will offset the effects of these constraints to make the patient more autonomous. It is not clear that all of Ackerman's examples involve paternalism, since they do not all involve the usurpation of patients' decision making. In any event, physicians who act as Ackerman recommends run the danger exemplified by the second kind of case, when they fail to see that a disagreement with a patient about some course of treatment may be due, not to the constraining effects of illness on autonomy, but to a disagreement about values.

TRUTH TELLING

Traditional codes of medical ethics have little to say about lying, other forms of deception, or truth telling. Yet some of the most widely disputed issues in biomedical ethics center on physicians' obligation to be truthful with patients. Until fairly recently, it was not unusual for physicians to lie to patients about their illnesses for paternalistic reasons. Nor was it unusual for physicians to prescribe alternating injections of sterilized water with injections of painkilling drugs for patients who were told that all the injections contained an opiate. In the first kind of case, physicians often argued that patients did not want to know the truth or that the truth could seriously harm patients. In the second kind of case, physicians often argued that the deceptive practices were justified because water can have a psychotherapeutic effect but is much less dangerous to the patient than overly frequent injections of opiates.[1] Are physicians ever morally justified in paternalistic lies or deceptive practices? If so, under what conditions?

One way to approach these questions is to begin with more general questions. Is it always morally wrong to lie? Is it always right to tell the truth? If it is *always* wrong to lie or to deceive others, then it is wrong for anyone, including physicians, to do so. If lies and intentional deception are *sometimes* morally acceptable, we should attempt to specify the conditions that make them acceptable. Once these conditions are determined, we can then explore the particular physician-patient encounter to see if it satisfies them.

Rule-utilitarians, for example, faced with deciding under what conditions, if any, lies and deceptive practices are justified, would have to consider the possible consequences of adopting and following a particular rule. In the medical context, they would ask, "What would be the effect on the physician-patient relationship if physicians followed the rule, 'Lie to your patients whenever you believe that doing so is in the patient's best interests'?" In weighing the potential consequences of following such a rule, they would have to account for the erosive effect that following it would have on patients' trust of physicians.

Suppose a physician argued as follows: Physicians ought to lie to patients because (1) it is extremely difficult to convey the technical facts and uncertainties inherent in a medical situation to persons who lack medical training, (2) most patients do not want to know the truth, and (3) the truth can harm patients. In responding to this argument, a rule-utilitarian would have to examine the three factual claims underpinning this view, a task carried out by Roger Higgs in this chapter (though without special reference to rule-utilitarianism). In response to (1), Higgs argues that (a) while communicating the patient's medical situation to the patient may be difficult, it is generally not impossible, and (b) the admission "'I do not know' can be a major piece of honesty." In response to (2), Higgs cites studies suggesting that most patients *do* want the truth. In response to (3), Higgs contends the following: (a) While the truth can sometimes harm patients, such cases are less common than physicians have claimed; (b) the manner of disclosure is crucial to the likelihood of harm; and (c) lying can also be harmful by preventing a patient from being able to plan appropriately for the future and by weakening patient trust of physicians.

The rule-utilitarian who agreed with Higgs's findings would still have to determine whether exceptions should be built into a rule against lying to patients. These exceptions would probably be designed to cover cases with strong evidence to show that a patient does not want to know or would be seriously harmed by knowing. The rule-utilitarian would then have to determine whether the harm done to these patients would be outweighed by the overall good consequences of following a rule that prohibits all lying to patients.

Deontologists, of course, take a different approach. Immanuel Kant, whose deontological position is discussed in Chapter 1, is usually read as defending an "absolutist" position: All lies, including those told out of altruistic motives, are wrong. Not all deontologists agree with this absolutist position. As noted in Chapter 1, W. D. Ross maintains, for example, that there is a prima facie obligation not to lie or intentionally deceive, but that this obligation can sometimes be overridden by some other prima facie obligation. In medicine, the overriding obligation might sometimes be the physician's duty to promote the patient's medical well-being.

In the end, perhaps the kind of situation in which it is most plausible to argue that physicians may lie or deceive is one in which truthfulness seems likely to destroy a patient's hope. An example is that of a critically ill patient who might be devastated by the disclosure that her cancer is inoperable; without hope, she might quickly succumb to her disease. But we must not assume prematurely that truthful disclosure would have this effect, because hope may prove to be highly resilient. Moreover, it has been argued that disclosing the truth is usually compatible with inspiring hope, by responding to important patient concerns other than survival—such as the patient's hope that death will be relatively painless, the hope that he or she will not be abandoned before death, and the hope that loved ones will maintain contact in the time remaining.[2]

The question of whether physicians may ever lie or otherwise deceive their patients represents one aspect of the more general issue of what truth telling requires of physicians. Another aspect of this general issue concerns *nondisclosure* as opposed to active deception. Is it ever morally acceptable for a physician not to disclose a patient's diagnosis to him or her? There is broad agreement that, in emergencies, patients may receive medical treatment without prior disclosure of their condition and without other elements of informed consent (as discussed in the next section). But, after the emergency has passed, is it ever acceptable not to disclose information about the patient's medical condition, information that may have emerged for the first time during the emergency?

Or suppose, in another sort of case, that a patient's family insists, for reasons related to their cultural background, that a patient not be informed of his or her diagnosis. The patient, let us suppose, has inoperable colon cancer. Her family insists that, in their culture, treatment decisions are left to family members and physicians while medical "death sentences" are withheld from unknowing patients. Such a scenario is likely to create a dilemma for the physician (or at least for any physician working in a culture where truthful disclosure is the prevailing norm). On the one hand, the physician recognizes that the patient has a right to truthful disclosure about his or her medical condition. On the other hand, the physician appreciates the value of respecting other cultures and their moral practices. In an article reprinted in this chapter, Benjamin Freedman addresses this sort of dilemma. He defends an approach that steers a middle path between the poles of (1) *imposing* the truth on patients who may not want to receive it and (2) deferring completely to a family's cultural expectations even when doing so seems morally misguided. The approach he recommends involves gradually and sensitively *offering* a patient the opportunity to learn the truth, at whatever level of detail the patient wishes.

INFORMED CONSENT

Discussions about truth telling in medical ethics frequently arise in conjunction with discussions of the requirements of informed consent. It is now widely accepted that competent adult patients have a moral and legal right not to be subjected to medical interventions without their informed and voluntary consent.[3] But lying to patients or withholding information from them can seriously undermine their ability to make informed decisions and, therefore, to give informed consent. To be able to give such consent, and thereby exercise their right of self-determination, patients must have access to relevant information, and physicians are usually in the best position to supply it. Judge Spotswood W. Robinson III affirms this point in a judicial opinion reprinted in this chapter, *Canterbury v. Spence*, when he argues that physicians have a duty to "satisfy the vital informational needs of the patient."

The informed consent requirement is a relatively recent addition to the recognized ethical constraints governing the physician-patient relationship. Traditional codes of medical ethics recognize no physician obligation to inform patients about their diagnoses and the risks and benefits of alternative treatments. There is some controversy about when exactly the doctrine of informed consent was introduced into case law. But the 1972 *Canterbury* decision firmly established the doctrine and language of informed consent (even if the doctrine was introduced earlier), and great attention has been given in biomedical ethics to informed consent since that time. For example, Congress assigned the task of determining the ethical and legal implications of the informed consent requirement to the President's Commission for the Study of Ethical Problems in Medicine and Biomedical and Behavioral Research. In its 1982 report, a selection from which is reprinted here, the commission describes informed consent "as an ethical obligation that involves a process of shared decisionmaking based upon the mutual respect and participation ([of patients and health-care professionals)][4] and identifies two values as providing the ethical foundation of the requirement: respect for the patient's autonomy, or self-determination, and promotion of the patient's well-being."

Much of the literature on informed consent focuses on several difficulties that affect the application of the requirement. (1) Who is *competent* to give consent? (2) When is consent *informed*? That is, how much information must a patient receive and understand before his or her consent is considered adequately informed? (3) When is consent *voluntary*? Each of these questions will be briefly examined in order to show some of the difficulties that affect the application of the requirement. It is important to note that the problems here are both conceptual and empirical. The meaning of the concepts *competent*, *informed*, and *voluntary* must be explicated so that it can be determined just what counts as voluntary and informed consent. Then in a particular case, it must be determined whether the individual in question is, in fact, capable of giving voluntary and informed consent.

(1) Who is *competent* to give consent? At a general conceptual level, we might say that *to be competent to give consent is to be capable of consenting autonomously*. In view of the analysis of autonomous action presented in Chapter 1, a patient who is capable of consenting autonomously would be capable of consenting intentionally, with sufficient understanding of what consent entails in the circumstances, and with sufficient freedom from internal and external constraints. A sick patient in a hospital or institution may not be functioning normally enough to be competent. Patients who are under great emotional stress, who are frightened or in severe pain, are often incapable of making important decisions autonomously.

Recent work on competence stresses that it is not "all or nothing." Still, for practical purposes in medical decision making, some threshold must be used to determine who counts as competent and who does not. The commission's report maintains that individuals should be judged incapable of decision making only when they lack the ability to make decisions that promote their well-being in keeping with their own previously expressed values and preferences.

(2) How much *information* must patients receive—and understand—before their consent is informed? Suppose a patient suffering from breast cancer agrees to have a radical mastectomy. But she has not been told that studies indicate that this radical surgery is no more effective, in circumstances like hers, than much less radical surgery. Presumably, the patient has not been given sufficient information for her decision to count as an informed

one. But what general criteria must the physician use in determining when sufficient information has been given? And is more information always better than less? Studies have shown that patients receiving long, detailed explanations of the risks and purposes of a procedure may understand and retain little of the significant information. In contrast, those who are given less detailed information may be able to comprehend and retain more of the important information.[5]

(3) When is consent really *voluntary*, or sufficiently free of internal and external constraints? It is often argued that it is easy to manipulate even clearly competent patients into giving consent when someone in a position of authority makes the request. For example, it has been shown that physicians, whose patients sometimes see them as "god" figures, and psychiatrists, whose judgments patients generally trust, find it easy to get the consent they request. When patients are influenced in this way, is their consent sufficiently voluntary? How about patients who are strongly pressured by family members to consent to treatment?

In consideration of these criteria for informed consent, leading work on this topic, such as that of the President's Commission, stresses the importance of the process of communication and of the patient's information processing. Studies have been undertaken both to understand and to improve the procedures used to get consent.[6] For genuine informed consent, it is often insufficient simply to transmit information to patients via a form or a short conversation listing possible risks and alternatives; it may be necessary to assess the degree of patient understanding, and perhaps some of the other factors that may affect the patient's decision, such as concern about a physician's reaction to a refusal.

Take the example of a terminally ill, diabetic, cancer-ridden patient who, after repeatedly rejecting amputation of his gangrenous left foot, suddenly consented. His consent appeared both voluntary and informed. However, given his history and the staff's knowledge of his values, an ethics consultant was called in to determine the reasons for the patient's change of mind. After a long conversation with the patient, the consultant learned that the patient had consented to the amputation only because he erroneously believed that without his consent the physician and the hospital would refuse to continue their care—raising questions about how informed and voluntary his decision was. Once the patient understood that this belief was incorrect, he withdrew his consent to the amputation. This case illustrates that informed consent requires more than forms and cursory rituals. It also shows the need for medical professionals to have insight into the communication processes they use to achieve informed consent.

But what extent, or quality, of communication can be reasonably expected, legally and morally, as a standard of informed consent? Whatever the answer, is it compatible with good medical practice? In one of this chapter's readings, Howard Brody criticizes the prevailing legal standards of informed consent for encouraging the impression that informed consent is separate from, and even interferes with, sound medical care. In his view, part of the problem stems from the fact that most physician-patient encounters occur in the context of primary care, whereas the courts and many commentators appear to take surgery and other risky procedures as the paradigm of such encounters. Brody discusses the advantages of a "conversation" standard of informed consent (which is illustrated in the case described previously), but argues that this demanding standard is probably not feasible legally. As a compromise between prevailing legal standards and the conversation standard, Brody recommends a "transparency" standard: A physician has provided adequate disclosure when his or her essential thinking about the medical situation has been made transparent to the patient.

THE PRACTICE OF MEDICINE IN A MULTICULTURAL SOCIETY

A cluster of issues regarding the physician-patient relationship may be somewhat loosely collected together under the term *multicultural*. The physician-patient encounter often brings together individuals who come from different countries with distinct cultures (or different subcultures within the same country) and who may speak different languages. For this reason, a physician and patient may have different cultural understandings of ethically appropriate practices and even different views about the governance of the universe (e.g., a universe governed by natural, causal laws versus one featuring the supernatural effects of spirit or magic).

A physician and patient who have different cultural perspectives may disagree significantly on *ethical* matters. For example, they may have different views regarding who possesses legitimate decision-making authority, the importance of truth telling in medical practice, the role of family in decisions primarily affecting a patient, and the proper treatment of children.

A physician and patient associated with different cultural traditions may also differ on *factual or metaphysical* questions that bear on patient care. A patient may, for example, believe that discussing the possibility of negative medical outcomes—such as succumbing to cancer—increases the likelihood of these possibilities coming to pass; or a patient may believe that rituals that cause great pain to children are necessary to eradicate evil spirits from their bodies. With a different view of causation, a Western physician may consider such beliefs irrational and potentially harmful if taken seriously—yet may feel ethically conflicted due to an awareness of the importance of respecting patients' cultural beliefs and traditions. In a reading reprinted in this chapter, Ruth Macklin explores several types of conflicts that can arise for physicians in multicultural settings and recommends ways of resolving some of these conflicts.

Distinct issues arise when a physician encounters a patient whose treatment preferences are crucially affected by a racial, ethnic, or national prejudice. Think, for example, of a white patient who does not want to be treated by Hispanic health-care professionals. Analyzing a case of a Korean patient who did not want to be treated by a Japanese physician— a preference rooted in long-felt suspicion of the Japanese due to their occupation of Korea during part of the twentieth century—Kenneth Kipnis addresses this type of conflict in one of this chapter's readings.

CONTESTED THERAPIES WITHIN THE PHYSICIAN-PATIENT RELATIONSHIP

Some services that physicians are capable of providing to patients test the boundaries of the appropriate practice of medicine, adding a layer of ethical complexity to the physician-patient relationship. Primary care, emergency medicine, certain types of surgery, and psychiatric treatment for psychiatric illnesses furnish uncontroversial examples of appropriate medical care. Another type of intervention that is widely (though far from universally) regarded as appropriate is gene therapy—or, inasmuch as this area of medicine is in its clinical infancy, gene therapy *research*. Certain other services and interventions that physicians may be capable of providing are more controversial. For example, if research in genetics leads to the ability to *enhance* human traits by genetic means—beyond what is necessary for normal health and functioning—such genetic enhancement will be enormously controversial. (Chapter 8 explores ethical issues connected with gene therapy and genetic enhancement.) Should physicians be permitted to employ their skills in a medical setting for purposes other than the treatment or prevention of disease, impairment, or dysfunction? Or does such employment of medical expertise transgress the appropriate boundaries of medicine? And how are we to determine these boundaries? Do they include the full range of services that patients want and physicians are willing to provide, as suggested by a free market model of health-care delivery? Or are the boundaries of appropriate medical practice determined by moral values inherent in medicine?

While the prospect of genetic enhancement raises these questions for possible future scenarios, many currently available services make these issues immediately relevant. One example is cosmetic surgery—surgery undertaken primarily for cosmetic purposes, such as breast augmentation and "nose jobs." In an article reprinted in this chapter, Franklin G. Miller, Howard Brody, and Kevin C. Chung argue that medicine is governed by a moral framework that identifies the appropriate goals of medical practice. In view of this "internal morality of medicine," which is contrasted with the more minimal ethics of the marketplace, the authors contend that cosmetic surgery is ethically questionable, located at best on the periphery of medical practice.

While cosmetic surgery has been available for decades, some means of medical enhancement are relatively new. "Cosmetic psychopharmacology," for example, emerged in the early 1990s. *Cosmetic psychopharmacology* is a term that was coined by psychiatrist Peter Kramer in his landmark book, *Listening to Prozac*, to refer to the use of psychiatric medications for certain patients who lacked any diagnosable psychiatric disorder or illness).[7] Kramer had noticed that, among "the worried well"—patients who were not clinically depressed or anxious, for example, but who struggled with fairly ordinary psychological issues—some not only felt much better when taking Prozac, but also functioned more successfully at work, in relationships, and in other respects. Quite a few of these patients experienced personality changes—becoming more trusting, outgoing, and confident, for example—and welcomed these transformations. Hence the term *cosmetic* psychopharmacology. Since the publication of Kramer's book, other SSRIs (selective serotonin reuptake inhibitors) besides Prozac, such as Paxil and Zoloft, have had similar effects on some patients who have no diagnosable disorder or illness. Naturally, the prescription of psychiatric medications for enhancement purposes tests the boundaries of appropriate medical practice.

Another trend raising such concerns is the increasing prescription of stimulants such as Ritalin for children—mostly boys—who have trouble concentrating, sitting still, and completing homework but may not meet clinical criteria for ADHD (Attention Deficit/Hyperactivity Disorder) or any other disorder for which stimulants are normally prescribed. Are these children being drugged as an alternative to improving teacher-student ratios, making helpful changes in the home environment, or introducing other remedies to fairly normal, if inconvenient, juvenile behavior? Rather than taking stimulants on a regular basis, some children and teenagers take them to improve concentration during important exams or while completing especially taxing assignments. Is their reliance on a medication in such contexts in their best interests? Is such discretionary use of stimulants fair to those children who lack access to them? Moreover, what is our society doing to childhood when pressures to behave and/or excel lead so many parents to seek stimulants for cognitively and behaviorally normal youngsters? These and other issues redound to a question raised earlier: Can physicians responsibly prescribe medications for patients who enjoy normal health and functioning? Claudia Mills addresses such questions as these in one of this chapter's selections.

CONFLICTS OF INTEREST, PROBLEMS OF CONSCIENCE, AND MANAGED CARE

A final cluster of issues pertaining to the physician-patient relationship involves *conflicts of interest* and *problems of conscience*—areas of concern that have become especially urgent in the present era of managed care. Medical tradition has long recognized *promotion of patient well-being* as the overarching end or goal of medicine; a more contemporary articulation would add the phrase "within constraints of respecting patient autonomy." More specific goals of medicine that have been traditionally recognized include the preservation of life, relief of pain and suffering, restoration of physical and mental functioning, and care for the dying, among other goals. While there is some dispute about exactly which specific goals can be subsumed under promotion of patient well-being, more intense controversy attends the competition of other incentives with the physician's focus on patient welfare. These competing incentives create conflicts of interest for physicians.

One type of conflict of interest pits *patient well-being against the health-related interests of physicians*. Do physicians have an obligation, stemming from their professional roles, to provide health care when doing so puts them at physical risk? For example, are physicians duty-bound to care for patients infected with the human immunodeficiency virus (HIV)? A second, closely related type of conflict of interest pits *patient well-being against the financial interests of physicians*. Can the latter legitimately compete with patient well-being?

A third type of conflict of interest pits *patient well-being against society's financial interests*. Marcia Angell, in a reading reprinted in this chapter, examines the relatively recent American expectation that doctors act as "double agents." In addition to the traditional expectation that doctors serve patients in addressing their medical needs, in recent decades there has been at least some expectation that doctors respond to society's need to curtail medical costs. But does responding to this societal need constitute a legitimate objective within medical practice?

A final type of conflict of interest to be considered here pits *patient well-being against the financial interests of an insurer*. The insurer may be a private company, such as a managed care organization, or a public program, such as Medicare or Medicaid. Can the financial health of an insurer legitimately compete in importance with patient well-being? Is a physician an agent of the insurer and not just of the patient? If the insurer is a for-profit company, the physician arguably becomes an agent of company stockholders, whose primary interest is maximizing earnings.

These questions became especially acute in the 1990s as managed care became the dominant model for health care delivery and finance in the United States and, at least to some extent, in many other countries. The somewhat vague term *managed care* may be understood to designate any carefully organized and integrated system of health-care delivery that is designed to control costs; it covers health maintenance organizations, preferred provider organizations, and other insurance schemes that carefully limit expenditures on patient care. Typically, managed care arrangements attempt to control costs at least in part by providing physicians with incentives—often financial incentives—for limiting expenditures by limiting care. Thus, a conflict of interest of the fourth type, as just discussed, typically creates for physicians a conflict of the second type, which makes patient well-being compete with the physician's own financial interests. Understanding the goals of medicine in a largely traditional, patient-centered way, Daniel Callahan in this chapter explores in detail the tension between these goals and managed care.

When physicians face conflicts of interest created by the tension between their traditional patient-centered focus and the financial pressures of managed care, they may experience *problems of conscience*. Conscience involves an agent's awareness of the moral value of his or her actions. A physician's conscience may be troubled by decisions, whether already taken or merely contemplated for the future, that feel morally compromised. In this chapter's final reading, James F. Childress presents a framework that physicians may use to identify and clarify options grounded in conscience as a way of responding to unacceptable pressures from managed care organizations.

D.D.

NOTES

1 See, e.g., J. Sice, "Letter to the Editor," *The Lancet* 2 (1972), p. 651.
2 This viewpoint is forcefully articulated in Howard Brody, "Hope," *JAMA* 246 (September 25, 1981), pp. 1411–1412.
3 Some commentators prefer the language of "decision-making capacity" to that of "competence" outside of legal contexts, but we are not persuaded that "competence" is exclusively a legal term.
4 President's Commission for the Study of Ethical Problems in Medicine and Biomedical and Behavioral Research, *Making Health Care Decisions: The Ethical and Legal Implications of Informed Consent in the Patient-Practitioner Relationship*, Vol. 1: *Report* (Washington, DC: U.S. Government Printing Office, 1982), p. 2.
5 On this point, see Ralph J. Alfidi, "Controversy, Alternatives, and Decisions in Complying with the Legal Doctrine of Informed Consent," *Radiology* 114 (January 1975), pp. 231–234.
6 Barrie R. Cassileth et al., "Informed Consent—Why Are Its Goals Imperfectly Realized?" *New England Journal of Medicine* 302 (1980), pp. 896–900; and T. M. Grundner, "On the Readability of Surgical Consent Forms," *ibid.*, pp. 900–902.
7 Peter D. Kramer, *Listening to Prozac* (New York: Viking, 1993).

PHYSICIANS' OBLIGATIONS AND VIRTUES

THE HIPPOCRATIC OATH

Little is known about the life of Hippocrates, a Greek physician born about 460 B.C. A collection of documents known as the *Hippocratic Writings* (largely written from the fifth to the fourth century B.C.) is believed to represent the remains of the Hippocratic school of medicine. Some of the works in this collection are credited to Hippocrates. The oath reprinted here, however, is believed to have been written by a philosophical sect known as the Pythagoreans in the latter part of the fourth century B.C. For the Middle Ages and later centuries, the Hippocratic Oath embodied the highest aspirations of the physician. It sets forth two sets of duties: (1) duties to the patient and (2) duties to the other members of the guild (profession) of medicine. In regard to the patient, it includes a set of absolute prohibitions (e.g., against abortion and euthanasia) as well as a statement of the physician's obligation to help and not to harm the patient.

I swear by Apollo Physician and Asclepius and Hygieia and Panaceia and all the gods and goddesses, making them my witnesses, that I will fulfill according to my ability and judgment this oath and this covenant:

To hold him who has taught me this art as equal to my parents and to live my life in partnership with him, and if he is in need of money to give him a share of mine, and to regard his offspring as equal to my brothers in male lineage and to teach them this art—if they desire to learn it—without fee and covenant; to give a share of precepts and oral instruction and all the other learning to my sons and to the sons of him who has instructed me and to pupils who have signed the covenant and have taken an oath according to the medical law, but to no one else.

I will apply dietetic measures for the benefit of the sick according to my ability and judgment; I will keep them from harm and injustice.

I will neither give a deadly drug to anybody if asked for it, nor will I make a suggestion to this effect. Similarly I will not give to a woman an abortive remedy. In purity and holiness I will guard my life and my art.

I will not use the knife, not even on sufferers from stone, but will withdraw in favor of such men as are engaged in this work.

Whatever houses I may visit, I will come for the benefit of the sick, remaining free of all intentional injustice, of all mischief and in particular of sexual relations with both female and male persons, be they free or slaves.

What I may see or hear in the course of the treatment or even outside of the treatment in regard to the life of men, which on no account one must spread abroad, I will keep to myself holding such things shameful to be spoken about.

If I fulfill this oath and do not violate it, may it be granted to me to enjoy life and art, being honored with fame among all men for all time to come; if I transgress it and swear falsely, may the opposite of all this be my lot.

FUNDAMENTAL ELEMENTS OF THE PATIENT-PHYSICIAN RELATIONSHIP
Council on Ethical and Judicial Affairs, American Medical Association

This statement asserts (1) the collaborative nature of the patient-physician relationship and (2) a set of patient rights. Regarding the collaborative relationship, patients are said to have a responsibility to work cooperatively with physicians in addressing health-related needs. Patients' rights include the right to accept or refuse recommended medical treatments, the right to confidentiality, and the right to "have available adequate health care."

From ancient times, physicians have recognized that the health and well-being of patients depend upon a collaborative effort between physician and patient. Patients share with physicians the responsibility for their own health care. The patient-physician relationship is of greatest benefit to patients when they bring medical problems to the attention of their

physicians in a timely fashion, provide information about their medical condition to the best of their ability, and work with their physicians in a mutually respectful alliance. Physicians can best contribute to this alliance by serving as their patients' advocates and by fostering these rights:

1. The patient has the right to receive information from physicians and to discuss the benefits, risks, and costs of appropriate treatment alternatives. Patients should

receive guidance from their physicians as to the optimal course of action. Patients are also entitled to obtain copies or summaries of their medical records, to have their questions answered, to be advised of potential conflicts of interest that their physicians might have, and to receive independent professional opinions.

2. The patient has the right to make decisions regarding the health care that is recommended by his or her physician. Accordingly, patients may accept or refuse any recommended medical treatment.

3. The patient has the right to courtesy, respect, dignity, responsiveness, and timely attention to his or her needs.

4. The patient has the right to confidentiality. The physician should not reveal confidential communications or information without the consent of the patient, unless provided for by law or by the need to protect the welfare of the individual or the public interest.

5. The patient has the right to continuity of health care. The physician has an obligation to cooperate in the coordination of medically indicated care with other health care providers treating the patient. The physician may not discontinue treatment of a patient as long as further treatment is medically indicated, without giving the patient reasonable assistance and sufficient opportunity to make alternative arrangements for care.

6. The patient has a basic right to have available adequate health care. Physicians, along with the rest of society, should continue to work toward this goal. Fulfillment of this right is dependent on society providing resources so that no patient is deprived of necessary care because of an inability to pay for the care. Physicians should continue their traditional assumption of a part of the responsibility for the medical care of those who cannot afford essential health care. Physicians should advocate for patients in dealing with third parties when appropriate.

THE VIRTUOUS PHYSICIAN AND THE ETHICS OF MEDICINE
Edmund D. Pellegrino

Pellegrino defends a vision of medical ethics in which virtue ethics and duty-based ethics are each essential components. Citing several important codes of medical ethics, including the Hippocratic Oath, Pellegrino argues for a three-tiered system of obligations incumbent upon physicians. In "ascending order of ethical sensitivity," they are (1) obedience to the law, (2) the observance of moral rights and fulfillment of moral duties, and (3) the practice of virtue. According to Pellegrino, physicians' practice of virtue distinguishes itself less in the avoidance of clearly unethical actions than in the avoidance of actions at the ambiguous margin of moral responsibility, where altruism is pitted against self-interest. Examples of practices at this moral margin include investing in for-profit hospitals, selling services for whatever the market will bear, and making referrals on the basis of friendship and reciprocity rather than skill.

. . . In most professional ethical codes, virtue and duty-based ethics are intermingled. The Hippocratic Oath, for example, imposes certain duties like pro-

From *Virtue and Medicine: Explorations in the Character of Medicine*, edited by Earl E. Shelp, pp. 248–253. © 1985 by D. Reidel Publishing Company. Reprinted by permission of Kluwer Academic Publishers.

tection of confidentiality, avoiding abortion, not harming the patient. But the Hippocratic physician also pledges: ". . . in purity and holiness I will guard my life and my art." This is an exhortation to be a good person and a virtuous physician, in order to serve patients in an ethically responsible way.

Likewise, in one of the most humanistic statements in medical literature, the first century A.D. writer, Scribonius Largus, made *humanitas* (compassion) an essential virtue. It is thus really a role-specific duty. In doing so he was applying the Stoic doctrine of virtue to medicine [1, 5].

The latest version (1980) of the AMA 'Principles of Medical Ethics' similarly intermingles duties, rights, and exhortations to virtue. It speaks of 'standards of behavior,' 'essentials of honorable behavior,' dealing 'honestly' with patients and colleagues and exposing colleagues 'deficient in character.' The *Declaration of Geneva*, which must meet the challenge of the widest array of value systems, nonetheless calls for practice 'with conscience and dignity' in keeping with 'the honor and noble traditions of the profession.' Though their first allegiance must be to the Communist ethos, even the Soviet physician is urged to preserve 'the high title of physician,' 'to keep and develop the beneficial traditions of medicine' and to 'dedicate' all his 'knowledge and strength to the care of the sick.'

Those who are cynical of any protestation of virtue on the part of physicians will interpret these excerpts as the last remnants of a dying tradition of altruistic benevolence. But at the very least, they attest to the recognition that the good of the patient cannot be fully protected by rights and duties alone. Some degree of supererogation is built into the nature of the relationship of those who are ill and those who profess to help them.

This too may be why many graduating classes, still idealistic about their calling, choose the Prayer of Maimonides (not by Maimonides at all) over the more deontological Oath of Hippocrates. In that 'prayer' the physician asks: ". . . may neither avarice nor miserliness, nor thirst for glory or for a great reputation engage my mind; for the enemies of truth and philanthropy may easily deceive me and make me forgetful of my lofty aim of doing good to thy children." This is an unequivocal call to virtue and it is hard to imagine even the most cynical graduate failing to comprehend its message.

All professional medical codes, then, are built of a three-tiered system of obligations related to the special roles of physicians in society. In the ascending order of ethical sensitivity they are: observance of the laws of the land, then observance of rights and fulfillment of duties, and finally the practice of virtue.

A legally based ethic concentrates on the minimum requirements—the duties imposed by human laws which protect against the grosser aberrations of personal rights. Licensure, the laws of torts and contracts, prohibitions against discrimination, good Samaritan laws, definitions of death, and the protection of human subjects of experimentation are elements of a legalistic ethic.

At the next level is the ethics of rights and duties which spells out obligations beyond what law defines. Here, benevolence and beneficence take on more than their legal meaning. The ideal of service, of responsiveness to the special needs of those who are ill, some degree of compassion, kindliness, promise-keeping, truth-telling, and non-maleficence and specific obligations like confidentiality and autonomy, are included. How these principles are applied, and conflicts among them resolved in the patient's best interests, are subjects of widely varying interpretation. How sensitively these issues are confronted depends more on the physician's character than his capability at ethical discourse or moral casuistry.

Virtue-based ethics goes beyond these first two levels. We expect the virtuous person to do the right and the good even at the expense of personal sacrifice and legitimate self-interest. Virtue ethics expands the notions of benevolence, beneficence, conscientiousness, compassion, and fidelity well beyond what strict duty might require. It makes some degree of supererogation mandatory because it calls for standards of ethical performance that exceed those prevalent in the rest of society [6].

At each of these three levels there are certain dangers from over-zealous or misguided observance. Legalistic ethical systems tend toward a justification for minimalistic ethics, a narrow definition of benevolence or beneficence, and a contract-minded physician-patient relationship. Duty- and rights-based ethics may be distorted by too strict adherence to the letter of ethical principles without the modulations and nuances the spirit of those principles implies. Virtue-based ethics, being the least specific, can more easily lapse into self-righteous paternalism or an unwelcome over-involvement in the personal life of the patient. Misapplication of any moral system even with good intent converts benevolence into maleficence. The virtuous person might be expected to be more sensitive to these aberrations than someone whose ethics is more deontologically or legally flavored.

The more we yearn for ethical sensitivity the less we lean on rights, duties, rules, and principles, and the more we lean on the character traits of the moral agent. Paradoxically, without rules, rights, and duties specifically spelled out, we cannot predict what form a particular person's expression of virtue will take. In a pluralistic society, we need laws, rules, and principles to assure a dependable minimum level of moral conduct. But that minimal level is insufficient in the complex and often unpredictable circumstances of decision-making, where technical and value desiderata intersect so inextricably.

The virtuous physician does not act from unreasoned, uncritical intuitions about what feels good. His dispositions are ordered in accord with that 'right reason' which both Aristotle and Aquinas considered essential to virtue. Medicine is itself ultimately an exercise of practical wisdom—a right way of acting in difficult and uncertain circumstances for a specific end, i.e., the good of a particular person who is ill. It is when the choice of a right and good action becomes more difficult, when the temptations to self-interest are most insistent, when unexpected nuances of good and evil arise and no one is looking, that the differences between an ethics based in virtue and an ethics based in law and/or duty can most clearly be distinguished.

Virtue-based professional ethics distinguishes itself, therefore, less in the avoidance of overtly immoral practices than in avoidance of those at the margin of moral responsibility. Physicians are confronted, in today's morally relaxed climate, with an increasing number of new practices that pit altruism against self-interest. Most are not illegal, or, strictly speaking, immoral in a rights- or duty-based ethic. But they are not consistent with the higher levels of moral sensitivity that a virtue-ethics demands. These practices usually involve opportunities for profit from the illness of others, narrowing the concept of service for personal convenience, taking a proprietary attitude with respect to medical knowledge, and placing loyalty to the profession above loyalty to patients.

Under the first heading, we might include such things as investment in and ownership of for-profit hospitals, hospital chains, nursing homes, dialysis units, tie-in arrangements with radiological or laboratory services, escalation of fees for repetitive, high-volume procedures, and lax indications for their use, especially when third party payers 'allow' such charges.

The second heading might include the ever decreasing availability and accessibility of physicians, the diffusion of individual patient responsibility in group practice so that the patient never knows whom he will see or who is on call, the itinerant emergency room physician who works two days and skips three with little commitment to hospital or community, and the growing over-indulgence of physicians in vacations, recreation, and 'self-development.'

The third category might include such things as 'selling one's services' for whatever the market will bear, providing what the market demands and not necessarily what the community needs, patenting new procedures or keeping them secret from potential competitor-colleagues, looking at the investment of time, effort, and capital in a medical education as justification of 'making it back,' or forgetting that medical knowledge is drawn from the cumulative experience of a multitude of patients, clinicians, and investigators.

Under the last category might be included referrals on the basis of friendship and reciprocity rather than skill, resisting consultations and second opinions as affronts to one's competence, placing the interest of the referring physician above those of the patients, looking the other way in the face of incompetence or even dishonesty in one's professional colleagues.

These and many other practices are defended today by sincere physicians and even encouraged in this era of competition, legalism, and self-indulgence. Some can be rationalized even in a deontological ethic. But it would be impossible to envision the physician committed to the virtues assenting to these practices. A virtue-based ethics simply does not fluctuate with what the dominant social mores will tolerate. It must interpret benevolence, beneficence, and responsibility in a way that reduces self interest and enhances altruism. It is the only convincing answer the profession can give to the growing perception clearly manifest in the legal commentaries in the FTC ruling that medicine is nothing more than business and should be regulated as such.

A virtue-based ethic is inherently elitist, in the best sense, because its adherents demand more of themselves than the prevailing morality. It calls forth that extra measure of dedication that has made the best physicians in every era exemplars of what the human spirit can achieve. No matter to what depths a society may fall, virtuous persons will always be the beacons that light the way back to moral sensitivity; virtuous physicians are the beacons that show the way back to moral credibility for the whole profession.

Albert Jonsen, rightly I believe, diagnoses the central paradox in medicine as the tension between self-interest and altruism [4]. No amount of deft juggling of rights, duties, or principles will suffice to resolve that tension. We are all too good at rationalizing what we want to do so that personal gain can be converted from vice to virtue. Only a character formed by the virtues can feel the nausea of such intellectual hypocrisy.

To be sure, the twin themes of self-interest and altruism have been inextricably joined in the history of medicine. There have always been physicians who reject the virtues or, more often, claim them falsely. But, in addition, there have been physicians, more often than the critics of medicine would allow, who have been truly virtuous both in intent and act. They have been, and remain, the leaven of the profession and the hope of all who are ill. They form the sea-wall that will not be eroded even by the powerful forces of commercialization, bureaucratization, and mechanization inevitable in modern medicine.

We cannot, need not, and indeed must not, wait for a medical analogue of MacIntyre's 'new St. Benedict' to show us the way. There is no new concept of virtue waiting to be discovered that is peculiarly suited to the dilemmas of our own dark age. We must recapture the courage to speak of character, virtue, and perfection in living a good life. We must encourage those who are willing to dedicate themselves to a "higher standard of self effacement" [2].

We need the courage, too, to accept the obvious split in the profession between those who see and feel the altruistic imperatives in medicine, and those who

do not. Those who at heart believe that the pursuit of private self-interest serves the public good are very different from those who believe in the restraint of self-interest. We forget that physicians since the beginnings of the profession have subscribed to different values and virtues. We need only recall that the Hippocratic Oath was the Oath of physicians of the Pythagorean school at a time when most Greek physicians followed essentially a craft ethic [3]. A perusal of the Hippocratic Corpus itself, which intersperses ethics and etiquette, will show how differently its treatises deal with fees, the care of incurable patients, and the business aspects of the craft.

The illusion that all physicians share a common devotion to a high-flown set of ethical principles has done damage to medicine by raising expectations some members of the profession could not, or will not, fulfill. Today, we must be more forthright about the differences in value commitment among physicians. Professional codes must be more explicit about the relationships between duties, rights, and virtues. Such explicitness encourages a more honest relationship between physicians and patients and removes the hypocrisy of verbal assent to a general code, to which an individual physician may not really subscribe. Explicitness enables patients to choose among physicians on the basis of their ethical commitments as well as their reputations for technical expertise.

Conceptual clarity will not assure virtuous behavior. Indeed, virtues are usually distorted if they are the subject of too conscious a design. But conceptual clarity will distinguish between motives and provide criteria for judging the moral commitment one can expect from the profession and from its individual members. It can also inspire those whose virtuous inclinations need reinforcement in the current climate of commercialization of the healing relationship.

To this end the current resurgence of interest in virtue-based ethics is altogether salubrious. Linked to a theory of patient good and a theory of rights and duties, it could provide the needed groundwork for a reconstruction of professional medical ethics as that work matures. Perhaps even more progress can be made if we take Shakespeare's advice in *Hamlet*: "Assume the virtue if you have it not. . . . For use almost can change the stamp of nature."

BIBLIOGRAPHY

[1] Cicero: 1967, *Moral Obligations,* J. Higginbotham (trans.), University of California Press, Berkeley and Los Angeles.

[2] Cushing, H.: 1929, *Consecratio Medici and Other Papers,* Little, Brown and Co., Boston.

[3] Edelstein, L.: 1967, "The Professional Ethics of the Greek Physician," in O. Temkin (ed.), *Ancient Medicine: Selected Papers of Ludwig Edelstein,* Johns Hopkins University Press, Baltimore.

[4] Jonsen, A.: 1983, "Watching the Doctor," *New England Journal of Medicine* 308: 25, 1531–1535.

[5] Pellegrino, E.: 1983, "Scribonius Largus and the Origins of Medical Humanism," address to the American Osler Society.

[6] Reader, J.: 1982, "Beneficence, Supererogation, and Role Duty," in E. Shelp (ed.), *Beneficence and Health Care,* D. Reidel, Dordrecht, Holland, pp. 83–108.

PHYSICIAN-PATIENT MODELS AND PATIENT AUTONOMY

METAPHORS AND MODELS OF DOCTOR-PATIENT RELATIONSHIPS: THEIR IMPLICATIONS FOR AUTONOMY

James F. Childress and Mark Siegler

Childress and Siegler examine five models, or metaphors, for the physician-patient relationship: (1) *paternalism* (the physician as caring parent, the patient as child); (2) *partnership* (both parties as collaborating in pursuit of the shared goal of the patient's health); (3) *contract* (physician and patient as related to each other by specific contracts, detailing their obligations and rights); (4) *friendship* (physician and patient as intimately related due to the highly personal nature of health); and (5) *technical assistance* (the physician as technician, the patient as customer). The authors then explore the relative advantages and disadvantages of regarding the physician-patient relationship as a relationship between *intimates* or as one between *strangers,* before examining the implications of each for patient autonomy. They conclude by developing the metaphor of *negotiations* as a way to understand many interactions between physicians and patients.

INTRODUCTION

Many metaphors and models have been applied to relationships between patients and physicians. One example is an interpretation of physician-patient relationships as paternalistic. In this case, the physician is regarded as a parent and the patient is regarded as a child. Opponents of such a paternalistic view of medicine rarely reject the use of metaphors to interpret medical relationships; rather, they simply offer alternative metaphors, for example, the physician as partner or the patient as rational contractor.

Theoretical Medicine, vol. 5 (1984), pp. 17–30. © 1984 by D. Reidel Publishing Company. Reprinted by permission of Kluwer Academic Publishers.

Metaphors may operate even when patients and physicians are unaware of them. Physician-patient conflicts may arise if each party brings to their encounter a different image of medicine, as, for example, when the physician regards a paternalistic model of medicine as appropriate, but the patient prefers a contractual model.

As these examples suggest, metaphors involve seeing something as something else, for example, seeing a lover as a red rose, human beings as wolves, or medical therapy as warfare. Metaphors highlight some features and hide other features of their principal subject.[1] Thus, thinking about a physician as a parent highlights the physician's care for dependent others and his or her control over them, but it conceals the patient's payment of fees to the physician. Metaphors and models may be used to describe relationships as they exist, or to indicate what those relationships ought to be. In either the descriptive or the prescriptive use of metaphors, this highlighting and hiding occurs, and it must be considered in determining the adequacy of various metaphors. When metaphors are used to describe roles, they can be criticized if they distort more features than they illuminate. And when they are used to direct roles, they can be criticized if they highlight one moral consideration, such as care, while neglecting others, such as autonomy.

Since there is no single physician-patient relationship, it is probable that no single metaphor can adequately describe or direct the whole range of relationships in health care, such as open heart surgery, clinical research, and psychoanalysis. Some of the most important metaphors that have shaped health care in recent years include: parent-child, partners, rational contractors, friends, and technician-client. We want to determine the adequacy of these metaphors to describe and to direct doctor-patient relationships in the real world. In particular, we will assess them in relation to patient and physician autonomy.

METAPHORS AND MODELS OF RELATIONSHIPS IN HEALTH CARE

(1) The first metaphor is *paternal* or *parental,* and the model is paternalism. For this model, the locus of decision-making is the health care professional, particularly the physician, who has 'moral authority' within an asymmetrical and hierarchical relationship. (A variation on these themes appear in a model that was especially significant earlier—the priest-penitent relationship.)

Following Thomas Szasz and Marc Hollender, we can distinguish two different versions of paternalism, based on two different prototypes.[2] If we take the *parent-infant relationship* as the prototype, the physician's role is active, while the patient's role is passive. The patient, like the infant, is primarily a dependent recipient of care. This model is applied easily to such clinical situations as anesthesia and to the care of patients with acute trauma, coma, or delirium. A second version takes the *parent-adoles-*

cent child relationship as the prototype. Within this version, the physician guides the patient by telling him or her what to expect and what to do, and the patient co-operates to the extent of obeying. This model applies to such clinical situations as the outpatient treatment of acute infectious diseases. The physician instructs the patient on a course of treatment (such as antibiotics and rest), but the patient can either obey or refuse to comply.

The paternalist model assigns moral authority and discretion to the physician because good health is assumed to be a value shared by the patient and the physician and because the physician's competence, skills, and ability place him or her in a position to help the patient regain good health. Even if it was once the dominant model in health care and even if many patients and physicians still prefer it, the paternalist model is no longer adequate to describe or to direct all relationships in health care. Too many changes have occurred. In a pluralistic society such as ours, the assumption that the physician and patient have common values about health may be mistaken. They may disagree about the *meaning* of health and disease (for example, when the physician insists that cigarette smoking is a disease, but the patient claims that it is merely a nasty habit) or about the *value* of health relative to other values (for example, when the physician wants to administer a blood transfusion to save the life of a Jehovah's Witness, but the patient rejects the blood in order to have a chance of heavenly salvation).

As a normative model, paternalism tends to concentrate on care rather than respect, patients' needs rather than their rights, and physicians' discretion rather than patients' autonomy or self-determination. Even though paternalistic actions can sometimes be justified, for example, when a patient is not competent to make a decision and is at risk of harm, not all paternalistic actions can be justified.[3]

(2) A second model is one of *partnership,* which can be seen in Eric Cassell's statement: "Autonomy for the sick patient cannot exist outside of a good and properly functioning doctor-patient relation. And the relation between them is inherently a *partnership.*"[4] The language of collegiality, collaboration, association, co-adventureship, and covenant is also used. This model stresses that health care

professionals and their patients are partners or colleagues in the pursuit of the shared value of health. It is similar to the paternalist model in that it emphasizes the shared general values of the enterprise in which the participants are involved. But what makes this model distinctive and significant is its emphasis on the equality of the participants' interpretations of shared values such as health, along with respect for the personal autonomy of all the participants.[5] The theme of equality does not, however, cancel a division of competence and responsibility along functional lines within the relationship.

Szasz and Hollender suggest that the prototype of the model of 'mutual participation' or partnership is the adult-adult relationship. Within this model the physician helps the patient to help himself, while the patient uses expert help to realize his (and the physician's) ends. Some clinical applications of this model appear in the care of chronic diseases and psychoanalysis. It presupposes that "the participants (1) have approximately equal power, (2) be mutually interdependent (i.e., need each other), and (3) engage in activity that will be in some ways satisfying to both." Furthermore, "the physician does not know what is best for the patient. The search for this becomes the essence of the therapeutic interaction. The patient's own experiences furnish indispensable information for eventual agreement, under otherwise favorable circumstances, as to what 'health' might be for him."[6]

Although this model describes a few practices, it is most often offered as a normative model, indicating the morally desirable and even obligatory direction of practice and research.[7] As a normative model, it stresses the equality of value contributions and the autonomy of both professionals and other participants, whether sick persons or volunteers for research.

(3) A third model is that of *rational contractors.* Health care professionals and their patients are related or should be related to each other by a series of specific contracts. The prototype of this model is the specific contract by which individuals agree to exchange goods and services, and the enforcement of such contracts by governmental sanctions. According to Robert Veatch, one of the strongest proponents of the contractual model in health care, this model is the best compromise between the *ideal of partnership,* with its emphasis on both equality and autonomy, and the *reality* of medical care, where mutual trust cannot be presupposed. If we could realize mutual trust, we could develop partnerships. In the light of a realistic assessment of our situation, however, we can only hope for contracts. The model of rational contracts, according to Veatch, is the only realistic way to share responsibility, to preserve both equality and autonomy under less than ideal circumstances, and to protect the integrity of various parties in health care (e.g., physicians are free not to enter contracts that would violate their consciences and to withdraw from them when they give proper notice).[8]

Such a model is valuable but problematic both descriptively and normatively. It neglects the fact that sick persons do not view health care needs as comparable to other wants and desires, that they do not have sufficient information to make rational contracts with the best providers of health services, and that current structure of medicine obstructs the free operation of the marketplace and of contracts.[9] This model may also neglect the virtues of benevolence, care, and compassion that are stressed in other models such as paternalism and friendship.

(4) A fourth attempt to understand and direct the relationships between health care professionals and patients stresses *friendship.* According to P. Lain Entralgo,

> Insofar as man is a part of nature, and health an aspect of this nature and therefore a natural and objective good, the *medical relation* develops into comradeship, or association for the purpose of securing this good by technical means. Insofar as man is an individual and his illness a state affecting his personality, the medical relation ought to be more than mere comradeship—in fact it should be a friendship. All dogma apart, a good doctor has always been a friend to his patient, to all his patients.[10]

For this version of 'medical philia,' the patient expresses trust and confidence in the physician while the doctor's "friendship for the patient should consist above all in a desire to give effective technical help—benevolence conceived and realised in technical terms."[11] Technical help and generalized benevolence are 'made friendly' by explicit reference to the patient's personality.

Charles Fried's version of 'medical philia' holds that physicians are *limited, special-purpose friends* in relation to their patients. In medicine as well as in other professional activities such as law, the client may have a relationship with the professional that is analogous to friendship. In friendship and in these relationships, one person assumes the interests of another. Claims in both sets of relationships are intense and demanding, but medical friendship is more limited in scope.[12]

Of course, this friendship analogy is somewhat strained, as Fried recognizes, because needs (real and felt) give rise to medical relationships, even if professionals are free not to meet them unless they are emergencies, because patients pay professionals for their 'personal care,' and because patients do not have reciprocal loyalties. Nevertheless, Fried's analysis of the medical relationship highlights the equality, the autonomy, and the rights of both parties—the 'friend' and the 'befriended.' Because friendship, as Kant suggested, is "the union of two persons through equal and mutual love and respect," the model of friendship has some ingredients of both paternalism (love or care) and anti-paternalism (equality and respect).[13] It applies especially well to the same medical relationships that fit partnership; indeed, medical friendship is very close to medical partnership, except that the former stresses the intensity of the relationship, while the latter stresses the emotional reserve as well as the limited scope of the relationship.

(5) A fifth and final model views the health care professional as a *technician.* Some commentators have referred to this model as plumber, others as engineer; for example, it has been suggested that with the rise of scientific medicine the physician was viewed as "the expert engineer of the body as a machine."[14] Within this model, the physician 'provides' or 'delivers' technical service to patients who are 'consumers.' Exchange relations provide images for this interpretation of medical relations.

This model does not appear to be possible or even desirable. It is difficult to imagine that the health care professional as technician can simply present the 'facts' unadorned by values, in part because the major terms such as health and disease are not value-free and objective. Whether the 'technician' is in an organization or in direct relation to clients, he or she serves some values. Thus, this model may collapse into the contractual model or a bureaucratic model (which will not be discussed in this essay). The professional may be thought to have only technical authority, not moral authority. But he or she remains a moral agent and thus should choose to participate or not in terms of his or her own commitments, loyalties, and integrity. One shortcoming of the paternalist and priestly models, as Robert Veatch notes, is the patient's "moral abdication," while one shortcoming of the technician model is the physician's "moral abdication."[15] The technician model offers autonomy to the patient, whose values dominate (at least in some settings) at the expense of the professional's moral agency and integrity. In other models such as contract, partnership, and friendship, moral responsibility is shared by all the parties in part because they are recognized, in some sense, as equals.

RELATIONS BETWEEN INTIMATES AND BETWEEN STRANGERS

The above models of relationships between physicians and patients move between two poles: intimates and strangers.[16] In relations of intimacy, all the parties know each other very well and often share values, or at least know which values they do not share. In such relations, formal rules and procedures, backed by sanctions, may not be necessary; they may even be detrimental to the relationships. In relations of intimacy, trust rather than control is dominant. Examples include relationships between parents and children and between friends. Partnerships also share some features of such relationships, but their intimacy and shared values may be limited to a specific set of activities.

By contrast, in relations among strangers, rules and procedures become very important, and control rather than trust is dominant.[17] Of course, in most relations there are mixtures of trust and control. Each is present to some degree. Nevertheless, it is proper to speak about relations between strangers as structured by rules and procedures because the parties do not know each other well enough to have mutual trust. Trust means confidence in and reliance upon the other to act in accord with moral principles and rules or at least in accord with his or her publicly manifested principles and rules, whatever they might be. But if the other is a stranger, we do not know whether he or she accepts what we would count as moral principles and rules. We do not know whether he or she is worthy of trust. In the absence of intimate knowledge, or of shared values, strangers resort to rules and procedures in order to establish some control. Contracts between strangers, for example, to supply certain goods, represent instances of attempted control. But contractual relations do not only depend on legal sanctions; they also presuppose confidence in a shared structure of rules and procedures. As Talcott Parsons has noted, "transactions are actually entered into in accordance with a body of binding rules which are not part of the ad hoc agreement of the parties."[18]

Whether medicine is now only a series of encounters between strangers rather than intimates, medicine is increasingly regarded by patients and doctors, and by analysts of the profession—such as philosophers, lawyers, and sociologists—as a practice that is best understood and regulated *as if it were* a practice among strangers rather than among intimates. Numerous causes can be identified: first, the pluralistic nature of our society; second, the decline of close, intimate contact over time among professionals and patients and their families; third, the decline of contact with the 'whole person,' who is now parcelled out to various specialists; fourth, the growth of large, impersonal, bureaucratically structured institutions of care, in which there is discontinuity of care (the patient may not see the same professionals on subsequent visits).[19]

In this situation, Alasdair MacIntyre contends, the modern patient "usually approaches the physician as stranger to stranger: and the very proper fear and suspicion that we have of strangers extends equally properly to our encounters with physicians. We do not and cannot know what to expect of them . . . ."[20] He suggests that one possible response to this situation is to develop a rule-based bureaucracy in which "we can confront *any* individual who fills a given role with exactly the same expectation of exactly the same outcomes . . .". Our encounters with

physicians and other health care professionals are encounters between strangers precisely because of our pluralistic society: several value systems are in operation, and we do not know whether the physicians we encounter share our value systems. In such a situation, patient autonomy is "a solution of last resort" rather than "a central moral good." Finally patients have to decide for themselves what will be done to them or simply delegate such decisions to others, such as physicians.

Just as MacIntyre recognizes the value of patient autonomy in our pluralistic society, so John Ladd recognizes the value of the concept of rights among strangers.[21] He notes that a legalistic, rights-based approach to medicine has several important advantages because rules and rights "serve to define our relationships with strangers as well as with people whom we know . . . In the medical context . . . we may find ourselves in a hospital bed in a strange place, with strange company, and confronted by a strange physician and staff. The strangeness of the situation makes the concept of rights, both legal and moral, a very useful tool for defining our relationship to those with whom we have to deal."

Rules and rights that can be enforced obviously serve as ways to control the conduct of others when we do not know them well enough to be able to trust them. But all of the models of health care relationships identified above depend on some degree of trust. It is too simplistic to suppose that contracts, which can be legally enforced, do away with trust totally. Indeed, as we have argued, a society based on contracts depends to a very great extent on trust, precisely because not everything is enforceable at manageable cost. Thus, the issue is not simply whether trust or control is dominant, but, in part, the basis and extent of trust. Trust, at least limited trust, may be possible even among strangers. There may be a presumption of trust, unless the society is in turmoil. And there may be an intermediate notion of 'friendly strangers.' People may be strangers because of differences regarding values or uncertainty regarding the other's values; they may be friendly because they accept certain rules and procedures, which may ensure that different values are respected. If consensus exists in a pluralistic society, it is primarily about rules and procedures, some of which protect the autonomy of agents, their freedom to negotiate their own relationships.

PHYSICIAN-PATIENT INTERACTIONS AS NEGOTIATIONS

It is illuminating, both descriptively and prescriptively, to view some encounters and interactions between physicians and patients as negotiations. The metaphor of negotiation has its home in discussions to settle matters by mutual agreement of the concerned parties. While it frequently appears in disputes between management and labor and between nations, it does not necessarily presuppose a conflict of interests between the parties. The metaphor of negotiation may also illuminate processes of reaching agreement regarding the terms of continuing interaction even when the issue is mainly the determination of one party's interests and the means to realize those interests. This metaphor captures two important characteristics of medical relationships: (1) it accents the autonomy of both patient and physician, and (2) it suggests a process that occurs over time rather than an event which occurs at a particular moment.

The model of negotiation can both explain what frequently occurs and identify what ought to occur in physician-patient interactions. An example can make this point: A twenty-eight-year-old ballet dancer suffered from moderately severe asthma. When she moved from New York to Chicago, she changed physicians and placed herself in the hands of a famed asthma specialist. He initiated aggressive steroid therapy to control her asthma, and within several months he had managed to control her wheezing. But she was distressed because her dancing had deteriorated. She suspected that she was experiencing muscle weakness and fluid accumulation because of the steroid treatment. When she attempted to discuss her concerns with the physician, he maintained that "bringing the disease under complete control—achieving a complete remission of wheezes—will be the best thing for you in the long run." After several months of unhappiness and failure to convince the physician of the importance of her personal goals as well as her medical goals, she sought another physician, insisting that she didn't live just to breathe, but breathed so that she could dance.[22]

As in this case—and despite the claims of several commentators—people with medical needs generally do not confront physicians as strangers and as adversaries in contemporary health care. As we suggested earlier, even if they can be viewed as strangers in that they often do not know each other prior to the encounter, both parties may well proceed with a presumption of trust. Patients may approach physicians with some trust and confidence in the medical profession, even though they do not know the physicians before them. Indeed, codes of medical ethics have been designed in part to foster this trust by indicating where the medical profession stands and by creating a climate of trust. Thus, even if patients approach individual physicians as strangers, they may have some confidence in these physicians as members of the profession as they negotiate the particular terms of their relationship. At the other extreme, some patients may approach physicians as adversaries or opponents. But for negotiation to proceed, some trust must be present, even if it is combined with some degree of control, for example, through legal requirements and the threat of legal sanctions.

The general public trust in the medical profession's values and skills provides the presumptive basis for trust in particular physicians and can facilitate the process of negotiation. But, as we noted earlier, in a pluralistic society, even people who are strangers, i.e., who share very few substantive values, may be 'friendly' if they share procedural values. Certain procedural values may provide the most important basis for the trust that is necessary for negotiation; indeed, procedural principles and rules should structure the negotiation in order to ensure equal respect for the autonomy of all the parties.

First, the negotiation should involve adequate disclosure by both parties. In this process of communication—much broader and richer than most doctrines of informed consent recognize—both parties should indicate their values as well as other matters of relevance. Without this information, the negotiation cannot be open and fair. Second, the negotiation should be voluntary, i.e., uncoerced. Insofar as critical illness can be viewed as 'coercing' individuals through the creation of fear, etc., it may be difficult to realize this condition for patients with certain problems. However, for the majority of patients this condition is achievable. Third, the accommodation reached through the negotiation should be mutually acceptable.[23]

What can we say about the case of the ballet dancer in the light of these procedural requirements for negotiation? It appears that the relationship foundered not because of inadequate disclosure at the outset, or along the way, but because of the patient's change in or clarification of her values and the physician's inability to accommodate these other values. The accommodation reached at the outset was mutually acceptable for a time. Initially their values and their metaphors for their relationship were the same. The physician regarded himself as a masterful scientist who was capable technically of controlling a patient's symptoms of wheezing. In fact, he remarked on several occasions: "I have never met a case of asthma I couldn't help." The patient, for her part, selected the physician initially for the same reasons. She was unhappy that her wheezing persisted, and she was becoming discouraged by her chronic health problem. Because she wanted a therapeutic success, she selected an expert who would help her achieve that goal. Both the patient and the physician made several voluntary choices. The patient chose to see *this* physician and to see him for several months, and the physician chose to treat asthma aggressively with steroids.

In a short time, the patient reconsidered or clarified her values, discovering that her dancing was even more important to her than the complete remission of wheezing, and she wanted to renegotiate her relationship so that it could be more mutual and participatory. But her new metaphor for the relationship was incompatible with the physician's nonnegotiable commitment to his metaphor—which the patient had also accepted at the outset. Thus, the relationship collapsed. This case illustrates both the possibilities and the limitations of the model of negotiation. Even when the procedural requirements are met, the negotiation may not result in a satisfactory accommodation over time, and the negotiation itself may proceed in terms of the physician's and the patient's metaphors and models of the relationships, as well as the values they affirm.

Autonomy constrains and limits the negotiations and the activities of both parties: Neither party may violate the autonomy of the other or use the other merely as a means to an end. But respecting autonomy as a constraint and a limit does not imply seeking it as a *goal* or praising it as an *ideal*.[24] This point has several implications. It means, for exam-

ple, that patients may exercise their autonomy to turn their medical affairs completely over to physicians. A patient may instruct the physician to do whatever he or she deems appropriate: "You're the doctor; whatever you decide is fine." This relationship has been characterized as "paternalism with permission,"[25] and it is not ruled out by autonomy as a constraint or a limit. It might, however, be ruled out by a commitment to autonomy as an ideal. Indeed, commitment to autonomy as an ideal can even be paternalistic in a negative sense; it can lead the health care professional to try to force the patient to be free and to live up to the ideal of autonomy. But our conception of autonomy as a constraint and a limit prevents such actions toward competent patients who are choosing and acting voluntarily. Likewise, maintenance, restoration, or promotion of the patient's autonomy may be, and usually is, one important goal of medical relationships. But its importance can only be determined by negotiation between the physician and the patient. The patient may even subordinate the goal of autonomy to various other goals, just as the ballet dancer subordinated freedom from wheezing to the power to dance.

This view of autonomy as a limit or a constraint, rather than an ideal or a goal, permits individuals to define the terms of their relationship. Just as it permits the patient to acquiesce in the physician's recommendations, it permits the physician to enter a contract as a mere technician to provide certain medical services, as requested by the patient. In such an arrangement, the physician does *not* become a mere means or a mere instrument to the patient's ends. Rather, the physician exercises his or her autonomy to enter into the relationship to provide technical services. Such actions are an expression of autonomy, not a denial of autonomy. If, however, the physician believes that an action requested by the patient—for example, a specific mode of therapy for cancer or a sterilization procedure—is not medically indicated, or professionally acceptable, or in the patient's best interests, he or she is not obligated to sacrifice autonomy and comply. In such a case, the professional refuses to be an instrument of or to carry out the patient's wishes. When the physician cannot morally or professionally perform an action (not legally prohibited by the society) he or she may have a duty to inform the patient of other physicians who might be willing to carry out the patient's wishes. A refusal to be an instrument of another's wishes is very different from trying to prevent another from realizing his or her goals.

Negotiation is not always possible or desirable. It is impossible, or possible only to a limited extent, in certain clinical settings in which the conditions for a fair, informed, and voluntary negotiation are severely limited, often because one party lacks some of the conditions for autonomous choices. First, negotiation may be difficult if not impossible with some types of patients, such as the mentally incompetent. Sometimes paternalism may be morally legitimate or even morally obligatory when the patient is not competent to negotiate and is at risk. In such cases, parents, family members, or others may undertake negotiation with the physician, for example, regarding defective newborns or comatose adults. But health care professionals and the state may have to intervene in order to protect the interests of the patient who cannot negotiate directly. Second, the model of negotiation does not fit situations in which patients are forced by law to accept medical interventions such as compulsory vaccination, involuntary commitment, and involuntary psychiatric treatment. In such situations, the state authorizes or requires treatment against the wishes of the patient; the patient and the physician do not negotiate their relationship. Third, in some situations physicians have dual or multiple allegiances, some of which may take priority over loyalty to the patient. Examples include military medicine, industrial medicine, prison medicine, and university health service. The physician is not free in such settings to negotiate in good faith with the patient, and the patient's interests and rights may have to be protected by other substantive and procedural standards and by external control. Fourth, negotiation may not be possible in some emergencies in which people desperately need medical treatment because of the risk of death or serious bodily harm. In such cases, the physician may *presume* consent, apart from a process of negotiation, if the patient is unable to consent because of his/her condition or if the process of disclosing information and securing consent would consume too much time and thus endanger the patient. Finally, procedural standards are important for certain types of patients, such as the poor, the uneducated, or those with 'unattractive medical problems' (e.g., drug addiction, obesity, and hypochondriasis). In such cases, there is a tendency—surely not a universal one—to limit the degree of negotiation with the patient because of social stigmatization. A patient advocate may even be appropriate.

In addition to the procedural requirements identified earlier, there are societal constraints and limits on negotiation. Some actions may not be negotiable. For example, the society may prohibit 'mercy killing,' even when the patient requests it and the physician is willing to carry it out.[26] Such societal rules clearly limit the autonomy of both physicians and patients, but some of these rules may be necessary in order to protect important societal values. However, despite such notable exceptions as 'mercy killing,' current societal rules provide physicians and patients with considerable latitude to negotiate their own relationship and actions within that relationship.

If negotiation is a process, its accommodations at various points can often be characterized in terms of the above models—parent-child, friends, partners, contractors, and technician-consumer. Whatever accommodation is reached through the process of negotiation is not final or irrevocable. Like other human interactions, medical relationships change over time. They are always developing or dissolving. For example, when a patient experiencing anginal chest pain negotiates a relationship with a cardiologist, he may not have given or even implied consent to undergo coronary angiography or cardiac surgery if the cardiologist subsequently believes that it is necessary. Medical conditions change, and people change, often clarifying or modifying their values over time. In medical relationships either the physician or the patient may reopen the negotiation as the relationship evolves over time and may even terminate the relationship. For example, the ballet dancer in the case discussed above elected to terminate the relationship with the specialist. That particular relationship had not been fully negotiated in the first place. But even if it had been fully negotiated, she could have changed her mind and terminated it. Such an option is essential if the autonomy of the patient is to be protected over time. Likewise, the physician should have the option to renegotiate or to withdraw from the relationship (except in emergencies), as long as he or she gives adequate notice so that the patient can find another physician.

NOTES

1 On metaphors, see George Lakoff and Mark Johnson, *Metaphors We Live By* (Chicago: University of Chicago Press, 1980).

2 See Thomas S. Szasz and Marc H. Hollender, 'A contribution to the philosophy of medicine: The basic models of the doctor-patient relationship,' *Archives of Internal Medicine* 97, (1956) 585–92; see also, Thomas S. Szasz, William F. Knoff, and Marc H. Hollender, 'The doctor-patient relationship and its historical context,' *American Journal of Psychiatry* 115, (1958) 522–28.

3 For a fuller analysis of paternalism and its justification, see James F. Childress, *Who Should Decide?: Paternalism in Health Care* (New York: Oxford University Press, 1982).

4 Eric Cassell, 'Autonomy and ethics in action,' *New England Journal of Medicine* 297, (1977) 333–34. Italics added. Partnership is only one of several images and metaphors Cassell uses, and it may not be the best one to express his position, in part because he tends to view autonomy as a goal rather than as a constraint.

5 According to Robert Veatch, the main focus of this model is "an equality of dignity and respect, an equality of value contributions". Veatch, 'Models for ethical medicine in a revolutionary age,' *Hastings Center Report* 2, (June 1972) 7. Contrast Eric Cassell who disputes the relevance of notions of "equality" and "inequality." *The Healer's Art: A New Approach to the Doctor-Patient Relationship* (Philadelphia: J. B. Lippincott Company, 1976), pp. 193–94.

6 Thomas S. Szasz and Marc H. Hollender, 'A contribution to the philosophy of medicine: The basic models of the doctor-patient relationship,' pp. 586–87. (See Note 2.)

7 See, for example, Paul Ramsey, 'The ethics of a cottage industry in an age of community and research medicine,' *New England Journal of Medicine* 284, (1971) 700–706; *The Patient as Person: Explorations in Medical Ethics* (New Haven: Yale University Press, 1970), esp. Chap. 1; and Hans Jonas, 'Philosophical reflections on experimenting with human subjects,' Ethical Aspects of Experimentation with Human Subjects, *Daedalus* 98, (1969) 219–47.

8 Robert Veatch, 'Models for ethical medicine in a revolutionary age,' p. 7. (See Note 5.)

9 See Roger Masters, 'Is contract an adequate basis for medical ethics?,' *Hastings Center Report* 5, (December 1975) 24–28. See also May, 'Code and covenant or philanthropy and contract?' in *Ethics in Medicine: Historical Perspectives and Contemporary Concerns*, ed. by Stanley Joel Reiser, Arthur J. Dyck, and William J. Curran (Cambridge, Mass.: The MIT Press, 1977), pp. 65–76.

10 P. Lain Entralgo, *Doctor and Patient*, trans. from the Spanish by Frances Partridge (New York: McGraw-Hill Book Co., World University Library, 1969), p. 242.

11 *Ibid.*, p. 197.

12 See Charles Fried, *Medical Experimentation: Personal Integrity and Social Policy* (New York: American Elsevier Publishing Co., Inc., 1974), p. 76. Our discussion of Fried's position is drawn from that work, *Right and Wrong* (Cambridge, Mass.: Harvard University Press, 1978), Chap. 7, and 'The lawyer as friend: The moral foundations of the lawyer-client relation,' *The Yale Law Journal* 85, (1976) 1060–89.

13 Immanuel Kant, *The Doctrine of Virtue*, Part II of *The Metaphysic of Morals*, trans. by Mary J. Gregor (New York: Harper and Row, Harper Torchbook, 1964), p. 140.

14 Thomas S. Szasz, William F. Knoff, and Marc H. Hollender, 'The doctor-patient relationship and its historical context,' p. 525. See also Robert Veatch, 'Models for ethical medicine in a revolutionary age,' p. 5, and Leon Kass, 'Ethical dilemmas in the care of the ill: I. What is the physician's service?' *Journal of the American Medical Association* 244, (1980) 1815 for criticisms of the technical model (from very different normative positions).

15 Veatch, 'Models for ethical medicine in a revolutionary age,' p. 7.

16 See Stephen Toulmin, 'The tyranny of principles,' *Hastings Center Report* 11, (December 1981) 31–39.

17 On trust and control, see James F. Childress, 'Non-violent resistance: Trust and risk-taking,' *Journal of Religious Ethics* 1, (1973) 87–112.

18 Talcott Parsons, *The Structure of Social Action* (New York: The Free Press, 1949), p. 311.

19 On the factors in the decline of trust, see Michael Jellinek, 'Erosion of patient trust in large medical centers,' *Hastings Center Report* 6, (June 1976) 16–19.

20 Alasdair MacIntyre, 'Patients as agents,' in *Philosophical Medical Ethics: Its Nature and Significance*, ed. by Stuart F. Spicker and H. Tristram Engelhardt, Jr. (Boston: D. Reidel Publishing Co., 1977).

21 John Ladd, 'Legalism and medical ethics,' *The Journal of Medicine and Philosophy* 4, (March 1979) 73.

22 This case has been presented in Mark Siegler, 'Searching for moral certainty in medicine: A proposal for a new model of the doctor-patient encounter,' *Bulletin of the New York Academy of Medicine* 57, (1981) 56–69.

23 See *ibid.* for a discussion of negotiation. Other proponents of a model of negotiation include Robert A. Burt, *Taking Care of Strangers: The Rule of Law in Doctor-Patient Relations* (New York: Free Press, 1979) and Robert J. Levine, *Ethics and Regulation of Clinical Research* (Baltimore: Urban and Schwarzenberg, 1981).

24 See the discussion in Childress, *Who Should Decide?*, Chap. 3.

25 Alan W. Cross and Larry R. Churchill, 'Ethical and cultural dimensions of informed consent,' *Annals of Internal Medicine* 96, (1982) 110–13.

26 See Oscar Thorup, Mark Siegler, James Childress, and Ruth Roettinger, 'Voluntary exit: Is there a case of rational suicide?' *The Pharos* 45, (Fall 1982) 25–31.

WHY DOCTORS SHOULD INTERVENE

Terrence F. Ackerman

Ackerman criticizes the notion of respect for autonomy that identifies it with noninterference. He argues that noninterference fails to respect patient autonomy because it does not take account of the transforming effects of illness. Ackerman's major contention is that the autonomy of those who are ill is limited by all kinds of constraints—physical, cognitive, emotional, and social. Ackerman argues in favor of sometimes overriding patients' treatment-related preferences, maintaining that real respect for the autonomy of patients requires physicians actively to attempt to neutralize the impediments that interfere with patients' choices, helping them restore control over their lives.

Patient autonomy has become a watchword of the medical profession. According to the revised 1980 AMA Principles of Medical Ethics,[1] no longer is it permissible for a doctor to withhold information from a patient, even on grounds that it may be harmful. Instead the physician is expected to "deal honestly with patients" at all times. Physicians also have a duty to respect the confidentiality of the doctor-patient relationship. Even when disclosure to a third party may be in the patient's interests, the doctor is instructed to release information only when required by law. Respect for the autonomy of patients has given rise to many specific patient rights—among them the right to refuse treatment, the right to give informed consent, the right to privacy, and the right to competent medical care provided with "respect for human dignity."

While requirements of honesty, confidentiality, and patients' rights are all important, the underlying moral vision that places exclusive emphasis upon these factors is more troublesome. The profession's notion of respect for autonomy makes noninterference its essential feature. As the Belmont Report has described it, there is an obligation to "give weight to autonomous persons' considered opinions and choices while refraining from obstructing their actions unless they are clearly detrimental to others."[2] Or, as Tom Beauchamp and James Childress have suggested, "To respect autonomous agents is to rec-

ognize with due appreciation their own considered value judgments and outlooks even when it is believed that their judgments are mistaken." They argue that people "are entitled to autonomous determination without limitation on their liberty being imposed by others."[3]

When respect for personal autonomy is understood as noninterference, the physician's role is dramatically simplified. The doctor need be only an honest and good technician, providing relevant information and dispensing professionally competent care. Does noninterference really respect patient autonomy? I maintain that it does not, because it fails to take account of the transforming effects of illness.

"Autonomy," typically defined as self-governance, has two key features. First, autonomous behavior is governed by plans of action that have been formulated through deliberation or reflection. This deliberative activity involves processes of both information gathering and priority setting. Second, autonomous behavior issues, intentionally and voluntarily, from choices people make based upon their own life plans.

But various kinds of constraints can impede autonomous behavior. There are physical constraints—confinement in prison is an example—where internal or external circumstances bodily prevent a person from deliberating adequately or acting on life plans. Cognitive constraints derive from either a lack of information or an inability to understand that information. A consumer's ignorance regarding the merits or defects of a particular product fits the description.

Reprinted with permission of the author and the publisher from *Hastings Center Report*, vol. 12 (August 1982), pp. 14–17.

Psychological constraints, such as anxiety or depression, also inhibit adequate deliberation. Finally, there are social constraints—such as institutionalized roles and expectations ("a woman's place is in the home," "the doctor knows best") that block considered choices.

Edmund Pellegrino suggests several ways in which autonomy is specifically compromised by illness:

> In illness, the body is interposed between us and reality—it impedes our choices and actions and is no longer fully responsive. . . . Illness forces a reappraisal and that poses a threat to the old image; it opens up all the old anxieties and imposes new ones—often including the real threat of death or drastic alterations in life-style. This ontological assault is aggravated by the loss of . . . freedoms we identify as peculiarly human. The patient. . .lacks the knowledge and skills necessary to cure himself or gain relief of pain and suffering. . . . The state of being ill is therefore a state of "wounded humanity," of a person compromised in his fundamental capacity to deal with his vulnerability.[4]

The most obvious impediment is that illness "interposes" the body or mind between the patient and reality, obstructing attempts to act upon cherished plans. An illness may not only temporarily obstruct long-range goals; it may necessitate permanent and drastic revision in the patient's major activities, such as working habits. Patients may also need to set limited goals regarding control of pain, alteration in diet and physical activity, and rehabilitation of functional impairments. They may face considerable difficulties in identifying realistic and productive aims.

The crisis is aggravated by a cognitive constraint—the lack of "knowledge and skills" to overcome their physical or mental impediment. Without adequate medical understanding, the patient cannot assess his or her condition accurately. Thus the choice of goals is seriously hampered and subsequent decisions by the patient are not well founded.

Pellegrino mentions the anxieties created by illness, but psychological constraints may also include denial, depression, guilt, and fear. I recently visited an eighteen-year-old boy who was dying of a cancer that had metastasized extensively throughout his ab-

domen. The doctor wanted to administer further chemotherapy that might extend the patient's life a few months. But the patient's nutritional status was poor, and he would need intravenous feedings prior to chemotherapy. Since the nutritional therapy might also encourage tumor growth, leading to a blockage of the gastrointestinal tract, the physician carefully explained the options and the risks and benefits several times, each time at greater length. But after each explanation, the young man would say only that he wished to do whatever was necessary to get better. Denial prevented him from exploring the alternatives.

Similarly, depression can lead patients to make choices that are not in harmony with their life plans. Recently, a middle-aged woman with a history of ovarian cancer in remission returned to the hospital for the biopsy of a possible pulmonary metastasis. Complications ensued and she required the use of an artificial respirator for several days. She became severely depressed and soon refused further treatment. The behavior was entirely out of character with her previous full commitment to treatment. Fully supporting her overt wishes might have robbed her of many months of relatively comfortable life in the midst of a very supportive family around which her activities centered. The medical staff stalled for time. Fortunately, her condition improved.

Fear may also cripple the ability of patients to choose. Another patient, diagnosed as having a cerebral tumor that was probably malignant, refused lifesaving surgery because he feared the cosmetic effects of neurosurgery and the possibility of neurological damage. After he became comatose and new evidence suggested that the tumor might be benign, his family agreed to surgery and a benign tumor was removed. But he later died of complications related to the unfortunate delay in surgery. Although while competent he had agreed to chemotherapy, his fears (not uncommon among candidates for neurosurgery) prevented him from accepting the medical intervention that might have secured him the health he desired.

Social constraints may also prevent patients from acting upon their considered choices. A recent case involved a twelve-year-old boy whose rhabdomyosarcoma had metastasized extensively. Since all therapeutic interventions had failed, the only remaining option was to involve him in a phase 1 clinical trial. (A phase 1 clinical trial is the initial test-ing of a drug in human subjects. Its primary purpose is to identify toxicities rather than to evaluate ther-apeutic effectiveness.) The patient's course had been very stormy, and he privately expressed to the staff his desire to quit further therapy and return home. However, his parents denied the hopeless-ness of his condition, remaining steadfast in their belief that God would save their child. With deep re-gard for his parents' wishes, he refused to openly object to their desires and the therapy was adminis-tered. No antitumor effect occurred and the patient soon died.

Various social and cultural expectations also take their toll. According to Talcott Parsons, one fea-ture of the sick role is that the ill person is obligated ". . . to seek *technically competent* help, namely, in the most usual case, that of a physician and to *coop-erate* with him in the process of trying to get well."[5] Parsons does not describe in detail the elements of this cooperation. But clinical observation suggests that many patients relinquish their opportunity to de-liberate and make choices regarding treatment in deference to the physician's superior educational achievement and social status ("Whatever you think, doctor!"). The physical and emotional demands of illness reinforce this behavior.

Moreover, this perception of the sick role has been socially taught from childhood—and it is not easily altered even by the physician who ardently tries to engage the patient in decision making. In-deed, when patients are initially asked to participate in the decision-making process, some exhibit con-siderable confusion and anxiety. Thus, for many per-sons, the institutional role of patient requires the physician to assume the responsibilities of making decisions.

Ethicists typically condemn paternalistic prac-tices in the therapeutic relationship, but fail to in-vestigate the features that incline physicians to be paternalistic. Such behavior may be one way to as-sist persons whose autonomous behavior has been impaired by illness. Of course, it is an open moral question whether the constraints imposed by illness ought to be addressed in such a way. But only by coming to grips with the psychological and social di-mensions of illness can we discuss how physicians can best respect persons who are patients.

RETURNING CONTROL TO PATIENTS

In the usual interpretation of respect for personal autonomy, noninterference is fundamental. In the medical setting, this means providing adequate in-formation and competent care that accords with the patient's wishes. But if serious constraints upon au-tonomous behavior are intrinsic to the state of being ill, then noninterference is not the best course, since the patient's choices will be seriously limited. Under these conditions, real respect for autonomy entails a more inclusive understanding of the relationship be-tween patients and physicians. Rather than restrain-ing themselves so that patients can exercise whatever autonomy they retain in illness, physicians should actively seek to neutralize the impediments that in-terfere with patients' choices.

In *The Healer's Art*, Eric Cassell underscored the essential feature of illness that demands a revi-sion in our understanding of respect for autonomy:

> If I had to pick the aspect of illness that is most de-structive to the sick, I would choose the loss of con-trol. Maintaining control over oneself is so vital to all of us that one might see all the other phenomena of illness as doing harm not only in their own right but doubly so as they reinforce the sick person's percep-tion that he is no longer in control.[6]

Cassell maintains, "The doctor's job is to return control to his patient." But what is involved in "re-turning control" to patients? Pellegrino identifies two elements that are preeminent duties of the physician: to provide technically competent care and to fully in-form the patient. The noninterference approach em-phasizes these factors, and their importance is clear. Loss of control in illness is precipitated by a physical or mental defect. If technically competent therapy can fully restore previous health, then the patient will again be in control. Consider a patient who is treated with antibiotics for a routine throat infection of strep-tococcal origin. Similarly, loss of control is fueled by lack of knowledge—not knowing what is the matter, what it portends for life and limb, and how it might be dealt with. Providing information that will enable the patient to make decisions and adjust goals enhances personal control.

If physical and cognitive constraints were the only impediments to autonomous behavior, then

Pellegrino's suggestions might be adequate. But providing information and technically competent care will not do much to alter psychological or social impediments. Pellegrino does not adequately portray the physician's role in ameliorating these.

How can the doctor offset the acute denial that prevented the adolescent patient from assessing the benefits and risk of intravenous feedings prior to his additional chemotherapy? How can he deal with the candidate for neurosurgery who clearly desired that attempts be made to restore his health, but feared cosmetic and functional impairments? Here strategies must go beyond the mere provision of information. Crucial information may have to be repeatedly shared with patients. Features of the situation that the patient has brushed over (as in denial) or falsely emphasized (as with acute anxiety) must be discussed in more detail or set in their proper perspective. And the physician may have to alter the tone of discussions with the patient, emphasizing a positive attitude with the overly depressed or anxious patient, or a more realistic, cautious attitude with the denying patient, in order to neutralize psychological constraints.

The physician may also need to influence the beliefs or attitudes of other people, such as family members, that limit their awareness of the patient's perspective. Such a strategy might have helped the parents of the dying child to conform with the patient's wishes. On the other hand, physicians may need to modify the patient's own understanding of the sick role. For example, they may need to convey that the choice of treatment depends not merely upon the physician's technical assessment, but on the quality of life and personal goals that the patient desires.

Once we admit that psychological and social constraints impair patient autonomy, it follows that physicians must carefully assess the psychological and social profiles and needs of patients. Thus, Pedro Lain-Entralgo insists that adequate therapeutic interaction consists in a combination of "objectivity" and "cooperation." Cooperation "is shown by psychologically reproducing in the mind of the doctor, insofar as that is possible, the meaning the patient's illness has for him."[7] Without such knowledge, the physician cannot assist patients in restoring control over their lives. Ironically, some critics have insisted that physicians are not justified in acting for the well-being of patients because they possess no "expertise" in securing the requisite knowledge about the patient.[8] But knowledge of the patient's psychological and social situation is also necessary to help the patient to act as a fully autonomous person.

BEYOND LEGALISM

Current notions of respect for autonomy are undergirded by a legal model of doctor-patient interaction. The relationship is viewed as a typical commodity exchange—the provision of technically competent medical care in return for financial compensation. Moreover, physicians and patients are presumed to have an equal ability to work out the details of therapy, *provided that* certain moral rights of patients are recognized. But the compromising effects of illness, the superior knowledge of physicians, and various institutional arrangements are also viewed as giving the physician an unfair power advantage. Since the values and interests of patients may conflict with those of the physician, the emphasis is placed upon noninterference.[9]

This legal framework is insufficient for medical ethics because it fails to recognize the impact of illness upon autonomous behavior. Even if the rights to receive adequate information and to provide consent are secured, affective and social constraints impair the ability of patients to engage in contractual therapeutic relationships. When people are sick, the focus upon equality is temporally misplaced. The goal of the therapeutic relationship is the "development" of the patient—helping to resolve the underlying physical (or mental) defect, and to deal with cognitive, psychological, and social constraints in order to restore autonomous functioning. In this sense, the doctor-patient interaction is not unlike the parent-child or teacher-student relationship.

The legal model also falls short because the therapeutic relationship is not a typical commodity exchange in which the parties use each other to accomplish mutually compatible goals, without taking a direct interest in each other. Rather, the status of patients as persons whose autonomy is compromised constitutes the very stuff of therapeutic art. The physician is attempting to alter the fundamental ability of patients to carry through their life plans. To accomplish this delicate task requires a personal knowledge about and interest in the patient. If we accept these points, then we must reject the narrow focus of medical ethics upon noninterference and emphasize patterns of interaction that free patients from constraints upon autonomy.

I hasten to add that I am criticizing the legal model only as a *complete* moral framework for therapeutic interaction. As case studies in medical ethics suggest, physicians and patients *are* potential adversaries. Moreover, the disability of the patient and various institutional controls provide physicians with a distinct "power advantage" that can be abused. Thus, a legitimate function of medical ethics is to formulate conditions that assure noninterference in patient decision making. But various positive interventions must also be emphasized, since the central task in the therapeutic process is assisting patients to reestablish control over their own lives.

In the last analysis, the crucial matter is how we view the patient who enters into the therapeutic relationship. Cassell points out that in the typical view ". . . the sick person is seen simply as a well person with a disease, rather than as qualitatively different, not only physically but also socially, emotionally, and even cognitively." In this view, ". . . the physician's role in the care of the sick is primarily the application of technology . . . and health can be seen as a commodity."[10] But if, as I believe, illness renders sick persons "qualitatively different," then respect for personal autonomy requires a therapeutic interaction considerably more complex than the noninterference strategy.

Thus the current "Principles of Medical Ethics" simply exhort physicians to be honest. But the crucial requirement is that physicians tell the truth in a way, at a time, and in whatever increments are necessary to allow patients to effectively use the information in adjusting their life plans.[11] Similarly, respecting a patient's refusal of treatment maximizes autonomy only if a balanced and thorough deliberation precedes the decision. Again, the "Principles" suggest that physicians observe strict confidentiality. But the more complex moral challenge is to use confidential information in a way that will help to give the patient more freedom. Thus, the doctor can keep a patient's report on family dynamics private, and still use it to modify attitudes or actions of family members that inhibit the patient's control.

At its root, illness is an evil primarily because it compromises our efforts to control our lives. Thus, we must preserve an understanding of the physician's art that transcends noninterference and addresses this fundamental reality.

REFERENCES

1 American Medical Association, *Current Opinions of the Judicial Council of the American Medical Association* (Chicago, Illinois: American Medical Association, 1981), p. ix. Also see Robert Veatch, "Professional Ethics: New Principles for Physicians?," *Hastings Center Report* 10 (June 1980), 16–19.
2 The National Commission for the Protection of Human Subjects of Biomedical and Behavioral Research, *The Belmont Report: Ethical Principles and Guidelines for the Protection of Human Subjects of Research* (Washington, D.C.: U.S. Government Printing Office, 1978), p. 58.
3 Tom Beauchamp and James Childress, *Principles of Biomedical Ethics* (New York: Oxford University Press, 1980), p. 59.
4 Edmund Pellegrino, "Toward a Reconstruction of Medical Morality: The Primacy of the Act of Profession and the Fact of Illness," *The Journal of Medicine and Philosophy* 4 (1979), 44–45.
5 Talcott Parsons, *The Social System* (Glencoe, Illinois: The Free Press, 1951), p. 437.
6 Eric Cassell, *The Healer's Art* (New York: Lippincott, 1976), p. 44. Although Cassell aptly describes the goal of the healer's art, it is unclear whether he considers it to be based upon the obligation to respect the patient's autonomy or the duty to enhance the well-being of the patient. Some parts of his discussion clearly suggest the latter.
7 Pedro Lain-Entralgo, *Doctor and Patient* (New York: McGraw-Hill, 1969), p. 155.
8 See Allen Buchanan, "Medical Paternalism," *Philosophy and Public Affairs* 7 (1978), 370–90.
9 My formulation of the components of the legal model differs from, but is highly indebted to, John Ladd's stimulating analysis in "Legalism and Medical Ethics," in John Davis et al, editors, *Contemporary Issues in Biomedical Ethics* (Clifton, N.J.: The Humana Press, 1979), pp. 1–35. However, I would not endorse Ladd's position that the moral principles that define our duties in the therapeutic setting are of a different logical type from those that define our duties to strangers.
10 Eric Cassell, "Therapeutic Relationship: Contemporary Medical Perspective," in Warren Reich, editor, *Encyclopedia of Bioethics* (New York: Macmillan, 1978), p. 1675.
11 Cf. Norman Cousins, "A Layman Looks at Truth-telling," *Journal of the American Medical Association* 244 (1980), 1929–30. Also see Howard Brody, "Hope," *Journal of the American Medical Association* 246 (1981), pp. 1411–12.

TRUTH TELLING

ON TELLING PATIENTS THE TRUTH
Roger Higgs

Higgs argues for the paramount importance of physicians' telling patients the truth, before taking on the complex issue of whether this rule has exceptions. He considers and rejects most of the arguments commonly offered to justify lying to patients or otherwise deceiving them. In the end, he maintains, "there are *some* circumstances in which the health professions are probably exempted from society's general requirement for truthfulness," but these are very rare circumstances in which there are clearly no acceptable alternatives.

. . . [T]hose with experience, either as patients or professionals, will immediately recognize the situation. Although openness is increasingly practised, there is still uncertainty in the minds of many doctors or nurses faced with communicating bad news; as for instance when a test shows up an unexpected and probably incurable cancer, or when meeting the gaze of a severely ill child, or answering the questions of a mother in mid-pregnancy whose unborn child is discovered to be badly handicapped. What should be said? There can be few who have not, on occasions such as these, told less than the truth. Certainly the issue is a regular preoccupation of nurses and doctors in training. Why destroy hope? Why create anxiety, or something worse? Isn't it 'First, do no harm'?[1]

The concerns of the patient are very different. For many, fear of the unknown is the worst disease of all, and yet direct information seems so hard to obtain. The ward round goes past quickly, unintelligible words are muttered—was I supposed to hear and understand? In the surgery the general practitioner signs his prescription pad and clearly it's time to be gone. Everybody is too busy saving lives to give explanations. It may come as a shock to learn that it is policy, not just pressure of work, that prevents a patient learning the truth about himself. If truth is the first casualty, trust must be the second. 'Of course they wouldn't say, especially if things were bad,' said the elderly woman just back from outpatients, 'they've got that

Reprinted from Michael Lockwood, ed., *Moral Dilemmas in Modern Medicine* (1985), pp. 187–191, 193–202, by permission of Oxford University Press. © Roger Higgs 1985.

Oath, haven't they?' She had learned to expect from doctors, at the best, silence; at the worst, deception. It was part of the system, an essential ingredient, as old as Hippocrates. However honest a citizen, it was somehow part of the doctor's job not to tell the truth to his patient. . . .

[I]t is easier to decide what to do when the ultimate outcome is clear. It may be much more difficult to know what to say when the future is less certain, such as in the first episode of what is probably multiple sclerosis, or when a patient is about to undergo a mutilating operation. But even in work outside hospital, where such dramatic problems arise less commonly, whether to tell the truth and how much to tell can still be a regular issue. How much should this patient know about the side effects of his drugs? An elderly man sits weeping in an old people's home, and the healthy but exhausted daughter wants the doctor to tell her father that she's medically unfit to have him back. The single mother wants a certificate to say that she is unwell so that she can stay at home to look after her sick child. A colleague is often drunk on duty, and is making mistakes. A husband with venereal disease wants his wife to be treated without her knowledge. An outraged father demands to know if his teenage daughter has been put on the pill. A mother comes in with a child to have a boil lanced. 'Please tell him it won't hurt.' A former student writes from abroad needing to complete his professional experience and asks for a reference for a job he didn't do.[2] Whether the issue is large or small, the truth is at stake. What should the response be?

Discussion of the apparently more dramatic situations may provide a good starting point. Recently a small group of medical students, new to clinical experience, were hotly debating what a patient with cancer should be told. One student maintained strongly that the less said to the patient the better. Others disagreed. When asked whether there was any group of patients they could agree should never be told the truth about a life-threatening illness, the students chose children, and agreed that they would not speak openly to children under six. When asked to try to remember what life was like when they were six, one student replied that he remembered how his mother had died when he was that age. Suddenly the student who had advocated non-disclosure became animated. 'That's extraordinary. My mother died when I was six too. My father said she'd gone away for a time, but would come back soon. One day he said she was coming home again. My younger sister and I were very excited. We waited at the window upstairs until we saw his car drive up. He got out and helped a woman out of the car. Then we saw. It wasn't mum. I suppose I never forgave him—or her, really.'[3]

It is hard to know with whom to sympathize in this sad tale. But its stark simplicity serves to highlight some essential points. First, somehow more clearly than in the examples involving patients, not telling the truth is seen for what it really is. It is, of course, quite possible, and very common in clinical practice, for doctors (or nurses) to engage in deliberate deceit without actually *saying* anything they believe to be false. But, given the special responsibilities of the doctor, and the relationship of trust that exists between him and his patient, one could hardly argue that this was morally any different from telling outright lies. Surely it is the *intention* that is all important. We may be silent, tactful, or reserved, but if we intend to deceive, what we are doing is tantamount to lying. The debate in ward or surgery is suddenly stood on its head. The question is no longer 'Should we tell the truth?' but 'What justification is there for telling a lie?' This relates to the second important point, that medical ethics are part of general morality, and not a separate field of their own with their own rules. Unless there are special justifications, health-care professionals are working within

the same moral constraints as lay people. A lie is a lie wherever told and whoever tells it.

But do doctors have a special dispensation from the usual principles that guide the conduct of our society? It is widely felt that on occasion they do, and such a dispensation is as necessary to all doctors as freedom from the charge of assault is to a surgeon. But if it is impossible to look after ill patients and always be open and truthful, how can we balance this against the clear need for truthfulness on all other occasions? If deception is like a medicine to be given in certain doses in certain cases, what guidance exists about its administration?

. . . Although the writer of the 'Decorum' in the Hippocratic corpus advises physicians of the danger of telling patients about the nature of their illness '. . . for many patients through this cause have taken a turn for the worse,'[4] the Oath itself is completely silent on this issue. This extraordinary omission is continued through all the more modern codes and declarations. The first mention of veracity as a principle is to be found in the American Medical Association's 'Principles of Ethics' of 1980, which states that the physician should 'deal honestly with patients and colleagues and strive to expose those physicians deficient in character or competence, or who engage in fraud and deception.'[5] Despite the difficulties of the latter injunction, which seems in some way to divert attention from the basic need for honest communication with the patient, here at last is a clear statement. This declaration signally fails, however, to provide the guidance that we might perhaps have expected for the professional facing his or her individual dilemma.

The reticence of these earlier codes is shared, with some important exceptions, by medical writing elsewhere. Until recently most of what had been usefully said could be summed up by the articles of medical writers such as Thomas Percival, Worthington Hooker, Richard Cabot, and Joseph Collins, which show a wide scatter of viewpoints but do at least confront the problems directly.[6] There is, however, one widely quoted statement by Lawrence Henderson, writing in the *New England Journal of Medicine* in 1955.[7] 'It is meaningless to speak of telling the truth, the whole truth and nothing but the truth to a patient . . . because it is . . . a sheer impossibility . . . Since telling the truth is impossible, there can be no sharp distinction between what is true and what is false.' . . .

But we must not allow ourselves to be confused, as Henderson was, and as so many others have been, by a failure to distinguish between truth, the abstract concept, of which we shall always have an imperfect grasp, and *telling* the truth, where the intention is all important. Whether or not we can ever fully grasp or express the whole picture, whether we know ultimately what the truth really is, we must speak truthfully, and intend to convey what we understand, or we shall lie. In Sissela Bok's words 'The moral question of whether you are lying or not is not *settled* by establishing the truth or falsity of what you say. In order to settle the question, we must know whether you *intend your statement to mislead.*'[8] . . .

Most modern thinkers in the field of medical ethics would hold that truthfulness is indeed a central principle of conduct, but that it is capable of coming into conflict with other principles, to which it must occasionally give way. On the other hand, the principle of veracity often receives support from other principles. For instance, it is hard to see how a patient can have autonomy, can make a free choice about matters concerning himself, without some measure of understanding of the facts as they influence the case; and that implies, under normal circumstances, some open, honest discussion with his advisers.[9] . . .

Once the central position of honesty has been established, we still need to examine whether doctors and nurses really do have, as has been suggested, special exemption from being truthful because of the nature of their work, and if so under what circumstances. . . . It may finally be decided that in a crisis there is no acceptable alternative, as when life is ebbing and truthfulness would bring certain disaster. Alternatively, the moral issue may appear so trivial as not to be worth considering (as, for example, when a doctor is called out at night by a patient who apologizes by saying, 'I hope you don't mind me calling you at this time, doctor,' and the doctor replies, 'No, not at all.'). However, . . . occasions of these two types are few, fewer than those in which deliberate deceit would generally be regarded as acceptable in current medical practice, and should

regularly be debated 'in public' if abuses are to be avoided.[10] To this end it is necessary now to examine critically the arguments commonly used to defend lying to patients.

First comes the argument that it is enormously difficult to put across a technical subject to those with little technical knowledge and understanding, in a situation where so little is predictable. A patient has bowel cancer. With surgery it might be cured, or it might recur. Can the patient understand the effects of treatment? The symptom she is now getting might be due to cancer, there might be secondaries, and they in turn might be suppressible for a long time, or not at all. What future symptoms might occur, how long will she live, how will she die—all these are desperately important questions for the patient, but even for her doctor the answers can only be informed guesses, in an area where uncertainty is so hard to bear.

Yet to say we do not know anything is a lie. As doctors we know a great deal, and *can* make informed guesses or offer likelihoods. The whole truth may be impossible to attain, but truthfulness is not. 'I do not know' can be a major piece of honesty. To deprive the patient of honest communication because we cannot know everything is, as we have seen, not only confused thinking but immoral. Thus deprived, the patient cannot plan, he cannot choose. If choice is the crux of morality, it may also, as we have argued elsewhere, be central to health. If he cannot choose, the patient cannot ever be considered to be fully restored to health.[11]

This argument also raises another human failing—to confuse the difficult with the unimportant. Passing information to people who have more restricted background, whether through lack of experience or of understanding, can be extremely difficult and time-consuming, but this is no reason why it should be shunned. Quite the reverse. Like the difficult passages in a piece of music, these tasks should be practiced, studied, and techniques developed so that communication is efficient and effective. For the purposes of informed consent, the patient must be given the information he needs, as a reasonable person, to make a reasoned choice.

The second argument for telling lies to patients is that no patient likes hearing depressing or frightening news. That is certainly true. There must be few who do. But in other walks of life no professional would normally consider it his or her duty to suppress information simply in order to preserve happiness. No accountant, foreseeing bankruptcy in his client's affairs, would chat cheerfully about the budget or a temporarily reassuring credit account. Yet such suppression of information occurs daily in wards or surgeries throughout the country. Is this what patients themselves want?

In order to find out, a number of studies have been conducted over the past thirty years.[12] In most studies there is a significant minority of patients, perhaps about a fifth, who, if given information, deny having been told. Sometimes this must be pure forgetfulness, sometimes it relates to the lack of skill of the informer, but sometimes with bad or unwelcome news there is an element of what is (perhaps not quite correctly) called 'denial.' The observer feels that at one level the news has been taken in, but at another its validity or reality has not been accepted. This process has been recognized as a buffer for the mind against the shock of unacceptable news, and often seems to be part of a process leading to its ultimate acceptance.[13] But once this group has been allowed for, most surveys find that, of those who have had or who could have had a diagnosis made of, say, cancer, between two-thirds and three-quarters of those questioned were either glad to have been told, or declared that they would wish to know. Indeed, surveys reveal that most *doctors* would themselves wish to be told the truth, even though (according to earlier studies at least) most of those same doctors said they would not speak openly to their patients—a curious double standard! Thus these surveys have unearthed, at least for the present, a common misunderstanding between doctors and patients, a general preference for openness among patients, and a significant but small group whose wish not to be informed must surely be respected. We return once more to the skill needed to detect such differences in the individual case, and the need for training in such skills.

Why doctors have for so long misunderstood their patients' wishes is perhaps related to the task itself. Doctors don't want to give bad news, just as patients don't want it in abstract, but doctors have the choice of withholding the information, and in so do-

ing protecting themselves from the pain of telling, and from the blame of being the bearer of bad news. In addition it has been suggested that doctors are particularly fearful of death and illness. Montaigne suggested that men have to think about death and be prepared to accept it, and one would think that doctors would get used to death. Yet perhaps this very familiarity has created an obsession that amounts to fear. Just as the police seem over-concerned with violence, and firemen with fire, perhaps doctors have met death in their professional training only as the enemy, never as something to come to terms with, or even as a natural force to be respected and, when the time is ripe, accepted or even welcomed. . . .

. . . Paternalism may be justifiable in the short term, and to 'kid' someone, to treat him as a child because he is ill, and perhaps dying, may be very tempting. Yet true respect for that person (adult or child) can only be shown by allowing him allowable choices, by granting him whatever control is left, as weakness gradually undermines his hold on life. If respect is important then at the very least there must be no acceptable or effective alternative to lying in a particular situation if the lie is to be justified.

. . . However, a third argument for lying can be advanced, namely, that truthfulness can actually do harm. 'What you don't know can't hurt you' is a phrase in common parlance (though it hardly fits with concepts of presymptomatic screening for preventable disease!). However, it is undeniable that blunt and unfeeling communication of unpleasant truths can cause acute distress, and sometimes long-term disability. The fear that professionals often have of upsetting people, of causing a scene, of making fools of themselves by letting unpleasant emotions flourish, seems to have elevated this argument beyond its natural limits. It is not unusual to find that the fear of creating harm will deter a surgical team from discussing a diagnosis gently with a patient, but not deter it from performing radical and mutilating surgery. Harm is a very personal concept. Most medical schools have, circulating in the refectory, a story about a patient who was informed that he had cancer and then leapt to his death. The intended moral for the medical student is, keep your mouth shut and do no harm. But that may not be the correct lesson to be learned from such cases (which I believe, in any case, to be less numerous than is commonly supposed). The style of telling could have been brutal, with no follow-up or support. It may have been the suggested treatment, not the basic illness, that led the patient to resort to such a desperate measure. Suicide in illness is remarkably rare, but, though tragic, could be seen as a logical response to an overwhelming challenge. No mention is usually made of suicide rates in other circumstances, or the isolation felt by ill and warded patients, or the feelings of anger uncovered when someone takes such precipitate and forbidden action against himself. What these cases do, surely, is argue, not for no telling, but for better telling, for sensitivity and care in determining how much the patient wants to know, explaining carefully in ways the patient can understand, and providing full support and 'after-care' as in other treatments.

But even if it is accepted that the short-term effect of telling the truth may sometimes be considerable psychological disturbance, in the long term the balance seems definitely to swing the other way. The effects of lying are dramatically illustrated in 'A Case of Obstructed Death?'[14] False information prevented a woman from returning to healthy living after a cancer operation, and robbed her of six months of active life. Also, the long-term effect of lies on the family and, perhaps most importantly, on society, is incalculable. If trust is gradually corroded, if the 'wells are poisoned,' progress is hard. Mistrust creates lack of communication and increased fear, and this generation has seen just such a fearful myth created around cancer.[15] Just how much harm has been done by this 'demonizing' of cancer, preventing people coming to their doctors, or alternatively creating unnecessary attendances on doctors, will probably never be known.

There are doubtless many other reasons why doctors lie to their patients; but these can hardly be used to justify lies, even if we should acknowledge them in passing. Knowledge is power, and certainly doctors, though usually probably for reasons of work-load rather than anything more sinister, like to remain 'in control.' Health professionals may, like others, wish to protect themselves from confrontation, and may find it easier to coerce or manipulate than to gain permission. There may be a desire to avoid any pressure for change. And there is the constant problem of lack of time. . . .

If the importance of open communication with the patient is accepted, [however,] we need to know when to say what. If a patient is going for investigations, it may be possible at that time, before details are known, to have a discussion about whether he would like to know the details. A minor 'contract' can be made. 'I promise to tell you what I know, if you ask me.' Once that time is past, however, it requires skill and sensitivity to assess what a patient wants to know. Allowing the time and opportunity for the patient to ask questions is the most important thing, but one must realize that the patient's apparent question may conceal the one he really wants answered. 'Do I have cancer?' may contain the more important questions 'How or when will I die?' 'Will there be pain?' The doctor will not necessarily be helping by giving an extended pathology lesson. The informer may need to know more: 'I don't want to avoid your question, and I promise to answer as truthfully as I can, but first . . .' It has been pointed out that in many cases the terminal patient will tell the doctor, not vice versa, if the right opportunities are created and the style and timing is appropriate. Then it is a question of not telling but listening to the truth.[16]

If in spite of all this there still seems to be a need to tell lies, we must be able to justify them. That the person is a child, or 'not very bright,' will not do. Given the two ends of the spectrum of crisis and triviality, the vast middle range of communication requires honesty, so that autonomy and choice can be maintained. If lies are to be told, there really must be no acceptable alternative. . . . If we break an important moral principle, that principle still retains its force, and its 'shadow' has to be acknowledged. As professionals we shall have to ensure that we follow up, that we work through the broken trust or the disillusionment that the lie will bring to the patient, just as we would follow up and work through bad news, a major operation, or a psychiatric 'sectioning.' This follow-up may also be called for in our relationship with our colleagues if there has been major disagreement about what should be done.

In summary, there are *some* circumstances in which the health professions are probably exempted from society's general requirement for truthfulness.

But not telling the truth is usually the same as telling a lie, and a lie requires strong justification. Lying must be a last resort, and we should act as if we were to be called upon to defend the decision in public debate, even if our duty of confidentiality does not allow this in practice. We should always aim to respect the other important principles governing interactions with patients, especially the preservation of the patient's autonomy. When all is said and done, many arguments for individual cases of lying do not hold water. Whether or not knowing the truth is essential to the patient's health, telling the truth is essential to the health of the doctor-patient relationship.

NOTES

1 *Primum non nocere*—this is a latinization of a statement which is not directly Hippocratic, but may be derived from the *Epidemics* Book 1 Chapter II: 'As to diseases, make a habit of two things—to help, or at least do no harm.' *Hippocrates,* 4 Vols. (London: William Heinemann, 1923–31), Vol. I. Translation W. H. S. Jones.

2 Cases collected by the author in his own practice.

3 Case collected by the author.

4 Quoted in Reiser, Dyck, and Curran (eds), *Ethics in Medicine, Historical Perspectives and Contemporary Concerns* (Cambridge, Mass.: MIT Press, 1977).

5 American Medical Association, 'Text of the American Medical Association New Principles of Medical Ethics.' *American Medical News* (August 1–8, 1980), 9.

6 To be found in Reiser *et al.*, op. cit. (see n. 4 above).

7 Lawrence Henderson, 'Physician and Patient as a Social System,' *New England Journal of Medicine,* 212 (1935).

8 Sissela Bok, *Lying: Moral Choice in Public and Private Life* (London: Quartet, 1980).

9 Alastair Campbell and Roger Higgs, *In That Case* (London: Darton, Longman and Todd, 1982).

10 John Rawls, *A Theory of Justice* (Cambridge, Mass.: Harvard University Press, Belknap Press, 1971).

11 Op. cit. (see n. 9 above).

12 Summarized well in Robert Veatch, 'Truth-telling I' in Warren T. Reich (ed.), *Encyclopaedia of Bioethics* (New York: Free Press, 1978).

13 The five stages of reacting to bad news, or news of dying, are described in *On Death and Dying* by Elizabeth Kübler-Ross (London: Tavistock, 1970). Not everyone agrees with her model. For another view see a very stimulating article 'Therapeutic Uses of Truth' by Michael Simpson in E. Wilkes (ed.), *The Dying Patient* (Lancaster: MTP Press, 1982). 'In my model there are only two stages—the stage when you believe in the Kübler-Ross five and the stage when you do not.'

14 Roger Higgs, 'Truth at the Last—A Case of Obstructed Death?', *Journal of Medical Ethics,* 8 (1982), 48–50, and Roger Higgs, 'Obstructed Death Revisited,' *Journal of Medical Ethics,* 8 (1982), pp. 154–56.

15 Susan Sontag, *Illness as Metaphor* (New York: Farrar, Straus and Giroux, 1978).

16 Cicely Saunders, 'Telling Patients,' *District Nursing* (now *Queens Nursing Journal*) (September 1963), pp. 149–50, 154.

OFFERING TRUTH: ONE ETHICAL APPROACH TO THE UNINFORMED CANCER PATIENT

Benjamin Freedman

Freedman addresses a conflict that arises with some patients who are unaware that they have cancer. The conflict arises, he explains, from two widely accepted moral assumptions: (1) that patients have a right to know their medical diagnoses, and (2) that physicians should be respectful of the cultural values of patients and their families. These two assumptions clash when a patient's family insists, citing cultural reasons, that the patient not be informed of having cancer. Freedman argues that an approach of offering truth to such patients—providing them the opportunity to learn the truth at whatever level of detail they desire—affords a way to satisfy ethical and legal norms of patient autonomy, reduce conflicts between families and physicians, and acknowledge the cultural values that underlie family requests.

Medical and social attitudes toward cancer have evolved rapidly during the last 20 years, particularly in North America.[1,2] Most physicians, most of the time, in most hospitals, accept the ethical proposition that patients are entitled to know their diagnosis. However, there remains in my experience a significant minority of cases in which patients are never informed that they have cancer or, although informed of the diagnosis, are not informed when disease progresses toward a terminal phase. Although concealment of diagnosis can certainly occur in cases of other terminal or even nonterminal serious illnesses, it seems to occur more frequently and in more exacerbated form with cancer because of the traditional and cultural resonances of dread associated with cancer.

These cases challenge our understanding of and commitment to an ethical physician-patient relationship. In addition, they are observably a significant source of tension between healthcare providers. When the responsible physician persists in efforts to conceal the truth from patients, consultant physicians, nurses, social workers, or others may believe that they cannot discharge their functions responsibly until the patient has been told. Alternatively, when a treating physician decides to inform the patient of his or her diagnosis, strong resistance from family members who have instigated a conspiracy of silence may be anticipated.

This article outlines one approach, employed in my own ethical consultations and at some palliative care services or specialized oncology units. This approach, offering truth to patients with cancer, affords a means of satisfying legal and ethical norms of patient autonomy, ameliorating conflicts between families and physicians, and acknowledging the cultural norms that underlie family desires.

COMMON FEATURES OF CASES

Mrs A is a woman in her 60s with colon cancer, with metastatic liver involvement and a mass in the abdomen. She is not expected to survive longer than weeks. Other than a course of antibiotics, which she

Reprinted with permission of the publisher from *Archives of Internal Medicine*, vol. 153 (March 8, 1993), pp. 572–576. Copyright © 1993, American Medical Association.

was just about to complete, no active treatment is indicated or intended. She is alert. She knows that she has an infection: her family refuses to inform her that she has cancer. The precipitating cause of the ethical consultation, requested by the newly assigned treating physician (Dr H), is his ethical discomfort with treating Mrs A in this manner.

When one is confronted with a case of concealment, it is worth wondering how it came about that everyone but the patient has been told of the diagnosis, so that similar situations may be avoided in the future. Often, a diagnosis is defined in the course of surgery and disclosed to waiting relatives; this may most appropriately be handled by a prior understanding with the patient, communicated to the family, as to whether and how much they will be told before the patient awakens. But there are at least two other major ways in which a situation of concealment might develop.

A patient might be admitted in medical crisis, at a time when he or she is obtunded and incapable of being informed of his or her condition and treatment options. Law and ethics alike require that the medical team inform and otherwise deal with the person who is most qualified to speak on the patient's behalf (usually, the next of kin), until the patient has recovered enough to speak for himself or herself. Unfortunately for this plan, though, a patient will often fail to cross, at one moment, the bright line from incompetent to competent. Consequently, patterns of communicating with the relative instead of with the patient may persist beyond the intended period. Such situations have their own momentum. Later disclosure to the patient will need to deal both with the burden of providing bad news and with the fact that this information has been concealed from the patient up to that point.

A second typical way in which concealment develops is the following. A patient with close family ties is always attended by a relative (commonly, spouse or child) at medical appointments. Before a firm diagnosis is established, that relative manages to elicit a promise from the physician not to tell the patient should the tests show that the patient has cancer. Faced with a distraught and deeply caring relative, the physician goes along, at least as a temporizing tactic, only to discover, as described above, how the situation develops its own inertia. The cycle may be broken in a number of ways. Sometimes the physician simply decides to call a halt to concealment; often the patient's care is transferred to another physician who has not been a party to the conspiracy, as had happened with Mrs A.

> As clinical ethicist, I met with Dr H and the relevant family members (husband, daughter, and son). Most of the discussion was held with the son; the husband, a first-generation Greek-Canadian immigrant, knows little English and was at any rate somewhat withdrawn. As expected, they are a close family, deeply solicitous of the patient, and convinced that she will suffer horribly were she to be told she has cancer. They confirmed my sense that the Greek cultural significance of cancer equals death—something that in this case is in all likelihood true.
>
> At this time the family was willing to sign any document we wanted them to, assuming all responsibility for the decision to conceal the truth from Mrs A. "Do us this one favor" was a plea that punctuated the discussion.

Although other factors, such as the context of treatment and the patient's own idiosyncratic personality, may cause the same kind of problem in communication, my experience suggests the situation is often, as here, mediated by cultural factors. As one text on ethnic factors in family counseling puts it, "Greek Americans do not believe that the truth shall make you free, and the therapist should not attempt to impose the love of truth upon them."[3] (And compare Dalla-Vorgia et al.[4]) I often find other immigrant families of Mediterranean or Near Eastern origin reacting similarly, for example, Italian families and those of Sephardic Jews who have immigrated from Morocco. In all cases, in my experience, there is a special plea on the part of families to respect their cultural pattern and tradition. Health-care providers often feel the force of this claim and its corollary: informing the patient would be an act of ethical and cultural imperialism. Moreover, the family not uncommonly feels strongly enough that legal action is threatened unless their wishes are respected. Mrs A's family, in fact, threatened to sue at one point when they were told that Mrs A's diagnosis would be revealed.

TELLING FAMILIES WHY THE PATIENT SHOULD BE INFORMED

By the time a clinical ethical consultation is requested, the situation has often become highly charged emotionally. In addition to the unpleasantness of threats of legal action, there may have been some physical confrontation.

> Mrs S was a Sephardic woman in her 70s with widespread metastatic seedings in the pleura and pericardium from an unknown primary tumor. Her family insisted that she not be informed of her diagnosis and prognosis. Suffering from a subjective experience of apnea, she was to have a morphine drip begun to alleviate her symptoms. The family physically expelled the nurse from the room. If their mother were to learn she was getting morphine, they said, she would deduce that her situation was grave.

Such aberrant behavior cannot fairly be understood without realizing that these families may be acting out of uncommonly deep concern for the well-being of the patient, as they (perhaps misguidedly) understand it. The health-care team shares the same ultimate goal, to care for the patient in a humane, decent, caring manner. This commonality can serve as the basis for continuing discussion, as in the above case of Mrs A, the Greek patient.

> Discussion with the family was long and meandering. The usual position of the health-care team was explained in some detail: patients in our institution are generally told their diagnosis; we are accustomed to telling patients that they have cancer, and we know how to handle the varied normal patient reactions to this bad news; patients do not (generally) kill themselves immediately on being told, or die a voodoo death, in spite of the family's fears and cultural beliefs about patient reaction to this diagnosis. Patients have a right to this information and may have the need to attend to any number of tasks pending death: to say goodbye, to make arrangements, to complete unfinished business. As her illness progresses, decisions will likely need to be made about further treatment, for example, of infections or blockages that develop. Already, one of Mrs A's kidneys is blocked and her urine is backing up. If the mass should obstruct her other kidney, for example, should a catheter be placed directly into the kidney or not?

These decisions of treatment management for dying patients are dreadful and should if possible be made by the patient, with awareness of her choices and prospects. In addition, Mrs A is very likely already suspicious that she is gravely ill, and we have no means of dealing with her fears without the ability to speak to her openly. Finally, the fears that the family expresses about the manner of informing her—"How can we tell our mother. 'You have cancer, it will kill you in weeks' "—are groundless: she must be told that she is very ill, but we would never advise telling her she has a period of x weeks to live—a statement that is never wise or medically sound—nor will we try to remove her hope.

The physician or other health-care provider may be primarily motivated by the ethical principle of respect for patient autonomy, grounding a patient's right to know of his or her situation, choices, and likely fate. Connected with this may be the correct belief that any consent to treatment that the patient provides without having an opportunity to learn the reason for that treatment is legally invalid. To be properly informed, consent must be predicated on information about the nature and consequences of treatment, which must in turn be understood in the context of the patient's illness. A patient cannot validly consent to the passing of a tube into the kidney without being informed that her urinary tract is blocked, or of the reason for that blockage.

These reasons, so determinative for the physician, often carry no weight with the family. In Mrs A's case, for example, the family pledged to sign anything we would like to free us of liability. Our response, that their willingness cannot affect either our moral or legal obligation, which vests in the patient directly, was similarly unpersuasive; nonetheless, it was a fact and had to be said.

The direct negative impact on the patient's care and comfort that results from her being left in the dark represents more in the way of common ground between family and health-care provider. It is often quite clear that failure to reveal the truth causes a variety of unfortunate psychosocial results. As in all such cases, we high-lighted for Mrs A's family the strong possibility that she already suspects she is ill and dying of cancer but is unable to speak about this with them because all of us, in our concealment and

evasions, had not given her "permission" to broach the topic. Mrs A is dying, but there are things worse than dying, for example, dying in silence when one needs to speak.

It is also important to emphasize to families that the patient may have "unfinished business" that he or she would like to complete. For example, after one of my earliest consultations of this nature, the patient in question chose to leave the hospital for several weeks to revisit his birthplace in Greece.

Finally, it is sometimes the case that the failure to discuss with the patient his or her diagnosis can directly result in inadequate or inappropriate medical care. Mrs S, above, was denied adequate comfort measures because the institution of morphine might tip her off to her condition. In another case, the son and daughter-in-law of a patient insisted that she not receive chemotherapy for an advanced but treatable blood cancer so that she would be spared the knowledge of her disease and the side effects of treatment. In such cases, great injury is added to the insult of withholding the truth from a patient. Often, it is this prospect that serves as the trigger to mobilize the health-care team to seek an ethical consultation.

OFFERING TRUTH TO THE UNINFORMED PATIENT WITH CANCER

A patient's knowledge of diagnosis and prognosis is not all-or-nothing. It exists along a continuum, anchored at one end by the purely theoretical "absolute ignorance" and at the other by the unattainable "total enlightenment." Actual patients are to be found along this continuum at locations that vary in response to external factors (verbal information, nonverbal clues, etc) as well as internal dynamics, such as denial.

The approach called here "offering truth" represents a brief dance between patient and health-care provider, a pas de deux, that takes place within that continuum. When offering truth to the patient with cancer, rather than simply ascertaining that the patient is for the moment lucid, and then proceeding to explain all aspects of his or her condition and treatment, both the physician(s) and I attempt repeatedly to ascertain from the patient how much he or she wants to know. In dealing with families who insist that the patient remain uninformed, I explain this approach, a kind of compromise between the polar stances. I also explain that sometimes the results are surprising, as indeed happened with Mrs A.

> In spite of all the explanations we provided to Mrs A's family of the many reasons why it might be best to speak with her of her illness, they continued to resist. Mrs A, the son insisted, would want all the decisions that arise to be made by the physicians, whom they all trusted, and the family itself.
>
> If their assessment of Mrs A is correct, I pointed out, we have no problem. Dr H agrees with me that while Mrs A has a *right* to know, she does not have a *duty* to know. We would not force this information on her—indeed, we cannot. Patients who do not want to know will sometimes deny ever having been told, however forthrightly they have been spoken to. So Mrs A will be offered this information, not have it thrust on her—and if they are right about what she wants, and her personality, she will not wish to know.
>
> Mrs A was awake and reasonably alert, although not altogether free of discomfort (nausea). She was told that she had had an infection that was now under control, but that she remains very ill, as she herself can tell from her weakness. Does she have any questions she wants to ask; does she want to talk? She did not. We repeated that she remains very ill and asked if she understands that—she did. Some patients, it was explained to her, want to know all about their disease—its name, prognosis, treatment choices, famous people who have had the disease, etc.—while others do not want to know so much, and some want to leave all of the decisions in the hands of their family and physicians. What would she like? What kind of patient is she? She whispered to her daughter that she wants to leave it alone for now.
>
> That seemed to be her final word. We repeated to her that treatment choices would need to be made shortly. She was told that we would respect her desire, but that if she changed her mind we could talk at any time; and that, in any event, she must understand that we would stay by her and see to her comfort in all possible ways. She signified that she understood and said that we should deal with her children. Both Dr H and I understood this as explicitly authorizing her children to speak for her with respect to treatment decisions.

The above approach relies on one simple tactic: a patient will be offered the opportunity to learn the truth, at whatever level of detail that patient desires. The most important step in these attempts is to ask questions of the patient and then listen closely to the patient's responses. Since the discussion at hand concerns how much information the patient would like to receive, here, unlike most physician-patient interchanges, the important decisions will need to be made by the patient.

Initiating discussion is relatively easy if the patient is only recently conscious and responsive; it is more difficult if a conspiracy of silence has already taken effect. The conversation with the patient might be initiated by telling him or her that at this time the medical team has arrived at a fairly clear understanding of the situation and treatment options. New test results may be alluded to; this is a fairly safe statement, since new tests are always being done on all patients. These conversational gambits signal that a fresh start in communication can now be attempted. (At the same time it avoids the awkwardness of a patient's asking, "Why haven't you spoken to me before?")

The patient might then be told that, before we talk about our current understanding of the medical situation, it is important to hear from the patient himself or herself, so that we can confirm what he or she knows or clear up any misunderstanding that may have arisen. The patient sometimes, with more than a little logic, responds, "Why are you asking me what is wrong? You're the doctor, you tell me what's wrong." A variety of answers are possible. A patient might be told that we have found that things work better if we start with the patient's understanding of the illness; or that time might be saved if we know what the patient understands, and go from there; or that whenever you try to teach someone, you have to start with what they know. Different approaches may suggest themselves as more fitting to the particular patient in question. The important thing is to begin to generate a dynamic within which the patient is speaking and the physician responding, rather than vice versa. Only then can the pace of conversation and level of information be controlled by the patient. The structure of the discussion, as well as the content of what the physician says, must reinforce the message: We are now establishing a new opportunity to talk and question, but you as the patient will have to tell us how much you want to know about your illness.

The chief ethical principle underlying the idea that patients should be offered the truth is, of course, respect for the patient's personal autonomy. By holding the conversation, the patient is given the opportunity to express autonomy in its most robust, direct fashion: the clear expression of preference. Legal systems that value autonomy will similarly protect a physician who chooses to offer truth and to respect the patient's response to that offer; "a medical doctor need not make disclosure of risks when the patient requests that he not be so informed."[5] A patient's right to information vests in that patient, to exercise as he or she desires; so that a patient's right to information is respected no less when the patient chooses to be relatively uninformed as when full information is demanded.[6] This stance is entirely consistent with the recent adoption of the widely noted (and even more widely misconstrued) Patient Self-Determination Act.[7] The major innovation this entails has been to involve institutions in the process of informing patients of their rights. However, the Patient Self-Determination Act has not changed state laws about informed consent to treatment in any way,[8] and as such the basic question here addressed—a physician's responsibility to inform patients of their diagnoses—remains entirely unaffected.

When offering truth, we are forced to recognize that patients' choices should be respected not because we or others agree with those choices (still less, respected *only* when we agree with those choices), but simply because those are the patient's choices. Indeed, the test of autonomy comes precisely when we personally disagree with the path the patient had chosen. If, for example, patient choice is respected only when the patient chooses the most effective treatment, when respecting those choices we would be respecting only effective therapeutics, not the person who has chosen them.

Many physicians hold to the ideal of an informed, alert, cooperative, and intelligent patient. But the point of offering truth—rather than inflicting it—is to allow the patient to choose his or her own path. As a practical matter, of course, it could scarcely be otherwise. A physician with fanatic devotion to informing patients can lecture, explain, even harangue, but cannot force the patient to attend to what the physician is saying, or think about it, or remember it.

Families need to confront the same point. Ambivalence and conflict are often observed among family members concerning whether the patient who has not been informed "really" knows (or suspects, etc), and by offering the patient the opportunity to speak, this issue may be settled. More fundamentally, though, the concealing family—which is after all characterized by deep concern for the patient's well-being—will rarely (has never, in my experience to date) maintain that even if the patient demands to know the truth, the secret should still be kept. The family rather relies on the patient's failure to make this explicit demand as his or her tacit agreement to remain ignorant. Families can be helped to see that there may be many reasons for the patient's failure to demand the truth (including the fact that the patient may believe the lies that have been offered). If the patient wishes to remain in a state of relative ignorance, he or she will tell us that when asked; and if the patient states an explicit desire to be informed, families will find it hard to deny his or her right to have that desire respected.

Some families, naturally enough, suspect chicanery, that this approach is rigged to get the patient to ask for the truth. To them I respond that my experience proves otherwise: to my surprise and that of the physicians, some patients ask to leave this in the family's hands; to the surprise of families, some patients who seemed quietistic in fact strongly wish to be told the truth (which many of them had already suspected). We cannot know what the patient wants until we ask, I tell them, and we all want to do what the patient wants.

Having held the discussion, it is important to move on to its resolution as soon as possible.

> I met with Mrs S's children, together with a nurse, medical resident, and medical student, for about an hour and a half; the treating oncologist also made a brief appearance. The discussion featured a lengthy and eloquent exposition by the resident of why Mrs S needs to be spoken to, and a passionate and equally eloquent appeal by one son to respect the different culture from which they come. Finally, I introduced the idea that we offer her the truth, and then follow her lead. This was agreed to by the family, and I left.

The medical student thanked me some days later and told me the rest of the story. The tension that had existed between health-care team and family had largely dissipated; as the student put it, "People were able to look each other in the eye again." Mrs S was lucid but fatigued that evening; for that reason, and probably because they had already spent so much time talking at our meeting, the family delayed the agreed-on discussion. Unexpectedly, Mrs S did not survive the night.

CONCLUSION

The problem of the uninformed patient with cancer can be described in many different ways, for example, as faulty physician-patient communication; as an obstacle to good medical care; as a cause of stress among hospital staff; and as a failure to respect patient autonomy. A dimension at least as important as these, but rarely acknowledged, is the clash it may represent between diverse cultures and their basic moral commitments.

The approach presented above reflects an effort to maintain accepted standards of the physician-patient relationship while respecting the cultural background and requirements of families. This form of respect involves reasonable accommodation to these cultural expectations but should not be confused with uncritical acquiescence. The critical question is, perhaps, this: How should we react to a family that refuses to allow the patient an offering of truth, that maintains that discussion itself to be contrary to cultural norms? Under those circumstances, I believe the offering must be made notwithstanding family demands. My reasons have as much to do with my beliefs about the nature of ethnic and religious moral norms themselves as with the view that in cases of conflict, our public morality (as concretized in law) should prevail.

First, I believe that members of a cultural community are as prone to mistaking what their own norms require of them as we within the broader culture are to mistaking our own moral obligations. The norm of protecting the patient clearly requires rather than prohibits disclosure in some cases, including some described above, to prevent physical or psychological damage or to enable some final task to be consummated. All of the factors that we recognize sometimes to derange our own moral judgments—inertia, ill-grounded prejudices and generalizations,

lack of the courage to confront unpleasant situations, and many more—may operate as powerfully in deranging the views of those from another culture. Their initial sense of what ethics require may, that is, be mistaken, from the point of view of their own norms as well as those of modern, Western, secular culture.

Second, even if a family's judgment of what their culture requires is accurate, we must not presume that a patient like Mrs A will choose, in extremis, to abide by her own cultural norms. Like any immigrant, she may have adopted the norms of broad society, or, acculturated to some lesser degree, she may act according to some hybrid set of values. Concretely, the offering of truth is about her diagnosis; symbolically, it is a process that allows her to declare her own preference regarding which norms shall be respected and how.

A last word is in order about the view implicit in this approach regarding the nature of a bioethical consultation. As these cases illustrate, patients, families, and health-care professionals come to a meeting from different moral worlds, as well as different backgrounds and biographies; and these worlds involve not simply rights and privileges, but duties as well. A successful consultation attempts to clarify on behalf of the different parties their own moral principles and associated moral commitments. It needs to proceed from the premise that all present ultimately share a common goal: the well-being of the patient.

I am grateful to Eugene V. Bareza, MD, CM, and to Charles Weijer, MD, for valuable advice in the preparation of the manuscript. All errors are my own.

REFERENCES

1 Oken D. What to tell cancer patients: a study of medical attitudes. *JAMA*. 1961;175:1120–1128.

2 Novack DH, Plumer R. Smith R. L, Ochitil H. Morrow G. R, Bennett J. M. Changes in physicians' attitudes toward telling the cancer patient. *JAMA*. 1979;241:897–900.

3 Welts E. P. The Greek family. In: McGoldrick, M. M. Pearce J. K, Giordano J. *Ethnicity and Family Therapy*. New York, NY: Guilford Press; 1982:269–288.

4 Dalla-Vorgia P. Katsouyanni K. Garanis T. N, et al. Attitudes of a Mediterranean population to the truth-telling issue. *J Med Ethics*. 1992; 18:67–74.

5 *Cobbs v Grant*, 502 P2d 1 (Cal 1972) (a similar provision for a patient's right to waive being informed was established by the Supreme Court of Canada in *Reibl v Hughes* 2SCR 880 [1980]).

6 Freedman B. The validity of ignorant consent to medical research. *IRB Rev Hum Subjects Res.* 1982; 4(2):1–5.

7 The Patient Self Determination Act, sections 4206 and 4751 of the Omnibus Reconciliation Act of 1990. Pub L 101–508.

8 McCloskey E. Between isolation and intrusion: The Patient Self Determination Act. *Law Med Health Care.* 1991; 19:80–82.

INFORMED CONSENT

OPINION IN *CANTERBURY V. SPENCE*

Judge Spotswood W. Robinson III

A 19-year-old man, John W. Canterbury, developed paraplegia after a laminectomy (a surgical procedure). Prior to the surgery, his physician, William Thornton Spence, did not inform Canterbury that the operation involved the risk of paralysis. Canterbury brought an action against the physician and the hospital. In defending his decision to withhold the information from the patient, Dr. Spence testified that communicating the 1 percent risk "is not good medical practice because it might deter patients from undergoing needed surgery and might produce adverse psychological reactions which could preclude the success of the operation." In this selection, Judge Robinson argues that an adult patient of sound mind has the right to determine what should be done to his or her body. Because of this right, a physician has the duty to inform the patient about those dangers that "are material" to the patient's decision. The court allows two exceptions to this rule of disclosure. It holds, however, that a physician cannot remain silent simply because divulgence might prompt the patient to forgo therapy that the physician perceives as necessary.

Suits charging failure by a physician adequately to disclose the risks and alternatives of proposed treatment are not innovations in American law. They date back a good half-century, and in the last decade they have multiplied rapidly. There is, nonetheless, disagreement among the courts and the commentators on many major questions, and there is no precedent of our own directly in point. For the tools enabling resolution of the issues on this appeal, we are forced to begin at first principles.

The root premise is the concept, fundamental in American jurisprudence, that "[e]very human being of adult years and sound mind has a right to determine what shall be done with his own body. . . ." True consent to what happens to one's self is the informed exercise of a choice, and that entails an opportunity to evaluate knowledgeably the options available and the risks attendant upon each. The average patient has lit-

U.S. Court of Appeals, District of Columbia Circuit; May 19, 1972. 464 Federal Reporter, 2nd Series, 772. Reprinted with permission of West Publishing Company.

tle or no understanding of the medical arts, and ordinarily has only his physician to whom he can look for enlightenment with which to reach an intelligent decision.[1] From these almost axiomatic considerations springs the need, and in turn the requirement, of a reasonable divulgence by physician to patient to make such a decision possible.[2]

A physician is under a duty to treat his patient skillfully, but proficiency in diagnosis and therapy is not the full measure of his responsibility. The cases demonstrate that the physician is under an obligation to communicate specific information to the patient when the exigencies of reasonable care call for it. Due care may require a physician perceiving symptoms of bodily abnormality to alert the patient to the condition. It may call upon the physician confronting an ailment which does not respond to his ministrations to inform the patient thereof. It may command the physician to instruct the patient as to any limitations to be presently observed for his own welfare, and as to any precautionary therapy he should seek in the future. It may oblige the physician to advise the patient of the need for or desirability of any alternative treatment promising greater benefit than that being pursued. Just as plainly, due care normally demands that the physician warn the patient of any risks to his well-being which contemplated therapy may involve.

The context in which the duty of risk-disclosure arises is invariably the occasion for a decision as to whether a particular treatment procedure is to be undertaken. To the physician, whose training enables a self-satisfying evaluation, the answer may seem clear, but it is the prerogative of the patient, not the physician, to determine for himself the direction in which his interests seem to lie. To enable the patient to chart his course understandably, some familiarity with the therapeutic alternatives and their hazards becomes essential.

A reasonable revelation in these respects is not only a necessity but, as we see it, is as much a matter of the physician's duty. It is a duty to warn of the dangers lurking in the proposed treatment, and that is surely a facet of due care. It is, too, a duty to impart information which the patient has every right to expect.[3] The patient's reliance upon the physician is a trust of the kind which traditionally has exacted obligations beyond those associated with arms-length transactions. His dependence upon the physician for information affecting his well-being, in terms of contemplated treatment, is well-nigh abject. As earlier noted, long before the instant litigation arose, courts had recognized that the physician had the responsibility of satisfying the vital informational needs of the patient. More recently, we ourselves have found "in the fiducial qualities of [the physician-patient] relationship the physician's duty to reveal to the patient that which in his best interests it is important that he should know." We now find, as a part of the physician's overall obligation to the patient, a similar duty of reasonable disclosure of the choices with respect to proposed therapy and the dangers inherently and potentially involved. . . .

Once the circumstances give rise to a duty on the physician's part to inform his patient, the next inquiry is the scope of the disclosure the physician is legally obliged to make. The courts have frequently confronted this problem but no uniform standard defining the adequacy of the divulgence emerges

from the decisions. Some have said "full" disclosure, a norm we are unwilling to adopt literally. It seems obviously prohibitive and unrealistic to except physicians to discuss with their patients every risk of proposed treatment—no matter how small or remote—and generally unnecessary from the patient's viewpoint as well. Indeed, the cases speaking in terms of "full" disclosure appear to envision something less than total disclosure, leaving unanswered the question of just how much.

The larger number of courts, as might be expected, have applied tests framed with reference to prevailing fashion within the medical profession. Some have measured the disclosure by "good medical practice," others by what a reasonable practitioner would have bared under the circumstances, and still others by what medical custom in the community would demand. We have explored this rather considerable body of law but are unprepared to follow it. The duty to disclose, we have reasoned, arises from phenomena apart from medical custom and practice. The latter, we think, should no more establish the scope of the duty than its existence. Any definition of scope in terms purely of a professional standard is at odds with the patient's prerogative to decide on projected therapy himself. That prerogative, we have said, is at the very foundation of the duty to disclose, and both the patient's right to know and the physician's correlative obligation to tell him are diluted to the extent that its compass is dictated by the medical profession.[4]

In our view, the patient's right of self-decision shapes the boundaries of the duty to reveal. That right can be effectively exercised only if the patient possesses enough information to enable an intelligent choice. The scope of the physician's communications to the patient, then, must be measured by the patient's need, and that need is the information material to the decision. Thus the test for determining whether a particular peril must be divulged is its materiality to the patient's decision: all risks potentially affecting the decision must be unmasked. And to safeguard the patient's interest in achieving his own determination on treatment, the law must itself set the standard for adequate disclosure.

Optimally for the patient, exposure of a risk would be mandatory whenever the patient would deem it significant to his decision, either singly or in combination with other risks. Such a requirement, however, would summon the physician to second-guess the patient, whose ideas on materiality could hardly be known to the physician. That would make an undue demand upon medical practitioners, whose conduct, like that of others, is to be measured in terms of reasonableness. Consonantly with orthodox negligence doctrine, the physician's liability for nondisclosure is to be determined on the basis of foresight, not hindsight; no less than any other aspect of negligence, the issue on nondisclosure must be approached from the viewpoint of the reasonableness of the physician's divulgence in terms of what he knows or should know to be the patient's informational needs. If, but only if, the fact-finder can say that the physician's communication was unreasonably inadequate is an imposition of liability legally or morally justified.

Of necessity, the content of the disclosure rests in the first instance with the physician. Ordinarily it is only he who is in position to identify particular dangers; always he must make a judgment, in terms of materiality, as to whether and to what extent revelation to the patient is called for. He cannot know with complete exactitude what the patient would consider important to his decision, but on the basis of his medical training and experience he can sense how the average, reasonable patient expectably would react. Indeed, with knowledge of, or ability to learn, his patient's background and current condition, he is in a position superior to that of most others—attorneys, for example—who are called upon to make judgments on pain of liability in damages for unreasonable miscalculation.

From these considerations we derive the breadth of the disclosure of risks legally to be required. The scope of the standard is not subjective as to either the physician or the patient; it remains objective with due regard for the patient's informational needs and with suitable leeway for the physician's situation. In broad outline, we agree that "[a] risk is thus material when a reasonable person, in what the physician knows or should know to be the patient's position, would be likely to attach significance to the risk or cluster of risks in deciding whether or not to forgo the proposed therapy."

The topics importantly demanding a communication of information are the inherent and potential hazards of the proposed treatment, the alternatives to that treatment, if any, and the results likely if the patient remains untreated. The factors contributing significance to the dangerousness of a medical technique are, of course, the incidence of injury and the degree of the harm threatened. A very small chance of death or serious disablement may well be significant; a potential disability which dramatically outweighs the potential benefit of the therapy or the detriments of the existing malady may summon discussion with the patient.

There is no bright line separating the significant from the insignificant; the answer in any case must abide a rule of reason. Some dangers—infection, for example—are inherent in any operation; there is no obligation to communicate those of which persons of average sophistication are aware. Even more clearly, the physician bears no responsibility for discussion of hazards the patient has already discovered, or those having no apparent materiality to patients' decision on therapy. The disclosure doctrine, like others marking lines between permissible and impermissible behavior in medical practice, is in essence a requirement of conduct prudent under the circumstances. Whenever nondisclosure of particular risk information is open to debate by reasonable-minded men, the issue is for the finder of the facts.

Two exceptions to the general rule of disclosure have been noted by the courts. Each is in the nature of a physician's privilege not to disclose, and the reasoning underlying them is appealing. Each, indeed, is but a recognition that, as important as is the patient's right to know, it is greatly outweighed by the magnitudinous circumstances giving rise to the privilege. The first comes into play when the patient is unconscious or otherwise incapable of consenting, and harm from a failure to treat is imminent and outweighs any harm threatened by the proposed treatment. When a genuine emergency of that sort arises, it is settled that the impracticality of conferring with the patient dispenses with need for it. Even in situations of that character the physician should, as current law requires, attempt to secure a relative's consent if possible. But if time is too short to accommodate discussion, obviously the physician should proceed with the treatment.

The second exception obtains when risk-disclosure poses such a threat of detriment to the patient as to become unfeasible or contraindicated from a medical point of view. It is recognized that patients occasionally become so ill or emotionally distraught on disclosure as to foreclose a rational decision, or complicate or hinder the treatment, or perhaps even pose psychological damage to the patient. Where that is so, the cases have generally held that the physician is armed with a privilege to keep the information from the patient, and we think it clear that portents of that type may justify the physician in action he deems medically warranted. The critical inquiry is whether the physician responded to a sound medical judgment that communication of the risk information would present a threat to the patient's well-being.

The physician's privilege to withhold information for therapeutic reasons must be carefully circumscribed, however, for otherwise it might devour the disclosure rule itself. The privilege does not accept the paternalistic notion that the physician may remain silent simply because divulgence might prompt the patient to forgo therapy the physician feels the patient really needs. That attitude presumes instability or perversity for even the normal patient, and runs counter to the foundation principle that the patient should and ordinarily can make the choice for himself. Nor does the privilege contemplate operation save where the patient's reaction to risk information, as reasonably foreseen by the physician, is menacing. And even in a situation of that kind, disclosure to a close relative with a view to securing consent to the proposed treatment may be the only alternative open to the physician. . . .

NOTES

1 Patients ordinarily are persons unlearned in the medical sciences. Some few, of course, are schooled in branches of the medical profession or in related fields. But even within the latter group variations in degree of medical knowledge specifically referable to particular therapy may be broad, as for example, between a specialist and a general practitioner, or between a physician and a nurse. It may well be, then, that it is only in the unusual case that a court could safely assume that the patient's insights were on a parity with those of the treating physician.

2 The doctrine that a consent effective as authority to perform therapy can arise only from the patient's understanding of

alternatives to and risks of the therapy is commonly denominated "informed consent." The same appellation is frequently assigned to the doctrine requiring physicians, as a matter of duty to patients, to communicate information as to such alternatives and risks. See, *e.g.,* Comment, Informed Consent in Medical Malpractice, 55 Calif. L. Rev. 1396 (1967). While we recognize the general utility of shorthand phrases in literary expositions, we caution that uncritical use of the "informed consent" label can be misleading. See, *e.g.,* Plante, An Analysis of "Informed Consent," 36 Ford. L. Rev. 639, 671–72 (1968).

In duty-to-disclose cases, the focus of attention is more properly upon the nature and content of the physician's divulgence than the patient's understanding or consent. Adequate disclosure and informed consent are, of course, two sides of the same coin—the former a *sine qua non* of the latter. But the vital inquiry on duty to disclose relates to the physician's performance of an obligation, while one of the difficulties with analysis in terms of "informed consent" is its tendency to imply that what is decisive is the degree of the patient's comprehension. As we later emphasize, the physician discharges the duty when he makes a reasonable effort to convey sufficient information although the patient, without fault of the physician, may not fully grasp it. Even though the factfinder may have occasion to draw an inference on the state of the patient's enlightenment, the fact-finding process on performance of the duty ultimately reaches back to what the physician actually said or failed to say. And while the factual conclusion on adequacy of the revelation will vary as between patients—as, for example, between a lay patient and a physician-patient—the fluctuations are attributable to the kind of divulgence which may be reasonable under the circumstances.

3 Some doubt has been expressed as to the ability of physicians to suitably communicate their evaluations of risks and the advantages of optional treatment, and as to the lay patient's ability to understand what the physician tells him. Karchmer, Informed Consent: A Plaintiff's Medical Malpractice "Wonder Drug," 31 Mo. L. Rev. 29, 41 (1966). We do not share these apprehensions. The discussion need not be a disquisition, and surely the physician is not compelled to give his patient a short medical education; the disclosure rule summons the physician only to a reasonable explanation. That means generally informing the patient in non-technical terms as to what is at stake: the therapy alternatives open to him, the goals expectably to be achieved, and the risks that may ensue from particular treatment and no treatment. So informing the patient hardly taxes the physician, and it must be the exceptional patient who cannot comprehend such an explanation at least in a rough way.

4 For similar reasons, we reject the suggestion that disclosure should be discretionary with the physician.

THE VALUES UNDERLYING INFORMED CONSENT

*President's Commission for the Study of Ethical Problems
in Medicine and Biomedical and Behavioral Research*

The commission identifies and discusses two values that should guide decision making in the health-care provider-patient relationship: the promotion of a patient's well-being and respect for a patient's self-determination. The Commission locates the ethical foundation of informed consent in the promotion of these two values and makes recommendations intended to ensure that these values are respected and enhanced. In making its recommendations, the Commission rejects the idea that obtaining informed consent is simply a matter of reciting the contents of a form and getting a signature. It sees ethically valid consent as a *process* of shared decision making based on mutual respect and participation. Although stressing the importance of self-determination, the commission recognizes that some people may be permanently incapable of making their own decisions and that others may be temporarily unable to exercise their right of self-determination. It, therefore, provides some recommendations about making decisions for those unable to do so.

What are the values that ought to guide decision-making in the provider-patient relationship or by which the success of a particular interaction can be judged? The Commission finds two to be central: promotion of a patient's well-being and respect for a patient's self-determination.

SERVING THE PATIENT'S WELL-BEING

Therapeutic interventions are intended first and foremost to improve a patient's health. In most circumstances, people agree in a general way on what "improved health" means. Restoration of normal functioning (such as the repair of a fractured limb) and avoidance of untimely death (such as might occur without the use of antibiotics to control life-threatening infections in otherwise healthy persons) are obvious examples. Health care is, in turn, usually a means of promoting patients' well-being. The connection between a particular health care decision and an individual's well-being is not perfect, however. First, the definition of health can be quite controversial: does wrinkled skin or uncommonly short

Reprinted from President's Commission for the Study of Ethical Problems in Medicine and Biomedical and Behavioral Research, *Making Health Care Decisions,* Volume One: Report (1982), pp. 2–6, 41–46.

stature constitute impaired health, such that surgical repair or growth hormone is appropriate? Even more substantial variation can be found in ranking the importance of health with other goals in an individual's life. For some, health is a paramount value; for others—citizens who volunteer in time of war, nurses who care for patients with contagious diseases, hang-glider enthusiasts who risk life and limb—a different goal sometimes has primacy.

Absence of Objective Medical Criteria Even the most mundane case—in which there is little if any disagreement that some intervention will promote health—may well have no objective medical criteria that specify a single best way to achieve the goal. A fractured limb can be repaired in a number of ways; a life-threatening infection can be treated with a variety of antibiotics; mild diabetes is subject to control by diet, by injectable natural insulin, or by oral synthetic insulin substitutes. Health care professionals often reflect their own value preferences when they favor one alternative over another; many are matters of choice, dictated neither by biomedical principles or data nor by a single, agreed-upon professional standard.

In the Commission's survey it was clear that professionals recognize this fact: physicians maintained that decisional authority between them and their patients should depend on the nature of the decision at hand. Thus, for example, whether a pregnant woman over 35 should have amniocentesis was viewed as largely a patient's decision, whereas the decision of which antibiotic to use for strep throat was seen as primarily up to the doctor. Furthermore, on the question of whether to continue aggressive treatment for a cancer patient with metastases in whom such treatment had already failed, two-thirds of the physicians felt it was not a scientific, medical decision, but one that turned principally on personal values. And the same proportion felt the decision should be made jointly (which 64% of the doctors claimed it usually was).

Patients' Reasonable Subjective Preferences Determining what constitutes health and how it is best promoted also requires knowledge of patients' subjective preferences. In pursuit of the other goals and interests besides health that society deems legitimate, patients may prefer one type of medical intervention to another, may opt for no treatment at all, or may even request some treatment when a practitioner would prefer to follow a more conservative course that involved, at least for the moment, no medical intervention. For example, a slipped disc may be treated surgically or with medications and bed rest. Which treatment is better can be unclear, even to a physician. A patient may prefer surgery because, despite its greater risks, in the past that individual has spent considerable time in bed and become demoralized and depressed. A person with an injured knee, when told that surgery has about a 30% chance of reducing pain but almost no chance of eliminating it entirely, may prefer to leave the condition untreated. And a baseball pitcher with persistent inflammation of the elbow may prefer to take cortisone on a continuing basis even though the doctor suggests that a new position on the team would eliminate the inflammation permanently. In each case the goals and interests of particular patients incline them in different directions not only as to how, but even as to whether, treatment should proceed.

Given these two considerations—the frequent absence of objective medical criteria and the legitimate subjective preferences of patients—ascertain-

ing whether a health care intervention will, if successful, promote a patient's well-being is a matter of individual judgment. Societies that respect personal freedom usually reach such decisions by leaving the judgment to the person involved.

The Boundaries of Health Care This does not mean, however, that well-being and self-determination are really just two terms for the same value. For example, when an individual (such as a newborn baby) is unable to express a choice, the value that guides health care decisionmaking is the promotion of well-being—not necessarily an easy task but also certainly not merely a disguised form of self-determination.

Moreover, the promotion of well-being is an important value even in decisions about patients who can speak for themselves because the boundaries of the interventions that health professionals present for consideration are set by the concept of well-being. Through societal expectations and the traditions of the professions, health care providers are committed to helping patients and to avoiding harm. Thus, the well-being principle circumscribes the range of alternatives offered to patients: informed consent does not mean that patients can insist upon anything they might want. Rather, it is a choice among medically accepted and available options, all of which are believed to have some possibility of promoting the patient's welfare, including always the option of no further medical interventions, even when that would not be viewed as preferable by the health care providers.

In sum, promotion of patient well-being provides the primary warrant for health care. But, as indicated, well-being is not a concrete concept that has a single definition or that is solely within the competency of health care providers to define. Shared decisionmaking requires that a practitioner seek not only to understand each patient's needs and develop reasonable alternatives to meet those needs but also to present the alternatives in a way that enables patients to choose one they prefer. To participate in this process, patients must engage in a dialogue with the practitioner and make their views on well-being clear. The majority of physicians (56%) and the public (64%) surveyed by the Commission felt that increasing the patient's role in medical decision-making would improve the quality of health care.[1]

Since well-being can be defined only within each individual's experience, it is in most circumstances congruent to self-determination, to which the Report now turns.

RESPECTING SELF-DETERMINATION

Self-determination (sometimes termed "autonomy") is an individual's exercise of the capacity to form, revise, and pursue personal plans for life. Although it clearly has a much broader application, the relevance of self-determination in health care decisions seems undeniable. A basic reason to honor an individual's choices about health care has already emerged in this Report: under most circumstances the outcome that will best promote the person's well-being rests on a subjective judgment about the individual. This can be termed the instrumental value of self-determination.

More is involved in respect for self-determination than just the belief that each person knows what's best for him- or herself, however. Even if it could be shown that an expert (or a computer) could do the job better, the worth of the individual, as acknowledged in Western ethical traditions and especially in Anglo-American law, provides an independent—and more important—ground for recognizing self-determination as a basic principle in human relations, particularly when matters as important as those raised by health care are at stake. This noninstrumental aspect can be termed the intrinsic value of self-determination.

Intrinsic Value of Self-Determination The value of self-determination readily emerges if one considers what is lost in its absence. If a physician selects a treatment alternative that satisfies a patient's individual values and goals rather than allowing the patient to choose, the absence of self-determination has not interfered with the promotion of the patient's well-being. But unless the patient has requested this course of conduct, the individual will not have been shown proper respect as a person nor provided with adequate protection against arbitrary, albeit often well-meaning, domination by others. Self-determination can thus be seen as both a shield and a sword.

Freedom from Interference Self-determination as a shield is valued for the freedom from outside control it is intended to provide. It manifests the wish to be an instrument of one's own and "not of other men's acts of will."[2] In the context of health care, self-determination overrides practitioner-determination even if providers were able to demonstrate that they could (generally or in a specific instance) accurately assess the treatment an informed patient would choose. To permit action on the basis of a professional's assessment rather than on a patient's choice would deprive the patient of the freedom not to be forced to do something—whether or not that person would agree with the choice. Moreover, denying self-determination in this way risks generating the frustration people feel when their desires are ignored or countermanded. . . .

SUMMARY OF CONCLUSIONS AND RECOMMENDATIONS

. . . The ethical foundation of informed consent can be traced to the promotion of two values: personal well-being and self-determination. To ensure that these values are respected and enhanced, the Commission finds that patients who have the capacity to make decisions about their care must be permitted to do so voluntarily and must have all relevant information regarding their condition and alternative treatments, including possible benefits, risks, costs, other consequences, and significant uncertainties surrounding any of this information. This conclusion has several specific implications:

1. Although the informed consent doctrine has substantial foundations in law, it is essentially an ethical imperative.

2. Ethically valid consent is a process of shared decisionmaking based upon mutual respect and participation, not a ritual to be equated with reciting the contents of a form that details the risks of particular treatments.

3. Much of the scholarly literature and legal commentary about informed consent portrays it as a highly rational means of decisionmaking about health care matters, thereby suggesting that it may only be suitable for and applicable to well-educated,

articulate, self-aware individuals. Whether this is what the legal doctrine was intended to be or what it has inadvertently become, it is a view the Commission unequivocally rejects. Although subcultures within American society differ in their views about autonomy and individual choice and about the etiology of illness and the roles of healers and patients,[3] a survey conducted for the Commission found a universal desire for information, choice, and respectful communication about decisions.[4] Informed consent must remain flexible, yet the process, as the Commission envisions it throughout this Report, is ethically required of health care practitioners in their relationships with all patients, not a luxury for a few.

4.   Informed consent is rooted in the fundamental recognition—reflected in the legal presumption of competency—that adults are entitled to accept or reject health care interventions on the basis of their own personal values and in furtherance of their own personal goals. Nonetheless, patient choice is not absolute.

•   Patients are not entitled to insist that health care practitioners furnish them services when to do so would violate either the bounds of acceptable practice or a professional's own deeply held moral beliefs or would draw on a limited resource on which the patient has no binding claim.

•   The fundamental values that informed consent is intended to promote—self-determination and patient well-being—both demand that alternative arrangements for health care decisionmaking be made for individuals who lack substantial capacity to make their own decisions. Respect for self-determination requires, however, that in the first instance individuals be deemed to have decisional capacity, which should not be treated as a hurdle to be surmounted in the vast majority of cases, and that incapacity be treated as a disqualifying factor in the small minority of cases.

•   Decisionmaking capacity is specific to each particular decision. Although some people lack this capacity for all decisions, many are incapacitated in more limited ways and are capable of making some decisions but not others. The concept of capacity is best understood and applied in a functional manner. That is, the presence or absence of capacity does not depend on a person's status or on the decision reached, but on that individual's actual functioning in situations in which a decision about health care is to be made.

•   Decisionmaking incapacity should be found to exist only when people lack the ability to make decisions that promote their well-being in conformity with their own previously expressed values and preferences.

•   To the extent feasible people with no decisionmaking capacity should still be consulted about their own preferences out of respect for them as individuals.

5.   Health care providers should not ordinarily withhold unpleasant information simply because it is unpleasant. The ethical foundations of informed consent allow the withholding of information from patients only when they request that it be withheld or when its disclosure per se would cause substantial detriment to their well-being. Furthermore, the Commission found that most members of the public do not wish to have "bad news" withheld from them.

6.   Achieving the Commission's vision of shared decisionmaking based on mutual respect is ultimately the responsibility of individual health care professionals. However, health care institutions such as hospitals and professional schools have important roles to play in assisting health care professionals in this obligation. The manner in which health care is provided in institutional settings often results in a fragmentation of responsibility that may neglect the human side of health care. To assist in

guarding against this, institutional health care providers should ensure that ultimately there is one readily identifiable practitioner responsible for providing information to a particular patient. Although pieces of information may be provided by various people, there should be one individual officially charged with responsibility for ensuring that all the necessary information is communicated and that the patient's wishes are known to the treatment team.

7. Patients should have access to the information they need to help them understand their conditions and make treatment decisions. To this end the Commission recommends that health care professionals and institutions not only provide information but also assist patients who request additional information to obtain it from relevant sources, including hospital and public libraries.

8. As cases arise and new legislation is contemplated, courts and legislatures should reflect this view of ethically valid consent. Nevertheless, the Commission does not look to legal reforms as the primary means of bringing about changes in the relationship between health care professionals and patients.

9. The Commission finds that a number of relatively simple changes in practice could facilitate patient participation in health care decisionmaking. Several specific techniques—such as having patients express, orally or in writing, their understanding of the treatment consented to—deserve further study. Furthermore, additional societal resources need to be committed to improving the human side of health care, which has apparently deteriorated at the same time there have been substantial gains in health care technology. The Department of Health and Human Services, and especially the National Institutes of Health, is an appropriate agency for the development of initiatives and the evaluation of their efficacy in this area.

10. Because health care professionals are responsible for ensuring that patients can participate effectively in decisionmaking regarding their care, educators have a responsibility to prepare physicians and nurses to carry out this obligation. The Commission therefore concludes that:

    • Curricular innovations aimed at preparing health professionals for a process of mutual decisionmaking with patients should be continued and strengthened, with careful attention being paid to the development of methods for evaluating the effectiveness of such innovations.

    • Examinations and evaluations at the professional school and national levels should reflect the importance of these issues.

    • Serious attention should be paid to preparing health professionals for team practice in order to enhance patient participation and well-being.

11. Family members are often of great assistance to patients in helping to understand information about their condition and in making decisions about treatment. The Commission recommends that health care institutions and professionals recognize this and judiciously attempt to involve family members in decisionmaking for patients, with due regard for the privacy of patients and for the possibilities for coercion that such a practice may entail.

12. The Commission recognizes that its vision of health care decisionmaking may involve greater commitments of time on the part of health professionals. Because of the importance of shared decisionmaking based on mutual trust, not only for the promotion of patient well-being and self-determination but also for the therapeutic gains that can be realized, the Commission recommends that all medical and surgical interventions be thought of as including appropriate discussion with patients. Reimbursement to the professional should

therefore take account of time spent in discussion rather than regarding it as a separate item for which additional payment is made.

13. To protect the interests of patients who lack decisionmaking capacity and to ensure their well-being and self-determination, the Commission concludes that:

- Decisions made by others on patients' behalf should, when possible, attempt to replicate the ones patients would make if they were capable of doing so. When this is not feasible, decisions by surrogates on behalf of patients must protect the patients' best interests. Because such decisions are not instances of personal self-choice, limits may be placed on the range of acceptable decisions that surrogates make beyond those that apply when a person makes his or her own decisions.

- Health care institutions should adopt clear and explicit policies regarding how and by whom decisions are to be made for patients who cannot decide.

- Families, health care institutions, and professionals should work together to make health care decisions for patients who lack decisionmaking capacity. Recourse to courts should be reserved for the occasions when concerned parties are unable to resolve their disagreements over matters of substantial import, or when adjudication is clearly required by state law. Courts and legislatures should be cautious about requiring judicial review of routine health care decisions for patients who lack capacity.

- Health care institutions should explore and evaluate various informal administrative arrangements, such as "ethics committees," for review and consultation in nonroutine matters involving health care decisionmaking for those who cannot decide.

- As a means of preserving some self-determination for patients who no longer possess decisionmaking capacity, state courts and legislatures should consider making provision for advance directives through which people designate others to make health care decisions on their behalf and/or give instructions about their care.

The Commission acknowledges that the conclusions contained in this Report will not be simple to achieve. Even when patients and practitioners alike are sensitive to the goal of shared decisionmaking based on mutual respect, substantial barriers will still exist. Some of these obstacles, such as longstanding professional attitudes or difficulties in conveying medical information in ordinary language, are formidable but can be overcome if there is a will to do so. Others, such as the dependent condition of very sick patients or the ever-growing complexity and subspecialization of medicine, will have to be accommodated because they probably cannot be eliminated. Nonetheless, the Commission's vision of informed consent still has value as a measuring stick against which actual performance may be judged and as a goal toward which all participants in health care decisionmaking can strive. . . .

NOTES

1 Many physicians and patients said they believed an increased patient role would give the patient a better understanding of the medical condition and treatment, would improve physician performance in terms of the honesty and scope of discussion, and would generally improve the doctor-patient relationship. However, a number of physicians claimed that greater patient involvement would improve the quality of care because it would improve compliance and would make patients more cooperative and willing to accept the doctor's judgment.

2 Isaiah Berlin, "Two Concepts of Liberty," in *Four Essays on Liberty*, Clarendon Press, Oxford (1969) at 118–38.

3 Robert A. Hahn, *Culture and Informed Consent: An Anthropological Perspective* (1982), Appendix F, in Volume Three of this Report.

4 The Commission's survey of the public broke down these responses on the basis of variables such as age, gender, race, education, and income.

TRANSPARENCY: INFORMED CONSENT IN PRIMARY CARE
Howard Brody

Brody argues that accepted legal standards of informed consent, as commonly employed by the courts, give physicians the unhelpful message that informed consent is essentially a legalistic exercise intruding upon good medical care—an impression especially likely in the context of primary-care medicine. An alternative that would send physicians the right message, a "conversation" standard, is probably not legally workable, according to the author. Brody contends that a compromise, the "transparency" standard, sets reasonable obligations for physicians and permits courts to review appropriately. According to this standard, disclosure is considered adequate when the physician's basic thinking has been made transparent to the patient.

While the patient's right to give informed consent to medical treatment is now well-established both in U.S. law and in biomedical ethics, evidence continues to suggest that the concept has been poorly integrated into American medical practice, and that in many instances the needs and desires of patients are not being well met by current policies.[1] It appears that the theory and the practice of informed consent are out of joint in some crucial ways. This is particularly true for primary care settings, a context typically ignored by medical ethics literature, but where the majority of doctor-patient encounters occur. Indeed, some have suggested that the concept of informed consent is virtually foreign to primary care medicine where benign paternalism appropriately reigns and where respect for patient autonomy is almost completely absent.[2]

It is worth asking whether current legal standards for informed consent tend to resolve the problem or to exacerbate it. I will maintain that accepted legal standards, at least in the form commonly employed by courts, send physicians the wrong message about what is expected of them. An alternative standard that would send physicians the correct message, a conversation standard, is probably unworkable legally. As an alternative, I will propose a transparency standard as a compromise that gives physicians a doable task and allows courts to review

appropriately. I must begin, however, by briefly identifying some assumptions crucial to the development of this position even though space precludes complete argumentation and documentation.

CRUCIAL ASSUMPTIONS

Informed consent is a meaningful ethical concept only to the extent that it can be realized and promoted within the ongoing practice of good medicine. This need not imply diminished respect for patient autonomy, for there are excellent reasons to regard respect for patient autonomy as a central feature of good medical care. Informed consent, properly understood, must be considered an essential ingredient of good patient care, and a physician who lacks the skills to inform patients appropriately and obtain proper consent should be viewed as lacking essential medical skills necessary for practice. It is not enough to see informed consent as a nonmedical, legalistic exercise designed to promote patient autonomy, one that interrupts the process of medical care.

However, available empirical evidence strongly suggests that this is precisely how physicians currently view informed consent practices. Informed consent is still seen as bureaucratic legalism rather than as part of patient care. Physicians often deny the existence of realistic treatment alternatives, thereby attenuating the perceived need to inform the patient of meaningful options. While patients may be informed, efforts are seldom made to assess accurately the patient's actual need or desire for information, or what the patient then proceeds to do with

Reprinted with permission of the author and the publisher from *Hastings Center Report*, vol. 19 (September–October 1989), pp. 5–9. © The Hastings Center.

the information provided. Physicians typically under-estimate patients' desire to be informed and overestimate their desire to be involved in decision-making. Physicians may also view informed consent as an empty charade, since they are confident in their abilities to manipulate consent by how they discuss or divulge information.[3]

A third assumption is that there are important differences between the practice of primary care medicine and the tertiary care settings that have been most frequently discussed in the literature on informed consent. The models of informed consent discussed below typically take as the paradigm case something like surgery for breast cancer or the performance of an invasive and risky radiologic procedure. It is assumed that the risks to the patient are significant, and the values placed on alternative forms of treatment are quite weighty. Moreover, it is assumed that the specialist physician performing the procedure probably does a fairly limited number of procedures and thus could be expected to know exhaustively the precise risks, benefits, and alternatives for each.

Primary care medicine, however, fails to fit this model. The primary care physician, instead of performing five or six complicated and risky procedures frequently, may engage in several hundred treatment modalities during an average week of practice. In many cases, risks to the patient are negligible and conflicts over patient values and the goals of treatment or non-treatment are of little consequence. Moreover, in contrast to the tertiary care patient, the typical ambulatory patient is much better able to exercise freedom of choice and somewhat less likely to be intimidated by either the severity of the disease or the expertise of the physician; the opportunities for changing one's mind once treatment has begun are also much greater. Indeed, in primary care, it is much more likely for the full process of informed consent to treatment (such as the beginning and the dose adjustment of an anti-hypertensive medication) to occur over several office visits rather than at one single point in time.

It might be argued that for all these reasons, the stakes are so low in primary care that it is fully appropriate for informed consent to be interpreted only with regard to the specialized or tertiary care setting.

I believe that this is quite incorrect for three reasons. First, good primary care medicine ought to embrace respect for patient autonomy, and if patient autonomy is operationalized in informed consent, properly understood, then it ought to be part and parcel of good primary care. Second, the claim that the primary care physician cannot be expected to obtain the patient's informed consent seems to undermine the idea that informed consent could or ought to be part of the daily practice of medicine. Third, primary care encounters are statistically more common than the highly specialized encounters previously used as models for the concept of informed consent.[4]

ACCEPTED LEGAL STANDARDS

Most of the literature on legal approaches to informed consent addresses the tension between the community practice standard and the reasonable patient standard, with the latter seen as the more satisfactory, emerging legal standard.[5] However, neither standard sends the proper message to the physician about what is expected of her to promote patient autonomy effectively and to serve the informational needs of patients in daily practice.

The community practice standard sends the wrong message because it leaves the door open too wide for physician paternalism. The physician is instructed to behave as other physicians in that specialty behave, regardless of how well or how poorly that behavior serves patients' needs. Certainly, behaving the way other physicians behave is a task we might expect physicians to readily accomplish; unfortunately, the standard fails to inform them of the end toward which the task is aimed.

The reasonable patient standard does a much better job of indicating the centrality of respect for patient autonomy and the desired outcome of the informed consent process, which is revealing the information that a reasonable person would need to make an informed and rational decision. This standard is particularly valuable when modified to include the specific informational and decisional needs of a particular patient.

If certain things were true about the relationship between medicine and law in today's society, the reasonable patient standard would provide acceptable guidance to physicians. One feature would be that physicians esteem the law as a positive force in guiding their practice, rather than as a threat to their well-being that must be handled defensively. Another element would be a prospective consideration by the law of what the physician could reasonably have been expected to do in practice, rather than a retrospective review armed with the foreknowledge that some significant patient harm has already occurred.

Unfortunately, given the present legal climate, the physician is much more likely to get a mixed or an undesirable message from the reasonable patient standard. The message the physician hears from the reasonable patient standard is that one must exhaustively lay out all possible risks as well as benefits and alternatives of the proposed procedure. If one remembers to discuss fifty possible risks, and the patient in a particular case suffers the fifty-first, the physician might subsequently be found liable for incomplete disclosure. Since lawsuits are triggered when patients suffer harm, disclosure of risk becomes relatively more important than disclosure of benefits. Moreover, disclosure of information becomes much more critical than effective patient participation in decisionmaking. Physicians consider it more important to document what they said to the patient than to document how the patient used or thought about that information subsequently.

In specialty practice, many of these concerns can be nicely met by detailed written or videotaped consent documents, which can provide the depth of information required while still putting the benefits and alternatives in proper context. This is workable when one engages in a limited number of procedures and can have a complete document or videotape for each.[6] However, this approach is not feasible for primary care, when the number of procedures may be much more numerous and the time available with each patient may be considerably less. Moreover, it is simply not realistic to expect even the best educated of primary care physicians to rattle off at a moment's notice a detailed list of significant risks attached to any of the many drugs and therapeutic modalities they recommend.

This sets informed consent apart from all other aspects of medical practice in a way that I believe is widely perceived by nonpaternalistic primary care physicians, but which is almost never commented upon in the medical ethics literature. To the physician obtaining informed consent, *you never know when you are finished.* When a primary care physician is told to treat a patient for strep throat or to counsel a person suffering a normal grief reaction from the recent death of a relative, the physician has a good sense of what it means to complete the task at hand. When a physician is told to obtain the patient's informed consent for a medical intervention, the impression is quite different. A list of as many possible risks as can be thought of may still omit some significant ones. A list of all the risks that actually have occurred may still not have dealt with the patient's need to know risks in relation to benefits and alternatives. A description of all benefits, risks, and alternatives may not establish whether the patient has understood the information. If the patient says he understands, the physician has to wonder whether he really understands or whether he is simply saying this to be accommodating. As the law currently *appears* to operate (in the perception of the defensively minded physician), there never comes a point at which you can be certain that you have adequately completed your legal as well as your ethical task.

The point is not simply that physicians are paranoid about the law; more fundamentally, physicians are getting a message that informed consent is very different from any other task they are asked to perform in medicine. If physicians conclude that informed consent is therefore not properly part of medicine at all, but is rather a legalistic and bureaucratic hurdle they must overcome at their own peril, blame cannot be attributed to paternalistic attitudes or lack of respect for patient autonomy.

THE CONVERSATION MODEL

A metaphor employed by Jay Katz, informed consent as conversation, provides an approach to respect for patient autonomy that can be readily integrated within primary care practice.[7] Just as the specific needs of an individual patient for information, or the meaning that patient will attach to the information as it is presented, cannot be known in advance, one cannot always tell in advance how a conversation is going to turn out. One must follow the process along and take one's cues from the un-folding conversation itself. Despite the absence of any formal rules for carrying out or completing a conversation on a specific subject, most people have a good intuitive grasp of what it means for a conversation to be finished, what it means to change the subject in the middle of a conversation, and what it means to later reopen a conversation one had thought was completed when something new has just arisen. Thus, the metaphor suggests that informed consent consists not in a formal process carried out strictly by protocol but in a conversation designed to encourage patient participation in all medical decisions to the extent that the patient wishes to be included. The idea of informed consent as physician-patient conversation could, when properly developed, be a useful analytic tool for ethical issues in informed consent, and could also be a powerful educational tool for highlighting the skills and attitudes that a physician needs to successfully integrate this process within patient care.

If primary care physicians understand informed consent as this sort of conversation process, the idea that exact rules cannot be given for its successful management could cease to be a mystery. Physicians would instead be guided to rely on their own intuitions and communication skills, with careful attention to information received from the patient, to determine when an adequate job had been done in the informed consent process. Moreover, physicians would be encouraged to see informed consent as a genuinely mutual and participatory process, instead of being reduced to the one-way disclosure of information. In effect, informed consent could be demystified, and located within the context of the everyday relationships between physician and patient, albeit with a renewed emphasis on patient participation.[8]

Unfortunately, the conversation metaphor does not lend itself to ready translation into a legal standard for determining whether or not the physician has satisfied her basic responsibilities to the patient. There seems to be an inherently subjective element to conversation that makes it ill-suited as a legal standard for review of controversial cases. A conversation in which one participates is by its nature a very different thing from the same conversation described to an outsider. It is hard to imagine how a

jury could be instructed to determine in retrospect whether or not a particular conversation was adequate for its purposes. However, without the possibility for legal review, the message that patient autonomy is an important value and that patients have important rights within primary care would seem to be severely undermined. The question then is whether some of the important strengths of the conversation model can be retained in another model that does allow better guidance.

THE TRANSPARENCY STANDARD

I propose the transparency standard as a means to operationalize the best features of the conversation model in medical practice. According to this standard, adequate informed consent is obtained when a reasonably informed patient is allowed to participate in the medical decision to the extent that patient wishes. In turn, "reasonably informed" consists of two features: (1) the physician discloses the basis on which the proposed treatment, or alternative possible treatments, have been chosen; and (2) the patient is allowed to ask questions suggested by the disclosure of the physician's reasoning, and those questions are answered to the patient's satisfaction.

According to the transparency model, the key to reasonable disclosure is not adherence to existing standards of other practitioners, nor is it adherence to a list of risks that a hypothetical reasonable patient would want to know. Instead, disclosure is adequate when the physician's basic thinking has been rendered transparent to the patient. If the physician arrives at a recommended therapeutic or diagnostic intervention only after carefully examining a list of risks and benefits, then rendering the physician's thinking transparent requires that those risks and benefits be detailed for the patient. If the physician's thinking has not followed that route but has reached its conclusion by other considerations, then what needs to be disclosed to the patient is accordingly different. Essentially, the transparency standard requires the physician to engage in the typical patient-management thought process, only to *do it out loud in language understandable to the patient.*[9]

To see how this might work in practice, consider the following as possible general decision-making strategies that might be used by a primary physician:

1. The intervention, in addition to being presumably low-risk, is also routine and automatic. The physician, faced with a case like that presented by the patient, almost always chooses this treatment.

2. The decision is not routine but seems to offer clear benefit with minimal risk.

3. The proposed procedure offers substantial chances for benefit, but also very substantial risks.

4. The proposed intervention offers substantial risks and extremely questionable benefits. Unfortunately, possible alternative courses of action also have high risk and uncertain benefit.

The exact risks entailed by treatment loom much larger in the physician's own thinking in cases 3 and 4 than in cases 1 and 2. The transparency standard would require that physicians at least mention the various risks to patients in scenarios 3 and 4, but would not necessarily require physicians exhaustively to describe risks, unless the patient asked, in scenarios 1 and 2.

The transparency standard seems to offer some considerable advantages for informing physicians what can legitimately be expected of them in the promotion of patient autonomy while carrying out the activities of primary care medicine. We would hope that the well-trained primary care physician generally thinks before acting. On that assumption, the physician can be told exactly when she is finished obtaining informed consent—first, she has to share her thinking with the patient; secondly, she has to encourage and answer questions; and third, she has to discover how participatory he wishes to be and facilitate that level of participation. This seems a much more reasonable task within primary care than an exhaustive listing of often irrelevant risk factors.

There are also considerable advantages for the patient in this approach. The patient retains the right to ask for an exhaustive recital of risks and alternatives. However, the vast majority of patients, in a primary care setting particularly, would wish to sup-

plement a standardized recital of risks and benefits of treatment with some questions like, "Yes, doctor, but what does this really mean for me? What meaning am I supposed to attach to the information that you've just given?" For example, in scenarios 1 and 2, the precise and specific risk probabilities and possibilities are very small considerations in the thinking of the physician, and reciting an exhaustive list of risks would seriously misstate just what the physician was thinking. If the physician did detail a laundry list of risk factors, the patient might very well ask, "Well, doctor, just what should I think about what you have just told me?" and the thoughtful and concerned physician might well reply, "There's certainly a small possibility that one of these bad things will happen to you; but I think the chance is extremely remote and in my own practice I have never seen anything like that occur." The patient is very likely to give much more weight to that statement, putting the risks in perspective, than he is to the listing of risks. And that emphasis corresponds with an understanding of how the physician herself has reached the decision.

The transparency standard should further facilitate and encourage useful questions from patients. If a patient is given a routine list of risks and benefits and then is asked "Do you have any questions?" the response may well be perfunctory and automatic. If the patient is told precisely the grounds on which the physician has made her recommendation, and then asked the same question, the response is much more likely to be individualized and meaningful.

There certainly would be problems in applying the transparency standard in the courtroom, but these do not appear to be materially more difficult than those encountered in applying other standards; moreover, this standard could call attention to more important features in the ethical relationship between physician and patient. Consider the fairly typical case, in which a patient suffers harm from the occurrence of a rare but predictable complication of a procedure, and then claims that he would not have consented had he known about that risk. Under the present "enlightened" court standards, the jury would examine whether a reasonable patient would have needed to know about that risk factor prior to making a decision on the proposed intervention. Under the transparency standard, the question would instead be whether the physician thought about that risk factor as a relevant consideration prior to recommending the course of action to the patient. If the physician did seriously consider that risk factor, but failed to reveal that to the patient, he was in effect making up the patient's mind in advance about what risks were worth accepting. In that situation, the physician could easily be held liable. If, on the other hand, that risk was considered too insignificant to play a role in determining which intervention ought to be performed, the physician may still have rendered his thinking completely transparent to the patient even though that specific risk factor was not mentioned. In this circumstance, the physician would be held to have done an adequate job of disclosing information.[10] A question would still exist as to whether a competent physician ought to have known about that risk factor and ought to have considered it more carefully prior to doing the procedure. But that question raises the issue of negligence, which is where such considerations properly belong, and removes the problem from the context of informed consent. Obviously, the standard of informed consent is misapplied if it is intended by itself to prevent the practice of negligent medicine.

TRANSPARENCY IN MEDICAL PRACTICE

Will adopting a legal standard like transparency change medical practice for the better? Ultimately only empirical research will answer this question. We know almost nothing about the sorts of conversations primary care physicians now have with their patients, or what would happen if these physicians routinely tried harder to share their basic thinking about therapeutic choices. In this setting it is possible to argue that the transparency standard will have deleterious effects. Perhaps the physician's basic thinking will fail to include risk issues that patients, from their perspective, would regard as substantial. Perhaps how physicians think about therapeutic choice will prove to be too idiosyncratic and variable to serve as any sort of standard. Perhaps disclosing basic thinking processes will impede rather than promote optimal patient participation in decisions.

But the transparency standard must be judged, not only against ideal medical practice, but also against the present-day standard and the message it sends to practitioners. I have argued that that message is, "You can protect yourself legally only by guessing all bad outcomes that might occur and warning each patient explicitly that he might suffer any of them." The transparency standard is an attempt to send the message, "You can protect yourself legally by conversing with your patients in a way that promotes their participation in medical decisions, and more specifically by making sure that they see the basic reasoning you used to arrive at the recommended treatment." It seems at least plausible to me that the attempt is worth making.

The reasonable person standard may still be the best way to view informed consent in highly specialized settings where a relatively small number of discrete and potentially risky procedures are the daily order of business. In primary care settings, the best ethical advice we can give physicians is to view informed consent as an ongoing process of conversation designed to maximize patient participation after adequately revealing the key facts. Because the conversation metaphor does not by itself suggest measures for later judicial review, a transparency standard, or something like it, may be a reasonable way to operationalize that concept in primary care practice. Some positive side-effects of this might be more focus on good diagnostic and therapeutic decision-making on the physician's part, since it will be understood that the patient will be made aware of what the physician's reasoning process has been like, and better documentation of management decisions in the patient record. If these occur, then it will be clearer that the standard of informed consent has promoted rather than impeded high quality patient care.

ACKNOWLEDGMENTS

I plan to develop these ideas at somewhat greater length, with special emphasis on the duty to disclose remote risks, in a volume to be titled *The Healer's Power* (in preparation). I am grateful to Margaret Wallace and Stephen Wear for their insightful comments during the preparation of this manuscript.

REFERENCES

1 Charles W. Lidz *et al.,* "Barriers to Informed Consent," *Annals of Internal Medicine* 99:4 (1983), 539–43.

2 Tom L. Beauchamp and Laurence McCullough, *Medical Ethics: The Moral Responsibilities of Physicians* (Englewood Cliffs, NJ: Prentice-Hall, 1984).

3 For a concise overview of empirical data about contemporary informed consent practices, see Ruth R. Faden and Tom L. Beauchamp, *A History and Theory of Informed Consent* (New York: Oxford University Press, 1986), 98–99 and associated footnotes.

4 For efforts to address ethical aspects of primary care practice, see Ronald J. Christie and Barry Hoffmaster, *Ethical Issues in Family Medicine* (New York: Oxford University Press, 1986); and Harmon L. Smith and Larry R. Churchill, *Professional Ethics and Primary Care Medicine* (Durham, NC: Duke University Press, 1986).

5 Faden and Beauchamp, *A History and Theory of Informed Consent,* 23–49 and 114–50. I have also greatly benefited from an unpublished paper by Margaret Wallace.

6 For a specialty opinion to the contrary, see W. H. Coles *et al.,* "Teaching Informed Consent," in *Further Developments in Assessing Clinical Competence,* Ian R. Hart and Ronald M. Harden, eds. (Montreal: Can-Heal Publications, 1987), 241–70. This paper is interesting in applying to specialty care a model very much like the one I propose for primary care.

7 Jay Katz, *The Silent World of Doctor and Patient* (New York: Free Press, 1984).

8 Howard Brody, *Stories of Sickness* (New Haven: Yale University Press, 1987), 171–81.

9 For an interesting study of physicians' practices on this point, see William C. Wu and Robert A. Pearlman, "Consent in Medical Decisionmaking: The Role of Communication," *Journal of General Internal Medicine* 3:1 (1988), 9–14.

10 A court case that might point the way toward this line of reasoning is *Precourt v. Frederick,* 395 Mass. 689 (1985). See William J. Curran, "Informed Consent in Malpractice Cases: A Turn Toward Reality," *New England Journal of Medicine* 314:7 (1986), 429–31.

THE PRACTICE OF MEDICINE IN A MULTICULTURAL SOCIETY

ETHICAL RELATIVISM IN A MULTICULTURAL SOCIETY
Ruth Macklin

Macklin explores ethical problems that sometimes arise when a physician and a patient come from different cultural backgrounds. Respect for cultural diversity requires physicians to be generally tolerant or respectful of patients' differing beliefs and practices, according to Macklin. But in some cases tolerance can lead to harm of patients or their family members, while in other cases tolerance apparently conflicts with what mainstream Western ethics regards as the autonomy-based rights of the patient (e.g., the right to disclosure of medical information). In analyzing these ethical problems, Macklin attempts to determine which of the values involved are culturally relative and which are based on universal ethical principles.

Cultural pluralism poses a challenge to physicians and patients alike in the multicultural United States, where immigrants from many nations and diverse religious groups visit the same hospitals and doctors. Multiculturalism is defined as "a social-intellectual movement that promotes the value of diversity as a core principle and insists that all cultural groups be treated with respect and as equals" (Fowers and Richardson 1996, p. 609). This sounds like a value

Reprinted with permission of the publisher from *Kennedy Institute of Ethics Journal,* vol. 8, no. 1 (March 1998), pp. 1–2, 4–15, 17–22. Copyright © 1998 by The Johns Hopkins University Press.

that few enlightened people could fault, but it produces dilemmas and leads to results that are, at the least, problematic if not counterintuitive.

Critics of mainstream bioethics within the United States and abroad have complained about the narrow focus on autonomy and individual rights. Such critics argue that much—if not most—of the world embraces a value system that places the family, the community, or the society as a whole above that of the individual person. The prominent American sociologist Renée Fox is a prime example of such critics: "From the outset, the conceptual framework of bioethics has accorded paramount status to the value-complex of individualism, underscoring the principles of individual rights, autonomy, self-determination, and their legal expression in the jurisprudential notion of privacy" (Fox 1990, p. 206).

The emphasis on autonomy, at least in the early days of bioethics in the United States, was never intended to cut patients off from their families by focusing monistically on the patient. Instead, the intent was to counteract the predominant and longstanding paternalism on the part of the medical profession. In fact, there was little discussion of where the family entered in and no presumption that a family-centered approach to sick patients was somehow a violation of the patient's autonomy. Most patients want and need the support of their families, regardless of whether they seek to be autonomous agents regarding their own care. Respect for autonomy is perfectly consistent with recognition of the important role that families play when a loved one is ill. Autonomy has fallen into such disfavor among some bioethicists that the pendulum has begun to swing in the direction of families, with urgings to "take families seriously" (Nelson 1992) and even to consider the interests of family members equal to those of the competent patient (Hardwig 1990). . . .

A circumstance that arises frequently in multicultural urban settings is one that medical students bring to ethics teaching conferences. The patient and family are recent immigrants from a culture in which physicians normally inform the family rather than the patient of a diagnosis of cancer. The medical students wonder whether they are obligated to follow the family's wish, thereby respecting their cultural custom, or whether to abide by the ethical requirement at least to explore with patients their desire to receive information and to be a participant in their medical care. When medical students presented such a case in one of the conferences I co-direct with a physician, the dilemma was heightened by the demographic picture of the medical students themselves. Among the 14 students, 11 different countries of origin were represented. Those students either had come to the United States themselves to study or their parents had immigrated from countries in Asia, Latin America, Europe, and the Middle East.

The students began their comments with remarks like, "Where I come from, doctors never tell the patient a diagnosis of cancer" or "In my country, the doctor always asks the patient's family and abides by their wishes." The discussion centered on the question of whether the physician's obligation is to act in accordance with what contemporary medical ethics dictates in the United States or to respect the cultural difference of their patients and act according to the family's wishes. Not surprisingly, the medical students were divided on the answer to this question.

Medical students and residents are understandably confused about their obligation to disclose information to a patient when the patient comes from a culture in which telling a patient she has cancer is rare or unheard of. They ask: "Should I adhere to the American custom of disclosure or the Argentine custom of withholding the diagnosis?" That question is miscast, since there are some South Americans who want to know if they have cancer and some North Americans who do not. It is not, therefore, the cultural tradition that should determine whether disclosure to a patient is ethically appropriate, but rather the patient's wish to communicate directly with the physician, to leave communications to the family, or something in between. It would be a simplistic, if not unethical response on the part of doctors to reason that "This is the United States, we adhere to the tradition of patient autonomy, therefore I must disclose to this immigrant from the Dominican Republic that he has cancer."

Most patients in the United States do want to know their diagnosis and prognosis, and it has been amply demonstrated that they can emotionally and psychologically handle a diagnosis of cancer. The same may not be true, however, for recent immigrants from other countries, and it may be manifestly untrue in certain cultures. Although this, too, may change in time, several studies point to a cross-cultural difference in beliefs and practice regarding disclosure of diagnosis and informed consent to treatment.

One survey examined differences in the attitudes of elderly subjects from different ethnic groups toward disclosure of the diagnosis and prognosis of a terminal illness and regarding decision making at the end of life (Blackhall et al. 1995). This study found marked differences in attitudes between

Korean Americans and Mexican Americans, on the one hand, and African Americans and Americans of European descent, on the other. The Korean Americans and Mexican Americans were less likely than the other two groups to believe that patients should be told of a prognosis of terminal illness and also less likely to believe that the patient should make decisions about the use of life-support technology. The Korean and Mexican Americans surveyed were also more likely than the other groups to have a family-centered attitude toward these matters; they believed that the family and not the patient should be told the truth about the patient's diagnosis and prognosis. The authors of the study cite data from other countries that bear out a similar gap between the predominant "autonomy model" in the United States and the family-centered model prevalent in European countries as well as in Asia and Africa.

The study cited was conducted at 31 senior citizen centers in Los Angeles. In no ethnic group did 100 percent of its members favor disclosure or nondisclosure to the patient. Forty-seven percent of Korean Americans believed that a patient with metastatic cancer should be told the truth about the diagnosis, 65 percent of Mexican Americans held that belief, 87 percent of European Americans believed patients should be told the truth, and 89 percent of African Americans held that belief.

It is worth noting that the people surveyed were all 65-years-old or older. Not surprisingly, the Korean and Mexican American senior citizens had values closer to the cultures of their origin than did the African Americans and European Americans who were born in the United States. Another finding was that among the Korean American and Mexican American groups, older subjects and those with lower socioeconomic status tended to be opposed to truth telling and patient decision making more strongly than the younger, wealthier, and more highly educated members of these same groups. The authors of the study draw the conclusion that physicians should ask patients if they want to receive information and make decisions regarding treatment or whether they prefer that their families handle such matters.

Far from being at odds with the "autonomy model," this conclusion supports it. To ask patients

how much they wish to be involved in decision making does show respect for their autonomy: patients can then make the autonomous choice about who should be the recipient of information or the decision maker about their illness. What would fail to show respect for autonomy is for physicians to make these decisions without consulting the patient at all. If doctors spoke only to the families but not to the elderly Korean American or Mexican American patients without first approaching the patients to ascertain their wishes, they would be acting in the paternalistic manner of the past in America, and in accordance with the way many physicians continue to act in other parts of the world today. Furthermore, if physicians automatically withheld the diagnosis from Korean Americans because the majority of people in that ethnic group did not want to be told, they would be making an assumption that would result in a mistake almost 50 percent of the time.

INTOLERANCE AND OVERTOLERANCE

A medical resident in a New York hospital questioned a patient's ability to understand the medical treatment he had proposed and doubted whether the patient could grant truly informed consent. The patient, an immigrant from the Caribbean islands, believed in voodoo and sought to employ voodoo rituals in addition to the medical treatment she was receiving. "How can anyone who believes in that stuff be competent to consent to the treatment we offer?" the resident mused. The medical resident was an observant Jew who did not work, drive a car, or handle money on the sabbath and adhered to Kosher dietary laws. Both the Caribbean patient and the Orthodox Jew were devout believers in their respective faiths and practiced the accepted rituals of their religions.

The patient's voodoo rituals were not harmful to herself or to others. If the resident had tried to bypass or override the patient's decision regarding treatment, the case would have posed an ethical problem requiring resolution. Intolerance of another's religious or traditional practices that pose no threat of harm is, at least, discourteous and at worst, a prejudicial attitude. And it does fail to show respect for persons and their diverse religious and cultural practices. But it does not (yet) involve a failure to respect persons at a more fundamental level, which would occur if the doctor were to deny the patient her right to exercise her autonomy in the consent procedures.

At times, however, it is the family that interferes with the patient's autonomous decisions. Two brothers of a Haitian immigrant were conducting a conventional Catholic prayer vigil for their dying brother at his hospital bedside. The patient, suffering from terminal cancer and in extreme pain, had initially been given the pain medication he requested. Sometime later a nurse came in and found the patient alert, awake, and in excruciating pain from being undermedicated. When questioned, another nurse who had been responsible for the patient's care said that she had not continued to administer the pain medication because the patient's brothers had forbidden her to do so. Under the influence of the heavy dose of pain medication, the patient had become delirious and mumbled incoherently. The brothers took this as an indication that evil spirits had entered the patient's body and, according to the voodoo religion of their native culture, unless the spirit was exorcised it would stay with the family forever, and the entire family would suffer bad consequences. The patient manifested the signs of delirium only when he was on the medication, so the brothers asked the nurse to withhold the pain medication, which they believed was responsible for the entry of the evil spirit. The nurse sincerely believed that respect for the family's religion required her to comply with the patient's brothers' request, even if it contradicted the patient's own expressed wish. The person in charge of pain management called an ethics consultation, and the clinical ethicist said that the brothers' request, even if based on their traditional religious beliefs, could not override the patient's own request for pain medication that would relieve his suffering.

There are rarely good grounds for failing to respect the wishes of people based on their traditional religious or cultural beliefs. But when beliefs issue in actions that cause harm to others, attempts to prevent those harmful consequences are justifiable. An example that raises public health concerns is a ritual practiced among adherents of the religion known as Santería, practiced by people from Puerto Rico and other groups of Caribbean origin. The ritual involves scattering mercury around the household to ward off

bad spirits. Mercury is a highly toxic substance that can harm adults and causes grave harm to children. Shops called "botánicas" sell mercury as well as herbs and other potions to Caribbean immigrants who use them in their healing rituals.

The public health rationale that justifies placing limitations on people's behavior in order to protect others from harm can justify prohibition of the sale of mercury and penalties for its domestic use for ritual purposes. Yet the Caribbean immigrants could object: "You are interfering with our religious practices, based on your form of scientific medicine. This is our form of religious healing and you have no right to interfere with our beliefs and practices." It would not convince this group if a doctor or public health official were to reply: "But ours is a well-confirmed, scientific practice while yours is but an ignorant, unscientific ritual." It may very well appear to the Caribbean group as an act of cultural imperialism: "These American doctors with their Anglo brand of medicine are trying to impose it on us." This raises the difficult question of how to implement public health measures when the rationale is sufficiently compelling to prohibit religious or cultural rituals. Efforts to eradicate mercury sprinkling should enlist members of the community who agree with the public health position but who are also respected members of the cultural or religious group.

BELIEF SYSTEM OF A SUBCULTURE

Some widely held ethical practices have been transformed into law, such as disclosure of risks during an informed consent discussion and offering to patients the opportunity to make advanced directives in the form of a living will or appointing a health care agent. Yet these can pose problems for adherents of traditional cultural beliefs. In the traditional culture of Navajo Native Americans, a deeply rooted cultural belief underlies a wish not to convey or receive negative information. A study conducted on a Navajo Indian reservation in Arizona demonstrated how Western biomedical and bioethical concepts and principles can come into conflict with traditional Navajo values and ways of thinking (Carrese and Rhodes 1995). In March 1992, the Indian Health Service adopted the requirements of the Patient

Self-Determination Act, but the Indian Health Service policy also contains the following proviso: "Tribal customs and traditional beliefs that relate to death and dying will be respected to the extent possible when providing information to patients on these issues" (Carrese and Rhodes 1995, p. 828).

The relevant Navajo belief in this context is the notion that thought and language have the power to shape reality and to control events. The central concern posed by discussions about future contingencies is that traditional beliefs require people to "think and speak in a positive way." When doctors disclose risks of a treatment in an informed consent discussion, they speak "in a negative way," thereby violating the Navajo prohibition. The traditional Navajo belief is that health is maintained and restored through positive ritual language. This presumably militates against disclosing risks of treatment as well as avoiding mention of future illness or incapacitation in a discussion about advance care planning. Western-trained doctors working with the traditional Navajo population are thus caught in a dilemma. Should they adhere to the ethical and legal standards pertaining to informed consent now in force in the rest of the United States and risk harming their patients by "talking in a negative way"? Or should they adhere to the Navajo belief system with the aim of avoiding harm to the patients but at the same time violating the ethical requirement of disclosure to patients of potential risks and future contingencies?

The authors of the published study draw several conclusions. One is that hospital policies complying with the Patient Self-Determination Act are ethically troublesome for the traditional Navajo patients. Since physicians who work with that population must decide how to act, this problem requires a solution. A second conclusion is that "the concepts and principles of Western bioethics are not universally held" (Carrese and Rhodes 1995, p. 829). This comes as no surprise. It is a straightforward statement of the thesis of descriptive ethical relativism, the evident truth that a wide variety of cultural beliefs about morality exist in the world. The question for normative ethics endures: What follows from these particular facts of cultural relativity? A third conclusion the authors draw, in light of their find-

ings, is that health care providers and institutions caring for Navajo patients should reevaluate their policies and procedures regarding advance care planning.

This situation is not difficult to resolve, ethically or practically. The Patient Self-Determination Act does not mandate patients to actually make an advance directive; it requires only that health care institutions provide information to patients and give them the opportunity to make a living will or appoint a health care agent. A physician or nurse working for the Indian Health Service could easily fulfill this requirement by asking Navajo patients if they wish to discuss their future care or options, without introducing any of the negative thinking. This approach resolves one of the limitations of the published study. As the authors acknowledge, the findings reflect a more traditional perspective and the full range of Navajo views is not represented. So it is possible that some patients who use the Indian Health Service may be willing or even eager to have frank discussions about risks of treatment and future possibilities, even negative ones, if offered the opportunity.

It is more difficult, however, to justify withholding from patients the risks of proposed treatment in an informed consent discussion. The article about the Navajo beliefs recounts an episode told by a Navajo woman who is also a nurse. Her father was a candidate for bypass surgery. When the surgeon informed the patient of the risks of surgery, including the possibility that he might not wake up, the elderly Navajo man refused the surgery altogether. If the patient did indeed require the surgery and refused because he believed that telling him of the risk of not waking up would bring about that result, then it would be justifiable to withhold that risk of surgery. Should not that possibility be routinely withheld from all patients, then, since the prospect of not waking up could lead other people—Navajos and non-Navajos alike—to refuse the surgery? The answer is no, but it requires further analysis.

Respect for autonomy grants patients who have been properly informed the right to refuse a proposed medical treatment. An honest and appropriate disclosure of the purpose, procedures, risks, benefits, and available alternatives, provided in terms the patient can understand, puts the ultimate decision in the hands of the patient. This is the ethical standard according to Western bioethics. A clear exception exists in the case of patients who lack decisional capacity altogether, and debate continues regarding the ethics of paternalistically overriding the refusal of marginally competent patients. This picture relies on a key feature that is lacking in the Navajo case: a certain metaphysical account of the way the world works. Western doctors and their patients generally do not believe that talking about risks of harm will produce those harms (although there have been accounts that document the "dark side" of the placebo effect). It is not really the Navajo values that create the cross-cultural problem but rather, their metaphysical belief system holding that thought and language have the power to shape reality and control events. In fact, the Navajo values are quite the same as the standard Western ones: fear of death and avoidance of harmful side effects. To understand the relationship between cultural variation and ethical relativism, it is essential to distinguish between cultural relativity that stems from a difference in values and that which can be traced to an underlying metaphysics or epistemology.

Against this background, only two choices are apparent: insist on disclosing to Navajo patients the risks of treatment and thereby inflict unwanted negative thoughts on them; or withhold information about the risks and state only the anticipated benefits of the proposed treatment. Between those two choices, there is no contest. The second is clearly ethically preferable. It is true that withholding information about the risks of treatment or potential adverse events in the future radically changes what is required by the doctrine of informed consent. It essentially removes the "informed" aspect, while leaving in place the notion that the patient should decide. The physician will still provide some information to the Navajo patient, but only the type of information that is acceptable to the Navajos who adhere to this particular belief system. True, withholding certain information that would typically be disclosed to patients departs from the ethical ideal of informed consent, but it does so in order to achieve the ethically appropriate goal of beneficence in the care of patients.

The principle of beneficence supports the withholding of information about risks of treatment from

Navajos who hold the traditional belief system. But so, too, does the principle of respect for autonomy. Navajos holding traditional beliefs can act autonomously only when they are not thinking in a negative way. If doctors tells them about bad contingencies, that will lead to negative thinking, which in their view will fail to maintain and restore health. The value of both doctor and patient is to maintain and restore health. A change in the procedures regarding the informed consent discussion is justifiable based on a distinctive background condition: the Navajo belief system about the causal efficacy of thinking and talking in a certain way. The less-than-ideal version of informed consent does constitute a "lower" standard than that which is usually appropriate in today's medical practice. But the use of a "lower" standard is justified by the background assumption that that is what the Navajo patient prefers.

What is relative and what is nonrelative in this situation? There is a clear divergence between the Navajo belief system and that of Western science. That divergence leads to a difference in what sort of discussion is appropriate for traditional Navajos in the medical setting and that which is standard in Western medical practice. According to one description, "always disclose the risks as well as the benefits of treatment to patients," the conclusion points to ethical relativism. But a more general description, one that heeds today's call for cultural awareness and sensitivity, would be: "Carry out an informed consent discussion in a manner appropriate to the patient's beliefs and understanding." That obligation is framed in a nonrelative way. A heart surgeon would describe the procedures, risks, and benefits of bypass surgery in one way to a patient who is another physician, in a different way to a mathematician ignorant of medical science, in yet another way to a skilled craftsman with an eighth grade education, and still differently to a traditional Navajo. The ethical principle is the same; the procedures differ.

OBLIGATIONS OF PHYSICIANS

The problem for physicians is how to respond when an immigrant to the United States acts according to the cultural values of her native country, values that differ widely from accepted practices in American

Suppose an African immigrant asks an ___ to perform genital surgery on her baby girl. Or imagine that a Laotian immigrant from the Iu Mien culture brings her four-month-old baby to the pediatrician for a routine visit and the doctor discovers burns on the baby's stomach. The African mother seeks to comply with the tradition in her native country, Somalia, where the vast majority of women have had clitoridectomies. The Iu Mien woman admits that she had used a traditional folk remedy to treat what she suspected was her infant's case of a rare folk illness.

What is the obligation of physicians in the United States when they encounter patients in such situations? At one extreme is the reply that in the United States, physicians are obligated to follow the ethical and cultural practices accepted here and have no obligation to comply with patients' requests that embody entirely different cultural values. At the other extreme is the view that cultural sensitivity requires physicians to adhere to the traditional beliefs and practices of patients who have emigrated from other cultures.

A growing concern on the part of doctors and public health officials is the increasing number of requests for genital cutting and defense of the practice by immigrants to the United States and European countries. A Somalian immigrant living in Houston said he believed his Muslim faith required him to have his daughters undergo the procedure; he also stated his belief that it would preserve their virginity. He was quoted as saying, "It's my responsibility. If I don't do it, I will have failed my children" (Dugger 1996, p. 1). Another African immigrant living in Houston sought a milder form of the cutting she had undergone for her daughter. The woman said she believed it was necessary so her daughter would not run off with boys and have babies before marriage. She was disappointed that Medicaid would not cover the procedure, and planned to go to Africa to have the procedure done there. A New York City physician was asked by a father for a referral to a doctor who would do the procedure on his three-year-old daughter. When the physician told him this was not done in America, the man accused the doctor of not understanding what he wanted (Dugger 1996, pp. 1, 9).

However, others in our multicultural society consider it a requirement of "cultural sensitivity" to accommodate in some way to such requests of African immigrants. Harborview Medical Center in Seattle sought just such a solution. A group of doctors agreed to consider making a ritual nick in the fold of skin that covers the clitoris, but without removing any tissue. However, the hospital later abandoned the plan after being flooded with letters, postcards, and telephone calls in protest (Dugger 1996).

A physician who conducted research with East African women living in Seattle held the same view as the doctors who sought a culturally sensitive solution. In a talk she gave to my medical school department, she argued that Western physicians must curb their tendency to judge cultural practices different from their own as "rational" or "irrational." Ritual genital cutting is an "inalienable" part of some cultures, and it does a disservice to people from those cultures to view it as a human rights violation. She pointed out that in the countries where female genital mutilation (FGM) is practiced, circumcised women are "normal." Like some anthropologists who argue for a "softer" linguistic approach (Lane and Rubinstein 1996), this researcher preferred the terminology of "circumcision" to that of "female genital mutilation."

One can understand and even have some sympathy for the women who believe they must adhere to a cultural ritual even when they no longer live in the society where it is widely practiced. But it does not follow that the ritual is an "inalienable" part of that culture, since every culture undergoes changes over time. Furthermore, to contend that in the countries where FGM is practiced, circumcised women are "normal" is like saying that malaria or malnutrition is "normal" in parts of Africa. That a human condition is statistically normal implies nothing whatever about whether an obligation exists to seek to alter the statistical norm for the betterment of those who are affected.

Some Africans living in the United States have said they are offended that Congress passed a law prohibiting female genital mutilation that appears to be directed specifically at Africans. France has also passed legislation, but its law relies on general statutes that prohibit violence against children (Dugger 1996). In a recent landmark case, a French court sent a Gambian woman to jail for having had the genitals of her two baby daughters mutilated by a midwife. French doctors report an increasing number of cases of infants who are brought to clinics hemorrhaging or with severe infections. . . .

Another case vignette describes a Laotian woman from the Mien culture who immigrated to the United States and married a Mien man. When she visited her child's pediatrician for a routine four-month immunization, the doctor was horrified to see five red and blistered quarter-inch round markings on the child's abdomen (Case Study: Culture, Healing, and Professional Obligations 1993). The mother explained that she used a traditional Mien "cure" for pain, since she thought the infant was experiencing a rare folk illness among Mien babies characterized by incessant crying and loss of appetite, in addition to other symptoms. The "cure" involves dipping a reed in pork fat, lighting the reed, and passing the burning substance over the skin, raising a blister that "pops like popcorn." The popping indicates that the illness is not related to spiritual causes; if no blisters appear, then a shaman may have to be summoned to conduct a spiritual ritual for a cure. As many as 11 burns might be needed before the end of the "treatment." The burns are then covered with a mentholated cream.

The Mien woman told the pediatrician that infection is rare and the burns heal in a week or so. Scars sometimes remain but are not considered disfiguring. She also told the doctor that the procedure must be done by someone skilled in burning, since if a burn is placed too near the line between the baby's mouth and navel, the baby could become mute or even retarded. The mother considered the cure to have been successful in the case of her baby, since the child had stopped crying and regained her appetite. Strangely enough, the pediatrician did not say anything to the mother about her practice of burning the baby, no doubt from the need to show "cultural sensitivity." She did, however, wonder later whether she should have said something since she thought the practice was dangerous and also cruel to babies. . . .

[In commentaries on these cases, one often finds] a great reluctance to criticize, scold, or take le-

gal action against parents from other cultures who employ painful and potentially harmful rituals that have no scientific basis. This attitude of tolerance is appropriate against the background knowledge that the parents do not intend to harm the child and are simply using a folk remedy widely accepted in their own culture. But tolerance of these circumstances must be distinguished from a judgment that the actions harmful to children should be permitted to continue. What puzzles me is the notion that "cultural sensitivity" must extend so far as to refrain from providing a solid education to these parents about the potential harms and the infliction of gratuitous pain. In a variety of other contexts, we accept the role of physicians as educator of patients. Doctors are supposed to tell their patients not to smoke, to lose weight, to have appropriate preventive medical checkups such as pap smears, mammograms, and proctoscopic examinations.

Pediatricians are thought to have an even more significant obligation to educate the parents of their vulnerable patients: inform them of steps that minimize the risks of sudden infant death syndrome, tell them what is appropriate for an infant's or child's diet, and give them a wide array of other social and psychological information designed to keep a child healthy and flourishing. Are these educational obligations of pediatricians only appropriate for patients whose background culture is that of the United States or Western Europe? Should a pediatrician not attempt to educate parents who, in their practice of the Santería religion, sprinkle mercury around the house? The obligation of pediatricians to educate and even to urge parents to adopt practices likely to contribute to the good health and well being of their children, and to avoid practices that will definitely or probably cause harm and suffering, should know no cultural boundaries.

My position is consistent with the realization that Western medicine does not have all the answers. This position also recognizes that some traditional healing practices are not only not harmful but may be as beneficial as those of Western medicine. The injunction to "respect cultural diversity" could rest on the premise that Western medicine sometimes causes harm without compensating benefits (which is true) or on the equally true premise that traditional practices such as acupuncture and herbal remedies, once scorned by mainstream Western medicine, have come to be accepted side-by-side with the precepts of scientific medicine. Typically, however, respect for multicultural diversity goes well beyond these reasonable views and requires toleration of manifestly painful or harmful procedures such as the burning remedy employed in the Mien culture. We ought to be able to respect cultural diversity without having to accept every single feature embedded in traditional beliefs and rituals.

The reluctance to impose modern medicine on immigrants from a fear that it constitutes yet another instance of "cultural imperialism" is misplaced. Is it not possible to accept non-Western cultural practices side by side with Western ones, yet condemn those that are manifestly harmful and have no compensating benefit except for the cultural belief that they are beneficial? [Two] commentators who urged respect for the Mien woman's burning treatment on the grounds that it is practiced widely, the reasons for it are widely understood among the Mien, and the procedure works, from a Mien point of view [Brown and Jameton 1993, p. 17], seemed to be placing that practice on a par with practices that "work" from the point of view of Western medicine. Recall that if the skin does not blister, the Mien belief holds that the illness may be related to spiritual causes and a shaman might have to be called. Should the pediatrician stand by and do nothing, if the child has a fever of 104° and the parent calls a shaman because the skin did not blister? Recall also that the Mien woman told the pediatrician that if the burns are not done in the right place, the baby could become mute or even retarded. Must we reject the beliefs of Western medicine regarding causality and grant equal status to the Mien beliefs? To refrain from seeking to educate such parents and to not exhort them to alter their traditional practices is unjust, as it exposes the immigrant children to health risks that are not borne by children from the majority culture.

It is heresy in today's postmodern climate of respect for the belief systems of all cultures to entertain the notion that some beliefs are demonstrably false and others, whether true or false, lead to manifestly harmful actions. We are not supposed to talk about the evolution of scientific ideas or about progress in the Western world, since that is a colonialist way of thinking. If it is simply "the white man's burden, medicalized" (Morsy 1991) to urge African families living in the United States not to genitally mutilate their daughters, or to attempt to educate Mien mothers about the harms of burning their babies, then we are doomed to permit ethical relativism to overwhelm common sense.

Multiculturalism, as defined at the beginning of this paper, appears to embrace ethical relativism and yet is logically inconsistent with relativism. The second half of the definition states that multiculturalism "insists that all cultural groups be treated with respect and as equals." What does this imply with regard to cultural groups that oppress or fail to respect other cultural groups? Must the cultural groups that violate the mandate to treat all cultural groups with respect and as equals be respected themselves? It is impossible to insist that all such groups be treated with respect and as equals, and at the same time accept any particular group's attitude toward and treatment of another group as inferior. Every cultural group contains subgroups within the culture: old and young, women and men, people with and people without disabilities. Are the cultural groups that discriminate against women or people with disabilities to be respected equally with those that do not?

What multiculturalism does not say is whether all of the beliefs and practices of all cultural groups must be equally respected. It is one thing to require that cultural, religious, and ethnic groups be treated as equals; that conforms to the principle of justice as equality. It is quite another thing to say that any cultural practice whatever of any group is to be tolerated and respected equally. This latter view is a statement of extreme ethical relativism. If multiculturalists endorse the principle of justice as equality, however, they must recognize that normative ethical relativism entails the illogical consequence of toleration and acceptance of numerous forms of injustice in those cultures that oppress women and religious and ethnic minorities.

REFERENCES

Blackhall, Leslie; Murphy, Sheila T.; Frank, Gelya; Michel, Vicki; and Azen, Stanley. 1995. Ethnicity and Attitudes Toward Patient Autonomy. *Journal of the American Medical Association* 274: 820–25.

Brown, Kate, and Jameton, Andrew. 1993. Culture, Healing, and Professional Obligations: Commentary. *Hastings Center Report* 23 (4): 17.

Carrese, Joseph, and Rhodes, Lorna A. 1995. Western Bioethics on the Navajo Reservation: Benefit or Harm? *Journal of the American Medical Association* 274: 826–29.

Case Study: Culture, Healing, and Professional Obligations. 1993. *Hastings Center Report* 23 (4): 15.

Dugger, Celia W. 1996. Tug of Taboos: African Genital Rite vs. U.S. Law. *New York Times* (28 December): 1, 9.

Fowers, Blaine J., and Richardson, Frank C. 1996. Why Is Multiculturalism Good? *American Psychologist* 51: 609–21.

Fox, Renée C. 1990. The Evolution of American Bioethics: A Sociological Perspective. In *Social Science Perspectives on*

Medical Ethics, ed. George Weisz, pp. 201–20. Philadelphia: University of Pennsylvania Press.

Hardwig, John. 1990. "What About the Family?" *Hastings Center Report* 20 (2): 5–10.

Lane, Sandra D., and Rubinstein, Robert A. 1996. Judging the Other: Responding to Traditional Female Genital Surgeries. *Hastings Center Report* 26 (5): 31–40.

Morsy, Soheir A. 1991. Safeguarding Women's Bodies: The White Man's Burden Medicalized. *Medical Anthropology Quarterly* 5 (1): 19–23.

Nelson, James Lindemann. 1992. Taking Families Seriously. *Hastings Center Report* 22 (4): 6–12.

QUALITY CARE AND THE WOUNDS OF DIVERSITY
Kenneth Kipnis

Presenting a case of a Korean patient who did not want to be treated by Japanese physicians, Kipnis raises the question of when, if ever, it is appropriate to accommodate a patient's prejudice. He examines a variety of possible answers to this question, including the view that medical staff should accommodate only those prejudicial beliefs that result from past victimization. Kipnis tentatively concludes that if efforts to change a patient's thinking are unsuccessful, his or her wishes should be honored.

Since 1982 I have done ethics consultation at a number of hospitals in the state of Hawaii. Uniquely separate from the Mainland, situated in an isolated part of the Mid-Pacific, many of us who have been transplanted here find ourselves developing something of a planetary perspective. Heretofore accustomed to being a majority, Caucasians like myself represent only about a third of the population. There are about as many Japanese-Americans. The balance is a cosmopolitan blend of Chinese, Filipinos, Hawaiians, Samoans, Koreans, Puerto Ricans, Native Americans, African-Americans and other groups. About 40% of our current marriages are interracial and all of us are minorities. It is an unusual place to be doing ethics.

Several years ago I was called to a hospital to assist in a case involving an older Korean gentle-

man. He had had a difficult medical condition—hard to diagnose and treat—and had steadily gotten worse despite the vigorous efforts of the medical and nursing staffs. At last the doctors had felt they knew what the problem was and offered the patient a treatment plan that promised a better than 50% chance of recovery with only minimal risks. Nonetheless the patient had refused further treatment. He said that, having suffered enough already, he did not want the doctors to do anything else. Though there had been an earlier history of mental illness, there was no evidence that it was playing any role in this refusal. He had understood his options as these had been explained and he had appreciated the consequences of his choice. This refusal was properly charted and the staff awaited the expected terminal trajectory.

Had nothing else occurred, I would not have been called in and the Korean patient would likely have expired as expected. But when he was asked the hospital's routine questions about code status, his request for full support generated the call for an

Reprinted with permission of the author from "Newsletter on Philosophy and Medicine," in *APA Newsletters,* vol. 97, no. 2 (Spring 1998), pp. 112–114.

ethics consult. Following a telephone conversation with the patient's attending physician, I went to the bedside and joined up with a hospital ethics consultant, a very experienced nurse who had just finished reviewing his chart. The task for the two of us was to understand the glaring discrepancy between his informed refusal of potentially life-saving treatment and his firm request for cardioversion if he went into arrest. The latter was a burdensome procedure that could prolong his life for only a brief interval. Why was he rejecting the promising treatment but requesting the code? What was making the difference for him?

For at least 40 minutes the two of us conversed with the patient, questioned him, gently pressed him, and still the discrepancy remained opaque. Finally, perhaps caving in to our persistence, he quietly asked if we would mind if he said something embarrassing. We encouraged him to go on. In the most timorous of voices, the Korean gentleman asked if we had noticed that all of his doctors had been Japanese?

I was stunned by an instantaneous appreciation of what was going on. For most of the first half of the 20th century, Imperial Japan had ruthlessly tyrannized Korea much as Nazi Germany had oppressed Poland during World War II. Exploited as inferiors, many Koreans still retain powerful anti-Japanese sentiments. This unfortunate man perceived himself as exquisitely vulnerable, surrounded by his too-familiar oppressors.

As it happened, neither of us at the bedside had noticed that the gentleman's doctors had been Japanese. The physician I had spoken with on the telephone was a woman with an unexceptional accent and a non-Japanese last name. The nurse working with me had never met her. We did, however, know enough recent Korean-Japanese history to appreciate the patient's concerns. He "knew" why he kept getting worse. The Japanese doctors were not trying to make him better. What we were seeing as failures to improve, he saw as successful attempts to cause his death. To make things even worse, he was familiar enough with Western ideals of toleration, equality, and individualism to know that, in Hawaii, it was improper to offer his candid opinion of Japanese physicians. There was a cryptic note in the chart

that he had once asked a nurse if he could have a doctor in a three-piece suit. He had noticed, we later learned, that while Japanese doctors on the unit wore white coats, many of the others wore three-piece suits. When this ploy failed, he had then tried to evade the deadly ministrations of his Japanese physicians by refusing their offers of treatment. Of course he would want a prompt emergency response if he went into an immediately life-threatening condition. After all, he wanted to live. Paradoxically, he was refusing life-saving treatment in order to save his life.

Clearly the patient needed to see a non-Japanese physician. The nurse-ethicist relayed our findings to a very cooperative attending who readily agreed with our recommendation. Within a few hours another doctor—a non-Japanese physician wearing a three-piece suit—was at the bedside persuading the patient to accept treatment.

In the years since, I have often reflected on what happened that afternoon. On many occasions I have recounted the story to medical and nursing students and to clinical staff. I have used the case to show that ethics consultation can be critically important in patient care. Here was an instance in which a patient's life may have been saved by an ethics consult. I have used it to illustrate the importance of understanding the patient's underlying value commitments. There are times when our job isn't done until the patient's decision makes sense against the background of the patient's reasonably stable personal values. Here the two of us kept up the questioning until the patient's process of decision came into focus. In retrospect it was critically important that we took the time we needed. And I have used the case to illustrate the importance of understanding cultural differences. Perhaps the two of us—and the hospital staff as well—should have been more appreciative of Korean cultural sensibilities.

But more recently I have been troubled by another aspect of this case.

The history of the United States can easily be read as a dramatic succession of cultural collisions. From the prototypical "Columbian encounter," to the expansion into lands occupied by Native Americans, to our social and political responses to race-based slavery, and up to our current divisions around immigration and affirmative action, we have wrestled mightily with the painful legacies—the wounds—of cultural diversity. While much of this history is unbecoming, there is some credit we can take for the progress that has been made in overcoming prejudice and eliminating discrimination. Schools that formerly barred the entry of women and minority groups now strive for diversity. Social institutions now commonly express and often honor their commitments to nondiscrimination. Prejudicial slurs and racial stereotypes, when they are advanced, are frequently challenged. These familiar features of American life are new. For many—perhaps most of us—they are welcome.

Even so, clinicians still see patients who demand accommodation on the basis of racist beliefs and attitudes. Prejudice and stereotypical thinking patterns may be dominating a patient's preferences when, for example, a Southern white male in an emergency room refuses to be treated by a black resident, or a Vietnam veteran objects to being attended by a Southeast Asian doctor. While, on the one hand, clinicians have a professional concern to help make the patient comfortable, that value can be in conflict both with the civic obligation to refrain from becoming an instrument of invidious discrimination and the collegial obligation to stand up for the professional dignity of one's colleagues.

What has bothered me about my role in the case of the Korean gentleman was that, until recently, those aspects of the case had completely escaped my attention. Notwithstanding the history of Japan and Korea during the first half of the 20th century, I had no reason to believe that physicians of Japanese ancestry, currently practicing in Hawaii, had it in for their Korean patients. Both the nurse-ethicist and I viewed the gentleman's misgivings as wholly baseless. Although we did not discuss the matter with the patient (as perhaps we should have), we took it for granted that even though Japanese occupation forces had historically mistreated Korean nationals, it did not follow that Japanese doctors in Hawaii were now mistreating Korean patients. Yet instead of challenging the patient's beliefs on the basis of our own experience, the two of us left them unquestioned. Not only that: despite the absence of any reason to doubt the fidelity and honor of the gentleman's Japanese

physician, we successfully effected her withdrawal in keeping with what we believed to be the patient's baseless prejudices. Was it right for us to do this? If it was, when is it appropriate to accommodate patient prejudice and when is it not?

One route might be to distinguish between prejudicial beliefs that are the consequence of past victimization and those that emerge purely as an integral aspect of the processes of oppression. It seems easy to sympathize with a Jewish survivor of the Nazi concentration camps who is severely distressed at the prospect of being treated by a German physician. It seems difficult to sympathize with an anti-Semitic skinhead who does not want to be seen or touched by a Jewish physician. In similar fashion, one might suppose that the Korean gentleman's sentiments are grounded in his painful memories of the brutal Japanese occupation and, with that pedigree, perhaps worthy of accommodation. But the Vietnam veteran's objection to treatment by a Southeast Asian points up the difficulty with this approach. Is the veteran a victim or an oppressor? Strong cases might be made both ways. Without in the least diminishing the seriousness of the damage they may do, racists themselves may lead profoundly diminished lives, spiritually and socially crippled by the attitudes they have absorbed. Alas, the world does not divide nearly into victims and oppressors; and, accordingly, a refusal to accommodate a prejudice-based preference may merely reflect the limits of our moral imagination.

At least one colleague has asked me whether I knew—really knew—that the Japanese physicians were not trying to harm the Korean patient. In related discussions I have encountered vigorous disagreement about whether women who routinely ask for female gynecologists are merely prejudiced against men or merely knowledgeable about the relative merits of women. Although there was agreement in that debate that some male ob-gyns were sensitive and considerate and some female ob-gyns were not, there appeared also to be consensus (among those in a position to know) that female ob-gyns were a better bet. Is this a prejudice or not? Having never been a Korean patient of a Japanese physician (or, for that matter, a female patient of an ob-gyn), my experience is an inferior source of data.

Perhaps on this basis, we should routinely defer to patient preferences. Maybe they know something we do not.

On the other hand, these preferences are very like those that have historically created institutionalized practices of sexism and racism. Until the 1960s many American owners of hotels and restaurants assumed—perhaps reasonably—that white customers would not want to dine and lodge with black customers. The presence of widespread prejudice can have the result of excluding stigmatized groups from careers and opportunities that are routinely open to others. Perhaps the distinction between accommodatable and unaccommodatable prejudice turns on the severity of the cumulative effects of accommodation. The Japanese doctors working at the hospital were not, it seemed, suffering discernable losses as a consequence of Korean prejudice. For all I know, my case may have been unique. However, the historically broad reticence among white patients to accept the ministrations of black physicians may have contributed to unjust exclusionary practices. We may be better off as a consequence of holding that the preferences of others cannot be used to justify hiring on the basis of sex or race. Notwithstanding male modesty, female sports reporters now have equal access to men's locker rooms. The societal need to overcome damaging discrimination can, it seems, give us a weighty reason to refuse to accommodate prejudice-based preferences. Perhaps it is this social injustice that should properly limit accommodation.

But recollect that the Korean gentleman was existentially prepared to die rather than accept treatment by his Japanese doctor. One supposes that, besides Koreans, other groups may be equally willing to live out equally firm commitments to prejudice-based preferences. Consider for the moment only those cases in which the accommodation to prejudice-based preference does significant damage to the interests of stigmatized groups. Should HMOs, hospitals and health-care professionals be prepared to sacrifice the lives of vulnerable patients on the altar of tolerance and nondiscrimination? One can perhaps envision an institutional or professional commitment to offer high quality services, but if a vulnerable patient refuses these on the basis of a health-care professional's race, sex, religion, etc.,

that is the patient's choice: the death that ensues is not our responsibility.

And yet a commitment to quality care can involve a commitment to providing that care in ways that patients can accept. In these cases one cannot evade responsibility by showing that quality care was offered but refused. Responsibility seems to be there when (1) the reason the care was refused had to do with how it was offered, and (2) the care could have been offered in a way that would have led to acceptance. How do we deal with vulnerable patients whose prejudice-based existential preferences are damaging to our deepest senses of justice and human dignity? The dilemma involves a conflict between the clear duty to minister as best one can to the patient's pressing health care needs and the equally clear prohibition on becoming an instrument of injustice. Vulnerable patients with societally damaging, prejudice-based existential preferences force us to make a choice.

I confess I am not confident about how these values should be prioritized. While it is sometimes a mark of success merely to have stated a problem clearly, a few tentative suggestions can be made in closing. In the first place, it would surely be ethically prudent to try to finesse the dilemma. Perhaps the Southern white male in the ER could be persuaded to accept treatment from the black resident. And it seems that there is good reason to confront the patient directly: at a minimum to defend the capabilities and integrity of one's black colleague and to make clear for the record that one does not share the patient's opinion. Perhaps in some cases this tactic will suffice to make the problem disappear.

But if it does not and one has to choose, I believe it should be on behalf of the patient and his or her physical well-being. For it is that value that, above all, informs the practices of health care: its distinctive skills, knowledge, and technologies. Conversely, professional training programs in medical and nursing schools are not even peripherally concerned with assessing the claims of those who have been aggrieved and wounded by history. It is inevitable that health care—like all human pursuits—will be practiced in a profoundly imperfect world and that these imperfections will implicate practitioners and clients alike. In the face of all of these shortcomings, there is something to be said for mindfully striving to treat vulnerable patients with dignity and respect, even when their values are hateful.

The author is indebted to the contributors to the *Bioethics Discussion Forum at the Medical College*

of Wisconsin for helpful and illuminating commentary on some of the issues raised by this case. An earlier version of this piece appeared in Clinical Ethics Report, *Fall/Winter, 1996, pp. 5–8.*

CONTESTED THERAPIES WITHIN THE PHYSICIAN-PATIENT RELATIONSHIP

COSMETIC SURGERY AND THE INTERNAL MORALITY OF MEDICINE
Franklin G. Miller, Howard Brody, and Kevin C. Chung

The authors confront the issue of whether cosmetic surgery is a legitimate medical practice. Medicine, they argue, is "governed by a moral framework consisting of goals proper to medicine, role-specific duties, and clinical virtues"; professional integrity requires adherence to this "internal morality of medicine." Underscoring the distinction between consumer sovereignty in the business world and patient autonomy in medicine, the authors argue that advertising for cosmetic surgery routinely violates the Code of Ethics for the American Society of Plastic and Reconstructive Surgeons. They conclude that, from the standpoint of the internal morality of medicine, cosmetic surgery is ethically questionable, located at best at the periphery of acceptable medical practice.

Cosmetic surgery is a fast-growing medical practice. In 1997 surgeons in the United States performed the four most common cosmetic procedures—liposuction, breast augmentation, eyelid surgery, and facelift—443,728 times, an increase of 150% over the comparable total for 1992.[1] Estimated total expenditures for cosmetic surgery range from $1 to $2 billion.[2] As managed care cuts into physicians' income and autonomy, cosmetic surgery, which is not covered by health insurance, offers a financially attractive medical specialty.

Although increasingly popular, cosmetic surgery is a most unusual medical practice. Invasive surgical operations performed on healthy bodies for the sake of improving appearance lie far outside the core domain of medicine as a profession dedicated to saving lives, healing, and promoting health. These cosmetic procedures are not medically indicated for

a diagnosable medical condition. Yet they pose risks, cause side effects, and are subject to complications, including pain, bruising, swelling, discoloration, infections, formation of scar tissue, nerve damage, hardening of implants, etc.[3] Moreover, cosmetic surgery is a consumer-oriented entrepreneurial practice, heavily promoted by advertising in newspapers, magazines, the yellow pages of the telephone directory, and by marketing on the World Wide Web. The remarkable nature of cosmetic surgery is reflected on in the following comments of a plastic surgeon: "But then on top of it all we actually operate on people who are normal. It's amazing that we're allowed to do that, the idea that we can get a permit to operate on someone who is totally normal is an unbelievable privilege."[4]

Is cosmetic surgery a medical privilege or an abuse of medical knowledge and skill? With the exception of feminist scholarship, which focuses on the personal and social meaning and value of cosmetic surgery for the lives of women, the bioethics literature has neglected to pay attention to moral

Reprinted with the permission of Cambridge University Press from *Cambridge Quarterly of Healthcare Ethics*, vol. 9, no. 3 (July 2000), pp. 353–364. Copyright © 2000 Cambridge University Press.

issues posed by cosmetic surgery.[5] In this article we examine cosmetic surgery from the perspective of professional integrity and the internal morality of medicine—a perspective that we have explicated and defended in two previous essays[6]

THE INTERNAL MORALITY OF MEDICINE

All members of our society are likely to become patients, vulnerable to life-threatening or disrupting conditions and in need of medical attention and treatment to cure, prevent, or ameliorate disease, injury, or bodily dysfunction. Owing to this vulnerability and need for professional care, medicine is not a morally neutral technique. Rather, it is a professional practice governed by a moral framework consisting of goals proper to medicine, role-specific duties, and clinical virtues. We call this framework "the internal morality of medicine." The professional integrity of physicians is constituted by loyalty and adherence to this internal morality.

A variety of formulations have been proposed for the goals of medicine. A recent report of an international group of scholars, convened by The Hastings Center, recommended a comprehensive list of four goals: (i) "the prevention of disease and injury and promotion and maintenance of health"; (ii) "the relief of pain and suffering caused by maladies"; (iii) "the care and cure of those with a malady, and the care of those who cannot be cured"; and (iv) "the avoidance of premature death and the pursuit of a peaceful death."[7] For our inquiry into the ethics of cosmetic surgery, this list is noteworthy in two respects. The designation of multiple goals signifies that medicine is too complex and diverse in its legitimate scope to be encompassed by any single, essential goal, such as healing or promoting health. If healing is the single essential goal of medicine, then it is obvious that cosmetic surgery does not belong within legitimate medical practice. But this essentialist perspective would also rule out a variety of medical practices, such as contraception and sterilization, which prima facie are not devoted to healing or promoting health but are widely accepted as medically appropriate. The diversity of goals proper to medicine, and their openness to interpretation, makes mapping the moral domain of

medicine complex and contested. Though broad in its scope, this list of goals is subject to limits. The central goal of relief of pain and suffering is confined to conditions that qualify as "maladies." What counts as a malady warranting medical attention may be subject to conflicting interpretations and may change over time. The important qualification, however, means that it is not within the purview of physicians to attempt to relieve any and all pain and suffering that may afflict human beings.

Specification of the goals of medicine is necessary but not sufficient for mapping the normative domain of medicine. In addition to being oriented to a set of proper goals, medicine is guided and constrained by a set of internal duties that pertain to the legitimacy of practices in pursuit of medical goals. We have identified four internal duties incumbent on physicians of integrity: (i) competence in the technical and humanistic skills required to practice medicine; (ii) avoiding disproportionate harms that are not balanced by the prospect of compensating medical benefits; (iii) refraining from the fraudulent misrepresentation of medicine as a scientific practice and clinical art; and (iv) fidelity to the therapeutic relationship with patients in need of care.[8] The internal morality of medicine also encompasses a set of clinical virtues—dispositions of character and conduct facilitating excellence in pursuit of the goals of medicine and the performance of professional duties. We hope to specify and explicate the medical virtues in a future undertaking, but this is not required for our purpose of critical examination of cosmetic surgery.

THE DISTINCTION BETWEEN BUSINESS AND MEDICINE

From the time of the ancient Greeks to the present, medicine as a professional practice has been distinguished from business.[9] Governance by an internal morality underlies this distinction. Business, to be sure, does not lie outside the domain of morality. But medicine is subject to specialized and more stringent ethical constraints than are characteristic of and appropriate to business enterprise. The distinction between consumers and patients and the use of advertising are two key aspects of the traditional contrast between business and professional medical practice; and both are relevant to the evaluation of cosmetic surgery in the light of the internal morality of medicine.

Central to business in a market economy is the doctrine of consumer sovereignty: that subjective preferences and money determine access to commodities in the marketplace. In medicine consumer sovereignty is attenuated, if not foreign to the domain. Medical care is provided by physicians who diagnose presenting problems and recommend medically indicated treatment or preventive interventions. Patients may demand specific medical interventions, particularly in the context of intense public attention to health and ready access to health information. But interventions that patients request or demand are medically appropriate only if they are consistent with diagnostic criteria, medical indications, and professional judgment.

Patient autonomy is not the same as consumer sovereignty. Ethical medical treatment depends on the informed consent of patients, who have a right to refuse treatment, including medically indicated life-saving interventions. Patient autonomy, however, falls short of consumer sovereignty because patients do not have a right to receive whatever treatments they demand and are prepared to pay for. Preference and the ability to pay may be necessary for access to medical care in our society, but they are not sufficient. The extent to which cosmetic surgery is oriented toward and dependent on consumer demand is relevant to its moral assessment from the perspective of professional integrity.

In business, advertising functions as a standard means of linking sellers and buyers of products and services. Medical ethics, however, traditionally has prohibited advertising by physicians.[10] This traditional prohibition may have reflected, in part, a concern for status: marketing by advertising was considered beneath the dignity of learned professionals as distinct from tradesmen. The traditional prohibition eroded in the wake of the successful legal challenge by the Federal Trade Commission in 1978 of the American Medical Association's ban on physician advertising. Nevertheless, the vulnerability of patients and the imbalance of knowledge and power between physicians and patients continue to make advertising by physicians ethically problem-

atic. Here the truism applies that what is legal is not necessarily ethical.

Insofar as advertising by physicians is informational, it may alert individuals to unattended medical needs and appropriate treatments. But if it aims at stimulating demand for interventions that are not medically indicated, it potentially compromises professional integrity. Advertising cosmetic surgery puts physicians in the position of selling invasive procedures for which there is no medical need. Demand-stimulating advertising is especially problematic in medicine, since the willingness of physicians to provide treatments may operate as a legitimation in the mind of patients. That professionally qualified physicians are prepared to offer invasive procedures may encourage ambivalent patients to submit to medical intervention. Accordingly, advertising for interventions that are not medically needed to promote health is ethically suspect. What is acceptable business practice for selling consumer products and services is not necessarily appropriate for medical treatment. We argue below that the prevalence and unprofessional character of advertising contributes significantly to making the practice of cosmetic surgery ethically problematic.

MAPPING THE NORMATIVE DOMAIN OF MEDICINE

One of the major purposes of a conception of the internal morality of medicine is normative evaluation of practices by physicians to determine or question whether they belong within the proper domain of medicine. Violations of the internal morality of medicine consist of practices that are not supported by the goals of medicine and/or conflict with one or more of the internal duties of physicians. Examples include physician participation in capital punishment by lethal injection and prescribing anabolic steroids for athletes. Since these practices have nothing to do with treating or preventing a disease, injury, or malady, they do not serve the goals of medicine. Both involve causing or risking harms that are not compensated by medical benefits. Their performance by physicians fraudulently misrepresents medical practice by suggesting that it is proper for a physician to execute criminals or prescribe drugs to enhance athletic prowess. In addition, capital punishment is inconsistent with the context of a therapeutic relationship between physician and patient. Surgical procedures performed by a physician on close family members offer another example of a violation of the internal morality of medicine. Here the violation does not concern the goals of medicine, assuming that the procedure is medically indicated. However, the close family relationship has the potential to interfere substantially with competence (by impairing objectivity, clinical judgment, and thoroughness of medical inquiry) and with the therapeutic relationship between physician and patient.

In a previous essay we discussed a number of "borderline" medical practices, which belong within the legitimate domain of medicine but are not clearly supported by the goals of medicine and seem to conflict to some extent with one or more of the internal duties.[11] Examples include contraception and sterilization. On further reflection, we suggest that it is preferable to describe such procedures and practices as "peripheral" rather than borderline, since there are no precise, specifiable borders circumscribing unqualifiedly legitimate medical practices and defining violations. Among the definitions of "periphery" is "a zone constituting an imprecise boundary," which we think aptly characterizes the normative terrain. Thus we suggest a normative mapping of medicine that encompasses a core of legitimate medical practice, consistent with the goals and internal duties of medicine, a periphery of more or less acceptable procedures and practices outside the core, and a range of violations beyond the pale of medical legitimacy. Designating the zone within which a procedure or practice belongs is a matter of judgment based on coherence or fit with the internal morality of medicine.

Reasonable differences of opinion are likely with respect to mapping practices and procedures as within the core or the periphery. Consider the case of contraception and sterilization. Although not a disease or a malady, pregnancy is a condition that in our society brings women under medical attention. Unwanted pregnancy can be understood as a disability, which interferes with the ability of women to function normally in social life. This suggests the conclusion that contraception promotes the health of women. The health promotion rationale for contraception or sterilization is stronger in the case of women who are likely to experience serious health risks from becoming pregnant, which would support including these procedures within the core of medicine in these circumstances. Male sterilization via vasectomy, in contrast, would seem to lie more clearly in the periphery. If undertaken to prevent unwanted pregnancy, the pregnancy it prevents belongs to another person, not to the one sterilized. Unwanted paternity, unlike unwanted pregnancy, does not qualify as a medical condition to be prevented. Vasectomy, then, appears more like a "lifestyle" procedure than tubal ligation—a medical means of permitting sexual intercourse without risking pregnancy and paternity. This surgical procedure does pose some risks and complications not compensated by medical benefits. Yet we consider it an acceptable peripheral medical practice that does not threaten or violate professional integrity.

Is Cosmetic Surgery Compatible with the Internal Morality of Medicine? From the perspective of the ethics of the marketplace, governed by consumer sovereignty and honesty and fair play on the part of providers of commercial services, there appears to be nothing wrong with cosmetic surgery. It falls within the vast domain of commercial and consumer activity devoted to enhancing appearance. Cosmetic surgery involves certain risks and complications, but so does a range of other legitimate consumer activities, such as driving cars and engaging in recreational sports. In a "free society" what grounds are there for restricting the freedom of adults to purchase, and of medical practitioners to sell, cosmetic surgery? According to business ethics there are no ethical objections to cosmetic surgery as long as patients are adequately informed about risks and complications and are not subject to fraudulent marketing, and practitioners are technically competent. "Shaping up" by liposuction, for example, would seem to be an ethically acceptable, though less virtuous, alternative to jogging and working out, which are not without risks and potential complications.

Outside the minimalist ethics of the marketplace, a variety of value considerations are relevant to ethical appraisal of cosmetic surgery. The practice of cosmetic surgery may be criticized on the grounds that it is fueled by vanity and narcissistic fixation on bodily appearance. It reinforces intense concern with body image and culturally prescribed standards of beauty, especially among women, who are the major "consumers" of cosmetic surgery. It contributes to a youth culture that disdains and stigmatizes aging and the elderly. Cosmetic surgery upholds culturally specific standards of beauty— Caucasian, Anglo-Saxon, or Northern European— that stigmatize the appearance of ethnic groups that deviate from this standard. Finally, it promotes inequality between those who have and those who lack the resources to purchase the marketplace advantages of enhanced appearance via cosmetic surgery. None of these considerations, however, is relevant to the internal morality of medicine.

How, then, does cosmetic surgery stand with respect to the internal morality of medicine and professional integrity? It is difficult to find any solid support for cosmetic surgery within the goals of medicine. Those who seek to enhance their appearance by cosmetic surgery do not suffer from a diagnosable disease or injury. The qualifier "cosmetic" signifies that the surgery is not medically indicated or needed to promote health.

It might be objected that the description of cosmetic surgery as an appearance enhancement fails to do justice to the real, often prolonged, suffering from a negative body image that typically precedes choice of cosmetic surgery.[12] The point is well taken, but it does not follow that the suffering involved belongs within the purview of medicine. As discussed above, the goals of medicine concern not all human suffering, but only that suffering connected with a malady. "Malady" in the medical context suggests an objectively diagnosable condition calling for medical treatment; and this is precisely what is lacking in the case of cosmetic surgery. The "need" for cosmetic surgery is a function entirely of subjective preference.

Kathy Davis conducted fieldwork in the Netherlands to study individuals who sought cosmetic surgery during a time in which it was covered by national health insurance. She observed 55 individuals who were examined by an official medical inspector to determine eligibility for cosmetic surgery. Davis observes,

With one exception, a man with a cauliflower nose, I was never able to guess what the person had come in for. In some cases, I had a suspicion, as, for example, when a woman with a rather prominent nose appeared, only to have them dashed when she explained that she wanted an eyelid correction because her five-year-old son was always asking her 'why she had been crying.' My first impression confirmed that applicants for cosmetic surgery looked no different than the run-of-the-mill woman (or man) on the street and some were even decidedly attractive. Their appearance did not seem to warrant corrective measures as drastic as cosmetic surgery.[13]

Davis's inability to perceive the deficit in appearance prompting a request for cosmetic surgery was matched by a similar inability on the part of the responsible medical inspector. "Despite attempts to develop objective criteria for appearance, my observations of the Inspector's difficulties in actually making decisions about who should have cosmetic surgery presented a different picture. In practice, he routinely complained that he was unable to see why the applicant wanted cosmetic surgery."[14]

Whether all cosmetic surgery falls outside the core domain of medicine may be subject to conflicting interpretations. Reconstructive plastic surgery to correct ravages of disease and injuries as well as gross physical abnormalities constitutes a core medical practice. Reconstructive procedures, however, lie along a continuum, without any clear boundary between therapeutic reconstructive surgery for a diagnosable problem and purely cosmetic surgery. In addition, reconstructive surgery in response to deformity is guided by aesthetic considerations. Yet compare, for example, plastic surgery to remove a port-wine stain causing severe facial disfigurement, but without any functional impairment, with liposuction to produce a trimmer appearance or a facelift to "rejuvenate" facial features. The former appearance problem qualifies as a malady that is objectively discernable by all observers, and it is reasonable to describe corrective surgery as medically indicated. In the latter cases the appearance problems giving rise to a request for cosmetic surgery are a matter entirely of subjective judgment. If surgery to remove a disfiguring port-wine stain is regarded as in part cosmetic, then at least some cosmetic procedures belong within the core of medical practice. This conclusion has no bearing, however, on the vast majority of purely cosmetic surgery procedures performed on normal bodies, which are not supported by the goals of medicine.

To give an aura of standard medical legitimacy to cosmetic surgery, cosmetic surgeons have concocted diagnostic categories warranting cosmetic surgical intervention, most notably, the "inferiority complex."[15] The extent to which this disposition to construct diagnostic categories can be taken is exemplified by Davis's account of a case conference by an eminent Dutch plastic surgeon, who described a rhinoplasty for a 15-year-old Moroccan girl. The rationale for surgery was explained in terms of a new syndrome: "inferiority complex due to racial characteristics."[16] Although on critical reflection such a medical diagnosis is apt to appear blatantly bogus, the felt need to invoke some diagnostic category to warrant cosmetic surgery testifies to the point that objective diagnosis underlies legitimate medical treatment.

Let us imagine for a moment what would be required of cosmetic surgery if we really believed that dissatisfaction with one's bodily appearance was a legitimate medical diagnosis. We have a model for such a state of affairs in the surgical treatment of transsexuals, who find their body appearance totally at odds with their perceived gender identity, and suffer considerable anguish as a result. It is considered a legitimate surgical practice to operate on such persons to change their secondary sexual characteristics. But it is important to note how this is done in centers that can claim to be competent and comprehensive in their care. In particular, it is common to have sex change surgeons working very closely with teams of psychiatrists and other mental health workers, who do intensive screening of each applicant before the team decides that surgery should be performed. If the mental health assessment uncovers any evidence of psychological problems, so that managing those problems might relieve the gender dysphoria without doing surgery, then surgery is withheld and the appropriate psychotherapy is recommended instead.

This model suggests that if cosmetic surgeons truly believed that they were treating "real" psychiatric "maladies," then in order to provide minimally competent care, they ought to be working in tandem with mental health teams of this sort, and offering nonsurgical options to at least some of their patients. To our knowledge, very few if any cosmetic surgery offices and clinics are run in this fashion, which tends to suggest that cosmetic surgeons themselves do not take very seriously the claim that their practices are legitimated by the reality of psychiatric disease.

In addition to lacking support by the goals of medicine, cosmetic surgery is also ethically questionable with respect to the internal medical duties. These procedures pose risks of harm and have the potential for complications that are not compensated by any medical benefits. Furthermore, it is arguable that the willingness of physicians to perform cosmetic surgery on bodies that are not diseased, injured, or grossly abnormal fraudulently misrepresents medicine. This practice suggests a medical need and rationale for intervention, when in fact there is no diagnosable condition warranting medical treatment.

These considerations lead to the hardly surprising conclusion that cosmetic surgery lies outside the core of normative medical practice. But they leave open the question whether cosmetic surgery is a legitimate practice within the periphery of medicine or should be considered a violation of the internal morality of medicine. It is interesting to note that some of the early leaders of plastic surgery in the 1920s and 1930s expressed ethical concerns about cosmetic surgery.[17] They distinguished ethically appropriate reconstructive surgery in response to deformity and injury from purely cosmetic surgery, which they saw as the province of unprofessional "beauty doctors." For example, in an influential 1926 article published in *Annals of Surgery*, John Staige Davis wrote: "What is the ethical difference between doing an abdominal operation and removing wrinkles from a sagging face? The abdominal operation is necessary to the health of the patient, the operation for removal of wrinkles is unessential and is simply decorative surgery. True plastic surgery without question . . . is absolutely distinct and separate from what is known as cosmetic or decorative surgery."[18] Although a persuasive argument might be advanced that purely cosmetic surgery, not associated with any diagnosable deformity, violates the internal morality of medicine, we do not take this position. The continuum between reconstructive and cosmetic surgery, which makes it difficult to determine where the former ends and the latter begins, casts doubt on a blanket judgment that cosmetic surgery lies outside the domain of legitimate medical practice.

The Ethical Relevance of Advertising for Cosmetic Surgery Professional integrity concerns the fit between commitment to the norms of the internal morality of medicine and medical practice. All peripheral medical procedures and practices challenge professional integrity, since they are at best weakly supported by the goals of medicine, and they are apt to conflict with one or more of the internal duties. We submit that professional integrity is threatened, and potentially compromised, when peripheral procedures are not isolated or occasional occurrences within practice dedicated to core medical activities but are the predominant or exclusive focus of medical practice, as commonly characterizes cosmetic surgery. Moreover, the consumer-oriented, business context of cosmetic surgery risks compromising professional integrity, particularly insofar as it makes use of demand-stimulating marketing.

Advertisements for cosmetic surgery are prevalent in newspapers and the yellow pages of the telephone directory. Hundreds of sites on the World Wide Web are devoted to cosmetic surgery. For example, in the October 1997 yellow pages for suburban Washington, D.C., seven of the eight largest ads for physicians are for cosmetic surgery; and of those ads that take up one-quarter of a page or more, 18 of 31 are for cosmetic surgery. The weekly Health section of the *Washington Post* routinely contains ads placed by physicians for cosmetic surgery. These ads typically feature pictures of scantily clad, well-proportioned women and slogans such as "Bikini Time," "Let your mirror image be a masterpiece," "Reshape your future," "Spring into summer with a new look," "A New You for The New Millennium." In the *Washington Post Magazine* glossy ads have appeared recently for cosmetic surgery focusing on large-breasted women, with the slogans "Big and

Believable," and "A Bustline for the Shoreline." These ads also feature the names, medical degrees, and board certification of plastic surgeons. Such advertisements juxtapose the lowest common denominator of marketing—sex sells—with markers of professional competence. The role of physician as salesman is displayed by the frequent offer in cosmetic surgery ads of free consultations, often with the aid of computer imaging. Targeted at women, these ads play on, and possibly contribute to, widespread dissatisfaction with body image and foster unrealistic expectations of what can be achieved by cosmetic surgery. Moreover, they give no indication of risks or complications from cosmetic surgery or the chance of less than fully satisfying outcomes.

The marketing of cosmetic surgery to consumers as a commercial service is particularly accentuated in a recent ad in the *Washington Post* health section. Under the bold headline, "Body Sculpting," it depicts the silhouette of a nude woman with an hourglass figure. Also in bold is the announcement of "100% Financing" followed by a list of cosmetic procedures offered and the following sales pitch: "Call today to arrange for a free consultation with one of our experienced plastic surgeons who'll use computer imaging to demonstrate how you could look after cosmetic surgery. You'll also learn about our finance plan with no down payment and low monthly payments."

It is revealing to evaluate the professional appropriateness of cosmetic surgery marketing by comparing samples of advertisements for cosmetic surgery, such as those described above, with statements from the Code of Ethics for the American Society of Plastic and Reconstructive Surgeons, approved in 1992.[19] Under the heading of Specific Principles, conditions are listed under which "Each member may be subject to disciplinary action, including expulsion." The category pertaining to advertising is the following: "The member . . . uses or participates in the use of any form of communication (including computer imaging and electronic communications) containing a false, fraudulent, deceptive, or misleading statement or claim." Included among unethical communication is a statement or claim that "[i]s intended or is likely to create false or unjustified expectations of favorable results";

"[a]ppeals primarily to layperson's fears, anxieties, or emotional vulnerabilities"; and "[i]s intended or likely to attract patients by use of puffery or exaggerated claims."

We contend that advertisements for cosmetic surgery routinely violate these professional ethical guidelines. They purvey misleading images and slogans, appeal to emotional vulnerabilities, and foster unrealistic expectations, rather than convey useful information about cosmetic surgery. These advertisements suggest that there is "a quick fix" for bodily improvement. They trade on glamour and dreams without drawing attention to risks and complications. Unprofessional advertising aimed at stimulating demand for invasive surgical procedures that are not medically indicated threatens, if not violates, professional integrity. Moreover, apart from the unprofessional character of much advertising for cosmetic surgery, the very use of advertising for cosmetic surgery is ethically problematic. Physicians should not be in the business of promoting medically unnecessary surgery on normal individuals.

It is a very basic component of the internal morality of medicine that physicians not be involved in the deliberate creation of disease just so that they can expand their practices and increase their earnings. For example, sprinkling resistant microorganisms into the town water supply would be the grossest possible violation of the internal morality of medicine. Yet if we imagine that an individual's dissatisfaction with his or her own bodily appearance is the (so-called) "disease" that cosmetic surgery is designed to treat, then it is arguable that the most extreme and misleading advertisements are analogous to this physician-as-Typhoid-Mary example. The ads are deliberately designed to convince people who might previously have thought that their appearance was acceptable that they are in fact seriously inadequate unless they seek a surgical correction for their newly discovered "problem."

An obvious rejoinder is that a medical "problem" can never be defined completely in isolation from the state of the art of medical therapy. On this view, advertising does not create a new perception of a problem that did not previously exist. Instead, people who all along had problems, but imagined that nothing practically could be done, are now being informed that a relatively safe and effective treatment exists so that they can be encouraged to come forward and seek relief. But this response seems disingenuous when we reflect how dependent body image is on the prevailing social norms of beauty. The more extreme ads for cosmetic surgery convey the message that the models shown in the ads represent the standard of beauty to which all sensible people should aspire, and that these models have achieved that standard of beauty precisely because they have themselves submitted to cosmetic surgery (perhaps numerous times). By promoting *dis-ease* and thus stimulating demand for cosmetic surgery, such advertisements clearly violate the internal morality of medicine.

IMPLICATIONS

Our argument suggests that cosmetic surgery is ethically questionable from the perspective of the internal morality of medicine, which makes it at best a peripheral medical practice. Ethical concern is heightened by the organization of cosmetic surgery as a consumer-oriented business supported by heavy use of marketing, much of which is misleading and unprofessional. Accordingly, we conclude that the current state of cosmetic surgery practice threatens professional integrity. Some might go further and conclude that cosmetic surgery does not belong within medicine.[20] This rigorist position may seem appealing theoretically but is unlikely to have any practical effect. More importantly, if cosmetic surgery should be ruled out of medicine because it does not serve the goals of medicine, then other widely endorsed procedures and practices that also are not supported by the goals of medicine, such as contraception and sterilization, may be ethically imperiled. We contend that the marketing of cosmetic surgery raises especially serious concern from the perspective of professional ethics—concern that ought to be addressed in practice. Cosmetic surgeons who engage in misleading or fraudulent advertising appear to want to have it both ways. In marketing cosmetic surgery, they use standard, but contextually objectionable, techniques of consumer advertising, coupled with drawing attention to their professional medical credentials. The incoherence between projection of professional competence and trust, and the reliance on sleazy advertising techniques, compromises professional integrity.

Those wishing to defend the ethics of cosmetic surgery as consistent with the internal morality of medicine may take comfort in our labeling of the practice as "peripheral" rather than as outside the boundaries. But the preceding discussion suggests that a price is paid when a practice is accepted as peripheral within medicine. The more a practice occupies a peripheral rather than a central position in relation to the goals and duties internal to medicine, the more physicians are obligated to free that practice from any association with potentially distracting or corrupting influences such as a profit motive. To see what this entails, recall how surgical sterilization was often handled by many physicians 20 or 30 years ago, when there tended to be more moral unease than there is today about the peripheral position of that practice. In a day when concern about informed consent had not yet been felt in most of medical practice, physicians went to great lengths to assure that patients were fully informed and had carefully thought about sterilization before being willing to do the procedure. It was as if these physicians were bending over backwards to demonstrate that it was not a desire to expand their practices and make more money that stimulated them to do those surgeries.

On this view, if cosmetic surgeons took the internal morality of medicine seriously, they would scrupulously refrain from ethically suspect advertising and minimize the profit-making orientation of their practice—even more so than physicians whose daily work was more safely nestled within the core of medicine. By contrast, in the practice of cosmetic surgery we find the coexistence of two factors: (i) a practice within medicine that is demonstrably quite peripheral; and (ii) heavy reliance on questionable advertising and other signs that an ethic of business rather than of medicine is operating. We conclude that a serious threat to the internal morality of medicine exists in the way this practice is conducted, even though we do not contend that the practice itself is totally outside the bounds of allowable medical activity.

Leaders of the medical profession, particularly those connected with the practice of plastic surgery, should take steps to curb unethical marketing of invasive procedures that are not medically indicated. In addition, they should promote attention to professional ethics in the context of specialty training of plastic surgeons. More broadly, teaching the internal morality of medicine, by precept and example, may discourage medical students and physicians in training from diverting their careers to a peripheral and ethically problematic practice, outside the core domain of medicine.

On the theoretical level we suggest that the critical evaluation of cosmetic surgery from the perspective of the internal morality of medicine demonstrates the significance of this ethical approach. Focus on the internal morality of medicine brings to light ethical considerations and concerns that lie beneath the surface of the mainstream of bioethics. As new interventions are developed that are aimed at enhancing human abilities and subjective well-being, in contrast to treating disease, injury, or dysfunction—e.g., growth hormone to combat the effects of aging, "cosmetic psychopharmacology," drugs to enhance sexual performance, and genetic engineering—attention to the internal morality of medicine and professional integrity is likely to grow more prominent, and this perspective is likely to achieve greater refinement and depth.

NOTES

1 American Society of Plastic and Reconstructive Surgeons (www.plasticsurgery.org).

2 Gillespie R. Women, the body and brand extension in medicine: Cosmetic surgery and the paradox of choice. *Women & Health* 1996;24:75.

3 Davis K. *Reshaping the Female Body: The Dilemma of Cosmetic Surgery.* New York: Routledge 1995:27–8.

4 Siebert C. The cuts that go deeper. *New York Times Magazine* 1996; July 7:24.

5 Sherwin S. Feminism and bioethics. In: Wolf S. M., ed. *Feminism & Bioethics.* New York: Oxford University Press, 1996:59.

6 Miller F. G., Brody H. Professional integrity and physician-assisted death. *Hastings Center Report* 1995;25(3):8–17; Brody H. Miller F. G. The internal morality of medicine: explication and application to managed care. *Journal of Medicine and Philosophy* 1998; 23:384–410.

7 Callahan D. The goals of medicine: Setting new priorities [Special Supplement]. *Hastings Center Report* 1996; 25(6):S1–S26.

8 See note 6, Miller. Brody 1995.

 9 Plato, *The Republic*. trans. HDP Lee. Harmondsworth, U.K.:
    Penguin, 1955:69–70.
10 Dyer A. R. Ethics, advertising and the definition of a
    profession. *Journal of Medical Ethics* 1985;11:72–8.
11 See note 6, Brody. Miller 1998;23:384–410.
12 See note 3, Davis 1995.
13 See note 3, Davis 1995:70.
14 See note 3, Davis 1995:72.
15 Haiken E. *Venus Envy: A History of Cosmetic Surgery*.
    Baltimore: Johns Hopkins University Press, 1997:90–130.

16 See note 3, Davis 1995:2.
17 See note 15, Haiken 1997:50–2, 93–103.
18 See note 15, Haiken 1997:93.
19 American Society of Plastic and Reconstructive Surgeons.
    Code of Ethics, rev. 1992.
20 Hyman D. A. Aesthetics and ethics: the implications of
    cosmetic surgery. *Perspectives in Biology and Medicine*
    1990; 33:190–202.

ONE PILL MAKES YOU SMARTER: AN ETHICAL APPRAISAL OF THE RISE OF RITALIN
Claudia Mills

Responding to the explosive growth in American children's use of the stimulant Ritalin since the early 1990s, Mills notes that the drug is now often prescribed for children who exhibit fairly normal childlike behaviors such as making careless errors in schoolwork, failing to pay attention, and squirming in their seats. The thought that we are increasingly drugging our children in order to get them to conform to adult expectations tends to disturb us, she argues, although it is difficult to say exactly what about this trend is genuinely disturbing. In the end, what is most troubling about the rise of Ritalin use in children, according to Mills, is neither the means of improving performance—a pill—nor the inequitable distribution of this means, but the goal of hyper-achievement. Our society's relentless pursuit of this goal, she concludes, may rob our children of their opportunity to be children.

The statistics at least *seem* alarming. The production of Ritalin, an amphetamine derivative used for the treatment of attention deficit disorder in children (and, lately, in adults as well), has risen a whopping 700 percent since 1990. According to figures given by Lawrence Diller in *Running on Ritalin*, over the decade, the number of Americans using Ritalin has soared from 900,000 to almost 5 million—the vast majority children from the ages of 5 to 12, though there is a significant rise in Ritalin use among teens and adult as well. No comparable rise is reported in other countries, though a much smaller surge has taken place in Canada and Australia. In Virginia

Beach, Va. (perhaps the most egregious example), 17 percent of fifth-grade boys were taking Ritalin in 1996 to control behavior problems and improve school performance. (Boys on Ritalin outnumber girls in a ratio of 3.5 to 1; when I was recently complaining to another mother about my own son's academic difficulties, she said simply, "Welcome to the world of boys.")

Stimulants have been used to treat behavior problems in children since 1937; Ritalin itself appeared on the market in the 1960s to treat what was then called "hyperactivity" — impulsive, disruptive behavior by children who just "couldn't sit still." In recent years, however, the root problem has been identified as "attention deficit disorder" (ADD), either with or without attendant hyperactivity.

Symptoms of ADD, according to the standard survey used in its diagnosis, include: "often fails to

Report from the Institute for Philosophy & Public Policy, vol. 18, no. 4
(1988), pp. 13–17. Also in Verna Gehring and William Galston, eds.,
Philosophical Dimensions in Public Policy (Transaction, 2002).
Copyright © 2002 by Transaction Publishers. Reprinted by permission of
Transaction Publishers.

give close attention to details or makes careless mistakes in schoolwork," "often has difficulty organizing tasks and activities, and "often avoids, dislikes, or is reluctant to engage in tasks that require mental effort (such as schoolwork or homework)." Symptoms of ADD-H (the variant with hyperactivity) include: "often fidgets with hands or feet or squirms in seat" and "often has difficulty playing or engaging in leisure activities quietly." Ritalin, by most accounts, is remarkably effective in getting such children to settle down and pay attention, with resultant (at least short-term) gains in parental sanity and academic achievement.

The fear, stated quite baldly, is that as a society we are drugging our children in ever-larger numbers to get them to conform to adult expectations. Dislikes homework? Makes careless mistakes? Squirms in seat? To many it seems that we are drugging our children to get them to stop being *children*. I myself feel profoundly troubled by the rise of Ritalin — and by my own temptation to use it for my child, who, yes, makes careless mistakes and has been known to fidget. But, I will argue, it is surprisingly difficult to pinpoint any justifiable sources of discomfort here — both harder than one might think, and more illuminating. The effort to do so will lead us into an exploration of a range of issues about how we view our children and ourselves.

Here, then, are some possible responses to our concerns about the rise of Ritalin, followed by some speculations about the deeper—and legitimate— fears that fuel these concerns.

RATIONALES FOR TREATMENT

On some accounts, the rise in Ritalin simply reflects our commendably growing willingness to treat a serious and common disorder that has too long been left untreated. That there is soaring use of any drug is not itself a problem, if the drug is treating a genuine medical condition that responds favorably to treatment. If there is some real disorder in the area of children's brains that controls their ability to pay attention (current research is focusing on the prefrontal cortex), and this disorder is causing problems in school and home, and it can be easily treated, *shouldn't* it be treated? Why should children have to struggle with their schoolwork, and parents struggle with discipline, if

the root cause of disappointing academic performance and poor behavior is a medical one that can be easily treated? On one expert's estimate attention deficient disorder is even now underdiagnosed, and so we should expect—and welcome—a further doubling of Ritalin use in response.

However, it is unclear that there really is any one, clearly identified "thing" that "is" attention deficit disorder. Diller argues persuasively that when parents or doctors speak of a child as "having" ADD, this tends to mean only that the child in fact scored positively on a certain number of questions on the kind of survey described earlier. Certainly diagnosis of ADD is inexact, to say the least—often based largely on reported frustration by parents and teachers sometimes made (as admitted by some teachers I've spoken to in my own local schools) by prescribing Ritalin on a trial basis and seeing if it works.

The trouble with the latter approach is that Ritalin almost always "works," in that it almost always enhances performance, at least in the short term (Diller reports that there is no evidence of long-term improvement in children taking Ritalin). According to one study cited by Diller, "stimulants had essentially the same effects on normal children as on children with attention or behavior problems." Diller notes an increasing amount of what has been called "diagnostic bracket creep," as the criteria for diagnosis become ever more loose and generous, allowing more borderline ADD children to benefit from drug treatment.

Now, it can be argued that it shouldn't matter whether children receiving Ritalin have some underlying "brain disorder" that causes inattention, or whether they are inattentive for other, less physiologically based reasons. Why is the *cause* of a condition relevant to whether or not we have reason to try to treat it? For example, if parents are debating whether or not to treat an abnormally short child with growth hormone, David B. Allen and Norman Fost have argued that it shouldn't matter whether the child's height is caused by a hormone deficiency or by his genetic endowment: What should matter is whether this is causing a problem for him, and whether it can be successfully treated.

With the diagnosis of attention deficit disorder so elastic, however, one begins to wonder whether the "disorder" in question is simply that the child places at the lower end of the spectrum for behavior or achievement—that is, that parents, clinging stubbornly to Lake Wobegon fantasies, insist that all children generally and their own children in particular should be "above average," or certainly not below average. (I have discovered from my own experience that teachers are also quick to suggest an ADD evaluation for a child with any academic difficulties.) If attention or behavior problems interfere with a child's achieving his or her "full potential," parents and teachers may be increasingly tempted to turn to medication, even where this can mean not just allowing their children to perform "normally," but raising them significantly above the norm. Diller mentions one student whose use of Ritalin allowed him to become his high school's valedictorian: Off the drug, he still performed well, but his grades slipped, from straight A's to A's intermingled with B's.

Some of us will be troubled by using Ritalin in such cases. But why shouldn't every child be able to use whatever means are available to improve his or her performance, whatever his starting point? If we were to raise poor performers to the mean, but refuse to raise average performers above the mean, this could seem unfair to the superior performers. Why shouldn't they have a chance at enhancement, too?

RITALIN AS A MEANS OF ENHANCEMENT

As Ronald Cole-Turner points out, in his article in this issue, most of us are already "enhancement enthusiasts." We not only strive to improve our children all the time, but would criticize parents who neglected to do so. If we give children Ritalin to enhance their academic performance—well, don't we send them to school in the first place for the same reason? It doesn't seem all that problematic to want our children to be more attentive, more responsive, better behaved, better able to learn: Isn't better, by definition, *better*? Cole-Turner argues, however, that while the goal of enhancement may be a legitimate one (I will raise doubts about this below), we need also to look at the means. Means *do* matter.

First, some means may be problematic in themselves, including the use of drugs. A friend with whom I was discussing the rise in Ritalin use voiced

the reactions of many in saying, "Putting kids on drugs? Uh-uh." Now, drugs of any kind are often attended with a myriad of negative (and perhaps not yet discovered) side effects. But stimulants like Ritalin have been used to treat behavior problems in children for six decades with few observed ill effects. Ritalin causes insomnia, which can be avoided by not taking it in the evening; some children experience suppressed appetite. But the vast majority experience no distressing side effects at all.

The term "drugs" generally carries with it a stigma: When we think of "children on drugs," we think first of illegal drug use; when we talk about "drugging our children," we visualize children wandering through the day in a dopey, feel-good haze. It is important to free Ritalin from such unwarranted associations. Its use is legal, although controlled, and, far from inducing a fuzzy "drugged" state, it works to increase the ability to pay attention. With Ritalin, children don't "tune out," but "tune in." Or so we might claim.

Second, as Cole-Turner argues, some means to an end may be valued for their own sake and in their own right—either because they also represent ends that we value, or because we value reaching the end only after an experience of striving and struggle. If we choose a "quick fix" to solve our problems and achieve our goals, we may end up achieving different goals altogether, or, at the least, give up the long and ultimately more rewarding journey to our destination. In the case of Ritalin, the fear is that we will be content to give "problem children" a couple of little pills every day, rather than put in the extra effort as parents and teachers to reach them and teach them, to help ther learn and grow in a more messy and non-medicalized way. Specifically, the fear is that we will see Ritalin as a means of bypassing tough and loving parental discipline or real (and expensive) commitments to shouldering the rising costs of effective public education.

Now, clearly we value parental love and discipline and the long journey of education as ends in themselves, not just as means to producing more successful children. Focusing for the moment on education, we don't send children to school simply to get them to acquire a certain body of knowledge and master a certain body of skills, but because the process of learning is itself valuable. I still remember the thrill the first time I really "got" long division. Or the shock of joy with which I first learned, from my high school American history teacher, that there really are two sides to every question. We may worry that Ritalin provides an easy way out of facing the challenge—and reward—of truly educating our children. For teachers who can teach and classroom environments in which children can learn cost vastly more than daily doses of Ritalin.

To this concern about Ritalin, I have two responses. First, Ritalin could be defended as a means, not of bypassing the journey of education, but of permitting certain children to engage in the journey more fully, to pay attention to the journey in all its richness. Ritalin doesn't substitute for learning; it at best assists in providing one of the preconditions for learning—the ability to pay attention to what is being taught. Ritalin or no Ritalin, we will still need to teach our children, both how to behave and how to learn, in the most creative ways possible.

This suggests, second, that when it comes to parents and to teaching, we do not need to fear that we will take the easy way out, because, quite simply, there *is* no easy way out. Cole-Turner points out correctly that while new means "may relocate our human struggle, they do not eliminate it." Even if we are what Gerald Klerman has called "pharmacological calvinists," who reject drug-based solutions as too easy, who value the hard way just because it's hard, this gives us no reason to resist Ritalin. Anyone who is a parent or teacher knows that there will be no shortage of hard work in raising and educating children. If hard is what we want, we're home free: however hard we want parenting and teaching to be, it will be hard enough.

EQUALITY AND COMPETITIVENESS

As I approach what I take to be the most serious worry about Ritalin, let me mention one other objection that is sometimes raised to it and other programs of medical enhancement. This objection concedes that Ritalin can provide genuine and legitimate advantages for those who use it, but charges that these advantages are not distributed fairly. Responsible diagnoses of attention deficit disorder are expensive and beyond the budget of many families, who are already poorly served by an inadequate health care system. With the rise of Ritalin, whose use is con-

centrated among white, upper-middle-class families, the children of the rich get cognitively richer, and the children of the poor fall ever further behind.

This objection, if it stands on its merits, could be met by efforts to equalize provision of Ritalin (as well as access to medical care generally). If racial or class disparities in Ritalin use were our chief concern, the solution would be obvious. But in my view, the biggest problem with Ritalin lies not with the kids who don't get it, but with (at least some of) those who do.

The real reason that I remain uncomfortable with the rise of Ritalin concerns not the means of enhancement, but the goal itself—what our motives are for seeking enhancement so diligently and desperately, and, even more, what we as a society are currently counting as enhancement. What, in the end, are we trying to gain?

Now, there are clear advantages to being able to pay attention, clear advantages to being able to learn. Dan Brock notes that often our efforts at enhancement are meant to provide us with "intrinsic goods" that we value for their own sake. If these are what we are seeking in putting our children on Ritalin, this doesn't seem particularly troubling. But it seems to me, chiefly as an observer of my own life in one white, upper-middle-class American neighborhood, that many of us want more than this. We don't want to be better than our own imperfect selves; we want to be better than somebody else. We don't want Garrison Keillor's vision of a world where all the children are above average—we want a world where our own children are more above average than anybody else's. A friend of mine who is a principal in an affluent suburban elementary school says that in his school there are only three kinds of children: gifted, very gifted, and extremely gifted. We have grade inflation because so many students and parents insist on getting top grades that now teachers give top grades to almost everybody. And we give our children Ritalin in part because we cannot bear that they be below average; indeed, we cannot bear that they not be above average. This goal itself is troubling to me independent of any questions about the means to achieve it.

Of course, as Brock observes, such a goal is ultimately self-defeating: once everyone achieves the same relative enhancement, the competitive benefit of the enhancement disappears. But it may be a long time before we figure this out. And in the meantime we have to live in the world that we have been creating.

The concerns that I am raising now are targeted not only against Ritalin use, but against other, more familiar and widely accepted means of enhancement as well. For I don't think that our non-pharmaceutical strategies to produce better, brighter children are themselves beyond reproach. When I compare my own childhood experiences with those of my children, I feel a sorrow that I think runs deeper than mere nostalgia for a sentimentalized version of one's own past.

When I was a child, competitive sports didn't begin until fairly late in elementary school; now they begin for some children in kindergarten or even preschool. Children who wait until third or fourth grade to join a soccer or basketball team find themselves at an insuperable competitive disadvantage. In fact, in my neighborhood, a number of the children have already burned out on a sport and decided to drop it by the age at which children a generation age were just beginning. I began piano lessons in third grade; my own children began in kindergarten. How else can they keep up with everyone else's children who have also been studying music from the cradle—indeed, with children who listened to tapes of Mozart in utero?

And so middle-class children have childhoods in which they are chauffeured by their ever-more-frantic parents from one enrichment activity to another: two sports, two musical instruments, Scouts, Odyssey of the Mind, after-school language programs, science discovery programs, theater workshops. Parents who have a different vision of what childhood might be are reluctant to pursue it, for fear that their children will be left too far behind. One parenting magazine recently published an article about a family that actually chose not to participate in any after-school activities, where this was considered sufficiently unusual to merit a feature article in a national magazine.

The irony in all this is that Ritalin is prescribed for attention deficit disorder. Yet as we struggle to enhance our children faster than our neighbors manage to enhance theirs, we fill our lives with an even greater level of distractions. Diller speculates that if Huck Finn and Tom Sawyer walked out of Twain's pages and into a suburban American school today, they might well find themselves on Ritalin. He worries about our inability to tolerate and appreciate a range of temperaments and personality styles. I worry about this, too, but more about whether we are losing the ability to let children be children—or at least to let them be average children, not gifted, very gifted, or extremely gifted, savoring childhood as it slips by all too quickly.

If we want our kids to pay attention, maybe we have to begin paying attention to what it is that's worth paying attention *to*.

SOURCES

Lawrence H. Diller, *Running on Ritalin: A Physician Reflects on Children, Society, and Performance in a Pill* (Bantam Books, 1998), and "The Run on Ritalin: Attention Deficit Disorder and Stimulant Treatment in the 1990s," *Hastings Center Report*, vol. 26, no. 2 (1996); Erik Parens, "Is Better Always Good? The Enhancement Project," *Hastings Center Report*, vol. 28, no. 1 (1998) (Parens quotes Dan Brock and David B. Allen and Norman Fost Peter J. Whitehouse, Eric Juengst, Maxwell Mehlman, and Thomas H. Murray, "Enhancing Cognition in the Intellectually Intact," *Hastings Center Report*, vol. 27, no. 3 (1997) (this article cites Gerald Klerman on "pharmacological calvinism").

CONFLICTS OF INTEREST, PROBLEMS OF CONSCIENCE, AND MANAGED CARE

THE DOCTOR AS DOUBLE AGENT

Marcia Angell

Angell examines the contemporary expectation that American doctors should function as "double agents"—with conflicting allegiances to patients' medical needs and to society's financial interests. Because this situation is a result of rapidly increasing medical costs, themselves the result of an inherently inflationary health-care finance system, the solution, Angell argues, is to restructure the system to remove the inflationary pressures. Failure to do so, she concludes, is to endanger the patient-centered ethic at the moral core of medicine.

In earlier times—that is, before 1980—it was generally agreed that the doctor's sole obligation was to take care of each patient. The doctor was the patient's fiduciary or agent, and the doctor was to act only in the patient's interest. Now all that has changed. Many of us—economists, governmental officials, corporate executives, even ethicists, and yes, even many doctors themselves—now believe that doctors have other obligations that compete with their obligation to the patient. In particular, they believe that doctors have acquired an obligation to save resources for society. Doing so requires doctors to practice with one eye on costs, which may mean sometimes denying beneficial care that they would surely have provided in earlier times.

According to the new view, doctors are no longer simply agents for their patients. They are now agents for society's needs as well. They are, in short, *double agents*, expected to decide whether the benefits of treatment to their patients are worth the costs to society. Many distinguished ethicists have enthusiastically embraced this new ethic (Callahan 1990; Morreim 1991). To them, keeping an eye on the price tag means saving scarce resources for other, more important uses.

How did this extraordinary shift in our view of doctors' obligations come about? Is it just coincidence that it began with our first realization—roughly in the mid-1970s—that our seemingly endless resources were in fact finite? And is it just coincidence that it accorded with the wishes of the third-party payers—who discovered during the 1980s that they had severe and growing budgetary problems? In short, can it be that the ethical underpinnings of the practice of medicine have been scrapped in a single decade for financial reasons? Is economics driving ethics?

I'll begin with my conclusions. I believe that doctors *are* now asked to be double agents and that their dual obligation is a recent construct, which arose out of the economic difficulties of the large third-party payers. I will argue that we embrace this new ethic at our peril. Even if we as a society decide that health care should take a smaller piece of the national economic pie, there are ways to do this that do not entail rebuilding—and perhaps destroying—almost overnight, the ethical underpinnings of the profession.

HISTORICAL REVIEW

First, a quick review of how we got here. This requires an economic analysis, since my thesis is that economics is now driving ethics. The economic history of health care in the United States can be divided into three phases. First, there was the phase of the true market, lasting until roughly World War II. Patients paid doctors out-of-pocket for their medical care. If the price was too high, the doctor was confronted with an unhappy patient. Even after private insurance companies began to flourish in the 1930s, the premiums were still paid out-of-pocket and so patients continued to feel the costs, although the pain was blunted. Fortunately, medical care was fairly inexpensive. Unfortunately, it was also relatively ineffective, compared with the power of modern medicine.

The second phase was marked by the entry of big business into the health care picture. Big business began to offer health insurance as a fringe benefit in order to evade the wage and price controls in effect during World War II. Offering health insurance was tantamount to increasing wages, and furthermore, it was not taxed. The connection between employment and health insurance was thus an historical accident that haunts us still. But the important effect of this connection for the discussion here is that it insulates patients from the costs of medical care. Neither doctors nor patients had to worry any

Reprinted with permission of the publisher from *Kennedy Institute of Ethics Journal*, vol. 3 (September 1993), pp. 279–286.

longer about the costs of medical care. With the enactment of Medicare and Medicaid in 1966, this insulation from costs spread to the poor and, most importantly, to the elderly—a politically powerful group. By the end of the 1960s, anything resembling a true market in health care had vanished. Nearly everyone was covered by third-party payers—government, business, and private insurance companies. And medical care was becoming both more expensive and more effective. Despite the increasing costs, the third parties happily paid the charges, with few questions asked.

The third phase began with the realization that health care costs were consistently rising far more rapidly than the GNP. Now that patients and doctors and hospitals were insulated from accountability, there were no limits on the expansion of the health care industry in this country. It was open-ended and nearly risk-free, absorbing an ever greater share of our domestic spending. While national expenditures for other social goods, such as education, stagnated or declined, expenditures for health care rose rapidly—from roughly 6 percent of the GNP in 1965 to nearly 10 percent in 1980 to 13 percent in 1991 (Stoline and Weiner 1993).

Not only was there nothing to stop the inflation, but there were features that virtually guaranteed it. These included the piecework, fee-for-service reimbursement system that is greatly skewed toward high-technology procedures and specialists. Doctors, of course, act as both providers and purchasing agents, so these highly paid specialists could easily generate their own business. For example, the cardiologist who recommends coronary angiography to a patient also bills for it.

COST CONTAINMENT

In the 1970s, the Arab oil embargo made Americans realize that our resources were finite. Health care costs began to occupy the attention of some experts and policymakers. By the 1980s, it became clear to nearly everyone that we could not indefinitely sustain rising health care costs, and for the first time, efforts were made to control them. "Cost containment" crept into the lexicon, and by the end of the 1980s the *New England Journal of Medicine* probably received more manuscripts about cost containment than about can-

cer. The efforts to control costs were spearheaded by the major third parties—government and big business. They were responding essentially to budgetary problems, not to moral problems. They went about cost containment in a number of ad hoc, uncoordinated ways, as briefly mentioned below. None of them was notably successful. In fact health care costs rose even faster—I believe, *because* of cost containment efforts, not despite them.

Regulation by third parties, including managed care, simply led to the growth of an expensive and intrusive new bureaucracy. Efforts to foster competition led to increased marketing, not to lower prices. And attempts to limit demand through higher deductibles and copayments simply shifted costs and limited care, primarily to the most vulnerable. Efforts by insurers to avoid risks also shifted costs. In general, savings to one part of the system were costs to another. In fact, the dominant characteristic of the American health care system is that there is no system. There is just a hodge-podge of arrangements, existing independently, often working at cross purposes, and generating enormous administrative costs. Indeed, administrative costs—billing, marketing, underwriting, claims processing, utilization review—now consume more than 20 cents of the health care dollar (Woolhandler and Himmelstein 1991).

Why do I recapitulate this sorry history of the economics of the American health care system? I do so because it is important to understand the context in which doctors are being invited to act as double agents. They are invited to do so in an open-ended, inherently inflationary system (or, rather, nonsystem) that spends roughly 40 percent more per citizen on health care than the next most expensive health care system in the world and at least twice as much on administrative costs. Further, this system is embedded in a society that routinely spends billions and billions on such goods as tobacco, television ads, and cosmetics. Clearly, we as a society are not facing scarcity; instead we are facing the inefficient and frivolous use of vast resources.

SAVING FOR THIRD PARTIES

What precisely is the doctor supposed to do as double agent? In a nutshell, doctors are supposed to tailor their care of patients to save money for third parties.

For example, under the DRG system of hospital reimbursement for Medicare patients, doctors are supposed to be agents for the hospital, discharging patients as rapidly as possible and keeping services to a minimum so that the hospital can game the system. In many HMOs doctors are expected to keep costs as low as possible, and some HMOs even directly reward doctors with bonuses when the HMO comes out ahead. They may also withhold a portion of doctors' salaries if they refer patients to specialists too often or use too many tests and procedures. Thus, doctors are agents for the HMO and have a direct incentive to undertreat their patients, just as in the fee-for-service system they have an incentive to overtreat them. Other forms of managed care also deter doctors from delivering care. Those that require utilization review often make it so complicated and difficult to get approval for hospitalization or procedures that the doctor is reluctant even to try. And it should be noted that nearly all medical care these days is managed in one way or another, by which I mean it is subject to efforts of insurers to limit care.

In essence, then, doctors are increasingly being asked, in one way or another, to save money for a third party—and sometimes for themselves—by scrimping on the medical care they deliver. But the pressure is seldom described in these terms. Instead, it is described as practicing "cost-effective" medicine. "Cost-effective" is the new watchword. It used to be a technical term that referred to the least expensive of two equally effective alternatives, or to the most effective of two equally costly ones. Now it is simply a shorthand for any attempt to save money. The word sounds fine, and who can object to it?

JUSTIFICATION FOR DOUBLE AGENTS

But how can we justify asking doctors to deprive their patients of care, including clearly beneficial care that in other circumstances they would not hesitate to provide? Just as the problem is new, so are the ethical justifications.

First, it is claimed that limiting care is what society wishes, and that the medical profession has an obligation not only to accept the will of society but to further it. Doctors are simply anticipating and delivering what is expected of them by the body politic, despite the fact that individual patients may want something else when they are sick.

Second, it is argued that because third parties now pay for nearly all medical care, they have gained a legitimate voice—indeed, the overriding voice—in how much medical care patients should receive. I find this a peculiarly American argument. Essentially the message is that whoever pays the piper calls the tune. The purest example of this view is the Oregon plan for rationing the care received by Medicaid patients. This is often described as a decision to allocate scarce resources rationally and justly, but it is, of course, nothing of the sort. It is instead a matter of taxpayers deciding to limit the care received by the poor, on the grounds that the taxpayers are funding it. Those who drew up the priority list of medical services are not those to whom it would apply. Even if we were to accept the idea that paying for medical care confers the right to limit it, we should remember that most patients do in fact still pay for their medical care, just as they always did. They simply pay in advance and indirectly, through their work or their taxes. The third parties are not using their own money.

The third justification for doctors to be double agents is the most compelling. It appeals to the doctor as good citizen or, more dramatically, to the doctor as occupant of a metaphorical lifeboat with limited supplies. According to this view, resources saved in denying patients expensive medical care could be used to provide less expensive care to a larger number of patients. Or it could be used for even more important public purposes, such as education. This line of argument has been put forward most persuasively by Dan Callahan (1990) who contends that Americans have overvalued individual health care compared with other social goods.

ARGUMENTS AGAINST DOUBLE AGENTS

Despite these justifications, I see five serious problems with the view that doctors should act to contain costs, patient by patient. First and most simply, this view of the role of doctors is based on the premise that resources in our health care system are in fact scarce. But, of course, they aren't. The mere fact that we spend so much more on health care than all other advanced nations is proof that our health care resources are plentiful. Given that in 1990 we spent about $2,566 on every man, woman, and child in the United States, and Canada spent only $1,770, we can hardly claim inadequate resources (Schieber, Poullier, and Greenwald 1992). And since Americans and Canadians are subject to the same ailments and have roughly the same outcomes, we must assume that our system is grossly inefficient. Clearly, the answer to an inefficient system is not to stint on care, but rather to restructure the system to make it more efficient.

Second, enlisting doctors as ad hoc rationers presumes that resources saved by denying health care would be put to better use. But in our system there is absolutely no reason to think that it would. As Norman Daniels (1986) has pointed out, in the United Kingdom or Canada, resources saved by denying care would be used for presumably more valuable health care, but that is not the case here. In the U.S., we do not have a closed system in which funds taken from one form of health care are diverted to another that is deemed to be more important. Instead, funds not used for health care may find their way into any sector of the larger economy, to be used for anything—e.g., defense, education, farm subsidies, or personal savings. Furthermore, even funds that remain within the health care system might not be used for more effective care; instead, money saved on, say, heart transplantation may very well find its way to a hospital's public relations office or to higher salaries for administrators. Under these circumstances, it is very difficult to sustain an ethical argument for doctors acting as double agents. The only principled way to ration health care is to close the system and establish limits that apply to everyone—not just to the poor.

Third, asking doctors to be double agents overlooks an important symbolic function of health care. Our society was founded on the principle that individuals enjoy a set of basic rights that cannot be denied them. As medicine has become increasingly effective in preserving life, medical care has come to be counted among these rights. Thus, doctors are seen to preserve a basic human right, namely life, just as criminal lawyers are seen to preserve liberty by defending their clients. Lawyers do not decide part way through a trial to call it quits because it's just too expensive to go on with it. In both situations, there has been a consensus that the single-minded focus on the patient or the client serves the broader interests of society. This argument is particularly compelling in a society as unequal as ours. People will tolerate the vast inequities in income and privilege in this country only if they feel assured that their irreducible set of rights is truly protected. It has been suggested that high technology medicine may serve precisely such a reassuring function in our society. And public opinion polls tend to support this view (Blendon 1991). The public, in contrast to the third-party payers, does not feel that we are spending too much on health care, only that we are not getting our money's worth.

Fourth, when doctors act as double agents, they are merely acting on their own particular prejudices. They are deciding that this or that medical service costs too much. This is not a medical judgment, but a political or philosophical one. Another doctor (or a plumber or electrician) might make quite a different judgment. This is no way to allocate health care.

And fifth and perhaps most important, the doctor as double agent is not honest. Sick people need and expect their doctors' single purpose to be to heal them. The doctor-patient relationship would not survive a candid statement by the doctor that only care that seems to the doctor to be worth the money will be provided. Anything short of full efforts to heal the individual patient, then, must involve a hidden agenda—an ethically indefensible position.

CONCLUSION

In sum, we should be loath to abandon or modify the patient-centered ethic, and we should be wary of ethical justifications for doing so. Unfortunately, history shows us that ethics in practice are often highly malleable, *justifying* political decisions rather than *informing* them. Necessity is the mother of invention, in ethics as well as in other aspects of life. For example, in 1912, when the AMA thought salaried practice was a threat to the autonomy of the profession, its Code of Ethics pronounced it unethical for physicians to join group practices. Now, some 80 years later, we are again hearing that it is a matter of ethics for the medical profession to carry out what is essentially a political agenda. But ethics should be a little more stable than that. Ethics should be based on fundamental moral principles governing our behavior and obligations toward one another. If a doctor is ethically committed to care for the individual patient, that commitment should not be abridged lightly. And it should not be nullified by a budgetary crunch. Doctors should continue to care for each patient unstintingly, even while they join with other citizens to devise a more efficient and just health care system. To control costs effectively will in my view require a coherent national health care system, with a global cap and a single payer (Angell 1993). Only in this way can we have an affordable health care system that does not require doctors to be double agents.

ACKNOWLEDGMENT

This article is based on the annual Edmund D. Pellegrino Lecture at the Kennedy Institute of Ethics.

REFERENCES

Angell, Marcia. 1993. How Much Will Health Care Reform Cost? *New England Journal of Medicine* 328: 1778–79.

Blendon, Robert J. 1991. The Public View of Medicine. *Clinical Neurosurgery* 37: 2563–65.

Callahan, Daniel. 1990. *What Kind of Life? The Limits of Medical Progress.* New York: Simon & Schuster.

Daniels, Norman. 1986. Why Saying No to Patients in the United States Is So Hard: Cost Containment, Justice, and Provider Autonomy. *New England Journal of Medicine* 314: 1380–83.

Morreim, E. Haavi. 1991. *Balancing Act: The New Medical Ethics of Medicine's Economics.* Boston: Kluwer Academic Publishers.

Schieber, George J.; Poullier, Jean-Pierre; and Greenwald, Leslie M. 1992. U.S. Health Expenditure Performance: An International Comparison and Data Update. *Health Care Financing Review* 13 (4): 1–15.

Stoline, Anne M., and Weiner, Jonathan p. 1993. *The New Medical Marketplace: A Physician's Guide to the Health Care System in the 1990s.* Baltimore: Johns Hopkins University Press.

Woolhandler, Steffie, and Himmelstein, David. 1991. The Deteriorating Administrative Efficiency of the U.S. Health Care System. *New England Journal of Medicine* 324: 1253–58.

MANAGED CARE AND THE GOALS OF MEDICINE
Daniel Callahan

Callahan confronts the question of whether managed care—a system of integrated health-care delivery designed to control costs—is compatible with the goals of medicine. He understands the goals of medicine to include the promotion of health and the prevention of disease, the relief of pain and suffering, the cure of those who are ill and the care of those who cannot be cured, and the forestalling of death and pursuit of a peaceful death. Managed care, Callahan argues, is in principle compatible with the goals of medicine but in practice may not be, depending upon such factors as whether profit is sought and whether the integrity of physicians' medical judgment is preserved.

The recent dramatic increase in managed care plans, the increase in the number of people affected by these plans, and the post-1994 enthusiasm generated by them in some quarters raise a basic question. Are some means of financing and delivering health care more (or less) compatible with the goals of medi-

Reprinted with permission of Blackwell Publishing Ltd. from *Journal of the American Geriatrics Society,* vol. 46, no. 3 (March 1998), pp. 385–388.

cine? Or, to add a slightly different twist, are some means more open, in practice, to corrupting the goals of medicine even if, in principle, they are compatible with those goals?

I ask these questions because, as I will argue, there is no reason, *in principle,* that managed care cannot be harmonious with the goals of medicine, but there is every reason to worry that, *in practice,* there will be significant conflict. In the end, much will depend on (1) the place managed care attains in the American healthcare system, (2) the way its programs are organized and administered, and (3) the extent to which market and profit motives come to dominate the programs.

In addition to making that particular argument, however, I want also to press the claim that when debating the meaning and possibilities of managed care, we should also engage in a parallel debate about the goals of medicine. Just as we would do well to assume that much is still ambiguous and uncertain about the nature and future of managed care, we should also recognize that the goals of medicine are not—in our contemporary context—clear or self-evident. A general problem with most recent healthcare debates, both in the United States and abroad, has been a dissociation of ends and means: the debates are almost entirely about means—organizational, financial, political—and too little about what medicine should now be seeking. Procedural questions have come to dominate substantive ones. I will first discuss the goals of medicine and then move on to the relationship between these goals and managed care.

THE GOALS OF MEDICINE

Modern scientific medicine has been ambitious in its aims and expansionary in its scope. It has believed in the value and necessity of constant medical progress, in the superiority of scientific medicine and a reductionistic organically oriented methodology, and in serving human needs that transcend the narrow confines of health as it has been traditionally conceived. In recent years, this set of medical values has been combined with a number of important cultural values. These include the right of autonomy and self-determination and the need for an equitable distribution of healthcare resources.

All of these values, medical and social, have had their critics, and I do not want to paint a monochromatic picture. Scepticism has been expressed about the possibilities of medical progress, and there have been calls for a medical paradigm that is biopsychosocial rather than reductionistic and some worries about the medicalization of all of life's problems. Autonomy has by no means been embraced by

all physicians, or by all patients, and the struggles over equitable resource distribution have seen market proponents arrayed against those who believe in a more centrally organized and government-oriented system.

Despite these arguments, however, there has been much common agreement about the central importance of the doctor-patient relationship, the necessity of high quality medical care, and the need for medicine to maintain its internal integrity. Given the earlier cited assorted disagreements, however—some of them profound—one might well ask if some goals of medicine could now command general assent and, if so, whether it will be possible for managed care to serve them well.

Let me address the first question by listing the goals that were specified by a recent international project on the goals of medicine of which I was a part:

- The prevention of disease and injury and the promotion and maintenance of health
- The relief of pain and suffering caused by maladies
- The care and cure of those with a malady, and the care of those who cannot be cured
- The avoidance of premature death and the pursuit of a peaceful death

I do not believe there would be much dispute about these four goals as listed. The problem arises when one wants to know whether some are more important than, or should take priority over, others; what the meaning of those goals might be in different cultural and social contexts; and whether age, gender, and other social characteristics should make a difference in the interpretation of those goals. I will not pursue those questions here because they are explored at length in *The Goals of Medicine: Setting New Priorities.*[1] Instead, I will examine the goals stated above and ask, generally, about their compatibility with managed care.

First the aims of managed care must be specified. I believe it fair to say that managed care is meant to be the provision of health care in a way that integrates the various elements of health care while controlling the costs of that care. In short, managed care has both a medical goal, the integration of care, and a financial goal, controlling the costs of that care. That is the theory and the ideal. At the same time, proponents of managed care have also espoused a commitment to the welfare of patients, to a grounding in the best scientific information, and to high quality of care. For-profit organizations have added the further specification that they seek a decent financial return to their shareholders.

Now if one is interested only in comparing the ideal goals of medicine with the ideal goals of managed care, no apparent conflicts exist. Do not managed care organizations espouse the value of health promotion and disease prevention? Do they not espouse the relief of pain and suffering? Do they not pursue the cure of those who can be cured and the care of those who cannot? Do they not espouse the avoidance of a premature death and the pursuit of a peaceful death?

THE REAL AND THE IDEAL WORLD

What about the ways things are, that real world that so commonly impinges on our ideals? Everything is not so clear there. Whereas health promotion and disease prevention are ideals, the time pressures on physician gatekeepers are frequently such that they have little time to do the kind of counseling necessary for good health promotion. There is no evidence that the relief of pain and suffering is handled better by managed care organizations than by earlier financial and organizational arrangements; medicine as a whole has not done well with this kind of care. Managed care, by common agreement, has not done well with chronic illness and disability; in fact, it seems to be doing quite poorly. In regard to the care of the dying, managed care has yet to make any special mark although there is some, but not much, evidence to suggest it is going to do a better job in the near future than the rest of medicine has in the past, which has not been exemplary.

Nevertheless, the managed care world is now complex, diverse, and changing rapidly. One can find grist for any mill, with good examples and bad, horror stories and uplifting stories. Just how managed care will shake out in the long run is anything but clear, and, thus, it is probably premature to take either the good reports or the unsettling ones as symbols of models of the future. Much will depend on the responsiveness of managed care organizations to public and professional criticism, the effects of market competition, the extent to which the organizations are able (and not just willing) to change their ways, and the degree and kind of government regulations that develop concerning the quality of the care they provide.

It is all too easy to forget the kinds of abuses that fee-for-service medicine spawned, not only in generating excessive costs and flagrant waste but also in exposing patients to the hazards of unnecessary and even harmful treatments, treatments generated by that most noxious of combinations an infatuation with technology and action wedded to a belief that it is just fine if doctors, particularly specialists, do well even as they do good. What managed care has going for it at the moment is that even those members of the public who are critical still, on the whole, accept the trade-off between the kind of quality they would like and the amount of money that are willing to pay for it. A lower quality, if the price is right, seems not unacceptable to the public.

FORMS OF CARE, FORMS OF ORGANIZATION

However, I am still skimming what I take to be the surface of the problem. I asked at the outset whether some forms of delivering health care are more or less compatible with the goals of medicine and whether some are more open than others to corrupting the goals of medicine. On the surface, there seems no inherent conflict between the ideal goals of medicine and the ideals of managed care. Even if numerous complaints abound about some of the actual practices of managed care, they may turn out to be correctable when the dust of the present rapid change settles a bit.

There are three serious soft spots—real points of hazard—that need closer examination: (1) the profit motive in managed care; (2) the effect on physician integrity of managerial oversight and practice guidelines; and (3) the effect of the present emphasis on managed care on the American health system as a whole. It is not easy to show the kind of compatibility between the goals of medicine and those of managed care to which I have so far pointed.

Profits, the Market, and Managed Care Managed care comes in two economic forms, nonprofit and for-profit. Because I have spent my entire career in the nonprofit world, I am under no illusion that altruism and economic self-denial are always the norm there. Many people make a very good living from nonprofit medicine—think of the salaries of those who manage large systems or hospitals—and few of those who do will tell those with money to give them less of it. Even so, the purpose of nonprofit organizations is not making money or pleasing outside stockholders. There is in that sense no fundamental conflict between the altruistic goals of medicine as an institution and the altruistic goals of (most) nonprofit organizations, including those in health care. That some or many individuals in those organizations are not swept away personally by fits of altruism does not conflict with the general organizational point.

It is a different matter with for-profit organizations. Conflict of interest is built in at the heart of their enterprise: the good of the organization and those who own it against the good that medicine would do. Even worse, actually, the principal aim of for-profit medicine (or so I believe) is to make money. The ethics, goals, and ethos of medicine may be operative in that context, but more as a secondary aim than as an equally competitive primary value.

Now I do not doubt that some, perhaps many, people in for-profit medicine may have chosen that field for their entrepreneurial ventures because they could combine doing good and doing (very) well. Many of us want to find means of succeeding both ways in this world, of doing something valuable for others while, at the same time, doing something for ourselves. In this case, however, the controlling principle of for-profit organizations has to be their capacity to turn a profit. Why? The answer is not simply to keep everyone in the organization happy and well-fed, which nonprofits can do, but also to turn a profit for those who have invested their money in the organization and who expect not just to feel good but to get a good financial return on their investment.

Whereas a good excuse in the nonprofit world might be that no money was made, that the organization just broke even for the year (which is in fact

what it should do), this is intolerable in the for-profit world. Few investors would be happy to know that their money was doing many wonderful things but not making them any money. That's fine with their personal eleemosynary contributions but not their financial investments.

In short, an inherent and fundamental conflict exists between the goals of medicine and the goals of for-profit managed care organizations. Because the latter might occasionally accomplish some or even much good while turning a profit does not eliminate the conflict. In hard times, or in highly competitive situations, those organizations will have to make a choice about their moral and financial priorities. It is hard to see how a responsible for-profit manager could justify harming the stake of his or her investors in the name of the higher goals of medicine. That is not what he is supposed to do. It would be a form of managerial irresponsibility in the context of the purpose for which he was hired. We might salute that person for personal courage and integrity, but there would be no management prizes.

It seems no less obvious that when financial or other incentives exist for physicians to hold down costs, the same fundamental conflict arises. The situation is not different from the one that applied earlier in fee-for-service medicine, in which there was at least a tacit financial incentive to treat patients (by calling for more tests, more visits, more shifting of therapies, etc.). In that situation, however, the conflict of interest was self-imposed: the physicians did not have to do what, absent compelling medical reasons, they did not see a need to do. In the case of managed care incentives, however, they are built into the system, allowing no choice of escape.

Managerial Oversight and Physician Integrity
The problem of financial incentives for physicians touches directly on a broader issue, the effect of managerial oversight on physician integrity. This oversight can take the form of pressures to stay within certain parameters in treatment patterns, to withhold referrals to specialists, and to gain permission for certain forms of diagnostic or therapeutic interventions. There are two separate issues here. The first is whether, speaking objectively, there is any necessary harm to patients as a result of such pressures. The

second is whether the subjective harm to her integrity that a physician might feel constitutes a moral real harm.

On the first issue, the answer, I believe, is that patients will not necessarily be harmed by managerial oversight of their physicians. Those pressures may force a physician to practice better medicine than he otherwise might on his own, might protect patients from unnecessary diagnostic and therapeutic procedures, and might ensure that the most scientifically based medicine is practiced. I say "not necessarily" because there is nothing in managerial oversight per se that threatens harm to patients. Everything will depend on how that oversight is managed as well as its general quality, which can be good or bad.

On the second issue, a different kind of judgment is necessary. If by "physician integrity" one means the notion that a physician should be free to practice medicine in a way that is in accord with her considered medical and moral judgment, then managerial oversight can pose a threat to that integrity. This threat would be possible even in those cases where, in fact, the patient might be better off because of the oversight. However, that is irrelevant where integrity is concerned for medical integrity concerns how a physician evaluates the competence and correctness of her actions. The importance of the ancient Socratic maxim that one should "know oneself" is matched by the more modern notion that one should be "true to oneself," but that may be impossible if managerial decisions force conduct that one would not choose oneself.

Managed Care and the American Health System
In 1993 and 1994, there was a strong push for some form of universal health care. That push failed, abysmally so, opening the way for a powerful private sector turn toward managed care. However, the purpose of managed care is to organize the operation and procedures of a healthcare system, not to extend health care to those who do not have it. The way it has worked out is that managed care is being applied to those who already have or can afford coverage, not to those who have none at all. Whereas managed care organizations have financial incentives to increase their membership, those incentives do not apply to those who cannot pay (or are poorly subsidized

by government) or to those who might increase costs significantly.

I have not heard of any managed care organization whose ambition is to capture the entire population and, thus, to achieve universal care, nor do I expect to in this or any other world. If this comment is true of nonprofit managed care organizations, it will be true in spades for for-profit managed care organizations. Indeed, so strong are the financial incentives *not* to enroll an unlimited number of people indiscriminately that one can say an inherent conflict exists between the goal of universal care and the actual operation of managed care organizations.

However, could it happen that, with sufficient competition and a truly free market, universal care might—by a kind of ink-blot creep—eventually cover everyone? That is not likely, at least without government subvention, because a large group of people would remain who could not pay out of their own pockets or have employers who could pay for them. Managed care, in any event, is designed not to be a form of equitable national health care allocation but to be a way of organizing the inner life of a particular system.

MEDICAL GOALS, ECONOMIC MEANS

I have pointed to three places where an achievement of the goals of medicine could be compromised by managed care, particularly in its for-profit manifestation. Unlike other problems with managed care, those I have pointed to appear to be intrinsic to that form of care and would not be overcome easily. The attempt to mix the altruistic aims of medicine as an institution with the self-seeking that is native to a profit motive poses the most fundamental conflict. The only possible guard against this kind of conflict—impossible to imagine—would be some kind of corporate dedication to risk financial ruin rather than compromise medical goals. If ever a manager were tempted to go in that direction, one could well imagine a quick objection from his colleagues, but will our patients be better off if we go under altogether? The tyranny of survival would no doubt take over at that point.

The only way to overcome the threat to the subjective sense of physician integrity is to give physicians an active and cooperative role in fashioning the incentives and pressures under which they would live. Even if this role were of some help, however, there would still be some individual physicians whose judgment would deviate from that of their peers and the common consensus. There would be no obvious relief for them, except for an organization that would tolerate some deviance. But how much deviance could an organization tolerate if it began posing a threat to the bottom line or, more benignly, allowed some physicians to flaunt the standards by which their peers agreed to live?

Finally, what more might be said about managed care and universal health coverage? It would be a fool's mission to look to the managed care fraternity and industry to take the lead in a new drive for universal healthcare coverage. That kind of coverage also faces a general legislative and taxpayer unwillingness to see taxes raised in any significant way to provide universal care. In a universal health care system, the techniques of managed care might well insure the most efficient kind of care, but only government support, over and beyond those techniques, would bring about the needed universality.

We seem, then, to be stuck where we began in 1994. Managed care is sweeping the land, mainly because it has seemed the best way to control costs, whether those of government entitlement programs or those of private employers providing benefits for their employees. Nevertheless, it has left unaddressed, and will continue to leave unaddressed, the needs of those who cannot pay. At this point, only some kind of moral or entitlement revolution seems sufficient to bring universal health care. There is, unhappily, little evidence that any such revolution is brewing. In the meantime, as we wait, great creativity will be needed to find ways for managed care to overcome its practical problems, reassure its legitimate critics, and ameliorate the intrinsic conflict it poses for a proper pursuit of the goals of medicine.

REFERENCE

1 The goals of medicine: Setting new priorities. Hastings Cent Rep 1992 (special supplement); 26:1–27.

CONSCIENCE AND CONSCIENTIOUS ACTIONS IN THE CONTEXT OF MCOS
James F. Childress

After examining the concepts of conscience and conscientious action, Childress explores the ways in which managed care organizations (MCOs) often exert pressures on clinicians that create conflicts of interest and problems of conscience. He then describes a range of acts of non-cooperation—including conscientious objection or refusal, withdrawal, and whistle blowing—that may express and protect a clinician's conscience. Finally, he calls for the development of public policies in medicine that will reduce the demands on conscience, reduce conflicts of interest that create problems of conscience, and reduce the risks faced by those who act conscientiously.

Conscience is an agent's mode of consciousness and awareness of his or her own acts and their value or disvalue, their goodness or badness, their rightness or wrongness. It is often retrospective. It often emerges as agents look back over their acts. And it is often negative—a bad conscience or feelings of guilt and shame that accompany an awareness of one's own acts as bad or wrong. We often describe a good conscience as quiet, clean, and easy and refer to this state of affairs as one of peace, wholeness, and integrity. (For a more complete discussion, see Chil-

Reprinted with permission of the publisher from *Kennedy Institute of Ethics Journal*, vol. 17, no. 4 (1997), pp. 403–411. Copyright © 1997 by The Johns Hopkins University Press.

dress 1979.) Acts are conscientious when they are rooted in this consciousness, this awareness, and when they are efforts to abide by the standards or realize the ideals that give conscience its content.

Sometimes we also appeal to our consciences to explain and justify our actions. We say: "We can't do that because it would violate our consciences." It would violate standards we affirm in conscience and would thus subvert our integrity and our sense of wholeness and harmony in the self, as well create unpleasant feelings such as guilt and shame. Appeals to conscience, in short, express an agent's sense of moral limits, particularly against institutional, social, legal, and political authorities.

However, the dictates of conscience are formal—conscience demands that agents do what they believe to be right *or else*, where "or else" indicates the threat of the kinds of negative experiences already noted. Conscience thus demands consistency between belief and action. When agents anticipate a loss of integrity if they act in certain ways, they refer to fundamental, core beliefs, ones that define their character, but these may vary from one person to another.

Agents who appeal to their consciences to explain and justify their conduct often indicate that they would suffer a severe sanction—the loss of integrity or wholeness—if they violated their moral limits. They frequently express this fear in dramatic ways: "I couldn't live with myself if I did that." "I have to answer to myself first." "I must protect my sense of myself." "I could not look at myself in the mirror." "I would hate myself in the morning." "I couldn't sleep at night."

With this brief sketch of conscience and conscientious actions, including appeals to conscience to explain and justify actions, I now will examine how managed care organizations (MCOs) sometimes create conflicts of conscience. However, my discussion in no way supposes that MCOs are ethically unjustifiable arrangements for health care. (For a more complete discussion of ethical issues in managed care, see Childress, forthcoming.)

MANAGED CARE ORGANIZATIONS AND CONFLICTS OF CONSCIENCE

The following case, which was prepared by physician Elena Gates (ASLME 1995, 30 September),

Associate Clinical Professor of Obstetrics and Gynecology at the University of California in San Francisco, offers one way into some of the conflicts of conscience that may arise in MCOs.

The faculty obstetric practice at a large urban medical center is in the process of negotiating contracts for prenatal care and delivery. Most of the health plans with which the group has contracts are interested in shortening the length of stay for delivery. One of the plans makes the following offer:

The plan will reimburse $1400.00 per patient for prenatal care and delivery (about 30% below their current reimbursement rate). As an incentive to achieve a shorter length of stay, the plan will raise the reimbursement rate to $1500.00 per patient if the group is able to bring its length of stay for uncomplicated births down from 1.8 days to 1.3 days.

This health plan brings with it about 25% of the total number of obstetric patients cared for by the faculty practice each year. Declining to contract with this plan would clearly hurt the practice (as well as the teaching program at the medical school, which benefits from the faculty private practice in terms of patient volume).

As they discuss the health plan's offer, several members of the group indicate that they feel that obstetric length of stay can safely be decreased as part of the overall effort to responsibly decrease the cost of medical care. They are pleased at the opportunity to increase reimbursements. Other members of the group are concerned about what appears to be clear conflict of interest: get the patient out sooner and take home more money. One individual points out that if such an incentive were agreed to, it would have to be disclosed to patients. There ensues a discussion about how best to rationalize such an incentive plan to the group's pregnant patients. No acceptable approach is arrived at. A fundamental disagreement remains between those who believe that accepting the health plan's offer is reasonable and those who feel that it is clearly inappropriate.

Some of the participants in this case worried about apparent and real conflicts of interest and conflicts of obligation. *Conflicts of obligation* occur when a physician has an obligation to the patient and an obligation to persons or entities other than the patient. For example, a physician may have an obligation to the patient and an obligation to the MCO (among other entities). These obligations *to* the patient and *to* the MCO may not in fact conflict, according to one interpretation, because the physician's contract with the MCO may specify his/her obligation to the patient so that it does not conflict with the obligation to MCO. However, in reality, especially when traditional expectations are changing, patients may and often do believe that traditional physician obligations to patients still stand and still have priority.

So there may be a conflict between traditional profession-based obligations to patients and new organization-based obligations. Similar conflicts emerge in other institutional and organizational settings, such as the military, prisons, certain companies, and sports medicine. They also arise in research and teaching and anywhere else the physician serves as a "double agent" (Angell 1993). In an extreme form of conflict, the clinician may find it both obligatory to do X and obligatory not to do X. Here the physician faces a genuine dilemma. Such a dilemma may arise in certain rationing schemes adopted by MCOs.

Managed care organizations ration health care in the sense of limiting access to some forms of potentially beneficial care on the basis of cost. Rationing may occur, for instance, when a primary care provider, who serves as a gatekeeper to various forms of health care, determines that a particular patient's medical complaint does not merit referral to a costly specialist. Such a judgment may reflect the particular rationing scheme the MCO has designed to serve its own goals in health care without substantial input from physicians or patients. Constraints on physicians' abilities to act on behalf of their patients pose serious ethical problems for medical gatekeepers and others. Physicians sometimes may be able to act effectively on their patients' behalf without "gaming the system," but some "gaming" actions may threaten, perhaps unfairly, the MCO's allocation pattern. Hence their dilemma.

A few years ago, Dennis Novack and colleagues (1989) wanted to determine how physicians respond to situations in which deception offers one way, perhaps the only way, to accomplish some morally significant ends. Following is one of the scenarios the researchers used in the study:

You are seeing Mrs. Lewis, a 52-year-old patient of yours, for her annual physical, which reveals no abnormalities. You tell her that everything looks normal and that you are going to order routine blood tests and her annual screening mammography, which you feel is important for women of her age. She is against the mammography, saying that the last time you ordered it, she had to pay for it herself. You know she is of modest means and cannot easily afford it. You are surprised that her health insurance did not cover it. Upon asking your secretary, you learn that the insurance covers the cost of mammography only if there is a breast mass or objective clinical evidence of the possibility of cancer. The secretary tells you that the way to get around this [problem] is to put down "rule out cancer" instead of "screening mammography" on the form.

Almost 70 percent of the physicians in the survey said they would put "rule out cancer," even though, for the insurance company, that designation indicates a breast mass or other objective clinical evidence of the possibility of cancer, neither of which is present in this case. Most were willing to represent a screening test as a diagnostic test. Furthermore, and quite interestingly, 85 percent of this group insisted that their act would not involve "deception." Even 53 percent of the physicians who elsewhere in the survey indicated they never deceive would put "rule out cancer." In such cases, physicians have to determine when one obligation (to help the patient) outweighs another obligation (not to deceive).

Conflicts of interest appear when physicians or other health care professionals have personal (often financial) interests at odds with fidelity or loyalty to the patient. Here the patient's interests conflict with the professional's own interests. Conflicts of interest do not necessarily involve breaches of obligations. As Marc Rodwin (1993) notes, conflicts of interest refer to circumstances, situations, states of affairs, and conditions that create incentives of some kind for professionals to breach their obligations of fidelity, their fiduciary obligations, to the patient or client. They provide the incentives for acts, but are not themselves acts. They create the risk of breached obligations, especially by weakening the agent's conscience.

Of course, conflicts of interest also mark fee-for-service medicine, not only in such practices as fee-splitting, self-referral, and the like, but in its very temptation to overdiagnose and overtreat for additional fees. The new incentives offered to physicians to limit services are attempts to correct the problems of fee-for-service medicine. After all, since the incentives of fee-for-service are partly responsible for the run-a-way costs, reverse incentives could conceivably curtail those costs. "Only one thing was overlooked," Rodwin (1993, p. 9) observes, "rewarding physicians for using resources frugally does not eliminate financial conflicts of interests. It creates new conflicts with different effects."

For example, most health maintenance organizations (HMOs) hold back a portion of the primary physician's income—10 to 30 percent with the higher figures appearing in for-profit HMOs. Part or all of that amount is returned at the end of the year, depending on the overall financial condition of the HMO and, in some cases, the particular physician's productivity and frugality. Such an arrangement clearly creates incentives for physicians to limit their care to patients and thus establishes a troubling conflict of interest. It is all the more troubling when the financial incentives are direct and substantial, when, for instance, the particular physician's salary is substantially affected by his or her productivity and frugality rather than by the overall productivity and frugality of the practice group. Two critics charge that MCOs in effect pressure "doctors to exploit patients' trust for financial gain" or, perhaps more accurately, financial survival (Woolhandler and Himmelstein 1995).

CONSCIENTIOUS NON-COOPERATION

A fundamental question of conscience emerges when physicians and other health care professionals have to determine whether and to what extent they will participate in practices they consider unethical—for instance, in MCOs that create conflicts of interest and conflicts of obligation. Traditionally Roman Catholic moral theology has distinguished between formal and material cooperation in evil. In formal cooperation, the agent both consents to and actively participates in the wrongdoing of others, while in material cooperation the agent does not consent but nevertheless through an action that is good or indifferent somehow contributes to the evil action (see Maguire 1986, p. 129). Although not unproblematic, this traditional doctrine at least, as Daniel Maguire

(1986, p. 129) notes, "face[d] the fact that in a complex world of sinful persons, total detachment from evil is impossible." However impossible total detachment is, conscientious persons may attempt to detach themselves from certain acts, practices, and policies.

One sort of detachment is the refusal to do what one considers morally wrong or bad. For instance, an individual may refuse to comply with a "gag" rule. In this sort of case, the agent is expected to perform an act that he or she takes to be morally wrong under the circumstances and conscientiously refuses to do so. Suppose that in the case presented earlier the plan insists that physicians not disclose the incentives to the patient. Or suppose the MCO reviews a patient's chart and insists that a particular obstetrics patient be discharged even though her physician believes that it is in her best medical interest to remain a day or two longer. Conscientious refusals to act as the MCO dictates in some cases may raise moral questions because agents have made contracts with, and thus promises to, the organization or because the acts involve deception and other acts that are considered prima facie though not absolutely wrong.

A second kind of detachment involves efforts to avoid complicity in others' wrongdoing. Suppose the clinician is able to avoid directly doing what she considers unethical. She may, nevertheless, be aware that the MCO's morally shady practices affect her patients adversely even though they do not directly affect her clinical decisions. Then questions may arise about whether her participation (if she hasn't signed on yet) or continued participation (if she has already signed on) may (1) appear to signal silent approval, or (2) even help to legitimate the institution or organization, and thus constitute a kind of complicity with evil practices.

A third kind of detachment involves efforts to effect change from within the existing structure. In many cases, agents argue that they are remaining in an unethical institution, organization, or practice in order to improve it from within. For example, some U.S. government officials made this argument during the war in Vietnam. Similarly, a clinician may conscientiously view this as an option—to remain within a particular MCO to try to improve its policies and practices. This is often a difficult matter of conscience: How far can one compromise and get one's hands "dirty" in order to bring about change?

A fourth possibility is whistle blowing. While remaining within the MCO, a clinician may "blow the whistle," protesting unethical practices and calling for their reform. For instance, Steffie Woolhandler and David Himmelstein (1995, p. 1707) wrote an exposé of MCO practices in the *New England Journal of Medicine*:

> Until [needed] reforms are carried out, many physicians scrambling to preserve their careers will be tempted or forced into the corporate embrace. But if we shun the sick or withhold information to benefit ourselves, we conspire in the demise of our profession. Let us not end up like tobacco-company executives, who, repenting their sins, find that their contracts forbid confessing them.

Dr. Himmelstein was fired by his MCO after this exposé appeared, but the company said he was not dismissed because of his efforts for government-financed health care or this exposé. He was subsequently rehired. Yet another possibility is to blow the whistle in conjunction with withdrawal or disassociation from evil. This possibility combines voice and exit. (See the classic work by Hirschman 1970. In addition, see Weisband and Franck 1975).

Whistle blowing is often justified on the grounds that it may effectively alter objectionable practices. However, where change appears to be impossible or at least highly unlikely—or the agent fears certain repercussions and yet is unable to continue to participate in the practice—he or she may choose to withdraw or resign silently. For instance, a clinician may be unable in conscience to continue to participate in an MCO and may choose to withdraw without signaling her reasons and thus making a moral issue. Her concern is to protect her conscience, not to try to bring about change.

But even where efforts to effect change would probably be futile, agents may still choose to disassociate themselves symbolically from certain practices—they may choose to put themselves on record without expecting positive results. They choose to express and bear witness to important values (see Hill 1979).

CONCLUDING REFLECTIONS

Without proposing where individuals should draw lines or set limits of conscience, I have explored a few themes in conscience and conscientious actions and examined how some problems of conscience may arise in conflicts of obligation and conflicts of interest in MCOs. In this context, I considered a range of acts of non-cooperation that may express and protect an individual's conscience—conscientious objection or refusal, withdrawal, whistle blowing, and so forth. Some forms of non-cooperation—for example, deceptively gaming the system—are themselves morally problematic. In other cases, the moral decisions may be quite difficult—for instance, an obstetrician in the case presented earlier may have difficulty determining the responsible course of action if the group accepts the contract and decides not to disclose to patients the plan's financial incentives.

In addition, the personal and professional costs of some conscientious acts may be quite significant. It is not fair to expect individual professionals to bear all the moral burdens and risks. Managed care is important and it embodies important values, but it also sometimes creates situations of moral risk. It may take what Bernard Williams (1981) calls "moral luck" to avoid unmanageable moral conflicts—where we inevitably sacrifice some value we affirm. But we cannot and should not count on "moral luck" (or what some religious traditions might call "providence") or on personal and professional virtue in response to such risk. Public policies can also play an important role.

Public policies are important to ensure certain minimum standards of conduct—it is not possible to rely completely on professional virtue in the context of managed care. Public policies need to prohibit, regulate, and mandate certain forms of organizational structure and professional action. For example, public policies should require adequate disclosure at the time of enrollment and during care, and they should prohibit "gag clauses," as some states have done.

Beyond such information requirements, public policies also should regulate MCOs by limiting what they may do. In the obstetrics case, under the new contract the group would have to try to bring the length of stay for uncomplicated births down from 1.8 days to 1.3 days, and they would have a strong financial incentive to do so. Several states have set a standard for the length of stays in hospital following uncomplicated deliveries, and this legislative action is symbolically as well as actually important.

In short, it is important not to put all the moral burden on the individual professional's conscience. We should praise morally heroic actions, but as a society we should enact public policies to reduce the demands on conscience, to reduce conflicts of interest that create incentives for breaches of conscience, and to reduce the risks for conscientious actions—for example, the risks of being dismissed.

REFERENCES

Angell, Marcia. 1993. The Doctor as Double Agent. *Kennedy Institute of Ethics Journal* 3: 279–86.

ASLME. American Society of Law, Medicine, and Ethics. 1995. *Managed Care, Integrated Delivery Systems, and Consolidation—Law, Medicine, and Ethics.* Proceedings of the Annual Meeting, 29–30 September, Boston, MA.

Childress, James F. 1979. Appeals to Conscience. *Ethics* 89: 315–35.

———. Forthcoming. Managed Care: Some Basic Ethical Issues.

Hill, Thomas E., Jr. 1979. Symbolic Protest and Calculated Silence. *Philosophy and Public Affairs* 9: 83–102.

Hirschman, Albert O. 1970. *Exit, Voice, and Loyalty: Responses to Decline in Firms, Organizations, and States.* Cambridge, MA: Harvard University Press.

Maguire, Daniel C. 1986. Cooperation with Evil. In *Dictionary of Christian Ethics*, 2d ed., ed. James F. Childress and John Macquarrie, p. 129. Philadelphia: The Westminster Press.

Novack, Dennis H.; Detering, Barbara J.; Arnold, Robert; et al. 1989. Physicians' Attitudes Toward Using Deception to Resolve Difficult Ethical Problems. *Journal of the American Medical Association* 261: 2980–85.

Rodwin, Marc A. 1993. *Medicine, Money, and Morals: Physicians' Conflicts of Interest.* New York: Oxford University Press.

Weisband, Edward, and Franck, Thomas A. 1975. *Resignation in Protest: Political and Ethical Choices between Loyalty to Team and Loyalty to Conscience in American Public Life.* New York: Grossman Publishers.

Williams, Bernard. 1981. Moral Luck. In *Moral Luck: Philosophical Papers 1973–1980*, pp. 20–39. Cambridge: Cambridge University Press.

Woolhandler, Steffie, and Himmelstein, David U. 1995. Extreme Risk—The New Corporate Proposition for Physicians. *New England Journal of Medicine* 333: 1706–8.

ANNOTATED BIBLIOGRAPHY

Beauchamp, Tom L.: "The Promise of the Beneficence Model for Medical Ethics," *Journal of Contemporary Health Law and Policy 6* (Spring 1990), pp. 145–155. Beauchamp presents a historical and conceptual overview of the beneficence and autonomy models of the physician-patient relationship, before critically evaluating the effort of Edmund D. Pellegrino to reconcile the two in a reconstructed beneficence model.

Bok, Sissela: *Lying: Moral Choice in Public and Private Life* (New York: Random House, 1978). In this classic book, Bok provides a highly detailed examination of ethical issues connected with lying.

Buchanan, Allen E., and Dan W. Brock: *Deciding for Others: The Ethics of Surrogate Decision Making* (Cambridge: Cambridge University Press, 1989). Part I of this influential work develops a general theory of medical decision making for incompetent patients. Part II applies this theoretical framework to the distinctive problems raised by minor, elderly, and psychiatric patients.

Council on Ethical and Judicial Affairs, American Medical Association: "Conflicts of Interests: Physician Ownership of Medical Facilities," *JAMA* 267 (May 6, 1992), pp. 2366–2369. This position paper by the American Medical Association argues that physicians generally should not refer patients to medical facilities at which they do not directly provide care if they have a financial interest in the facility. An exception is made, however, for cases in which the community has a demonstrated need for the facility, and there is no alternative way to finance the facility.

Edelstein, Ludwig: *Ancient Medicine* (Baltimore, MD: Johns Hopkins, 1967). Edelstein discusses the Hippocratic Oath and identifies two distinct sets of obligations—those to the patient and those to the physician's teacher and the teacher's progeny.

Elliott, Carl, and Tod Chambers, eds.: *Prozac as a Way of Life* (Chapel Hill, NC: University of North Carolina Press, 2004). The eleven essays in this volume offer groundwork for a philosophical discussion of the ethical and cultural dimensions of the selective serotonin reuptake inhibitor antidepressants. Focusing on the growing use of medication as a means of enhancement (as opposed to treatment), authors from the fields of bioethics, psychiatry, and psychology addresses issues connected with personal identity, the elasticity of psychiatric diagnosis, and aggressive marketing by drug companies.

Faden, Ruth R., and Tom L. Beauchamp: *A History and Theory of Informed Consent* (New York: Oxford University Press, 1986). This ambitious work spans the history, theory, and practice of informed consent in medicine, human behavioral research, philosophy, and law.

Green, Ronald M.: "Medical Joint-Venturing: An Ethical Perspective," *Hastings Center Report* 20 (July–August 1990), pp. 22–26. Green considers and rejects leading arguments offered in defense of medical joint-venturing, in which physicians refer patients to facilities (e.g., surgery centers) in which they have financial interests. Arguing that such joint-venturing fails even to meet ethical standards appropriate to business, he concludes that the practice is ethically indefensible.

Grisso, Thomas, and Paul S. Appelbaum: *Assessing Competence to Consent to Treatment: A Guide for Physicians and Other Health Professionals* (New York: Oxford University Press, 1998). The product of an eight-year study of patients' decision-making capacities, this book describes the role of competence in the doctrine of informed consent, analyzes the elements of decision making, and shows how determinations of competence can be made in varied medical settings.

Lidz, Charles W., Paul S. Appelbaum, and Alan Meisel: "Two Models of Implementing Informed Consent," *Archives of Internal Medicine* 148 (June 1988), pp. 1385–1389. The authors provide detailed, contrasting descriptions of two ways of implementing the doctrine of informed consent: the event model and the process model. They argue in favor of the process model before noting some of its limitations.

Parens, Erik, ed.: *Enhancing Human Traits: Ethical and Social Implications* (Washington, DC: Georgetown University Press, 1998). This anthology serves as an excellent introduction to such biomedical enhancements as cosmetic surgery, antidepressants for "the worried well," and genetic enhancements. The thirteen essays explore conceptual, ethical, policy-related, and cultural issues provoked by efforts to enhance human traits with biomedical means.

Pellegrino, Edmund D.: "Managed Care at the Bedside: How Do We Look in the Moral Mirror?" *Kennedy Institute of Ethics Journal* 7 (December 1997), pp. 321–330. Focussing on ethical issues that arise at the bedside, Pellegrino argues that while managed care is morally neutral in principle, in practice it often creates significant conflicts for physicians and forces compromises in the caring dimensions of the physician-patient relationship.

President's Commission for the Study of Ethical Problems in Medicine and Biomedical and Behavioral Research: *Making Health Care Decisions: The Ethical and Legal Implications of Informed Consent in the Patient-Practitioner Relationship*, Vol. 1: *Report* (Washington, DC: U.S. Government Printing Office, 1982). This report presents the commission's conclusions and recommendations regarding both the role of informed consent in the patient-practitioner relationship and the means to promote a fuller understanding by patients and professionals of their common enterprise.

_____: *Making Health Care Decisions*, Vol. 2: *Appendices: Empirical Studies of Informed Consent*. This volume contains the empirical studies used by the President's Commission in formulating its conclusions.

_____: *Making Health Care Decisions*, Vol. 3: *Studies in the Foundations of Informed Consent*. Viewpoints represented in this volume are those of a psychologist, a historian, an anthropologist, a sociologist, a pediatrician-oncologist, a philosopher, and a medical student.

President's Council on Bioethics: *Beyond Therapy: Biotechnology and the Pursuit of Happiness* (Washington, DC: President's Council on Bioethics, 2003). This report investigates the potential implications of using biotechnology "beyond therapy" in seeking better children, superior individual performance, avoidance of the effects of aging, and happiness. The PCB intends with this report "to advance the nation's awareness and understanding of a critical set of bioethical issues and to bring them beyond the narrow circle of bioethics professionals into the larger public arena."

Rodwin, Marc A.: *Medicine, Money, and Morals: Physicians' Conflicts of Interests* (New York: Oxford University Press, 1993). After providing a historical overview of the American medical profession's response to conflicts of interest from 1890 to 1992, Rodwin examines incentives to increase services, incentives to decrease services, and the profession's ineffective responses to both types of incentive. In the final two chapters, he draws inferences for effective public policy.

White, Becky Cox: *Competence to Consent* (Washington, DC: Georgetown University Press, 1994). In addition to offering a concise introduction to major philosophical and ethical issues involved in competence to consent, this book presents White's own theory of competence and a set of practical suggestions.

Wicclair, Mark R.: "Patient Decision-Making Capacity and Risk," *Bioethics* 5 (April 1991), pp. 91–104. Wicclair criticizes "risk-related standards" of decision-making capacity (competence). His main target is the standard defended by Allen E. Buchanan and Dan W. Brock, which requires balancing the values of (1) respecting a patient's self-determination and (2) protecting his or her well-being.

CHAPTER 3

HOSPITALS, NURSES, FAMILIES, AND MEDICAL CONFIDENTIALITY

INTRODUCTION

Today a great deal of medical care is provided in hospitals, nursing homes, clinics, and other institutions. Providers of this care include nurses, social workers, staff physicians, operating room technicians, and other professionals and paraprofessionals. Many medical care providers are not private practitioners but employees of these institutions. Meanwhile, as contemporary biomedical ethics continues to evolve as a field, the proper role of patients' family members in medical decision making receives increasing attention. This attention to the family's role is especially focused when parents face difficult, even agonizing, decisions affecting the long-term welfare of their infants or young children. Institutional settings, the involvement of professionals in addition to physicians, and the participation of family are all factors that extend our discussion of medical decision making well beyond the moral considerations raised in Chapter 2, which center on the physician-patient relationship. This chapter examines the rights of hospital patients, the role and responsibilities of nurses, issues connected with the family's involvement in medical decision making, and issues concerning the protection of patient confidentiality.

PROFESSIONAL STATEMENTS REGARDING PATIENTS' RIGHTS AND PROFESSIONALS' OBLIGATIONS

What can hospital patients reasonably expect during their stay in a hospital? What are their rights and responsibilities? The American Hospital Association's (AHA) "The Patient Care Partnership: Understanding Expectations, Rights and Responsibilities," reprinted in this chapter, addresses these questions at a general level. An earlier AHA document, "The Patient's Bill of Rights," focused much more on patients' rights than does the present statement, which supersedes the earlier one.[1] Statements of patients rights serve as reminders to hospital patients and health professionals that patients have certain specific rights and must be treated as persons with dignity; they are neither "mere objects" to be manipulated by professionals nor subservient individuals who have waived their rights simply by becoming hospital patients.

In partial contrast, the "Patient Care Partnership" indicates at a more general level what patients can reasonably expect during a hospital stay. For example, patients can expect hospital staff to maintain a commitment to high-quality care and a safe environment. Patients can also expect an informed consent process that includes a discussion of the patient's diagnosis, appropriate treatment options, the risks and expected benefits of each option, and the patient's health care priorities. To facilitate this communication process, patients have a responsibility to be forthcoming about their medical histories, allergies, current medications, and other matters. Finally, patients can expect conscientious protection of their rights, including their rights to informed consent, to designate a surrogate decision maker, and to medical confidentiality.

Whether in the hospital setting or elsewhere, patients' rights entail obligations on the part of health-care professionals. For example, the idea that patients have a right to confidentiality implies that professionals are obliged to respect their patients' confidentiality. But professionals often see themselves as having obligations not only to patients, but to other persons or groups as well. For example, the American Nurses Association Code of Ethics for Nurses, reprinted in this chapter, articulates nurses' obligations to the nursing profession and to the public as well as to patients. Interestingly, while other codes of nursing ethics have generally asserted an obligation to carry out physicians' orders, this code does not. The omission is consistent with the priority given in the code to the patient's rights and welfare: "The nurse's primary commitment is to the patient."

THE ROLE AND RESPONSIBILITIES OF NURSES

Nurses face moral problems similar to those faced by physicians as well as moral problems uniquely related to their professional role. Like physicians, nurses must sometimes choose between doing what they believe will promote patients' well-being and respecting patients' self-determination. Various models of the nurse-patient relationship are possible, including a paternalistic model and a very different contracted-clinician model, which respects both a patient's right of self-determination and a nurse's right of conscientious refusal.[2]

But nurses also face dilemmas that physicians do not face. These dilemmas result from the nurse's position within the system or unit in which nurses work—which may be regarded as a *hierarchy* or as a *team,* depending on which features are emphasized. Nurses in hospitals care for patients and supervise others providing care. Usually, they are directly responsible both for patient care and implementing therapy. At the same time, nurses often have little influence in decision making regarding patients. Furthermore, they are generally regarded as subordinate to doctors, who make diagnoses and issue orders that nurses are expected to carry out. Under these circumstances, nurses are sometimes confronted with situations in which their obligations to patients seem to conflict with their obligations to physicians. The following questions exemplify the kinds of problems nurses face: Should nurses follow physicians' orders when nurses have good reason to believe that the orders are mistaken, the physicians refuse to admit that they might be mistaken, and following orders seems likely to jeopardize patients' safety? What should nurses do if they have good reason to believe that physicians are violating one or more of their patients' rights? For example, what should a nurse do when a physician lies to or withholds important information from a patient?

Developing themes emphasized in feminist ethics (as discussed in Chapter 1), some commentators have emphasized the difficulties nurses face when protecting patients' interests requires them to "buck" the system. Joy Kroeger-Mappes, for example, underscores the hierarchical nature of this system and attributes a large part of the difficulty to classist and sexist forces in society.[3] She defends the increasingly prominent ideal of the nurse as an autonomous professional who is prepared, under some circumstances, to challenge physicians' authority in advocating for patients' interests.

In response to this emerging ideal, Lisa H. Newton, in an article reprinted in this chapter, defends the traditional ideal of the nurse, whose role requires submission to the authority of physicians. In defending the traditional nurse, Newton argues that hospitals can function properly only if professionals' roles are clearly recognized; since only physicians have the training required to deal with many medical situations, their authority must be respected. (Her arguments suggest viewing the doctor much as a quarterback. From this perspective, a player who questions and interferes with the quarterback's play calling is unlikely to help the team.) Moreover, hospital patients have emotional needs that are best met by nurses, who in their traditional role can act as surrogate mothers to patients.

Helga Kuhse in this chapter directly challenges the claim that the nature of nursing demands submission and subservience, rebutting a variety of arguments—including some advanced by Newton—that have been offered in support of this claim. For example, according to Kuhse, the idea that nurses' subservience is required for efficient handling of patients' medical needs rests on two dubious assumptions: that most or all medical decision making is characterized by great urgency and that maximal efficiency is achieved by nurses' adopting an absolute rule (as opposed to a presumption) of following doctors' orders. She also contends that the surrogate mother role for nurses would be unnecessary and condescending to many patients, demoralizing to nurses, and overly deferential to physicians' views about the goals of treatment. She concludes that the proper role for nurses is one of advocacy for patients rather than subservience to physicians. Indeed, in her view, subservience would harm patients more than it would benefit them.

That nurses should advocate for patients is assumed by Amy M. Haddad, who in this chapter focuses on the details of nurse-physician interactions in ethical decision making. Reflecting themes from the ethics of care (as discussed in Chapter 1), Haddad suggests that some common differences in the ethical perspectives of men and women may sometimes contribute to ethical conflicts that arise between physicians and nurses; she also highlights their differing degrees of power and authority. Haddad uses a case to illustrate strategies for protecting patients' interests without unnecessarily damaging professional relationships or compromising nurses' self-respect.

FAMILIES AND MEDICAL DECISION MAKING

As we have seen, professional obligations cannot be adequately addressed if we examine only the role of the physician in medical decision making. Nurses and other health professionals also have important roles. On the other side of the professional-patient relationship, it is surely insufficient to examine the patient's standpoint, because family members and others who are close to the patient sometimes figure importantly in medical decision making.

To put these questions into proper perspective, it will help to consider what may be the most significant breakthrough in contemporary biomedical ethics: the substantial moral authority now conferred on patients with decision-making capacity (see the introduction to Chapter 2). This newfound respect for patient autonomy has helped to generate a widely accepted hierarchy of decision-making standards. According to this hierarchy of standards, in cases where patients are competent (that is, where they have decision-making capacity), their *informed consent* is needed to justify medical interventions on them.[4] The standard of informed consent, however, does not meaningfully apply in the case of patients who are at the relevant time incompetent and therefore incapable of mature, responsible decision making. In the case of formerly competent patients, however, if there is significant evidence supporting a particular *substituted judgment,* then that standard applies. A substituted judgment is a judgment about what a patient would have wanted for the current situation in which he or she is incompetent.[5] In the case of patients who have never been competent, such as children and some severely mentally retarded adults, and in the case of formerly competent patients for whom there is insufficient evidence regarding what they would have wanted in the present circumstances, it is apparently impossible to respect their autonomy— either present or past. Thus, medical decisions for these patients are to be guided by consideration of their *best interests.* The hierarchy of decision-making standards therefore has this structure:

1. Informed Consent

2. Substituted Judgment

3. Best Interests

A striking feature of this picture is how patient-centered it is. Either the *patient's* informed consent is obtained, or an attempt is made to determine what the *patient* would have wanted, or one attempts to determine the *patient's* best interests. For reasons explored in detail in Chapter 2, such a patient-centered approach seems greatly preferable to the over-reaching paternalism that characterized traditional medical ethics.[6] But might the currently dominant picture of decision-making standards confer too much authority on the patient's preferences and interests?

The possibility of an affirmative answer emerges when we consider the patient's *family* in a variety of scenarios. (The term "family" need not be limited to those individuals whom the law recognizes as family; for example, a patient's closest friend might count as family.) Let us briefly examine four kinds of cases. In the first two kinds of cases, a conflict between the patient's interests and the family's interests is only apparent, not real, so serious consideration of the family's interests would not genuinely threaten the patient-centered approach. (1) Sometimes a patient's medical decision making is significantly responsive to family interests. In an example discussed by Thomas A. Mappes and Jane S. Zembaty in a reading reprinted in this chapter, a competent, terminally ill man is prepared to "let go" of life and refuse all life supports, but his wife is not yet ready to live without him. Out of love for his wife, such a man might give informed consent to life-extending treatment. In cases of this sort, the standard of informed consent appears to be consistent with recognition of the importance of family members' interests.

(2) A second kind of case involves surrogate decision making for incompetent patients. Suppose an incompetent, cancer-stricken woman could live another year or two

with aggressive treatment (where the burdens of treatment are not so great as to make treatment contrary to her medical interests). Her husband understands that while consideration of her medical interests alone appears to favor treatment, his wife would prefer *not* to be treated in the present situation for this simple reason: The costs of aggressive treatment and other medical costs accumulating over one or two years would exhaust family savings that she wanted very much to devote to their daughter's medical school education. In this case, because the woman is so responsive to family members' interests (in a sense, making them part of her own interests), a substituted judgment would be compatible with a significant appreciation of family interests.

Two remaining kinds of cases feature real conflicts between family interests and the widely accepted patient-centered hierarchy of decision-making standards. (3) In one of these kinds of cases, patients' decisions are contrary to family members' interests. Mappes and Zembaty describe the case of an elderly man who has suffered a stroke, yet remains competent, and now requires significant nursing care. His doctor suggests that he enter a nursing home but he refuses, citing the availability of his wife to care for him. His frail wife, however, feels unable to provide such care for him without seriously threatening her own health. Nevertheless, he insists that she meet his nursing needs—and she appears psychologically unable to refuse in the face of his insistence. In this case, the standard of informed consent suggests that he should be permitted to refuse nursing home care. Yet the burden such a refusal would place on his wife raises the question of whether this standard is morally adequate in cases like this, or whether, as Mappes and Zembaty argue, family interests need to enter the ethical analysis.

(4) In a final type of case to be considered here, family members who serve as surrogate decision makers for incompetent patients have interests that conflict with patients' interests. Suppose, for example, that an elderly woman with progressive Alzheimer's disease (which is cognitively disabling) and other medical problems is hospitalized with what may be terminal illness. Her husband rejects further aggressive treatments for his wife. To a significant extent, his decision is driven by his own interests in being free from the financial and emotional burdens imposed by his wife's long-term illness.[7] Cases like this raise the question of whether the substituted-judgment standard is too patient-centered when patient and family have conflicting interests.

It is increasingly doubtful that the "conventional wisdom" represented in the patient-centered hierarchy of standards is entirely adequate. Appropriate consideration of family interests seems to complicate the moral picture in at least some cases of medical decision making. How to adjudicate between the patient's and the family's interests, where the two sets of interests diverge, is one major area of controversy connected with the family's role in medical decision making. Equally controversial are parents' judgments regarding their children's best interests in certain medical contexts. Providing two examples are (1) parental decisions regarding cochlear implant surgery for their deaf children and (2) parental decisions regarding surgery and gender assignment for their intersex children.

Cochlear implants are surgically implanted devices that can partially enable hearing and speech comprehension for many deaf individuals. It may seem obvious that it is in a deaf child's best interests to have this surgery—even though it might not prove effective in his or her case and "successful" surgeries, so far, have been only partially effective. After all, one might naturally assume, deafness is a major disability so we should embrace any intervention that offers a chance of reducing the effects of deafness.

Matters are not so simple, however. First, for deaf children who have undergone cochlear implant surgery, learning to recognize and produce spoken language while depending on these devices is likely to be a long, arduous process—again, with no guarantee of success. More fundamentally, according to some commentators, enthusiasm about this type of surgery reflects the hearing majority's prejudice against deafness. Indeed, some have argued, cochlear implants represent a threat to a unique culture, the Deaf (with a capital D) culture. As Bonnie Tucker explains in a reading reprinted in this chapter, champions of Deaf culture regard deafness as a cultural identity rather than a disability. Deaf culturists define their community partly in terms of a shared language, American Sign Language (ASL). From their perspective, cochlear implant surgery represents an effort to assimilate deaf persons into the hearing mainstream, at best devaluing Deaf culture and at worst threatening cultural genocide. Responding to this position, Tucker, who is deaf, contends that deafness poses substantial objective disadvantages and that learning a spoken language in addition to ASL is the most promising approach to overcoming these disadvantages. Accordingly, she criticizes parents who refuse to authorize cochlear implant surgeries—a choice that, she thinks, constricts the opportunities available to deaf children—as well as Deaf culturists who oppose the use of these devices while demanding costly accommodations for their deafness.

Parental decisions for intersex children are, if anything, even more difficult and controversial than parental decisions about cochlear implant surgery for deaf children. Some infants are born intersex—that is, with one of various conditions that make it difficult to determine from outward appearance whether the infants are boys or girls. Intersex conditions include a wide variety of genital anomalies, such as a very large clitoris, a very small penis, or an underdeveloped vagina or testes. The most common intersex condition is congenital adrenal hyperplasia, in which an excess of androgen in infants who are genetically female causes the genitals to appear more masculine. Whereas removal of the entire clitoris used to be common in such cases, today it is more common to trim down excess tissue while preserving nerve-rich tissue. A rarer condition is that of a genetically male infant who is born with a "micropenis." Surgically creating a larger penis is extremely complicated, so many infants with this condition have undergone surgery that created a vagina and were raised as girls. In one of this chapter's readings, Sherri A. Groveman explains her intersex condition, Androgen Insensitivity Syndrome, which is characterized by XY (male) chromosomes and testes, but, due to an androgen receptor defect, an inability of the body to respond to testosterone in the testes and thereby acquire masculine-looking characteristics. Groveman's parents consented to a gonadectomy (removal of the testes) and female gender assignment; they also hid the truth of Groveman's condition from her, leaving her to discover the truth as an adult.

At least until recently, the standard medical approach to intersex was to perform "normalizing" surgery on the infant with a long-term strategy of shielding the growing child from the truth about his and/or her condition.[8] Lately this strategy has been challenged by many mature intersex individuals who have expressed anger and dismay at having been surgically modified before they could consent and then deceived about their condition. On the whole, the medical profession has been highly paternalistic in pressuring parents to consent to the standard approach ("normalizing" surgery and gender assignment without disclosure), has known little about the long-term effects of different approaches, and has arguably expressed their own discomfort about ambiguous genitalia in favoring the standard approach.

According to Groveman, what parents of intersex children need is emotional support, education about intersex, and the freedom to make well-informed, voluntary decisions for their children. While this assertion addresses the circumstances of the parents' decision making, there remains the question of what the intersex child's best interests require. Groveman implicitly addresses this question by arguing that intersex children need the truth about their ambiguous sexuality, need social acceptance, and (at least before they can competently decide for themselves) need no more surgery than is necessary for physical health.

CONFIDENTIALITY AND CONFLICTING OBLIGATIONS

Among patients' rights, the rights to privacy and confidentiality deserve special discussion along with the ethical principle of confidentiality. This chapter focuses on confidentiality rather than privacy. However, a clear understanding of confidentiality is best achieved in view of the distinction between confidentiality and privacy.

A person enjoys *privacy* when other individuals do not without permission invade what may be called his or her "sphere of privacy": a realm of intimate or sensitive information about the person that he or she generally does not wish to share with others or wishes to share with only a small circle of persons. Thus, sensitive medical information about Mr. Ramirez lies within his sphere of privacy. Since he would approve of his attending physician and other health professionals closely involved in his care learning details of his medical history, Mr. Ramirez would not consider their examining his medical record a violation of his privacy. By contrast, if another patient examined Mr. Ramirez's medical record without his permission, Mr. Ramirez would no doubt regard this intrusion as a violation of his privacy (an unauthorized entering of his sphere of privacy). To take another example, how Ms. Robbins appears while undressed lies within her sphere of privacy. Thus, if a stranger goes to great lengths to peer through Ms. Robbins's bedroom window while she is undressing, Ms. Robbins would almost certainly consider this unauthorized viewing an invasion of her privacy.

While privacy involves others not entering a person's sphere of privacy without permission, *confidentiality* involves those who have legitimate access to private information not bringing it out of that sphere and sharing it with others without permission. Thus, a doctor may legitimately enter (or access) large segments of a patient's sphere of privacy: his or her medical history, the appearance of his or her naked body if a physical examination or other procedure requires undressing, aspects of the patient's social history that bear directly on the patient's medical situation (e.g., concerning a history of alcoholism), and so on. If a doctor lacking permission discloses sensitive information to individuals other than health professionals who are closely involved with the patient's care, such disclosure constitutes a breach of confidentiality.

The importance of the principle of confidentiality in medicine has long been recognized. It is affirmed in the Hippocratic Oath as well as in more recent professional codes and statements such as those of the American Medical Association and the American Hospital Association. It is also recognized by the ethical codes of medical record librarians and social workers. The law further recognizes, in two ways, the importance of the patient's right to control information held by health professionals. First, physicians and psychotherapists are subject to legal sanctions if they reveal confidential information about patients. Second, physicians and psychotherapists are ordinarily exempt from giving testimony about their patients before a court of law. Most discussions of the moral significance of the principle of confidentiality in health care stress either respect for patient autonomy or the importance of protecting the trust undergirding the professional-patient relationship.

While the importance of medical confidentiality is broadly appreciated, some commentators hold that the duty to respect confidentiality is a prima facie one—that is, one that is sometimes justifiably overridden in conflicts with other moral duties. In this chapter the opinions in *Tarasoff v. Regents of the University of California* focus on the moral dilemmas posed for health-care professionals when such conflicts arise. Some of these conflicts take graphic form in the case (with commentaries) about HIV and confidentiality included in this chapter. The general issue this case provokes is, "Under what conditions, if any, may health-care professionals disclose confidential information about patients infected with HIV, in order to prevent harm to others?" In the *Tarasoff* case, the conflict at issue was between a psychologist's duty to respect the confidence of a patient, Prosenjit Poddar, and the psychologist's possible duty to warn a young woman, Tatiana Tarasoff, that Poddar might try to kill her. He did not warn the woman or her family, and Poddar did kill her. Did the psychologist have a duty to warn someone who was not his patient? If he did, should this duty have taken precedence over his duty to respect Poddar's confidences? The contrast between the majority and the dissenting opinions in the case serves to heighten awareness of the moral dilemmas raised for the professional who must choose between violating confidentiality and failing to perform an act that might save the life of another human being or otherwise prevent serious harm.

D.D.

NOTES

1 American Hospital Association, "A Patient's Bill of Rights" (first published 1973; revised 1992).
2 Sheri Smith, "Three Models of the Nurse-Patient Relationship," in Stuart F. Spicker and Sally Gadow (eds.), *Nursing: Images and Ideals* (New York: Springer Publishing Company, 1980), pp. 176–188.
3 Joy Kroeger-Mappes, "Ethical Dilemmas for Nurses: Physicians' Orders Versus Patients' Rights" (originally published in Thomas A. Mappes and Jane S. Zembaty, eds., *Biomedical Ethics* [New York: McGraw-Hill, 1981], pp. 75–102).
4 Exceptions in the case of emergencies, in which there is insufficient time for obtaining informed consent, are generally accepted and may be justified by the assumption that patients *would* consent to interventions in such circumstances if they had the opportunity to do so. Such presumed consent may also justify other exceptions to the rule requiring (explicit) informed consent, but we need not consider them for present purposes.
5 One form of evidence that can be especially useful in attempting to determine what a formerly competent patient would have wanted in the present situation is an *advance directive* that offers some specific directions for treatment decisions. Allen E. Buchanan and Dan W. Brock have argued, however, that there are several good reasons to conceptualize the honoring of advance directives as a distinct decision-making standard that is appropriately located between the informed-consent and substituted-judgment standards within the hierarchy discussed. See *Deciding for Others* (Cambridge: Cambridge University Press, 1989), Chapter 2.
6 Traditional paternalism is also patient-centered insofar as the patient's best interests are the focus of decision making. The more recent approach makes the patient's *decisions and priorities* the central concern.
7 John Hardwig presents this case in "The Problem of Proxies with Interests of Their Own: Toward a Better Theory of Proxy Decisions," *Journal of Clinical Ethics* 4 (Spring 1993), pp. 20–27.
8 Lisa Melton, "New Perspectives on the Management of Intersex," *The Lancet* 357 (June 30, 2001), p. 2110.

THE PATIENT CARE PARTNERSHIP: UNDERSTANDING EXPECTATIONS, RIGHTS AND RESPONSIBILITIES

American Hospital Association

This statement, issued by the American Hospital Association (AHA) in 2003, supersedes the AHA's "A Patient's Bill of Rights." The present statement indicates at a general level what patients can expect during a hospital stay. These expectations include the following: (1) a commitment on the part of hospital staff to high-quality care and a safe environment; (2) a decision-making process, involving both physician and patient, that includes a discussion of the patient's medical condition, appropriate treatment options, the risks and expected benefits of each option, and the patient's health-care priorities; and (3) protection of the patient's rights to informed consent, to designate a surrogate decision maker, and to medical confidentiality.

When you need hospital care, your doctor and the nurses and other professionals at our hospital are committed to working with you and your family to meet your health care needs. Our dedicated doctors and staff serve the community in all its ethnic, religious and economic diversity. Our goal is for you and your family to have the same care and attention we would want for our families and ourselves.

The sections explain some of the basics about how you can expect to be treated during your hospital stay. They also cover what we will need from you to care for you better. If you have questions at any time, please ask them. Unasked or unanswered questions can add to the stress of being in the hospital. Your comfort and confidence in your care are very important to us.

WHAT TO EXPECT DURING YOUR HOSPITAL STAY

- **High quality hospital care.** Our first priority is to provide you the care you need, when you need it, with skill, compassion, and respect. Tell your caregivers if you have concerns about your care or if you have pain. You have the right to know the identity of doctors, nurses and others involved in your

care, and you have the right to know when they are students, residents or other trainees.

- **A clean and safe environment.** Our hospital works hard to keep you safe. We use special policies and procedures to avoid mistakes in your care and keep you free from abuse or neglect. If anything unexpected and significant happens during your hospital stay, you will be told what happened, and any resulting changes in your care will be discussed with you.

- **Involvement in your care.** You and your doctor often make decisions about your care before you go to the hospital. Other times, especially in emergencies, those decisions are made during your hospital stay. When decision-making takes place, it should include:

Discussing your medical condition and information about medically appropriate treatment choices. To make informed decisions with your doctor, you need to understand:

The benefits and risks of each treatment.
Whether your treatment is experimental or part of a research study.
What you can reasonably expect from your treatment and any long-term effects it might have on your quality of life.
What you and your family will need to do after you leave the hospital.

The financial consequences of using uncovered services or out-of-network providers. Please tell your caregivers if you need more information about treatment choices.

Discussing your treatment plan. When you enter the hospital, you sign a general consent to treatment. In some cases, such as surgery or experimental treatment, you may be asked to confirm in writing that you understand what is planned and agree to it. This process protects your right to consent to or refuse a treatment. Your doctor will explain the medical consequences of refusing recommended treatment. It also protects your right to decide if you want to participate in a research study.

Getting information from you. Your caregivers need complete and correct information about your health and coverage so that they can make good decisions about your care. That includes:

Past illnesses, surgeries or hospital stays.
Past allergic reactions.
Any medicines or dietary supplements (such as vitamins and herbs) that you are taking.
Any network or admission requirements under your health plan.

Understanding your health care goals and values. You may have health care goals and values or spiritual beliefs that are important to your well-being. They will be taken into account as much as possible throughout your hospital stay. Make sure your doctor, your family and your care team know your wishes.

Understanding who should make decisions when you cannot. If you have signed a health care power of attorney stating who should speak for you if you become unable to make health care decisions for yourself, or a "living will" or "advance directive" that states your wishes about end-of-life care; give copies to your doctor, your family and your care team. If you or your family need

help making difficult decisions, counselors, chaplains and others are available to help.

- **Protection of your privacy.** We respect the confidentiality of your relationship with your doctor and other caregivers, and the sensitive information about your health and health care that are part of that relationship. State and federal laws and hospital operating policies protect the privacy of your medical information. You will receive a Notice of Privacy Practices that describes the ways that we use, disclose and safeguard patient information and that explains how you can obtain a copy of information from our records about your care.

- **Preparing you and your family for when you leave the hospital.** Your doctor works with hospital staff and professionals in your community. You and your family also play an important role in your care. The success of your treatment often depends on your efforts to follow medication, diet and therapy plans. Your family may need to help care for you at home.

  You can expect us to help you identify sources of follow-up care and to let you know if our hospital has a financial interest in any referrals. As long as you agree that we can share information about your care with them, we will coordinate our activities with your caregivers outside the hospital. You can also expect to receive information and, where possible, training about the self-care you will need when you go home.

- **Help with your bill and filing insurance claims.** Our staff will file claims for you with health care insurers or other programs such as Medicare and Medicaid. They also will help your doctor with needed documentation. Hospital bills and insurance coverage are often confusing. If you have questions about your bill, contact our business office. If you need help understanding your insurance coverage or health plan, start with your insurance company or health benefits manager. If you do not have health coverage, we will try to help you and your family find financial help or make other arrangements. We need your help with collecting needed information and other requirements to obtain coverage or assistance.

While you are here, you will receive more detailed notices about some of the rights you have as a hospital patient and how to exercise them. We are always interested in improving. If you have questions, comments, or concerns, please contact _____.

CODE OF ETHICS FOR NURSES
American Nurses Association

In 2001 the American Nurses Association House of Delegates approved the principles enumerated here as part of a revised Code of Ethics for Nurses. The principles articulate some of the obligations nurses have to their patients, the nursing profession, and the public. Especially significant are the statement that "[t]he nurse's primary commitment is to the patient . . ." and the absence of any statement to the effect that nurses have an obligation to follow physicians' orders.

1. The nurse, in all professional relationships, practices with compassion and respect for the inherent dignity, worth and uniqueness of every individual, unrestricted by considerations of social or economic status, personal attributes, or the nature of health problems.

2. The nurse's primary commitment is to the patient, whether an individual, family, group, or community.

3. The nurse promotes, advocates for, and strives to protect the health, safety, and rights of the patient.

4. The nurse is responsible and accountable for individual nursing practice and determines the appropriate delegation of tasks consistent with the nurse's obligation to provide optimum patient care.

5. The nurse owes the same duties to self as to others, including the responsibility to pre-serve integrity and safety, to maintain competence, and to continue personal and professional growth.

6. The nurse participates in establishing, maintaining, and improving healthcare environments and conditions of employment conducive to the provision of quality healthcare and consistent with the values of the profession through individual and collective action.

7. The nurse participates in the advancement of the profession through contributions to practice, education, administration, and knowledge development.

8. The nurse collaborates with other health professionals and the public in promoting community, national, and international efforts to meet health needs.

9. The profession of nursing, as represented by associations and their members, is responsible for articulating nursing values, for maintaining the integrity of the profession and its practice, and for shaping social policy.

THE ROLE AND RESPONSIBILITIES OF NURSES

IN DEFENSE OF THE TRADITIONAL NURSE
Lisa H. Newton

Newton counters the emerging ideal of the nurse as an autonomous professional who is prepared to challenge doctors' authority and advocate for patients' interests. In its place she urges "the traditional ideal of the skilled and gentle caregiver, whose role in health care requires submission to authority as an essential component." In defending the traditional nurse, Newton argues the following: (1) to run properly, hospital bureaucracies require clear roles and lines of authority; (2) only physicians are properly trained to handle serious medical situations that arise without warning; and (3) the vulnerable, compromised situation of hospital patients gives rise to emotional needs that can be met only by nurses, who serve (in some respects) as surrogate mothers. After exploring limits of the nurse-mother analogy, Newton responds to objections motivated by a feminist perspective. In this discussion, she emphasizes that being an autonomous person is compatible with choosing a nonautonomous professional role, such as that of the nurse, and that support for men's participation in nursing would be liberating for them.

When a truth is accepted by everyone as so obvious that it blots out all its alternatives and leaves no respectable perspectives from which to examine it, it becomes the natural prey of philosophers, whose essential activity is to question accepted opinion. A case in point may be the ideal of the "autonomous professional" for nursing. The consensus that this ideal and image are appropriate for the profession is becoming monolithic and may profit from the presence of a full-blooded alternative ideal to replace the cardboard stereotypes it routinely condemns. That alternative, I suggest, is the traditional ideal of the skilled and gentle caregiver, whose role in health care requires submission to authority as an essential component. We can see the faults of this traditional ideal very clearly now, but we may perhaps also be able to see virtues that went unnoticed in the battle to displace it. It is my contention that the image and ideal of the traditional nurse contain virtues that can be found nowhere else in the health care professions, that perhaps make an irreplaceable contribution to

the care of patients, and that should not be lost in the transition to a new definition of the profession of nursing. . . .

ROLE COMPONENTS

The first task of any philosophical inquiry is to determine its terminology and establish the meanings of the key terms for its own purposes. To take the first term, a *role* is a norm-governed pattern of action undertaken in accordance with social expectations. The term is originally derived from the drama, where it signifies a part played by an actor in a play. In current usage, any ordinary job or profession (physician, housewife, teacher, postal worker) will do as an example of a social role; the term's dramatic origin is nonetheless worth remembering, as a key to the limits of the concept.

Image and ideal are simply the descriptive and prescriptive aspects of a social role. The *image* of a social role is that role as it is understood to be in fact, both by the occupants of the role and by those with whom the occupant interacts. It describes the character the occupant plays, the acts, attitudes, and expectations normally associated with the role. The *ideal* of

Reprinted from *Nursing Outlook,* vol. 29 (June 1981), pp. 348–354, with permission from Mosby-Year Book, Inc.

a role is a conception of what that role could or should be—that is, a conception of the norms that should govern its work. It is necessary to distinguish between the private and public aspects of image and ideal.

Since role occupants and the general public need not agree either on the description of the present operations of the role or on the prescription for its future development, the private image, or self-image of the role occupant, is therefore distinct from the public image or general impression of the role maintained in the popular media and mind. The private ideal, or aspiration of the role occupant, is distinct from the public ideal or normative direction set for the role by the larger society. Thus, four role-components emerge, from the public and private, descriptive and prescriptive, aspects of a social role. They may be difficult to disentangle in some cases, but they are surely distinct in theory, and potentially in conflict in fact.

TRANSITIONAL ROLES

In these terms alone we have the materials for the problematic tensions within transitional social roles. Stable social roles should exhibit no significant disparities among images and ideals: what the public generally gets is about what it thinks it should get; what the job turns out to require is generally in accord with the role-occupant's aspirations; and public and role-occupant, beyond a certain base level of "they-don't-know-how-hard-we-work" grumbling, are in general agreement on what the role is all about. On the other hand, transitional roles tend to exhibit strong discrepancies among the four elements of the role during the transition; at least the components will make the transition at different times, and there may also be profound disagreement on the direction that the transition should take. . . .

BARRIERS TO AUTONOMY

The first contention of my argument is that the issue of autonomy in the nursing profession lends itself to misformulation. A common formulation of the issue, for example, locates it in a discrepancy between public image and private image. On this account, the public is asserted to believe that nurses are ill-educated, unintelligent, incapable of assuming responsibility,

and hence properly excluded from professional status and responsibility. In fact they are now prepared to be truly autonomous professionals through an excellent education, including a thorough theoretical grounding in all aspects of their profession. Granted, the public image of the nurse has many favorable aspects—the nurse is credited with great manual skill, often saintly dedication to service to others, and, at least below the supervisory level, a warm heart and gentle manners. But the educational and intellectual deficiencies that the public mistakenly perceives outweigh the "positive" qualities when it comes to deciding how the nurse shall be treated, and are called upon to justify not only her traditionally inferior status and low wages, but also the refusal to allow nursing to fill genuine needs in the health care system by assuming tasks that nurses are uniquely qualified to handle. For the sake of the quality of health care as well as for the sake of the interests of the nurse, the public must be educated through a massive educational campaign to the full capabilities of the contemporary nurse; the image must be brought into line with the facts. On this account, then, the issue of nurse autonomy is diagnosed as a public relations problem: the private ideal of nursing is asserted to be that of the autonomous professional and the private image is asserted to have undergone a transition from an older subservient role to a new professional one but the public image of the nurse ideal is significantly not mentioned in this analysis.

An alternative account of the issue of professional autonomy in nursing locates it in a discrepancy between private ideal and private image. Again, the private ideal is that of the autonomous professional. But the actual performance of the role is entirely slavish, because of the way the system works—with its tight budgets, insane schedules, workloads bordering on reckless endangerment for the seriously ill, bureaucratic red tape, confusion, and arrogance. Under these conditions, the nurse is permanently barred from fulfilling her professional ideal, from bringing the reality of the nurse's condition into line with the self-concept she brought to the job. On this account, then, the nurse really is not an autonomous professional, and total reform of the power structure of the health care industry will be necessary in order to allow her to become one.

A third formulation locates the issue of autonomy in a struggle between the private ideal and an altogether undesirable public ideal: on this account, the public does not want the nurse to be an autonomous professional, because her present subservient status serves the power needs of the physicians; because her unprofessional remuneration serves the monetary needs of the entrepreneurs and callous municipalities that run the hospitals; and because the low value accorded her opinions on patient care protects both physicians and bureaucrats from being forced to account to the patient for the treatment he receives. On this account, the nurse needs primarily to gather allies to defeat the powerful interest groups that impose the traditional ideal for their own unworthy purposes, and to replace that degrading and dangerous prescription with one more appropriate to the contemporary nurse.

These three accounts, logically independent, have crucial elements of content in common. Above all, they agree on the objectives to be pursued: full professional independence, responsibility, recognition, and remuneration for the professional nurse. And as corollary to these objectives, they agree on the necessity of banishing forever from the hospitals and from the public mind that inaccurate and demeaning stereotype of the nurse as the Lady with the Bedpan: an image of submissive service, comforting to have around and skillful enough at her little tasks, but too scatterbrained and emotional for responsibility.

In none of the interpretations above is any real weight given to a public ideal of nursing, to the nursing role as the public thinks it ought to be played. Where public prescription shows up at all, it is seen as a vicious and false demand imposed by power alone, thoroughly illegitimate and to be destroyed as quickly as possible. The possibility that there may be real value in the traditional role of the nurse, and that the public may have good reasons to want to retain it, simply does not receive any serious consideration on any account. It is precisely that possibility that I take up in the next section.

DEFENDING THE "TRADITIONAL NURSE"

As Aristotle taught us, the way to discover the peculiar virtues of any thing is to look to the work that it accomplishes in the larger context of its environment. The first task, then, is to isolate those factors of need or demand in the nursing environment that require the nurse's work if they are to be met. I shall concentrate, as above, on the hospital environment, since most nurses are employed in hospitals.

The work context of the hospital nurse actually spans two societal practices or institutions: the hospital as a bureaucracy and medicine as a field of scientific endeavor and service. Although there is enormous room for variation in both hospitals bureaucracies and medicine, and they may therefore interact with an infinite number of possible results, the most general facts about both institutions allow us to sketch the major demands they make on those whose function lies within them.

To take the hospital bureaucracy first: its very nature demands that workers perform the tasks assigned to them, report properly to the proper superior, avoid initiative, and adhere to set procedures. These requirements are common to all bureaucracies, but dramatically increase in urgency when the tasks are supposed to be protective of life itself and where the subject matter is inherently unpredictable and emergency prone. Since there is often no time to re-examine the usefulness of a procedure in a particular case, and since the stakes are too high to permit a gamble, the institution's effectiveness, not to mention its legal position, may depend on unquestioning adherence to procedure.

Assuming that the sort of hospital under discussion is one in which the practice of medicine by qualified physicians is the focal activity, rather than, say, a convalescent hospital, further contextual requirements emerge. Among the prominent features of the practice of medicine are the following: it depends on esoteric knowledge, which takes time to acquire and which is rapidly advancing; and, because each patient's illness is unique, it is uncertain. Thus, when a serious medical situation arises without warning, only physicians will know how to deal with it (if their licensure has any point), and they will not always be able to explain or justify their actions to nonphysicians, even those who are required to assist them in patient care.

If the two contexts of medicine and the hospital are superimposed, three common points can be seen. Both are devoted to the saving of life and health; the atmosphere in which that purpose is carried out is inevitably tense and urgent; and, if the purpose is to be accomplished in that atmosphere, all participating activities and agents must be completely subordinated to the medical judgments of the physicians. In short, those, other than physicians, involved in medical procedures in a hospital context have no right to insert their own needs, judgments, or personalities into the situation. The last thing we need at that point is another autonomous professional on the job, whether a nurse or anyone else.

PATIENT NEEDS: THE PRIME CONCERN

From the general characteristics of hospitals and medicine, that negative conclusion for nursing follows. But the institutions are not, after all, the focus of the endeavor. If there is any conflict between the needs of the patient and the needs of the institutions established to serve him, his needs take precedence and constitute the most important requirements of the nursing environment. What are these needs?

First, because the patient is sick and disabled, he needs specialized care that only qualified personnel can administer, beyond the time that the physician is with him. Second, and perhaps most obviously to the patient, he is likely to be unable to perform simple tasks such as walking unaided, dressing himself, and attending to his bodily functions. He will need assistance in these tasks, and is likely to find this need humiliating; his entire self-concept as an independent human being may be threatened. Thus, the patient has serious emotional needs brought on by the hospital situation itself, regardless of his disability. He is scared, depressed, disappointed, and possibly, in reaction to all of these, very angry. He needs reassurance, comfort, someone to talk to. The person he really needs, who would be capable of taking care of all these problems, is obviously his mother, and the first job of the nurse is to be a mother surrogate.

That conclusion, it should be noted, is inherent in the word "nurse" itself: it is derived ultimately from the Latin *nutrire,* "to nourish or suckle"; the first meaning of "nurse" as a noun is still, according to *Webster's New Twentieth Century Unabridged*

Dictionary "one who suckles a child not her own." From the outset, then, the function of the nurse is identical with that of the mother, to be exercised when the mother is unavailable. And the meanings proceed in logical order from there: the second definitions given for both noun and verb involve caring for children, especially young children, and the third, caring for those who are childlike in their dependence—the sick, the injured, the very old, and the handicapped. For all those groups—infants, children, and helpless adults—it is appropriate to bring children's caretakers, surrogate mothers, nurses, into the situation to minister to them. It is especially appropriate to do so, for the sake of the psychological economies realized by the patient: the sense of self, at least for the Western adult, hangs on the self-perception of independence. Since disability requires the relinquishing of this self-perception, the patient must either discover conditions excusing his dependence somewhere in his self-concept, or invent new ones, and the latter task is extremely difficult. Hence the usefulness of the maternal image association: it was, within the patient's understanding of himself "all right" to be tended by mother; if the nurse is (at some level) mother, it is "all right" to reassume that familiar role and to be tended by her.

LIMITS ON THE "MOTHER" ROLE

The nurse's assumption of the role of mother is therefore justified etymologically and historically but most importantly by reference to the psychological demands of and on the patient. Yet the maternal role cannot be imported into the hospital care situation without significant modification—specifically, with respect to the power and authority inherent in the role of mother. Such maternal authority includes the right and duty to assume control over children's lives and make all decisions for them; but the hospital patient most definitely does not lose adult status even if he is sick enough to want to. The ethical legitimacy as well as the therapeutic success of his treatment depend on his voluntary and active cooperation in it and on his deferring to some forms of power and authority—the hospital rules and the physician's sapiential authority, for example. But these very partial, conditional, restraints are nowhere near the threat to patient autonomy that the real presence of a mother would be; maternal authority, total, diffuse, and unlimited, would be incompatible with the retention of moral freedom. And it is just this sort of total authority that the patient is most tempted to attribute to the nurse, who already embodies the nurturant component of the maternal role. To prevent serious threats to patient autonomy, then, the role of nurse must be from the outset, as essentially as it is nurturant, unavailable for such attribution of authority. Not only must the role of nurse not include authority; it must be incompatible with authority: essentially, a subservient role.

The nurse role, as required by the patient's situation, is the nurturant component of the maternal role and excludes elements of power and authority. A further advantage of this combination of maternal nurturance and subordinate status is that, just as it permits the patient to be cared for like a baby without threatening his autonomy, it also permits him to unburden himself to a sympathetic listener of his doubts and resentments, about physicians and hospitals in general, and his in particular, without threatening the course of his treatment. His resentments are natural, but they lead to a situation of conflict, between the desire to rebel against treatment and bring it to a halt (to reassert control over his life), and the desire that the treatment should continue (to obtain its benefits). The nurse's function speaks well to this condition: like her maternal model, the nurse is available for the patient to talk to (the physician is too busy to talk), sympathetic, understanding, and supportive; but in her subordinate position, the nurse can do absolutely nothing to change his course of treatment. Since she has no more control over the environment than he has, he can let off steam in perfect safety, knowing that he cannot do himself any damage.

The norms for the nurse's role so far derived from the patient's perspective also tally, it might be noted, with the restrictions on the role that arise from the needs of hospitals and medicine. The patient does not need another autonomous professional at his bedside, any more than the physician can use one or the hospital bureaucracy contain one. The conclusion so far, then, is that in the hospital environment, the traditional (nurturant and subordinate) role of the nurse seems more adapted to the nurse function than the new autonomous role.

PROVIDER OF HUMANISTIC CARE

So far, we have defined the hospital nurse's function in terms of the specific needs of the hospital, the physician, and the patient. Yet there is another level of function that needs to be addressed. If we consider the multifaceted demands that the patient's family, friends, and community make on the hospital once the patient is admitted, it becomes clear that this concerned group cannot be served exclusively by attending to the medical aspect of care, necessary though that is. Nor is it sufficient for the hospital-as-institution to keep accurate and careful records, maintain absolute cleanliness, and establish procedures that protect the patient's safety, even though this is important. Neither bureaucracy nor medical professional can handle the human needs of the human beings involved in the process.

The general public entering the hospital as patient or visitor encounters and reacts to that health care system as an indivisible whole, as if under a single heading of "what the hospital is like." It is at this level that we can make sense of the traditional claim that the nurse represents the "human" as opposed to "mechanical" or "coldly professional" aspect of health care, for there is clearly something terribly missing in the combined medical and bureaucratic approach to the "case": they fail to address the patient's fear for himself and the family's fear for him, their grief over the separation, even if temporary, their concern for the financial burden, and a host of other emotional components of hospitalization.

The same failing appears throughout the hospital experience, most poignantly obvious, perhaps, when the medical procedures are unavailing and the patient dies. When this occurs, the physician must determine the cause and time of death and the advisability of an autopsy, while the bureaucracy must record the death and remove the body; but surely this is not enough. The death of a human being is a rending of the fabric of human community, a sad and fearful time; it is appropriately a time of bitter regret, anger, and weeping. The patient's family, caught up in the institutional context of the hospital, cannot assume alone the burden of discovering and expressing the emotions appropriate to the occasion; such expression, essential for their own regeneration after their loss, must originate somehow within the hospital context itself. The hospital system must, somehow, be able to share pain and grief as well as it makes medical judgments and keeps records.

The traditional nurse's role addresses itself directly to these human needs. Its derivation from the maternal role classifies it as feminine and permits ready assumption of all attributes culturally typed as "feminine": tenderness, warmth, sympathy, and a tendency to engage much more readily in the expression of feeling than in the rendering of judgment. Through the nurse, the hospital can be concerned, welcoming, caring, and grief-stricken; it can break through the cold barriers of efficiency essential to its other functions and share human feeling.

The nurse therefore provides the in-hospital health care system with human capabilities that would otherwise be unavailable to it and hence unavailable to the community in dealing with it. Such a conclusion is unattractive to the supporters of the autonomous role for the nurse, because the tasks of making objective judgments and of expressing emotion are inherently incompatible; and since the nurse shows grief and sympathy on behalf of the system, she is excluded from decision-making and defined as subordinate.

However unappealing such a conclusion may be, it is clear that without the nurse role in this function, the hospital becomes a moral monstrosity, coolly and mechanically dispensing and disposing of human life and death, with no acknowledgment at all of the individual life, value, projects, and relationships of the persons with whom it deals. Only the nurse makes the system morally tolerable. People in pain deserve sympathy, as the dead deserve to be grieved; it is unthinkable that the very societal institution to which we generally consign the suffering and the dying should be incapable of sustaining sympathy and grief. Yet its capability hangs on the presence of nurses willing to assume the affective functions of the traditional nursing role, and the current attempt to banish that role, to introduce instead an autonomous professional role for the nurse, threatens to send the last hope for a human presence in the hospital off at the same time.

THE FEMINIST PERSPECTIVE

From this conclusion it would seem to follow automatically that the role of the traditional nurse should be retained. It might be argued, however, that the value of autonomy is such that any nonautonomous role ought to be abolished, no matter what its value to the current institutional structure.

Those who aimed to abolish black slavery in the United States have provided a precedent for this argument. They never denied the slave's economic usefulness; they simply denied that it could be right to enslave any person and insisted that the nation find some other way to get the work done, no matter what the cost. On a totally different level, the feminists of our own generation have proposed that the traditional housewife and mother role for the woman, which confined women to domestic life and made them subordinate to men, has been very useful for everyone except the women trapped in it. All the feminists have claimed is that the profit of others is not a sufficient reason to retain a role that demeans its occupant. As they see it, the "traditional nurse" role is analogous to the roles of slave and housewife—it is derived directly, in fact, as we have seen, from the "mother" part of the latter role—exploitative of its occupants and hence immoral by its very nature and worthy of abolition.

But the analogy does not hold. A distinction must be made between an autonomous person—one who, over the course of adult life, is self-determining in all major choices and a significant number of minor ones, and hence can be said to have chosen, and to be responsible for, his own life—and an autonomous *role*—a role so structured that its occupant is self-determining in all major and most minor role-related choices. An autonomous person can certainly take on a subordinate role without losing his personal autonomy. For example, we can find examples of slaves (in the ancient world at least) and housewives who have claimed to have, and shown every sign of having, complete personal integrity and autonomy with their freely chosen roles.

Furthermore, slave and housewife are a very special type of role, known as "life-roles." They are to be played 24 hours a day, for an indefinite period of time; there is no customary or foreseeable respite from them. Depending on circumstances, there may be de facto escapes from these roles, permitting their occupants to set up separate personal identities (some of the literature from the history of American slavery suggests this possibility), but the role-definitions do not contemplate part-time occupancy. Such life-roles are few in number; most roles are the part-time "occupational roles," the jobs that we do eight hours a day and have little to do with the structuring the rest of the twenty-four. An autonomous person can, it would seem, easily take up a subordinate role of this type and play it well without threat to personal autonomy. And if there is excellent reason to choose such a role—if, for example, an enterprise of tremendous importance derives an essential component of its moral worth from that role—it would seem to be altogether rational and praiseworthy to do so. The role of "traditional nurse" would certainly fall within this category.

But even if the traditional nurse role is not inherently demeaning, it might be argued further, it should be abolished as harmful to the society because it preserves the sex stereotypes that we are trying to overcome. "Nurse" is a purely feminine role, historically derived from "mother," embodying feminine attributes of emotionality, tenderness, and nurturance, and it is subordinate—thus reinforcing the link between femininity and subordinate status. The nurse role should be available to men, too, to help break down this unfavorable stereotype.

This objective to the traditional role embodies the very fallacy it aims to combat. The falsehood we know as sexism is not the belief that some roles are autonomous, calling for objectivity in judgment, suppression of emotion, and independent initiative in action, but discouraging independent judgment and action and requiring obedience to superiors; the falsehood is the assumption that only men are eligible for the first class and only women are eligible for the second class.

One of the most damaging mistakes of our cultural heritage is the assumption that warmth, gentleness, and loving care, such as are expected of the nurse, are simply impossible for the male of the species, and that men who show emotion, let alone those who are ever known to weep, are weaklings, "sissies," and a disgrace to the human race. I suspect that this assumption has done more harm to the culture than its more publicized partner, the assumption that women are (or should be) incapable of objective judgment or executive function. Women will survive without leadership roles, but it is not clear that a society can retain its humanity if all those eligible for leadership are forbidden, by virtue of that eligibility, to take account of the human side of human beings: their altruism, heroism, compassion, and grief, their fear and weakness, and their ability to love and care for others.

In the words of the current feminist movement, men must be liberated as surely as women. And one of the best avenues to such liberation would be the encouragement of male participation in the health care system, or other systems of the society, in roles like the traditional nursing role, which permit, even require, the expressive side of the personality to develop, giving it a function in the enterprise and restoring it to recognition and respectability.

CONCLUSIONS

In conclusion, then, the traditional nurse role is crucial to health care in the hospital context; its subordinate status, required for its remaining features, is neither in itself demeaning nor a barrier to its assumption by men or women. It is probably not a role that everyone would enjoy. But there are certainly many who are suited to it, and should be willing to undertake the job.

One of the puzzling features of the recent controversy is the apparent unwillingness of some of the current crop of nursing school graduates to take on the assignment for which they have ostensibly been prepared, at least until such time as it shall be redefined to accord more closely with their notion of professional. These frustrated nurses who do not want the traditional nursing role, yet wish to employ their skills in the health care system in some way, will clearly have to do something else. The health care industry is presently in the process of very rapid expansion and diversification, and has created significant markets for those with a nurse's training and the capacity, and desire, for autonomous roles. Moreover, the nurse in a position which does not have the "nurse" label, does not need to combat the "traditional nurse" image and is ordinarily accorded greater freedom of action. For this reason alone it would appear that those nurses intent on occupying autonomous roles and tired of fighting stereotypes that they find degrading and unworthy of their abilities, should seek out occupational niches that do not bear the label, and the stigma, of "nurse."

I conclude, therefore: that much of the difficulty in obtaining public acceptance of the new "autonomous professional" image of the nurse may be due, not to public ignorance, but to the opposition of a vague but persistent public ideal of nursing; that the ideal is a worthy one, well-founded in the hospital context in which it evolved; and that

the role of traditional nurse, for which that ideal sets the standard, should therefore be maintained and held open for any who would have the desire and the personal and professional qualifications, to assume it. Perhaps the current crop of nursing school graduates do not desire it, but there is ample room in the health care system for the sort of "autonomous professional" they wish to be, apart from the hospital nursing role. Wherever we must go to fill this role, it is worth going there, for the traditional nurse is the major force remaining for humanity in a system that will turn into a mechanical monster without her.

ADVOCACY OR SUBSERVIENCE FOR THE SAKE OF PATIENTS?
Helga Kuhse

Kuhse addresses the question of whether nurses, whose primary professional obligation is to serve the interests of patients, should conduct themselves as patient advocates or assume a role of subservience to physicians (as Newton argues). Against the claim that the role of the nurse is *naturally* subservient to the doctor's role, Kuhse argues that professional roles evolve over time and have no fixed essences (natures); moreover, there is considerable overlap between contemporary nursing functions and the functions traditionally performed by physicians. She next casts doubt, with a variety of arguments, on the thesis that, because nursing and medicine have fundamentally different philosophical commitments, nurses should accept a subservient role. Taking up specific arguments advanced by Newton, Kuhse contends (1) that the claim that nurses' subservience is required for proper handling of serious medical situations is based on dubious assumptions and (2) that there are several good reasons to reject the surrogate mother role for nurses. She concludes that nurses' subservience to physicians would likely harm patients more than it would help them.

. . . The view that doctors were gods whose commands must always be obeyed was beginning to be seriously questioned in the 1960s and 1970s. There had always been courageous nurses who had occasionally challenged orders,[1] but it is almost as if nurses needed a new metaphor to capture their new

understanding of their role before they could finally attempt to free themselves from the shackles of the past. This new focus was provided by the metaphor of the nurse as patient advocate. Whereas the old metaphors had focused attention on such virtues as submissiveness and unquestioning obedience and loyalty to those in command, the new metaphor of patient advocate highlighted the virtues of assertiveness and courage, and marked a revolutionary shift in the self-perception of nurses and their role. The nurse's first loyalty, the metaphor suggested, is owed not to the doctor but to the patient. In thus focusing on the nurse's responsibilities to patients, that is, on the *recipients* rather than the *providers* of medical care, the metaphor of the nurse as patient advocate made it possible for nurses to see themselves as *professionals*. No longer were they, as the old metaphors had suggested, the loyal handmaidens of medical men: they were professionals whose primary responsibility—like that of all professionals—was to their clients or patients.[2] . . .

NURSING—A NATURALLY SUBSERVIENT PROFESSION?

. . . Our first question must be this: *should* nurses reject their traditional largely subservient role and act as patient advocates? . . .

. . . I shall, without argument, assume that a profession such as medicine or nursing does not exist for the sole or even primary purpose of benefiting its members. This view is widely shared and is implicit in most if not all professional codes;[3] it is also regarded as one of the necessary conditions for an organization to claim professional status.[4] For the purposes of our discussion, then, I shall assume that both nursing and medicine are professions which are, or ought to be, aiming at the welfare of others, where those others are patients or clients.

This raises the question of the relationship between medicine and nursing, and between doctors and nurses. Might it not be the case that the subordinate role of nurses has its basis not in objectionable sexism but rather in a natural hierarchy between the professions, a hierarchy that serves patients best?

Robert Baker is among those who have pointed out that we cannot simply assume that the nurse's subservient role has a sexist basis. He does not deny that sexism exists or that the subservient nursing role has traditionally been seen as a feminine one; but, he writes,

it is not at all clear whether the role of the nurse is seen as dependent because it is filled by females, who are held to be incapable of independent action by a male-dominated, sexist society . . . *or* whether females have been channelled into nursing because the profession, *by its very nature,* requires its members to

play a dependent and subservient role (i.e., the traditional female role in a sexist society).[5]

In other words, the facts that almost all nurses are women, that the traditional nurse's role has been a subservient one and that most societies were and are male-dominated and sexist, cannot lead us to the conclusion that the nurse's role necessarily rests on objectionable sexism. The nurse's role may, 'by its very nature,' be a subservient one. But is nursing 'by its very nature' subservient to medicine—is it a naturally subservient profession?

There is clearly something odd about speaking of the 'natural subservience' of nursing to medicine, or for that matter of 'the natural subservience' of any profession in relation to another. To speak of 'natural subservience' suggests that the subservient or dominant character of the relevant profession is somehow naturally given and in that sense fixed and largely unchangeable. But is this view correct? . . . [N]ursing has developed in a very particular social and historical context, in response to the then prevailing goals and purposes of medicine on the one hand and the social roles of women and men on the other. Would this not make it more appropriate to view the character of the two health-care professions, and the tasks and privileges that attach to them, as a historically contingent accident or social construct, rather than as a compelling natural necessity?[6]

It seems to me the answer must be 'yes.' There are no natural professional hierarchies that exist independently of human societies, and we should reject the idea that professions have fixed natures and instead view them as changing and changeable social institutions. When looking at professions in this way we may, of course, still want to think of them as having particular characteristics by which they can be defined ('social natures,' if you like), but we would now view these characteristics as socially constructed, in much the same way as the institution itself is a social and historical construct.

How, then, might one go about capturing the 'social nature' or characteristics of a profession? One might do this in one of two ways: either by focusing on the functions or roles performed by members of the profession or by focusing on the profession's philosophical presuppositions or goals.

Function or Role What is the function or role of a nurse? What is a nurse? The clear and neat boundaries and distinctions presupposed by our everyday language and by the terms we use rarely accord with the real world.[7] We often speak of 'the role' or 'the function' of the nurse, or of the 'the role' or 'the function' of the doctor. These terms are problematical because nurses and doctors working in different areas of health care perform very different functions and act in many different roles, and there is a considerable degree of overlap between the changeable and changing functions performed by members of the two professions.

The expansion of knowledge, of nursing education, and of medical science and technology has resulted in the redefinition and scope of nursing practice. Nurses now carry out a range of procedures that were formerly exclusively performed by doctors. Some nurses give injections, take blood samples, administer medication, perform diagnostic procedures, do physical examinations, respond to medical emergencies and so on.

Take diagnosis and medical treatment. The diagnosis and treatment of medical problems had always been regarded as the realm solely of doctors. But, as Tristram H. Engelhardt notes, if one looks closely at the diagnostic activities performed by nurses, it is difficult to see them as essentially different from medical diagnoses. Nursing diagnoses such as ' "Airway clearance, ineffective;" "Bowel elimination, alteration in: Diarrhoea;" "Cardiac output, alteration in, decrease;" "Fluid volume deficit,"' Engelhardt points out, all have their medical equivalents; and the diagnosis of psychological or psychiatric disturbances, such as ' "Coping, ineffective individual," or "Thought processes, alteration in" can be given analogues in the *Diagnostic and Statistical Manual of Mental Disorders* of the American Psychiatric Association.'[8]

Nurses are not permitted by law to perform any 'medical acts,' but in practice the line between medical and nursing acts has become rather blurred[9] and is, in any case, the result of social and historical choice. Moreover, as nurses have become more assertive and conscious of their own knowledge and expertise, there has been a broadening of the definitions of nursing practice. In 1981 the American Nursing Association thus produced a model definition of nursing practice, which included 'diagnosis . . . in the promotion and maintenance of health.' By 1984, 23 US states had included [nursing] diagnoses, or similar terms, in their nursing practice acts.[10]

To conclude, then, the fact that nurses work in very different areas of health care, where they perform very different functions, and the fact that there are considerable overlaps between contemporary nursing functions and the functions traditionally performed by doctors makes it difficult to see how it would be possible to define nursing in terms of a particular function or role performed by nurses. If we thus think of 'the nature' of nursing in terms of some specific function or role performed by all nurses, this suggests not only that nursing lacks a particular nature, but also makes it difficult to claim that nursing is 'naturally subservient' to medicine.

It is true, of course, that nurses frequently work under the direction of doctors, and that control over many of the functions performed by them is retained by the medical profession. It is also true that only doctors may, by law, perform operations, prescribe medical treatments and authorize access to certain drugs. This might lead one to the conclusion that nursing and medicine can be distinguished by the range of socially and legally sanctioned tasks and privileges that members of one but not of the other profession may lawfully engage in. Such a distinction would, of course, be possible. But it is not a distinction that allows one to infer anything about the subservient or dominant 'nature' of either one of the two professions. The distribution of socially and legally sanctioned privileges and powers between medicine and nursing is itself a historically contingent fact, and there is nothing to suggest that the current distribution of powers and privileges is either natural or that it is the one that we should, upon reflection, adopt.[11] . . .

Philosophical Commitment Is it possible to distinguish the two professions by their philosophical commitment, that is, by the philosophical presuppositions that guide their respective health-care endeavours? It is, again, not easy to see how this might be done. Someone intent on rejecting the view that nursing is naturally subservient to medicine might point out that there is no essential difference between the philosophical commitment of the two professions that would allow one to speak of one of them as being subservient to the other. Both nursing and medicine are other-directed and committed to the welfare of clients or patients; members of both professions have a similar understanding of pain and of suffering, of well-being and of health, and both accept the same scientific presuppositions. If there are differences between individual doctors and nurses, these are no more pronounced than those found between individuals from the same professions. Hence, one might conclude, nursing does not have a nature which is different from that of medicine and can therefore not be said to be naturally subservient to medicine.

Another, diametrically opposed avenue is sometimes chosen by those writing in the field to prove wrong the claim that the nurse's role is a naturally subservient one. Rather than trying to show that the nurse's role is—either functionally or in terms of its philosophical commitment—*indistinguishable* from that of doctors, this second group of nurses claims that the nursing commitment is fundamentally *different* from that of medicine. In other words, those who take this approach start with the premise that medicine and nursing have different philosophical commitments or 'natures,' and then go on to deny that this will necessarily lead to the conclusion that nursing ought to be playing a subservient role to medicine.[12]

This is generally done in one of two ways. The first involves drawing a distinction in terms of a commitment to 'care' and to 'cure.' Whereas medicine is said to be directed at 'cure,' the therapeutic commitment or moral end of nursing is identified as 'care.' Medicine and doctors, it is said, often focus on treating or curing the patient's medical condition; nursing, on the other hand, is based on holistic care, where patients are treated as complex wholes. . . . The second way of attempting to draw a distinction between nursing and medicine involves an appeal to two different ethics. Whereas medicine is said to be based on principles and rules (a so-called [male] ethics of justice), nursing is said to be based on relational caring (a so-called [female] ethics of care).

This means, very roughly, that doctors will put ethical principles or rules before the needs or wants of individual patients, whereas nurses regard the needs or wants of individual patients as more important than adherence to abstract principles or rules.

These two views do not deny that nursing is context-dependent or that nurses perform very different functions in different health-care settings; they also acknowledge that nurses and doctors sometimes perform very similar or identical functions and act in very similar roles. Nonetheless, those who take this view assume that nursing is different from medicine because it has a different philosophical commitment or end—that of care. 'Care'—the nurture, the physical care, and the emotional support provided by nurses to preserve the 'human face' of medicine and the dignity of the patient—cannot, the suggestion is, 'be absent if nursing is present.'[13]

There are a number of reasons why I am pessimistic about the endeavour of distinguishing nursing from medicine and nurses from doctors in this way. . . . Here the following [summary] will suffice: it seems very difficult, in a straightforward and practical sense, to make philosophical commitments, such as the commitment to care, the defining characteristic of a profession. Such a definition would presumably include all nurses who have this commitment, but would exclude all those who do not. A registered nurse, who has all the relevant professional knowledge and expertise, who performs her nursing functions well, but—let us assume—subscribes to 'the scientific medical model' or to an 'ethics of justice' would now, presumably, no longer *be* a nurse. Would her philosophical commitment make her a doctor? And would a doctor, who subscribes to 'care' now more appropriately be described as a nurse?

The problem is raised particularly poignantly in settings, such as intensive care units (ICUs), where the emphasis is on survival and 'cure.' After Robert Zussman, a sociologist, had observed doctors and nurses in two American ICUs for some time, he reached the conclusion that ICU nurses were not 'gentle carers' but technicians. Zussman does not deny that other nurses may well be differently motivated, but in the ICU, he says, they are 'mini-interns.' 'They are not patient advocates. They are not "angels of mercy." Like physicians, they have become technicians.'[14] . . .

. . . Even if a sound distinction in the philosophical or ethical commitments of nursing and medicine could be drawn, this would not settle the question of whether nursing is or is not a naturally subservient profession. The fact (if it is a fact) that medicine has one philosophical commitment or nature and nursing another is quite independent of the further question of whether one of the professions is, or ought to be, subservient to the other. Further argument would be needed to show that, for nothing of substance follows from establishing that one thing, or one profession, is different from another.

SUBSERVIENCE FOR THE SAKE OF LIFE OR LIMB?

What arguments could be provided to show that nurses and nursing ought to adopt a subservient role to doctors and medicine? In accordance with our assumption that nursing is an other-directed profession, a profession that primarily aims at the good of patients, such arguments would have to show that nurses' subservience would benefit patients more than nurses' autonomy. . . .

. . . [O]ur main focus will be hospital-based nurses. Most nurses work in hospitals, and it is part of their role to carry out the treatment plans of doctors. Here a powerful argument is sometimes put that, regardless of what is true for other nurses, it is essential that nurses who work in acute-care settings adopt a subservient role. Those who take this view do not necessarily deny that it may be quite appropriate for some nurses, in some contexts, to play an autonomous role; but, they insist, when we are talking about hospitals matters are different.[15]

Hospitals are bureaucratic institutions and bureaucratic institutions, so a typical argument goes, rely for efficient functioning on vertical structures of command, on strict adherence to procedure and on avoidance of initiative by those who have been charged with certain tasks. While this is true of all bureaucratic institutions, strict adherence to rules and to chains of command becomes critically important when we are focusing on hospitals. In such a setting much is at stake. A patient's health, and even

her life, will often depend on quick and reliable responses by members of the health-care team to the directions of the person in charge.[16]

Let us accept that efficiency will often depend on some of the central criteria identified above. This does not, however, answer questions regarding the proper relationship between nurses and doctors. Take the notion of a bureaucratic hierarchy. A simple appeal to that notion does not tell us how the bureaucratic hierarchy should be arranged.[17] Here it is generally assumed that it is appropriate for doctors to be in charge and appropriate for nurses to follow the doctors' orders. But why should this be so? Why is it so widely assumed that doctors should perform the role of 'captain of the ship'[18] and nurses those of members of the crew?

The Argument from Expertise The reason most commonly given for this type of arrangement is that doctors, but not nurses, have the relevant medical knowledge and expertise to deal with the varied and often unique medical conditions that afflict patients, and the different emergencies that might arise. Just as it would not do to put crew-members with only a limited knowledge of navigation in charge of a ship traversing unpredictable and potentially dangerous waters, so it would not do to put nurses with only a limited knowledge of medicine in charge of the treatment plans of patients. Many a ship and many a patient would be lost as a result of such an arrangement. Hence, if we want ships and patients to be in good hands, it follows that those with expertise—doctors and captains—must be in charge.

Such an argument is put by Lisa H. Newton, a vocal critic of nursing's quest for autonomy. If the purpose of saving life and health is to be accomplished in an atmosphere which is often tense and urgent, then, Newton argues,

all participating activities and agents must be completely subordinated to the medical judgements of the physician . . . [T]hose other than physicians, involved in medical procedures in a hospital context, have no right to insert their own needs, judgements, or personalities into the situation. The last thing we need at that point is another autonomous professional on the job, whether a nurse or anyone else.[19]

There is something right and something wrong about the above kind of argument. To see this, the argument needs untangling.

Shared Goals, Urgency and Medical Authority

In her argument Newton implicitly assumes that the therapeutic goals of doctors are morally worthy ones, and that the ethical question of whether a doctor should, for example, prolong a patient's life or allow her to die is not in dispute. This assumption is inherent in her observation that the tasks at hand are, or ought to be 'protective of life itself.'[20] While we know that this very question is frequently in dispute, let us, for the purpose of our initial discussion, accept and work with that assumption. We shall question it later.

There is no doubt that doctors have special medical expertise that is relevant to the achievement of various therapeutic goals, including the goal of saving or prolonging life. Extensive medical studies and registration or licensing procedures ensure that doctors are experts in medical diagnosis and medical therapy. Their education equips them well to act quickly and decisively in complicated and unforeseen medical circumstances. As a general rule (but only as a general rule—there could be exceptions to this rule) doctors would thus be better equipped than nurses to respond to a range of medical emergencies. In emergency situations, then, where urgent action is required, it is likely that the best outcome for patients as a whole will be achieved if doctors are in charge. Moreover, since the outcome of medical measures in such contexts often depends crucially on the practical assistance of nurses, it is important that nurses will, as a general rule, quickly and unquestioningly respond to the doctor's orders. . . .

In addition to those cases where urgent action by a medical expert is required to achieve the desired therapeutic goal, there are also some other specialized contexts, such as the operating room, where it is appropriate for doctors to exercise and for nurses to recognize medical authority. . . . There is a connection, then, between the possession of particular expertise and authority. Expertise can be crucial to the achievement of goals and, provided the goals are shared, it will frequently be appropriate for people who are authorities in a particular field to also be *in* authority.

If we accept this argument, it follows that doctors ought, other things being equal, to be in charge in medical emergencies and in other specialized contexts that are characterized by an element of urgency. They ought to be in charge because this arrangement best ensures that the therapeutic goal will be reached.

Acceptance of this view has, however, less far-reaching consequences than might be assumed. First, even if particular therapeutic treatment goals are most likely to be achieved if a single medically trained person is in charge *during,* for example, operations or resuscitation procedures, this does not entail that the doctor should have overall authority as far as the patient's treatment is concerned. The authority to decide on an operation or on the desirability of implementing resuscitation procedures might, for example, rest with the patient or her relatives, and the nurse could conceivably be in charge of the overall treatment plan of the patient.[21]

Second, it does not follow that nurses must, even during emergency procedures, *blindly* follow a doctor's order. Doctors, like the rest of us, are fallible human beings and sometimes make mistakes. This means that the nurse's obligation to follow a doctor's order, even in these specialized contexts, cannot be absolute and may at times be overridden by other considerations, such as the avoidance of harm to patients. . . .

. . . Given, then, that doctors will occasionally make mistakes and that nurses frequently have the professional knowledge to detect them, it will be best if nurses do not understand their duty to follow a doctor's order as an absolute and exceptionless one. If the doctor's order is, in the nurse's professional judgement, clearly wrong, then the nurse must bring her 'professional intelligence' into play and question it. . . .

Does a nurse who subscribes to the general proposition or rule that there are times when it will best serve the interests of patients that she accept the authority of doctors thereby necessarily adopt a subservient or non-autonomous role? Does she abrogate her autonomy? I think not. As long as a nurse does not *surrender* her autonomy or judgement, that is, does not blindly follow every order she is given, but rather *decides,* after reflection, to adopt a general rule that it will be best to accept and act on the doctor's authority under certain circumstances, then she is not a subservient tool in the doctor's hands. She is not, as was once proposed, simply 'an intelligent machine.'[22] She is a moral agent who, in distinction from a mere machine, *chooses* to act in one way rather than another.

To sum up, then: the argument that nurses should—for the sake of achieving certain worthy therapeutic goals such as the saving of life—adopt a subservient role to doctors typically rests on at least two rather dubious assumptions. The first assumption is that all or most decision-making is characterized by great urgency. The second assumption is that the therapeutic goal is best achieved by nurses adopting an absolute rather than a prima facie rule to carry out the doctor's orders. But, as we have seen, both assumptions must be rejected, on the grounds outlined above. . . .

DO PATIENTS NEED SUBSERVIENT MOTHER SURROGATES?

A different kind of argument is sometimes put to show that nurses should, for the sake of patients, adopt a subservient role to doctors. Only then, the argument asserts, will nurses be able to meet the emotional needs of patients. To examine that claim, we shall once again focus on an argument provided by Lisa H. Newton. In her defence of the traditional role of the nurse, Newton appeals to an argument based on the patient's needs. Because a patient may not be able to take care of himself, Newton points out,

> his entire self-concept of an independent human being may be threatened . . . He needs comfort, reassurance, someone to talk to. The person he really needs, who would be capable of taking care of all these problems, is obviously his mother, and the first job of the nurse is to be a mother surrogate.[23]

But, Newton continues her argument, mothers are not only figures of considerable authority; it is also ordinarily part of the mother's role to take control of various aspects of her dependent children's lives, and to make important decisions for them. Patients are, however, not children. Their autonomy must be protected from the threatening authority of the mother surrogate. This requires, Newton asserts, that

the role of the nurse must be from the outset, as essentially as it is nurturant, unavailable for such attribution of authority. Not only must the role of the nurse not include authority; it must be incompatible with authority: essentially, a subservient role.[24]

This non-threatening caring function, performed by the nurse, would not only permit the patient 'to be cared for like a baby,' but would also allow patients to unburden themselves and to express their doubts and resentments about doctors and the treatments prescribed by them. Patients, Newton notes, may sometimes be torn between the desire to discontinue treatment (to reassert control over their lives) and a desire to continue treatment (to reap its benefits). The nurse will be there as a sympathetic listener 'but in her subordinate position . . . can do absolutely nothing to change the course of treatment,' that is, both nurse and patient are subject to what she calls the 'sapiential authority' of the physician.[25]

The traditional subordinate role of the nurse is thus justified by the needs of patients. Patients, Newton holds, need the emotional support of a mother surrogate but, to protect the patient's autonomy and to ensure compliance with the medical treatment plan, the nurse must completely surrender her autonomy.

Should we accept this type of argument? The first point to be noted is this: Newton's claims about humiliating treatment, about strong emotional needs and about the threatened loss of the patient's self-concept as an independent human being, while undoubtedly correct in some cases, do not apply to all patients and in all circumstances. Many patients enter hospital for relatively minor treatments or observations and do not feel that their self-concept is threatened in any way by their status of patient. They do not need or want a mother surrogate. Rather, their needs are much more likely to be met by a nurse who not only provides them with professional nursing care, but who also refuses to surrender her professional intelligence and autonomy to the doctor to protect the patient from potential harm.

Then there are the patients who are seriously ill and whose self-concept may indeed be threatened by the medical treatment they are receiving or by their incapacitated state. Many of these patients will undoubtedly benefit from the presence of a caring and sympathetic nurse, who will listen to them with warmth and understanding. But would they want the subservient nurse Newton holds in store for them? Would their emotional needs really be satisfied by talking to a self-effacing health-care professional who, afraid of either posing a threat to the patient's autonomy or the 'sapiential authority' of the doctor, would be making sympathetic clucking noises, but would not engage with the patient in any meaningful way? I doubt it very much. By refusing to engage with patients in a meaningful way, she would be signalling to them that she does not take their concerns seriously, no more seriously than a well-meaning mother would take the incoherent babbling of her sick baby. This would not only be extremely upsetting to many patients, but would also enforce their sense of powerlessness, the feeling that they have lost control over their lives—as indeed they may have. . . .

As we noted above, Newton recognizes that a patient may wish to discontinue treatment so as to 'reassert control over his life.'[26] Would supporting the patient in this desire—assuming that it is a reasonable one—really threaten his autonomy? And is not the nurse's refusal ever to take the patient's desire seriously tantamount to abandoning him to another authority—the authority of the doctor? While we should not ignore the possibility that a powerful mother figure might pose a threat to the patient's autonomy, why should we assume that a powerful father figure—that of the doctor—might not pose a similar or a greater threat?

Newton simply assumes that the therapeutic success of treatment presupposes that the patient defer to the 'physician's sapiential authority.' What she does not explain, however, is why the physician's ends or goals—therapeutic success or prolongation of life, for example—should count for more than, say, the judgement of the patient or the nurse. In other words, we are not told where the doctor's moral authority comes from or why we should regard his decisions as sound. . . .

The adoption by nurses of a subservient role of the kind envisaged by Newton would most likely harm patients more than it would benefit them; it would also be an utterly demoralizing role for many contemporary nurses, even if it would be compatible with some understanding of autonomy. Nurses would be required to stand by, doing nothing, while doctors make the occasional mistake, or provide treatment to unwilling but disempowered patients. To conclude, then, I can see no good reason why nurses should adopt a subservient mother surrogate role for the sake of patients. On the contrary, there are a number of strong reasons why nurses should reject it. . . .

NOTES

[1] See, for example, 'Where does loyalty to the physician end?' (editorial), *American Journal of Nursing,* 10 (Jan. 1910), pp. 230–1; 'Where does loyalty to the physician end?' (letters), *American Journal of Nursing,* 10 (Jan. 1910), pp. 274, 276. (I owe these reference to Gerald R. Winslow, 'From loyalty to advocacy: a new metaphor for nursing,' *Hastings Center Report,* 14 (June 1984), p. 34.)

[2] Parts of this chapter have greatly benefited from Gerald R. Winslow, 'From loyalty to advocacy.'

[3] See, for example, the 1973 International Council of Nurses *Code for Nurses,* which holds that '[t]he nurse's primary responsibility is to those people who require nursing care.' See also the 1980 report on revisions to the Principles of Medical Ethics endorsed by the American Medical Association, which states that '[t]he profession does not exist for itself; it exists for a purpose and increasingly that purpose will be defined by society.' (As quoted by Robert M. Veatch, 'Medical ethics: an introduction,' in R. M. Veatch (ed.), *Medical Ethics* (1989), p. 22.)

[4] See, for example, Carolla A. Quinn and Michael D. Smith, *The Professional Commitment: Issues and ethics in nursing* (1987), ch. 1.

[5] Robert Barker, 'Care of the sick and cure of the disease: comment on "The Fractured Image," ' in Stuart F. Spicker and Sally Gadow (eds), *Nursing: Images and ideals— Opening dialogue with the humanities* (1980), pp. 42–3. See also James L. Muyskens, *Moral Problems in Nursing: A philosophical investigation* (1982), pp. 31ff.

[6] On this point, see also H. Tristram Engelhardt, Jr, 'Physicians, patients, health care institutions—and the people in between: nurses,' in Anne Bishop and John R. Scudder, Jr, *Caring, Curing, Coping* (1985), p. 63.

[7] Ibid., p. 62.

[8] American Psychiatric Association, *Diagnostic and Statistical Manual of Mental Disorders,* 3rd edn (1980), as cited by Engelhardt, ibid., p. 71.

[9] See Martin Benjamin and Joy Curtis, *Ethics in Nursing,* 3rd edn (1992), pp. 91–5.

[10] Ibid., p. 92.

[11] H. Tristram Engelhardt, Jr, 'Physicians, patients, health care institutions—and the people in between: nurses,' pp. 62–79.

[12] See, for example, Jean Watson, 'Introduction: an ethic of caring/curing/nursing *qua* nursing,' in *The Ethics of Care and the Ethics of Cure: Synthesis in Chronicity*, ed. Jean Watson and Marilyn A. Ray (1988), pp. 1–3.

[13] James L. Muyskens, *Moral Problems in Nursing*, p. 36.

[14] Robert Zussman, *Intensive Care: Medical ethics and the medical profession* (1992), ch. 5, at p. 80.

[15] Lisa Newton, 'In defense of the traditional nurse,' *Nursing Outlook*, 29 (June 1981), pp. 348–54. See also Lisa H. Newton, 'A vindication of the gentle sister: comment on "The Fractured Image," '' in Stuart F. Spicker and Sally Gadow (eds), *Nursing: Images and ideals*, pp. 34–40.

[16] Lisa H. Newton, 'In defense of the traditional nurse,' p. 350.

[17] Of course, it also leaves open the question of whether bureaucratic, hierarchical structures are the ones we should adopt in the first place. While I believe that there might well be other and more satisfactory arrangements, I will set this question aside and not discuss it any further.

[18] As H. Tristram Engelhardt, Jr, notes ('Physicians, patients, health care institutions' p. 68), the now famous phrase by which doctors were construed as 'captain of the ship,' was used in the case of *McConnel* v. *Williams*, 361 Pa. 355, 65 A. 2nd 243 (1959).

[19] Lisa H. Newton, 'In defense of the traditional nurse,' p. 351.

[20] Ibid.

[21] This point is made by Andrew Jameton, *Nursing Practice: The ethical issues*, p. 46. There might, however, be some advantage in having doctors—on account of their expertise—in charge of the treatment plans of emergency-prone patients *if* the agreed goal is to save life. This would ensure that the person most qualified to conduct the relevant procedure would not have to defer to the authority in charge of the overall treatment plan before implementing a procedure.

[22] Sarah Dock, 'The relation of the nurse to the doctor and the doctor to the nurse,' *American Journal of Nursing*, 17 (1917), p. 394.

[23] Lisa H. Newton, 'In defense of the traditional nurse,' p. 351.

[24] Ibid., p. 352.

[25] Ibid.

[26] Ibid.

THE NURSE/PHYSICIAN RELATIONSHIP AND ETHICAL DECISION MAKING

Amy M. Haddad

Haddad explores the nurse-physician relationship in the context of ethical decision making. After describing differences in power and authority between physicians and nurses, Haddad argues that the divergent ways in which these professionals approach ethical problems may reflect differences in the characteristic ethical problem-solving styles of men and women (as stressed in the ethics of care). Haddad then explores a case involving a man of uncertain competence. She uses this case to illustrate the importance of (1) direct, nondeferential communication by nurses to physicians and (2) a vivid awareness of the effects of particular decisions on relationships within the health-care team and on the patient's quality of life.

FACTORS AFFECTING THE NURSE/PHYSICIAN RELATIONSHIP

In 1967, Leonard I. Stein, MD identified a basic communication pattern that physicians and nurses used. He called it the "Doctor-Nurse Game."[1] The game is still played daily in many surgery departments. The object of the game is for the nurse to be bold, have initiative, and be responsible for making significant recommendations while appearing to be doing none of this. It should appear that it was the physician who made the recommendations.

Both the nurse and physician need to be acutely aware of subtle nonverbal cues and verbal nuances in the conversation. The major rule of the game is that open disagreement must be avoided at all costs. Nurses learn to make suggestions and ask for recommendations in a way that sounds like they are not

Reprinted with permission of the publisher from *AORN Journal*, vol. 53 (January 1991), pp. 151–156.

doing so. It is interesting that Dr Stein and his colleagues revisited the Doctor-Nurse Game in 1990.[2] Twenty-three years later, they found only minor changes in the way the game is played.

Consequences of this indirect method of communication are that it is inefficient and stifles open communication that is essential in ethical decision making. The doctor-nurse game is similar to the superior-subordinate game that occurs in almost all organizational hierarchies. Subordinates often use the passive voice to make suggestions to superiors within the organization.

Stereotypes are oversimplified, unvarying conceptions about a person or a group. Traditional gender stereotypes in nursing, both positive (eg, ministering, self-sacrificing angels, nurturing mothers) and negative (eg, sexpots, battle axes), add a new dimension to the superior-subordinate game. Positive (eg, noble, decisive leaders; captain of the ship) and negative (eg, egotistical, arrogant dictators) stereotypes in medicine have the same effect. Unfortunately, negative stereotypes in nursing and medicine tend to mirror those of women and men in society at large.

Another influencing factor in the nurse/physician relationship arises from the inherent inequity in power and authority that each discipline exercises. Physicians exercise a great deal of direct power in the health care system. Even though some reimbursement systems have begun to erode the physician's role as gatekeeper, physicians still tend to determine who is admitted and what type of treatments and procedures are to be performed. These decisions translate directly into revenue for the hospital.

Nurses are not a direct source of revenue for the hospital, but the hospital would not be able to function without them. Nurses' work is largely unseen but essential. Therefore, nurses, like others in traditionally female jobs, exercise little direct authority regarding decisions that affect their work or welfare. They generally receive little pay for the amount of responsibility associated with their work, and they receive little recognition and respect for their contribution to the enterprise as a whole.

Physicians, especially surgeons, earn more and generally are self-employed. The difference in income and employment status result in class barriers between physicians and nurses. The two groups rarely socialize with each other, which limits opportunities for informal discussions outside of the work setting. Informal discussions over coffee, at lunch, or during social activities help individuals understand each other's values and motivations, which inevitably affect how the people work together.

Physicians and nurses also differ in educational preparation. Nurses generally have fewer years of formal education, which puts them at a disadvantage. Efforts to increase entry-level education in nursing have been strongly resisted by organized medicine. Physicians argue that increased education pulls nurses away from patient care. The more education a nurse has, however, the more she or he threatens the status quo and the authority of the physician. All of these factors influence the ability to collaborate and resolve ethical problems. The process becomes even more difficult because nurses and physicians usually do not perceive ethical problems in the same way.

APPROACHES TO ETHICAL DECISION MAKING

Carol Gilligan, PhD, noted some significant differences in how males and females reason morally.[3] One view predominant in females acknowledges that people's lives are embedded in relationships and that the relationships are central to moral decision making. People with this interdependent view are concerned about being responsible and responsive to others. They consider the specifics of a situation when making a decision. This view is most clearly reflected in the concept of mercy and commonly is used by nurses in making ethical decisions.

A counter view of moral reasoning consists of a rights and rules perspective and is directed toward justice and fair play. Males tend to use this type of moral reasoning. They seek a general rule that can be applied to specific situations. Physicians often take this approach when making ethical decisions.

These different attitudes affect ethical decision making. Nurses may appear unsure. They may seem overly concerned with details and the specifics of a situation and, therefore, slow to come to decisions. Nurses will identify interrelationships and include these as important factors when coming to a decision. They will ask how people are related and who will be affected by the decision and how. Often, nurses will consider quality of life and ability to function in ethical decision making.

Physicians, on the other hand, may have difficulty seeing the need for details and ambiguity. This is particularly true of surgeons who are rewarded, both financially and professionally, for their decisiveness and ability to act quickly under pressure. Because physicians are still trained in a reductionistic framework, they are likely to use a "rule out" approach to analyze ethical problems. Therefore, they have a tendency to break down the problem to its essential elements and dispense with all the extraneous details that nurses seem to believe are important. It is common for physicians to confuse professional expertise for moral authority. They often take it upon themselves to make ethical decisions with little or no collaboration or input.

CASE STUDY

The following case illustrates these different perspectives in action and how they affect ethical decision making. Dorothy Donahoe, RN, is assigned to complete the preoperative assessment on Wilford Cook, a 77-year-old patient in the intensive care unit. He is scheduled for spinal fusion. Dorothy reads through Wilford's clinical record and is overwhelmed at Wilford's course of treatment since he was admitted.

Wilford had no living relatives and had lived in a state institution for the mentally handicapped most of his life. With deinstitutionalization, he was placed in a group living setting in the community. To everyone's surprise, he surpassed all expectations regarding his functional abilities. Wilford learned to read and write, and he was able to work independently in the community.

Wilford had been admitted one month earlier for evaluation of chronic respiratory insufficiency and recurrent bronchitis and pneumonia. Dorothy notes that Wilford had carefully signed each permit for the various tests and procedures performed since his admission. Wilford had not, however, signed the surgical permit for removal of a mediastinal mass. On the line where his signature should have been are the words, "No, No, No." Below these words is the signature of the surgeon who had operated on Wilford and removed not only a malignant mediastinal mass but several vertebrae.

Since the surgery two weeks ago, Wilford has remained on a ventilator and in a semiconscious state. The head of the bed can be elevated only slightly because of the possibility of compressing the spinal cord. Dorothy decides to speak to the nurse in the critical care unit. He tells Dorothy the following:

Wilford didn't want the initial surgery. I believe he understood the risks and alternatives to surgery. I guess the surgeon thought Wilford wasn't capable of giving consent. Because Wilford doesn't have any family, I guess the surgeon thought he was acting in Wilford's best interest. Wilford hasn't done well since surgery.

Now the surgeon wants to put in Harrington rods to help support the spine so we can get Wilford up. If you ask me, I think that's too aggressive. However, when I suggested to Dr Anton that a tracheostomy would be easier to manage and more comfortable for Wilford, he told me that a tracheostomy was too aggressive!

Dorothy goes in to see Wilford. He has an endotracheal tube attached to the ventilator. Wilford responds to Dorothy's touch. Dorothy introduces herself and asks Wilford if he understands that the surgeon wants to take him back to the operating room and place support rods in his spine in place of the bones that were removed. Wilford nods. Dorothy asks, "Wilford, do you want to have this surgery?" Wilford shakes his head "no" slowly but purposefully.

Dorothy returns to the surgery department to speak to Dr Anton. She knows it is against hospital policy for a surgeon to sign a consent form unless it is an emergency procedure. She also thinks that Wilford needs someone to speak for him, but she is not certain how to go about finding someone. Dorothy finds Dr Anton and speaks to him. "Dr Anton, I have just been up to see Mr Cook in the critical care unit. Have you spoken to him about surgery?"

Dr Anton responds,

I see no point in talking to him. He has a long history of mental retardation. Without the support of Harrington rods, he'll never be able to sit up, let alone walk. He definitely needs the operation.

Dorothy has assisted with this type of procedure before. She knows it is an extremely complicated and lengthy operation that is hard on healthy adolescents, much less a terminally ill man who obviously does not want to go through the procedure. Dorothy hesitantly continues,

When I went in to see Mr Cook, he seemed to understand me and responded negatively when I brought up the surgery. I also noticed that the oncologist on the case doesn't think any treatment would be helpful at this point. The prognosis is very poor.

Dr Anton responds, "Just what are you saying? Are you suggesting that this operation is not indicated?"

What is Dorothy saying? She is using indirect communication patterns of the doctor-nurse game. Dr Anton has picked up on the underlying theme of her concerns and is directly challenging her.

Dorothy and the critical care nurse have demonstrated many characteristics of the interdependent view of ethical decision making. They are concerned about honoring the patient's wishes and about his quality of life. Hence, the critical care nurse saw the need for a tracheostomy to improve Wilford's quality of life. Dorothy expressed concern about a procedure that offered little benefit but would surely increase Wilford's pain and suffering in whatever time he has left.

The surgeon is concerned about Wilford's life and may believe that quality of life applies only if there is life. The surgeon has not only made a medical decision but an ethical one. He has decided what kind of life Wilford will have during his last days. It is obvious that the surgeon will do what he thinks is necessary to help this questionably competent patient, and he is willing to override any concerns expressed by the patient.

Neither Dorothy nor Dr Anton are completely right or wrong. To come to a decision that draws on the strengths of both perspectives, some fundamental changes must occur in the way they work together. The following changes in the nurse's attitude may help improve the nurse-physician relationship.

AREAS FOR CHANGE

Nurses must learn to be credible, articulate, knowledgeable, and strong. This means anticipating arguments and heated exchanges. One place to begin is with language. Nurses must practice assertiveness and avoid over-qualifying and hesitancy. This requires direct communication and an abandonment of the doctor-nurse game.

For example, in the exchange between Dr Anton and Dorothy, Dr Anton responded, "Just what are you saying? Are you suggesting that this operation is not indicated?"

Dorothy wants to avoid a confrontation about the efficacy of the surgery so she could respond with, "No, I'm not suggesting that. I am saying that Mr Cook has clearly communicated that he does not want to undergo surgery." This response is assertive and direct. Dorothy has focused her response on Mr Cook's expressed wishes, not the appropriateness of the operation. Now the discussion revolves around Mr Cook's competency. Since there is a disagreement regarding Mr Cook's competency, Dorothy could then pursue guardianship to protect Mr Cook's interests.

Other types of language that discredit the speaker, such as, "I think this is probably wrong, but . . ." or "I know you're terribly busy and I hate to bother you, but . . ." also should be eliminated. These phrases interpret for the listener and give the listener permission to discount what follows. Nurses' observations about the specific details of a patient's life are important and should be shared with clarity and conviction. Nursing contributions to the decision-making process must not be lost in deferential language. One way to change language is to listen to peers and correct usage that undermines the speaker's intent.

In addition to direct communication, nurses should use every available opportunity to teach physicians about their roles and responsibilities within the health care system. It is ironic, but frequently true, that health care professionals who work in close proximity are not remotely aware of what the other members of the team do.

Education can occur in interdisciplinary committees, during workshops and in-service programs, and especially during one-to-one interactions. On a more formal basis, a surgery department could set up an interdisciplinary ethics committee to review particularly troublesome cases and to establish guidelines for common ethical problems in surgery. The shared authority of the group process allows for better decisions to emerge. There also is greater commitment to the decision by those involved. The establishment of such a group can be an excellent source of support for nurses and physicians.

Finally, nurses must realize that the patterns of interaction highlighted throughout this discussion are large trends and not just personal, isolated experiences. It is important for nurses to recognize the personal and structural aspects of people and situations at work. By doing this, they will learn to cut their losses and focus energy on relationships that are amenable to change. Because of their roles and expertise, nurses have access to information regarding patients' responses to health problems and the

meaning patients give to the phrase *quality of life.* Both are major factors in all ethical decisions.

Because of their roles, physicians have expertise in diagnosis, prognosis, and treatment of disease and disability. Both aspects of these two essential health care professionals are necessary for humane and competent ethical decision making.

NOTES

1 L. I. Stein, "The doctor-nurse game," *Archives of General Psychiatry* 16 (June 1967) 699–703.

2 L. I. Stein, D. T. Watts, T. Howell, "The doctor-nurse game revisited," *The New England Journal of Medicine* 322 (Feb 22, 1990) 546–549.

3 C. Gilligan, *In a Different Voice: Psychological Theory and Women's Development* (Cambridge, Mass.: Harvard University Press, 1982).

FAMILIES AND MEDICAL DECISION MAKING

PATIENT CHOICES, FAMILY INTERESTS, AND PHYSICIAN OBLIGATIONS

Thomas A. Mappes and Jane S. Zembaty

Mappes and Zembaty address two major questions regarding physicians' obligations vis-à-vis family interests in the context of medical decision making. First, what are a physician's obligations when the exercise of patient autonomy threatens to be inconsistent with the patient's moral obligations to family members? Departing from an exclusively patient-centered approach, the authors argue that physicians are sometimes obliged to act in an effort to protect family interests. Second, does respect for patient autonomy generally require that physicians try to prevent patients' treatment decisions from being influenced by family considerations? Drawing from a series of clarifications about the concept of autonomy, Mappes and Zembaty answer negatively, contending that patient decisions that are responsive to family interests are often compatible with patient autonomy. Nevertheless, according to the authors, respect for autonomy sometimes requires physicians to attempt to create meaningful alternatives for patients through communication with the family.

Much has been written on the subject of the physician-patient relationship and the moral principles that are relevant to it (see, e.g., Veatch 1972; President's Commission 1982; Beauchamp and Childress 1989; Ackerman 1982; Brody 1987; Brock 1991). Suggested models of the physician-patient relationship typically have focused on physicians' obligations to patients and, for the most part, have not raised questions about the relevance of family interests to treatment decisions. When family interests in

Reprinted with permission of the publisher from *Kennedy Institute of Ethics Journal,* vol. 4, no. 1 (March 1994), pp. 27–46. Copyright © 1994 by The Johns Hopkins University Press.

treatment decisions have been recognized, they have sometimes been regarded merely as "threats" to patient autonomy. However, it is a mistake to conceptualize family interests as forces that necessarily compromise patient autonomy, and it is a mistake to think that family interests are systematically irrelevant in treatment decisions.

Recently, the relevance of family interests in treatment decisions and the resultant ramifications for physicians' obligations to patients have received more attention (see, e.g., Hardwig 1990; Doukas 1991; Loewy 1991; Nelson 1992; Blustein 1993). This emerging literature raises a number of important questions, and we will consider two especially important ones, each of which addresses the obligations of physicians vis-à-vis family interests. (1) What should a physician do when an exercise of patient autonomy threatens to negate the patient's moral obligations to others in his or her family? (2) Does respect for patient autonomy typically require efforts on the part of a physician to keep a patient's treatment decisions from being influenced by family considerations? . . .

Since a proper response to our two questions depends upon avoiding misconceptions about autonomy, we begin our discussion with a series of clarifications about this central concept. In the light of these clarifications, we then present a response to the second question and ultimately return to the first.

AUTONOMY

[John] Hardwig's discussion of autonomy [in a groundbreaking article on the relevance of family interests in medical decision making (Hardwig 1990)] provides a useful starting point for exploring the ways in which incorrect thinking about autonomy can lead to mistaken conclusions about physicians' obligations vis-à-vis family interests. While we agree with Hardwig regarding the relevance of family considerations in treatment decisions, we are sharply critical of his claims about autonomy. Hardwig discusses two conceptions of autonomy. In the first, which we shall call A1, autonomy is "the patient's freedom or right to choose the treatment he believes is best for himself" (Hardwig 1990, p. 8). Having identified A1 as the "accepted meaning" of patient autonomy in biomedical ethics, Hardwig rejects it and calls for a basic conceptual shift in which

autonomy is "the *responsible* use of freedom;" we shall call this conception A2. To use freedom responsibly is to make choices that are consistent with one's moral responsibilities; autonomy is "diminished whenever one ignores, evades, or slights one's responsibilities" (Hardwig 1990, p. 8).

Autonomy as A1 Although Hardwig does not develop A1 in any detail, his formulation conveys the impression that mainstream thinking in biomedical ethics necessarily incorporates an egoistic understanding of autonomy, so that acts that are primarily other-regarding might be construed as nonautonomous. Some of his remarks reflect this egoistic interpretation:

> Our present individualistic medical ethics is isolating and destructive. For by implicitly suggesting that patients make "their own" treatment decisions on a self-regarding basis and supporting those who do so, such an ethics encourages each of us to see our lives as simply our own. (Hardwig 1990, p. 7).

But Hardwig's account of the accepted sense of autonomy cannot be sustained. At the very least, there is a need to distinguish between understanding the accepted sense as the patient's right to make a treatment decision and, as Hardwig presents it, the right to choose what one believes is literally *best for oneself.* It is one thing to say that a patient has a right to determine which treatment, all things considered, he or she prefers and it is another, much narrower and egoistic thing to say that one has a right to choose the treatment that one believes is best for oneself. Surely, the right of self-determination so widely accepted in biomedical ethics does not preclude one's choosing a less than optimal treatment because, on balance, one sees it as the best choice given many considerations, including factors such as cost and family interests. Indeed, one line of argument often advanced in biomedical ethics stresses the right of autonomous patients to make choices for themselves even when their choices are foolish or potentially harmful to self.

To the extent that A1 reflects an exaggeratedly egoistic, individualistic understanding of autonomy, Hardwig is right to complain about it. But it is far from clear that he is right to assert that A1, understood in this characteristically egoistic way, is the accepted meaning of autonomy in biomedical ethics. . . .

It is, of course, even doubtful that there is such a thing as *the* accepted view of autonomy in biomedical ethics. The literature in biomedical ethics contains numerous, very careful analyses of autonomy, many of which do not entail an oversimplified, egoistic understanding of the concept (Childress 1990; Beauchamp and Childress 1989; Dworkin 1988; Miller 1981). One prominent approach is to see autonomy as rational self-determination. But autonomy understood as rational self-determination is open to what are usually described as altruistic, moral concerns. Although autonomy, on this view, is compatible with egoistic thinking, it does not require it. Rather it is neutral with respect to egoistic and altruistic concerns.

Consider, as well, the three-condition analysis of autonomous action presented by Tom L. Beauchamp and James F. Childress (1989, p. 69) in the third edition of *Principles of Biomedical Ethics,* certainly a work as "mainstream" as one is likely to find in biomedical ethics: "Accordingly, we analyze autonomous action in terms of normal choosers who act (1) intentionally, (2) with understanding, and (3) without controlling influences that determine the action." Since condition (3) is calculated to exclude various forms of manipulation and coercion, there is no plausible basis, on this analysis, for excluding as nonautonomous those actions motivated primarily by regard or loving concern for the interests of others. Thus, in keeping with a broader tradition that views autonomy as rational self-determination, this particular mainstream analysis of autonomous action is neutral with respect to egoistic and altruistic concerns.

Writers inclined to conceptualize autonomy along exaggeratedly individualistic lines share a common mistake. They draw a sharp and false dichotomy between self-regarding and other-regarding actions and concerns, labeling the former "egoistic" and the latter "altruistic." When this sharp dichotomy goes unquestioned, it is easy to think of self-interest along purely egoistic lines. But it is only on one, very narrow, egoistic understanding of self-interest . . . that it is correct to contrast all other-regarding actions as altruistic. While some writers in

biomedical ethics in particular and ethical theory in general may be committed implicitly or explicitly to a narrow, egoistic conception of . . . self-interest, many others are not. . . .

. . . [On a broader conception of self-interest, one's own interests may include those of others.] When one identifies with the interests of others and acts [to further those interests], one is *also* acting in one's self-interest. Rational self-determination in such cases does not generate decisions that are selfishly individualistic; nor is there anything odd in describing such a choice as one that serves one's best interests, all things considered.

Hardwig realizes that for many patients, "the interests of their family are *part* of their interests" (Hardwig 1990, p. 8). However, by his misdescription of the dominant conception of autonomy in biomedical ethics, he presents us with a false dilemma: either A1, understood in a selfish, grossly individualistic way, or A2, a conception of autonomy from which it follows that any action not in keeping with one's moral obligations is nonautonomous.

Autonomy as A2 As Hardwig formulates A2, patients inclined to make morally inappropriate decisions may be seen as lacking the sort of autonomy that entitles them to be viewed as autonomous moral agents—i.e., individuals "empowered" to make their own decisions: "For autonomy is the *responsible* use of freedom and is therefore diminished whenever one ignores, evades, or slights one's responsibilities. . . ." . . . (Hardwig 1990, p. 8). In keeping with his account of A2, Hardwig (1990, pp. 8–9) then identifies a potential conflict for a patient advocate:

> The responsibilities of patients imply that there is often a conflict between patient autonomy and the patient's interests. . . . Does the patient advocate try to promote the patient's (self-defined) *interests?* Or does she promote the patient's *autonomy* even at the expense of those interests?

As Hardwig (1990, p. 9) sees the implications of A2, physicians dedicated to promoting patient autonomy would do so by "encouraging their patients to sacrifice health, happiness, sometimes even life itself" when necessary for patients to meet their moral responsibilities.

There are at least two important reasons, however, why it is unwise to reconceptualize autonomy as A2. First, the ramifications for our understanding of informed consent seem thoroughly unpalatable. Protection of patient autonomy is usually thought to be the primary (though not the only) justification for the informed consent requirement. If we adopt A2, it seems that we also would have to change our conception of what is required for informed consent. We would either have to add a "moral competence" requirement or be required to amend our notions of competency so that the moral element becomes a part of the usual competence requirement. In either case, patients who were deemed incapable of making a morally correct decision could be labeled incompetent to make their own decisions. The potential for abuse in this regard is staggering, especially insofar as this revisionary program ignores one of the most important reasons for our society's emphasis on the principle of respect for autonomy and the related requirement of informed consent.

Ours is a pluralistic society. Since patients and physicians may have very different value systems, one function of the principle of respect for autonomy is to restrict the imposition of physician values upon patients. The literature in biomedical ethics repeatedly stresses the "unequal relationship" between physicians and patients and the need to guard against medical paternalism, including paternalistically-motivated coercion and manipulation. Let us suppose that A2 becomes the accepted sense of autonomy in biomedical ethics. Moralistically motivated physicians might then appeal to the principle of respect for autonomy to justify actions that, on [mainstream views] of autonomy, would be considered coercive or manipulative.

On Hardwig's approach, the following scenario is possible. A patient opts for an extremely expensive form of therapy that offers only a very slight chance of survival. Paying for this therapy requires the expenditure of funds that could be used to support the college educations of his three children. On the one hand, the physician might view the patient's decision as morally irresponsible. On the other hand, the patient, perhaps because he worked his way through college, might see nothing irresponsible in his decision. He might argue that his children, too, can make their own way in the world, but without the therapy, he has no chance of survival. Who is to be the moral "expert" in such a case? Who should be responsible for determining the "moral competence" of the patient?

Years ago, Isaiah Berlin (1969, pp. 145–54) addressed the dangers of conceptualizing freedom in such a way that individuals would be unfree if they did not consciously accept some ideal of rationality and would be free only when they were "forced" to live up to that ideal in the interests of their own freedom. A conception of autonomy from which it follows that any moral failure renders one less than autonomous and, therefore, as not having the right to make one's own decisions is equally problematic.

The second reason for rejecting A2 appeals to the demands of analytic clarity. The supposed advantage of adopting A2 is that patient autonomy can never really conflict with a patient's moral obligations to family members. Since a genuine exercise of patient autonomy will never negate a patient's moral obligations to family members, a physician will never face a situation in which the principle of respect for autonomy will have to be compromised in order to prevent the patient from acting in a way that entails an immoral disregard for family interests. Thus, if A2 is adopted, the "dilemma" of the physician evaporates. In our view, however, the dilemma is real and must be confronted directly. It should not be defined out of existence simply by manipulating the concept of autonomy. We are better off acknowledging that the principle of respect for autonomy can genuinely conflict with other moral principles and that these other principles are sometimes overriding, rather than "camouflaging the justification" for overriding the patient's expressed wishes as one of respect for autonomy (Childress 1990, p. 16).

Our major claim in this section is that two mistakes about autonomy must be avoided. On the one hand, we must not make the mistake (associated with A1) of thinking that patient autonomy is incompatible with responsiveness to family interests. On the other hand, we must not make the mistake (associated with A2) of thinking that patient autonomy is incompatible with nonresponsiveness to family interests, even when such nonresponsiveness involves a failure to act in accordance with some moral obligation to one's family. The point to be emphasized is that patient autonomy is compatible with both responsiveness and nonresponsiveness to family interests. It all depends upon the type of person the patient is and the values and concerns with which the patient identifies.

WHEN PATIENT DECISIONS ARE RESPONSIVE TO FAMILY INTERESTS

Consider the case of a terminally ill patient who is asked by her physician whether she wants resuscitation if she experiences cardiac arrest (Case 1). The patient rejects the idea of resuscitation saying, "My husband and children have been through so much already, I just don't want to put them through any more." The patient might even say, "If I had only myself to consider, I might choose resuscitation, but it's time for them to get on with their lives." Assuming that the physician believes that the patient should opt for resuscitation, should the physician attempt to persuade the patient to change her mind? The correct answer would seem to be no, although the physician should certainly communicate clearly his or her recommendation to elect resuscitation and the grounds on which it is based. What is ultimately at stake is the patient's best interest, all things considered, a judgment that is not properly a matter of medical expertise but of patient self-determination.

Suppose, however, that the physician argues that respect for patient autonomy entails an effort on the physician's part to persuade the patient to make the resuscitation decision independently of any impact it might have on the family. In our view, a physician who embraces this line of thought risks interfering with patient autonomy while simultaneously claiming to be protecting it. As previously discussed, a patient's treatment decision is not rendered nonautonomous simply because it is motivated primarily by regard for the interests of family members. There is no sound basis for thinking that the patient's rejection of resuscitation is anything less than a substantially autonomous decision. The patient identifies with the interests of her husband and children; their interests are also *her* interests. Her concern about their well-being is part of who

she is, and her rejection of resuscitation is a choice that expresses who she is. Thus, an effort to persuade her to make treatment decisions independently of these connections is an effort to persuade her to make decisions as if she were someone other than who she is, and this cannot coherently be done in the name of respect for patient autonomy.

Now consider the case of a terminally ill patient who has come to terms with his impending death (Case 2). His pain is adequately controlled, but he finds the aggressive treatment that sustains his life to be burdensome and pointless. The patient is ready to "let go," but his wife is not; she is adamant that aggressive treatment be continued. Consequently the patient is confronted with a desperate dilemma: Either reject the continuation of aggressive treatment and cause intense distress for his wife or accept the burden of a continued life. Responsive to his wife's wishes, the patient decides to continue the treatment.

In our view, the health care providers in this case should respond to the patient's dilemma by counseling his wife in the hope of creating a climate in which the patient is not forced to choose between two of his most powerful interests—his interest in terminating a burdensome existence and his interest in his wife's well-being. This is not to say, however, that his decision to accept aggressive treatment is rendered nonautonomous simply by its responsiveness to the perceived needs of his wife. Because their lives are interconnected, her interests are also his interests, and yet there is something terribly regrettable in the present state of affairs. If she were better able to come to terms with the situation, the dilemma would evaporate, and the patient could be spared the continuation of a life that has become unduly burdensome. Considerations of beneficence, then, should motivate the health care providers to offer counseling to the patient's wife.

The principle of respect for autonomy also supports counseling in this case. Although it is incorrect to interpret the patient's decision to accept aggressive treatment as nonautonomous, it is nevertheless true that the patient finds himself in a tragically unfortunate dilemma. Since counseling the patient's wife could eradicate the dilemma, this course of action has the potential for creating an extremely meaningful option for the patient, namely, choosing, with his wife's blessing, to reject the continuation of aggressive treatment. Insofar as one's autonomy is promoted by the construction of alternatives that better serve one's interests, the creation of this option can be seen as promoting the patient's autonomy. By understanding, rather than trying to change, the patient's interests as he perceives them and by attempting to create a situation in which the patient can make a decision that is responsive to *all* of his most pressing interests, the health care providers would demonstrate a genuine commitment to the principle of respect for patient autonomy.

Let us turn now to a case (Case 3) that was originally constructed by [James Lindemann] Nelson in "Taking Families Seriously":

> Imagine a patient suffering from a kidney stone. She would prefer to have the stone removed via lithotripsy, a benign, noninvasive, but very expensive procedure; her family, whose insurance does not cover lithotripsy, is certainly anxious that she receive the best care, but is also very concerned about the $12,000 or so the procedure would cost. . . . Insurance will cover the more traditional procedure, which is safe and effective but does involve anesthesia and the insertion of a catheter through the urethra. (Nelson 1992, p. 9).

The money at issue has special significance for the family because it would have to be taken from savings that were intended to be the down payment on a house located in a neighborhood with high-quality schools. Although Nelson discusses some aspects of this case that we presently cannot explore, one of his central concerns, understandably, relates to the requirement of voluntary informed consent.

> If the family's interest in enhancing educational opportunity is allowed to prevail over the patient's interest in lithotripsy, then it is hard to say that the patient's acceptance of the violation of her physical integrity is an instance of a fully free and informed consent. . . .
>
> . . . [I]f the urologist's patient were to say "I'd much prefer lithotripsy, but my family is so against using the money that way that I guess I'll have to go along with the surgery," it is far from clear that the urologist has what counts as a free and informed consent, and therefore lacks what her professional ethics

construes as the authorization for an invasive procedure. (Nelson 1992, pp. 9–10).

Since the patient's consent is presumably informed, the issue that Nelson raises is really whether the patient's consent is sufficiently voluntary. Does the fact that the patient makes the treatment decision with evident reluctance seriously compromise the voluntary nature of the choice?

In an effort to clarify this matter, let us consider Case 3.1, which is a variation on Case 3. Suppose that the kidney stone patient has no family and reluctantly decides against lithotripsy because, although she much prefers this noninvasive procedure, she is ultimately unwilling to spend the money that she is saving for a down payment on a new house. No one would argue that her consent to the traditional procedure failed to be sufficiently voluntary, even though her decision was attended by a significant measure of regret or reluctance. But just as this patient has clearly made an autonomous decision based on a consideration of her various interests, so too, at least on one construction, has the patient in Nelson's original case (Case 3). So long as the first patient sufficiently identifies with the educational interests of her family, their interests are her interests as well. She would rather have lithotripsy than the traditional procedure, but on balance, and with understandable reluctance, she chooses (voluntarily and autonomously) the traditional procedure.

But now let us consider Case 3.2, which is another variation on Case 3. When push comes to shove, the patient and the family simply disagree. The patient has an investment in the educational interests of her family, but sees her medical needs as the overriding concern. Thus, when she says to the urologist, "my family is so against using the money [for lithotripsy] that I guess I'll have to go along with the surgery," she really is not saying that after discussions with her family, she has decided that the best decision is the one that is responsive to her family's educational interests. Nor is she saying that although she and her family still disagree about the best resolution of this conflict, she is deeply committed to democratic decision making in all family matters. It is easy to see, therefore, why a urologist, at least initially, would feel uneasy about proceeding with the traditional procedure.

In an important way, the patient's situation in Case 3.2 is analogous to that of a kidney stone patient who prefers lithotripsy, but does not have the money to pay for it. Presumably inability to pay for lithotripsy would not, in itself, cast doubt on the voluntariness of consent to the traditional procedure. Many decisions involve a range of alternatives that is restricted by features more or less implicit in the context within which a decision must be made, but these preexisting constraints (financial and otherwise) do not typically undermine the possibility of substantially voluntary action. If they did, few human decisions and actions would qualify as voluntary; thus, few would qualify as autonomous.

But should we say that the patient's decision to accept the traditional procedure is substantially autonomous when she is at odds with her family in the way described in Case 3.2? Because her situation is relevantly similar to that of the kidney stone patient who consents to the traditional procedure simply because he or she cannot afford lithotripsy, we believe so. However, respect for autonomy might well require reasonable efforts on the part of the urologist or other health care professionals to create a wider range of choice for the patient. For example, it may be possible through some form of family mediation to break the impasse between the patient and her family. Mediation efforts in this case might explore whether the patient and family accurately understand the risks and discomforts of the traditional procedure. Perhaps the family is not taking these risks and discomforts seriously enough, or perhaps the patient is more fearful than necessary about the traditional procedure. If these and other relevant matters are processed by the patient and her family with the assistance of a skilled mediator, there is a reasonable chance that the conflict can be resolved. Whatever the choice collectively agreed upon—whether lithotripsy or surgery—the patient would be able to make it without compromising the solidarity of the family.

The cases discussed in this section lead us to three tentative conclusions. First, treatment decisions made by patients responsive to family interests do not typically fail to qualify as substantially autonomous; thus, physicians should not, in the name of patient autonomy, encourage patients to disregard such considerations. Second, it is nevertheless possible, in some cases, for physicians or other health care professionals to create meaningful alternatives for patients through interaction or communication with the family. Third, when the creation of such alternatives is a realistic goal, respect for patient autonomy requires a good-faith effort to do so, assuming of course that appropriate resources—time, energy, and expertise—are available.

WHEN PATIENT DECISIONS ARE NONRESPONSIVE TO FAMILY INTERESTS

In the original lithotripsy case, the urologist was faced with a patient who agreed, albeit reluctantly, to place her family's educational interests above her own preferred treatment choice. But what happens when a patient adamantly insists on a course of action that is contrary to family interests? Consider the following case (Case 4). An elderly patient has been paralyzed by a stroke, but is deemed competent to make his own decisions. There is no real chance that the paralysis can be reversed, and his doctor believes that the patient should enter a nursing home after leaving the hospital. The patient, however, wants to go home even though his only caretaker would be his rather frail, elderly wife who suffers from a heart ailment. His wife knows both that she is incapable of the physically demanding work required to care for him and that he will not accept nursing help in their home. She explains to her husband that if her health fails, not only will he eventually have to go into a nursing home, but she may become bedridden or die. When her husband remains adamant, she pleads with his physician to intercede on her behalf. It occurs to the physician that he could threaten to terminate his relationship with the patient, and since the patient has a great deal of faith in his doctor and would be frightened at a change of physician, this threat might be sufficient to change his mind. What, if anything, should the physician do?

In this case it seems reasonable to maintain that the patient's decision is morally incorrect. . . . Knowing that if he goes home, his wife will do everything in her power to help him, he is willing to put his wife's well-being in serious jeopardy in order to facilitate what he takes to be his own well-being. The physician has several options: (1) refuse the wife's request and release the patient from the hospital; (2) try to convince the patient to change his mind; (3) ask supporting health care professionals to speak with the patient in an effort to change his mind; or (4), if neither (2) nor (3) is effective, threaten the patient with the withdrawal of his future services.

It might be argued that it is never appropriate for a physician to attempt to persuade a patient against a course of action that seems to embody an immoral disregard for the interests of others. It is thought, on this view, that persuasion in any such case is incompatible with the principle of respect for patient autonomy and that this principle is of such great importance that no competing moral considerations are sufficient to override it. But such a systematic rejection of physician efforts to persuade cannot be sustained.

In ordinary life we tend to resent people who instruct us in our moral duties. However, if one person requires the cooperation of another in order to undertake an immoral course of action, both the articulation of a moral criticism by the latter and an effort to dissuade the first person seem entirely appropriate. Moreover, efforts to persuade someone that it would be morally wrong to perform a certain action can be compatible with respect for individual autonomy. Moral argument, like other forms of reasoned argument, does not typically threaten a person's autonomy, but rather reaffirms that the person being addressed is considered to be an autonomous agent. Still, it may be argued that while this is well and good in ordinary life, the situation is very different within the framework of the physician-patient relationship.

In many ways illness renders patients extremely vulnerable, especially to the physicians upon whom their well-being depends (Ackerman 1982; Ingelfinger 1972; Cassell 1991). Even though influence—e.g., efforts at persuasion—exerted on a person in good health may be entirely benign with respect to their impact on autonomous decision making, the same type of influence may be overwhelming when exerted by a physician on an individual with a significant illness or disability. This is difficult territory, and we cannot do full justice to the subtlety of

judgment needed to determine whether a particular form of influence exerted by a physician on a particular patient in a particular situation would be likely to undermine patient autonomy in some significant way. It is our belief, however, that many patients, even very sick ones, are not likely to be overwhelmed or controlled by a physician's persuasive efforts. This is not to say that patients will not be persuaded by a physician. The point is that even if they decide to follow the course of action promoted by the physician, the decision that has been made is substantially autonomous. The will of the patient in such cases has been influenced, but not controlled, by the physician.

In our view, a physician may be morally obligated in certain cases to attempt to persuade a patient against a treatment choice or, more generally, a course of action that seems to embody an immoral disregard for the interests of others. Furthermore, we mean for this judgment to apply even in cases in which it is likely that persuasion would seriously compromise patient autonomy. Of course, the range of cases in which attempts at persuasion would seriously compromise autonomy and yet be morally acceptable must be carefully delimited if we are not to run afoul of the informed consent requirement. Thus coercing a patient to accept a particular form of medical treatment seems much more problematic than, for example, coercing the elderly stroke victim to enter a nursing home. Our point is not that the principle of respect for patient autonomy is unimportant but that a physician might be required in some cases to compromise patient autonomy in order to protect family interests.

It is understandable that the elderly stroke victim in Case 4 has an intense desire to return home, but there is also good reason to think that his decision would have an extremely negative impact on his wife's well-being. We believe that the physician should strongly urge the patient to consent to be transferred to a nursing home, and we make this judgment even if there is good reason to believe that the patient, who is very attached to and dependent upon his physician, would be overwhelmed by the persuasive power of the physician.

Our acceptance of physician persuasion when it is necessary to protect compelling family interests is open to the charge that we are willing to tolerate a form of moral imperialism. One might argue that the only way to prevent patients from having the moral views of their physicians imposed upon them is to adopt a rule that systematically prohibits physicians from persuasion based on their moral judgments. . . . [But there] is a difference between a physician's attempt to persuade a patient against a course of action that clearly entails an unacceptable level of harm to other people and, for example, an attempt to persuade a patient against sterilization because the physician believes sterilization is incompatible with the will of God. We believe that persuasion in the first case is justified whereas persuasion in the second case is not. The difference is that the physician's moral judgment in the first case is based on a factor—protection of third party interests—whose moral relevance is uncontroversial, whereas the basis of the physician's moral judgment in the second case is not. However, given the potential for abuse, it might be best if the physician were expected to engage in some sort of consultation process—perhaps, where available, utilizing the resources of an ethics committee—before deciding that persuasion would be legitimate in any case where the patient's autonomy might be seriously compromised by the physician's persuasive efforts.

If the elderly stroke victim adheres to his resolution to return home despite attempts by the physician or other health care professionals to dissuade him, should the physician, in a further attempt to get the patient to "do the right thing," threaten to terminate the relationship? This is a very difficult question, despite the fact that we believe physicians ordinarily have a right to withdraw from cases if they are asked to participate in a course of action that they believe to be morally irresponsible.[1] The stroke victim's dependency on a particular physician is such that the threat of withdrawal would be perceived by the patient as a serious threat to his well-being. Thus, if the physician were to issue such a threat, it would likely have a very substantial coercive force and would thereby violate the principle of respect for autonomy.

Two distinct rationales might be advanced to justify the physician's threat to terminate his relationship with the elderly stroke victim, even though this course of action entails a violation of the principle of respect for autonomy. The physician might appeal to the principle of beneficence and argue that a threat to withdraw is justified in this case because *the patient himself* will be much better off in the long run if he agrees to enter a nursing home. But to phrase the justification in this way immediately reminds us of the potential dangers of generalizing this approach. We would fall back into a way of thinking that makes it too easy to justify physician interference with patient autonomy, thereby returning to the excesses of paternalism that the principle of respect for autonomy was intended to tame. But suppose the physician simply maintains that it is not the necessity of protecting patient well-being that is at issue, but the necessity of protecting the patient's wife from an immoral disregard for her interests. It is consistent with our earlier reasoning to say that a threat to withdraw might be justified on this basis. However, a great deal depends on the psychological and physical state of the patient. Could a threat to withdraw be made without risking serious harm to the patient? If not, given the overriding importance of the principle of nonmaleficence with regard to the patient, such a threat would not be justified. And if a threat, though justified, ultimately proved unsuccessful in changing the patient's mind, the physician's actual withdrawal—i.e., the actualization of the threat—would probably not be justified because of its seriously detrimental impact on patient welfare.

The case of the elderly stroke victim leads us to a number of tentative conclusions. First, in certain cases it is morally appropriate for physicians to attempt to persuade their patients against a course of action that the physician believes to embody an immoral disregard for family interests. Second, although some such efforts at persuasion violate the principle of respect for autonomy, others do not. Third, in those cases where efforts at persuasion do constitute violations of the principle of respect for autonomy, the prima facie obligation to respect autonomy may be overridden when the need to protect family interests is sufficiently compelling. Fourth, other actions by physicians, such as threats to withdraw, when calculated to deter patients from acting in a way that embodies an immoral disregard for family interests, may be morally appropriate even when they are not in keeping with the principle of respect for autonomy.

CONCLUSION

Discussion of the relevance of family interests in treatment decisions and the possible ramifications for physicians' obligations to patients is still in its initial stages. In this article, we have attempted to further the discussion in useful ways. In countering possible misconceptions of autonomy, we have shown in particular that patient decisions that are responsive to family interests are often entirely compatible with patient autonomy. Although respect for autonomy in such cases may sometimes require that physicians attempt to create meaningful alternatives for patients, it does not require that physicians attempt to guard patients against the influence of family considerations. We also have explored the tensions that emerge for physicians when the exercise of patient autonomy seems to embody an immoral disregard for family interests. In committing ourselves to the view that the protection of family interests may sometimes be a morally decisive factor in determining what a physician should do, we clearly depart from an exclusively patient-centered approach to medical decision making. The time has come to factor a new layer of complexity into the already complex picture of medical decision making.

We are grateful for suggestions made by David DeGrazia on earlier versions of this article. We have also benefitted from the helpful comments of three anonymous reviewers.

NOTE

1 We are visualizing situations in which the care of a patient would be transferred from one physician to another. Presumably the literal abandonment of a patient by a physician is neither morally nor legally permissible.

REFERENCES

Ackerman, Terrence F. 1982. Why Doctors Should Intervene. *Hastings Center Report* 12 (4): 14–17.

Beauchamp, Tom L., and Childress, James F. 1989. *Principles of Biomedical Ethics.* 3d ed. New York: Oxford University Press.

Berlin, Isaiah. 1969. *Four Essays on Liberty.* Oxford: Oxford University Press.

Blustein, Jeffrey. 1993. The Family in Medical Decisionmaking. *Hastings Center Report* 23 (3): 6–13.

Brock, Dan. 1991. The Ideal of Shared Decision Making Between Physicians and Patients. *Kennedy Institute of Ethics Journal* 1: 28–47.

Brody, Howard. 1987. The Physician-Patient Relationship: Models and Criticisms. *Theoretical Medicine* 8: 205–20.

Cassell, Eric J. 1991. The Importance of Understanding Suffering for Clinical Ethics. *Journal of Clinical Ethics* 2: 81–82.

Childress, James F. 1990. The Place of Autonomy in Bioethics. *Hastings Center Report* 20 (1): 12–17.

Doukas, David J. 1991. Autonomy and Beneficence in the Family: Describing the Family Covenant. *Journal of Clinical Ethics* 2: 145–48.

Dworkin, Gerald. 1988. *The Theory and Practice of Autonomy.* New York: Cambridge University Press.

Hardwig, John. 1990. What About the Family? *Hastings Center Report* 20 (2): 5–10.

Ingelfinger, Franz J. 1972. Informed (But Uneducated) Consent. *New England Journal of Medicine* 287: 465–66.

Loewy, Erich H. 1991. Families, Communities, and Making Medical Decisions. *Journal of Clinical Ethics* 2: 150–53.

Miller, Bruce. 1981. Autonomy and the Refusal of Lifesaving Treatment. *Hastings Center Report* 11 (4): 25–28.

Nelson, James Lindemann. 1992. Taking Families Seriously. *Hastings Center Report* 22 (4): 6–12.

President's Commission for the Study of Ethical Problems in Medicine and Biomedical and Behavioral Research. 1982. *Making Health Care Decisions.* Washington, DC: U.S. Government Printing Office.

Veatch, Robert M. 1972. Models for Ethical Medicine in a Revolutionary Age. *Hastings Center Report* 3 (2): 5–7.

DEAF CULTURE, COCHLEAR IMPLANTS, AND ELECTIVE DISABILITY

Bonnie Poitras Tucker

In this excerpt from a longer article, Tucker addresses the claim that cochlear implants represent a threat to Deaf (with a capital D) culture by enabling partial hearing in deaf persons. Proponents of Deaf culture, she explains, understand deafness as a cultural identity rather than a disability, express pride in their shared use of

American Sign Language (ASL), and reject efforts, such as the use of cochlear implants, to assimilate deaf persons into the hearing mainstream. In response to this position, Tucker, who is deaf, argues that inability to hear is genuinely disadvantageous, that learning English as well as ASL better overcomes these disadvantages than does learning ASL alone, and that cochlear implants expand the range of opportunities available to deaf children whereas hostility to mainstream hearing culture narrows those opportunities. She also criticizes those who reject cochlear implants yet demand costly accommodations for their deafness.

During the past decade, a growing concept of Deaf culture has taken root. Under this concept, people who cannot hear are viewed as either deaf (with a small d) or Deaf (with a capital D). Persons who view themselves as deaf are those who, although impaired in their ability to hear, have assimilated into hearing society and do not view themselves as members of a separate culture. People who call themselves "Deaf," however, view and define deafness as a cultural identity rather than as a disability for some purposes; they insist that their culture and separate identity must be nourished and maintained.[1]

A cochlear implant is a surgically implanted device that is capable of restoring hearing and speech understanding to many individuals who are severely or profoundly deaf. Numerous studies show both the ability of profoundly deaf individuals to hear speech with cochlear implants and the ability of implanted deaf children to develop age-appropriate spoken and receptive language skills.[2] As reported in May 1998 to the Advisory Council of the National Institute on Deafness and Other Communication Disorders: "It has now been demonstrated that the long-term benefits of cochlear implants in children are not limited to speech recognition but extend into dramatically improved language learning and language skills."[3] In a recent survey, parents of 176 implanted children perceived that: (1) 44 percent of the children had greater than 70 percent open speech discrimination (using sound alone with no visual clues), (2) 61 percent of the children had greater than 50 percent open speech discrimination, and (3) 84 percent of the children had greater than 40 percent open speech discrimination.[4]

Because cochlear implants have the potential to ameliorate or eliminate ramifications of deafness, they are opposed by Deaf culturists, who view efforts to "cure" deafness or ameliorate its effects as an immoral means of killing Deaf culture.

The theory of Deaf culture is primarily premised on a shared language—American Sign Language (ASL). Individuals who communicate via ASL clearly *do* speak a different language. American Sign Language is visual rather than spoken, with its own syntax and grammar. ASL is quite different from signed English, which involves signing each English word as it is spoken, using English grammar and structure. In addition, some members of the Deaf cultural community claim to be part of a separate culture as a result of attending segregated (often residential) schools for Deaf children,[5] or as a result of their participation in Deaf clubs or wholly Deaf environments in which they socialize or work.

According to the leaders of the National Association of the Deaf (NAD), Deaf people like being Deaf, want to be Deaf, and are proud of their Deafness. Deaf culturists claim the right to their own "ethnicity, with [their] own language and culture, the same way that Native Americans or Italians [or blacks] bond together."[6] They claim the right to "personal diversity," which is "something to be cherished rather than fixed and erased." In short, they claim the right to their "birthright of silence."

Many individuals who are deaf, however, do not agree that these facts give rise to a true culture. The now deceased Larry G. Stewart, a leading member of the signing deaf community (a strong proponent and user of sign language), noted that " '[D]eaf culture' was not discovered; it was created for political purposes. The term has yet to be satisfactorily defined."[7] Dr. Stewart went on to say that "[i]n the larger sense of world cultures, the meaning of culture is so powerful and complex that to apply it so narrowly to a group of highly diverse deaf American citizens, whose members are as heterogeneous as the general population, simply makes no sense" (p. 129).

Although Deaf culturists equate being deaf to being a member of a racial or tribal minority, many deaf people find the analogy nonsensical. Deaf people lack one of the five critical senses. True deaf people such as this author are physically incapable of talking on the telephone alone. We have to use the phone with the aid of a third party—an interpreter or a relay service, both of which present extremely awkward situations. Most of us would *love* to be able to pick up the telephone and make a personal or business call when and how we feel like it without having to scramble to find an interpreter and without having to make the call with a third person privy to every word. We'd like to be able to go to a movie or a play regardless of whether captioning or interpreters are available. We'd like to be able to participate in group conversations, to hear the conversation at the dinner table. We'd like to be able to hear music; to hear our children and grandchildren laugh and cry; to listen to the radio when we are driving; to have a car phone; to be able to use the drive-up window at McDonald's; to hear the announcements at the airport; to be able to talk to the person in front of or behind us on a hiking trail; to be able to go to a professional meeting on the spur of the moment; to be able to get any job we want without having to consider how our deafness will interfere with the job duties. We'd particularly like to hear our own voices and to be able to control the tone and pitch and loudness of our voices. The list is endless. Why would any human being *want* to deny such pleasures to herself or her children?

Many members of the Deaf cultural community strongly desire to have Deaf children, who will be a part of their parents' Deaf culture. Some expectant Deaf parents visit geneticists for the purpose of determining whether their children are likely to be born deaf. As explained by Jamie Israel, a genetic counselor at Gallaudet University's genetic services center, "[m]any of our [Deaf] families are not interested in fixing or curing deaf genes . . . [m]any . . .

couples come in and want . . . [D]eaf children."[8] If their children are *not* likely to be born deaf, Deaf parents may choose not to have children, or to abort children in gestation, just as hearing or deaf people who determine through genetic research that their children *are* likely to be born deaf may choose not to have children or to abort children in gestation.

The desire of parents to have children who will be like them and fit into their world is certainly understandable. But most parents want more for their children than they have. While this author's parents, for example, never went to college, they wanted all their children to have that opportunity. Similarly, although we cannot hear, most people who are deaf want our children and grandchildren to have that ability.

Dena S. Davis notes that "the primary argument against deliberately seeking to produce deaf children is that it violates the child's own autonomy and narrows the scope of her choices when she grows up; in other words, it violates her right to an 'open future.'"[9] Insisting that children who are deaf be raised in a Deaf cultural community denies these children the right to choose for themselves whether to accept or reject the larger hearing world.

Deaf culturists argue that parents should not make decisions about cochlear implants for their deaf children, that the children should be allowed to make such decisions for themselves when they are old enough to do so. However, experience has proven that early implantation is necessary for maximum efficacy of a cochlear implant. Thus, waiting ten or fifteen years to make the decision for a child to have a cochlear implant is the same as deciding that the child will *not* have an implant. If a child who is deaf is going to learn to talk, he or she must begin learning at a *very* early age. A person who is deaf does not learn to speak at the age of twelve or older, the age at which the child is arguably old enough to decide for herself how she wants to live her life. But a child who is deaf who learns to speak and is part of the hearing world during childhood *can* learn to sign later in life and join the Deaf world.

Many of the leaders of the Deaf culture movement can speak, as a result of early oral training (or in a few cases because they became deaf later in life), and the majority of those leaders know perfect

English—although they know ASL as well. Indeed, it is their oral skills that have enabled them to argue for Deaf isolationism so persuasively. Many of these leaders of Deaf culture, however, do not want today's deaf children to learn spoken English. Rather, they believe that spoken English should be rejected by Deaf people, and that Deaf people should use only ASL as their mode of "spoken" (actually signed) language. This is known as the "bi-bi," or "bilingual-bicultural" approach.[10] Under this approach, Deaf children are to learn ASL only, and not spoken *or* signed English. Bi-bi advocates believe that children who are deaf should be taught their "natural language" of ASL, which they consider to be the "birthright of all deaf children" (p. 60). Their rationale is expressed as follows:

> Natural sign not only serves deaf children as a means of communication between other sign language users but can support intellectual development and the acquisition of ideas in the same way that spoken language serves hearing people. It is, therefore, a folly, say bilingualists, to create an artificial sign system, such as SE [signed English] . . . , when a bona fide sign language already exists. It is not only a folly but, say most supporters of bilingualism, a moral crime to attempt to force young deaf children to do something they cannot do, that is, learn spoken language as a first language. . . . (p. 63)

The contention on the part of the Deaf culture movement that children who are deaf are unable to "learn spoken language as a first language" is, of course, belied by the thousands of deaf children, including this author, who have learned spoken language as a first (and in many cases only) language. Nevertheless, advocates of biculturalism espouse the view that once a child who is deaf has acquired a strong "natural" language (ASL), the child can then be taught *written* (but not spoken) English as a second language. What biculturists do not explain, at least in any satisfactory manner, is why even if one accepts the proposition that sign language is more natural to deaf children than speech, learning ASL is more "natural" than learning signed English. Nor do biculturists explain why a child who is deaf should have to struggle with learning to read and write English as a second language, when even if the child is

taught to sign only, it would be so much easier for the child to learn and sign English, and then apply those English signing skills when learning how to read and write.

The leaders of Deaf culture who espouse the most radical interpretation of the "bi-bi" movement and want to deny children who are deaf both spoken and signed English, would deny deaf children the very skills that allow many of the Deaf culture leaders to perform successfully in this hearing world. One oral deaf leader, Kevin Nolan, noted that "nearly all" the Deaf culture leaders he knows "have had the benefit of early oral education."[11] Mr. Nolan asks:

> Why should they deny children who are deaf the opportunity to realize the same oral successes that they themselves have experienced? . . . Having benefited from oral education in their own childhoods, why do they . . . deny their oral backgrounds—those very backgrounds that helped them to become the leaders that they are today? (p. T3)

When this author and many of the leaders of the Deaf culture movement were growing up, technology was very limited. Most people of our generation (born at least between 1940 and 1960) who are profoundly deaf were not able to obtain much, if any, benefit from hearing aids. (This author, for example, has never been able to wear a hearing aid.) The times have changed, drastically! Technology has *vastly* improved. Today's deaf children are able to wear much-improved hearing aids or to have cochlear implants. And the technology is still improving rapidly. It is very likely that in ten to fifteen years, perhaps less, cochlear implants will have improved to the point where almost all children who are deaf could benefit very substantially from an implant.

Deaf culture advocates, however, are strongly opposed to research geared at "curing" deafness and are particularly opposed to placing cochlear implants in children. They assert that members of their minority group "are in no more need of a cure for their condition than are Haitians or Hispanics."[12] To many members of the Deaf cultural community, cochlear implants represent "the ultimate denial of deafness, the ultimate refusal to let deaf children be Deaf" (p. 40). As stated by Roz Rosen, former president of NAD, since "[h]earing is not a life or death matter . . . [it is] consequently not worth the medical, moral and ethical risk of altering a child."[13] In accord with this reasoning, Deaf culturists have strongly criticized the National Institute of Health's National Institute on Deafness and Other Communication Disorders, which gives federal grants for research geared at the prevention and treatment of deafness and other communication disorders.[14]

Gallaudet students and their families or friends have informed this author that cochlear implants are greatly frowned upon at Gallaudet, and that implanted individuals who attend Gallaudet are usually pressured (often by their peers rather than by staff or faculty members) to remove them or at least not to wear their processors. As one reporter succinctly stated:

> As anyone at Gallaudet knows, a student with a [cochlear implant] device . . . runs the risk of being shunned. "I have some friends with implants," says Scott Mohan, a sixth generation deaf senior at Gallaudet. "They just don't use them anymore."
>
> "You can understand why," says Keith Muller, Executive Director of the League for the Hard of Hearing in New York City. "Kids who try to speak in deaf schools are ridiculed. And the greater their oral success, the more they are criticized."[15]

The hatred with which Deaf culturists view cochlear implants is expressed in the ASL sign for a cochlear implant, which contains a two-fingered stab to the back of the neck, indicating a "vampire" in the cochlea.

One individual seeking information about cochlear implants sent a list of questions to selected cochlear implant recipients and parents of children with cochlear implants.[16] Questions asked included the following:

> (1) Do you think that having a cochlear implant takes away your Deaf pride?
> (2) Do you think that cochlear implants remove you as a member of Deaf culture?
> (3) Do you think that cochlear implants are a way for hearing people to break down Deaf society?
> (4) Do you think that a person should be allowed to choose whether or not to have a cochlear implant or should it be left up to the parents to decide? (Take into consideration that the longer you wait, the less likely it is that [the implant] will work).

At least several recipients of that questionnaire were angered by these questions. The responses of three individuals are illustrative.

To the question about whether cochlear implants take away "your Deaf pride," one respondent, Bill Boyle, noted, ". . . what the hell is deaf pride? Proud not to hear your child's voice, pianos, the birds in the trees? That's not pride, it's bull-headedness and selfishness. . . . I feel the implant enhances my pride. I am proud to be overcoming what was considered a severe handicap, proud to be part of the community as a whole, not to a 'club' of narrow minded people."[17]

To the question about whether cochlear implants "remove you as a member of Deaf culture," another recipient, Melissa Chaikof, responded:

> If the cochlear implant has removed my daughters from "[D]eaf culture," and it probably has, then that is fine by me. The [D]eaf culturists' opportunities in life are so limited, and my daughters' are not. Furthermore, it has been the choice of those in the "[D]eaf culture" to exclude those with implants from their group. . . .[18]

To the question about whether cochlear implants are a way for hearing people to break down Deaf society, Ms. Chaikof stated: "In obtaining implants for our daughter, we did not have the ulterior motive of 'breaking down Deaf society.' If that is an indirect result . . . [m]y concern for my daughters' futures is far greater than for the future of 'Deaf society.' "

The three respondents replied to the question about whether a person should be allowed to choose whether to have a cochlear implant or whether parents should make that decision as follows:

> (i) Mildred Oberkotter replied: "for young children, it is essential that parents choose what is best for their child's interest and [the child's ability to] function in his/her culture in which s/he is born. So much time and possible maximum value would be lost in language and auditory development if and when the child is cognitively ready to make such a decision for him/herself."[19]
> (ii) Melissa Chaikof replied: "I absolutely think that the decision as to whether or not to implant should be in the hands of the parents . . . and the implant team. Some children and some families make better

candidates. For example, one implant team here will not implant children in total communication [sign and some speech] or manual [sign language only] programs . . . [T]he kids whose parents are committed to an auditory-verbal approach [learning to listen], as we are, stand a very high chance of success." (iii) Bill Boyle replied: "If this [question] is about children, it is an enormous responsibility for the parents to decide. *But*—it is a decision [for] the parents who truly believe that their decision will be in the best interest of their child, and not a decision [for] NAD or others to decide. Yes, the longer you wait, the less benefit, so leave the parents alone and let them decide. . . ."

. . . Cochlear implants do not, and likely will not, eliminate deafness altogether. An individual who has an implant is still deaf. The difference is, however, that the ramifications of deafness are significantly reduced. At the present time, it is known that most children, and people who become deaf later in life and have memory of normal hearing, do very well with cochlear implants, thus reducing (if not eliminating) the need for special schools, interpreters, and other costly accommodations. Such individuals who refuse today to have cochlear implants, yet demand costly accommodations, should, in this author's opinion, be viewed as acting unethically.

In spite of all that is said above, it is impossible not to recognize the source and validity of the anger, hostility, and solidarity expressed by the Deaf culturists who choose to reject hearing society and who do not wish to be "hearing" to any degree. Any individual with any compassion who knows anything of the history of people who are deaf must understand how the concept of Deaf culture came into existence. Many people who are deaf continue to live as second class citizens, as indicated not only by the rejection of deaf people by most hearing people but by the facts that:

The average deaf person today reads at a fourth grade level. One in three drops out of high school. Only one in five who starts college gets a degree. Deaf adults make 30 percent less than the general population. Their unemployment rate is high, and when they are employed, it is usually in manual jobs such as kitchen workers, janitors, machine operators, tailors and car-

penters, for which a strong command of English is not required . . .[20]

Rejecting hearing society, technology that will alleviate the ramifications of deafness, and the potential eradication of most deafness, however, is not the solution to the problems of deaf people. Rather, deaf people with cochlear implants, particularly children, have a wealth of opportunities and potential life experiences available to them. To deny such opportunities based on theories of segregation is indeed illogical.

REFERENCES

1 For an article explaining the view-point of Deaf culture, see Edward Dolnick, "Deafness as Culture," *Atlantic* 272, no. 3 (1993): 37–53.
2 See, for example, Susan B. Waltzman, Noel L. Cohen, Railey H. Gomolin, Janet E. Green, William H. Shapiro et al., "Open-Set Speech Perception in Congenitally Deaf Children Using Cochlear Implants," *American Journal of Otology* 18, no. 3 (1997): 342–49; "Progress Report, Outcomes for Paediatric Cochlear Implantation in Nottingham: Safe—Effective—Efficient," Nottingham Paediatric Cochlear Programme, University Hospital NHS Trust, Queens Medical Centre, Nottingham, England (May 1997); T.A. Zwolan, P. R. Kileny, S. A. Telian, "Self-Report of Cochlear Implant Use and Satisfaction by Prelingually Deafened Adults," *Ear & Hearing* 17, no. 3 (1996): 198–210; Amy M. Robbins, "Implanted Children Can Speak, But Can They Communicate?" Paper Presented at the Sixth Symposium on Cochlear Implants in Children, University of Miami School of Medicine, Miami, Florida, February 1996; N. M. Young, J. C. Johnson, M. B. Mets, T. C. Hain, "Cochlear Implants in Young Children with Usher's Syndrome," *Annals of Otology, Rhinology & Laryngology* Suppl. 166, No. 9, Part 2 (1995): 342–45; Anne E. Geers and Jean S. Moog, eds., "Effectiveness of Cochlear Implants and Tactile Aids for Deaf Children: The Sensory Aids Study at Central Institute for the Deaf," *The Volta Review* 96, no. 5 (1994).
3 Report of Dr. Robert F. Naunton, Director, Division of Human Communications, National Institute of Deafness and Other Communication Disorders, 7 May 1998 (in the author's files).
4 Bonnie P. Tucker, *Cochlear Implants: A Handbook* (Jefferson, N.C.: McFarland & Co., 1998, forthcoming).
5 The vast majority of deaf children in the United States no longer attend such schools; the Individuals with Disabilities Education Act—enacted in 1973 for the purpose of providing children with disabilities with a free appropriate public education, primarily alongside children without disabilities—has resulted in sharp declines in special school enrollments. See, for example, Felicity Barringer, "Pride in a

Soundless World: Deaf Oppose a Hearing Aid," *New York Times,* 16 May 1993.

6 Roslyn Rosen, "President Rosen on Cochlear Implants," *NAD Broadcaster,* December 1992, p. 6; see also, "The President Signs On," *NAD Broadcaster,* January 1991, p. 3.

7 Larry G. Stewart, "Debunking the Bilingual/Bicultural Snow Job in the American Deaf Community," *A Deaf American Monograph* 42 (1992): 129–42.

8 Abigail Trafford, "The Brave New World of Genetic Planning," *Washington Post,* 15 November 1994.

9 Dena S. Davis, "Genetic Dilemmas and the Child's Right to an Open Future," *Hastings Center Report* 27, no. 2 (1997): 7–15, at 9.

10 See, for example, Wendy Lynas, *Communication Options in the Education of Deaf Children* (London: Whurr Publishers, 1994).

11 Kevin Nolan, "Communication Chores: A Parent's Perspective," *Clarke Speaks* (Winter/Spring 1997): T3.

12 Dolnick, "Deafness as Culture," p. 37.

13 Rosen, "President Rosen on Cochlear Implants."

14 The author is a member of the National Advisory Council to the National Institute on Deafness and Other Communication Disorders and has personal knowledge of such criticism.

15 M. Arana Ward, "As Technology Advances, A Bitter Debate Divides the Deaf," *Washington Post,* 11 May 1997.

16 E-mail by Kate T. Kubey of November 1996, submitted to the author by Mildred Oberkotter and Melissa K. Chaikof (in the author's files).

17 Response of Bill Boyle (in the author's files).

18 Response of Melissa K. Chaikof (in the author's files).

19 Response of Mildred Oberkotter (in the author's files).

20 Ward, "As Technology Advances."

THE HANUKKAH BUSH: ETHICAL IMPLICATIONS IN THE CLINICAL MANAGEMENT OF INTERSEX

Sherri A. Groveman

Presenting her own experiences as an intersex individual—a person born with ambiguous genitalia—Groveman confronts the mainstream medical view that intersex is "a tragedy—a mistake of nature to be corrected, to the maximum possible extent, by medicine." She strongly criticizes physicians' (until recently standard) practice of pressuring parents of an intersex newborn to consent to surgery that will make the infant appear more normal (either male- or female-looking) and to hide the truth from the intersex individual for as long as possible. What parents need in these situations, Groveman contends, is emotional support, resources for education about intersex, and the freedom to make unpressured medical decisions for their child. What the intersex individual needs over the years, she argues, is the truth about his and/or her ambiguous sexuality, acceptance of his and/or her condition, and—before reaching the age of consent—no more surgery than is necessary for physical health. Groveman concludes by expressing the joy she felt upon discovering a support group for persons with her particular form of intersex, Androgen Insensitivity Syndrome, and her hope that other intersex individuals will find similar support.

As a young child of a conservative, but unobservant, Jewish household, I viewed Christmas as being about the large, aromatic firs and spruces adorning my friends' apartments, decorated with dazzling or-naments and surrounded by a profusion of foil-wrapped packages. Hanukkah, by contrast, was embodied in our home by only a small menorah on our window sill. Is it any wonder that I begged, pleaded, and cajoled my parents for a Christmas tree? Wisely, they would not relent.

Soon I discovered that the parents of some Jewish friends had instituted a custom of "Hanukkah bushes," which, to any honest observer, were clearly Christmas trees in drag. Seeing one for the first time it felt fake, hollow, half of something but all of nothing. My friends' parents, uncomfortable about their minority status, had been co-opted by the overwhelming pressure to make life "easier" for their children by diluting their heritage while assimilating to the dominant culture.

With the benefit of hindsight, I am glad my parents did not yield to such pressure even as I regret they did not do more to educate me about my roots. Having now learned the history of my religion I have discovered all that is rich and precious about Hanukkah, dissipating any desire for a Christmas tree. My "Hanukkah bush" friends, by contrast, derive no such meaning from the Festival of Lights, but at the same time feel like frauds if they lay claim to actual Christmas trees. Did their parents' response to societal pressure, though well-intentioned to help these children "fit in," simply leave my friends incapable of functioning comfortably in either world? Can the same be said of doctors who importune parents to manage their intersex children with surgery and secrets?

I might mention, as a footnote to this parable, that the population of Jews in the world is no larger than the population of intersex persons. Thus, I suppose it is fortunate that pediatric endocrinologists are not the stewards of the world's religions, because with the same rationale they use to support surgery and secrecy in managing intersex— that is, that it is unfair to leave children's ambiguous genitals in their natural state, or even openly acknowledge to them that they are intersexed, because this will render them outcasts to the majority of society—these doctors might argue that it is unfair to obligate children to live with a religion shared by only a tiny fraction of the world's population. As a practical matter, of course, religious tolerance is an accepted norm in our society, whereas doctors perceive something inherently intolerable about intersex.

Intersex is a subject near and dear to my heart (and other parts of my anatomy). But it is also my personal history inflected by the burden of having lived almost all of my 40 years with the shame, secrecy, and isolation that are an inevitable byproduct of how my case was managed by the medical profession.

I have complete Androgen Insensitivity Syndrome (AIS), which is characterized by XY chromosomes and testes, but a complete inability, due to an androgen receptor defect, of the body to respond to the testosterone produced by the testes. Unable to virilize, my body, by preordination, simply developed along a female path. In my case, this was discovered 10 days after my birth, when my pediatrician noticed a swelling in my groin, suggesting a hernia. Exploratory surgery performed at two weeks revealed the presence of what seemed to be a testis. When the lab report confirmed this, my parents were told that it was medically necessary for them to consent to immediate gonadectomy. Lacking any better insight, they of course gave their consent.

In fact, there was no urgent medical necessity; my testes could have remained safely intact until puberty, at which time they should have been removed to prevent any risk of cancer. But I strongly suspect that there were pressing "psychological" necessities for their removal in infancy: (1) my doctors' desire to rid me of any vestige of a male anatomy and render my body "congruent"; (2) the equal desire to avoid the need at puberty to explain the nature of the surgery that would have to be performed, raising questions the doctors did not want to have to answer; and (3) shards of a superstitious fear that, despite what medicine knew in 1958 about "testicular feminization" (as it was then called), I might somehow virilize if my troublesome gonads were left intact.

Unlike Hanukkah, where my parents were sufficiently inculcated with the traditions of their religion to inoculate them against the pressure to conform to the dominant messages surrounding them, my parents are not, alas, intersexed, and so to learn the "culture" of what this meant to their child they had to rely on doctors to translate the language and meaning of words such as "chromosomes" and "gonads" and "pseudohermaphrodite." Unfortunately, like most doctors even today, my doctors were steeped in a tradition that viewed intersexuality as a tragedy—a mistake of nature to be corrected, to the maximum extent possible, by medicine. This culture had been handed down to them without any concern for the long-term outcome of the recipients of such treatment protocols. Thus, they became self-appointed tour guides to a foreign country when they themselves had not bothered to ever communicate with the natives.

My experience over the past three years assisting families affected by AIS informs me that the most critical variable to achieving a better outcome for intersex patients is not surgical management followed up with platitudes and half-truths, but instead is the provision of resources for parents to be thoroughly educated about what intersex is, and to work through any anxiety or guilt they feel about having an intersex child. When parents are able to communicate their comfort and acceptance, the child's self-esteem can develop from a solid foundation. When parents are, by contrast, apprehensive, fearful, or ignorant about intersex, their child is left to flounder in a sea of confusion without support. Regrettably medicine has seen fit to "correct" what is between the child's legs while offering limited educational assistance and psychological support to either the child or her/his family.

Indeed, the sole instruction my parents received from my endocrinologists was one of "damage control," calculated to confirm a solid image that I was their daughter in the same breath that doctors enjoined them that they should not disclose my true diagnosis to anyone, least of all me. While informing my parents that I was "just like a normal female," my doctors offered no suggestions other than fabrication about how they should help me cope with the reality of having XY chromosomes and testes while lacking ovaries, a uterus, fallopian tubes, or fertility.

Fortuitously, my surgeon failed to diagnose that I have a vagina incapable of intromission; had he done so he likely would have suggested vaginoplasty, a procedure that continues to be recommended in childhood to this day, despite its nearly 80 percent failure rate when performed prior to adolescence. Had I had been born with more ambiguous looking genitals, the solution offered would have been more surgery, most likely to make my genitals appear "female," even at the expense of diminishing sexual sensation. Cultural imperative, masquerading as medical necessity, would have made such additional surgeries inevitable.

I spent my adolescence filled with shame, though I was never told the true details of my diagnosis. My trauma was needlessly compounded by my doctor's stony silence while examining me, and his asking me to lie naked on an examining table so that teams of interns and residents could inspect my genitals. Such experiences themselves, far more than the true facts I later learned about the nature of AIS, instilled a sense of freakishness that I have only recently shaken. It is, however, disheartening to hear that similar treatment of intersex adolescents continues to this day.

Ultimately, I unearthed the truth about having AIS in a medical school library when I was 20 by researching the possible causes for my primary amenorrhea and lack of pubic hair. It is disorienting when you have always considered yourself female to learn that you have XY chromosomes and once had testes. It is equally disorienting when you have always considered yourself loved and cared for to discover that your parents and doctors have lied and left you to your own devices to discover this truth.

I appreciate that because I am 40 years old my treatment protocol was a product of 1960s thinking. I am frightened, however, that as we approach the turn of the millennium conventional medical treatment continues to endorses a nearly identical protocol. Doctors continue to debate the patient's right to know the truth, seemingly oblivious to the idea that they do not "own" the patient's medical information. This conspiracy of silence stems from the same root as the continuing protocol to surgically alter intersex infants' anatomies—an inability to see intersex as anything other than shameful and pathologic. This, in turn, is communicated to the parents, whom I believe would be far less traumatized by the reality of intersex if they weren't receiving such negative cues from doctors.

Regrettably doctors fail to offer appropriate psychological support to parents or even communicate that the capacity to give and receive love is a function of the size of one's heart, not the size or appearance of one's genitals. Yet this capacity for healthy relationships is threatened at best, and more typically destroyed altogether, through the toxic mixture of silence and surgery which is offered up as the only "solution" to the child's intersex "problem."

In the aftermath of such surgery, doctors behave as though the "problem" has been cured ("you used to be intersexed but we fixed it")—as though being intersexed were an historic detail of the patient's life. Unfortunately, this too is communicated to the parents, who, in turn, assume that there is no need to offer their child a safe place to mourn and grieve what has occurred, or to help their child ascribe meaning to being intersexed. Often the parents are sufficiently uncomfortable and guilt-ridden about the whole affair that they are highly motivated to accept the doctor's revisionist history of the child's intersex state. Thus, the child has endured a personal holocaust while having to remain mute.

I believe, based upon my experiences overseeing the U.S. branch of the AIS Support Group, attending 10 AIS Support Group meetings in the U.S. and the U.K., and getting to know more than 100 intersex people, ranging in age from two months to 73 years, that under the best of circumstances learning the truth about being intersexed can be temporarily traumatic. But not knowing the truth culminates in experiences that are almost universally tragic. With limited inaccurate information, and in the face of an overarching sense of shame, the mind conjures a parade of horribles far worse than any truth. Indeed, of the more than 60 women with AIS whom I personally know, I have not heard of a single instance where someone has reported that it was worse to know the truth than to live with lies.

Fortunately, many pediatric endocrinologists are endorsing the approach of truthful disclosure at the same time that they are revisiting the wisdom of surgical management of intersex. Apart from the ethical implications of a protocol rooted in dissimulation, the paradigm of deceit is, quite simply, shortsighted. The reports of women affiliated with the AIS Support Group reveal that patients are driven to learn what it is about themselves that seems to cause a palpable silence whenever they are examined by doctors or broach the subject of their childhood/adolescent gonadectomies. To that end, some members of our support group became expert in reading their medical charts upside down, while others inspected their files when their doctors momentarily left the examining room.

But there are even more unusual, and often painful, ways this information is obtained. Some members report the "dreaded" information spilling out in the heat of arguments with stepparents or siblings. One woman in our U.K. group literally discovered she had AIS by buying a house. She applied for a mortgage which required that she provide proof of good health. To do so she had to sign a medical release. She had never been told she had AIS—just that she had an "ovarian" problem and couldn't have children, but that this had no bearing on her health.

She innocently signed the release. A few weeks later her mortgage company called her and said "Everything is fine but we need to know what this 'androgen insensitivity' thing is all about."

It is important to note that the significance of truth-telling has increased with the advent of intersex support groups, such as the AIS Support Group, the Intersex Society of North America, and the Coalition for Intersex Support Advocacy and Education. These support groups provide a culture for intersexuals as well as validation of feelings; they offer enormous psychological relief for parents of intersex children, as well as intersex adolescents and adults.

To illustrate, in the case of AIS, many parents are understandably concerned about how they will communicate to their daughters that they have XY chromosomes; these parents are typically uncomfortable about this fact themselves. However, at a recent meeting of the AIS Support Group our members decided to take a photograph with the adult women with AIS, and the fathers of children with AIS, forming "Y's" with their arms while the mothers of such children crossed their arms to form "X's." The ability to defuse tension about "the chromosome thing" quite visibly allowed these parents to feel more comfortable and accepting of the entire issue.

Perhaps it is fitting that I have used a holiday theme in this article. For it was the day after Christmas in 1994 when I first discovered, while researching in a medical school library, that an AIS Support Group had recently been founded in the U.K. No gift I will receive in this lifetime will ever be as precious to me as discovering that information. My subsequent involvement with the support group has, remarkably, allowed me to view having AIS as a blessing—after all, if I didn't have AIS I would not have developed into the woman I believe God and nature intended me to be. This was certainly not the outcome my doctors would have predicted on a chilly September day when they removed my gonads and implored my parents never to tell me the truth. The miracle of life, however, is that we can evolve; I hope, in this holiday season, that this same miracle can touch those who will be privileged to care for the intersex children born while this article was being read.

MAJORITY OPINION IN *TARASOFF V. REGENTS OF THE UNIVERSITY OF CALIFORNIA*

Justice Mathew O. Tobriner

Tatiana Tarasoff was murdered by Prosenjit Poddar, who was a patient of psychotherapists employed by the University of California Hospital. Her parents brought an action against the university regents, doctors, and campus police. The Tarasoffs complained that the doctors and police had failed to warn them that their daughter was in danger from Poddar. In finding for the Tarasoffs, Justice Tobriner argues that a doctor or psychotherapist treating a mentally ill patient has a duty to warn third parties of threatened dangers arising out of the patient's violent intentions. Responding to the defendants' appeal to the important role played by the principle of confidentiality in the psychotherapeutic situation, Tobriner argues that the public interest in safety from violent assault must be weighed against the patient's right to privacy.

On October 27, 1969, Prosenjit Poddar killed Tatiana Tarasoff. Plaintiffs, Tatiana's parents, allege that two months earlier Poddar confided his intention to kill Tatiana to Dr. Lawrence Moore, a psychologist employed by the Cowell Memorial Hospital at the University of California at Berkeley. They allege that on Moore's request, the campus police briefly detained Poddar, but released him when he appeared rational. They further claim that Dr. Harvey Powelson, Moore's superior, then directed that no further action be taken to detain Poddar. No one warned plaintiffs of Tatiana's peril. . . .

We shall explain that defendant therapists cannot escape liability merely because Tatiana herself was not their patient. When a therapist determines, or pursuant to the standards of his profession should determine, that his patient presents a serious danger of violence to another, he incurs an obligation to use reasonable care to protect the intended victim against such danger. The discharge of this duty may require the therapist to take one or more of various steps, depending upon the nature of the case. Thus it may call for him to warn the intended victim or others likely to apprise the victim of the danger, to notify the police, or to take whatever other steps are reasonably necessary under the circumstances. . . .

California Supreme Court; July 1, 1976. 131 California Reporter 14.
Reprinted with permission of West Publishing Co.

PLAINTIFFS' COMPLAINTS

. . . Plaintiffs' first cause of action, entitled "Failure to Detain a Dangerous Patient," alleges that on August 20, 1969, Poddar was a voluntary outpatient receiving therapy at Cowell Memorial Hospital. Poddar informed Moore, his therapist, that he was going to kill an unnamed girl, readily identifiable as Tatiana, when she returned home from spending the summer in Brazil. Moore, with the concurrence of Dr. Gold, who had initially examined Poddar, and Dr. Yandell, assistant to the director of the department of psychiatry, decided that Poddar should be committed for observation in a mental hospital. Moore orally notified Officers Atkinson and Teel of the campus police that he would request commitment. He then sent a letter to Police Chief William Beall requesting the assistance of the police department in securing Poddar's confinement.

Officers Atkinson, Brownrigg, and Halleran took Poddar into custody, but, satisfied that Poddar was rational, released him on his promise to stay away from Tatiana. Powelson, director of the department of psychiatry at Cowell Memorial Hospital, then asked the police to return Moore's letter, directed that all copies of the letter and notes that Moore had taken as therapist be destroyed, and "ordered no action to place Prosenjit Poddar in 72-hour treatment and evaluation facility."

Plaintiffs' second cause of action, entitled "Failure to Warn on a Dangerous Patient," incorporates the allegations of the first cause of action, but adds the assertion that defendants negligently permitted Poddar to be released from police custody without "notifying the parents of Tatiana Tarasoff that their daughter was in grave danger from Prosenjit Poddar." Poddar persuaded Tatiana's brother to share an apartment with him near Tatiana's residence; shortly after her return from Brazil, Poddar went to her residence and killed her.

Plaintiffs' third cause of action, entitled "Abandonment of a Dangerous Patient," seeks $10,000 punitive damages against defendant Powelson. Incorporating the crucial allegations of the first cause of action, plaintiffs charge that Powelson "did the things herein alleged with intent to abandon a dangerous patient, and said acts were done maliciously and oppressively."

Plaintiffs' fourth cause of action, for "Breach of Primary Duty to Patient and the Public," states essentially the same allegations as the first cause of action, but seeks to characterize defendants' conduct as a breach of duty to safeguard their patient and the public. Since such conclusory labels add nothing to the factual allegations of the complaint, the first and fourth causes of action are legally indistinguishable. . . .

. . . We direct our attention . . . to the issue of whether Plaintiffs' second cause of action can be amended to state a basis for recovery.

PLAINTIFFS CAN STATE A CAUSE OF ACTION AGAINST DEFENDANT THERAPISTS FOR NEGLIGENT FAILURE TO PROTECT TATIANA

The second cause of action can be amended to allege that Tatiana's death proximately resulted from defendants' negligent failure to warn Tatiana or others likely to apprise her of her danger. Plaintiffs contend that as amended, such allegations of negligence and proximate causation, with resulting damages, establish a cause of action. Defendants, however, contend that in the circumstances of the present case they owed no duty of care to Tatiana or her parents and that, in the absence of such duty, they were free to act in careless disregard of Tatiana's life and safety.

In analyzing this issue, we bear in mind that legal duties are not discoverable facts of nature, but merely conclusory expressions that, in cases of a particular type, liability should be imposed for damage done. "The assertion that liability must . . . be denied because defendant bears no 'duty' to plaintiff 'begs the essential question—whether the plaintiff's interests are entitled to legal protection against the defendant's conduct. . . . [Duty] is not sacrosanct in itself, but only an expression of the sum total of those considerations of policy which lead the law to say that the particular plaintiff is entitled to protection.' "

In the landmark case of *Rowland v. Christian* (1968), Justice Peters recognized that liability should be imposed "for an injury occasioned to another by his want of ordinary care or skill" as expressed in section 1714 of the Civil Code. Thus, Justice Peters, quoting from *Heaven v. Pender* (1883) stated: "Whenever one person is by circumstances placed in such a position with regard to another . . . that if he did not use ordinary care and skill in his own conduct . . . he would cause danger of injury to the person or property of the other, a duty arises to use ordinary care and skill to avoid such danger.' "

We depart from "this fundamental principle" only upon the "balancing of a number of considerations"; major ones "are the foreseeability of harm to the plaintiff, the degree of certainty that the plaintiff suffered injury, the closeness of the connection between the defendant's conduct and the injury suffered, the moral blame attached to the defendant's conduct, the policy of preventing future harm, the extent of the burden to the defendant and consequences to the community of imposing a duty to exercise care with resulting liability for breach, and the availability, cost and prevalence of insurance for the risk involved."

The most important of these considerations in establishing duty is foreseeability. As a general principle, a "defendant owes a duty of care to all persons who are foreseeably endangered by his conduct, with respect to all risks which make the conduct unreasonably dangerous." As we shall explain, however, when the avoidance of foreseeable harm requires a defendant to control the conduct of another person, or to warm of such conduct, the common law has traditionally imposed liability only if the defendant bears some special relationship to the dangerous person or to the potential victim. Since the relationship between a therapist and his patient satisfies this requirement, we need not here decide whether foreseeability alone is sufficient to create a duty to exercise reasonable care to protect a potential victim of another's conduct.

Although, as we have stated above, under the common law, as a general rule, one person owed no duty to control the conduct of another nor to warn those endangered by such conduct, the courts have carved out an exception to this rule in cases in which the defendant stands in some special relationship to either the person whose conduct needs to be controlled or in a relationship to the foreseeable victim of that conduct. Applying this exception to the present case, we note that a relationship of defendant therapists to either Tatiana or Poddar will suffice to establish a duty of care; as explained in section 315 of the Restatement Second of Torts, a duty of care may arise from either "(a) a special relation . . . between the actor and the third person which imposes a duty upon the actor to control the third person's conduct, or (b) a special relation . . . between the actor and the other which gives to the other a right of protection."

Although Plaintiffs' pleadings assert no special relation between Tatiana and defendant therapists, they establish as between Poddar and defendant therapists the special relation that arises between a patient and his doctor or psychotherapist. Such a relationship may support affirmative duties for the benefit of third persons. Thus, for example, a hospital must exercise reasonable care to control the behavior of a patient which may endanger other persons. A doctor must also warn a patient if the patient's condition or medication renders certain conduct, such as driving a car, dangerous to others.

Although the California decisions that recognize this duty have involved cases in which the defendant stood in a special relationship *both* to the victim and to the person whose conduct created the danger, we do not think that the duty should logically be constricted to such situations. Decisions of other jurisdictions hold that the single relationship of a doctor to his patient is sufficient to support the duty to exercise reasonable care to protect others

against dangers emanating from the patient's illness. The courts hold that a doctor is liable to persons infected by his patient if he negligently fails to diagnose a contagious disease, or having diagnosed the illness, fails to warn members of the patient's family.

Since it involved a dangerous mental patient, the decision in *Merchants Nat. Bank & Trust Co. of Fargo v. United States* (1967) comes closer to the issue. The Veterans Administration arranged for the patient to work on a local farm, but did not inform the farmer of the man's background. The farmer consequently permitted the patient to come and go freely during non-working hours; the patient borrowed a car, drove to his wife's residence and killed her. Notwithstanding the lack of any "special relationship" between the Veterans Administration and the wife, the court found the veterans Administration liable for the wrongful death of the wife.

In their summary of the relevant rulings Fleming and Maximov conclude that the "case law should dispel any notion that to impose on the therapists a duty to take precautions for the safety of persons threatened by a patient, where due care so requires, is in any way opposed to contemporary ground rules on the duty relationship. On the contrary, there now seems to be sufficient authority to support the conclusion that by entering into a doctor-patient relationship the therapist becomes sufficiently involved to assume some responsibility for the safety, not only of the patient himself, but also of any third person whom the doctor knows to be threatened by the patient." [Fleming & Maximov, *The Patient or His Victim: The Therapist's Dilemma* (1974) 62 Cal. L. Rev. 1025, 1030.]

Defendants contend, however, that imposition of a duty to exercise reasonable care to protect third persons is unworkable because therapists cannot accurately predict whether or not a patient will resort to violence. In support of this argument amicus representing the American Psychiatric Association and other professional societies cites numerous articles which indicate that therapists, in the present state of the art, are unable reliably to predict violent acts; their forecasts, amicus claims, tend consistently to overpredict violence, and indeed are more often wrong than right. Since predictions of violence are often erroneous, amicus concludes, the courts should not render rulings that predicate the liability of therapists upon the validity of such predictions.

The role of the psychiatrist, who is indeed a practitioner of medicine, and that of the psychologist who performs an allied function, are like that of the physician who must conform to the standards of the profession and who must often make diagnoses and predictions based upon such evaluations. Thus the judgment of the therapist in diagnosing emotional disorders and in predicting whether a patient presents a serious danger of violence is comparable to the judgment which doctors and professionals must regularly render under accepted rules of responsibility.

We recognize the difficulty that a therapist encounters in attempting to forecast whether a patient presents a serious danger of violence. Obviously we do not require that the therapist, in making the determination, render a perfect performance; the therapist need only exercise "that reasonable degree of skill, knowledge, and care ordinarily possessed and exercised by members of [that professional specialty] under similar circumstances." Within the broad range of reasonable practice and treatment in which professional opinion and judgment may differ, the therapist is free to exercise his or her own best judgment without liability; proof, aided by hindsight, that he or she judged wrongly is insufficient to establish negligence.

In the instant case, however, the pleadings do not raise any question as to failure of defendant therapists to predict that Poddar presented a serious danger of violence. On the contrary, the present complaints allege that defendant therapists did in fact predict that Poddar would kill, but were negligent in failing to warn.

Amicus contends, however, that even when a therapist does in fact predict that a patient poses a serious danger of violence to others, the therapist should be absolved of any responsibility for failing to act to protect the potential victim. In our view, however, once a therapist does in fact determine, or under applicable professional standards reasonably should have determined, that a patient poses a serious danger of violence to others, he bears a duty to exercise reasonable care to protect the foreseeable victim of that danger. While the discharge of this duty of due care will necessarily vary with the facts of each case, in each instance the adequacy of the therapist's conduct must be measured against the traditional negligence standard of the rendition of reasonable care under the circumstances. As explained in Fleming and Maximov, *The Patient or His Victim: The Therapist's Dilemma* (1974), "... the ultimate question of resolving the tension between the conflicting interests of patient and potential victim is one of social policy, not professional expertise. ... In sum, the therapist owes a legal duty not only to his patient, but also to his patient's would-be victim and is subject in both respects to scrutiny by judge and jury. ..."

The risk that unnecessary warnings may be given is a reasonable price to pay for the lives of possible victims that may be saved. We would hesitate to hold that the therapist who is aware that his patient expects to attempt to assassinate the President of the United States would not be obligated to warn the authorities because the therapist cannot predict with accuracy that his patient will commit the crime.

Defendants further argue that free and open communication is essential to psychotherapy; that "unless a patient . . . is assured that . . . information [revealed by him] can and will be held in utmost confidence, he will be reluctant to make the full disclosure upon which diagnosis and treatment . . . depends." The giving of a warning, defendants contend, constitutes a breach of trust which entails the revelation of confidential communications.

We recognize the public interest in supporting effective treatment of mental illness and in protecting the rights of patients to privacy and the consequent public importance of safeguarding the confidential character of psychotherapeutic communication. Against this interest, however, we must weigh the public interest in safety from violent assault. The Legislature has undertaken the difficult task of balancing the countervailing concerns. In Evidence Code section 1014, it established a broad rule of privilege to protect confidential communications between patient and psychotherapist. In Evidence Code section 1024, the Legislature created a specific and limited exception to the psychotherapist-patient privilege: "There is no privilege . . . if the psychotherapist has reasonable cause to believe that the patient is in such mental or emotional condition as to be dangerous to himself or to the person or property of another and that disclosure of the communication is necessary to prevent the threatened danger."

We realize that the open and confidential character of psychotherapeutic dialogue encourages patients to express threats of violence, few of which are ever executed. Certainly a therapist should not be encouraged routinely to reveal such threats; such disclosures could seriously disrupt the patient's relationship with his therapist and with the persons threatened. To the contrary, the therapist's obligations to his patient require that he not disclose a confidence unless such disclosure is necessary to avert danger to others, and even then that he do so discreetly, and in a fashion that would preserve the privacy of his patient to the fullest extent compatible with the prevention of the threatened danger.

The revelation of a communication under the above circumstances is not a breach of trust or a violation of professional ethics; as stated in the Principles of Medical Ethics of the American Medical Association (1957), section 9: "A physician may not reveal the confidence entrusted to him in the course of medical attendance . . . *unless he is required to do so by law or unless it becomes necessary in order to protect the welfare of the individual or of the community.*" (Emphasis added.) We conclude that the public policy favoring protection of the confidential character of patient-psychotherapist communications must yield to the extent to which disclosure is essential to avert danger to others. The protective privilege ends where the public peril begins.

Our current crowded and computerized society compels the interdependence of its members. In this risk-infested society we can hardly tolerate the further exposure to danger that would result from a concealed knowledge of the therapist that his patient was lethal. If the exercise of reasonable care to protect the threatened victim requires the therapist to warn the endangered party or those who can reasonably be expected to notify him, we see no sufficient societal interest that would protect and justify concealment. The containment of such risks lies in the public interest. For the foregoing reasons, we find that Plaintiffs' complaints can be amended to state a cause of action against defendants Moore, Powelson, Gold, and Yandell and against the Regents as their employer, for breach of a duty to exercise reasonable care to protect Tatiana. . . .

DISSENTING OPINION IN *TARASOFF V. REGENTS OF THE UNIVERSITY OF CALIFORNIA*

Justice William P. Clark

Justice Clark, dissenting from Justice Tobriner's majority opinion, argues that confidentiality in the psychiatrist-patient relationship must be assured for three reasons. (1) Without the promise of such confidentiality, people needing treatment will be deterred from seeking it. (2) Effective therapy requires the patient's full disclosure of his or her innermost thoughts. Without the assurance that the thoughts disclosed will not be revealed by the therapist, the patient could not overcome the psychological barriers standing in the way of such revelations. (3) Successful treatment itself requires a relationship of trust between psychiatrist and patient. In light of these three reasons, Clark argues that if a duty to warn is imposed on psychiatrists, the result will be an increase in violent acts by persons who either don't seek help or whose therapy is unsuccessful. Furthermore, Clark holds, imposing such a duty on psychiatrists will result in an increase in the involuntary civil commitment of patients.

Until today's majority opinion, both legal and medical authorities have agreed that confidentiality is essential to effectively treat the mentally ill, and that imposing a duty on doctors to disclose patient threats to potential victims would greatly impair treatment. Further, recognizing that effective treatment and society's safety are necessarily intertwined, the Legislature has already decided effective and confidential treatment is preferred over imposition of a duty to warn.

The issue whether effective treatment for the mentally ill should be sacrificed to a system of warnings is, in my opinion, properly one for the Legislature, and we are bound by its judgment. Moreover, even in the absence of clear legislative direction, we must reach the same conclusion because imposing the majority's new duty is certain to result in a net increase in violence. . . .

COMMON LAW ANALYSIS

Entirely apart from the statutory provisions, the same result must be reached upon considering both general tort principles and the public policies favoring effective treatment, reduction of violence, and justified commitment.

Generally, a person owes no duty to control the conduct of another. Exceptions are recognized only in limited situations where (1) a special relationship exists between the defendant and injured party, or (2) a special relationship exists between defendant and the active wrongdoer, imposing a duty on defendant to control the wrongdoer's conduct. The majority does not contend the first exception is appropriate to this case.

Policy generally determines duty. Principal policy considerations include foreseeability of harm, certainty of the plaintiff's injury, proximity of the defendant's conduct to the plaintiff's injury, moral blame attributable to defendant's conduct, prevention of future harm, burden on the defendant, and consequences to the community.

Overwhelming policy considerations weigh against imposing a duty on psychotherapists to warn

California Supreme Court; July 1, 1976. 131 California Reporter 14.
Reprinted with permission of West Publishing Co.

a potential victim against harm. While offering virtually no benefit to society, such a duty will frustrate psychiatric treatment, invade fundamental patient rights and increase violence.

The importance of psychiatric treatment and its need for confidentiality have been recognized by this court. "It is clearly recognized that the very practice of psychiatry vitally depends upon the reputation in the community that the psychiatrist will not tell." [Slovenko, *Psychiatry and a Second Look at the Medical Privilege* (1960) 6 Wayne L. Rev. 175, 188.]

Assurance of confidentiality is important for three reasons.

Deterrence from Treatment First, without substantial assurance of confidentiality, those requiring treatment will be deterred from seeking assistance. It remains an unfortunate fact in our society that people seeking psychiatric guidance tend to become stigmatized. Apprehension of such stigma—apparently increased by the propensity of people considering treatment to see themselves in the worst possible light—creates a well-recognized reluctance to seek aid. This reluctance is alleviated by the psychiatrist's assurance of confidentiality.

Full Disclosure Second, the guarantee of confidentiality is essential in eliciting the full disclosure necessary for effective treatment. The psychiatric patient approaches treatment with conscious and unconcious inhibitions against revealing his innermost thoughts. "Every person, however well-motivated, has to overcome resistances to therapeutic exploration. These resistances seek support from every possible source and the possibility of disclosure would easily be employed in the service of resistance." (Goldstein & Katz, *Psychiatrist-Patient Privilege: The GAP Proposal and the Connecticut Statute,* 36 Conn. Bar J., 175, 179; see also, 118 Am. J. Psych. 734, 735.) Until a patient can trust his psychiatrist not to violate their confidential relationship, "the unconscious psychological control mechanism of repression will prevent the recall of past experiences." [Butler, *Psychotherapy and Griswold: Is Confidentiality a Privilege or a Right?* (1971) 3 Conn. L. Rev. 599, 604.]

Successful Treatment Third, even if the patient fully discloses his thoughts, assurance that the confidential relationship will not be breached is necessary to maintain his trust in his psychiatrist—the very means by which treatment is effected. "[T]he essence of much psychotherapy is the contribution of trust in the external world and ultimately in the self, modelled upon the trusting relationship established during therapy" (Dawidoff, *The Malpractice of Psychiatrists,* 1966 Duke L. J. 696, 704). Patients will be helped only if they can form a trusting relationship with the psychiatrist. All authorities appear to agree that if the trust relationship cannot be developed because of collusive communication between the psychiatrist and others, treatment will be frustrated.

Given the importance of confidentiality to the practice of psychiatry, it becomes clear the duty to warn imposed by the majority will cripple the use and effectiveness of psychiatry. Many people, potentially violent—yet susceptible to treatment—will be deterred from seeking it; those seeking it will be inhibited from making revelations necessary to effective treatment; and, forcing the psychiatrist to violate the patient's trust will destroy the interpersonal relationship by which treatment is effected.

VIOLENCE AND CIVIL COMMITMENT

By imposing a duty to warn, the majority contributes to the danger to society of violence by the mentally ill and greatly increases the risk of civil commitment—the total deprivation of liberty—of those who should not be confined. The impairment of treatment and risk of improper commitment resulting from the new duty to warn will not be limited to a few patients but will extend to a large number of the mentally ill. Although under existing psychiatric procedures only a relatively few receiving treatment will ever present a risk of violence, the number making threats is huge, and it is the latter group—not just the former—whose treatment will be impaired and whose risk of commitment will be increased.

Both the legal and psychiatric communities recognize that the process of determining potential violence in a patient is far from exact, being fraught with complexity and uncertainty.[1]

In fact precision has not even been attained in predicting who of those having already committed violent acts will again become violent, a task recognized to be of much simpler proportions.

This predictive uncertainty means that the number of disclosures will necessarily be large. As noted above, psychiatric patients are encouraged to discuss all thoughts of violence, and they often express such thoughts. However, unlike this court, the psychiatrist does not enjoy the benefit of overwhelming hindsight in seeing which few, if any, of his patients will ultimately become violent. Now, confronted by the majority's new duty, the psychiatrist must instantaneously calculate potential violence from each patient on each visit. The difficulties researchers have encountered in accurately predicting violence will be heightened for the practicing psychiatrist dealing for brief periods in his office with heretofore nonviolent patients. And, given the decision not to warn or commit must always be made at the psychiatrist's civil peril, one can expect most doubts will be resolved in favor of the psychiatrist protecting himself.

Neither alternative open to the psychiatrist seeking to protect himself is in the public interest. The warning itself is an impairment of the psychiatrist's ability to treat, depriving many patients of adequate treatment. It is to be expected that after disclosing their threats, a significant number of patients, who would not become violent if treated according to existing practices, will engage in violent conduct as a result of unsuccessful treatment. In short, the majority's duty to warn will not only impair treatment of many who would never become violent but worse, will result in a net increase in violence.[2]

The second alternative open to the psychiatrist is to commit his patient rather than to warn. Even in the absence of threat of civil liability, the doubts of psychiatrists as to the seriousness of patient threats have led psychiatrists to overcommit to mental institutions. This overcommitment has been authoritatively documented in both legal and psychiatric studies. This practice is so prevalent that it has been estimated that "as many as twenty harmless persons are incarcerated for every one who will commit a violent act." [Steadman & Cocozza, *Stimulus/ Response: We Can't Predict Who Is Dangerous* (Jan. 1975) 8 Psych. Today 32, 35.]

Given the incentive to commit created by the majority's duty, this already serious situation will be worsened. . . .

NOTES

1 A shocking illustration of psychotherapists' inability to predict dangerousness . . . is cited and discussed in Ennis, *Prisoners of Psychiatry: Mental Patients, Psychiatrists, and the Law* (1972): "In a well-known study, psychiatrists predicted that 989 persons were so dangerous that they could not be kept even in civil mental hospitals, but would have to be kept in maximum security hospitals run by the Department of Corrections. Then, because of a United States Supreme Court decision, those persons were transferred to civil hospitals. After a year, the Department of Mental Hygiene reported that one-fifth of them had been discharged to the community, and over half had agreed to remain as voluntary patients. During the year, only 7 of the 989 committed or threatened any act that was sufficiently dangerous to require retransfer to the maximum security hospital. Seven correct predictions out of almost a thousand is not a very impressive record.

"Other studies, and there are many, have reached the same conclusion: psychiatrists simply cannot predict dangerous behavior." (*Id.* at p. 227.)

2 The majority concedes that psychotherapeutic dialogue often results in the patient expressing threats of violence that are rarely executed. The practical problem, of course, lies in ascertaining which threats from which patients will be carried out. As to this problem, the majority is silent. They do, however, caution that the therapist certainly "should not be encouraged routinely to reveal such threats; such disclosures could seriously disrupt the patient's

relationships, with his therapist and with the persons threatened."

Thus, in effect, the majority informs the therapists that they must accurately predict dangerousness—a task recognized as extremely difficult—or face crushing civil liability. The majority's reliance on the traditional standard of care for professionals that "therapist need only exercise 'that reasonable degree of skill, knowledge, and care ordinarily possessed and exercised by members of [that professional specialty] under similar circumstances' " is seriously misplaced. This standard of care assumes that, to a large extent, the subject matter of the specialty is ascertainable. One clearly ascertainable element in the psychiatric field is that the therapist cannot accurately predict dangerousness, which, in turn, means that the standard is inappropriate for lack of a relevant criterion by which to judge the therapist's decision. The inappropriateness of the standard the majority would have us use is made patent when consideration is given to studies, by several eminent authorities, indicating that "[t]he chances of a second psychiatrist agreeing with the diagnosis of a first psychiatrist 'are barely better than 50–50; or stated differently, there is about as much chance that a different expert would come to some different conclusion as there is that the other would agree.' " (Ennis & Litwack, *Psychiatry and the Presumption of Expertise: Flipping Coins in the Courtroom,* 62 Cal. L. Rev. 693, 701, quoting Ziskin, Coping with Psychiatric and Psychological Testimony, 126.) The majority's attempt to apply a normative scheme to a profession which must be concerned with problems that balk at standardization is clearly erroneous.

In any event, an ascertainable standard would not serve to limit psychiatrist disclosure of threats with the resulting impairment of treatment. However compassionate, the psychiatrist hearing the threat remains faced with potential crushing civil liability for a mistaken evaluation of his patient and will be forced to resolve even the slightest doubt in favor of disclosure or commitment.

PLEASE DON'T TELL!: A CASE ABOUT HIV AND CONFIDENTIALITY
(with commentaries by Leonard Fleck and Marcia Angell)

The case features a 21-year-old Hispanic male, Carlos, who is about to end his hospital stay for gunshot wounds and receive nursing care at home from his sister, Consuela. Secretly homosexual and concerned about disgrace within his family, Carlos pleads with the attending physician not to inform his sister that he (Carlos) is HIV-positive. Yet not informing Consuela would seem to increase her risk of contracting HIV while attending to his wounds. The case ends with the question of whether Carlos's physician would be justified in breaching confidentiality on the grounds that he has a "duty to warn."

In the first commentary, Fleck states his assumption that breaches of confidentiality are justified only when there is an imminent threat of serious, irreversible harm; there is no alternative way to avert that threat; and the harm that would thereby be averted is proportionate to the harm associated with breaching confidentiality. Citing a very remote risk of Carlos's infecting Consuela and identifying an alternative to informing her, Fleck argues that breaching confidentiality would be unjustified. In the second commentary, Angell argues that Consuela should be neither deceived nor further exploited by a health-care system that is encouraging her to provide a service it would otherwise be responsible for. Angell concludes that the doctor should give Carlos the choice of either telling his sister that he is HIV-positive or forfeiting her nursing care.

The patient, Carlos R., was a twenty-one year old Hispanic male who had suffered gunshot wounds to the abdomen in gang violence. He was uninsured. His stay in the hospital was somewhat shorter than might have been expected, but otherwise unremarkable. It was felt that he could safely complete his recovery at home. Carlos admitted to his attending physician that he was HIV-positive, which was confirmed.

At discharge the attending physician recommended a daily home nursing visit for wound care. However, Medicaid would not fund this nursing visit because a caregiver lived in the home who could adequately provide this care, namely, the patient's twenty-two-year-old sister Consuela, who in fact was willing to accept this burden. Their mother had died almost ten years ago, and Consuela had been a mother to Carlos and their younger sister since then. Carlos had no objection to Consuela's providing this care, but he insisted absolutely that she was not to know his HIV status. He had always been on good terms with Consuela, but she did not know he was actively homosexual. His greatest fear, though, was that his father would learn of his homosexual orientation, which is generally looked upon with great disdain by Hispanics.

Would Carlos's physician be morally justified in breaching patient confidentiality on the grounds that he had a "duty to warn"?

COMMENTARY

By Leonard Fleck If there were a home health nurse to care for this patient, presumably there would be no reason to breach confidentiality since the expectation would be that she would follow universal precautions. Of course, universal precautions could be explained to the patient's sister. In an ideal world this would seem to be a satisfactory response that protects both Carlos's rights and Consuela's welfare. But the world is not ideal.

We know that health professionals, who surely ought to have the knowledge that would motivate them to take universal precautions seriously, often fail to take just such precautions. It is easy to imagine that Consuela could be equally casual or careless, especially when she had not been specifically warned that her brother was HIV-infected. Given this possibility, does the physician have a duty to warn that would justify breaching confidentiality? I shall argue that he may not breach confidentiality but he must be reasonably attentive to Consuela's safety. Ordinarily the conditions that must be met to invoke a duty to warn are: (1) an imminent threat of serious and irreversible harm, (2) no alternative to averting that threat other than this breach of confidentiality, and (3) proportionality between the harm averted by this breach of confidentiality and the harm associated with such a breach. In my judgment, none of these conditions are satisfactorily met.

No one doubts that becoming HIV-infected represents a serious and irreversible harm. But, in reality, is that threat imminent enough to justify breaching confidentiality? If we were talking about two individuals who were going to have sexual intercourse on repeated occasions, then the imminence condition would likely be met. But the patient's sister will be caring for his wound for only a week or two, and wound care does not by itself involve any exchange of body fluids. If we had two-hundred and forty surgeons operating on two-hundred and forty HIV-infected patients, and if each of those surgeons nicked himself while doing surgery, then the likelihood is that only one of them would become HIV-infected. Using this as a reference point, the likelihood of this young woman seroconverting if her intact skin comes into contact with the blood of this patient is very remote at best.

Moreover in this instance there are alternatives. A frank and serious discussion with Consuela about the need for universal precautions, plus monitored, thorough training in correct wound care, fulfills what I would regard as a reasonable duty to warn in these circumstances. Similar instructions ought to be given to Carlos so that he can monitor her performance. He can be reminded that this is a small price for protecting his confidentiality as well as his sister's health. It might also be necessary to provide gloves and other such equipment required to observe universal precautions.

We can imagine easily enough that there might be a lapse in conscientiousness on Consuela's part, that she might come into contact with his blood. But even if this were to happen, the likelihood of her seroconverting is remote at best. This is where proportionality between the harm averted by the breach and the harm associated with it comes in. For if confidentiality were breached and she were informed of his HIV status, this would likely have very serious consequences for Carlos. As a layperson with no professional duty to preserve confidentiality herself, Consuela might inform other family members, which could lead to his being ostracized from the family. And even if she kept the information confidential, she might be too afraid to provide the care for Carlos, who might then end up with no one to care for him.

The right to confidentiality is a right that can be freely waived. The physician could engage Carlos in a frank moral discussion aimed at persuading him that the reasonable and decent thing to do is to inform his sister of his HIV status. Perhaps the physician offers assurances that she would be able to keep that information in strict confidence. The patient agrees. Then what happens? It is easy to imagine that Consuela balks at caring for her brother, for fear of infection.

Medicaid would still refuse to pay for home nursing care because a caregiver would still be in the home, albeit a terrified caregiver. Consuela's response may not be rational, but it is certainly possible. If she were to react in this way it would be an easy "out" to say that it was Carlos who freely agreed to the release of the confidential information so now he'll just have to live with those consequences. But the matter is really more complex than that. At the very least the physician would have to apprise Carlos of the fact that his sister might divulge his HIV status to some number of other individuals. But if the physician impresses this possibility on Carlos vividly enough, Carlos might be even more reluctant to self-disclose his HIV status to Consuela. In that case the physician is morally obligated to respect that confidentiality.

COMMENTARY

By Marcia Angell It would be wrong, I believe, to ask this young woman to undertake the nursing care of her brother and not inform her that he is HIV-infected.

The claim of a patient that a doctor hold his secrets in confidence is strong but not absolute. It can be overridden by stronger, competing claims. For example, a doctor would not agree to hold in confidence a diagnosis of rubella, if the patient were planning to be in the presence of a pregnant woman without warning her. Similarly, a doctor would be justified in acting on knowledge that a patient planned to commit a crime. Confidentiality should, of course, be honored when the secret is entirely personal, that is, when it could have no substantial impact on anyone else. On the other hand, when it would pose a major threat to others, the claim of confidentiality must be overridden. Difficulties arise when the competing claims are nearly equal in moral weight.

In this scenario, does Consuela have any claims on the doctor? I believe she does, and that her claims are very compelling. They stem, first, from her right to have information she might consider relevant to her decision to act as her brother's nurse, and, second, from the health care system's obligation to warn of a possible risk to her health. I would like to focus first on whether Consuela has a right to information apart from the question of whether there is in fact an appreciable risk. I believe that she has such a right, for three reasons.

First, there is an element of deception in *not* informing Consuela that her brother is HIV-infected. Most people in her situation would want to know if their "patient" were HIV-infected and would presume that they would be told if that were the case. (I suspect that a private nurse hired in a similar situation would expect to be told—and that she would be.) At some level, perhaps unconsciously, Consuela would assume that Carlos did not have HIV infection because no one said that he did. Thus, in keeping Carlos's secret, the doctor implicitly deceives Consuela—not a net moral gain, I think.

Second, Consuela has been impressed to provide nursing care in part because the health system is using her to avoid providing a service it would otherwise be responsible for. This fact, I believe, gives the health care system an additional obligation to her, which includes giving her all the information that might bear on her decision to accept this responsibility. It might be argued that the information about her brother's HIV infection is not relevant, but it is patronizing to make this assumption. She may for any number of reasons, quite apart from the risk of transmission, find it important to know that he is HIV-infected.

Finally, I can't help feeling that this young woman has already been exploited by her family and that the health care system should not collude in doing so again. We are told that since she was twelve, she has acted as "mother" to a brother only one year younger, presumably simply because she is female, since she is no more a mother than he is. Now she is

being asked to be a nurse, as well as a mother, again presumably because she is female. In this context, concerns about the sensibilities of the father or about Carlos's fear of them are not very compelling, particularly when they are buttressed by stereotypes about Hispanic families. Furthermore, both his father and his sister will almost certainly learn the truth eventually.

What about the risk of transmission from Carlos to Consuela? Many would—wrongly, I believe—base their arguments solely on this question. Insofar as they did, they would have very little to go on. The truth is that no one knows what the risk would be to Consuela. To my knowledge, there have been no studies that would yield data on the point. Most likely the risk would be extremely small, particularly if there were no blood or pus in the wound, but it would be speculative to say how small. We do know that Consuela has no experience with universal precautions and could not be expected to use them diligently with her brother unless she had some sense of why she might be doing so. In any case, the doctor has no right to decide for this young woman that she should assume a risk, even if he believes it would be remote. That is for her to decide. The only judgment he has a right to make is whether *she* might consider the information that her brother is HIV-infected to be relevant to her decision to nurse him, and I think it is reasonable to assume she might.

There is, I believe, only one ethical way out of this dilemma. The doctor should strongly encourage Carlos to tell his sister that he is HIV-infected or offer to do it for him. She could be asked not to tell their father, and I would see no problem with this. I would have no hesitation in appealing to the fact that Carlos already owes Consuela a great deal. If Carlos insisted that his sister not be told, the doctor should see to it that his nursing needs are met in some other way. In sum, then, I believe the doctor should pass the dilemma to the patient: Carlos can decide to accept Consuela's generosity—in return for which he must tell her he is HIV-infected (or ask the doctor to tell her)—or he can decide not to tell her and do without her nursing care.

ANNOTATED BIBLIOGRAPHY

Annas, George J.: *The Rights of Patients*, 2nd ed. (Carbondale, IL: Southern Illinois University Press, 1989). This American Civil Liberties Union handbook on the rights of hospital patients is a guide for those directly affected by the problems discussed in this chapter. Using a question-and-answer approach, the book provides a statement of the rights patients had under the law when the guidebook was written.

Bayer, Ronald, and Kathleen E. Toomey: "HIV Prevention and the Two Faces of Partner Notification," *American Journal of Public Health* 82 (August 1992), pp. 1158–1164. Bayer and Toomey begin by contrasting the respective histories and rationales of two approaches to notifying sexual or needle-sharing partners at risk—the moral "duty to warn" ethic and the contact-tracing approach. They then argue that confusing these approaches in the context of the AIDS epidemic can lead us to "mischaracterize processes that are fundamentally voluntary as mandatory, and processes that respect confidentiality as invasive of privacy."

Benjamin, Martin, and Joy Curtis: *Ethics in Nursing*, 3rd ed. (New York: Oxford University Press, 1992). The purpose of this book is to give nursing students and nurses an introduction to the identification and analysis of ethical issues in nursing. The book includes a large number of actual cases, many of which are explored in detail.

Blustein, Jeffrey: "The Family in Medical Decisionmaking," *Hastings Center Report* 23 May–June 1993), pp. 6–13. Blustein argues that the ethos of patient autonomy survives two important challenges that would shift some of the decision-making authority currently granted to patients to families instead: John Hardwig's fairness-based argument and a challenge stemming from communitarian theory. Nevertheless, he contends, medical practice and medical ethics are at fault for not giving the family a more prominent role in medical decision making for competent patients.

Cohen, Elliot D.: "Confidentiality, Counseling, and Clients Who Have AIDS," *Journal of Counseling & Development* 68 (January/February 1990), pp. 282–286. Cohen uses ethical theory in exploring the limits of confidentiality that mental health professionals should observe in dealing with sexually active clients who have AIDS. He proposes a model rule to guide such decisions.

Crouch, Robert A.: "Letting the Deaf Be Deaf: Reconsidering the Use of Cochlear Implants in Prelingually Deaf Children," *Hastings Center Report* 27 (July–August 1997), pp. 14–21. Crouch cautions against the hasty assumption that cochlear implant surgery will promote the best interests of deaf children. According to the author, the efficacy of these devices is modest while the burdens can be great; meanwhile, forgoing surgery permits the child to enter the Deaf community with its unique history, language, and value system.

Dreger, Alice Domurat: " 'Ambiguous Sex'—or Ambivalent Medicine? Ethical Issues in the Treatment of Intersexuality," *Hastings Center Report* 28 (May–June 1998), pp. 24–36. Examining the history and cultural meaning of the treatment of intersexuality, Dreger criticizes standard medical approaches to these conditions on ethical grounds and offers several suggestions toward a better approach.

Kuhse, Helga: "Clinical Ethics and Nursing: 'Yes' to Caring, But 'No' to a Female Ethics of Care," *Bioethics* 9 (July 1995), pp. 207–219. Kuhse argues that, while care—a sensitivity and responsiveness to the particularities of a situation and to people's needs—is necessary for nursing ethics, the "ethics of care" is seriously inadequate for nursing ethics and as a general moral theory.

Macklin, Ruth: "HIV-Infected Psychiatric Patients: Beyond Confidentiality," *Ethics & Behavior* 1 (1991), pp. 3–20. Macklin examines ethical issues concerning HIV-infected psychiatric patients. Devoting most of her analysis to professionals' conflicting obligations of confidentiality and protecting persons at risk, she defends some limits to the first obligation before turning to other kinds of ethical dilemmas.

Nelson, Hilde Lindemann, and James Lindemann Nelson: *The Patient in the Family* (New York: Routledge, 1995). This book explores the moral relationship between two major institutions of modern life: health care and family. Using a wide variety of examples based on actual encounters between families and medicine, the authors attempt to develop a robust ethics of the family and demonstrate how the latter can reframe and illuminate various issues in biomedical ethics.

Nelson, James Lindemann: "Taking Families Seriously," *Hastings Center Report* 22 (July–August 1992), pp. 6–12. Nelson defends a presumption that a competent patient's informed consent is necessary and sufficient to authorize treatment, but argues that consideration of the interests of family members and others intimately involved with the patient can justify overriding this presumption in some cases.

Pence, Terry: "Nursing's Most Pressing Moral Issue," *Bioethics Forum* 10 (Winter 1994), pp. 3–9. In defending the thesis that nurses' appropriate role is one of advocacy for patients, Pence offers an account of the concept of advocacy, argues that advocacy's ascendance as a moral metaphor was a major turning point in nursing history, and responds to leading criticisms of the advocacy model.

Salsberry, Pamela J.: "Caring, Virtue Theory, and a Foundation for Nursing Ethics," *Scholarly Inquiry for Nursing Practice* 6 (Summer 1992), pp. 155–167. Salsberry critically examines virtue ethics as a foundation for a nursing ethics based on the ideal of caring. She argues that while virtue ethics can meet some of the conditions of an adequate foundation, it ultimately fails to provide a viable alternative to a duty-based approach as a foundation for nursing ethics.

Wilson, Bruce E., and William G. Reiner: "Management of Intersex: A Shifting Paradigm," *Journal of Clinical Ethics* 9 (Winter 1998), pp. 360–369. After introducing the clinical phenomena of intersex and the multiple meanings of the terms *male* and *female*, the authors criticize the old treatment paradigm for intersex, which was paternalistic and favored early surgical interventions, with a new approach that affords parents and the intersex patient, as he or she matures, a greater role in decision making.

Winslow, Betty J., and Gerald R. Winslow: "Integrity and Compromise in Nursing Ethics," *Journal of Medicine and Philosophy* 16 (June 1991), pp. 307–323. The authors grapple with ethical issues that arise for nurses when they consider compromise as a means of resolving conflicts in which they are entangled. They argue that compromise is compatible with moral integrity if certain conditions are met.

CHAPTER 4

HUMAN AND ANIMAL RESEARCH

INTRODUCTION

This chapter focuses primarily on ethical issues in biomedical research using human subjects. Investigations of these issues employ some of the same ethical concepts and principles discussed in the previous two chapters. Here, too, one finds an emphasis on the value of individual autonomy and on the requirements of informed consent or, in the case of incompetent patients, proxy consent consistent with either the substituted-judgment standard or the best-interests standard. At the same time, a concern unique to research is its potential benefits to society as a whole. In addition to confronting issues related to the requirements of informed consent and (to a lesser extent) proxy consent, this chapter explores special issues that arise in connection with research involving certain "vulnerable" populations of patients including the elderly, children, racial minorities, and the mentally ill. It also features a discussion of randomized clinical trials in general and a closely related discussion of specific problems associated with research in developing countries.

In addition to examining these topics pertaining to human research, this chapter includes an extensive discussion of the ethics of biomedical research involving animal subjects. Animals lack the decision-making capacity required for informed consent and never have had such capacity (precluding meaningful substituted judgments); nor can it be plausibly argued, in most cases, that serving as a research subject promotes an animal's best interests. Is the use of animals as research subjects morally justified? If so, what is the justification for animal research, under what conditions can it be ethically conducted, and can the answers to these questions be integrated into a coherent overall account of research ethics that addresses human research subjects as well?

CONCEPTUAL ISSUES

Before examining some of the ethical issues raised by human research, we should clarify the meaning of *human research* (or *human experimentation*) and the distinction often drawn between therapeutic and nontherapeutic research. In the biomedical context, *therapy* ordinarily refers to a set of activities whose primary purpose is to relieve suffering, restore or maintain health, or prolong life. Therapy takes many forms. Medical treatment, diagnosis, and even some preventive measures (e.g., vaccine injections) are typically classified as forms of therapy. It is important to notice that the primary aim of therapy is to benefit the recipient. In contrast, *research* or *experimentation* refers to a set of scientific activities whose primary purpose is to contribute to generalizable knowledge about the chemical, physiological, or psychological processes involved in human (or sometimes animal) functioning. In human research, human beings serve as subjects.

A distinction has often been drawn between therapeutic and nontherapeutic research. As with all research, *therapeutic research* is concerned with the acquisition of generalizable knowledge. However, in therapeutic research the patient-subjects are themselves expected (or at least hoped) to benefit medically from the new drug, vaccine, treatment, or diagnostic procedure under investigation. For example, the first patients on kidney dialysis machines and the first recipients of coronary bypass surgery were participants in medical experiments. The techniques in question had never been tried on human subjects, so the use of these techniques on the patient-subjects was experimental. Furthermore, medical professionals gained information that furthered their research and contributed to generalizable knowledge. At the same time, the new techniques provided a form of therapy designed to alleviate the patient-subjects' own medical problems. They hoped to benefit from procedures that were thought to offer promise of proving more effective than any other therapy available. By contrast, *nontherapeutic research* is often characterized as research whose sole aim is to furnish data that contributes to generalizable knowledge. Providing therapy for the research subjects is not regarded as an aim of nontherapeutic research.

In practice, however, it is difficult to draw a clear line between therapeutic and nontherapeutic research. Therapeutic research is not conducted solely to benefit patient-subjects since the purpose of all research is to contribute to generalizable knowledge. Moreover, the therapeutic project may require patient-subjects to undergo additional procedures unrelated to their own therapy. They may have to give blood samples or undergo catheterization, for example. Such additional procedures are nontherapeutic for the patients and may carry risks unrelated to their own therapy. Nontherapeutic research, in turn, may indirectly provide medical benefits (such as a thorough medical checkup) for subjects.

Despite these complications, which somewhat obscure the distinction between therapeutic and nontherapeutic research, many commentators find the distinction helpful in exploring ethical issues pertaining to research. For example, it is commonly believed that in therapeutic research it is morally acceptable to impose somewhat higher risk to patient-subjects than would be acceptable in nontherapeutic research. The acceptance of the therapeutic/nontherapeutic distinction is reflected in codes of research ethics that continue to employ it. For example, the Declaration of Helsinki, reprinted in this chapter, implies the distinction by announcing, in addition to basic principles for all medical research, several principles for medical research combined with medical care. (Earlier versions of this ethical code more explicitly distinguished what it called *clinical research* and *nonclinical research*). Some commentators today find it clearer and more helpful to articulate a distinction between research that "offers the prospect of direct medical benefit" to subjects and research that does not.[1]

THE JUSTIFICATION OF RESEARCH USING HUMAN SUBJECTS

Many biomedical research projects entail some risk to subjects. New drugs may prove toxic, for example. Some studies involve deliberately exposing subjects to a disease such as malaria before they can be used to test the efficacy of a new treatment. What moral justification is available for research that puts human subjects at risk?

The most commonly offered justification for human research is utilitarian in character and features two main claims. First, human experimentation enhances the discovery of new diagnostic and therapeutic techniques. For example, past research has enabled the development of cardiovascular surgery, renal transplantation, and the control of poliomyelitis. Second, controlled experiments are necessary for sound medical practice. Iatrogenic illnesses (illnesses caused by medical interventions) are preventable only if clinical research provides necessary data about human reactions to specific therapies. In the past, physicians employed many techniques that were of no benefit and sometimes even harmed patients. For example, neither the blood-letting common in the eighteenth century nor the practice of freezing the stomachs of patients with ulcers in the twentieth century proved to have any therapeutic value. Yet both practices were believed to be therapeutic. Well-designed, controlled research projects, it is argued, will help to minimize the use of worthless or harmful procedures. The utilitarian conclusion is that human experimentation is not just morally permissible, but morally required, because its future benefits and prevention of harm to many will far outweigh its harmful consequences to some research subjects.

Sometimes a different sort of argument, based on considerations of fairness—or perhaps gratitude—is advanced to justify human research and to defend the view that individuals have a duty to participate as research subjects. The argument can be stated simply. We are the beneficiaries of advances that past biomedical research made possible. Without the use of human subjects, these advances would not have occurred. Having benefited from the sacrifices made by past research subjects, we have a fairness-based (or gratitude-based) obligation to reciprocate by serving as subjects ourselves. One possible reply to this argument is that current participation in research will primarily benefit individuals in the future; few persons who made sacrifices in the past will be alive to benefit from the so-called "reciprocity" of people today serving as research subjects. A proponent of the fairness-based argument might respond that what is important is not that particular subjects be "paid back" for their past services; the idea is rather that humanity has made sacrifices for presently living individuals, who should in turn be willing to make sacrifices for humanity. Another reply to the fairness-based argument claims that medical progress, while extremely important, is a moral goal. As such, it cannot compete with rights of an individual, including the right to decline to serve as a subject. Moral goals, no matter how important, may be pursued only within the constraints of respecting people's rights. Thus no one has a duty to participate in research.[2]

Discussions of whether or not individuals have a duty to serve as research subjects sometimes reflect what may be called *the protection model* of participation in research. This model emphasizes that research participation typically involves risks to subjects, highlighting the importance of adequate subject protection. The protection model is at least partly inspired by historical examples, some of which are discussed in this chapter, in which subjects were not adequately protected. In recent years, however, what may be called *the access model* of participation in research has emerged into prominence. This model stresses that participation in research can, in the absence of effective therapies for some illnesses, benefit subjects. AIDS activists argued in the 1980s and early 1990s—before there were effective treatments for HIV (human immunodeficiency virus) infection—that participation in clinical trials testing the efficacy of various treatments could benefit HIV-positive individuals. Activists often asserted that these patients have a right to participate in promising studies. Similar access-based claims have also been made on behalf of women, African Americans, children, and other groups who have been in some way under represented in research. Whether one views the ethics of research participation mainly in terms of the protection model or in terms of the access model, the requirements of informed consent and proxy consent remain matters of paramount concern.

THE INFORMED-CONSENT REQUIREMENT

Most of the literature on the ethics of human research is concerned with specifying the conditions under which research involving human subjects is ethically acceptable. Since World War II, more than thirty different guidelines and codes of ethics identifying these conditions have been formalized. Foremost among these are two codes included in this chapter, the Nuremberg Code and the Declaration of Helsinki. Common to all these documents is the principle that research may not be conducted on human subjects without their informed consent (or, as some codes allow, the consent—where appropriate—of a proxy). Discussions of this requirement are commonplace in the literature on human research, and some of the major topics connected with informed consent are treated in this chapter.

One major topic is the justification of the informed-consent requirement. Arguments in favor of requiring that human beings not be used as research subjects without their informed consent are similar to those favoring the requirement in the context of the physician-patient relationship. The primary argument, advanced from a deontological perspective, rests on the principle of respect for autonomy or the value of individual self-determination. Respect for human beings as persons requires protection and promotion of their autonomy. Research that uses human subjects without their consent violates that autonomy and is therefore morally unacceptable. One major proponent of this position, Paul Ramsey, holds that informed consent is the "chief canon of loyalty" between the biomedical researcher and the patient-subject. It serves as a deontological check on any attempt to justify the use of human subjects solely on utilitarian grounds, insofar as it affirms that human beings are not objects to be used, without their consent, for others' benefit. In Ramsey's view, only individuals who are (1) capable of knowingly involving themselves in a common cause with the researcher and (2) willing to participate as research subjects may serve in that capacity.[3]

Some of the literature on informed consent in research focuses on special causes for concern where individuals from certain "vulnerable" groups serve as subjects. These causes for concern often involve one or more of the following factors: (1) the fact of vulnerability itself, (2) egregious historical failures on the part of researchers to comply with the informed-consent requirement, and (3) cultural complexities in implementing this requirement.

Some groups of individuals are inherently vulnerable due to their incapacity to make informed decisions regarding their medical care and their dependence on others to protect their interests. In one of this chapter's readings, Barry F. Brown considers the conditions under which incompetent elderly patients may be enrolled in research that offers no direct medical benefit to them. In defending his view, he appeals to our society's experience with another area of research involving incompetent subjects whose welfare must be safeguarded by others: pediatric research. In another reading in this chapter, Alexander Morgan Capron discusses ethical issues in research on psychiatric and other mental disorders that may affect decision-making capacity. The subjects of this research are vulnerable on account of both the social stigma associated with these disorders and their significant potential for reducing or eliminating decision-making capacity.

Perhaps the most notorious historical example of ethical noncompliance with the informed-consent requirement is that of Nazi researchers who performed many gruesome experiments on nonconsenting adults without any regard for their interests. the Nuremberg Code was written in the wake of these atrocities. Somewhat less well-known are what have come to be called "the radiation experiments." During the Cold War with the Soviet Union, federal agencies in the United States funded and in some cases conducted research projects in which hundreds of Americans were exposed to high doses of radiation. Often the subjects were from such vulnerable groups as newborns, the terminally ill, prisoners, mentally retarded persons, racial minorities, or the indigent. Frequently, subjects had no opportunity to provide consent of any kind, much less informed consent.[4]

Another historical cause for concern is described briefly by Patricia A. King in this chapter: a federally funded, longitudinal study in Tuskegee, Alabama, of the consequences of untreated syphilis in which all of the subjects were black men. Among the shocking facts about this research is that, after penicillin was discovered, subjects were not informed of its availability, although it was known to be effective in treating syphilis. Because the violation of the subjects' right to self-determination was apparently related to racism, this episode also suggests cultural reasons for concern about the implementation of the informed-consent requirement. In fact, King's article uses the Tuskegee experience as a backdrop to a broader cultural concern regarding the use of minority research subjects, an uncomfortable tension between avoiding the perpetuation of negative stereotyping while being prepared to note racially correlated differences that may be medically significant.

Psychiatric research, as Capron's article demonstrates, presents in subtler ways both historical and cultural causes for concern. Available evidence suggests that for decades well-intentioned psychiatric researchers have frequently violated the rights of subjects. As Capron explains, one recurring problem is the regular absence of procedures that could ensure that supposedly competent patients have, in fact, provided voluntary and informed consent. While such ethical problems in psychiatric research may be viewed as a historical cause for concern, the reasons for concern are also cultural. For one thing, persisting societal prejudice against persons with mental illness probably makes it easier, in practice, for researchers and the public to overlook their rights. Furthermore, the culture of the biomedical research community is so strongly pro-research that it has proved unreliable in protecting subjects' rights against the tide of utilitarian efforts to use them as means to the end of biomedical progress. Capron suggests that this pro-research bias is especially evident in the work of institutional review boards, which are charged with the task of reviewing their own institutions' proposals for human research to ensure compliance with federal regulations. In his view, because these boards are dominated by researchers and have an inherent conflict of interest (representing the interests both of subjects and of the research institution), they often fail to prevent unethical research from receiving approval and funding.

PROXY CONSENT FOR RESEARCH SUBJECTS INCAPABLE OF INFORMED CONSENT

Since children, especially young children, cannot give informed consent due to their lack of decision-making capacity, any research that involves them as subjects may seem to violate the informed-consent requirement. The same may be said of adult patients who are incompetent due to mental illness, severe retardation, or dementia. Concerns are alleviated somewhat in the case of research that is reasonably expected to benefit the subject. In this case, as with validated therapies, it is usually agreed that proxies, such as parents or other legal guardians, can legitimately consent on the incompetent individual's behalf. However, when the procedure is not intended to benefit the subject directly but solely to acquire knowledge that will benefit future patients, the participation of the child or incompetent adult is more problematic. Is it ever right for proxies to permit incompetent subjects to participate in nontherapeutic research?

As Capron explains, it is widely accepted today that promising research offering no prospect of direct benefits for incompetent subjects may be acceptable if it entails no more than "minimal risk" for the subjects. Proponents of research using children cite its benefits to children as a group; results of studies on adults cannot be simply extrapolated to children because the bodies of children and adults are significantly different. In addition, some diseases, like infantile autism, are unique to children. Not to involve them in research would therefore greatly impoverish pediatric medicine, making children as a class "therapeutic orphans." (This argument assumes that what can be learned from therapeutic research is insufficient to solve this practical problem.) To some extent, similar arguments apply to mentally ill individuals and to elderly patients with Alzheimer's disease or other conditions that compromise mental functioning. Many of these individuals lack decision-making capacity occasionally, intermittently, or even permanently. Some research on their illnesses (e.g., studies of severe psychosis or late-stage Alzheimer's disease) would appear to require the use of incompetent subjects. If only persons who are capable of providing informed consent were used in research, we might never achieve sufficient understanding of some mentally compromising conditions to develop effective treatments for them. For these and other reasons, the use of certain classes of incompetent individuals as research subjects seems necessary for progress in pediatrics and in particular areas of psychiatry, geriatrics, and other subfields of medicine. In view of these potential gains, most commentators accept the validity of proxy consent under some circumstances.

It is worth noting, however, that the acceptance of proxy consent is not universal. Focusing on research in children, Ramsey has famously argued that it is always wrong to subject them to procedures that are not expected to benefit them directly. An experimental procedure holds the promise of directly benefiting a child if the procedure is (1) seen as the best means of achieving the child's recovery or (2) intended to protect the child against some greater risk. Using young children in experimental trials of polio vaccines, for example, at a time when children were at risk of contracting the crippling disease summer after summer, was morally acceptable in Ramsey's view, because the risks of the experimental procedure had to be weighed against the dangers posed for the experimental subjects themselves by polio epidemics. But Ramsey rejects the claim that using children as subjects in a nontherapeutic experiment is morally acceptable when the intended (eventual) beneficiaries are children as a group. His position is grounded in the claim that nontherapeutic human research must be a joint venture, freely undertaken by two autonomous persons—the researcher and the competent subject. He therefore refuses to recognize the validity of proxy consent to any nontherapeutic procedures. Challenging Ramsey's approach, Brown blurs the distinction between therapeutic and nontherapeutic research by defending some research on incompetent individuals that offers no prospect of immediate medical benefit to them so long as the research is *indirectly therapeutic*—potentially benefiting the subject's "community" (e.g., demented patients, children) with eventual prevention, mitigation, or cure of the relevant condition. Meanwhile, Capron's discussion of research on mental disorders that may affect decision-making capacity suggests a position somewhat more permissive than Ramsey's and somewhat more restrictive than Brown's.

EXPERIMENTAL DESIGN AND RESEARCH
IN DEVELOPING NATIONS

Questions about informed and proxy consent also arise in discussions of randomized clinical trials (RCTs). Considered the "gold standard" of clinical research, the RCT is a comparison of two or more treatment arms—scientifically controlled with random assignment of subjects—to study the efficacy of new therapies. In one of this chapter's readings, Samuel Hellman and Deborah S. Hellman argue that RCTs present an ethical dilemma admitting of no comfortable solution. Typically, at the beginning of a study or at some point during the study, they maintain, researchers have an opinion about which treatment arm is preferable in terms of the patient-subjects' best interests. But while sharing that opinion seems required out of fidelity to the patient—that is, promotion of his or her best interests—doing so would ruin the study, according to the authors.

Although today it is widely appreciated that RCTs can place researchers in conflicting roles, not all commentators consider the problem intractable. In a reading reprinted in this chapter, Don Marquis attempts to resolve this problem. For purposes of discussion, he focuses on decisions about inviting patients to enroll in a trial, not decisions connected with their best interests during a trial; and he focuses on studies that compare two treatments as opposed to studies that compare one or more treatments and a placebo. Marquis argues that the solution rests in a full appreciation of informed consent. On his proposal, a physician may be fully justified in (1) recommending the treatment he or she considers superior and (2) asking whether the patient would like to enroll in an RCT in which subjects may or may not receive the recommended treatment. Recommending a treatment permits the physician to fulfill the duty of fidelity while providing crucial information to the patient, who can then make an informed decision in response to the offer of enrolling in the study.

In recent years, issues about proper study design have been provoked with special urgency by a series of placebo-controlled studies, conducted in developing countries, to assess the efficacy of a particular regimen involving zidovudine (AZT). Some background information will help to clarify the issues. While AIDS is a major problem in "first-world" or developed countries, it is far more devastating in certain developing countries in which a frighteningly high percentage of the population is infected with HIV. Years ago an American clinical trial showed that the rate of transmission of HIV from pregnant women to fetuses is cut by two thirds through a specific regimen involving AZT. These experimental results sparked an interest in helping women and infants in developing countries. But the regimen that had already been proven effective was extremely expensive. Moreover, it required that women receive counseling and undergo HIV testing early in pregnancy, comply with an extensive oral regimen and with intravenous administration of AZT during labor and delivery, and refrain from breast-feeding. Such requirements struck many officials as virtually impossible to implement in developing countries; researchers, public health experts, and officials from Ivory Coast, Uganda, several other African countries, and Thailand agreed that a briefer course of oral AZT treatment for pregnant women, if it proved effective, would be a more realistic regimen in their nations. Trials were designed to study the efficacy of an oral regimen of AZT administered in the late stages of pregnancy, and all but one of these trails included a placebo arm.

A crucial ethical question emerged and remains with us retrospectively now that these studies have been completed: Considering what was known about the effectiveness of AZT in reducing transmission, was it ethically permissible to commence a trial including a placebo arm in which subjects did not receive AZT? According to one school of thought, such studies treated some subjects unjustly. Because researchers had good reason to believe that even a short course of oral AZT would be more effective than no treatment, willingness to include a placebo arm entailed a willingness to impose a serious disadvantage on subjects in that arm. (Some commentators called for an alternative study design that would have compared the effectiveness of the rigorous regimen validated by the American trial against the effectiveness of a short course of oral AZT; one study did in fact employ such a design.) Proponents of this school of thought have cited the Declaration of Helsinki, which asserts that in biomedical research, "considerations related to the well-being of the human subject should take precedence over the interests of science and society." Prior to a substantial revision of the code in 2000, these critics also cited another statement that no longer appears: "In any medical study, every patient—including those of a control group, if any—should be assured of the best proven diagnostic and therapeutic method."

An opposing school of thought maintains that placebo controls were necessary to ensure that short-course AZT was better than no treatment at all. From this perspective, it is irrelevant that effective preventive treatment for mother-fetus transmission of AZT was available elsewhere in the world, because it was not available in the developing countries in question. In a reading reprinted in this chapter, Baruch Brody defends a standard that he believes appropriate (and preferable to the statement from the Declaration of Helsinki just quoted): "All participants in the study, including those in the control group, should not be denied any treatment *that should otherwise be available to [them] in light of the practical realities of health care resources available in the country in question.*" In Brody's view, the AZT trials in question probably satisfied this standard.

These trials have provoked other ethical concerns in addition to those related to study design and the inclusion of a placebo arm. Another issue concerns the possibility of coercion. Some commentators have argued that subjects were unable to make a genuinely voluntary choice about enrollment. Living in extreme poverty and lacking access even to basic health care, pregnant women who were offered the choice of joining a study that provided some chance of receiving AZT treatment were in no position to decline. In response to this concern, Brody agrees that it was reasonable for the women, in their circumstances, to enroll in the study to gain possible benefit for themselves and their fetuses, but he denies that any coercion was involved. A coercive offer, he maintains, involves a threat to make someone worse off than he or she would have been without the offer—and this was not the case in these studies.

A third concern about the AZT trials in developing countries is that the citizens of these countries were exploited insofar as the short course of AZT, even if it proved effective, would not be available to them following the study. In a reading reprinted in this chapter, Leonard H. Glantz, George J. Annas, Michael A. Grodin, and Wendy K. Mariner argue that in order for such trials to be justified, the risks or burdens imposed on trial participants must be offset by the prospect of actual benefit to the citizens of the developing country. Thus, if the trial yields beneficial knowledge, benefits must actually reach individuals in the country in which the trial took place; otherwise, the subjects will have been exploited. A practical upshot of this approach is that those who plan trials in developing nations must identify, in advance of commencing a trial, the source and amount of funding for providing any benefits of the research to the local populace—a moral requirement that was not satisfied in the case of the African maternal-fetal HIV transmission studies. (This requirement goes somewhat beyond the following principle from the current version of the Declaration of Helsinki: "Medical research is only justified if there is *a reasonable likelihood* that the populations in which they are carried out stand to benefit from the results of the research" [emphasis added]). Although the short-course regimen did prove effective, and some efforts have been made to expand access to it in the countries in question, Glantz et al. are correct that the feasibility of providing access to local citizens was not established in advance. Moreover, access to the beneficial treatment has only been partial.

According to Brody, however, legitimate concerns about exploitation will be met if the subjects themselves—not necessarily the broader local community—are provided access to effective treatment following the study. The subjects, not other citizens in the same countries, bear any risks and burdens associated with participation in the trials. Brody's reasoning is consonant with another statement from the Helsinki code: "At the conclusion of the study, every patient entered into the study should be assured of access to prophylactic, diagnostic, and therapeutic methods identified by the study." The most recent amendment to the Declaration of Helsinki, addressing this very statement, adds a note specifying that "[p]ost-trial access arrangements or other care must be described in the study protocol so the ethical review committee can consider such arrangements during its review." This requirement addresses the concern of Glantz et al. regarding the prospective identification of means for providing post-trial access to any benefits identified in the study, but it applies only to study participants rather than to the broader local community.

ANIMAL RESEARCH

The use of animals in biomedical research intended to benefit humans raises its own set of troubling questions. Some questions concern the moral status of animals while others concern the importance of the research. Regarding the first set of issues, should animals be regarded as having any significant moral status? If so, is their moral status the same as that of humans, so that whatever is morally impermissible in the case of humans is also impermissible in the case of animals? If that is the case, then it would seem that animals, like humans, could be ethically used in very little nontherapeutic research that entails substantial risks or harm to the subjects. If, on the other hand, animals have moral status but less than that possessed by human beings, how is this judgment to be justified? In general, what characteristics must a being possess to be entitled to moral consideration? What is required for full moral status? Note that if one contends that humans have exclusive, or radically superior, moral status on the basis of certain characteristics—such as autonomy, moral agency, or some degree of rationality—one provokes the *problem of nonparadigm humans*. The problem is that any criterion that apparently excludes animals from the domain of moral status (or full moral status) will apparently also exclude certain human beings who lack the characteristic in question.

Regarding the importance of the research, is there a genuine need to use animals in experiments intended to benefit humans? More precisely, if animals' moral status does not preclude their use in nontherapeutic research that poses significant risks to the animal subjects, how valuable must the sought knowledge be to justify a particular experiment? Is the use of animals necessary to obtain that knowledge? Or could alternatives to animal research yield equally useful information?

In its "International Guiding Principles for Biomedical Research Involving Animals," reprinted in this chapter, the Council for International Organizations of Medical Sciences (CIOMS) apparently assumes that the moral status of animals does not preclude their use in research, including nontherapeutic research posing significant risks. At the same time, CIOMS asserts that researchers have a responsibility to minimize animal subjects' pain, distress, and discomfort and must use alternatives to animal research wherever feasible.

One might consider CIOMS's position a moderate view on animals' moral status and the ethics of animal research.

Representing a different view, Peter Singer has influentially argued that animals' interests must be given *equal consideration* to comparable human interests—so that, for example, a human's and an animal's interest in avoiding suffering should be considered equally morally important.[5] Failure to meet this standard, Singer contends, is *speciesism,* which is morally analogous to racism and sexism. Applying the principle of equal consideration, Singer condemns the vast bulk of animal experimentation for causing great harm to sentient animals while rarely achieving important research goals. He argues that the use of animals in research is justified only in those rare instances when using a human of comparable mental capacities would also be justified.

Responding to Singer's arguments and to what he calls "the animal rights view," Carl Cohen, in a reading reprinted in this chapter, argues against extending the principle of equal consideration to animals and in favor of speciesism. Because only members of the human community have moral rights, he contends, animals are appropriately used to advance biomedical research. Indeed, according to Cohen, we have an obligation to increase the total amount of animal research to protect human subjects and benefit future human patients. Edwin Converse Hettinger, also in this chapter, responds directly and in detail to each of Cohen's major arguments. He argues, among other things, that Cohen has not responded adequately to the problem of nonparadigm humans, that utilitarianism (which assumes equal consideration for humans and animals) supports relatively little animal research, and that the promise of alternative methods is much greater than Cohen allows. In the chapter's final reading, David DeGrazia sketches the general ethical perspectives of the biomedical community (to which Cohen gives voice) and the animal protection community (reflected in Hettinger's article) and argues that representatives of these two perspectives, perhaps surprisingly, can agree on some important ethical claims. He then identifies concrete steps that the biomedical and animal protection communities can take to foster better communication about the animal research issue and promote more defensible practices.

D.D.

NOTES

1 See, e.g., National Bioethics Advisory Commission (NBAC), *Research Involving Persons with Mental Disorders That May Affect Decisionmaking Capacity,* Vol. I: *Report and Recommendations of the National Bioethics Advisory Commission* (Rockville, MD: NBAC, 1998), pp. 44–46.

2 For an argument more or less along these lines, see Hans Jonas, "Philosophical Reflections on Experimenting with Human Subjects," in Paul Freund, ed., *Experimentation with Human Subjects* (New York: Braziller, 1970), pp. 1–31.

    A less frequently advanced but interesting line of argument in support of the claim that people sometimes have a duty to serve as research subjects runs as follows. Sometimes threats to the community are so grave that some people's interests must be sacrificed or, to put it another way, some people have to make sacrifices. In times of war, according to the argument, conscription into the military is justified if volunteers are not forthcoming in sufficient numbers. In times of famine, when not everyone can eat, those who have more than enough to eat may be required to relinquish some of their food, and some individuals (say, those who are extremely feeble and likely to die anyway) may have to suffer the consequences of not receiving food. In research, the argument continues, there may be times when individuals must be "conscripted" for research—say, to test a promising vaccine during an epidemic. (Note that this argument might be advanced from a utilitarian standpoint or from a deontological perspective.) Whatever its merits, it differs from the two more prominent sorts of argument just presented in that it applies only in rare circumstances (e.g., epidemics) and not generally.

3 Paul Ramsey, *The Patient as Person* (New Haven, CT: Yale University Press, 1970).

4 Advisory Committee on Human Radiation Experiments, *Final Report* (Washington, DC: U.S. Government Printing Office, 1995).

5 Peter Singer, *Animal Liberation* (New York: Avon Publishers, 1975; 2nd edition 1990).

ETHICAL CODES

THE NUREMBERG CODE

The Nuremberg Code of Ethics in Medical Research was developed by the Allies after the Second World War. During the war crimes trials in Germany, this code provided the standards against which the practices of Nazis involved in human experimentation were judged. The Nuremberg Code emphasizes the centrality of voluntary consent. Its first and longest article discusses consent in great detail. The code also sets forth other criteria that must be met before any experiment using human beings as subjects can be judged morally acceptable.

(1) The voluntary consent of the human subject is absolutely essential. This means that the person involved should have legal capacity to give consent; should be so situated as to be able to exercise free power of choice, without the intervention of any element of force, fraud, deceit, duress, overreaching, or other ulterior form of constraint or coercion; and should have sufficient knowledge and comprehension of the elements of the subject matter involved as to enable him to make an understanding and enlightened decision. This latter element requires that before the acceptance of an affirmative decision by the experimental subject there should be made known to him the nature, duration, and purpose of the experiment; the method and means by which it is to be conducted; all inconveniences and hazards reasonably to be expected; and the effects upon his health or person which may possibly come from his participation in the experiments.

The duty and responsibility for ascertaining the quality of the consent rests upon each individual who initiates, directs or engages in the experiment. It is a personal duty and responsibility which may not be delegated to another with impunity.

Reprinted from *Trials of War Criminals Before the Nuremberg Military Tribunals* (Washington, DC: U.S. Government Printing Office, 1948).

(2) The experiment should be such as to yield fruitful results for the good of society, unprocurable by other methods or means of study, and not random and unnecessary in nature.

(3) The experiment should be so designed and based on the results of animal experimentation and a knowledge of the natural history of the disease or other problem under study that the anticipated results [will] justify the performance of the experiment.

(4) The experiment should be so conducted as to avoid all unnecessary physical and mental suffering and injury.

(5) No experiment should be conducted where there is an a priori reason to believe that death or disabling injury will occur; except, perhaps, in those experiments where the experimental physicians also serve as subjects.

(6) The degree of risk to be taken should never exceed that determined by the humanitarian importance of the problem to be solved by the experiment.

(7) Proper preparations should be made and adequate facilities provided to protect the experimental subject against even remote possibilities of injury, disability, or death.

(8) The experiment should be conducted only by scientifically qualified persons. The highest degree of skill and care should be required through all

stages of the experiment of those who conduct or engage in the experiment.

(9) During the course of the experiment the human subject should be at liberty to bring the experiment to an end if he has reached the physical or mental state where continuation of the experiment seems to him to be impossible.

(10) During the course of the experiment the scientist in charge must be prepared to terminate the experiment at any stage, if he has probable cause to believe, in the exercise of good faith, superior skill and careful judgment required of him that a continuation of the experiment is likely to result in injury, disability, or death to the experimental subject.

DECLARATION OF HELSINKI
World Medical Association

In 1964 the Eighteenth World Medical Assembly, meeting in Helsinki, Finland, adopted an ethical code to guide physicians and other investigators who conduct medical research involving human subjects. This code has been amended seven times, most substantially in 2000; the version reprinted here is the most recent (2004) version. The Declaration of Helsinki has much in common with the Nuremberg Code, most fundamentally the requirement of informed consent. Two differences, however, are especially noteworthy. First, the Declaration of Helsinki notes that some, but not all, medical research is combined with medical care. Accordingly, it articulates, in addition to basic principles for all medical research, a set of principles for medical research combined with medical care (also known as *clinical research* or *therapeutic research*). Second, while the Nuremberg Code does not address research on subjects who are unable to provide informed consent, the Helsinki code addresses such research, asserting the ethical acceptability under certain conditions of what is usually called "proxy consent." Recent amendments include the additions (1) in 2002 of a note of clarification on paragraph 29, which concerns the circumstances in which use of placebo controls is justified, and (2) in 2004 a note of clarification on paragraph 30, which concerns subjects' post-trial access to procedures identified as beneficial during the course of the trial or to alternative medical care.

A. INTRODUCTION

1. The World Medical Association has developed the Declaration of Helsinki as a statement of ethical principles to provide guidance to physicians and other participants in medical research involving human subjects. Medical research involving human subjects includes research on identifiable human material or identifiable data.

2. It is the duty of the physician to promote and safeguard the health of the people. The physician's knowledge and conscience are dedicated to the fulfillment of this duty.

3. The Declaration of Geneva of the World Medical Association binds the physician with the words, "The health of my patient will be my first consideration," and the International Code of Medical Ethics declares that, "A physician shall act only in the patient's interest when providing medical care

which might have the effect of weakening the physical and mental condition of the patient."

4. Medical progress is based on research which ultimately must rest in part on experimentation involving human subjects.

5. In medical research on human subjects, considerations related to the well-being of the human subject should take precedence over the interests of science and society.

6. The primary purpose of medical research involving human subjects is to improve prophylactic, diagnostic and therapeutic procedures and the understanding of the aetiology and pathogenesis of disease. Even the best proven prophylactic, diagnostic, and therapeutic methods must continuously be challenged through research for their effectiveness, efficiency, accessibility, and quality.

7. In current medical practice and in medical research, most prophylactic, diagnostic, and therapeutic procedures involve risks and burdens.

8. Medical research is subject to ethical standards that promote respect for all human beings and protect their health and rights. Some research populations are vulnerable and need special protection. The particular needs of the economically and medically disadvantaged must be recognized. Special attention is also required for those who cannot give or refuse consent for themselves, for those who may be subject to giving consent under duress, for those who will not benefit personally from the research and for those for whom the research is combined with care.

9. Research Investigators should be aware of the ethical, legal and regulatory requirements for research on human subjects in their own countries as well as applicable international requirements. No national ethical, legal or regulatory requirement should be allowed to reduce or eliminate any of the protections for human subjects set forth in this Declaration.

B. BASIC PRINCIPLES FOR ALL MEDICAL RESEARCH

10. It is the duty of the physician in medical research to protect the life, health, privacy, and dignity of the human subject.

11. Medical research involving human subjects must conform to generally accepted scientific principles, be based on a thorough knowledge of the scientific literature, other relevant sources of information, and on adequate laboratory and, where appropriate, animal experimentation.

12. Appropriate caution must be exercised in the conduct of research which may affect the environment, and the welfare of animals used for research must be respected.

13. The design and performance of each experimental procedure involving human subjects should be clearly formulated in an experimental protocol. This protocol should be submitted for consideration, comment, guidance, and where appropriate, approval to a specially appointed ethical review committee, which must be independent of the investigator, the sponsor or any other kind of undue influence. This independent committee should be in conformity with the laws and regulations of the country in which the research experiment is performed. The committee has the right to monitor ongoing trials. The researcher has the obligation to provide monitoring information to the committee, especially any serious adverse events. The researcher should also submit to the committee, for review, information regarding funding, sponsors, institutional affiliations, other potential conflicts of interest and incentives for subjects.

14. The research protocol should always contain a statement of the ethical considerations involved and should indicate that there is compliance with the principles enunciated in this Declaration.

15. Medical research involving human subjects should be conducted only by scientifically qualified persons and under the supervision

of a clinically competent medical person. The responsibility for the human subject must always rest with a medically qualified person and never rest on the subject of the research, even though the subject has given consent.

16. Every medical research project involving human subjects should be preceded by careful assessment of predictable risks and burdens in comparison with foreseeable benefits to the subject or to others. This does not preclude the participation of healthy volunteers in medical research. The design of all studies should be publicly available.

17. Physicians should abstain from engaging in research projects involving human subjects unless they are confident that the risks involved have been adequately assessed and can be satisfactorily managed. Physicians should cease any investigation if the risks are found to outweigh the potential benefits or if there is conclusive proof of positive and beneficial results.

18. Medical research involving human subjects should only be conducted if the importance of the objective outweighs the inherent risks and burdens to the subject. This is especially important when the human subjects are healthy volunteers.

19. Medical research is only justified if there is a reasonable likelihood that the populations in which the research is carried out stand to benefit from the results of the research.

20. The subjects must be volunteers and informed participants in the research project.

21. The right of research subjects to safeguard their integrity must always be respected. Every precaution should be taken to respect the privacy of the subject, the confidentiality of the patient's information and to minimize the impact of the study on the subject's physical and mental integrity and on the personality of the subject.

22. In any research on human beings, each potential subject must be adequately informed of the aims, methods, sources of funding, any possible conflicts of interest, institutional affiliations of the researcher, the anticipated benefits and potential risks of the study, and the discomfort it may entail. The subject should be informed of the right to abstain from participation in the study or to withdraw consent to participate at any time without reprisal. After ensuring that the subject has understood the information, the physician should then obtain the subject's freely given informed consent, preferably in writing. If the consent cannot be obtained in writing, the non-written consent must be formally documented and witnessed.

23. When obtaining informed consent for the research project the physician should be particularly cautious if the subject is in a dependent relationship with the physician or may consent under duress. In that case the informed consent should be obtained by a well-informed physician who is not engaged in the investigation and who is completely independent of this relationship.

24. For a research subject who is legally incompetent, physically or mentally incapable of giving consent or is a legally incompetent minor, the investigator must obtain informed consent from the legally authorized representative in accordance with applicable law. These groups should not be included in research unless the research is necessary to promote the health of the population represented and this research cannot instead be performed on legally competent persons.

25. When a subject deemed legally incompetent, such as a minor child, is able to give assent to decisions about participation in research, the investigator must obtain that assent in addition to the consent of the legally authorized representative.

26. Research on individuals from whom it is not possible to obtain consent, including proxy or advance consent, should be done only if the physical/mental condition that

prevents obtaining informed consent is a necessary characteristic of the research population. The specific reasons for involving research subjects with a condition that renders them unable to give informed consent should be stated in the experimental protocol for consideration and approval of the review committee. The protocol should state that consent to remain in the research should be obtained as soon as possible from the individual or a legally authorized surrogate.

27. Both authors and publishers have ethical obligations. In publication of the results of research, the investigators are obliged to preserve the accuracy of the results. Negative as well as positive results should be published or otherwise publicly available. Sources of funding, institutional affiliations, and any possible conflicts of interest should be declared in the publication. Reports of experimentation not in accordance with the principles laid down in this Declaration should not be accepted for publication.

C. ADDITIONAL PRINCIPLES FOR MEDICAL RESEARCH COMBINED WITH MEDICAL CARE

28. The physician may combine medical research with medical care, only to the extent that the research is justified by its potential prophylactic, diagnostic, or therapeutic value. When medical research is combined with medical care, additional standards apply to protect the patients who are research subjects.

29. The benefits, risks, burdens, and effectiveness of a new method should be tested against those of the best current prophylactic, diagnostic, and therapeutic methods. This does not exclude the use of placebo, or no treatment, in studies where no proven prophylactic, diagnostic, or therapeutic method exists.[1]

30. At the conclusion of the study, every patient entered into the study should be assured of access to the best proven prophylactic, diagnostic, and therapeutic methods identified by the study.[2]

31. The physician should fully inform the patient which aspects of the care are related to the research. The refusal of a patient to participate in a study must never interfere with the patient-physician relationship.

32. In the treatment of a patient, where proven prophylactic, diagnostic, and therapeutic methods do not exist or have been ineffective, the physician, with informed consent from the patient, must be free to use unproven or new prophylactic, diagnostic, and therapeutic measures, if in the physician's judgement it offers hope of saving life, reestablishing health or alleviating suffering. Where possible, these measures should be made the object of research, designed to evaluate their safety and efficacy. In all cases, new information should be recorded and, where appropriate, published. The other relevant guidelines of this Declaration should be followed.

NOTES

1   Note of clarification on paragraph 29 of the WMA Declaration of Helsinki

The WMA hereby reaffirms its position that extreme care must be taken in making use of a placebo-controlled trial and that in general this methodology should only be used in the absence of existing proven therapy. However, a placebo-controlled trial may be ethically acceptable, even if proven therapy is available, under the following circumstances:

- Where for compelling and scientifically sound methodological reasons its use is necessary to determine the efficacy or safety of a prophylactic, diagnostic, or therapeutic method; or
- Where a prophylactic, diagnostic, or therapeutic method is being investigated for a minor condition and the patients who receive placebo will not be subject to any additional risk of serious or irreversible harm.

All other provisions of the Declaration of Helsinki must be adhered to, especially the need for appropriate ethical and scientific review.

2 Note of clarification on paragraph 30 of the WMA Declaration of Helsinki
The WMA hereby reaffirms its position that it is necessary during the study planning process to identify post-trial access by study participants to prophylactic, diagnostic, and therapeutic procedures identified as beneficial in the study or access to other appropriate care. Post-trial access arrangements or other care must be described in the study protocol so the ethical review committee may consider such arrangements during its review.

INTERNATIONAL GUIDING PRINCIPLES FOR BIOMEDICAL RESEARCH INVOLVING ANIMALS

Council for International Organizations of Medical Sciences

The Council for International Organizations of Medical Sciences (CIOMS) is an international organization that was established by the World Health Organization and Unesco in 1949. In this 1985 statement, CIOMS assumes both (1) that the use of animals in biomedical research is morally appropriate and (2) that such use of animals entails responsibility for their welfare. Reflecting these assumptions, CIOMS presents 11 principles that are intended to provide a framework for more specific policies in individual nations. These principles include an endorsement of the use of alternatives to animal research whenever feasible and the injunction to regard the minimization of animal subjects' pain, distress, and discomfort "as ethical imperatives."

BASIC PRINCIPLES

I. The advancement of biological knowledge and the development of improved means for the protection of the health and well-being both of man and of animals require recourse to experimentation on intact live animals of a wide variety of species.

II. Methods such as mathematical models, computer simulation and *in vitro* biological systems should be used wherever appropriate.

III. Animal experiments should be undertaken only after due consideration of their relevance for human or animal health and the advancement of biological knowledge.

IV. The animals selected for an experiment should be of an appropriate species and quality, and the minimum number required to obtain scientifically valid results.

V. Investigators and other personnel should never fail to treat animals as sentient, and should regard their proper care and use and the avoidance or minimization of discomfort, distress, or pain as ethical imperatives.

VI. Investigators should assume that procedures that would cause pain in human beings cause pain in other vertebrate species, although more needs to be known about the perception of pain in animals.

VII. Procedures with animals that may cause more than momentary or minimal pain or distress should be performed with appropriate sedation, analgesia, or anesthesia in accordance with accepted veterinary practice. Surgical or other painful procedures should not be performed on unanesthetized animals paralysed by chemical agents.

VIII. Where waivers are required in relation to the provisions of article VII, the decisions should not rest solely with the investigators directly concerned but should be made,

Reprinted with permission of the Council for International Organizations of Medical Sciences.

with due regard to the provisions of articles IV, V, and VI, by a suitably constituted review body. Such waivers should not be made solely for the purposes of teaching or demonstration.

IX. At the end of, or, when appropriate, during an experiment, animals that would otherwise suffer severe or chronic pain, distress, discomfort, or disablement that cannot be relieved should be painlessly killed.

X. The best possible living conditions should be maintained for animals kept for biomedical purposes. Normally the care of animals should be under the supervision of veterinarians having experience in laboratory animal science. In any case, veterinary care should be available as required.

XI. It is the responsibility of the director of an institute or department using animals to ensure that investigators and personnel have appropriate qualifications or experience for conducting procedures on animals. Adequate opportunities shall be provided for in-service training, including the proper and humane concern for the animals under their care. . . .

RESEARCH INVOLVING "VULNERABLE" POPULATIONS

PROXY CONSENT FOR RESEARCH ON THE INCOMPETENT ELDERLY

Barry F. Brown

Assuming the legitimacy of proxy consent for research involving incompetent elderly subjects who stand to benefit from their participation (paradigm cases of therapeutic research), Brown argues that certain indirect benefits should count in justifying such research. His argument rests on the conception of a common good that is broader than immediate benefit to the individual subject yet narrower than the good of society at large. On Brown's analysis, a subject who participates in research that will eventually benefit members of his or her "community"—say, elderly patients with Alzheimer's disease or children as a class—indirectly benefits from participation; the good of this community is, to some extent, his or her good. Ending on a cautionary note, Brown stresses the need for stringent protections of vulnerable research subjects.

In the past decade, the ethical issues of research with the elderly have become of increasing interest in gerontology, medicine, law, and biomedical ethics. In particular, the issue has been raised whether the elderly deserve special protection as a dependent group (Ratzan 1980). One of the most profound difficulties in this area of reflection is that of the justification of proxy consent for research on borderline or definitely incompetent patients.

Some diseases of the elderly, such as Alzheimer's disease, cause senile dementia: devastating for the patient and family and, in future, a considerable burden for society. This condition, in turn, renders a patient incapable of giving informed, voluntary consent to research procedures designed to learn about the natural history of the disease, to control it, and to find a cure. The research must be done on human subjects, since there is not as yet a suitable animal model; indeed some feel that there never can be such a model. A protection of the patient, rooted in concern for his best interests, from procedures to which he cannot give consent gives rise to a paradox: "If we can only perform senile dementia research using demented patients, but should not allow them to participate because they are incompetent, then we are left in a quandary. We cannot ethically conduct senile dementia research using demented patients because they are incompetent; but we cannot technically perform it using competent subjects because they are not demented" (Ratzan 1980: 36). Such a position seems to protect demented patients at the expense of their exposure, as a class, to prolonged misery or death.

If the patient cannot give consent, is the proxy consent of relatives ethically valid? That is, do the relatives have the moral right or capacity to give consent for procedures that may not offer much hope for the patient in that they may not offer a direct benefit to him?

Such procedures have by recent convention been called non-therapeutic. They might offer a possible benefit for other sufferers in the future, but little hope of benefit for *this* patient, here and now.

At present, an impasse has developed regarding such research. It appears that such procedures might be illegal under criminal laws on assault. If the research is strictly non-therapeutic, then no benefit is to be found for the patient-subject. If the requirement of therapeutic experimentation is that a direct, or fairly immediate, improvement in the patient's condition is the sole benefit that could count, then it is difficult to see how this could be discovered. For unlike the case of a curable disease or research on preventive measures for childhood diseases, such as polio, the Alzheimer's patients suffer from a presently terminal illness. Studies of the causation of this condition may hold little or no hope of alleviating the condition in them. There appears to be no present or future benefit directly accruing to them. Others may benefit, but they likely will not. Thus, it seems, there is no benefit in view.

If, in fact, such procedures, even relatively innocuous ones, are illegal, then such research cannot go ahead. If so, such persons will remain "therapeutic orphans" just as surely as infants and children unless proxy consent is valid. If proxy consent is also legally invalid, then the legal challenge to this im-

passe may be either legislative or judicial. In either case, ethical arguments must be offered as justification for the case that proxy consent is or ought to be legally valid. The following explorations are a contribution to that debate.

Can some kind of benefit for the demented be found in research that offers no immediate hope of improvement? I believe that it can, but the nature of that benefit will be unfamiliar or unacceptable to those who are sure that there are only two mutually exclusive alternatives: a utilitarian conception of the social good pitted against a deontological notion of the individual's rights.

Contemporary biomedical ethics routinely employs three principles in its effort to resolve such dilemmas (Reich 1978; Beauchamp & Childress 1983). These are the principle of beneficence, which demands that we do good and prevent harm; the principle of respect for persons (or the principle of autonomy), from which flows the requirement of informed consent; and the principle of justice, which demands the equitable distribution of the benefits and burdens of research. But the first two obviously conflict with each other in human experimentation: the principle of beneficence, which mandates research to save life and restore health, especially if this is seen as directed to the good of society, is in tension with the principle of respect for persons, which requires us to protect the autonomy of subjects. Moreover, the principle of beneficence requires us not only to benefit persons as patients through research, but also to avoid harming them as research subjects in the process. So there is an internal tension between moral demands created by the same principle. Finally, demented patients are no longer fully or sufficiently autonomous. Standard objections to paternalism do not apply. Consequently paternalism of the parental sort is not inappropriate, but rather necessary in order to protect the interest of the patient.

Simple application of these principles, therefore, will not provide a solution. Underlying the manner in which they are applied are radically different conceptions of the relationship of the individual good to the societal or common good.

In the present framework of philosophical opinion, there appear to be two major positions. On the one hand, some consequentialist arguments for nontherapeutic research justify non-consensual research procedures on the grounds that individual needs are subordinate to the general good conceived as an aggregate of individual goods. This good, that of the society as a whole, can easily be seen to take precedence over that of individuals. This is especially so if the disease being researched is conceptualized as an "enemy" of society. On the other hand, a deontological position argues that the rights of the individual take precedence over any such abstract general good as the advancement of science, the progress of medicine, or the societal good. In this view, to submit an individual incapable of giving or withholding consent to research procedures not for his own direct benefit is to treat him solely as a means, not as an end in himself. In this debate, one side characterizes the general good proposed by the other as much too broad and inimical to human liberty; the other sees the emphasis on individual rights as excessively individualistic or atomistic.

There are strengths and weaknesses in both approaches. The consequentialist rightly insists on a communal good, but justifies too much; the deontologist rightly protects individual interests, but justifies too little. I contend that if we are to resolve the dilemma concerning the incompetent "therapeutic orphan," it is necessary to go between these poles. In order to do so, I wish to draw upon and develop some recent explorations concerning non-therapeutic research with young children. In at least one important respect, that of incompetence, children and the demented are similar. We ought to treat similar cases similarly. I wish also to argue that research ethics requires: (1) a conception of the *common good* that is at once narrower than that of society as a whole and yet transcends immediate benefit to a single individual; and (2) a conception of the common good that sees it not in opposition to the individual good but including it, so that the good is seen as distributed to individuals.

THE LESSON OF RESEARCH WITH CHILDREN

As to the first, we may learn much from the discussions concerning research with children, particularly as they bear upon the distinction between therapeutic and non-therapeutic experimentation. In the 1970s a spirited debate took place between the noted

ethicists Paul Ramsey and Richard McCormick on the morality of experimentation with children (Ramsey 1970, 1976, 1977; McCormick 1974, 1976). Ramsey presented a powerful deontological argument against non-therapeutic experimentation with children. Since infants and young children cannot give consent, an essential requirement of the canon of loyalty between researcher and subject, they cannot be subjected ethically to procedures not intended for their own benefit. To do so, he contended, is to treat children solely as means to an end (medical progress), not as ends in themselves (Ramsey 1970).

McCormick, arguing from a natural law position similar to that developed in the next section, argued that since life and health are fundamental natural goods, even children have an obligation to seek to preserve them. Medical research is a necessary condition of ensuring health, and this is a desirable social goal. Consequently children, as members of society, have a duty in social justice to wish to accept their share of the burdens of participating in research that promises benefit to society and is of minimal or no risk. Thus the parents' proxy consent is a reasonable presumption of the child's wishes if he were able to consent (McCormick 1974).

There are two major puzzles generated by this debate over non-therapeutic research in children. First, Ramsey stressed that the condition to which a child may be at risk need not reside within his skin, but could be an epidemic dread disease. Thus, testing of preventive measures such as polio vaccine on children is justified; indeed it counts for Ramsey as therapeutic. This is interesting for several reasons. First, the therapeutic benefit may be indirect or remote, not necessarily immediate. Second, it embodies the concept of a group or population at risk smaller than society as a whole. Third, it apparently allows for considerable risk. There was a risk of contracting polio from the vaccine. Although the risk might have been slight statistically, the potential damage was grave. By Ramsey's own account, a slight risk of grave damage is a grave risk. Thus, he was prepared to go beyond the limit of minimal or no risk on the grounds that the polio vaccine was *therapeutic,* while McCormick attempted to justify *non-therapeutic* research on children, but confined the risk to minimal or none. It is odd that in the subsequent protracted debate, this difference was not contested.

The second major puzzle arises from McCormick's view that fetuses, infants, and children ought to participate in low or no-risk non-therapeutic research in order to share in the burden of social and medical progress in order that all may prosper. Note that only *burdens* are to be shared, not benefits. This is because the topic by definition was non-therapeutic experimentation. By putting it this way he seemed to many to be subordinating the interests of such subjects to a very broadly construed societal good. But let us remember that the argument for such research in the first place was that without it, infants and children would be "therapeutic orphans." That is, without pediatric research, there could be fewer and slower advances in pediatric therapy.

Although not of direct benefit, such research is intended for the long-term benefit of children, and is thus indirectly or remotely therapeutic. It is not conducted for "the benefit of society" or for "the advancement of medical science"; it is for children in the future. Otherwise, it could be carried out on adults. Thus, such research should be construed as done not in view of broad social benefit but for the benefit of children as a group or a sub-set of society. Of course, if advances are made in medicine for the sake of children, society benefits as well, but this is incidental and unnecessary. The sole justification is provided by the benefits now and to come for *children*. At the same time, such benefits set one of the limits for such research: it should be confined to children's conditions, and should not be directed at conditions for which the research may be done on competent persons.

THE COMMON GOOD OF A DISEASE COMMUNITY

Some of the hints arising from the foregoing debate can now be developed. It is indeed wrong to experiment on an incompetent person for "the benefit of society" if the research is unrelated to that person's disease and he is made a subject simply because he is accessible and unresistant. But is it necessarily unethical to conduct experiments on an incompetent person which attempt to discover the cause of the condition which causes the incompetence, and

which may cure it or prevent it in others, even if he will not himself be cured?

In a "third way" of conceptualizing the relation between the individual and the group, the good in view is neither that of society as a whole nor that of a single individual. It involves the group of persons with a condition, such as Alzheimer's disease. Here I turn to a conception of the common good articulated by John Finnis of Oxford. Finnis defines the common good not as the "greatest good for the greatest number" but as "a set of conditions which enables the members of a community to attain for themselves reasonable objectives, or to realize reasonably for themselves the value(s) for the sake of which they have reason to collaborate with each other (positively and/or negatively) in a community" (Finnis 1980: 155).

The community may be either the complete community or the political one, or it may be specialized, such as the medical community, the research community, or the community of children with leukemia, and so on. The common good is thus not the sum total of individual interests, but an ensemble of conditions which enable individuals to pursue their objectives or purposes, which enable them to flourish. The purposes are fundamental human goods: life, health, play, esthetic experience, knowledge, and others. Relevant to this discussion are life, health, especially mental integrity, and the consequent capacity for knowledge, all of which are threatened by diseases which cause dementia.

For my purposes, the community should be considered to be, at a minimum, those suffering from Alzheimer's disease. They have, even if they have never explicitly associated with each other, common values and disvalues: their lost health and the remaining health and vitality they possess. It could be said with McCormick that if they could do so, they would reasonably wish the good of preventing the condition in their relatives and friends.

But the community may be rightly construed more broadly than this. It naturally includes families with whom the patients most closely interact and which interact in voluntary agencies devoted to the condition, the physicians who treat them, the nurses, social workers, and occupational therapists who care for them, and the clinical and basic researchers who are working to understand, arrest, cure, and prevent the disease.

The participation of the patient, especially the demented patient, may be somewhat passive. He is a member of the specialized community by accident, not by choice, unless he has indicated his wish to become a research subject while still competent. Efforts to determine what a demented or retarded person would have wished for himself had he been competent have been made in American court decisions involving an incompetent patient's medical care. These "substituted judgment" approaches may have some worth, especially if the patient had expressed and recorded his wishes while still competent.

An individual might execute a document analogous to a human tissue gift—a sort of pre-dementia gift, in which he would officially and legally offer his person to medical research if and when he became demented. This might alleviate the problem of access to some extent, but it has its own difficulties. A pre-dementia volunteer cannot know in advance what types of research procedures will be developed in future, and so cannot give a truly informed consent except to either very specific procedures now known or to virtually anything. Such a precommitment may give some support to the decision to allow him to be a subject. But that decision, I contend, is justified by the claim, if valid, that it is for the common good of the dementia-care-research community, of which he is a member and to which, it is presumed, he would commit himself if he were capable of doing so at the time.

It is true, of course, that one might not ever have wished to participate in research procedures. In this case, the individual should be advised to register his or her objection in advance, along the lines that have been suggested for objection to organ donation in those countries that have a system of presumed consent for such donation. This can be achieved by carrying a card on which such an opt-out is recorded, or by placing one's name on a registry which might be maintained by support organizations. I suggest that unless one opt out in this manner, in the early stages of the disease, he or she be considered to have opted-in. That is, there should be a policy of presumed consent. In any event, as experience with organ retrieval has shown, in the final analysis it is the permission of relatives that is decisive in both those cases in which an individual has consented and those in which he or she has not made his or her wishes known.

The other members of the community may not all know each other. They do, however, have common values and, to a considerable degree, common objectives. There can be a high level of deliberate and active interaction, especially if there is close communication between the researchers, family, and volunteers in the voluntary health agencies.

What, then, is the ensemble of conditions which constitute the common good of the Alzheimer's community? Insofar as the purposes of collaboration include the effort to cure or to alleviate the disease, the common good would embrace, in addition to caring health professionals, a policy of promoting research, its ethical review, a sufficient number of committed clinical and scientific researchers, the requisite physical facilities and funding (some or all of which may be within other communities such as hospitals and medical schools), availability of volunteers for research, an atmosphere of mutual trust between researcher and subject, and finally ongoing research itself. This list is not exhaustive.

If access to the already demented is not allowed, and if this is essential for research on the disease to continue, it may well be impossible to find the answers to key questions about the disease. The common good of the Alzheimer's community would be damaged or insufficiently promoted. Since the goods of life and mental health are fundamental goods, this insufficiency would be profound.

One essential aspect of this common good is distributive justice. Each patient-subject shares not only in the burdens of research in order that all may prosper, but also the benefits. The benefits are not necessarily improved care or cure for the subject, but generally improved conditions for all such patient-subjects: a more aggressive approach to research, improved knowledge of the disease, increased probabilities for a cure, and others. Since the individual participates wholly in that good, he will be deprived of it in its entirety if it is not pursued. The common good is not so much a quantity of benefits as a quality of existence. It can therefore be distributed in its fullness to each member of the community. So, too, each can suffer its diminution.

Richard McCormick (1974) left his description of the common good unnecessarily broad and sweeping. According to some natural law theorists (Maritain 1947) the common good is always a distributed good, not simply the sum of parts. It is construed as flowing back upon the individual members of the community, who are not simply parts of a whole but persons, to whom the common good is distributed in its entirety. Thus, not only can the common good of which McCormick speaks be narrowed to that of children as a group (equivalent to Ramsey's population at risk) but the benefits of such research can be seen as redistributed to the individuals of the group. The benefits are not to be taken in the sense of an immediately available therapy, but in the sense of improved general conditions under which a cure, amelioration, or prevention for all is more likely.

CONCLUSION

Some of these observations can now be applied to the case of the elderly demented. First, the debate showed the inadequacy of the simple distinction between therapeutic and non-therapeutic experimentation, which has been challenged on several grounds in past years. For example, May (1976: 83) includes diagnostic and preventive types of research under therapeutic experimentation, whereas Reich (1978: 327) observes that the terms "therapeutic" and "non-therapeutic" are inadequate because they do not seem to include research on diagnostic and preventive techniques. In the area of the development of experimental preventive measures such as vaccines for epidemic diseases, and in the area of diseases in which research is carried out on terminal patients with little or no expectation of immediate benefit for these patients, the distinction is somewhat blurred. In each case, there is a defined population at risk: one without the disease but at great risk of contracting it, the other with a disease but with little hope of benefiting from the research.

Such types of research seem to constitute an intermediate category: the "indirectly therapeutic," involving the hope of either prevention or alleviation or cure. This category as applied to dementia shows some characteristics of therapeutic experimentation in the accepted sense, since it is carried out on persons who are ill and it is directed to their own illness. But it also shares some properties of non-therapeutic research, since it is not for their immediate treatment and, therefore, benefit. The good to be achieved is more remote, both in time and in application, since it is less sharply located in the individual than is therapy as such.

It must be admitted that there is a difference between the testing of a vaccine for prevention of disease in young, healthy children and research on elderly, seriously ill patients. In the former, the child-subjects will benefit if the vaccine is successful, or at least be protected from harm. In the latter, the subjects will not benefit by way of prevention or cure of their disease, but rather simply by being part of a community in which those goals are being actively pursued. The identification of the demented patient's good with that common good is doubtless less concrete than the identification of the child's good with that of his peers. But it seems to me that underlying both these cases is a notion of the common good required to justify all cases of research that do not promise a hope of direct benefit to a person who is, here and now, ill.

Years ago, Hans Jonas (1969) noted that a physician-researcher might put the following question to a dying patient: "There is nothing more I can do for you. But there is something you can do for me. Speaking no longer as your physician but on behalf of medical science, we could learn a great deal about future cases of this kind if you would permit me to perform certain experiments on you. It is understood that you yourself would not benefit from any knowledge we might gain; but future patients would." Although greatly vulnerable and deserving of maximum protection, such a patient might be ethically approached to be a research subject, because the benefits to future patients are in a way a value to him: "At least that residue of identification is left him that it is his own affliction by which he can contribute to the conquest of that affliction, his own kind of suffering which he helps alleviate in others; and so *in a sense it is his own cause*" (Jonas 1969: 532, emphasis mine).

In this case, the individual apprehends a good greater than his personal good, less than that of society: that of his disease class, which is *his* good. Of course, the identification of which Jonas speaks is psychological; he would likely not agree with the approach herein outlined and might require that such participation be through a conscious, free choice of the patient. Nevertheless, it is a real, objective good which justifies his choice and prevents us from asking him to participate in research unrelated to his disease. Can a relative, a son or daughter perhaps, ethically make that decision for an incompetent, demented Alzheimer's patient? If so, it is because, in a sense, it is the patient's cause, the patient's good as a member of a community which justifies that choice. It is not a matter of enforcing a social duty or minimal social obligation here, but seeking a good that lies in the relationship one has to others with the same disease. That same good, as noted above, limits the participation of the subject to research related precisely to his disease, not to anything else.

What is the implication of this for risk and the limits of risk? As has been seen, some wish to allow for exposure of subjects to greater than minimal risk provided only that it is classified as "therapeutic" (though the subjects are not ill). Others, in spite of the fact that the research is intended for the benefit of a group at risk, classify it as non-therapeutic and limit the acceptable risk to minimal levels. Are these the only alternatives? One advisory group has allowed, in the case of the mentally incompetent, for a "minor increase over minimal risk" in such circumstances (National Commission for the Protection of Human Subjects 1978: 16). This is presumably permitted because the research is "of vital importance for the understanding or amelioration of the type of disorder or condition of the subjects" or "may reasonably be expected to benefit the subjects in future" (17). But what counts as minor increase in risk? Proposed research into Alzheimer's might involve invasive procedures such as brain biopsies, implantation of electrodes, spinal taps, and injections of experimental drugs. Are these of greater risk than that specified by the National Commission simply because they are invasive of the human brain? Or is there clear statistical risk of serious added damage to the brain? These are matters for empirical study. The invasiveness per se should not rule out a procedure. The major limitations should be whether the procedure is painful, causes anxiety, or adds to the already

serious damage to the brain. If research involving procedures of greater risk than "minor increase over minimal" is ever to be justified, it must be so by the intent to avert the proportional evils of death or mental incapacity. If these are insufficient, then I fail to see what grounds might be available upon which to base a case for legislative change.

It is clear, then, that should such research be acceptable, it also demands that stringent protective procedures be established in order to ensure that the demented are not drafted into research unrelated to their disease class. This is because the standard, being broader than that of "direct or fairly immediate benefit," is open to an accordionlike expansion, and therefore to abuse. Such safeguards could include: rigorous assurance that the proxy's consent (in reality, simply a permission) is informed and voluntary, the provision of a consent auditor, and various layers of administrative review and monitoring, from a local institutional review board up to a judicial review with a guardian appointed to represent the patient-subject's rights. These procedures may prove to be onerous. But we are on dangerous ground, and as we try to avoid overprotection, which may come at the expense of improved therapy for all, we must also avoid opening up a huge door to exploitation.

REFERENCES

Beauchamp, T. L., & Childress, J. F. (1983). *Principles of biomedical ethics.* 2nd ed. New York: Oxford University Press.

Finnis, J. (1980). *Natural law and natural rights.* Oxford: Clarendon Press.

Jonas, H. (1969). Philosophical reflections on experimenting with human subjects. In T. Beauchamp and L. Walters (Eds.), *Contemporary issues in bioethics.* 2nd ed. Belmont, CA: Wadsworth.

Maritain, J. (1947). *The person and the common good.* New York: Charles Scribner's Sons.

May, W. (1976). Proxy consent to human experimentation. *Linacre Quarterly, 43,* 73–84.

McCormick, R. (1974). Proxy consent in the experimentation situation. *Perspectives in Biology and Medicine, 18,* 2–20

McCormick, R. (1976). Experimentation in children: sharing in sociality. *Hastings Center Report, 6,* 41–46.

National Commission for the Protection of Human Subjects (1978). *Report and recommendations: Research involving those institutionalized as mentally infirm.* Washington, DC.

Ramsey, P. (1970). *The patient as person.* New Haven: Yale University Press.

Ramsey, P. (1976). The enforcement of morals: Nontherapeutic research on children. *Hastings Center Report, 4,* 21–30.

Ramsey, P. (1977). Children as research subjects: a reply. *Hastings Center Report, 2,* 40–41.

Ratzan, R. (1980). "Being old makes you different": The ethics of research with elderly subjects. *Hastings Center Report, 5,* 32–42.

Reich, W. (1978). Ethical issues related to research involving elderly subjects. *Gerontologist, 18,* 326–37.

THE DANGERS OF DIFFERENCE

Patricia A. King

King cites the historically important case of the Tuskegee syphilis study—a federally funded study of the effects of untreated syphilis on African American men, in which subjects were not informed of the availability of penicillin—in exploring an ethical dilemma concerning racial differences in scientific studies. In King's view, the dilemma arises as follows. If racial differences are ignored and all groups are treated equally, harm may result from a failure to recognize racially correlated factors. On the other hand, if differences are recognized and efforts are made to respond to past injustices or unique burdens, harmful stereotypes may be reinforced. As a strategy for managing this dilemma, King recommends beginning with the defeasible presumption that whites and African Americans are biologically the same with respect to disease and treatment and looking for nonbiological factors before considering the possibility of biologically differentiated responses. As an example, she suggests that, "rather than trying to determine whether blacks and whites respond differently to AZT, attention should first be directed to learning whether response to AZT is influenced by social, cultural, or environmental conditions."

It has been sixty years since the beginning of the Tuskegee syphilis experiment and twenty years since its existence was disclosed to the American public. The social and ethical issues that the experiment poses for medicine, particularly for medicine's relationship with African Americans, are still not broadly understood, appreciated, or even remembered.[1] Yet a significant aspect of the Tuskegee experiment's legacy is that in a racist society that incorporates beliefs about the inherent inferiority of African Americans in contrast with the superior status of whites, any attention to the question of differences that may exist is likely to be pursued in a manner that burdens rather than benefits African Americans.

Reprinted with permission of the author and the publisher from *Hastings Center Report,* vol. 22 (November–December 1992), pp. 35–38. © The Hastings Center.

The Tuskegee experiment, which involved approximately 400 males with late-stage, untreated syphilis and approximately 200 controls free of the disease, is by any measure one of the dark pages in the history of American medicine. In this study of the natural course of untreated syphilis, the participants did not give informed consent. Stunningly, when penicillin was subsequently developed as a treatment for syphilis, measures were taken to keep the diseased participants from receiving it.

Obviously, the experiment provides a basis for the exploration of many ethical and social issues in medicine, including professional ethics,[2] the limitations of informed consent as a means of protecting research subjects, and the motives and methods used to justify the exploitation of persons who live in conditions of severe economic and social disadvantage. At bottom, however, the Tuskegee experiment is different from other incidents of abuse in clinical research because all the participants were black males. The racism that played a central role in this tragedy continues to infect even our current well-intentioned efforts to reverse the decline in health status of African Americans.[3]

Others have written on the scientific attitudes about race and heredity that flourished at the time that the Tuskegee experiment was conceived.[4] There has always been widespread interest in racial differences between blacks and whites, especially differences that related to sexual matters. These perceived differences have often reinforced and justified differential treatment of blacks and whites, and have done so to the detriment of blacks. Not surprisingly, such assumptions about racial differences provided critical justification for the Tuskegee experiment itself.

Before the experiment began a Norwegian investigator had already undertaken a study of untreated syphilis in whites between 1890 and 1910. Although there had also been a follow-up study of these untreated patients from 1925 to 1927, the original study was abandoned when arsenic therapy became available. In light of the availability of therapy a substantial justification for replicating a study of untreated syphilis was required. The argument that provided critical support for the experiment was that the natural course of untreated syphilis in blacks and whites was not the same.[5] Moreover, it was thought that the differences between blacks and whites were not merely biological but that they extended to psychological and social responses to the disease as well. Syphilis, a sexually transmitted disease, was perceived to be rampant among blacks in part because blacks—unlike whites—were not inclined to seek or continue treatment for syphilis.

THE DILEMMA OF DIFFERENCE

In the context of widespread belief in the racial inferiority of blacks that surrounded the Tuskegee experiment, it should not come as a surprise that the experiment exploited its subjects. Recognizing and taking account of racial differences that have historically been utilized to burden and exploit African Americans poses a dilemma.[6] Even in circumstances where the goal of a scientific study is to benefit a stigmatized group or person, such well-intentioned efforts may nevertheless cause harm. If the racial difference is ignored and all groups or persons are treated similarly, unintended harm may result from the failure to recognize racially correlated factors. Conversely, if differences among groups or persons are recognized and attempts are made to respond to past injustices or special burdens, the effort is likely to reinforce existing negative stereotypes that contributed to the emphasis on racial differences in the first place.

This dilemma about difference is particularly worrisome in medicine. Because medicine is pragmatic, it will recognize racial differences if doing so will promote health goals. As a consequence, potential harms that might result from attention to racial differences tend to be overlooked, minimized, or viewed as problems beyond the purview of medicine.

The question of whether (and how) to take account of racial differences has recently been raised in the context of the current AIDS epidemic. The participation of African Americans in clinical AIDS trials has been disproportionately small in comparison to the numbers of African Americans who have been infected with the Human Immunodeficiency Virus. Because of the possibility that African Americans may respond differently to drugs being developed and tested to combat AIDS,[7] those concerned about the care and treatment of AIDS in the African American community have called for greater participation by African Americans in these trials. Ironically, efforts to address the problem of under-representation must cope with the enduring legacy of the Tuskegee experiment—the legacy of suspicion and skepticism toward medicine and its practitioners among African Americans.[8]

In view of the suspicion Tuskegee so justifiably engenders, calls for increased participation by African Americans in clinical trials are worrisome. The question of whether to tolerate racially differentiated AIDS research testing of new or innovative therapies, as well as the question of what norms should govern participation by African Americans in clinical research, needs careful and thoughtful attention. A generic examination of the treatment of racial differences in medicine is beyond the scope of this article.

However, I will describe briefly what has occurred since disclosure of the Tuskegee experiment to point out the dangers I find lurking in our current policies.

INCLUSION AND EXCLUSION

In part because of public outrage concerning the Tuskegee experiment,[9] comprehensive regulations governing federal research using human subjects were revised and subsequently adopted by most federal agencies.[10] An institutional review board (IRB) must approve clinical research involving human subjects, and IRB approval is made contingent on review of protocols for adequate protection of human subjects in accordance with federal criteria. These criteria require among other things that an IRB ensure that subject selection is "equitable." The regulations further provide that:

> [i]n making this assessment the IRB should take into account the purposes of the research and the setting in which the research will be conducted and should be particularly cognizant of the special problems of research involving vulnerable populations, such as women, mentally disabled persons, or economically or educationally disadvantaged persons.[11]

The language of the regulation makes clear that the concern prompting its adoption was the protection of vulnerable groups from exploitation. The obverse problem—that too much protection might promote the exclusion or underrepresentation of vulnerable groups, including African Americans—was not at issue. However, underinclusion can raise as much of a problem of equity as exploitation.[12]

A 1990 General Accounting Office study first documented the extent to which minorities and women were underrepresented in federally funded research. In response, in December 1990 the National Institutes of Health, together with the Alcohol, Drug Abuse and Mental Health Administration, directed that minorities and women be included in study populations,

> so that research findings can be of benefit to all persons at risk of the disease, disorder or condition under study; special emphasis should be placed on the need for inclusion of minorities and women in studies of diseases, disorders and conditions that disproportionately affect them.[13]

If minorities are not included, a clear and compelling rationale must be submitted.

The new policy clearly attempts to avoid the perils of overprotection, but it raises new concerns. The policy must be clarified and refined if it is to meet the intended goal of ensuring that research findings are of benefit to all. There are at least three reasons for favoring increased representation of African Americans in clinical trials. The first is that there may be biological differences between blacks and whites that might affect the applicability of experimental findings to blacks, but these differences will not be noticed if blacks are not included in sufficient numbers to allow the detection of statistically significant racial differences. The second reason is that race is a reliable index for social conditions such as poor health and nutrition, lack of adequate access to health care, and economic and social disadvantage that might adversely affect potential benefits of new interventions and procedures. If there is indeed a correlation between minority status and these factors, then African Americans and all others with these characteristics will benefit from new information generated by the research. The third reason is that the burdens and benefits of research should be spread across the population regardless of racial or ethnic status.[14] Each of these reasons for urging that representation of minorities be increased has merit. Each of these justifications also raises concern, however, about whether potential benefits will indeed be achieved.

The third justification carries with it the obvious danger that the special needs or problems generated as a result of economic or social conditions associated with minority status may be overlooked and that, as a result, African Americans and other minorities will be further disadvantaged. The other two justifications are problematic and deserve closer examination. They each assume that there are either biological, social, economic, or cultural differences between blacks and whites.

THE WAY OUT OF THE DILEMMA

Understanding how, or indeed whether, race correlates with disease is a very complicated problem. Race itself is a confusing concept with both biological and social connotations. Some doubt whether race has biological significance at all.[15] Even if race is a biological fiction, however, its social significance remains.[16] As Bob Blauner points out, "Race is an essentially political construct, one that translates our tendency to see people in terms of their color or other physical attributes into structures that make it likely that people will act for or against them on such a basis."[17]

In the wake of Tuskegee and, in more recent times, the stigma and discrimination that resulted from screening for sickle cell trait (a genetic condition that occurs with greater frequency among African Americans), researchers have been reluctant to explore associations between race and disease. There is increasing recognition, however, of evidence of heightened resistance or vulnerability to disease along racial lines.[18] Indeed, sickle cell anemia itself substantiates the view that biological differences may exist. Nonetheless, separating myth from reality in determining the cause of disease and poor health status is not easy. Great caution should be exercised in attempting to validate biological differences in susceptibility to disease in light of this society's past experience with biological differences. Moreover, using race as an index for other conditions that might influence health and well-being is also dangerous. Such practices could emphasize social and economic differences that might also lead to stigma and discrimination.

If all the reasons for increasing minority participation in clinical research are flawed, how then can we promote improvement in the health status of African Americans and other minorities through participation in clinical research while simultaneously minimizing the harms that might flow from such participation? Is it possible to work our way out of this dilemma?

An appropriate strategy should have as its starting point the defeasible presumption that blacks and whites are biologically the same with respect to disease and treatment. Presumptions can be overturned of course, and the strategy should recognize the possibility that biological differences in some contexts are possible. But the presumption of equality acknowledges that historically the greatest harm has come from the willingness to impute biological differences rather than the willingness to overlook them. For some, allowing the presumption to be in

any way defeasible is troubling. Yet I do not believe that fear should lead us to ignore the possibility of biologically differentiated responses to disease and treatment, especially when the goal is to achieve medical benefit.

It is well to note at this point the caution sounded by Hans Jonas. He wrote, "Of the new experimentation with man, medical is surely the most legitimate; psychological, the most dubious; biological (still to come), the most dangerous."[19] Clearly, priority should be given to exploring the possible social, cultural, and environmental determinants of disease before targeting the study of hypotheses that involve biological differences between blacks and whites. For example, rather than trying to determine whether blacks and whites respond differently to AZT, attention should first be directed to learning whether response to AZT is influenced by social, cultural, or environmental conditions. Only at the point where possible biological differences emerge should hypotheses that explore racial differences be considered.

A finding that blacks and whites are different in some critical aspect need not inevitably lead to increased discrimination or stigma for blacks. If there indeed had been a difference in the effects of untreated syphilis between blacks and whites such information might have been used to promote the health status of blacks. But the Tuskegee experiment stands as a reminder that such favorable outcomes rarely if ever occur. More often, either racist assumptions and stereotypes creep into the study's design, or findings broken down by race become convenient tools to support policies and behavior that further disadvantage those already vulnerable.

REFERENCES

1 For earlier examples of the use of African Americans as experimental subjects, see Todd L. Savitt, "The Use of Blacks for Medical Experimentation and Demonstration in the Old South," *Journal of Southern History* 48, no. 3 (1982): 331–48.

2 David J. Rothman, "Were Tuskegee & Willowbrook 'Studies in Nature'?" *Hastings Center Report* 12, no. 2 (1982): 5–7.

3 For an in-depth examination of the health status of African Americans, see Woodrow Jones, Jr., and Mitchell F. Rice, eds., *Health Care Issues in Black America: Policies, Problems, and Prospects* (New York: Greenwood Press, 1987).

4 See, for example, Allan M. Brandt, "Racism and Research: The Case of the Tuskegee Syphilis Study," *Hastings Center Report* 8, no. 6 (1978): 21–29; and James H. Jones, *Bad Blood: The Tuskegee Syphilis Experiment* (New York: Free Press, 1981).

5 Jones, *Bad Blood*, p. 106.

6 Martha Minow, *Making All the Difference: Inclusion, Exclusion, and American Law* (Ithaca, N.Y.: Cornell University Press, 1990).

7 Wafaa El-Sadr and Linnea Capps, "The Challenge of Minority Recruitment in Clinical Trials for AIDS," *JAMA* 267, no. 7 (1992): 954–57.

8 See, for example, Stephen B. Thomas and Sandra Crouse Quinn, "Public Health Then and Now," *American Journal of Public Health* 81, no. 11 (1991): 1498–1505; Henry C. Chinn, Jr., "Remember Tuskegee," *New York Times,* 29 May 1992.

9 Tuskegee Syphilis Study Ad Hoc Advisory Panel, *Final Report of the Tuskegee Syphilis Study Ad Hoc Advisory Panel* (Washington, D.C.: U.S. Department of Health, Education and Welfare, Public Health Service, 1973).

10 Federal Policy for the Protection of Human Subjects; Notices and Rules, *Federal Register* 56, no. 117 (1991): 28002.

11 45 *Code of Federal Regulations*; sf 46.111(a)(3).

12 This problem is discussed in the context of research in prisons in Stephen E. Toulmin, "The National Commission on Human Experimentation: Procedures and Outcomes," in *Scientific Controversies: Case Studies in the Resolution and Closure of Disputes in Science and Technology,* ed. H. Tristram Engelhardt, Jr. and Arthur L. Caplan (New York: Cambridge University Press, 1987), pp. 602–6.

13 National Institutes of Health and Alcohol, Drug Abuse and Mental Health Administration, "Special Instructions to Applicants Using Form PHS 398 Regarding Implementation of the NIH/ADAMHA Policy Concerning Inclusion of Women and Minorities in Clinical Research Study Populations," December 1990.

14 Arthur L. Caplan, "Is There a Duty to Serve as a Subject in Biomedical Research?" *IRB: A Review of Human Subjects Research* 6, no. 5 (1984): 1–5.

15 See J. W. Green, *Cultural Awareness in the Human Services* (Englewood Cliffs, N.J.: Prentice-Hall, 1982), p. 59; Bob Blauner, "Talking Past Each Other: Black and White Languages of Race," *American Prospect* 61, no. 10 (1992): 55–64.

16 Patricia A. King, "The Past as Prologue: Race, Class, and Gene Discrimination," in *Using Ethics and Law as Guides,* ed. George J. Annas and Sherman Elias (New York: Oxford University Press, 1992), pp. 94–111.

17 Blauner, "Talking Past Each Other," p. 16.

18 See for example James E. Bowman and Robert F. Murray, Jr., *Genetic Variation and Disorders in People of African Origin* (Baltimore, Md.: Johns Hopkins University Press, 1981); Warren W. Leary, "Uneasy Doctors Add Race-Consciousness to Diagnostic Tools," *New York Times,* 15 September 1990.

19 Hans Jonas, "Philosophical Reflections on Experimenting with Human Subjects," in *Experimentation with Human Subjects,* ed. Paul A. Freund (New York: George Braziller, 1970), p. 1. Recent controversy in genetic research makes Jonas's warning particularly timely. See Daniel Goleman, "New Storm Brews on Whether Crime Has Roots in Genes," *New York Times,* 15 September 1992.

ETHICAL AND HUMAN-RIGHTS ISSUES IN RESEARCH ON MENTAL DISORDERS THAT MAY AFFECT DECISION-MAKING CAPACITY

Alexander Morgan Capron

Capron argues that a half-century after the Nuremberg Code was written and publicized, major ethical problems persist in connection with the local supervision of human research in general and with psychiatric research in particular—especially where subjects are children or others who are, or may be, unable to provide informed consent. Focusing on research on mental disorders that often affect decision-making capacity, Capron contends that even "therapeutic research" is fraught with risks that are often unacknowledged or minimized. In studies enrolling subjects who are allegedly able to consent, he argues, procedures necessary to confirm that consent is truly informed and voluntary are regularly absent. Capron next addresses ethical concerns connected with "minimal risk" research undertaken for the benefit of individuals other than the subjects. He concludes with the thesis that properly addressing these concerns will require establishing a highly visible review body that is independent of particular research institutions.

For research with human subjects, the more things change, the more they remain the same. In the 50-odd years since the 10 principles of the Nuremberg Code were set forth by the U.S. judges who convicted the Nazi concentration-camp physicians of crimes against humanity, the tensions inherent in using human beings as a means to advance biomedical knowledge have surfaced repeatedly. Ever more detailed codes and regulations from governments as well as professional bodies, such as the World Medical Association in its oft-revised Declaration of Helsinki,[1] have not put the subject to rest. Indeed, the lesson of the past half-century is that suffering, death, and violation of human rights can arise not only when dictators give inhumane scientists free rein to treat human beings as guinea pigs,[2, 3] but also when well-meaning physicians conduct research in a free and enlightened society.[4–6]

The most recent evidence of this phenomenon can be seen in two sets of problems: those associated with local supervision of research with human subjects in general and those that arise in psychiatric research, particularly that involving children and patients who are unable to make informed, voluntary decisions about their participation in such research. The two types of problems have come together in a number of instances, as investigators and institutions conducting research on mental disorders have been found by courts and federal bureaus, such as the Office for Protection from Research Risks at the National Institutes of Health, to have violated applicable statutes and regulations.

In a series of reports released in June 1998, the inspector general of the Department of Health and Human Services concluded that reforms were needed in the system of review by institutional review boards (IRBs) at both the local and the national level.[7] Since the passage of the 1974 National Research Act, universities and other research centers have been required to use IRBs to protect the rights and welfare of human subjects. Research institutions provide the Department of Health and Human Services with single- or multiproject assurances that their IRBs will apply the federal rules to all federally funded research conducted at the institution or by its employees; many assurances encompass all research with human subjects regardless of sponsorship. The inspector general concluded that the IRB system is in jeopardy because the local boards are overworked, they fail to oversee approved studies, their members lack sufficient training, and they face inherent conflicts of interest.[7] These problems persist because the Office for Protection from Research Risks and its counterparts in other departments have neither the resources nor the independence to provide adequate guidance to IRBs, much less to monitor their activities.

Nowhere have the problems with this delegation of federal authority been more apparent in recent times than in research on mental disorders. There have been press accounts of abuses at major institutions—particularly a series in the *Boston Globe* in November 1998[8] that concluded with an editorial calling on the Justice Department to conduct a criminal investigation—as well as congressional hearings on studies in which mental symptoms were provoked through either the withdrawal of medication or the administration of drug challenges to psychiatric patients or children.

The difficulties run deeper than inept review by IRBs or inadequate consent forms.[9] They involve not only the actions of individual researchers or the failings of their institutions but also conflicts over principles and objectives in the entire enterprise of medical research. These conflicts have not been—and may never be—resolved. Developing knowledge about human diseases and their treatment ultimately depends on using people as experimental animals. As articulated in the Nuremberg Code and reaffirmed since then, exposing people to risk in the name of science becomes licit only with their informed, voluntary consent. Today we add to that requirement the prior review of research protocols by IRBs to weed out projects whose scientific merit does not justify their risks and to ensure that accurate and understandable descriptions of the research will be conveyed to subjects. Yet even if IRBs did their job perfectly, their approval was never intended to substitute for consent freely provided by potential research subjects.

Reprinted by permission of the publisher from *The New England Journal of Medicine*, vol. 340 (May 6, 1999), pp. 1430–1434. Copyright © 1999 Massachusetts Medical Society. All rights reserved.

What, then, should happen when research focuses on conditions that interfere with a person's capacity to provide informed consent? Not too long ago, the prevailing view was that when consent could not be obtained (because of the mental incapacity of a child or a person with a mental disorder) "procedures which are of no direct benefit and which might carry risk of harm to the subject should not be undertaken."[10] Over the past 30 years, however, two exceptions have seriously eroded the prohibition against enrolling incapacitated subjects in research protocols. First, it now seems widely accepted that research would be unnecessarily impeded if such subjects could not be enrolled with the permission of their guardians when the research presents no more than minimal risk. Second, guardians may also enroll patients who lack decision-making capacity in riskier research that can reasonably be predicted to provide the patient with direct benefits that would otherwise be unattainable. Many of the problematic situations regarding research with mentally impaired subjects are connected to the second exception. It is the first, however, that actually raises graver issues.

THE PROBLEMS OF THERAPEUTIC RESEARCH

The Nuremberg Code—framed, as it was, in the context of research in concentration camps on unconsenting prisoners—made no exception for therapeutic intent in its consent requirements. The World Medical Association, however, reflected the prevailing medical view when it framed the 1964 Declaration of Helsinki around the "fundamental distinction . . . between clinical research in which the aim is essentially therapeutic for a patient, and clinical research the essential object of which is purely scientific and without therapeutic intent."[1] Although this articulation of the categories is seriously flawed,[11] the conclusion that "therapeutic research" should be subject to more relaxed standards of consent was incorporated into U.S. policies by the National Commission for the Protection of Human Subjects of Biomedical and Behavioral Research—for example, in its 1977 report on research involving children,[12] which led to federal regulations, and its 1978 report on institutionalized mentally infirm patients,[13] which never became part of the regulations regarding research on human subjects.

Yet the conventional formulation has it backwards. As a general rule, as I have written elsewhere, we should "set higher requirements for consent" and "impose additional safeguards on therapy combined with experimentation [than on research with normal volunteers], lest investigators even unwittingly expose 'consenting' patient-subjects to unreasonable risks."[14] The risk is not simply that patient who are recruited for research will become victims of what is called the therapeutic misconception—that is, construing research interventions as advantageous (especially when no other proven intervention exists) even when the prospect of benefit is in truth nonexistent or at best extremely remote.

The greater risk is that everyone involved, from the investigator to the members of the IRB to society at large, will allow this misconception to blind them to the reality that the entire rationale for supporting and pursuing research is that even the careful accumulation of observations derived from treatment interventions (in which choices are framed in terms of what is best for a particular patient) is not an adequate way to produce reliable, generalizable medical knowledge. Rather, the achievement of such knowledge requires a scientific approach in which, as Hans Jonas cogently observed, the subject of research is not an agent any longer but a "mere token or 'sample' . . . acted upon for an extraneous end without being engaged in a real relation."[15] Indeed, a collective therapeutic misconception may lie behind the shift in the paradigm over the past decade: today, many investigators, IRB members, and commentators alike apparently think the primary ethical requirement is no longer to protect research subjects from harm (especially in the case of those least able to protect themselves) but to avoid the perceived injustice of excluding potential subjects from studies.

There may be no medical field in which the limited effectiveness of available treatments generates more persistent despair among patients, their families, and physicians than mental illness. This despair is particularly evident with respect to conditions that radically compromise their victims' ability to function successfully in the world, to be themselves, and to enjoy the sense of safety and stability that most people take for granted. That sense of desperation has led to a willingness to permit research in which the potential for harm would lead any rational person to decline to participate. IRBs have, for example, approved "washout" studies, in which medications that successfully prevent symptoms in patients with schizophrenia are withdrawn, apparently on the basis of the investigators' suggestion that such studies offer the prospect of benefit because antipsychotic medication can have harmful side effects and some patients successfully stop medication after a while. But if the real purpose of the study is to develop criteria for predicting which patients are most likely to relapse, and if the manner and timing of the washout are dictated by the protocol rather than by the needs or preferences of individual patients, it is wrong to characterize the study as aiming to provide subjects with benefit, which will occur adventitiously if at all.[9]

ASSESSING THE CAPACITY TO CONSENT TO PARTICIPATE IN RESEARCH

The dangers in lowering standards of protection in therapeutic research are exacerbated for patients whose disorder may impair their capacity to make decisions. For this reason, the National Bioethics Advisory Commission, of which I am a member, recently recommended that IRBs "should require that an independent, qualified professional assess the potential subject's capacity to consent" to any protocol presenting more than minimal risk, unless the investigator provides good reasons for using less formal assessment procedures (recommendation 8).[16] This recommendation was criticized on the grounds that such assessments would stigmatize patients with mental disorders insofar as they are not routine for research on the medically ill. However, it would not stigmatize potential subjects in the world's eyes to tell them that the research design requires that their capacity to consent be evaluated, since that information would remain entirely within the confidential relationship between the potential subjects and those carrying out the research project. As any competent patient should quickly realize, such a requirement reflects no disrespect for potential subjects, though it may indicate some concern about the conflicting motives of researchers.

Nor are the norms of fairness violated by imposing such a requirement when none exists for re-

search in other areas. Even if empirical investigation showed that decision-making capacity is just as likely to be as compromised among patients suffering from other medical conditions as among those with mental illness, it is not prejudicial to insist that investigators take reasonable steps to make sure that subjects whose condition directly affects the brain can actually provide voluntary, informed consent. The objection based on unequal treatment would seem much more fitting if researchers on mental disorders already routinely used appropriate means to assess their subjects' decision-making capacity and were simply urging that investigators in other areas be held to the same standard. The National Bioethics Advisory Commission reviewed protocols for a number of recently published studies of mental disorders, all of which involved more than minimal risk to participants. Many involved patients with serious psychiatric conditions. Not a single protocol gave evidence of any effort on the part of the researchers to assess subjects' decision-making capacity. Nor was such a requirement apparently imposed by any IRB in approving these protocols.

The failures, if any, of researchers in other fields do not excuse the lack of attention on the part of psychiatric researchers to one of the basic prerequisites for ethical research. Insisting that the capacity to consent be appropriately assessed does not contradict the presumption, which applies to patients with mental disorders as to every other potential research subject, that all adults are competent. Ignoring the prima facie need for some evaluation of the ability to consent makes a mockery of that presumption by rendering it nothing more than a convenient rationale for ignoring the fact that the consent obtained from some subjects may not be valid.

The National Bioethics Advisory Commission further concluded that, whether or not the research offers the prospect of direct medical benefit to subjects, the enrollment of a subject depends on one of three procedures: informed consent, if the subject has decision-making capacity; "prospective authorization" for a particular class of research, given when the subject was still competent; or permission from a legally authorized representative chosen by the subject or from a concerned relative or friend who is available to monitor the subject's involvement in the research and who will base decisions about participation on "a best estimation of what the subject would have chosen if [still] capable of making a decision" (recommendations 11 through 14).[16] Moreover, even when research is intended to benefit subjects, objection by any subject (even one who lacks decision-making capacity) to enrolling or continuing in a protocol "must be heeded" (recommendation 7).[16]

THE USE OF PATIENTS IN RESEARCH TO BENEFIT OTHER PATIENTS

As compared with the harm that has arisen from the more lenient standards for therapeutic research, the other exception to the requirement of personal consent—namely, allowing guardians to enroll incapacitated subjects when the research presents no more than minimal risk of harm to the patient—may seem not to be problematic. Any difficulties this exception creates would seem to center around the vagueness of the term "minimal risk." Yet this exception has far-reaching, troubling effects.

The exception arose initially in the context of research with children. A flat prohibition against using children in research that provides them no direct benefit was seen as a barrier not only to conducting medical examinations and similar procedures to accumulate data on normal functioning, but also to using standard psychological tests or observational tools. Some theorists argued that guardians' permission should be honored as vicarious consent in such situations (on the presumption that, were they capable of deciding, children as reasonable people would recognize their obligation to aid the community) and as an exercise of appropriate paternalism (that is, a guardian by volunteering a child's participation is teaching the child the importance of sacrifice for the sake of others).[17] Even more important was the idea that parents' choice to expose their children to the risks of everyday life encompasses children's enrollment in research studies posing minimal risk. The same reasoning was then applied to other potential subjects who lacked the capacity to make decisions for themselves, including adults with various illnesses and injuries.

The exception for studies posing no more than minimal risk establishes the principle that it is acceptable to expose unconsenting people to some risk—not for their own direct good, but for the good of some larger group. But if minimal risk is acceptable, what about permitting participation when there is a minor increase over minimal risk? That is precisely what the National Commission for the Protection of Human Subjects recommended in 1977[12] and the Department of Health and Human Services adopted for research with children in 1983.[18] Furthermore, the regulations link the allowable interventions to those inherent in subjects' "actual or expected medical, dental, psychological, social, or educational situation," meaning that greater risks and burdens may be imposed on sick children than on healthy ones.

Psychiatric researchers urged the National Bioethics Advisory Commission to adopt a similar approach for people whose mental disorders prevented them from consenting to participate in research. This is what an advisory group in New York did when it recommended allowing surrogate decision makers to permit persons incapacitated with respect to decision making to participate in nonbeneficial research that presented a minor increase in risk over the minimal level.[19] The commission, however, rejected the creation of this intermediate category, whose nebulous nature only compounds the vagueness of minimal risk.

"Minor increase" is just the camel's head and neck following the nose of "minimal risk" into the tent. The flexible nature of these categories invites a relativist view, in which the addition of a little burden or risk to the lives of patients with chronic mental illnesses can easily be justified by the prospect of substantially advancing medical knowledge. Once IRBs become used to this way of thinking, it is easily applied not just to federally funded basic research but also to clinical trials of new drugs, which are less likely to advance scientific knowledge than to offer financial rewards to the pharmaceutical manufacturers that sponsor the trials and the clinicians who are paid to conduct them.

THE NEED TO CONFRONT PROBLEMS OPENLY AND SOLVE THEM

Occasionally, research may offer the prospect of developing critical knowledge about a disease or ways of treating it that cannot be obtained in any other way than by studying subjects who have the disease. If all who suffer from the condition are permanently unable to decide for themselves whether to participate in the research, and if it would be impossible for them to agree in advance to become subjects and to appoint a representative to make decisions on their behalf, then society may wish to ask whether this might be the rare case in which researchers may add the risk of injury to the insult of the illness that already burdens the patients.

An affirmative response to that question amounts to placing some especially vulnerable people in a role that, however worthy, is not one that they have chosen. If such a step is to receive the thoughtful attention it deserves, it should be confronted openly, not behind the doors of a local IRB but in a much more public forum. And the group that considers it must do what IRBs seldom do—namely, look at every aspect of the study design (has everything possible been done to reduce the chance of injury and to ameliorate any adverse event that does occur?), the selection of subjects (among all who suffer from the disease, why was this group chosen, and are no others available who are more able to assent or object to their participation?), the reliance on surrogate decision making (are the people asked to provide permission for these subjects actually able to do so in an informed, voluntary fashion?), and the claimed infeasibility of obtaining the subjects' consent (is the condition one in which prospective authorization is truly impossible, or is it merely inconvenient for the researchers?).

It seems likely that a body will be established to consider just such issues. Steven Hyman, the director of the National Institute of Mental Health (NIMH), has announced plans to create a new review panel to screen high-risk intramural and extramural studies funded by the institute. He also plans to eliminate "some of the repetitious 'me-too' studies in the intramural portfolio," in a separate initiative that is linked to the creation of the new review body "by a desire to make sure that the science in NIMH studies is good enough to justify the use of human subjects."[20]

Dr. Hyman may hope his move will blunt the effect of the recommendation by the National Bioethics Advisory Commission that the secretary of the Department of Health and Human Services appoint a special standing panel to review protocols that IRBs would be unable to approve on their own under the commission's proposed regulations (recommendation 2). The reason to assign this task to a national panel is to provide a process that is more visible, more knowledgeable, and more independent than can be expected from many IRBs. The special standing panel would review principally protocols that expose subjects to greater than minimal risk yet are not intended to benefit them directly and for which the subjects are not able to give informed consent and have not previously provided prospective authorization (recommendation 12). Besides approving studies employing methods that an IRB regards as posing more than minimal risk to participants, the special standing panel could in time reclassify some of these methods as ones that IRBs could approve for particular types of research with specified groups, without further review and approval by the panel. The guiding principle, as the commission puts it, is that the special standing panel should never "approve a protocol that reasonable, competent persons would decline to enter."[16] That principle does not resolve the tension inherent in research involving incapacitated persons, but at least it does not hide it.

Experience over the past two decades has made clear the need for special protection for patients with mental disorders. The regulations and official actions—as well as the recommendations for IRBs—of the National Bioethics Advisory Commission are the minimum needed. The federal government should adopt them without further delay.

REFERENCES

1 World Medical Association. Declaration of Helsinki. N Engl J Med 1964; 271:473–4.

2 Alexander L. Medical science under dictatorship. N Engl J Med 1949; 241:39–47.

3 Annas G. J, Grodin M. A. The Nazi doctors and the Nuremberg Code: human rights in human experimentation. New York: Oxford University Press, 1992.

4 Jones J. H. Bad blood: The Tuskegee syphilis experiment. Rev. ed. New York: Free Press, 1993.

5 United States Advisory Committee on Human Radiation Experiments. Final report on human radiation experiments. New York: Oxford University Press, 1996.

6 Hornblum A. M. Acres of skin: Human experiments at Holmesburg Prison: A true story of abuse and exploitation in the name of medical science. New York: Routledge, 1998.

7 Department of Health and Human Services, Inspector General. Institutional review boards: A time for reform. Washington, D.C.: Department of Health and Human Services, 1998.

8 Kong D., Whitaker R. Doing harm: research on the mentally ill. Boston Globe. November 15–18, 1998:A1.

9 Katz J. Human experimentation and human rights. St Louis Univ Law J 1993; 38:7–54.

10 British Medical Research Council. Responsibility in investigations on human subjects. In: Report of the British Medical Research Council for 1962–63. London: Her Majesty's Stationery Office (Cmnd. 2382), 1963: 23–4.

11 Levine R. J. Ethics and regulation of clinical research. 2nd ed. Baltimore: Urban & Schwarzenberg, 1986: 8–10.

12 National Commission for the Protection of Human Subjects of Biomedical and Behavioral Research. Report and recommendations: Research involving children. Washington, D.C.: Government Printing Office, 1977.

13 *Idem.* Report and recommendations: research involving those institutionalized as mentally infirm. Washington, D.C.: Government Printing Office, 1978.

14 Capron A. M. The law of genetic therapy. In: Hamilton M. P, ed. The new genetics and the future of man. Grand Rapids, Mich: Eerdmans, 1972: 133–56.

15 Jonas H. Philosophical reflections on experimenting with human subjects. In: Freund PA, ed. Experimentation with human subjects. New York: George Braziller, 1970: 1–31.

16 Research involving persons with mental disorders that may affect decisionmaking capacity. Rockville, Md.: National Bioethics Advisory Commission, November 12, 1998.

17 McCormick RA. Proxy consent in the experimental situation. Perspect Bio Med 1974; 18(1):2–20.

18 48 Fed Reg 9818, March 8, 1983, codified at 45 CFR § § 46.406–46.408, 1998.

19 New York State Advisory Work Group on Human Subject Research Involving the Protected Classes. Recommendation on the oversight of human subject research involving the protected classes. Albany: State of New York Department of Health, 1998. (App. D, Proposed regulations, p. D-56, §20 (b) & §20 (d).)

20 Marshall E. NIMH to screen studies for science and human risks. Science 1999; 283:464–5.

EXPERIMENTAL DESIGN AND RANDOMIZED CLINICAL TRIALS

OF MICE BUT NOT MEN: PROBLEMS OF THE RANDOMIZED CLINICAL TRIAL

Samuel Hellman and Deborah S. Hellman

Hellman and Hellman argue that an ethical dilemma confronts the use of randomized clinical trials, that is, controlled comparisons of two or more treatment arms (one of which may involve a placebo) in which subjects are randomly assigned to the different groups. According to the authors, such studies require researchers to enter into two largely incompatible roles. (1) As *physicians,* they are ethically required to act in their patients' best interests. (2) As *scientists,* they are expected to address rigorously the question of whether a particular therapy is effective, or how effective it is compared with others, in the hope of offering a genuine benefit to future patients. At some point in a study, the authors contend, researchers usually have an opinion about which treatment arm is more advantageous—but disclosing that judgment would ruin the study, while nondisclosure would mean failing to act in their patients' best interests. Hellman and Hellman conclude by suggesting that several research techniques might be sufficiently rigorous to offer viable alternatives to randomized clinical trials.

As medicine has become increasingly scientific and less accepting of unsupported opinion or proof by anecdote, the randomized controlled clinical trial has become the standard technique for changing diagnostic or therapeutic methods. The use of this technique creates an ethical dilemma.[1,2] Researchers participating in such studies are required to modify their ethical commitments to individual patients and do serious damage to the concept of the physician as a practicing, empathetic professional who is primarily concerned with each patient as an individual. Researchers using a randomized clinical trial can be described as physician-scientists, a term that expresses the tension between the two roles. The physician, by entering into a relationship with an individual patient, assumes certain obligations, including the commitment always to act in the patient's best interests. As Leon Kass has rightly maintained, "the physician must produce unswervingly the virtues of loyalty and fidelity to his patient."[3] Though the ethical requirements of this relationship have been modified by legal obligations to report wounds of a suspicious nature and certain infectious diseases, these obligations in no way conflict with the central ethical obligation to act in the best interests of the patient medically. Instead, certain nonmedical interests of the patient are preempted by other social concerns.

The role of the scientist is quite different. The clinical scientist is concerned with answering questions—i.e., determining the validity of formally constructed hypotheses. Such scientific information, it is presumed, will benefit humanity in general. The clinical scientist's role has been well described by Dr. Anthony Fauci, director of the National Institute of Allergy and Infectious Diseases, who states the goals of the randomized clinical trial in these words: "It's not to deliver therapy. It's to answer a scientific question so that the drug can be available for everybody once you've established safety and efficacy."[4] The demands of such a study can conflict in a number of ways with the physician's duty to minister to patients. The study may create a false dichotomy in

the physician's opinions: according to the premise of the randomized clinical trial, the physician may only know or not know whether a proposed course of treatment represents an improvement; no middle position is permitted. What the physician thinks, suspects, believes, or has a hunch about is assigned to the "not knowing" category, because knowing is defined on the basis of an arbitrary but accepted statistical test performed in a randomized clinical trial. Thus, little credence is given to information gained beforehand in other ways or to information accrued during the trial but without the required statistical degree of assurance that a difference is not due to chance. The randomized clinical trial also prevents the treatment technique from being modified on the basis of the growing knowledge of the physicians during their participation in the trial. Moreover, it limits access to the data as they are collected until specific milestones are achieved. This prevents physicians from profiting not only from their individual experience, but also from the collective experience of the other participants.

The randomized clinical trial requires doctors to act simultaneously as physicians and as scientists. This puts them in a difficult and sometimes untenable ethical position. The conflicting moral demands arising from the use of the randomized clinical trial reflect the classic conflict between rights-based moral theories and utilitarian ones. The first of these, which depend on the moral theory of Immanuel Kant (and seen more recently in neo-Kantian philosophers, such as John Rawls[5]), asserts that human beings, by virtue of their unique capacity for rational thought, are bearers of dignity. As such, they ought not to be treated merely as means to an end; rather, they must always be treated as ends in themselves. Utilitarianism, by contrast, defines what is right as the greatest good for the greatest number—that is, as social utility. This view, articulated by Jeremy Bentham and John Stuart Mill, requires that pleasures (understood broadly, to include such pleasures as health and well-being) and pains be added together. The morally correct act is the act that produces the most pleasure and the least pain overall.

A classic objection to the utilitarian position is that according to that theory, the distribution of pleasures and pains is of no moral consequence. This element of the theory severely restricts physicians from being utilitarians, or at least from following the theory's dictates. Physicians must care very deeply about the distribution of pain and pleasure, for they have entered into a relationship with one or a number of individual patients. They cannot be indifferent to whether it is these patients or others that suffer for the general benefit of society. Even though society might gain from the suffering of a few, and even though the doctor might believe that such a benefit is worth a given patient's suffering (i.e., that utilitarianism is right in the particular case), the ethical obligation created by the covenant between doctor and patient requires the doctor to see the interests of the individual patient as primary and compelling. In essence, the doctor-patient relationship requires doctors to see their patients as bearers of rights who cannot be merely used for the greater good of humanity.

As Fauci has suggested,[4] the randomized clinical trial routinely asks physicians to sacrifice the interests of their particular patients for the sake of the study and that of the information that it will make available for the benefit of society. This practice is ethically problematic. Consider first the initial formulation of a trial. In particular, consider the case of a disease for which there is no satisfactory therapy— for example, advanced cancer or the acquired immunodeficiency syndrome (AIDS). A new agent that promises more effectiveness is the subject of the study. The control group must be given either an unsatisfactory treatment or a placebo. Even though the therapeutic value of the new agent is unproved, if physicians think that it has promise, are they acting in the best interests of their patients in allowing them to be randomly assigned to the control group? Is persisting in such an assignment consistent with the specific commitments taken on in the doctor-patient relationship? As a result of interactions with patients with AIDS and their advocates, Merigan[6] recently suggested modifications in the design of clinical trials that attempt to deal with the unsatisfactory treatment given to the control group. The view of such activists has been expressed by Rebecca Pringle Smith of Community Research Initiative in New York: "Even if you have a supply of compliant martyrs, trials must have some ethical validity."[4]

If the physician has no opinion about whether the new treatment is acceptable, then random assignment is ethically acceptable, but such lack of enthusiasm for the new treatment does not augur well for either the patient or the study. Alternatively, the treatment may show promise of beneficial results but also present a risk of undesirable complications. When the physician believes that the severity and likelihood of harm and good are evenly balanced, randomization may be ethically acceptable. If the physician has no preference for either treatment (is in a state of equipoise[7,8]), then randomization is acceptable. If, however, he or she believes that the new treatment may be either more or less successful or more or less toxic, the use of randomization is not consistent with fidelity to the patient.

The argument usually used to justify randomization is that it provides, in essence, a critique of the usefulness of the physician's beliefs and opinions, those that have not yet been validated by a randomized clinical trial. As the argument goes, these not-yet-validated beliefs are as likely to be wrong as right. Although physicians are ethically required to provide their patients with the best available treatment, there simply is no best treatment yet known.

The reply to this argument takes two forms. First, and most important, even if this view of the reliability of a physician's opinion is accurate, the ethical constraints of an individual doctor's relationship with a particular patient require the doctor to provide individual care. Although physicians must take pains to make clear the speculative nature of their views, they cannot withhold these views from the patient. The patient asks from the doctor both knowledge and judgment. The relationship established between them rightfully allows patients to ask for the judgment of their particular physicians, not merely that of the medical profession in general. Second, it may not be true, in fact, that the not-yet-validated beliefs of physicians are as likely to be wrong as right. The greater certainty obtained with a randomized clinical trial is beneficial, but that does not mean that a lesser degree of certainty is without value. Physicians can acquire knowledge through methods other than the randomized clinical trial. Such knowledge, acquired over time and less formally than is required in a randomized clinical trial, may be of great value to a patient.

Even if it is ethically acceptable to begin a study, one often forms an opinion during its course—especially in studies that are impossible to conduct in a truly double-blinded fashion—that makes it ethically problematic to continue. The inability to remain blinded usually occurs in studies of cancer or AIDS, for example, because the therapy is associated by nature with serious side effects. Trials attempt to restrict the physician's access to the data in order to prevent such unblinding. Such restrictions should make physicians eschew the trial, since their ability to act in the patient's best interests will be limited. Even supporters of randomized clinical trials, such as Merigan, agree that interim findings should be presented to patients to ensure that no one receives what seems an inferior treatment.[6] Once physicians have formed a view about the new treatment, can they continue randomization? If random assignment is stopped, the study may be lost and the participation of the previous patients wasted. However, if physicians continue the randomization when they have a definite opinion about the efficacy of the experimental drug, they are not acting in accordance with the requirements of the doctor-patient relationship. Furthermore, as their opinion becomes more firm, stopping the randomization may not be enough. Physicians may be ethically required to treat the patients formerly placed in the control group with the therapy that now seems probably effective. To do so would be faithful to the obligations created by the doctor-patient relationship, but it would destroy the study.

To resolve this dilemma, one might suggest that the patient has abrogated the rights implicit in a doctor-patient relationship by signing an informed-consent form. We argue that such rights cannot be waived or abrogated. They are inalienable. The right to be treated as an individual deserving the physician's best judgment and care, rather than to be used as a means to determine the best treatment for others, is inherent in every person. This right, based on the concept of dignity, cannot be waived. What of altruism, then? Is it not the patient's right to make a sacrifice for the general good? This question must be considered from both positions—that of the patient and that of the physician. Although patients may decide to waive this right, it is not consistent with the role of a physician to ask that they do so. In asking, the doctor acts as a scientist instead. The physician's role here is to propose what he or she believes is best medically for the specific patient, not to suggest participation in a study from which the patient cannot gain. Because the opportunity to help future patients is of potential value to a patient, some would say physicians should not deny it. Although this point has merit, it offers so many opportunities for abuse that we are extremely uncomfortable about accepting it. The responsibilities of physicians are much clearer; they are to minister to the current patient.

Moreover, even if patients could waive this right, it is questionable whether those with terminal illness would be truly able to give voluntary informed consent. Such patients are extremely dependent on both their physicians and the health care system. Aware of this dependence, physicians must not ask for consent, for in such cases the very asking breaches the doctor-patient relationship. Anxious to please their physicians, patients may have difficulty refusing to participate in the trial the physicians describe. The patients may perceive their refusal as damaging to the relationship, whether or not it is so. Such perceptions of coercion affect the decision. Informed-consent forms are difficult to understand, especially for patients under the stress of serious illness for which there is no satisfactory treatment. The forms are usually lengthy, somewhat legalistic, complicated, and confusing, and they hardly bespeak the compassion expected of the medical profession. It is important to remember that those who have studied the doctor-patient relationship have emphasized its empathetic nature.

> [The] relationship between doctor and patient partakes of a peculiar intimacy. It presupposes on the part of the physician not only knowledge of his fellow men but sympathy. . . . This aspect of the practice of medicine has been designated as the art; yet I wonder whether it should not, most properly, be called the essence.[9]

How is such a view of the relationship consonant with random assignment and informed consent? The Physician's Oath of the World Medical Association affirms the primacy of the deontologic view of patients' rights: "Concern for the interests of the subject must always prevail over the interests of science and society."[10]

Furthermore, a single study is often not considered sufficient. Before a new form of therapy is generally accepted, confirmatory trials must be conducted. How can one conduct such trials ethically unless one is convinced that the first trial was in error? The ethical problems we have discussed are only exacerbated when a completed randomized clinical trial indicates that a given treatment is preferable. Even if the physician believes the initial trial was in error, the physician must indicate to the patient the full results of that trial.

The most common reply to the ethical arguments has been that the alternative is to return to the physician's intuition, to anecdotes, or to both as the basis of medical opinion. We all accept the dangers of such a practice. The argument states that we must therefore accept randomized, controlled clinical trials regardless of their ethical problems because of the great social benefit they make possible, and we salve our conscience with the knowledge that informed consent has been given. This returns us to the conflict between patients' rights and social utility. Some would argue that this tension can be resolved by placing a relative value on each. If the patient's right that is being compromised is not a fundamental right and the social gain is very great, then the study might be justified. When the right is fundamental, however, no amount of social gain, or almost none, will justify its sacrifice. Consider, for example, the experiments on humans done by physicians under the Nazi regime. All would agree that these are unacceptable regardless of the value of the scientific information gained. Some people go so far as to say that no use should be made of the results of those experiments because of the clearly unethical manner in which the data were collected. This extreme example may not seem relevant, but we believe that in its hyperbole it clarifies the fallacy of a utilitarian approach to the physician's relationship with the patient. To consider the utilitarian gain is consistent neither with the physician's role nor with the patient's rights.

It is fallacious to suggest that only the randomized clinical trial can provide valid information or that all information acquired by this technique is valid. Such experimental methods are intended to reduce error and bias and therefore reduce the uncertainty of the result. Uncertainty cannot be eliminated, however. The scientific method is based on increasing probabilities and increasingly refined approximations of truth.[11] Although the randomized clinical trial contributes to these ends, it is neither unique nor perfect. Other techniques may also be useful.[12]

Randomized trials often place physicians in the ethically intolerable position of choosing between the good of the patient and that of society. We urge that such situations be avoided and that other techniques of acquiring clinical information be adopted. For example, concerning trials of treatments for AIDS, Byar et al.[13] have said that "some traditional approaches to the clinical-trials process may be unnecessarily rigid and unsuitable for this disease." In this case, AIDS is not what is so different; rather, the difference is in the presence of AIDS activists, articulate spokespersons for the ethical problems created by the application of the randomized clinical trial to terminal illnesses. Such arguments are equally applicable to advanced cancer and other serious illnesses. Byar et al. agree that there are even circumstances in which uncontrolled clinical trials may be justified: when there is no effective treatment to use as a control, when the prognosis is uniformly poor, and when there is a reasonable expectation of benefit without excessive toxicity. These conditions are usually found in clinical trials of advanced cancer.

The purpose of the randomized clinical trial is to avoid the problems of observer bias and patient selection. It seems to us that techniques might be developed to deal with these issues in other ways. Randomized clinical trials deal with them in a cumbersome and heavy-handed manner, by requiring large numbers of patients in the hope that random assignment will balance the heterogeneous distribution of patients into the different groups. By observing known characteristics of patients, such as age and sex, and distributing them equally between groups, it is thought that unknown factors important in determining outcomes will also be distributed equally. Surely, other techniques can be developed to deal with both observer bias and patient selection.

Prospective studies without randomization, but with the evaluation of patients by uninvolved third parties, should remove observer bias. Similar methods have been suggested by Royall.[12] Prospective matched-pair analysis, in which patients are treated in a manner consistent with their physician's views, ought to help ensure equivalence between the groups and thus mitigate the effect of patient selection, at least with regard to known covariates. With regard to unknown covariates, the security would rest, as in randomized trials, in the enrollment of large numbers of patients and in confirmatory studies. This method would not pose ethical difficulties, since patients would receive the treatment recommended by their physician. They would be included in the study by independent observers matching patients with respect to known characteristics, a process that would not affect patient care and that could be performed independently any number of times.

This brief discussion of alternatives to randomized clinical trials is sketchy and incomplete. We wish only to point out that there may be satisfactory alternatives, not to describe and evaluate them completely. Even if randomized clinical trials were much better than any alternative, however, the ethical dilemmas they present may put their use at variance with the primary obligations of the physician. In this regard, Angell cautions, "If this commitment to the patient is attenuated, even for so good a cause as benefits to future patients, the implicit assumptions of the doctor-patient relationship are violated."[14] The risk of such attenuation by the randomized trial is great. The AIDS activists have brought this dramatically to the attention of the academic medical community. Techniques appropriate to the laboratory may not be applicable to humans. We must develop and use alternative methods for acquiring clinical knowledge.

REFERENCES

1 Hellman S. Randomized clinical trials and the doctor-patient relationship: and ethical dilemma. Cancer Clin Trials 1979; 2:189–93.

2 *Idem.* A doctor's dilemma: the doctor-patient relationship in clinical investigation. In: Proceedings of the Fourth National Conference on Human Values and Cancer, New York, March 15–17, 1984. New York: American Cancer Society, 1984:144–6.

3 Kass L. R. Toward a more natural science: biology and human affairs. New York: Free Press, 1985:196.

4 Palca J. AIDS drug trials enter new age. Science 1989; 246:19–21.

5 Rawls J. A theory of justice. Cambridge, Mass.: Belknap Press of Harvard University Press, 1971:183–92, 446–52.

6 Merigan T. C. You *can* teach an old dog new tricks—how AIDS trials are pioneering new strategies. N Engl J Med 1990; 323:1341–3.

7 Freedman B. Equipoise and the ethics of clinical research. N Engl J Med 1987; 317:141–5.

8 Singer P. A, Lantos J. D, Whitington PF, Broelsch C. E, Siegler M. Equipoise and the ethics of segmental liver transplantation. Clin Res 1988; 36:539–45.

9 Longcope W. T. Methods and medicine. Bull Johns Hopkins Hosp 1932; 50:4–20.

10 Report on medical ethics. World Med Assoc Bull 1949; 1:109, 111.

11 Popper K. The problem of induction. In: Miller D, ed. Popper selections. Princeton, N.J.: Princeton University Press, 1985:101–17.

12 Royall R. M. Ethics and statistics in randomized clinical trials. Stat Sci 1991; 6(1):52–62.

13 Byar D. P, Schoenfeld D. A, Green S. B, et al. Design considerations for AIDS trials. N Engl J Med 1990; 323:1343–8.

14 Angell M. Patients' preferences in randomized clinical trials. N Engl J Med 1984; 310:1385–7.

HOW TO RESOLVE AN ETHICAL DILEMMA
CONCERNING RANDOMIZED CLINICAL TRIALS
Don Marquis

Marquis addresses an apparent dilemma that arises when a physician considers enrolling patients in a randomized clinical trial and when the physician has an opinion about which treatment arm is preferable. (For the purpose of discussion, he focuses on trials that compare two treatments as opposed to one or more treatments and a placebo). On the one hand, the physician has a duty to promote the patient's best interests and so seemingly may not recommend enrollment in a study in which the patient might not receive the treatment the physician considers preferable. On the other hand, recognition of this duty and its apparent implication creates an obstacle to achieving sufficient enrollment for the study to generate significant results. After arguing against two popular strategies for resolving this problem, Marquis contends that "[t]aking informed consent seriously resolves the dilemma." On his proposal, a physician can both (1) recommend the treatment that he or she considers superior and (2) ask whether the patient would like to enroll in a randomized clinical trial in which he or she may or may not receive that treatment.

An apparent ethical dilemma arises when physicians consider enrolling their patients in randomized clinical trials. Suppose that a randomized clinical trial comparing two treatments is in progress, and a physician has an opinion about which treatment is better. The physician has a duty to promote the patient's best medical interests and therefore seems to be obliged to advise the patient to receive the treatment that the physician prefers. This duty creates a barrier to the enrollment of patients in randomized clinical trials.[1–10] Two strategies are often used to resolve the dilemma in favor of enrolling patients in clinical trials.

THE "EITHER YOU KNOW WHICH IS BETTER OR YOU DON'T" STRATEGY

According to one strategy, physicians should not recommend one treatment over another if they do not really know which one is better, and they do not really know which treatment is better in the absence of data from randomized clinical trials.[11] Data from uncontrolled studies are often influenced by the desire on both the investigator's part and the patient's part to obtain positive results.[12] Journal editors are more likely to publish reports of studies with positive results than reports of studies with negative results.[13] A treatment recommendation based on weaker evidence than that obtained from a randomized clinical trial is like a recommendation based on a mere hunch or an idiosyncratic preference.[14] Thus, according to this argument, in the absence of data

Reprinted by permission of the publisher from *The New England Journal of Medicine*, vol. 341 (August 26, 1999), pp. 691–693. © 1999 Massachusetts Medical Society. All rights reserved.

from a randomized clinical trial, evidence that provides an adequate basis for recommending a treatment rarely exists, and the enrollment dilemma is based on a mistake.

This strategy for resolving the dilemma is simplistic. It assumes that evidence available to physicians can be only one of two kinds: gold standard evidence or worthless prejudice. But clinical judgments may be based on evidence of intermediate quality, including physicians' experience with their own patients, their conversations with colleagues concerning their colleagues' experience, their evaluation of the results of nonrandomized studies reported in the literature, their judgment about the mechanism of action of one or both treatments, or their view of the natural history of a given disease. Evidence need not be conclusive to be valuable; it need not be definitive to be suggestive. Because all good physicians allow evidence of intermediate quality to influence their professional judgment when a relevant randomized clinical trial is not being conducted, it is unreasonable to claim that such evidence has no worth when a relevant randomized clinical trial is being conducted. Therefore, the "either you know which is better or you don't" strategy for dealing with the enrollment dilemma is not persuasive.

ADOPTING A LESS STRICT THERAPEUTIC OBLIGATION

The dilemma about enrolling patients in randomized clinical trials is generated by the claim that a physician has a strict therapeutic obligation to inform the patients of the physician's treatment preference, even when the preference is based on evidence that is not of the highest quality. The dilemma could be resolved if the physician's therapeutic obligation were less strict. This strategy was developed by Freedman.[14][15] He argued that the standard for determining whether a physician has engaged in medical malpractice or committed some other violation punishable by a professional disciplinary body is the standard of good practice as determined by a consensus of the medical community. There is no consensus about which of two treatments being compared in a randomized clinical trial is superior. (Otherwise, why conduct the trial?) Therefore, enrolling a patient in the trial does not violate the physician's therapeutic obligation to the patient, regardless of the physician's treatment preference. In addition, a patient who consults a physician with a preference for treatment. A could have consulted a physician who preferred treatment B. Therefore, enrolling a patient in a randomized clinical trial in order to be randomly assigned (perhaps) to treatment B does not make such a patient worse off than he or she would otherwise have been.

Despite these points, compelling arguments for the stricter interpretation of therapeutic obligation remain. In the first place, consider what physicians expect when they seek professional advice from their malpractice attorneys, their tax advisors, or for that matter, their own physicians. Surely they expect—and believe they have a right to expect—not merely minimally competent advice, but the best professional judgments of the professionals they have chosen to consult. In the second place, patients choose physicians in order to obtain medical advice that is, in the judgment of those physicians, the best available. If physicians do not provide such advice, then they tacitly deceive their patients, unless they disclose to their patients that they are not bound by this strict therapeutic obligation. Physicians should adopt the strict therapeutic obligation.

A RESOLUTION

The clash between a strict therapeutic obligation and a less strict one is only apparent. On the one hand, the less strict therapeutic obligation is supported by the argument that it is morally permissible to offer to enroll a patient in a randomized clinical trial. On the other hand, the strict therapeutic obligation is supported by the arguments concerning treatment recommendations. Recommending is different from offering to enroll. A recognition of this difference provides the basis for a solution to the dilemma.

Suppose that a randomized clinical trial is being conducted to compare treatments A and B and that a physician prefers A and informs the patient of this preference. All physicians have an obligation to obtain their patients' informed consent to treatment. A physician has respected this right only if he or she explains to the patient the risks and benefits of reasonable alternatives to the recommended treatment and offers the patient an opportunity to choose an alternative, if that is feasible. Either treatment B or enrollment in the trial comparing A and B is a reasonable alternative to treatment A, because presumably, A is not known to be superior to B: Indeed, there is some evidence that enrollment in a randomized clinical trial is a superior therapeutic alternative when a trial is available.[16] Respect for a patient's values is a central purpose of informed consent. A particular patient may place a greater value on participation in a study that will contribute to medical progress and to the well-being of patients in the future than on the unproved advantages of following the physician's recommendation. Therefore, a physician can both recommend a treatment and ask whether the patient is willing to enroll in the randomized clinical trial.

This resolution is based on the recognition that there can be evidence of the superiority of a treatment that falls short of the gold standard for evidence but is better than worthless. It also takes into account the good arguments for the view that physicians have a strict obligation to recommend the best treatment on the basis of their professional judgment, even when the recommendation is based on evidence that falls short of the gold standard. Nevertheless, because all physicians have an obligation to take informed consent seriously, because respect for informed consent entails offering a patient the reasonable alternatives to the recommended treatment, and because enrollment in an appropriate randomized clinical trial is often a reasonable therapeutic option, one could argue that offering a patient the opportunity to be enrolled in a clinical trial is not only morally permissible but, in many cases, also morally obligatory, if a relevant trial is being conducted and if enrollment in it is feasible. Taking informed consent seriously resolves the dilemma about whether to enroll patients in randomized clinical trials.

Is this analysis clinically realistic? Some may argue that if clinicians inform their patients that they prefer treatment A, then few of their patients will consent to participate in a trial comparing A with B. Furthermore, many clinicians may be unwilling to invest the time necessary to explain the option of enrollment in a trial, particularly if it seems unlikely that a patient, knowing the physician's preference for one of the treatments, will choose to participate in the trial.

On the other hand, in recent years the public has been exposed to a barrage of medical information and misinformation. Explaining to patients the difference between solid scientific evidence of the merits of a treatment and weaker evidence of its merits is worthwhile, whether or not a relevant randomized clinical trial is being conducted. When a relevant trial is being conducted, offering the patient enrollment in the trial should not impose on the physician a large, additional burden of explanation. Physicians can promote enrollment by explaining that their preference is based only on limited evidence, which may or may not be reliable. They can also explain that data from randomized clinical trials have often shown that the initial studies of new treatments were overly optimistic.[17]

In addition, using this informed-consent strategy to resolve the enrollment dilemma may not be morally optional. My analysis is based on two important obligations of physicians. The first is the strict obligation to recommend the treatment that is, in the physician's professional judgment, the best choice for the patient. The second is the obligation to obtain the patient's informed consent to the recommended treatment. The duty of obtaining informed consent implies that the physician is obligated to offer the patient the opportunity to enroll in a clinical trial when one is available, even if the physician has a treatment preference. The physician owes this duty to the individual patient, not simply to future patients who may benefit from advances in medical knowledge. Thus, the informed-consent strategy for resolving the dilemma about enrolling patients in randomized clinical trials leads to the conclusion that physicians have a greater duty to offer their patients enrollment in trials than has previously been realized. A strict, thoroughly defensible, therapeutic obligation need not interfere with the conduct of randomized clinical trials.

I am indebted to Erin Fitz-Gerald, Nina Ainslie, Stephen Williamson, Sarah Taylor, Jerry Menikoff, Don Hatton, and Ron Stephens for their criticisms.

REFERENCES

1 Chalmers T. C. The ethics of randomization as a decision-making technique and the problem of informed consent. Report of the 14th conference of cardiovascular training grant program directors, June 3–4, 1967. Bethesda, Md.: National Heart Institute, 1967:87–93.

2 Shaw L. W, Chalmers TC. Ethics in cooperative clinical trials. Ann N Y Acad Sci 1970; 169:487–95.

3 Kolata G. B. Clinical trials: methods and ethics are debated. Science 1977;198:1127–31.

4 Wikler D. Ethical considerations in randomized clinical trials. Semin Oncol 1981; 8:437–41.

5 Schafer A. The ethics of the randomized clinical trial. N Engl J Med 1982;307:719–24.

6 Marquis D. Leaving therapy to chance. Hastings Cent Rep 1983;13:40–7.

7 Gifford R. The conflict between randomized clinical trials and the therapeutic obligation. J Med Philos 1986; 11:347–66.

8 Hellman S, Hellman D. S. Of mice but not men: problems of the randomized clinical trial. N Engl J Med 1991; 324:1585–9.

9 Gifford R. Community equipoise and the ethics of randomized clinical trials. Bioethics 1995; 9:127–48.

10 Markman M. Ethical difficulties with randomized clinical trials involving cancer patients: examples from the field of gynecologic oncology. J Clin Ethics 1992; 3:193–5.

11 Spodick D. H. Ethics of the randomized clinical trial. N Engl J Med 1983; 308:343.

12 Passamani E. Clinical trials — are they ethical? N Engl J Med 1991; 324:1589–92.

13 Altman L. Negative results: a positive viewpoint. New York Times. April 29, 1986:B6.

14 Freedman B. Equipoise and the ethics of clinical research. N Engl J Med 1987; 317:141–5.

15 *Idem.* A response to a purported ethical difficulty with randomized clinical trials involving cancer patients. J Clin Ethics 1992; 3:231–4.

16 Davis S, Wright PW, Schulman S. F, et al. Participants in prospective, randomized clinical trials for resected non-small cell lung cancer have improved survival compared with nonparticipants in such trials. Cancer 1985; 56:1710–8.

17 Sacks H, Chalmers T. C, Smith H Jr. Randomized versus historical controls for clinical trials. Am J Med 1982; 72:233–40.

RESEARCH IN DEVELOPING COUNTRIES: TAKING BENEFIT SERIOUSLY

Leonard H. Glantz, George J. Annas, Michael A. Grodin, and Wendy K. Mariner

The authors confront the issue of whether it can be acceptable for researchers in wealthy countries to enroll citizens of developing countries in clinical trials. Citing guidelines published by the Council for International Organizations of Medical Sciences, the authors argue that to justify such trials, the risks or burdens imposed on trial participants must be offset by the prospect of actual benefit to the inhabitants of the developing country. Thus, if the trial yields beneficial knowledge, benefits must actually reach individuals in the country in which the trial took place; otherwise, the subjects will have been exploited. A practical implication of this approach is that "an essential prerequisite to designing ethical research in underdeveloped countries is identifying the source and amount of funding for providing the fruits of the research to the people of the developing country"—a moral requirement that was not satisfied in recent African AZT studies. The authors then consider and reply to a wide range of objections to the ethical standard they propose.

An April 1998 *New York Times Magazine* article described Ronald Munger's efforts to obtain blood samples from a group of extremely impoverished people in the Philippine Island of Cebu.[1] Munger sought the blood to study whether there was a genetic cause for this group's unusually high incidence of cleft lip and palate. One of many obstacles to the research project was the need to obtain the cooperation of the local health officer. It was not clear to Munger, or the reader, whether the health officer had a bona fide interest in protecting the populace or was looking for a bribe. The health officer asked Munger a few perfunctory questions about informed consent and the study's ethical review in the United States, which Munger answered. Munger also explained the benefits that mothers and children would derive from participating in the research. The mothers would learn their blood types (which they apparently desired) and whether they were anemic. If they were anemic, they would be given iron pills. Lunch would be served, and raffles arranged so that families could win simple toys and other small items.

Munger told the health officer that if his hypotheses were correct, the research would benefit the population of Cebu: if the research shows that increased folate and vitamin B6 reduces the risk of cleft lip and palate, families could reduce the risk of facial deformities in their future offspring. The reporter noted that the health officer "laughs aloud at the suggestion that much of what is being discovered in American laboratories will make it back to Cebu any time soon." Reflecting on his experience with another simple intervention, iodized salt, the health officer said that when salt was iodized, the price rose threefold "so those who need it couldn't afford it and those who didn't need it are the only ones who could afford it."

The simple blood collecting mission to Cebu illustrates almost all the issues presented by research in developing countries. First is the threshold question of the goal of the research and its importance to the population represented by the research subjects. Next is the quality of informed consent, including whether the potential subjects thought that participation in the research was related to free surgical care that was offered in the same facility (although it clearly was not) and whether one could adequately explain genetic hypotheses to an uneducated populace. Finally, there is the question whether the population from which subjects were drawn could benefit from the research. This research intervention is very low risk—the collection of 10 drops of blood from affected people and their family members. The risk of job or insurance discrimination that genetic research poses in this country did not exist for the Cebu population; ironically, they were protected from the risk of economic discrimination by the profound poverty in which they lived.

Even this simple study raises the most fundamental question: "Why is it acceptable for researchers in developed countries to use citizens of developing countries as research subjects?" A cautionary approach to permitting research with human subjects in underdeveloped countries has been recommended because of the risk of their inadvertent or deliberate exploitation by researchers from developed countries. This cautionary approach generally is invoked when researchers propose to use what are considered "vulnerable populations," such as prisoners and children, as research subjects.[2] Vulnerable populations are those that are less able to protect themselves, either because they are not capable of making their own decisions or because they are particularly susceptible to mistreatment.[3] For example, children may be incapable of giving informed consent or of standing up to adult authority, while prisoners are especially vulnerable to being coerced into becoming subjects. Citizens of developing countries are often in vulnerable situations because of their lack of political power, lack of education, unfamiliarity with medical interventions, extreme poverty, or dire need for health care and nutrition. It is the dire need of these populations that may make them both appropriate subjects of research and especially vulnerable to exploitation. This combination of need and vulnerability has led to the development of guidelines for the use of citizens of developing countries as research subjects.

CIOMS GUIDELINES

In 1992, the Council for International Organizations of Medical Sciences (CIOMS), in collaboration with the World Health Organization, published guide-lines for the appropriate use of research subjects from "underdeveloped communities."[4]

Like other human research codes, the CIOMS guidelines combine the protection of subjects' rights with protection of their welfare; as subjects become less able to protect their own rights (and therefore become more vulnerable), researchers and reviewers must increase their efforts to protect the welfare of subjects.[5] Perhaps the most important statement in these guidelines is what appears to be the injunction against using subjects in developing countries if the research could be carried out reasonably well in developed countries. Commentary to guideline 8 notes, for example, that there are diseases that rarely or never occur in economically developed countries, and that prevention and treatment research therefore needs to be conducted in the countries at risk for those diseases. The conclusion to be drawn from the substance of these guidelines is that in order for research to be ethically conducted, it must offer the potential of actual benefit to the inhabitants of that developing country.

In order for underdeveloped communities to derive potential benefit from research, they must have access to the fruits of such research. The CIOMS commentary to guideline 8 states that, "as a general rule, the sponsoring agency should ensure that, at the completion of successful testing, any product developed *will* be made reasonably available to inhabitants of the underdeveloped community in which the research was carried out: exceptions to this general requirement should be justified, and agreed to by all concerned parties before the research is begun."[6] This statement is directed at minimizing exploitation of the underdeveloped community that provides the research subjects. If developed countries use inhabitants of underdeveloped countries to create new products that would be beneficial to both the developed and the underdeveloped country, but the underdeveloped country cannot gain access to the product because of expense, then the subjects in the underdeveloped countries have been grossly exploited. As written, however, this CIOMS guideline is not strong or specific enough to prevent exploitation. Exemplifying this problem are recent short course zidovudine (AZT) studies in Africa that were approved and conducted despite the existence of the CIOMS guidelines.[7]

THE AFRICAN MATERNAL-FETAL HIV TRANSMISSION STUDIES

The goal of the short course AZT studies was to see if lower doses of the drug AZT than those used in the United States could reduce the rate of maternal-child transmission of HIV. It was well established that doses of AZT that cost $800 (not taking into account screening and other related costs) reduced maternal-fetal transmission of HIV by as much as two-thirds in the United States.[8, 9] If the developed countries had been willing to subsidize the cost of this regimen in Africa, no additional research would have been needed. But because many African countries could not afford this expense, the decision was made to attempt to see if lower (and therefore cheaper) doses would prevent maternal-fetal HIV transmission. Several impoverished countries were chosen as research sites. The justification for conducting research in those countries was not that they suffered from a disease that did not afflict people in developed countries, and not because no treatment existed, but because their impoverishment made an existing therapy unavailable to them (as long as developed countries refused to subsidize the costs).[10]

The issue, as always, is to determine the ethical acceptability of the proposed research *before* it is conducted. In a case like this, where the researchable problem exists *solely* because of economic reasons, the research hypothesis must contain an economic component. The research question should be formulated as follows:

(1) We know that a given regimen of AZT will reduce the rate of maternal-child transmission of HIV.

(2) Maternal-child transmission of HIV in many African countries is a serious problem but the effective AZT regimen is not available because it is too expensive.

(3) If an effective AZT regimen costs $X, then it will be made available in the country in which it is to be studied.

(4) Therefore, we will conduct trials in certain African countries to see if $X worth of AZT will effectively reduce maternal-child transmission of HIV in those countries.

The most important part of the development of this research question is number 3. Without knowing what dollar amount X actually represents, it is impossible to formulate a research question that can lead to any benefit to the citizens of the country in which the research is to be conducted. There is no way to determine what $X represents in the absence of committed funding. Therefore, an essential prerequisite to designing ethical research in underdeveloped countries is identifying the source and amount of funding for providing the fruits of the research to the people of the developing country in which it is to be studied as a condition of the research being approved.

If a study found, for example, that $50 worth of AZT has the same effect as $800 worth of AZT, it would greatly benefit the developed world. Developed countries, which currently spend $800 per case on drugs alone, could pay substantially less for this preventive measure, and, because the research was conducted elsewhere, none of their citizens would have been put at any risk. At the same time, if the underdeveloped country could not afford to spend $50 any more than it could spend $800, then it could not possibly derive information that would be of any benefit to its population. This is the definition of exploitation.[11]

It is only now that an effort is being made to determine how to raise the money to actually provide AZT to prevent maternal-child HIV transmission (as well as the other costly services that go with the appropriate administration of the drug) to the impoverished African countries that provided the human subjects.[12] These efforts began after parallel studies conducted in Thailand reported that lower doses of AZT reduced maternal-fetal transmission of HIV.[13] The Thai government had committed to providing the AZT before its trials began. In the African trials, however, no one "ensured" that at the completion of successful testing the product would be made reasonably available, thereby violating the CIOMS guidelines.[14] The guidelines say that there can be exceptions to this general requirement, but that exceptions must be "justified" and "agreed to by all concerned parties." It is not clear to whom the exception must be "justified" or on what grounds. Moreover, if the "concerned parties" are the sponsor and/or the investigator and the host country, they may not adequately represent the interests of the research subjects. The fact that representatives of the research community and officials of the host countries agree to exploit the population does not make the research any less exploitive.[15]

RULES FOR ETHICAL RESEARCH IN DEVELOPING COUNTRIES

We believe the standards for research in developing countries should include the following.

There should be a rebuttable presumption that researchers from developed countries will not conduct research in developing countries unless it can be shown that a direct benefit *will* be bestowed upon the residents of that country if the research proves to be successful. The person or entities proposing to conduct the study must demonstrate that there is a realistic plan, which includes identified funding, to provide the newly proven intervention to the population from which the potential pool of research subjects is to be recruited. In the absence of a realistic plan and identified funding, the population from which the research subjects will be drawn cannot derive benefit from the research. Therefore, the benefits cannot outweigh the risks, because there are, and will be, no benefits. Only by having committed funding and a plan to make a successful intervention available can it be determined that there will be sufficient benefit to justify conducting research on the target population. The distribution plan must be realistic. Where the health care infrastructure is so undeveloped that it would be impossible to deliver the intervention even if it were free, research would be unjustified in the absence of a plan to improve that country's health care delivery capabilities.

Some might argue that this standard is too strict and that it would reduce the amount of research that could be conducted in certain countries. The answer, of course, is that if the benefits of the research are not made available to the inhabitants of that country, they have lost nothing by the lack of such research. Others might argue that research in underdeveloped countries is justified if it might benefit the individual research subjects, even if it will not benefit anyone else in the population. However, research is, by definition, designed to create generalizable knowledge, and is legitimate in a developing country only if its purpose is to create generalizable knowledge that will benefit the citizens of that country. If the re-

search only has the potential to benefit the limited number of individuals who participate in the study, it cannot offer the benefit to the underdeveloped country that legitimizes the use of its citizens as research subjects. It should be emphasized that research whose goal is to prevent or treat large populations is fundamentally public health research, and public health research makes no sense (and thus should not be done) if its benefits are limited to the small population of research subjects.

It might be argued that there is no requirement that such a plan be devised prior to conducting research in the United States, and, therefore, that by adopting such a requirement we would be imposing a higher standard for research conducted in developing countries than we do for research conducted in the United States.

This argument only further demonstrates the differences between wealthy and poor countries. The reality in the United States is that regardless of the very significant gaps in insurance and Medicaid coverage and the health care discrepancies between the rich and poor, medical interventions are relatively widely available, especially when compared to developing countries. Upon the successful completion of the research that demonstrated the effectiveness of the 076 regimen in reducing maternal-child transmission, the primary beneficiaries of this new preventive intervention in the United States were poor women and their newborns. Unlike the United States, absent a plan to pay for a new intervention and lacking the infrastructure to deliver an intervention, it is virtually guaranteed that the intervention will not be generally available in a developing country.

The more accurate analogy to the African AIDS trials would be if investigators proposed the 076 protocol in the United States knowing that only poor women would be recruited as research subjects and that, if successful, the intervention would not be made generally available to poor women. Such research would be clearly unethical. Not only would this be a gross violation of the ethical principle of distributive justice, it would be a violation of the regulatory obligation of the equitable selection of subjects.[16]

A further objection is that one cannot always trust what a government or another potential funder promises. What is to prevent the promisor from reneging? The answer is, nothing. One can try to expose the funder to embarrassment and other pressures that might cause it to live up to the promise upon which researchers and subjects relied. However, the potential unethical behavior in the future by the funder is no excuse for not having a realistic plan at the outset. Furthermore, if we take this obligation seriously, this should only occur once per funder. After reneging once, they cannot be relied upon again to justify research in the future.

An additional objection to our position is that it will restrict access to new interventions because once a new intervention is developed, the price will come down and therefore the intervention will become available to the people of the impoverished country. The answer is to ask those who control the pricing of interventions if this will be the case in any particular instance. One could have asked Glaxo if it would reduce its price once it was shown that lower doses of AZT were effective. If the answer is yes, one can proceed. If the answer is no, or "we have not decided," there seems to be no justification to proceed if the current price would significantly restrict availability. There is nothing magical about pricing. Pricing is in the absolute control of manufacturers and there is no need to guess or speculate about what will happen to price. Indeed, this objection to our argument would justify conducting the full 076 trial itself in developing countries. The price *might* come down enough so that determining the efficacy of short course AZT regimens might not be needed at all. Such speculation should not be sufficient to put subjects at risk.

Finally, it might be argued that there are diseases that only affect people in developing countries for which there are no effective treatments, but that the treatments that might be discovered could be expensive. The argument continues that it is not right to fail to develop treatments that could benefit some affected people because it will not be available to most affected people. This objection raises quite a different issue from the one addressed in this article. The impetus for such research is the absence of effective treatment and not the absence of economic resources. We have discussed research intended to

determine whether effective but unaffordable interventions would work if used in lower, less expensive dosages. The researchable issue arises from an economic circumstance. The only way such research could offer any benefit is by "curing" the economic problem by establishing that the less expensive form of the intervention will be affordable and available. Absent knowledge of financial resources, one might well be creating a new unaffordable, and therefore useless, intervention. In contrast, in the case in which one is developing a new intervention, not because of poverty, but because no known effective intervention exists, and the disease is prevalent in a particular geographic area, the issue is quite different. In such a case one is not conducting research to try to "cure" the effects of poverty but rather because of the need to create new knowledge to treat a currently untreatable disease. However, even this case may raise problems similar to the ones addressed here. If one were to try to develop an intervention for such a condition and chose research subjects from impoverished segments of a society, knowing that only the richest segment of that society could benefit from that intervention, such subject selection would be unethical for many of the reasons we have discussed.

Our proposal to require researchers and their funders to develop realistic plans to make their interventions available to the relevant population of the developing country in which the research is proposed should not be controversial. It is well accepted in principle not only by groups like CIOMS, but by the funders of many of the African HIV trials, including the Centers for Disease Control and Prevention and the National Institutes of Health.[17] The principle is often honored in the breach, however. Research funders who hope that their studies will yield beneficial knowledge may neglect the steps necessary to ensure that the benefits will be made available. Ethical codes have not been sufficiently specific or enforceable to protect research subjects from exploitation. It is essential to replace vague promises with realistic plans that must be reviewed and approved before the research commences.

In at least one other instance it has been suggested that economic issues be addressed in the review of proposed research projects. The U.S. National Research Council's Committee on Human Genome Diversity recommended that "Arrangements regarding financial interests in the products or outcomes of the research should be negotiated as *part of the original project review* and informed-consent process."[18]

It is essential that the wealthier countries of the world use their resources, both financial and technological, to help resolve the health problems that afflict the poor of the world. Doing so will undoubtedly require research. But research is a means to solving health problems, not an end in itself. The goal must be to create interventions that will benefit the people of the countries in which the research is conducted. They will benefit only if the knowledge gained produces interventions that are affordable and accessible. This needs to be determined as a condition of approval before research is conducted so that limited research funds are not wasted, and research subjects are not drawn from populations that will not be able to benefit from the research.

REFERENCES

1 Lisa Belkin, "The Clues Are in the Blood," *New York Times Magazine,* 26 April 1998.

2 Michael Grodin and Leonard Glantz, eds., *Children as Research Subjects: Science. Ethics, and Law* (New York: Oxford University Press, 1994).

3 Wendy K. Mariner, "Distinguishing 'Exploitable' from 'Vulnerable' Populations: When Consent Is Not the Issue," in *Ethics and Research on Human Subjects: Proceedings,* ed. Zbigniew Bankowski and Robert J. Levine (Geneva: CIOMS, 1993), pp. 44–55.

4 Zbigniew Bankowski and Robert J. Levine. eds., *Ethics and Research on Human Subjects: International Guidelines* (Geneva: CIOMS. 1993), pp. 25–32. 43–46.

5 Sharon Perley, Sev S. Fluss, Zbigniew Bankowski, and Francoise Simon. "The Nuremberg Code: An International Overview," in *The Nazi Doctors and the Nuremberg Code,* ed. George J. Annas and Michael A. Grodin (New York: Oxford University Press, 1992), pp. 149–73.

6 Bankowski and Levine, *Ethics and Research,* p. 26. Emphasis added.

7 George Annas and Michael Grodin, "Human Rights and Maternal-Fetal HIV Transmission Prevention Trials in Africa," *American Journal of Public Health,* 88, no. 4 (1998): 560–63.

8 Edward Connor. Rhoda Sperling, Richard Gelber et al., "Reduction of Maternal-Infant Transmission of Human Immunodeficiency Virus Type 1 with Zidovudine Treatment," *NEJM* 331 (1994): 1173–80.

9 "Recommendation of the U.S. Public Health Service Task Force on the Use of Zidovudine to Reduce Prenatal Transmission of Human Immunodeficiency Virus," *MMWR Morbidity and Mortality Weekly Reports* 43 (1994): 1–20.

10 Harold Varmus and David Satcher, "Ethical Complexities of Conducting Research in Developing Countries," *NEJM* 337 (1997): 1003–1005.

11 The per capita health care expenditures of most of the African countries involved in mother-to-child HIV transmission prevention trials range from $5 to $22 U.S. *World Bank Sector Strategy Health Nutrition and Population,* 1997.

12 M. Bunce, "Chirac Seeks Worldwide Relief for AIDS in Africa," *Boston Globe,* 8 December 1997.

13 "Administration of Zidovudine During Late Pregnancy and Delivery to Prevent Perinatal HIV Transmission—Thailand 1996–1998," *MMWR Morbidity and Mortality Weekly Reports* 47, no. 8 (1998): 151–54. The editorial note states that "to implement these findings, ministries of health, donor agencies, and other interested agents *should* develop policies and practices to strengthen access to prenatal care, testing and counseling for HIV infections, and provision of ZDV for HIV-infected pregnant woman."

14 Bankowski and Levine, *Ethics and Research,* p. 45.

15 As the National Research Council's Committee on Human Genome Diversity properly put it, in the context of research on human subjects, "[s]ensitivity to the special practices and beliefs of a community cannot be used as a justification for violating universal human rights." Committee on Human Genetic Diversity, *Evaluating Human Genetic Diversity* (Washington, D.C.: National Academy Press, 1997), p. 65.

16 45 CFR 46.111(a)(3).

17 Varmus and Satcher, "Ethical Complexities of Conducting Research in Developing Countries."

18 *Evaluating Human Genetic Diversity,* at pp. 55–68. Emphasis added.

ETHICAL ISSUES IN CLINICAL TRIALS IN DEVELOPING COUNTRIES
Baruch Brody

Brody addresses three moral criticisms of recent clinical trials in developing countries that tested the efficacy of short-course AZT regimens in reducing maternal-fetal transmission of HIV: (1) that subjects who received placebos were treated unjustly; (2) that subjects' dire circumstances coerced them into agreeing to participate in the trials; and (3) that the developing countries in question were exploited insofar as they would not have access to the AZT regimens under study even if they proved effective (as argued by Glantz et al.). In response to the first criticism, Brody argues that the trials probably met the following appropriate standard of justice: "all participants in the study, including those in the control group, should not be denied any treatment *that should otherwise be available to [them] in light of the practical realities of health care resources available in the country in question.*" He responds to the second criticism by analyzing the concept of coercion and arguing that subjects were not coerced on any reasonable construal of this concept. Regarding the third criticism, Brody suggests that legitimate concerns about exploitation will be met if the subjects themselves—not necessarily the broader local community—are provided access to effective treatment following the study.

Since the publication of the results of AIDS Clinical Trials Group (ACTG) 076, it has been known that an extensive regimen of Zidovudine provided to the mother and to the newborn can drastically reduce (25.5 to 8.3%) the vertical transmission of HIV.[1] Unfortunately, the regimen in question is quite expensive and beyond the means of most developing countries, some of which are the countries most in need of effective techniques for reducing vertical transmission. This realization led to a series of important clinical trials designed to test the effectiveness of less extensive and less expensive regimens of antiretroviral drugs. These trials were conducted by researchers from developed countries in the developing countries which were in need of these less expensive regimens.

These new trials have been very successful. The Thai CDC trial showed a 50% reduction (18.9 to 9.4%) in transmission from a much shorter antepartum regimen of Zidovudine combined with a more modest intrapartum regimen.[2] The PETRA trial showed that Zidovudine and Lamivudine provided in modest intrapartum and postpartum regimens also significantly reduced transmission, whether or not they were provided antepartum.[3] There was a trend to more reduction of transmission if they were provided in a short antepartum regimen (16.5 to 7.8%) than if they were not (16.5 to 10.8%). Most crucially, there was no reduction (16.5 to 15.7%) if they were not provided postpartum. Finally, a single dose of nevirapine provided intrapartum and postpartum was shown in HIVNET 012 to significantly reduce transmission (21.3 to 11.9%).[4] In all cases except HIVNET 012, the control group received only a placebo. In HIVNET 012, the control group received a modest regimen of intrapartum and postpartum Zidovudine.

As a result of these trials, developing countries with some financial capabilities have the opportunity to drastically reduce vertical transmission by proven less expensive regimens. This constitutes an important contribution of these trials. Unfortunately, the poorest developing countries (including some in which these trials have been run) may not be able to afford even these shorter regimens unless the drugs in question are priced far less expensively for those countries. Efforts have begun to make that possible.[5]

Reprinted by permission of John Wiley & Sons Limited from *Statistics in Medicine,* vol. 21 (2002), pp. 2853–2858. © John Wiley & Sons Ltd.

There have been many critics of these trials who have argued that they were unethical. Some have gone on to attempt to explain how the information might have been obtained in other more ethical trials while others have not. My focus in this paper is not on that question. Instead, *I want to focus on the arguments offered in support of the claim that these trials were unethical.* I see the critics as advancing three very different criticisms, although the critics often do not carefully distinguish them. We will do so to enable each criticism to be analyzed. The *first criticism* is that an *injustice was done to the control group* in each of these trials (with perhaps the exception of HIVNET 012) since they were denied proven effective therapy as they only received a placebo. The *second criticism* is that the *participants in the trial were coerced* into participating, and did not give voluntary consent, because they had no real choice about participating since antiretroviral therapy was otherwise unavailable to them. The *third criticism* is that the *countries in question were exploited* by the investigators from the developed countries since they were testing the effectiveness of regimens that would not be available after the trial to the citizens of the countries in which the trials were conducted.

THE JUSTICE OF THE USE OF THE PLACEBO CONTROL GROUP

The scientific importance of the use of concurrent placebo control groups is well illustrated by the PETRA trial. If there had been no such control group, and the various regimens had been compared to the historical control group in ACTG 076, then the intrapartum only arm would have been judged a success, since its transmission rate was only 15.7% as compared to the 25.5% transmission rate in the control group in ACTG 076. But it actually was no better than the placebo control group in PETRA (16.5%). When the rate of transmission varies from one setting to another, you really cannot use historical control groups. Despite this scientific value, the critics have argued that it was wrong to use a placebo control arm because the patients in that arm were being denied a proven therapy (the 076 regimen) and were being offered nothing in its place.[6] The critics claim that this did not meet the standard found in

earlier versions of the Declaration of Helsinki: "In any medical study, every patient, including those of a control group, if any, should be assured of the best proven diagnostic and therapeutic method."[7]

Defenders of these trials quite properly note that none of the participants in these trials would otherwise have received any antiretroviral therapy, so nothing was being denied to them that they would otherwise have received. How then, ask the defenders, can the members of the control group have been treated unjustly? This led to a proposed, very controversial and eventually rejected, revision of the Declaration of Helsinki which read: "In any biomedical research protocol every patient-subject, including those of a control group, if any, should be assured that he or she will not be denied access to the best proven diagnostic, prophylactic, or therapeutic method that would otherwise be available to him or her."[8] The point is then that the justice or injustice of what is done to the control group depends on what the members of that group *would* have received if the trial had not been conducted.

While the reality of what the members of the control group would have received is obviously relevant, I am not satisfied that this proposed revision would have properly taken that into account. Would it be just, for example, to use such a placebo control group in a trial in a developed country where the antiretroviral therapy is widely available except to members of some persecuted minority, from whom the control group is drawn? They *would* not have received the treatment if the trial had not been conducted, although they *should* have given the resources available in the developed country. Their use in a placebo control group is not therefore justified. The proposed revision made too much reference to what would have occurred and not enough to what should have occurred.

A recent workshop proposed instead that "study participants should be assured the highest standard of care practically attainable in the country in which the trial is being carried out."[9] This seems better, although it may suggest too much. Suppose that the treatment is practically attainable but only by inappropriately cutting corners on other forms of health care which may have a higher priority. I would suggest therefore that the normative nature of the standard be made explicit. It would then read that all participants in the study, including those in the control group, should not be denied any treatment *that should otherwise be available to him or her in light of the practical realities of health care resources available in the country in question.* The question for IRBs reviewing proposals for such research is then precisely the question of justice.

On that standard, the trials in question were probably not unjust, although there is some debate about the Thai CDC trial in light of donated resources that became available in Thailand between its being planned and its being implemented.[10] Such trials will be harder to justify in the future given the current availability of proven much less expensive therapies which should be available even in some of the poorest countries. It is of interest to note that HIVNET 012 was not a placebo-controlled trial, but it was a superiority trial, and active controlled trials are less problematic scientifically when they are superiority trials. That may well be the way future transmission trials will be run.

COERCIVE OFFERS

It has been suggested by other critics that the participants in these trials were coerced into participating because of their desperation. "The very desperation of women with no alternatives to protect their children from HIV infection can be extremely coercive," argue one set of critics.[11] One of the requirements of an ethical trial is that the participants voluntarily agree to participate, and how can their agreement to participate be voluntary if it was coerced?

This line of thinking is analogous to the qualms that many have about paying research subjects substantial sums of money for their participation in research. Such inducements are often rejected on the grounds that they are coercive, because they are too good to refuse. The ICH [International Conference on Harmonization] Guidelines for Good Clinical Practice is one of many standards which incorporate this approach when it stipulates that the "IRB/IEC should review both the amount and method of payment to subjects to assure that neither present problems of coercion or undue influences on the research subject."[12]

Normally, coercion involves a threat to put someone below their baseline unless they cooperate

with the demands of the person issuing the threat.[13] As the researchers were not going to do anything to those who chose not to participate, they were clearly not threatening them. Further evidence of this comes from the reflection that threats are unwelcome to the parties being threatened, and there is no reason to suppose that the potential subjects saw the request to participate as something unwelcome. Even the critics recognize this. The potential subjects were being offered an opportunity that might improve their situation. This was an offer "too good to refuse," not a threat.

Should we expand the concept of coercion to include these very favorable offers? There are several reasons for thinking that we should not. First, it is widely believed that offering people valuable new opportunities is desirable. Moreover, the individuals in question want to receive these offers, and denying them the opportunity to receive them seems paternalistic or moralistic.[14] It is important that participants understand that what they are being offered is a chance to receive a treatment that may reduce transmission (since this is a randomized placebo-controlled trial of a new regimen), and ensuring that is essential for the consent to be informed. As long as care is taken to ensure that this information is conveyed in a culturally sensitive fashion, and is understood, then there seems to be little reason to be concerned about coercion simply because a good opportunity is being offered to those with few opportunities.

A colleague and I are currently working on one residual concern in this area. It has to do with studies in which there is a potential for long-term harms to subjects which they inappropriately discount because the very substantial short-term benefits cloud their judgment. This may be a ground for concern in some cases, but it is difficult to see how it would apply to the vertical transmission trials. For those trials, it is appropriate to conclude that concerns about coercion were unfounded.

EXPLOITATION OF SUBJECTS

The final criticism of the trials is that they are exploitative of developing countries and their citizens because the interventions in question, even if proven successful, will not be available in these countries.

To quote one of the critics: "To use a population as research subjects because of its poverty and its inability to obtain care, and then to not use that knowledge for the direct benefit of that population, is the very definition of exploitation. This exploitation is made worse by the fact that richer nations will unquestionably benefit from this research . . . [they] will begin to use these lower doses, thereby receiving economic benefit."[15]

There are really two claims being advanced in that quotation. The second, that the developed countries ran these trials to discover cheaper ways of treating their own citizens, is very implausible since pregnant women in developed countries are receiving even more expensive cocktails of drugs both to treat the woman and to reduce transmission. The crucial issue is whether the trials are exploitative of the developing countries.

There seems to be a growing consensus that they are exploitative unless certain conditions about future availability in the country in question are met. The Council for International Organizations of Medical Sciences (CIOMS) is the source of this movement, as it declared in its 1992 guidelines that "as a general rule, the initiating agency should insure that, at the completion of successful testing, any products developed will be made reasonably available to residents of the host community or country."[16] A slightly weaker version of this requirement was adopted by a recent workshop which concluded that "studies are only appropriate if there is a reasonable likelihood that the populations in which they are carried out stand to benefit from successful results."[17]

This growing consensus is part of what lies behind the effort to secure these benefits by negotiating more favorable prices for the use of the tested drugs in developing countries. It seems highly desirable that this goal be achieved. But I want to suggest that it should be viewed as an aspiration, rather than a requirement, and that a different, more modest requirement must be met to avoid charges of exploitation.

A good analysis of exploitation is that it is a wrong done to individuals who do not receive a fair share of the benefits produced by an activity in which they take part, even if they receive some benefit.[18] This is why a mutually beneficial activity, one from which both parties will be better off, can still be exploitative if one of the parties uses their greater bargaining power to harvest most of the benefits and the other party agrees because they need whatever modest benefit is being left for them.

As we apply this concept to the trials in question, we need to ask who needs to be protected from being exploited by the trials in question. It would seem that it is the participants. Are they getting a fair share of the benefits from the trial if it proves successful? This is a particularly troubling question when we consider those in the control group, whose major benefit from participation may have been an unrealized possibility of getting treated. If we judge that the participants have not received enough, then it is they who must receive more. An obvious suggestion is that they be guaranteed access to any regimen proved efficacious in any future pregnancies (or perhaps even that they be granted access to antiretroviral therapy for their own benefit). This would be analogous to familiar concepts of subjects receiving continued access to treatment after their participation in a trial is completed.

I certainly support every reasonable effort to increase access to treatments which will reduce vertical transmission. But imposing the types of community-wide requirements that have been suggested, but not necessarily justified if the above analysis is correct, may prevent important trials from being run because of the potential expense. Such proposals should be treated as moral aspirations, and exploitation should be avoided by focusing on what is owed to the subjects who have participated in the trials. It is they, after all, who are primarily at risk for being exploited.

These observations are about research in developing countries in general, and not just about research on vertical transmission. Three lessons have emerged. The standard for when a placebo control group is justified is a normative standard (what they should have received if they were not in the trial) rather than a descriptive standard (what they would have received if they were not in the trial). Coercion is not a serious concern in trials simply because attractive offers are made to the subjects. Legitimate concerns about exploiting subjects should be addressed by ensuring their future treatment, rather than by asking what will happen in their community at large.

NOTES

1 E. M. Connor, R. S. Sperling, R. Gelber, et al., "Reduction of Maternal-Infant Transmission of Human Immunodeficiency Virus Type I with Zidovudine Treatment," *New England Journal of Medicine,* 331 (1984): 1173–80.

2 N. Shaffer, R. Chuachoowong, P. A. Mock, et al., "Short-Course Zidovudine for Perinatal HIV Transmission in Bangkok, Thailand: A Randomised Controlled Trial," *Lancet,* 353 (1999): 773–80.

3 Conference data cited in K. DeCock, M. Fowler, E. Mercier, et al., "Prevention of Mother-to-Child HIV Transmission in Resource Poor Countries," *JAMA,* 283 (2000): 1175–82.

4 L. A. Guay, P. Musoke, T. Fleming, et al., "Intrapartum and Neonatal Single-Dose Nevirapine Compared with Zidovudine for Prevention of Mother-to-Child Transmission of HIV-1 in Kampala, Uganda," *Lancet,* 354 (2000): 795–802.

5 P. Brown, "Cheaper AIDS Drugs Due for Third World," *Nature,* 405 (2000): 263.

6 P. Lurie and S. M. Wolfe, "Unethical Trials of Interventions to Reduce Perinatal Transmission of the Human Immunodeficiency Virus in Developing Countries," *New England Journal of Medicine,* 337 (1997): 853–56.

7 World Medical Association, Declaration of Helsinki, Principle 11.3.

8 "Proposed Revision of the Declaration of Helsinki," *Bulletin of Medical Ethics,* 18–21 (1999).

9 Perinatal HIV Intervention Research in Developing Countries Workshop Participants, "Science Ethics and the Future of Research into Maternal Infant Transmission of HIV-1," *Lancet,* 353 (1999): 832–35.

10 P. Phanuphak, "Ethical Issues in Studies in Thailand of the Vertical Transmission of HIV," *New England Journal of Medicine,* 338 (1998): 834–35.

11 E. Tafesse and T. Murphy, Letter, *New England Journal of Medicine,* 338 (1998): 838.

12 ICH, *Guideline for Good Clinical Practice* (Geneva: IFPMA, 1996), guideline 3.1.8.

13 R. Nozick, "Coercion." In Morgenbesser S., ed. *Philosophy, Science, and Method* (New York: St. Martin's, 1969).

14 M. Wilkinson and A. Moore, "Inducement in Research," *Bioethics,* 11 (1997): 373–89.

15 I. Glantz and M. Grodin, Letter, *New England Journal of Medicine,* 338 (1998): 839.

16 CIOMS, *International Ethical Guidelines for Biomedical Research Involving Subjects* (Geneva: CIOMS, 1992), 68.

17 Perinatal HIV Intervention Research in Developing Countries Workshop Participants, "Science Ethics and the Future of Research into Maternal Infant Transmission of HIV-1," *Lancet,* 353 (1999): 832–35.

18 A. Wertheimer, *Exploitation* (Princeton, N.J.: Princeton University Press, 1996).

ANIMAL RESEARCH

THE CASE FOR THE USE OF ANIMALS IN BIOMEDICAL RESEARCH
Carl Cohen

Identifying himself as a speciesist, Cohen defends the extensive use of animals in biomedical research. Against the "animal rights" view, he contends that animals are incapable of moral agency and therefore lack moral rights. Against Peter Singer's view, which extends to animals the principle of equal consideration of interests, he maintains that animals' interests are not due equal consideration because animals lack the moral standing of humans; speciesism is therefore not analogous to racism and sexism. Indeed, Cohen argues, we have an obligation to expand animal research both to protect potential human subjects and to benefit future patients with advances in biomedicine. In his view, our obligations toward animals (e.g., not to be cruel to them) are minimal and do not compare in importance with our obligations to beings who have rights—namely, human beings.

Using animals as research subjects in medical investigations is widely condemned on two grounds: first, because it wrongly violates the *rights* of animals,[1] and second, because it wrongly imposes on sentient creatures much avoidable *suffering*.[2] Neither of these arguments is sound. The first relies on a mistaken understanding of rights; the second relies on a mistaken calculation of consequences. Both deserve definitive dismissal.

WHY ANIMALS HAVE NO RIGHTS

A right, properly understood, is a claim, or potential claim, that one party may exercise against another. The target against whom such a claim may be registered can be a single person, a group, a community, or (perhaps) all humankind. The content of rights claims also varies greatly: repayment of loans, nondiscrimination by employers, noninterference by the state, and so on. To comprehend any genuine right fully, therefore, we must know *who* holds the right, *against whom* it is held, and *to what* it is a right.

Alternative sources of rights add complexity. Some rights are grounded in constitutional law (e.g., the right of an accused to trial by jury); some rights are moral but give no legal claims (e.g., my right to your keeping the promise you gave me); and some rights (e.g., against theft or assault) are rooted both in morals and in law.

The differing targets, contents, and sources of rights, and their inevitable conflict, together weave a tangled web. Notwithstanding all such complications, this much is clear about rights in general: they are in every case claims, or potential claims, within a community of moral agents. Rights arise, and can be intelligibly defended, only among beings who actually do, or can, make moral claims against one another. Whatever else rights may be, therefore, they are necessarily human; their possessors are persons, human beings.

The attributes of human beings from which this moral capability arises have been described variously by philosophers, both ancient and modern: the

inner consciousness of a free will (Saint Augustine[3]); the grasp, by human reason, of the binding character of moral law (Saint Thomas[4]); the self-conscious participation of human beings in an objective ethical order (Hegel[5]); human membership in an organic moral community (Bradley[6]); the development of the human self through the consciousness of other moral selves (Mead[7]); and the underivative, intuitive cognition of the rightness of an action (Prichard[8]). Most influential has been Immanuel Kant's emphasis on the universal human possession of a uniquely moral will and the autonomy its use entails.[9] Humans confront choices that are purely moral; humans—but certainly not dogs or mice—lay down moral laws, for others and for themselves. Human beings are self-legislative, morally *autonomous*.

Animals (that is, nonhuman animals, the ordinary sense of that word) lack this capacity for free moral judgment. They are not beings of a kind capable of exercising or responding to moral claims. Animals therefore have no rights, and they can have none. This is the core of the argument about the alleged rights of animals. The holders of rights must have the capacity to comprehend rules of duty, governing all including themselves. In applying such rules, the holders of rights must recognize possible conflicts between what is in their own interest and what is just. Only in a community of beings capable of self-restricting moral judgments can the concept of a right be correctly invoked.

Humans have such moral capacities. They are in this sense self-legislative, are members of communities governed by moral rules, and do possess rights. Animals do not have such moral capacities. They are not morally self-legislative, cannot possibly be members of a truly moral community, and therefore cannot possess rights. In conducting research on animal subjects, therefore, we do not violate their rights, because they have none to violate.

To animate life, even in its simplest forms, we give a certain natural reverence. But the possession of rights presupposes a moral status not attained by the vast majority of living things. We must not infer, therefore, that a live being has, simply in being alive, a "right" to its life. The assertion that all animals, only because they are alive and have interests, also possess the "right to life"[10] is an abuse of that phrase, and wholly without warrant.

It does not follow from this, however, that we are morally free to do anything we please to animals. Certainly not. In our dealings with animals, as in our dealings with other human beings, we have obligations that do not arise from claims against us based on rights. Rights entail obligations, but many of the things one ought to do are in no way tied to another's entitlement. Rights and obligations are not reciprocals of one another, and it is a serious mistake to suppose that they are.

Illustrations are helpful. Obligations may arise from internal commitments made: physicians have obligations to their patients not grounded merely in their patients' rights. Teachers have such obligations to their students, shepherds to their dogs, and cowboys to their horses. Obligations may arise from differences of status: adults owe special care when playing with young children, and children owe special care when playing with young pets. Obligations may arise from special relationships: the payment of my son's college tuition is something to which he may have no right, although it may be my obligation to bear the burden if I reasonably can; my dog has no right to daily exercise and veterinary care, but I do have the obligation to provide these things for her. Obligations may arise from particular acts or circumstances: one may be obliged to another for a special kindness done, or obliged to put an animal out of its misery in view of its condition—although neither the human benefactor nor the dying animal may have had a claim of right.

Plainly, the grounds of our obligations to humans and to animals are manifold and cannot be formulated simply. Some hold that there is a general obligation to do no gratuitous harm to sentient creatures (the principle of nonmaleficence); some hold that there is a general obligation to do good to sentient creatures when that is reasonably within one's power (the principle of beneficence). In our dealings with animals, few will deny that we are at least obliged to act humanely—that is, to treat them with the decency and concern that we owe, as sensitive human beings, to other sentient creatures. To treat animals humanely, however, is not to treat them as humans or as the holders of rights.

A common objection, which deserves a response, may be paraphrased as follows:

> If having rights requires being able to make moral claims, to grasp and apply moral laws, then many humans—the brain-damaged, the comatose, the senile—who plainly lack those capacities must be without rights. But that is absurd. This proves [the critic concludes] that rights do not depend on the presence of moral capacities.[1, 10]

This objection fails; it mistakenly treats an essential feature of humanity as though it were a screen for sorting humans. The capacity for moral judgment that distinguishes humans from animals is not a test to be administered to human beings one by one. Persons who are unable, because of some disability, to perform the full moral functions natural to human beings are certainly not for that reason ejected from the moral community. The issue is one of kind. Humans are of such a kind that they may be the subject of experiments only with their voluntary consent. The choices they make freely must be respected. Animals are of such a kind that it is impossible for them, in principle, to give or withhold voluntary consent or to make a moral choice. What humans retain when disabled, animals have never had.

A second objection, also often made, may be paraphrased as follows:

> Capacities will not succeed in distinguishing humans from the other animals. Animals also reason; animals also communicate with one another; animals also care passionately for their young; animals also exhibit desires and preferences.[11, 12] Features of moral relevance—rationality, interdependence, and love—are not exhibited uniquely by human beings. Therefore [this critic concludes], there can be no solid moral distinction between humans and other animals.[10]

This criticism misses the central point. It is not the ability to communicate or to reason, or dependence on one another, or care for the young, or the exhibition of preference, or any such behavior that marks the critical divide. Analogies between human families and those of monkeys, or between human communities and those of wolves, and the like, are entirely beside the point. Patterns of conduct are not at issue. Animals do indeed exhibit remarkable behavior at times. Conditioning, fear, instinct, and intelligence all contribute to species survival. Membership in a community of moral agents nevertheless remains impossible for them. Actors subject to moral judgment must be capable of grasping the generality of an ethical premise in a practical syllogism. Humans act immorally often enough, but only they—never wolves or monkeys—can discern, by applying some moral rule to the facts of a case, that a given act ought or ought not to be performed. The moral restraints imposed by humans on themselves are thus highly abstract and are often in conflict with the self-interest of the agent. Communal behavior among animals, even when most intelligent and most endearing, does not approach autonomous morality in this fundamental sense.

Genuinely moral acts have an internal as well as an external dimension. Thus, in law, an act can be criminal only when the guilty deed, the actus reus, is done with a guilty mind, mens rea. No animal can ever commit a crime; bringing animals to criminal trial is the mark of primitive ignorance. The claims of moral right are similarly inapplicable to them. Does a lion have a right to eat a baby zebra? Does a baby zebra have a right not to be eaten? Such questions, mistakenly invoking the concept of right where it does not belong, do not make good sense. Those who condemn biomedical research because it violates "animal rights" commit the same blunder.

IN DEFENSE OF "SPECIESISM"

Abandoning reliance on animal rights, some critics resort instead to animal sentience—their feelings of pain and distress. We ought to desist from the imposition of pain insofar as we can. Since all or nearly all experimentation on animals does impose pain and could be readily forgone, say these critics, it should be stopped. The ends sought may be worthy, but those ends do not justify imposing agonies on humans, and by animals the agonies are felt no less. The laboratory use of animals (these critics conclude) must therefore be ended—or at least very sharply curtailed.

Argument of this variety is essentially utilitarian, often expressly so[13]; it is based on the calcula-

tion of the net product, in pains and pleasures, resulting from experiments on animals. Jeremy Bentham, comparing horses and dogs with other sentient creatures, is thus commonly quoted: "The question is not, Can they reason? nor Can they talk? but, Can they suffer?"[14]

Animals certainly can suffer and surely ought not to be made to suffer needlessly. But in inferring, from these uncontroversial premises, that biomedical research causing animal distress is largely (or wholly) wrong, the critic commits two serious errors.

The first error is the assumption, often explicitly defended, that all sentient animals have equal moral standing. Between a dog and a human being, according to this view, there is no moral difference; hence the pains suffered by dogs must be weighed no differently from the pains suffered by humans. To deny such equality, according to this critic, is to give unjust preference to one species over another; it is "speciesism." The most influential statement of this moral equality of species was made by Peter Singer:

> The racist violates the principle of equality by giving greater weight to the interests of members of his own race when there is a clash between their interests and the interests of those of another race. The sexist violates the principle of equality by favoring the interests of his own sex. Similarly the speciesist allows the interests of his own species to override the greater interests of members of other species. The pattern is identical in each case.[2]

This argument is worse than unsound; it is atrocious. It draws an offensive moral conclusion from a deliberately devised verbal parallelism that is utterly specious. Racism has no rational ground whatever. Differing degrees of respect or concern for humans for no other reason than that they are members of different races is an injustice totally without foundation in the nature of the races themselves. Racists, even if acting on the basis of mistaken factual beliefs, do grave moral wrong precisely because there is no morally relevant distinction among the races. The supposition of such differences has led to outright horror. The same is true of the sexes, neither sex being entitled by right to greater respect or concern than the other. No dispute here.

Between species of animate life, however—between (for example) humans on the one hand and cats or rats on the other—the morally relevant differences are enormous, and almost universally appreciated. Humans engage in moral reflection; humans are morally autonomous; humans are members of moral communities, recognizing just claims against their own interest. Human beings do have rights; theirs is a moral status very different from that of cats or rats.

I am a speciesist. Speciesism is not merely plausible; it is essential for right conduct, because those who will not make the morally relevant distinctions among species are almost certain, in consequence, to misapprehend their true obligations. The analogy between speciesism and racism is insidious. Every sensitive moral judgment requires that the differing natures of the beings to whom obligations are owed be considered. If all forms of animate life—or vertebrate animal life?—must be treated equally, and if therefore in evaluating a research program the pains of a rodent count equally with the pains of a human, we are forced to conclude (1) that neither humans nor rodents possess rights, or (2) that rodents possess all the rights that humans possess. Both alternatives are absurd. Yet one or the other must be swallowed if the moral equality of all species is to be defended.

Humans owe to other humans a degree of moral regard that cannot be owed to animals. Some humans take on the obligation to support and heal others, both humans and animals, as a principal duty in their lives; the fulfillment of that duty may require the sacrifice of many animals. If biomedical investigators abandon the effective pursuit of their professional objectives because they are convinced that they may not do to animals what the service of humans requires, they will fail, objectively, to do their duty. Refusing to recognize the moral differences among species is a sure path to calamity. (The largest animal rights group in the country is People for the Ethical Treatment of Animals; its codirector, Ingrid Newkirk, calls research using animal subjects "fascism" and "supremacism." "Animal liberationists do not separate out the *human* animal," she says, "so there is no rational basis for saying that a human being has special rights. A rat is a pig is a dog is a boy. They're all mammals."[15])

Those who claim to base their objection to the use of animals in biomedical research on their reckoning of the net pleasures and pains produced make a second error, equally grave. Even if it were true—as it is surely not—that the pains of all animate beings must be counted equally, a cogent utilitarian calculation requires that we weigh all the consequences of the use, and of the nonuse, of animals in laboratory research. Critics relying (however mistakenly) on animal rights may claim to ignore the beneficial results of such research, rights being trump cards to which interest and advantage must give way. But an argument that is explicitly framed in terms of interest and benefit for all over the long run must attend also to the disadvantageous consequences of not using animals in research, and to all the achievements attained and attainable only through their use. The sum of the benefits of their use is utterly beyond quantification. The elimination of horrible disease, the increase of longevity, the avoidance of great pain, the saving of lives, and the improvement of the quality of lives (for humans and for animals) achieved through research using animals is so incalculably great that the argument of these critics, systematically pursued, establishes not their conclusion but its reverse: to refrain from using animals in biomedical research is, on utilitarian grounds, morally wrong.

When balancing the pleasures and pains resulting from the use of animals in research, we must not fail to place on the scales the terrible pains that would have resulted, would be suffered now, and would long continue had animals not been used. Every disease eliminated, every vaccine developed, every method of pain relief devised, every surgical procedure invented, every prosthetic device implanted—indeed, virtually every modern medical therapy is due, in part or in whole, to experimentation using animals. Nor may we ignore, in the balancing process, the predictable gains in human (and animal) well-being that are probably achievable in the future but that will not be achieved if the decision is made now to desist from such research or to curtail it.

Medical investigators are seldom insensitive to the distress their work may cause animal subjects. Opponents of research using animals are frequently insensitive to the cruelty of the results of the restrictions they would impose.[2] Untold numbers of human beings—real persons, although not now identifiable—would suffer grievously as the consequence of this well-meaning but shortsighted tenderness. If the morally relevant differences between humans and animals are borne in mind, and if all relevant considerations are weighed, the calculation of long-term consequences must give overwhelming support for biomedical research using animals.

CONCLUDING REMARKS

Substitution The humane treatment of animals requires that we desist from experimenting on them if we can accomplish the same result using alternative methods—in vitro experimentation, computer simulation, or others. Critics of some experiments using animals rightly make this point.

It would be a serious error to suppose, however, that alternative techniques could soon be used in most research now using live animal subjects. No other methods now on the horizon—or perhaps ever to be available—can fully replace the testing of a drug, a procedure, or a vaccine, in live organisms. The flood of new medical possibilities being opened by the successes of recombinant DNA technology will turn to a trickle if testing on live animals is forbidden. When initial trials entail great risks, there may be no forward movement whatever without the use of live animal subjects. In seeking knowledge that may prove critical in later clinical applications, the unavailability of animals for inquiry may spell complete stymie. In the United States, federal regulations require the testing of new drugs and other products on animals, for efficacy and safety, before human beings are exposed to them.[16, 17] We would not want it otherwise.

Every advance in medicine—every new drug, new operation, new therapy of any kind—must sooner or later be tried on a living being for the first time. That trial, controlled or uncontrolled, will be an experiment. The subject of that experiment, if it is not an animal, will be a human being. Prohibiting the use of live animals in biomedical research, therefore, or sharply restricting it, must result either in the blockage of much valuable research or in the replacement of animal subjects with human sub-

jects. These are the consequences—unacceptable to most reasonable persons—of not using animals in research.

Reduction Should we not at least reduce the use of animals in biomedical research? No, we should increase it, to avoid when feasible the use of humans as experimental subjects. Medical investigations putting human subjects at some risk are numerous and greatly varied. The risks run in such experiments are usually unavoidable, and (thanks to earlier experiments on animals) most such risks are minimal or moderate. But some experimental risks are substantial.

When an experimental protocol that entails substantial risk to humans comes before an institutional review board, what response is appropriate? The investigation, we may suppose, is promising and deserves support, so long as its human subjects are protected against unnecessary dangers. May not the investigators be fairly asked, Have you done all that you can to eliminate risk to humans by the extensive testing of that drug, that procedure, or that device on animals? To achieve maximal safety for humans we are right to require thorough experimentation on animal subjects before humans are involved.

Opportunities to increase human safety in this way are commonly missed; trials in which risks may be shifted from humans to animals are often not devised, sometimes not even considered. Why? For the investigator, the use of animals as subjects is often more expensive, in money and time, than the use of human subjects. Access to suitable human subjects is often quick and convenient, whereas access to appropriate animal subjects may be awkward, costly, and burdened with red tape. Physician-investigators have often had more experience working with human beings and know precisely where the needed pool of subjects is to be found and how they may be enlisted. Animals, and the procedures for their use, are often less familiar to these investigators. Moreover, the use of animals in place of humans is now more likely to be the target of zealous protests from without. The upshot is that humans are sometimes subjected to risks that animals could have borne, and should have borne, in their place. To maximize the protection of human subjects, I conclude, the wide and imaginative use of live animal subjects should be encouraged rather than discouraged. This enlargement in the use of animals is our obligation.

Consistency Finally, inconsistency between the profession and the practice of many who oppose research using animals deserves comment. This frankly ad hominem observation aims chiefly to show that a coherent position rejecting the use of animals in medical research imposes costs so high as to be intolerable even to the critics themselves.

One cannot coherently object to the killing of animals in biomedical investigations while continuing to eat them. Anesthetics and thoughtful animal husbandry render the level of actual animal distress in the laboratory generally lower than that in the abattoir. So long as death and discomfort do not substantially differ in the two contexts, the consistent objector must not only refrain from all eating of animals but also protest as vehemently against others eating them as against others experimenting on them. No less vigorously must the critic object to the wearing of animal hides in coats and shoes, to employment in any industrial enterprise that uses animal parts, and to any commercial development that will cause death or distress to animals.

Killing animals to meet human needs for food, clothing, and shelter is judged entirely reasonable by most persons. The ubiquity of these uses and the virtual universality of moral support for them confront the opponent of research using animals with an inescapable difficulty. How can the many common uses of animals be judged morally worthy, while their use in scientific investigation is judged unworthy?

The number of animals used in research is but the tiniest fraction of the total used to satisfy assorted human appetites. That these appetites, often base and satisfiable in other ways, morally justify the far larger consumption of animals, whereas the quest for improved human health and understanding cannot justify the far smaller, is wholly implausible. Aside from the numbers of animals involved, the distinction in terms of worthiness of use, drawn with regard to any single animal, is not defensible. A given sheep is surely not more justifiably used to put lamb chops on the supermarket counter than to serve

in testing a new contraceptive or a new prosthetic device. The needless killing of animals is wrong; if the common killing of them for our food or convenience is right, the less common but more humane uses of animals in the service of medical science are certainly not less right.

Scrupulous vegetarianism, in matters of food, clothing, shelter, commerce, and recreation, and in all other spheres, is the only fully coherent position the critic may adopt. At great human cost, the lives of fish and crustaceans must also be protected, with equal vigor, if speciesism has been forsworn. A very few consistent critics adopt this position. It is the reductio ad absurdum of the rejection of moral distinctions between animals and human beings.

Opposition to the use of animals in research is based on arguments of two different kinds—those relying on the alleged rights of animals and those relying on the consequences for animals. I have argued that arguments of both kinds must fail. We surely do have obligations to animals, but they have, and can have, no rights against us on which research can infringe. In calculating the consequences of animal research, we must weigh all the long-term benefits of the results achieved—to animals and to humans— and in that calculation we must not assume the moral equality of all animate species.

REFERENCES

1 Regan T. The case for animal rights. Berkeley, Calif.: University of California Press, 1983.
2 Singer P. Animal liberation. New York: Avon Books, 1977.
3 St. Augustine. Confessions. Book Seven. 397 A.D. New York: Pocketbooks, 1957:104–26.
4 St. Thomas Aquinas. Summa theologica. 1273 A.D. Philosophic texts. New York: Oxford University Press, 1960:353–66.
5 Hegel GWF. Philosophy of right. 1821. London: Oxford University Press, 1952:105–10.
6 Bradley F. H. Why should I be moral? 1876. In: Melden AI, ed. Ethical theories. New York: Prentice-Hall, 1950:345–59.
7 Mead G. H. The genesis of the self and social control. 1925. In: Reck A. J, ed. Selected writings. Indianapolis: Bobbs-Merrill, 1964:264–93.
8 Prichard H. A. Does moral philosophy rest on a mistake? 1912. In: Cellars W, Hospers J, eds. Readings in ethical theory. New York: Appleton-Century-Crofts, 1952:149–63.
9 Kant I. Fundamental principles of the metaphysic of morals. 1785. New York: Liberal Arts Press, 1949.

10 Rollin B. E. Animal rights and human morality. New York: Prometheus Books, 1981.

11 Hoff C. Immoral and moral uses of animals. N Engl J Med 1980; 302:115–8.

12 Jamieson D. Killing persons and other beings. In: Miller H. B, Williams WH, eds. Ethics and animals. Clifton, N.J.: Humana Press, 1983:135–46.

13 Singer P. Ten years of animal liberation. New York Review of Books. 1985; 31:46–52.

14 Bentham J. Introduction to the principles of morals and legislation. London: Athlone Press, 1970.

15 McCabe K. Who will live, who will die? Washingtonian Magazine. August 1986:115.

16 U.S. Code of Federal Regulations, Title 21, Sect. 505(i). Food, drug, and cosmetic regulations.

17 U.S. Code of Federal Regulations, Title 16, Sect. 1500.40-2. Consumer product regulations.

THE RESPONSIBLE USE OF ANIMALS IN BIOMEDICAL RESEARCH
Edwin Converse Hettinger

Hettinger responds directly to Cohen's defense of animal research. Against Cohen's thesis that only human beings can have rights, Hettinger argues that one need not be a moral agent to possess rights, as suggested by the examples of human infants and severely retarded humans. Regarding Cohen's embrace of speciesism, Hettinger advances several arguments in an effort to demonstrate the incoherence of attributing moral status to a being on the basis of species membership rather than on the basis of the individual's characteristics. He goes on to argue that utilitarianism—which incorporates a principle of equal consideration of interests—supports animal research only in those cases where it also supports research on human beings whose mental capacities are comparable to those of animals. Hettinger next contends that the promise of alternatives to animal research is much greater than Cohen allows, before sketching an equal-consideration approach to the human use of animals.

Carl Cohen's defense of the use of animals for biomedical research in *The New England Journal of Medicine*[1] raises most of the major issues in the moral controversy concerning human treatment of nonhuman animals. It exhibits the major lines of attack against both animal rights advocates (such as Tom Regan)[2] and utilitarian animal-liberationists (such as Peter Singer).[3] It is also a showcase of the most common mistakes made by those who seek to defend the current human use of animals. . . .

DO ALL HUMANS BUT NO ANIMALS HAVE RIGHTS?

Cohen argues that only human beings can have rights.

Reprinted with permission of the author and the publisher from *Between the Species,* vol. 5, no. 3 (Summer 1989), pp. 123–31.

Rights arise, and can be intelligibly defended, only among beings who actually do, or can, make moral claims against one another. Whatever else rights may be, therefore, they are necessarily human; their possessors are persons, human beings. (p. 104)

Cohen is correct in maintaining that rights cannot arise unless there exist moral agents for whom these rights claims make sense. To say that some being has a right is to say (at least in part) that some other being has obligations to treat the right holder in certain ways specified by that right. So if there were no beings more cognitively and morally capable than pigs or dogs, there would be no rights.

However, the fact that rights claims require the existence of duty bearers does not imply that only those duty bearers can have rights. Even Cohen would grant that human infants have rights, yet they are not duty bearers. Thus, some creatures possess rights despite being unable to invoke them against others or to recognize and respect others' rights.

Cohen attempts to avoid this objection by shifting his criterion of rights possession to the *capacity* for being a moral agent, rather than actually being a moral agent.

> Animals . . . are not beings of a kind capable of exercising or responding to moral claims. Animals therefore have no rights, and they can have none. . . . The holders of rights must have the capacity to comprehend rules of duty. . . . (p. 104)

However, most people would grant that severely retarded humans have rights (Cohen does), and yet they do not have "the capacity to comprehend rules of duty." Thus if having the capacity to be a duty bearer is necessary for the possession of rights, then severely retarded humans cannot have rights.

Cohen responds to this point with his talk of "kinds."

> The capacity for moral judgment that distinguishes humans from animals is not a test to be administered to human beings one by one. Persons who are unable, because of some disability, to perform the full moral functions natural to human beings are certainly not for that reason ejected from the moral community. The issue is one of kind. Humans are of such a kind that they may be the subject of experiments only with their voluntary consent. The choices they make freely must be respected. Animals are of such a kind that it is impossible for them, in principle, to give or withhold voluntary consent or to make a moral choice. What humans retain when disabled, animals have never had. (p. 106)

Cohen seems to be claiming that the capacity for moral agency is essential to human beings and is necessarily lacking in other animals. Thus, severely retarded humans, because they are human, retain the capacity for moral agency even in their retarded state. Animals by their very nature lack this capacity. Since the capacity for moral agency confers rights, severely retarded humans have rights, whereas animals do not.

But many severely retarded humans could never carry out even the quasi-moral functions that some animals can perform. Dogs, for example, can be obedient, protective, and solicitous, while there are severely retarded humans who could not achieve these minimal moral abilities despite our best efforts. Given this fact, it just is not plausible to claim that severely retarded humans have the capacity for moral agency, while claiming that psychologically sophisticated animals do not. Cohen certainly has not given us any reason to accept this claim. He simply assumes that being a member of a biological species guarantees that one has certain capacities, despite overwhelming evidence that marginal members of species often lack capacities normal for that kind of creature. We need a strong argument before we should reject the obvious point that some animals have a greater capacity for moral behavior (however minimal) than do some severely retarded human beings.

Cohen might argue that severely retarded humans have the capacity for moral agency despite lacking the ability to realize that capacity. But why should we accept such an attenuated notion of capacity? Certainly capacities can be left unrealized, but if there is no possibility that they could ever be developed, what sense is there in claiming that the capacity is present? I see no reason to accept the notion that there can be unrealizable capacities.

IS SPECIESISM DEFENSIBLE?

Perhaps Cohen would agree that severely retarded humans lack the capacity for moral agency but thinks this is unimportant. He may be arguing that we should treat the severely retarded as human beings and that since human beings have rights (presumably because many of them are moral agents), severely retarded humans have rights as well. On this reading, Cohen is suggesting that we treat individuals according to their biological kind and ignore their individual characteristics. Moral status is to be determined by species membership, not individual qualities. This is "speciesism": the view that species membership is by itself a morally legitimate reason for treating individuals differently.

Peter Singer and others have argued that speciesism is "a form of prejudice no less objectionable than racism or sexism."[4] Cohen's speciesist perspective concerning the moral status of animals vis-à-vis humans does coincide uncomfortably with the outlook of racists and sexists toward blacks and women. Both judge according to class membership while ignoring individual qualities.

Cohen responds to this charge of speciesism by embracing it:

> I am a speciesist. Speciesism is not merely plausible; it is essential for right conduct, because those who will not make the morally relevant distinctions among species are almost certain, in consequence, to misapprehend their true obligations. The analogy between speciesism and racism is insidious. Every sensitive moral judgment requires that the differing natures of the beings to whom obligations are owed be considered. (p. 109)

This passage defends the truism that there often are differences between members of distinct species which are morally relevant in determining how we should treat them. But this is not what is at issue in the debate over speciesism. Singer, Regan, and other opponents of speciesism are not suggesting that we ignore morally relevant differences between members of different species and treat them all identically. (They are not suggesting, for example, that dogs be allowed at the dinner table or be allowed to vote.) What rejecting speciesism commits one to is being unwilling to use difference in species by itself as a reason for treating individuals differently. Similarly, rejecting racism and sexism commits one to not using race or sex by itself as a reason for differential treatment. Cohen's truism does not support speciesism in this problematic sense.

The analogy between speciesism and racism or sexism is deficient in one respect. Species classification marks broader differences between beings than does racial or sexual classification. Thus attempting to justify differential treatment on the basis of species membership alone (as Cohen does) is not *just* as morally objectionable as doing so on the basis of race or sex, since members of different species are more likely to require differential treatment than are members of different races or sexes (within a species). For example, in determining what sort of food or shelter to provide, it would be much more important to know a creature's species than it would be to know a person's race or sex.

But this does not imply that difference in species by itself is a morally legitimate reason for treating individuals differently, while difference in race or sex considered by itself is not. Arguing that a woman should be prohibited from combat because of her sex fails to provide a morally relevant reason for the recommendation. Arguing for this on the grounds that this woman lacks the required physical capacities is to provide a morally relevant reason. Similarly, arguing that a chimpanzee should be experimentally sacrificed rather than a human, simply because it is a chimpanzee, gives no morally relevant reason for the recommendation. However, arguing that the chimpanzee does not value or plan for its future life to the extent that the human does is to provide such a reason.

Thus even though considerations of species are frequently more closely correlated with morally relevant features than are considerations of race or sex, species membership by itself (like racial or sexual class membership) is not a morally legitimate reason for differential treatment. Speciesism is thus a moral mistake of the same sort as racism and sexism: it advocates differential treatment on morally illegitimate grounds.

The illegitimacy of judgments based on species membership alone becomes especially clear when comparing the moral status of a severely retarded human with that of psychologically sophisticated animals, since here the individual does not have what most members of the species have. The morally relevant differences which *usually* exist between individuals of two different biological kinds (and hence which would frequently justify treating them differently) are lacking when comparing severely retarded humans with psychologically sophisticated animals. Any plausible morally relevant characteristic—whether it be rationality, self-sufficiency, ability to communicate, free choice, moral agency, psychological sophistication, fullness of life, and so on—is possessed by some animals to a greater extent than by some severely retarded humans. In this case, to classify by biological kind and to argue for differential treatment on that basis alone obscures and ignores morally relevant features rather than relying on them. We should not treat individuals on the basis of group or kind membership when their individual characteristics are readily apparent and relevant.

Thus, Cohen's argument fails on this second interpretation, as well. His appeal to biological kind to justify differential moral status of severely retarded humans and psychologically sophisticated animals is an unjustified form of speciesism. Unless Cohen can show us that there is some morally relevant difference between severely retarded humans and psychologically sophisticated animals, his position is open to the following objection: if experimenting on severely retarded humans is a violation of their rights, then experimenting on psychologically sophisticated animals violates their rights, as well.

DOES UTILITARIANISM JUSTIFY ANIMAL EXPERIMENTATION?

Utilitarians hold that the right policy is the one whose consequences maximize the satisfaction of interests. In this calculation the interests of all affected parties are fairly taken into account. Utilitarians who oppose animal experimentation do so not on the grounds that animal rights are violated but because they think that the overall good resulting from these experiments is not sufficient to justify their negative consequences. The benefits which result from animal experimentation (such as an increase in scientific and medical knowledge) either do not outweigh the costs (e.g., animal pain and death) or could be achieved in a less costly fashion.

Cohen rejects the utilitarian critic's position that the like interests of humans and animals should be given equal moral weight. He denies that similar amounts of human and animal pain are equally morally significant.

> The first error is the assumption, often explicitly defended, that all sentient animals have equal moral standing. Between a dog and a human being, according to this view, there is no moral difference; hence the pains suffered by dogs must be weighed no differently from the pains suffered by humans. . . . If all forms of animate life . . . must be treated equally, and if therefore in evaluating a research program the pains of a rodent count equally with the pains of a human, we are forced to conclude (1) that neither humans nor rodents possess rights, or (2) that rodents possess all the rights that humans possess. . . . One or the other must be swallowed if the moral equality of all species is to be defended. (pp. 108–9)

This argument misses the mark. To claim that animals "have equal moral standing" and should have their like interests treated equally implies neither that there are no moral differences between humans and animals nor that we should treat animals in the same manner that we do humans.

From the utilitarian position that the right act is the one which maximizes the net satisfaction of interests it follows that it is morally preferable to give a human a slightly less amount of pain than to give an animal a slightly greater amount of pain (or *vice versa*). If the pains are of equal intensity and consequence, then one should be morally indifferent. The fact that one is the pain of a human and the other is the pain of an animal is not by itself morally relevant.

This is not to say that the same type of experiment on a human and an animal would cause each the same amount of pain and suffering and that we should be indifferent to which being we use. Giving a typical chimpanzee a deadly virus in order to test a vaccine is likely to cause less pain and suffering than giving a typical human the deadly virus for the same purpose. The greater psychological sophistication of the human, its greater intelligence and self-consciousness, makes possible a greater degree of pain and suffering. (Sometimes the reverse is true, however.)[5]

Even though pain and suffering would often be minimized by experimenting on an animal instead of a typical human, that does not show that we may morally discount the pain and suffering of animals. We must still count the pain and suffering of animals equally with the like pain and suffering of humans. But in cases where a human will suffer more, we should prefer the use of animals (and *vice versa*).

Cohen is thus mistaken in thinking that giving equal consideration to the like interests of animals and humans makes moral discriminations between the two impossible. For a utilitarian, equal consideration (or equal moral standing) does not imply identical treatment. Cohen has given us no cogent reason for rejecting the view that the like pains of humans and animals must be given equal moral weight. Since the pain of the animals on whom we experiment cannot be discounted, Cohen's utilitarian justification for the biomedical use of animals becomes far more difficult to achieve.

Cohen argues that even if "the pains of all animate beings must be counted equally" (p. 109), a utilitarian calculus would still come out in support of the biomedical use of animals:

> The sum of the benefits of their use is utterly beyond quantification. The elimination of horrible disease, the increase of longevity, the avoidance of great pain, the saving of lives, and the improvement of the quality of lives (for humans and for animals) achieved through research using animals is so incalculably great that the argument of these critics, systematically pursued, establishes not their conclusion but its reverse: to refrain from using animals in biomedical research is, on utilitarian grounds, morally wrong. (p. 110)

Substantial benefits have resulted (and continue to result) from biomedical experimentation, much of which involves the use of animals. And although a utilitarian benefit/cost analysis would reach the conclusion that it would be wrong to stop the use of animals entirely, it would not justify Cohen's call for an increase in the biomedical use of animals. Cohen can reach this conclusion only by abandoning utilitarianism (and its principle of equal consideration of like interests), by adopting the speciesist position which treats animal pain and distress as insignificant when it is a means to human benefit, and by being overly pessimistic about the possibility of alternatives to animal use.

THE POSSIBILITY OF SUBSTITUTION

Whether research using living creatures is justified on utilitarian grounds depends in large part on the availability of substitute procedures. A utilitarian benefit/cost analysis (which must consider alternative, less costly ways to achieve these benefits) would find that some, perhaps many but certainly not all experiments, using animals are morally justifiable. *Some* use of living beings continues to be

necessary and justifiable. Even developing alternatives to the biomedical use of animals often requires the use of animals. At present substitute techniques are not sufficiently developed to eliminate this use entirely (and they may never be).[6]

Nevertheless, Cohen is overly pessimistic about the possibility of alternatives to the current biomedical use of animals. His speciesism prevents him from appreciating or even acknowledging the numerous substitute procedures that are being developed. A recent report by the U.S. Congress' Office of Technology Assessment (OTA) on alternatives to animal use in research, testing, and education is much more encouraging about the potential for alternatives.[7] This study presents numerous suggestions involving the replacement, reduction, and refinement of the use of animals. In addition to the promising techniques of in vitro experimentation and computer simulation (which Cohen mentions), the OTA report suggests:

1. Coordinating investigations and sharing information (to reduce duplicative experiments when necessary for validating the original research);

2. Replacing the use of higher animals with lower animals (invertebrates for vertebrates and cold-blooded for warm-blooded animals);

3. Using plants instead of animals;

4. Sharing animals (e.g., getting several tissues from one animal);

5. Designing experiments which use statistical inferences and whose design provides reliable information despite the use of fewer animals;

6. Decreasing the pain and distress in animal experimentation by altering the experimental design and by using anesthetics and tranquilizers;

7. Using non-living chemical and physical systems that mimic biological functions;

8. Using human and animal cadavers; and

9. Teaching by demonstration instead of by individual student use of animals.

Recent amendments to the Animal Welfare Act[8] and the Public Health Service Act,[9] as well as legislation concerning the education of health professionals,[10] all encourage alternatives to the current methods of animal use.[11] Cohen's pessimistic assessment of these alternatives flies in the face of a growing trend of using already existing alternatives and of developing new substitute procedures. Experiments which cause animals pain, distress, or death are clearly not justifiable when such substitute procedures are available.

SHOULD WE INCREASE BIOMEDICAL ANIMAL USE?

Cohen argues that in order to achieve maximum safety for humans "the wide and imaginative use of live animal subjects should be encouraged rather than discouraged" (p. 112). Cohen is right that some experiments which subject humans to risk could be conducted using animals without loss in the significance of the results. Furthermore, risky experiments which are necessary *should* be performed on psychologically less sophisticated creatures. An increase in psychological sophistication brings with it a wider range of interests, a greater ability to experience satisfaction (and dissatisfaction), and the possibility of leading a fuller life. Inflicting suffering or death on these creatures causes greater harm.

In advocating an increase in the biomedical use of animals Cohen not only ignores the available alternatives but disregards the widespread experimental misuse of animals, as well. Numerous books and articles have persuasively documented that many experiments using animals have been unprofessional, of dubious scientific merit, repetitive, or cruel.[12] Two video tapes are especially persuasive; "Unnecessary Fuss," about head injury research involving baboons at the University of Pennsylvania,[13] and "Tools for Research," a general review of research using animals over the last twenty years.[14] The flurry of recent legislation concerning animal welfare cited above shows a growing public recognition of the misuse of laboratory animals. Government regulations for the care of laboratory animals have been developed to prevent these sorts of experiments, as well.[15] Cohen's suggestion that we encourage the wide and imaginative use of live animal subjects, instead of limiting this use and working to find substitute techniques, shows blatant disregard for this widely acknowledged problem.

CAN A CONSISTENT POSITION CONCERNING ANIMAL USE BE DEVELOPED?

Cohen charges his anti-speciesist opponents with inconsistency or absurdity: "Scrupulous vegetarianism, in matters of food, clothing, shelter, commerce, and recreation, and in all other spheres, is the only fully coherent position the critic may adopt" (p. 113). The person who eats veal and then strenuously objects to the killing of cats in relatively painless medical experiments *is* inconsistent. We do not *need* to eat animals for food (certainly not mammals); carefully chosen vegetarian diets are perfectly healthy. We do need the ongoing results of biomedical research and for some of this research the use of living creatures continues to be required.

Cohen is right that the use of animals in biomedical research is less difficult to defend than are other uses of animals. (Only one out of every hundred animals used is for this purpose.)[16] But the anti-speciesist critic of current biomedical uses of animals need not be committed to prohibiting all uses of animals. Since anti-speciesism allows for discriminating between animals, critics can consistently object to the raising, slaughtering, and consumption of veal calves while not objecting to commercial shrimp farming and shrimp consumption. A critic might also object to repeated surgery on healthy animals in the training of veterinarians and not object to the use of chick embryos for toxicity testing. The recommendation that experimenters substitute cold-blooded animals for warm-blooded ones or invertebrates for vertebrates is also perfectly consistent. These suggestions are not speciesist, since species membership *per se* is not the justification offered for differential treatment. Differences in the fullness of life, in psychological sophistication, and in the capacity for suffering are what motivates these suggestions.

Thus, one can argue for limiting animal use in biomedical research without embracing the extreme position prohibiting all uses of any animals for whatever reason. Cohen can successfully saddle only his most extreme opponents with this consequence. A more circumspect skepticism about the legitimacy of a significant portion of laboratory animal use is possible. Advocates of limiting the use of animals in biomedical research can consistently advocate the limited use of animals in other areas, as well. Both extremes—the absolute prohibition of all animal use, as well as Cohen's speciesist encouragement of such use—should be avoided. . . . [17]

NOTES

1 Carl Cohen, "The Case for the Use of Animals in Biomedical Research," *New England Journal of Medicine* 315 (1986): 865–70. [All page references are to section 10 of this volume]

2 Tom Regan, *The Case for Animal Rights* (Berkeley, Calif.: University of California Press, 1983).

3 Peter Singer, *Animal Liberation* (New York: Avon Books, 1975).

4 Peter Singer, "Animal Liberation" in *People, Penguins, and Plastics,* ed. Donald VanDeVeer and Christine Pierce (Belmont, Calif.: Wadsworth, 1986), p. 31.

5 Peter Singer, *Practical Ethics* (Cambridge: Cambridge University Press, 1979), p. 53.

6 Office of Technology Assessment (OTA), *Alternatives to Animal Use in Research, Testing, and Education,* publication no. OTA-BA-273 (Washington, D.C.: U.S. Government Printing Office, 1986), p. 138.

7 Ibid.

8 The Food Security Act of 1985 (Public Law 99–198).

9 The Health Research Extension Act of 1985 (Public Law 99–158).

10 The Health Professions Educational Assistance Amendments of 1985 (Public Law 99–129).

11 See OTA, *Alternatives to Animal Use in Research, Testing, and Education,* chap. 13.

12 See Singer, *Animal Liberation,* chap. 2; Richard Ryder, "Speciesism in the Laboratory" in *In Defense of Animals,* ed. Peter Singer (New York: Basil Blackwell, 1985) pp. 77–88; Dale Jamieson and Tom Regan, "On the Ethics of the Use of Animals in Science," in *And Justice for All* (Totowa, N.J.: Rowman and Littlefield, 1982), pp. 169–96; Bernard Rollin, *Animal Rights and Human Morality* (Buffalo, N.Y.: Prometheus Books, 1981), chap. 3.

13 Available from People for the Ethical Treatment of Animals, P.O. Box 42516, Washington, D.C. 20015.

14 Available from Bullfrog Films, Inc., Olney, Penn.

15 See National Institutes of Health, *Guidelines for the Care and Use of Laboratory Animals,* NIH publication no. 85-23 (Bethesda, Md.: National Institutes of Health, 1985).

16 See OTA, *Alternatives to Animal Use in Research, Testing, and Education,* p. 43.

17 I would like to thank Beverly Diamond, John Dickerson, Martin Perlmutter, and Hugh Wilder for helpful suggestions on earlier drafts of this paper.

THE ETHICS OF ANIMAL RESEARCH: WHAT ARE THE PROSPECTS FOR AGREEMENT?

David DeGrazia

After sketching the political background to the debate over animal research as well as the general ethical perspectives of the biomedical and animal protection communities, DeGrazia argues that representatives of these two groups can agree on some important ethical claims—and that further realistic steps can build on this common ground. First, he identifies and defends ten ethical claims on which reasonable members of both groups should, despite their differences, concur. Next, he identifies four issues on which disagreement between the two communities is likely to persist even if the discussion is open-minded, well informed, and honest. Finally, he enumerates ten concrete steps that the biomedical and/or animal protection communities can take to foster better communication about the animal research issue and more defensible practices.

Few human uses of nonhuman animals (hereafter simply "animals") have incited as much controversy as the use of animals in biomedical research. The political exchanges over this issue tend to produce much more heat than light, as representatives of both biomedicine and the animal protection community accuse opponents of being "Nazis," "terrorists," and the like. However, a healthy number of individuals within these two communities offer the possibility of a more illuminating discussion of the ethics of animal research.

One such individual is Henry Spira. Spira almost single-handedly convinced Avon, Revlon, and other major cosmetics companies to invest in the search for alternatives to animal testing. Largely due to his tactful but persistent engagement with these companies—and to their willingness to change—many consumers today look for such labels as "not tested on animals" and "cruelty free" on cosmetics they would like to buy.

Inspired by Spira, this paper seeks common ground between the positions of biomedicine and animal advocates. (The term "biomedicine" here refers to everyone who works in medicine or the life sciences, not just those conducting animal research. "Animal advocates" and "animal protection community" refer to those individuals who take a major interest in protecting the interests of animals and who believe that much current usage of animals is morally unjustified. The terms are not restricted to animal activists, because some individuals meet this definition without being politically active in seeking changes.) The paper begins with some background on the political and ethical debate over animal research. It then identifies important points of potential agreement between biomedicine and animal advocates; much of this common ground can be missed due to distraction by the fireworks of the current political exchange. Next, the paper enumerates issues on which continuing disagreement is likely. Finally, it concludes with concrete suggestions for building positively on the common ground.

Reprinted with the permission of Cambridge University Press from *Cambridge Quarterly of Healthcare Ethics,* vol. 8, no. 1 (Winter 1999), pp. 23–34. Copyright © 1999 Cambridge University Press.

My thanks to Arlene Klotzko and Peter Singer for their suggestions regarding this paper.

BACKGROUND ON THE DEBATE OVER ANIMAL RESEARCH

What is the current state of the debate over the ethics of animal research? Let us begin with the viewpoint of biomedicine. It seems fair to say that biomedicine has a "party line" on the ethics of animal research, conformity to which may feel like a political litmus test for full acceptability within the professional community. According to this party line, animal research is clearly justified because it is necessary for medical progress and therefore human health—and those who disagree are irrational, antiscience, misanthropic "extremists" whose views do not deserve serious attention. (Needless to say, despite considerable conformity, not everyone in biomedicine accepts this position.)

In at least some countries, biomedicine's leadership apparently values conformity to this party line more than freedom of thought and expression on the animal research issue. (In this paragraph, I will refer to the American situation to illustrate the point.) Hence the unwillingness of major medical journals, such as *JAMA* and *The New England Journal of Medicine,* to publish articles that are highly critical of animal research. Hence also the extraordinary similarity I have noticed in pro-research lectures by representatives of biomedicine. I used to be puzzled about why these lectures sounded so similar and why, for example, they consistently made some of the same philosophical and conceptual errors (such as dichotomizing animal welfare and animal rights, and taking the latter concept to imply identical rights for humans and animals). But that was before I learned of the "AMA [American Medical Association] Animal Research Action Plan" and the AMA's "White Paper." Promoting an aggressive pro-research campaign, these documents encourage AMA members to say and do certain things for public relations purposes, including the following: "Identify animal rights activists as anti-science and against medical progress"; "Combat emotion with emotion (eg [sic], 'fuzzy' animals contrasted with 'healing' children)"; and "Position the biomedical community as moderate—centrist—in the controversy, not as a polar opposite.[1]

It is a reasonable conjecture that biomedicine's party line was developed largely in reaction to fear—

both of the most intimidating actions of some especially zealous animal advocates, such as telephoned threats and destruction of property, and of growing societal concern about animals. Unfortunately, biomedicine's reaction has created a political culture in which many or most animal researchers and their supporters do not engage in sustained, critical thinking about the moral status of animals and the basic justification (or lack thereof) for animal research. Few seem to recognize that there is significant merit to the opposing position, fewer have had any rigorous training in ethical reasoning, and hardly any have read much of the leading literature on animal ethics. The stultifying effect of this cultural phenomenon hit home with me at a small meeting of representatives of biomedicine, in which I had been invited to explain "the animal rights philosophy" (the invitation itself being exceptional and encouraging). After the talk, in which I presented ideas familiar to all who really know the literature and issues of animal ethics, several attendees pumped my hand and said something to this effect: "This is the first time I have heard such rational and lucid arguments for the other side. I didn't know there were any."

As for the animal protection community, there does not seem to be a shared viewpoint except at a very general level: significant interest in animal welfare and the belief that much current animal usage is unjustified. Beyond that, differences abound. For example, the Humane Society of the United States opposes factory farming but not humane forms of animal husbandry, rejects current levels of animal use in research but not animal research itself, and condemns most zoo exhibits but not those that adequately meet animals' needs and approximate their natural habitats.[2] Meanwhile, the Animal Liberation Front, a clandestine British organization, apparently opposes all animal husbandry, animal research, and the keeping of zoo animals.[3] Although there are extensive differences within the animal protection community, as far as our paper topic goes, it seems fair to say that almost everyone in this group opposes current levels of animal research.

That's a brief sketch of the perspectives of biomedicine and animal advocates on the issue of animal research. What about the state of animal ethics itself? The leading book-length works in this field

exhibit a near consensus that the status quo of animal usage is ethically indefensible and that at least significant reductions in animal research are justified. Let me elaborate.

Defending strong animal rights positions in different ways, Tom Regan and Evelyn Pluhar advocate abolition of all research that involves harming animals.[4] Ray Frey and Peter Singer, by contrast, hold the use of animals to the very stringent utilitarian standard—accepting only those experiments whose benefits (factoring in the likelihood of achieving them) are expected to outweigh the harms and costs involved—where the interests of animal subjects (e.g., to avoid suffering) are given the same moral weight that we give comparable human interests.[5]

Without commiting either to a strong animal rights view or to utilitarianism, my own view shares with these theories the framework of equal consideration for animals: the principle that we must give equal moral weight to comparable interests, no matter who has those interests.[6] But unlike the aforementioned philosophers, I believe that the arguments for and against equal consideration are nearly equal in strength. I therefore have respect for progressive views that attribute moral standing to animals without giving them fully equal consideration. The unequal consideration view that I find most plausible gives moral weight to animals' comparable interests in accordance with the animals' cognitive, affective, and social complexity—a progressive, "sliding scale" view. Since I acknowledge that I might be mistaken about equal consideration, my approach tracks the practical implications both of equal consideration and of the alternative just described.

Arguing from pluralistic frameworks, which are developed in different ways, Steve Sapontzis, Rosemary Rodd, and Bernard Rollin support relatively little animal research in comparison with current levels.[7] Drawing significantly from feminist insights, Mary Midgley presents a view whose implications seem somewhat more accepting of the status quo of animal research but still fairly progressive.[8] Of the leading contributors to animal ethics, the only one who embraces the status quo of animal research and does not attribute significant moral status to animals is Peter Carruthers.[9] (It is ironic that while biomedicine characterizes those who are critical of animal research as irrational "extremists," nearly all of the most in-depth, scholarly, and respected work in animal ethics supports such a critical standpoint at a general level.)

In discussing the prospects for agreement between biomedicine and animal advocates, I will ignore political posturing and consider only serious ethical reflection. In considering the two sides of this debate, I will assume that the discussants are morally serious, intellectually honest, reflective, and well informed both about the facts of animal research and about the range of arguments that come into play in animal ethics. I will not have in mind, then, the researcher who urges audiences to dismiss "the animal rights view" or the animal activist who tolerates no dissent from an abolitionist position. The two representative interlocutors I will imagine differ on the issue of animal research, but their views result from honest, disciplined, well-informed ethical reflection. Clearly, their voices are worth hearing.

POINTS ON WHICH THE BIOMEDICAL AND ANIMAL PROTECTION COMMUNITIES CAN AGREE

The optimistic thesis of this paper is that the biomedical and animal protection communities can agree on a fair number of important points, and that much can be done to build upon this common ground. I will number and highlight (in bold) each potential point of agreement and then justify its inclusion by explaining how both sides can agree to it, without abandoning their basic positions, and why they should.

1. The use of animals in biomedical research raises ethical issues. Today very few people would disagree with this modest claim, and any who would are clearly in the wrong.[10] Most animal research involves harming animal subjects, provoking ethical concerns, and the leading goal of animal research, promotion of human health, is itself ethically important; even the expenditure of taxpayers' money on government-funded animal research raises ethical issues about the best use of such money. Although a very modest assertion, this point of agreement is important because it legitimates a process that is sometimes resisted: *discussing* the ethics of animal research.

It is worth noting a less obvious claim that probably enjoys strong majority support but not consensus: that animals (at least sentient ones, as defined below) have moral status. To say animals have moral status is to say that their interests have moral importance independently of effects on human interests. ("Interests" may be thought of as components of well-being. For example, sentient animals have an interest in avoiding pain, distress, and suffering.) If animals have moral status, then to brutalize a horse is wrong because of the harm inflicted on the horse, not simply because the horse is someone's property (if that is so) or because animal lovers' feelings may be hurt (if any animal lovers find out about the abuse). The idea is that gratuitously harming the horse *wrongs the horse*. Although nearly every leader in animal ethics holds that animals have moral status—and though most people, on reflection, are likely to find this idea commonsensical—Carruthers argues that it is mistaken.[11]

2. Sentient animals, a class that probably includes at least the vertebrates, deserve moral protection. Whether because they have moral status or because needlessly harming them strongly offends many people's sensibilities, sentient animals deserve some measure of moral protection. By way of definition, sentient animals are animals endowed with any sorts of feelings: (conscious) sensations such as pain or emotional states such as fear or suffering. But which animals are sentient? Addressing this complex issue implicates both the natural sciences and the philosophy of mind. Lately, strong support has emerged for the proposition that at least vertebrate animals are very likely sentient.[12] This proposition is implicitly endorsed by major statements of principles regarding the humane use of research animals, which often mention that they apply to vertebrates.[13] (Hereafter, the unqualified term "animals" will refer to sentient animals in particular.)

3. Many animals (at the very least, mammals) are capable of having a wide variety of aversive mental states, including pain, distress (whose forms include discomfort, boredom, and fear), and suffering. In biomedical circles, there has been some resistance to attributing suffering to animals, so government documents concerned with humane use of animals have often mentioned only pain, distress, and discomfort.[14] Because "suffering" refers to a *highly* unpleasant mental state (whereas pain, distress, and discomfort can be mild and transient), the attribution of suffering to animals is morally significant. An indication that resistance may be weakening is the attribution of suffering to sentient animals in the National Aeronautics and Space Administration's "Principles for the Ethical Care and Use of Animals."[15] Whatever government documents may say, the combined empirical and philosophical case for attributing suffering to a wide range of animals is very strong.[16]

4. Animals' experiential well-being (quality of life) deserves protection. If the use of animals raises ethical issues, meaning that their interests matter morally, we confront the question of what interests animals have. This question raises controversial issues. For example, do animals have an interest in remaining alive (life interests)? That is, does death itself—as opposed to any unpleasantness experienced in dying—harm an animal? A test case would be a scenario in which a contented dog in good health is painlessly and unwittingly killed in her sleep: Is she harmed?

Another difficult issue is whether animal well-being can be understood *entirely* in terms of experiential well-being—quality of life in the familiar sense in which (other things equal) pleasure is better than pain, enjoyment better than suffering, satisfaction better than frustration. Or does the exercise of an animal's natural capacities count positively toward well-being, even if quality of life is not enhanced? A test case would be a scenario in which conditioning, a drug, or brain surgery removes a bird's instinct and desire to fly without lowering quality of life: Does the bird's transformation to a new, nonflying existence represent a harm?

Whatever the answers to these and other issues connected with animal well-being, what is not controversial is that animals have an interest in experiential well-being, a good quality of life. That is why animal researchers are normally expected to use anesthesia or analgesia where these agents can reduce or eliminate animal subjects' pain, distress, or suffering.

5. Humane care of highly social animals requires extensive access to conspecifics. It is increasingly appreciated that animals have different needs based on what sorts of creatures they are.

Highly social animals, such as apes, monkeys, and wolves, need social interactions with conspecifics (members of their own species). Under normal circumstances, they will develop social structures, such as hierarchies and alliances, and maintain long-term relationships with conspecifics. Because they have a strong instinct to seek such interactions and relationships, depriving them of the opportunity to gratify this instinct harms these animals. For example, in some species, lack of appropriate social interactions impedes normal development. Moreover, social companions can buffer the effects of stressful situations, reduce behavioral abnormalities, provide opportunities for exercise, and increase cognitive stimulation.[17] Thus in the case of any highly social animals used in research, providing them extensive access to conspecifics is an extremely high moral priority.

6. Some animals deserve very strong protections (as, for example, chimpanzees deserve not to be killed for the purpose of population control). Biomedicine and animal advocates are likely to disagree on many details of ethically justified uses of animals in research, as we will see in the next section. Still, discussants can agree that there is an obligation to protect not just the experiential well-being, but also the lives, of at least some animals. This claim might be supported by the (controversial) thesis that such animals have life interests. On the other hand, it might be supported by the goal of species preservation (in the case of an endangered species), or by the recognition that routine killing of such animals when they are no longer useful for research would seriously disturb many people.[18]

Without agreeing on all the specific justifications, members of the National Research Council's Committee on Long-Term Care of Chimpanzees were able to agree (with one dissent) that chimps should not be killed for the purpose of population control, although they could be killed if suffering greatly with no alternative means of relief.[19] This recommended protection of chimps' lives is exceptional, because animal research policies generally state no presumption against killing animal subjects, requiring only that killings be as painless as possible.[20] Since this committee represents expert opinion in biomedicine, it seems correct to infer that biomedicine and the animal protection community can agree that at least chimpanzees should receive some very strong protections—of their lives and of certain other components of their well-being, such as their needs for social interaction, reasonable freedom of movement, and stimulating environments.[21]

7. Alternatives should now be used whenever possible and research on alternatives should expand. Those who are most strongly opposed to animal research hold that alternatives such as mathematical models, computer simulations, and in vitro biological systems should replace nearly all use of animals in research. (I say "nearly all" because, as discussed below, few would condemn animal research that does not harm its subjects.) Even for those who see the animal research enterprise more favorably, there are good reasons to take an active interest in alternatives. Sometimes an alternative method is the most valid way to approach a particular scientific question; often alternatives are cheaper.[22] Their potential for reducing animal pain, distress, and suffering is, of course, another good reason. Finally, biomedicine may enjoy stronger public support if it responds to growing social concern about animal welfare with a very serious investment in nonanimal methods. This means not just using alternatives wherever they are currently feasible, but also aggressively researching the possibilities for expanding the use of such methods.

8. Promoting human health is an extremely important biomedical goal. No morally serious person would deny the great importance of human health, so its status as a worthy goal seems beyond question. What is sometimes forgotten, however, is that a worthy goal does not automatically justify all the means thereto. Surely it would be unethical to force large numbers of humans to serve as subjects in highly painful, eventually lethal research, even if its goal were to promote human health. The controversy over animal research focuses not on the worthiness of its principal goal—promoting human health—but rather on the means, involving animal subjects, taken in pursuit of that goal.

9. There are some morally significant differences between humans and other animals. Many people in biomedicine are not aware that the views of animal advocates are consistent with this judgment. Indeed, some animal advocates might not re-

alize that their views are consistent with this judgment! So let me identify a couple of ideas, to which all should agree, that support it.

First, the principle of respect for autonomy applies to competent adult human beings, but to very few if any animals. This principle respects the self-regarding decisions of individuals who are capable of autonomous decisionmaking and action. Conversely, it opposes paternalism toward such individuals, who have the capacity to decide for themselves what is in their interests. Now, many sentient beings, including human children and at least most nonhuman animals, are not autonomous in the relevant sense and so are not covered by this principle.[23] Thus it is often appropriate to limit their liberty in ways that promote their best interests, say, preventing the human child from drinking alcohol, or forcing a pet dog to undergo a vaccination. We might say that where there is no autonomy to respect, the principles of beneficence (promoting best interests) and respect for autonomy cannot conflict; where there is autonomy to respect, paternalism becomes morally problematic.

Second, even if sentient animals have an interest, others things equal, in staying alive (as I believe), the moral presumption against taking human life is stronger than the presumption against killing at least some animals. Consider fish, who are apparently sentient yet cognitively extremely primitive in comparison with humans. I have a hard time imagining even very committed animal advocates maintaining that killing a fish is as serious a matter as killing a human being. Leaders in animal ethics consistently support—though in interestingly different ways—the idea that, ordinarily, killing humans is worse than killing at least some animals who have moral status. (It is almost too obvious to mention that it's worse to kill humans than to kill animals, such as amoebas, that *lack* moral status.[24])

The only notable exception seems to be Sapontzis, who tries to undermine the major arguments proffered to support such comparative claims. But the comparisons he opposes always involve humans and other mammals or birds.[25] The farther one goes down the phylogenetic scale, the more incredible it becomes to hold that it is equally prima facie wrong to kill humans and to kill other animals. At the very least, someone like Sapontzis will have to admit that killing humans tends to be worse than killing fish in that (1) humans tend to live much longer, so that untimely death generally robs them of more good years, and (2) untimely human death causes deep social sorrow and anguish to others in a way that is not paralleled in the fish world. So I believe that the comparative judgment I have made is well justified and embraceable by all parties to the present debate. There may be other morally interesting differences to which all should agree,[26] but these examples will suffice for present purposes.

10. Some animal research is justified. Many animal advocates would say that they disagree with this statement. But I'm not sure they do. Or, if they really do, they shouldn't. Let me explain by responding to the three likeliest reasons some animal advocates might take exception to the claim.

First, one might oppose all uses of animals that involve *harming them for the benefit of others* (even other animals)—as a matter of absolute principle—and overlook the fact that some animal research does not harm animal subjects at all. Although such nonharmful research represents a tiny sliver of the animal research enterprise, it exists. Examples are certain observational studies of animals in their natural habitats, some ape language studies, and possibly certain behavioral studies of other species that take place in laboratories but do not cause pain, distress, or suffering to the subjects. And if nonsentient animals cannot be harmed (in any morally relevant sense), as I would argue, then any research involving such animals falls under the penumbra of nonharming research.

Moreover, there is arguably no good reason to oppose research that imposes only *minimal* risk or harm on its animal subjects. After all, minimal risk research on certain human subjects who, like animals, cannot consent (namely, children) is permitted in many countries; in my view, this policy is justified. Such research might involve a minuscule likelihood of significant harm or the certainty of a slight, transient harm, such as the discomfort of having a blood sample taken.

Second, one might oppose all animal research because one believes that none of it actually benefits human beings. Due to physical differences between species, the argument goes, what happens to animal subjects when they undergo some biomedical intervention does not justify inferences about what will happen to humans who undergo that intervention. Furthermore, new drugs, therapies, and techniques must always be tried on human subjects before they can be accepted for clinical practice. Rather than tormenting animals in research, the argument continues, we should drop the useless animal models and proceed straight to human trials (with appropriate protections for human subjects, including requirements for informed or proxy consent).

Although I believe a considerable amount of current animal research has almost no chance of benefitting humans,[27] I find it very hard to believe that no animal research does. While it is true that human subjects must eventually be experimented on, evidence suggests that animal models sometimes furnish data relevant to human health.[28] If so, then the use of animal subjects can often decrease the risk to human subjects who are eventually involved in experiments that advance biomedicine, by helping to weed out harmful interventions. This by itself does not justify animal research, only the claim that it sometimes benefits humans (at the very least human subjects themselves and arguably the beneficiaries of biomedical advances as well).

Note that even if animal research never benefited humans, it would presumably sometimes benefit conspecifics of the animals tested, in sound veterinary research.[29] It can't be seriously argued that animal models provide no useful information about animals! Moreover, in successful *therapeutic* research (which aims to benefit the subjects themselves), certain animals benefit directly from research and are not simply used to benefit other animals. For that reason, blanket opposition to animal research, including the most promising therapeutic research in veterinary medicine, strikes me as almost unintelligible.

Almost unintelligible, but not quite, bringing us to the third possible reason for opposing all animal research. It might be argued that, whether or not it harms its subjects, all animal research involves *using animals (without their consent) for others' benefit,* since—qua research—it seeks *generalizable knowledge.* But to use animals in this way reduces them to *tools* (objects to be used), thereby *disrespecting* the animals.

Now the idea that we may never use nonconsenting individuals, even in benign ways, solely for the benefit of others strikes me as an implausibly strict ethical principle. But never mind. The fact that some veterinary research is intended to benefit the subjects themselves (as well as other animals or humans down the road) where no other way to help them is known shows that such research, on any reasonable view, is *not* disrespectful toward its subjects. Indeed, in such cases, the animals *would* consent to taking part, if they could, because taking part is in their interests. I fully grant that therapeutic veterinary research represents a minuscule portion of the animal research conducted today. But my arguments are put forward in the service of a goal that I think I have now achieved: demonstrating, beyond a shadow of a doubt, that some animal research is justified.

If animal advocates and representatives of biomedicine were aware of these ten points of potential agreement, they might perceive their opponents' views as less alien than they had previously taken them to be. This change in perception might, in turn, convince all parties that honest, open discussion of outstanding issues has a decent chance of repaying the effort.

POINTS ON WHICH AGREEMENT BETWEEN THE TWO SIDES IS UNLIKELY

Even if biomedicine and the animal protection community approach the animal research issue in good faith, become properly informed about animal ethics and the facts of research, and so forth, they are still likely to disagree on certain important issues. After all, their basic views differ. It may be worthwhile to enumerate several likely points of difference.

First, disagreement is likely on the issue of *the moral status of animals in comparison with humans*. While representatives of biomedicine may attribute moral status to animals, they hold that animals may justifiably be used in many experiments (most of which are nontherapeutic and harm the subjects) whose primary goal is to promote human health. But for animal advocates, it is not at all obvious that

much animal research is justified. This suggests that animal advocates ascribe higher moral status to animals than biomedicine does.[30]

Second, disagreement is likely to continue on the issue of *the specific circumstances in which the worthy goal of promoting human health justifies harming animals*. Biomedicine generally tries to protect the status quo of animal research. Animal advocates generally treat not using animals in research as a presumption, any departures from which would require careful justification. Clearly, animal advocates will have many disagreements with biomedicine over when it is appropriate to conduct animal research.

Third, in a similar vein, continuing disagreement is likely on the issue of *whether current protections for research animals are more or less adequate*. Biomedicine would probably answer affirmatively, with relatively minor internal disagreements over specific issues (e.g., whether apes should ever be exposed to diseases in order to test vaccines). Animal advocates will tend to be much more critical of current protections for research animals. They will argue, for example, that animals are far too often made to suffer in pursuit of less than compelling objectives, such as learning about behavioral responses to stress or trauma.

In the United States, critics will argue that the basic principles that are supposed to guide the care and use of animals in federally funded research ultimately provide very weak protection for research animals. That is because the tenth and final principle begins with implicit permission to make exceptions to the previous nine: "Where exceptions are required in relation to the provisions of these Principles, ..."[31] Since no limits are placed on permissible exceptions, this final principle precludes any absolute restraints on the harm that may be inflicted on research animals—an indefensible lack of safeguards from the perspective of animal advocates. (Although similar in several ways to these American principles, including some ways animal advocates would criticize, the *International Guiding Principles for Biomedical Research Involving Animals* avoids this pitfall of a global loophole. One of its relatively strong protections is Principle V: "Investigators and other personnel should never fail to treat animals as sentient, and should regard their proper care and use and the avoidance or minimization of discomfort, distress, or pain as ethical imperatives."[32])

Although protections of research animals are commonly thought of in terms of preventing unnecessary pain, distress, and suffering, they may also be thought of in terms of protecting animal life. A fourth likely area of disagreement concerns *whether animal life is morally protectable.* Return to a question raised earlier: whether a contented animal in good health is harmed by being painlessly killed in her sleep. Since government documents for the care and use of research animals generally require justification for causing pain or distress to animal subjects, but no justification for painless killing, it seems fair to infer that biomedicine generally does not attribute life interests to animals. Although I lack concrete evidence, I would guess that most animal advocates would see the matter quite differently, and would regard the killing of animals as a serious moral matter even if it is justified in some circumstances.

The four issues identified here as probable continuing points of difference are not intended to comprise an exhaustive list. But they show that despite the fact that the biomedical and animal protection communities can agree on an impressive range of major points, given their basic orientations they cannot be expected to agree on every fundamental question. Few will find this assertion surprising. But I also suggest, less obviously, that even if both sides cannot be entirely right in their positions, differences that remain after positions are refined through honest, open-minded, fully educated inquiry can be reasonable differences.

WHAT CAN BE DONE NOW TO BUILD UPON THE POINTS OF AGREEMENT

Let me close with a series of suggestions offered in the constructive yet critical-minded spirit of Henry Spira's work for how to build on the points of agreement identified above. For reasons of space, these suggestions will be stated somewhat tersely and without elaboration.

First, biomedical organizations and leaders in the profession can do the following: openly ac-

knowledge that ethical issues involving animals are complex and important; educate themselves or acquire education about the ethical issues; tolerate views departing from the current party line; open up journals to more than one basic viewpoint; and stop disseminating one-sided propoganda.

Second, the more "militant" animal advocates can acknowledge that there can be reasonable disagreement on some of the relevant issues and stop intimidating people with whom they disagree.

Third, biomedicine can openly acknowledge, as NASA recently did in its principles, that animals can suffer and invite more serious consideration of animal suffering.

Fourth, the animal protection community can give credit to biomedicine where credit is due—for example, for efforts to minimize pain and distress, to improve housing conditions, and to refrain from killing old chimpanzees who are no longer useful for research but are expensive to maintain.

Fifth, animal researchers and members of animal protection organizations can be required by their organizations to take courses in ethical theory or animal ethics to promote knowledgeable, skilled, broad-minded discussion and reflection.

Sixth, the animal protection community can openly acknowledge that some animal research is justified (perhaps giving examples to reduce the potential for misunderstanding).

Seventh, more animal research ethics committees can bring aboard at least one dedicated animal advocate who (unlike mainstream American veterinarians) seriously questions the value of most animal research.

Eighth, conditions of housing for research animals can be improved—for example, with greater enrichment and, for social animals, more access to conspecifics.

Ninth, all parties can endorse and support the goal of finding ways to *eliminate* animal subjects' pain, distress, and suffering.[33]

Tenth, and finally, governments can invest much more than they have to date in the development and use of alternatives to animal research, and all parties can give strong public support to the pursuit of alternatives.

NOTES

1 American Medical Association: Animal Research Action Plan. (June 1989), p. 6. See also American Medical Association. White Paper (1988).

2 See the Humane Society of the United States (HSUS). *Farm Animals and Intensive Confinement.* Washington, D.C.: HSUS, 1994; *Animals in Biomedical Research.* Washington, D.C.: HSUS, revised 1989; and *Zoos: Information Packet.* Washington, D.C.: HSUS, 1995.

3 Animal Liberation Front. Animal Liberation Frontline Information Service: the A.L.F. Primer. (website)

4 Regan T. *The Case for Animal Rights.* Berkeley: University of California Press, 1983; Pluhar E. *Beyond Prejudice.* Durham, North Carolina: Duke University Press, 1995.

5 Frey R. G. *Interests and Rights.* Oxford: Clarendon, 1980; Singer P. *Animal Liberation,* 2d ed. New York: New York Review of Books, 1990.

6 DeGrazia D. *Taking Animals Seriously.* Cambridge: Cambridge University Press, 1996.

7 Sapontzis S. F. *Morals, Reason, and Animals.* Philadelphia: Temple University Press, 1987; Rodd R. *Biology, Ethics, and Animals.* Oxford: Clarendon, 1990; and Rollin B. E. *Animal Rights and Human Morality,* 2d ed. Buffalo, New York: Prometheus, 1992.

8 Midgley M. *Animals and Why They Matter.* Athens, Georgia: University of Georgia Press, 1983.

9 Carruthers P. *The Animals Issue.* Cambridge: Cambridge University Press, 1992.

10 In a letter to the editor, Robert White, a neurosurgeon well known for transplanting monkeys' heads, asserted that "[a]nimal usage is not a moral or ethical issue . . ." (White R. Animal ethics? [letter]. *Hastings Center Report* 1990;20(6):43). For a rebuttal to White, see my letter, *Hastings Center Report* 1991;21(5):45.

11 See note 9, Carruthers 1992. For an attempt to undermine Carruthers' arguments, see note 6, DeGrazia 1996:53–6.

12 See Rose M., Adams D. Evidence for pain and suffering in other animals. In: Langley G., ed. *Animal Experimentation.* New York: Chapman and Hall, 1989:42–71; Smith J. A, Boyd K. M. *Lives in the Balance.* Oxford: Oxford University Press, 1991:ch. 4. See also note 7 Rodd 1990:ch. 3; and DeGrazia D., Rowan A. Pain, suffering, and anxiety in animals and humans. *Theoretical Medicine* 1991;12:193–211.

13 See, e.g., U.S. Government Principles for the Utilization and Care of Vertebrate Animals Used in Testing, Research, and Training. In: National Research Council. *Guide for the Care and Use of Laboratory Animals.* Washington, D.C.: National Academy Press, 1996:117–8; National Aeronautics and Space Administration. *Principles for the Ethical Care and Use of Animals.* NASA Policy Directive 8910.1, effective 23 March 1998; and Council for International Organizations of Medical Sciences. *International Guiding Principles for Biomedical Research Involving Animals.* Geneva: CIOMS, 1985:18.

14 See note 13, National Research Council 1996; CIOMS 1985.

15 See note 13, NASA 1998.

16 See note 12, Rose, Adams 1989; DeGrazia, Rowan 1991. And see note 7, Rodd 1990:ch. 3. There is also much evidence that at least mammals can experience anxiety. (See note 12, DeGrazia, Rowan 1991; note 12, Smith, Boyd 1991:ch. 4.)

17 See note 13, National Research Council 1996:37.

18 Note that the term "euthanasia," which means a death that is good for the one who dies, is inappropriate when animals are killed because they are costly to maintain or for similarly human-regarding reasons.

19 National Research Council Committee on Long-Term Care of Chimpanzees. *Chimpanzees in Research.* Washington, D.C.: National Academy Press, 1997:38.

20 Such policies typically state that animals who would otherwise experience severe or chronic pain or distress should be painlessly killed. See, e.g., note 13, National Research Council 1996:117; CIOMS 1985:19; and [British] Home Office. *Home Office Guidance on the Operation of the Animals; [Scientific Procedures] Act 1986.* London: Home Office, 1986. Although this directive addresses what to do with animals who could survive only in agony, it does not state any presumption against killing animals who could live well following research.

21 The committee addresses these chimpanzee interests in note 19, National Research Council 1997:ch. 3.

22 See note 12, Smith, Boyd 1991:334.

23 See note 6, DeGrazia 1996:204–10.

24 Admittedly, some unusual individuals would claim that amoebas have moral status, either because they think amoebas are sentient or because they think that sentience is unnecessary for moral status. I know of no one, however, who would claim that killing amoebas is as serious a matter as killing humans.

25 See note 7, Sapontzis 1987:216–22.

26 For example, if I am right, just as the moral presumption against taking life can differ in strength across species, so can the presumption against confining members of different species (the interest at stake being freedom). See note 6, DeGrazia 1996:254–6.

27 That is, except those humans who benefit directly from the conduct of research, such as researchers and people who sell animals and laboratory equipment.

28 See, e.g., note 12, Smith, Boyd 1991:ch. 3.

29 Peter Singer reminded me of this important point.

30 The idea of differences of moral status can be left intuitive here. Any effort to make it more precise will invite controversy. (See note 6, DeGrazia 1996:256–7.)

31 See note 13, National Research Council 1996:118.

32 See note 13, CIOMS 1985:18.

33 This is the stated goal of a new initiative of the Humane Society of the United States, which expects the initiative to expand to Humane Society International.

ANNOTATED BIBLIOGRAPHY

Appelbaum, Paul S., et al.: "False Hopes and Best Data: Consent to Research and the Therapeutic Misconception," *Hastings Center Report* 17 (April 1987), pp. 20–24. The authors focus on the potential conflict in randomized clinical trials between seeking generalizable knowledge and serving patients' best interests. After arguing that patient-subjects commonly labor under the "therapeutic misconception"—the denial of the possibility that one's participation in RCTs can be seriously disadvantageous to oneself—the authors maintain that proper educational efforts can dispel this misconception for many subjects.

Bateson, Patrick: "When to Experiment on Animals," *New Scientist* 20 (February 1986), pp. 30–32. Bateson proposes a framework for managing the conflict between the potential benefits of animal research and ethical concerns about using animals. His analysis of when animal research is justified is summarized in a decision cube that represents the dimensions of (1) quality of research, (2) certainty of medical benefit, and (3) animal suffering.

Brody, Baruch A.: *The Ethics of Biomedical Research: An International Perspective* (New York: Oxford University Press, 1998). This book analyzes major issues of research ethics through a review of differing policies throughout the world (especially North America, Western Europe, and the Pacific Rim). Topics covered include genetic research, reproductive research, research on vulnerable subjects, drug approval and the research process, and research on animals.

Buchanan, Allen: "Judging the Past: The Case of the Human Radiation Experiments," *Hastings Center Report* 26 (May–June 1996), pp. 25–30. Using the human radiation experiments as a case study, Buchanan argues for the legitimacy of retrospective moral judgments and traces implications of this thesis for how present practices and institutions should be judged.

DeGrazia, David: *Animal Rights: A Very Short Introduction* (Oxford: Oxford University Press, 2002). In this short volume, DeGrazia explores the mental life, interests, and moral status of animals before addressing the issues of meat-eating, the keeping of pets and zoo animals, and animal research.

Hellman, Deborah: "Trials on Trial," *Report from the Institute for Philosophy & Public Policy* 18 (Winter/Spring 1998), pp. 13–18. Hellman explores the ethical issues associated with placebo-controlled trials of the effectiveness of anti-retroviral drugs in reducing mother-to-infant transmission of HIV. In an exceptionally balanced and in-depth discussion, she examines the issues from the perspectives of the patient, the researcher, and the public health official, before concluding that in the context under discussion "the usual interpretations of both the equipoise principle and the standard of care principle are inapt."

Holmes, Helen Bequaert: "Can Clinical Research Be Both Ethical and Scientific?" *Hypatia* 4 (Summer 1989), pp. 154–165. Holmes argues that conflicts between physicians' therapeutic and research obligations in clinical research may result, in part, from excessive faith in the objectivity of science and in statistics. She contends that feminist approaches to clinical research hold promise for more satisfactorily dealing with the ethical and scientific issues involved.

Jonas, Hans: "Philosophical Reflections on Experimenting with Human Subjects," in Paul Freund, ed., *Experimentation with Human Subjects* (New York: Braziller, 1970), pp. 1–31. In this classic essay, Jonas challenges common arguments for the view that the use of human subjects in medical experimentation is morally justified. While Jonas does not argue that all such research is unjustified, he maintains that researchers and other scientists should be the first volunteers in justifiable research.

Journal of Medicine and Philosophy 11 (November 1986). This issue, entitled "Ethical Issues in the Use of Clinical Controls," is edited by Kenneth F. Schaffner. Schaffner provides a historical and methodological context for the essays in this volume, and the essays deal with some of the problems posed by clinical trials in general as well as by RCTs and prerandomized clinical trials in particular.

Kahn, Jeffrey, Anna C. Mastroianni, and Jeremy Sugarman, eds.: *Beyond Consent: Seeking Justice in Research* (New York: Oxford University Press, 1998). This edited volume examines the concept of justice and its application to human subjects research through the different lenses of important research populations: children, the vulnerable sick, captive and convenient populations, women, people of color, and subjects in international settings.

Kodish, Eric, John D. Lantos, and Mark Siegler: "The Ethics of Randomization," *CA—A Cancer Journal for Clinicians* 41 (May/June 1991), pp. 180–187. The authors explore ethical issues arising from the randomization of subjects in randomized clinical trials. Drawing from two important cases—the AZT study and a major study of breast-cancer patients—they argue for restrictive conditions on the use of RCTs.

Kopelman, Loretta M.: "Group Benefit and Protection of Pediatric Research Subjects: *Grimes v. Kennedy Krieger* and the Lead Abatement Study," *Accountability in Research* 9 (Summer 2002), pp. 177–192. Kopelman examines a legal case concerning a lead abatement study, drawing implications for the ethics of pediatric research.

Lurie, Peter, and Sidney M. Wolfe: "Unethical Trials of Interventions to Reduce Perinatal Transmission of the Human Immunodeficiency Virus in Developing Countries," *New England Journal of Medicine* 337 (September 18, 1997), pp. 853–856. The authors contend that because zidovudine has already been shown effective in reducing perinatal transmission of HIV, placebo-based trials in developing countries are unethical for failing to provide subjects in the placebo arm with the standard of care. In order to prevent the exploitation of vulnerable individuals, they argue, research ethics must embrace and maintain universal standards for the treatment of human subjects.

Macklin, Ruth: "International Research: Ethical Imperialism or Ethical Pluralism?" *Accountability in Research* 7 (Spring 1999), pp. 59–83. Against ethical relativism Macklin defends universal moral principles along with a pluralistic view about what specific research practices are appropriate in different cultural contexts. Employing this framework, she engages the ethics of placebo-controlled AZT trials in developing countries and ethical issues provoked by HIV vaccine trials.

National Bioethics Advisory Commission (NBAC): *Research Involving Persons with Mental Disorders That May Affect Decisionmaking Capacity,* vol. I: *Report and Recommendations of the National Bioethics Advisory Committee* (Bethesda, MD: NBAC, 1998). This report provides an overview of ethical issues in research involving subjects whose psychiatric conditions may affect their decision-making capacity. Attempting to reconcile the importance of progress in psychiatric research with the ethical imperative of protecting subjects' rights, the report includes numerous recommendations, including a call for a highly visible, independent panel that would review the most controversial research protocols in this area.

National Commission for the Protection of Human Subjects of Biomedical and Behavioral Research: *The Belmont Report: Ethical Principles and Guidelines for the Protection of Human Subjects of Research.* DHEW (OS) 78-0012. *The Belmont Report. Appendix,* vols. 1, 2. DHEW (OS) 78-0013, 78-0014. (Bethesda, MD, 1978). This report was produced by a commission established under the National Research Act (P.L. 93–348). The commission's purpose was to develop ethical guidelines for the conduct of research involving human subjects and to make recommendations for the application of these guidelines to research conducted or supported by the Department of Health, Education, and Welfare. *The Belmont Report* is the commission's final and most general report. Other reports, listed below, concern narrower topics. The appendices to this report and to the ones listed below contain many useful papers and other materials that were reviewed by the commission prior to formulating its recommendations.

_____: *Report and Recommendations: Research Involving Children.* DHEW (OS) 77-0004. *Appendix: Research Involving Children.* DHEW (OS) 77-0005. (Bethesda, MD: 1977).

_____: *Report and Recommendations: Research Involving Prisoners.* DHEW (OS) 76-131. *Appendix: Research Involving Prisoners.* DHEW (OS) 76-132. (Bethesda, MD: 1976).

_____: *Report and Recommendations: Research Involving Those Institutionalized as Mentally Infirm.* DHEW (OS) 78-0006. *Appendix: Research Involving Those Institutionalized as Mentally Infirm.* DHEW (OS) 78-0007. (Bethesda, MD, 1978).

Smith, Jane A., and Kenneth M. Boyd: *Lives in the Balance: The Ethics of Using Animals in Biomedical Research* (Oxford: Oxford University Press, 1991). This book is a report of a working party of the Institute of Medical Ethics (Great Britain) that met eighteen times to examine ethical issues related to animal research. Notable for both thoroughness and moderation, the book is especially helpful in addressing scientific aspects of the study of animals' mental states.

CHAPTER **5**

DEATH AND DECISIONS REGARDING LIFE-SUSTAINING TREATMENT

INTRODUCTION

Decisions regarding life-sustaining treatment frequently emerge from a complex dynamic involving physicians, patients, and families. A wide range of ethical questions and concerns can be raised about such decisions. This chapter begins by engaging some conceptual questions about death itself. Attention is then focused on the refusal of life-sustaining treatment by competent adults. A further concern is the ethics of do-not-resuscitate (DNR) orders, and discussion on this score leads to a consideration of more general questions related to the concept of medical futility. Next, in conjunction with a consideration of treatment decisions for incompetent adults, substantial attention is given to the topic of advance directives.

Most of the discussion in this chapter centers on adult patients who are facing the problems of death and dying at the end of a long life. However, the final issue under consideration is located near the other end of the spectrum of human life, where we are confronted with the severely impaired newborn child. Biomedical technology is sometimes sufficient to sustain or at least temporarily prolong the life of a severely impaired infant, depending upon the nature of the child's medical condition, but we must ask under what conditions continued treatment is morally appropriate.

THE DEFINITION AND DETERMINATION OF DEATH

Two groups of patients are at the center of controversy in recent discussions of the definition and determination of death. In the first group are patients whose *entire* brain has irreversibly ceased functioning. They are irreversibly unconscious, but cardiopulmonary function (heartbeat and respiration) is successfully maintained by a respirator and allied technology. These patients are usually identified either as "brain-dead" or "whole-brain-dead." Here they will be referred to as "brain-dead." In a second group of patients, brain-stem function is sufficient to sustain respiration and heartbeat, but brain damage—typically involving the cerebrum—is so severe that consciousness has been *irreversibly* lost. This group of patients includes those who are in a permanent coma and those whose "persistent vegetative state" (PVS) is permanent.[1] Are the patients in each of these groups alive or dead? In any case, what is the morally appropriate treatment for patients in each group?

The traditional standard for the determination of death is the permanent loss of respiration and heartbeat. According to this standard, brain-dead patients are alive so long as technological support systems sustain cardiopulmonary functioning. In 1968 an ad hoc committee of the Harvard Medical School issued an influential report. In this report, the ad hoc committee specified a set of tests for the identification of a permanently nonfunctioning (whole) brain—that is, the condition of brain death. In the view of the ad hoc committee, when this condition has been diagnosed, "death is to be declared and *then* the respirator turned off."[2] In essence, then, the ad hoc committee advanced a new standard for the determination of death. A brain-dead patient is a dead patient, even if cardiopulmonary function is being maintained by artificial means.

It is a matter of substantial importance whether brain-dead patients are alive or dead. For example, taking the vital organs of these patients for transplantation purposes is morally unproblematic if they are dead—presuming, of course, that appropriate consent procedures have been followed. If they are alive, however, taking their vital organs would presumably be the cause of their death. There are other important implications for the way we think and the way we talk. When a respirator is withdrawn from a brain-dead patient, how are we to conceptualize this action? If the patient is still alive, then it is appropriate to describe the removal of the respirator as the withdrawal of life-sustaining treatment, and it makes sense to say that we are allowing the patient to die. However, if the patient is already dead when we remove the respirator, it does not make sense to say that we are allowing the patient to die.

The substance of the Harvard proposal is reflected in the approach taken by the President's Commission for the Study of Ethical Problems in Medicine and Biomedical and Behavioral Research. In its 1981 report, *Defining Death,* the commission recommended that all states adopt the Uniform Determination of Death Act:

> An individual who has sustained either (1) irreversible cessation of circulatory and respiratory functions, or (2) irreversible cessation of all functions of the entire brain, including the brainstem, is dead. A determination of death must be made in accordance with accepted medical standards.

The whole-brain standard of death that is built into the Uniform Determination of Death Act has achieved widespread public acceptance in the United States, and yet the adequacy of the whole-brain standard continues to be challenged both on theoretical and clinical grounds.[3] Some of those who reject the whole-brain approach—including Martin Benjamin, in this chapter—argue for a higher-brain approach.

Charles M. Culver and Bernard Gert, in one of this chapter's selections, provide an analysis that ultimately factors out as an expression of the whole-brain approach. In their view, a patient who has undergone a permanent loss of functioning of the entire brain is dead, but a patient in a permanent vegetative state (or permanent coma) is not dead, even though, as they say, the organism has ceased to be a person. Indeed, insisting that "we must not confuse the death of an organism which was a person with an organism's ceasing to be a person," Culver and Gert explicitly argue against a higher-brain approach. In accordance with a higher-brain approach, the permanent loss of consciousness is sufficient for death; thus, it follows that a patient in a permanent vegetative state is already dead. Of course, if patients in a permanent vegetative state are already dead, then nothing that subsequently happens could be the cause of their death. In particular, it would be wrong to conceptualize the act of inducing cardiac arrest as killing the patient. Similarly, if the patient is already dead, the removal of organs for transplantation could not coherently be understood as an action tantamount to killing the patient.

Culver and Gert, committed to the more common view that a patient in a permanent vegetative state is still alive, also consider the issue of morally appropriate treatment. Although they are uncomfortable with the idea of killing a patient in a permanent vegetative state, they endorse allowing the patient to die by discontinuing all care, even "ordinary and routine care." Presumably, the discontinuance of ordinary and routine care would include the withholding of nutrition and hydration, that is, food and water.

COMPETENT ADULTS AND THE REFUSAL OF LIFE-SUSTAINING TREATMENT

Regarding the refusal of life-sustaining treatment by competent adults, there seem to be noteworthy differences among the following: (1) cases in which a patient, by accepting life-sustaining treatment, would return to a state of health; (2) cases in which a patient, by accepting life-sustaining treatment, would simply continue a severely compromised existence; and (3) cases in which a terminally ill patient, by accepting life-sustaining treatment, would merely *prolong the dying process.*

Refusal of treatment in cases of the first type is relatively uncommon but typically dramatic. The most discussed example involves a Jehovah's Witness who refuses to accept a blood transfusion for religious reasons. It is widely acknowledged, at least in theory, that respect for individual autonomy requires recognition of the right of a competent adult Jehovah's Witness to refuse a life-sustaining blood transfusion.[4]

In conjunction with ongoing developments in the courts, refusal of treatment in cases of the second type is probably becoming increasingly common. By and large, the law now recognizes the right of a competent adult—and not just one who is terminally ill or in the process of dying—to refuse life-sustaining treatment. Consider in this regard the example of a patient whose life is severely compromised by the presence of a painful and debilitating form of arthritis. This patient is coincidentally being treated for pneumonia and is temporarily dependent upon a respirator until the antibiotics have a chance to take effect. The pneumonia is entirely curable and the patient, however much compromised from a quality-of-life standpoint, is not in the process of dying. If the patient now decides to forgo the respirator, we cannot simply say that the patient has chosen not to prolong the dying process. Accordingly, although considerations of individual autonomy provide a strong moral warrant for the right to refuse life-sustaining treatment in general, some commentators would take issue with the right to refuse treatment in this kind of case because they are concerned about the implications of accepting quality-of-life considerations. It can also be argued that the refusal of life-sustaining treatment in this kind of case is tantamount to suicide,[5] an approach taken by Vicki Michel in one of this chapter's readings. Michel's discussion is also notable for its presentation of a disability-rights perspective on the issues at stake.

In another reading in this chapter, Tia Powell and Bruce Lowenstein focus attention on the case of a chronically disabled woman who chose to refuse life-sustaining treatment. The patient, who suffered a brain-stem stroke at the age of 37, remained mentally alert but was rendered quadriplegic and unable to speak. As described by Powell and Lowenstein, much of the ethical tension in the case can be traced to the fact that staff members working with the patient in a rehabilitation facility felt that she had decided too rapidly that she could not adjust to a life with serious disability.

Refusal of treatment in cases of the third type has a strong foundation in both morality and law and is certainly common. In many cases of terminal illness, "aggressive" treatment is capable of warding off death—for a time. However, it is often questionable whether such treatment is in a patient's best interest, and a competent adult is generally considered to have both a moral and a legal right to refuse treatment that would merely prolong the dying process.

Depending upon a patient's circumstances, life-sustaining treatment can take a variety of forms—for example, mechanical respiration, cardiopulmonary resuscitation, kidney dialysis, surgery, antiobiotics, and artificial nutrition and hydration. It is sometimes claimed that the provision of food and water is so fundamentally different from other forms of life-sustaining treatment that it may never be omitted. Those who systematically oppose withholding nutrition and hydration often call attention to the symbolic significance of food and water—their intimate connection with notions of care and concern. However, most commentators insist that there is no reason to apply a different standard to artificial nutrition and hydration. In their view, artificial nutrition and hydration—just like other life-sustaining treatments—will sometimes fail to offer a patient a net benefit, and the decision of a competent patient to refuse them must be respected.

In one of the selections in this chapter, the AMA Council on Ethical and Judicial Affairs acknowledges and endorses the right of competent patients to forgo life-sustaining treatment. The council explicitly argues against the view that it is never permissible to forgo artificial nutrition and hydration. One other issue discussed by the council is noteworthy. Although it is clear that medical decision making is sometimes influenced by the fact that many physicians are more comfortable with withholding a life-sustaining treatment to begin with rather than withdrawing it once it has been initiated, the council insists that there is no ethically significant distinction between withholding and withdrawing life-sustaining treatment.

DNR ORDERS AND MEDICAL FUTILITY

When a patient undergoes cardiac arrest, resuscitation techniques can sometimes restore heartbeat and thereby prolong life, yet in many cases a dying patient would not welcome attempts at cardiopulmonary resuscitation (CPR), and in some cases there is virtually no likelihood of success. In one of this chapter's readings, Tom Tomlinson and Howard Brody identify three distinct rationales for do-not-resuscitate (DNR) orders. Two of the identified rationales involve quality-of-life judgments. Insisting that quality-of-life judgments must ultimately be made by the patient or the patient's family (if the patient is incompetent), Tomlinson and Brody argue that it is inappropriate in such cases for a physician to write a DNR order without the permission of the patient or family. With regard to a third rationale, however, they contend that there is no need for the physician to secure the permission of the patient or family before writing a DNR order. They rely at this point on the concept of futility. In their view, sometimes "resuscitation would almost certainly not be successful," and the "decision that CPR is unjustified because it is futile is a judgment that falls entirely within the physician's expertise."

Although many patients and their families feel there is an ongoing need to assert a patient's right to refuse life-sustaining treatment against a perceived tendency among physicians to overtreat, it is also true that many physicians increasingly feel the need to assert a professional prerogative to limit treatment in the face of requests from patients and (more commonly) from families that "everything be done." If patients or their families desire treatments considered futile by physicians, are physicians justified in refusing to provide them? Clearly, Tomlinson and Brody would respond in the affirmative. However, the meaning of "futility" is presently the source of intense controversy in biomedical ethics, as is the ethical significance of the concept. Mark R. Wicclair, in this chapter, distinguishes various senses of futility and ultimately recommends that physicians avoid the language of futility in expressing their opposition to a given treatment.

ADVANCE DIRECTIVES AND TREATMENT DECISIONS FOR INCOMPETENT ADULTS

The rigors of incurable illness and the dying process frequently deprive previously competent patients of their decision-making capacity. How can a person best ensure that his or her personal wishes with regard to life-sustaining treatment (in various possible circumstances) will be honored even if decision-making capacity is lost? Although communication of one's attitudes and preferences to one's physician, family, and friends surely provides some measure of protection, it is frequently asserted that the most effective protection comes through the formation of advance directives.

There are two basic types of advance directives, and each has legal status in almost all, if not all, of the states. In executing an *instructional* directive, a person specifies instructions about his or her care in the event that decision-making capacity is lost. Such a directive, especially when it deals specifically with a person's wishes regarding life-sustaining treatment in various possible circumstances, is commonly called a *living will.* In executing a *proxy* directive, a person specifies a substitute decision maker to make health-care decisions for him or her in the event that decision-making capacity is lost. The legal mechanism for executing a proxy directive is often called a *durable power of attorney for health care.* Since purging ambiguities from even the most explicit written directives is difficult, as is foreseeing all the contingencies that might give rise to a need for treatment decisions, many commentators recommend the execution of a durable power of attorney for health care even if a person has already executed a living will.[6]

If a patient lacks decision-making capacity and has not executed a proxy directive, a surrogate decision maker must be identified; ordinarily this is a member of the family or a close personal friend. If the patient has provided an instructional directive, the surrogate is, of course, expected to follow the stated instructions. However, sometimes an instructional directive provides insufficient guidance for the treatment decision at hand, and frequently a surrogate decision maker must function in the absence of any instructional directive. In applying the *substituted-judgment* standard, the surrogate decision maker is expected to consider the patient's preferences and values and make the decision that the patient would have made if he or she had been able to choose. If no reliable basis exists to infer what the patient would have chosen, then the surrogate decision maker is expected to retreat to the *best-interests* standard. In applying the best-interests standard, the surrogate decision maker is expected to choose in accordance with the patient's best interests, which may reduce to choosing what a reasonable person in the patient's circumstances would choose.[7]

The Patient Self-Determination Act, passed by Congress in October 1990, requires all health-care institutions (e.g., hospitals and nursing homes) receiving federal funds to inform patients of their right to formulate advance directives. Nevertheless, advance directives remain problematic in many ways. Especially worrisome are concerns that can be raised about the construction, implementation, and force of instructional directives. For one thing, many of the standard-form living wills that have emerged in conjunction with state statutes can be activated only upon the diagnosis of a "terminal illness," a category that has usually been interpreted to exclude both a patient in a permanent vegetative state and one who is existing in a severely compromised state as a result of a progressively debilitating disease (e.g., Alzheimer's). Other phrases commonly found in living wills are also problematic. For example, suppose a patient signs a form that authorizes withholding or withdrawing life-sustaining treatment if there is "no reasonable expectation that I will regain a meaningful quality of life." Unless a person provides a further specification of what counts for him or her as "a meaningful quality of life," numerous problems of interpretation can arise. Another important question is whether physicians can ever be justified in refusing to honor the provisions of a patient's instructional directive.

In one of this chapter's selections, Thomas A. Mappes considers some of the many problems that can be raised about the construction and implementation of advance directives, especially instructional directives. In another selection, Norman L. Cantor explicitly confronts the task of constructing a highly personalized instructional directive. Mindful of the various inadequacies associated with "short-form" living wills, he provides a sophisticated example of an advance-directive document. Although Cantor refers to this document as his living will, it has been designed to include a proxy directive as well as an extensive instructional directive.

Also in this chapter, Rebecca Dresser focuses attention on patients who are incompetent, severely compromised, yet conscious and not terminally ill. The point of departure for her discussion is the *Wendland* case, in which the California Supreme Court refused to authorize the cessation of nutrition and hydration for Robert Wendland, a man who was left severely brain damaged as a result of an automobile accident. Dresser writes that "*Wendland* may signal a developing legal consensus," and she explores some of the implications of this consensus, especially in reference to advance directives.

THE TREATMENT OF IMPAIRED INFANTS

The selective nontreatment of severely impaired newborns is an issue that first made its way into the public consciousness in the early 1970s. In the 1980s, the issue gained an even higher profile. Media attention focused on a rash of "Baby Doe" cases, in which treatment was withheld from severely impaired newborns, and the Reagan administration was conspicuous in its effort to activate the machinery of government via the introduction of "Baby Doe" regulations.[8] As a result, the practice of selective nontreatment of severely impaired newborns has been subjected to intense scrutiny, with regard to both its legality and its morality.

The central moral question with regard to the treatment of impaired newborns may be identified as follows: Under what conditions, if any, is it morally acceptable to allow a severely impaired newborn to die? A closely related issue is embodied in a procedural question: Who should make the decision to treat or not treat? It has sometimes been argued that the decision is a medical one to be made by physicians. However, the more common view is that the parents are the appropriate decision makers, as informed by consultation with physicians and as limited by boundaries set by society at large. In this regard, it is often suggested that hospital ethics committees be assigned the responsibility of reviewing decisions to treat or not to treat severely impaired newborns.

Broadly speaking, there are three different views on the moral acceptability of allowing severely impaired newborns to die.

(1) It is morally acceptable to allow a severely impaired newborn to die if and only if death would be in the infant's best interests—that is, if and only if the infant would be better off dead. Defenders of this view are firmly committed to so-called quality-of-life judgments, but they systematically reject the contention that the cost (emotional and/or financial) of caring for severely impaired newborns is a relevant factor in the decision to treat or not treat. A similar but somewhat less restrictive view would endorse allowing a severely impaired newborn to die if and only if there is no significant potential for a meaningful human existence. In one of this chapter's selections, the members of The Hastings Center Research Project on the Care of Imperiled Newborns argue for the primacy of the best-interests standard, but they also insist that in some cases a "relational potential" standard comes into play. According to this standard, treatment is optional for an infant who lacks the potential for human relationships.

(2) It is morally acceptable to allow a severely impaired newborn to die if at least one of the following conditions is satisfied: (a) there is no significant potential for a meaningful human existence; (b) the emotional and/or financial hardship of caring for the impaired child would constitute a grave burden for the family. It is the introduction of the cost factor that distinguishes this second view from the first. Defenders of the second view often insist that the newborn child does not have the moral status of personhood, thereby defending the legitimacy of the cost factor.[9]

(3) It is never morally acceptable to allow a severely impaired newborn to die. More precisely, it would never be morally acceptable to withhold treatment from a severely impaired newborn unless it would be morally acceptable to withhold such treatment from a normal infant. Although there is no requirement to prolong the life of a dying infant, whatever medical treatment is considered appropriate for an otherwise normal infant must be provided for the seriously impaired newborn as well. For example, if antibiotics are indicated for an otherwise normal infant with pneumonia, then antibiotics may not be withheld in a case where pneumonia arises for an infant whose central nervous system is severely compromised. In this view, it is usually presumed that a newborn child has the status of personhood and, however severely compromised, has a right to life. Defenders of this view, such as John A. Robertson in one of this chapter's selections, often make arguments against the validity of quality-of-life judgments (as featured in both of the aforementioned views) as well as the validity of the cost factor (as featured exclusively in the second view).

T.A.M.

NOTES

1 The phrase *persistent vegetative state* (PVS) continues to be the source of confusion. When a patient's vegetative state is identified as "persistent," it is certainly implied that the vegetative state has endured for a significant period of time. (In fact, according to a reigning clinical standard, a vegetative state must last at least a month before it can be diagnosed as persistent.) Is it also implied in calling a vegetative state

"persistent" that it is irreversible, that is, permanent? Some writers in biomedical ethics speak of a patient's vegetative state as "persistent" only when it is believed that the condition is permanent. In this sense, a persistent vegetative state entails that the condition is permanent. More commonly, however, the phrase "persistent vegetative state" is used in a contrasting way. In this sense, a persistent vegetative state does not entail that the condition is permanent. When PVS is understood in this way, there is no contradiction in saying that a patient has recovered from PVS. Of course, whenever a patient has been in a vegetative state for a significant period of time, a medical determination of irreversibility is of central practical importance. For further clarification of PVS and the difference between permanent vegetative state and permanent coma, see Ronald E. Cranford, "Definition and Determination of Death: Criteria for Death," in Warren R. Reich, ed., *Encyclopedia of Bioethics,* rev. ed. (New York: Macmillan, 1995), pp. 531–533.

2 The Ad Hoc Committee of the Harvard Medical School to Examine the Definition of Brain Death, "A Definition of Irreversible Coma," *JAMA* 205 (August 6, 1968), p. 338.

3 See, for example, *Journal of Medicine and Philosophy* 26 (October 2001). The articles in this issue are grouped under the title "Revisiting Brain Death." Some critics of the whole-brain approach are opposed to the higher-brain approach as well. See, for example, Michael Potts et al., eds., *Beyond Brain Death: The Case Against Brain Based Criteria for Human Death* (Dordrecht: Kluwer, 2000).

4 See, for example, Ruth Macklin, "Consent, Coercion, and Conflicts of Rights," *Perspectives in Biology and Medicine* 20 (Spring 1977), pp. 360–371. For a discussion of added complexities, see Dena S. Davis, "Does 'No' Mean 'Yes'? The Continuing Problem of Jehovah's Witnesses and Refusal of Blood Products," *Second Opinion* 19 (January 1994), pp. 35–43.

5 The morality of suicide is discussed in Chapter 6.

6 Some commentators also recommend that patients complete a "values history," a document that is designed to provide background information on patient values and attitudes. A values history might function as a supplement to an instructional directive, intended to guide any necessary interpretation, or it could be intended as a resource for one's designated proxy or surrogate.

7 For one articulation of the "standard wisdom" regarding surrogate decision making for incompetent adults, see Dan W. Brock, "Surrogate Decision Making for Incompetent Adults: An Ethical Framework," *Mount Sinai Journal of Medicine* 58 (October 1991), pp. 388–392. In contrast, John Hardwig calls for a fundamental revision in the theory of surrogate (proxy) decision making. He challenges the appropriateness of exclusively patient-centered standards of surrogate decision making, and he argues that it is morally unsound to expect proxy decision makers to disregard their own interests and those of other family members. See John Hardwig, "The Problem of Proxies with Interests of Their Own: Toward a Better Theory of Proxy Decisions," *Journal of Clinical Ethics* 4 (Spring 1993), pp. 20–27.

8 The so-called final Baby Doe rule was published by the Department of Health and Human Services on April 15, 1985. For one interpretation of this rule, see Thomas H. Murray, "The Final, Anticlimactic Rule on Baby Doe," *Hastings Center Report* 15 (June 1985), pp. 5–9. For an alternative interpretation, see John C. Moskop and Rita L. Saldanha, "The Baby Doe Rule: Still a Threat," *Hastings Center Report* 16 (April 1986), pp. 8–14.

9 See, for example, H. Tristram Engelhardt, Jr., "Ethical Issues in Aiding the Death of Young Children," in Marvin Kohl, ed., *Beneficent Euthanasia* (Buffalo, NY: Prometheus, 1975), pp. 180–192.

THE DEFINITION AND DETERMINATION OF DEATH

WHY "UPDATE" DEATH?

President's Commission for the Study of Ethical Problems in Medicine and Biomedical and Behavioral Research

In this selection, taken from the first chapter of its report *Defining Death,* the commission provides a compact account of both (1) the interrelationships of brain, heart, and lung functions and (2) the loss of brain functions. Emphasis is placed on the difference between "whole-brain-death" and a "persistent vegetative state" in which brainstem function persists. Although reference is made to the commission's view that "the cessation of the vital functions of the entire brain [is] the only proper neurologic basis for declaring death," the analysis and argumentation the commission presents in support of this view is found only in subsequent chapters of the report.

For most of the past several centuries, the medical determination of death was very close to the popular one. If a person fell unconscious or was found so, someone (often but not always a physician) would feel for the pulse, listen for breathing, hold a mirror before the nose to test for condensation, and look to see if the pupils were fixed. Although these criteria have been used to determine death since antiquity, they have not always been universally accepted.

DEVELOPING CONFIDENCE IN THE HEART-LUNG CRITERIA

In the eighteenth century, macabre tales of "corpses" reviving during funerals and exhumed skeletons found to have clawed at coffin lids led to widespread fear of premature burial. Coffins were developed with elaborate escape mechanisms and speaking tubes to the world above, mortuaries employed guards to monitor the newly dead for signs of life, and legislatures passed laws requiring a delay before burial. . . .

. . . The invention of the stethoscope in the mid-nineteenth century enabled physicians to detect heartbeat with heightened sensitivity. The use of this instrument by a well-trained physician, together with other clinical measures, laid to rest public fears of premature burial. The twentieth century brought even more sophisticated technological means to determine death, particularly the electrocardiograph (EKG), which is more sensitive than the stethoscope in detecting cardiac functioning.

THE INTERRELATIONSHIPS OF BRAIN, HEART, AND LUNG FUNCTIONS

The brain has three general anatomic divisions: the cerebrum, with its outer shell called the cortex; the cerebellum; and the brainstem, composed of the midbrain, the pons, and the medulla oblongata. Traditionally, the cerebrum has been referred to as the "higher brain" because it has primary control of consciousness, thought, memory and feeling. The brainstem has been called the "lower brain," since it controls spontaneous, vegetative functions such as swallowing, yawning and sleep-wake cycles. It is important to note that these generalizations are not entirely accurate. Neuroscientists generally agree that such "higher brain" functions as cognition or consciousness probably are not mediated strictly by the cerebral cortex; rather, they probably result from complex interrelations between brainstem and cortex.

Respiration is controlled in the brainstem, particularly the medulla. Neural impulses originating in the respiratory centers of the medulla stimulate the diaphragm and intercostal muscles, which cause the lungs to fill with air. Ordinarily, these respiratory centers adjust the rate of breathing to maintain the correct levels of carbon dioxide and oxygen. In certain circumstances, such as heavy exercise, sighing, coughing or sneezing, other areas of the brain modulate the activities of the respiratory centers or even briefly take direct control of respiration.

Destruction of the brain's respiratory center stops respiration, which in turn deprives the heart of needed oxygen, causing it too to cease functioning. The traditional signs of life—respiration and heartbeat—disappear: the person is dead. The "vital signs" traditionally used in diagnosing death thus reflect the direct interdependence of respiration, circulation and the brain.

The artificial respirator and concomitant life-support systems have changed this simple picture. Normally, respiration ceases when the functions of the diaphragm and intercostal muscles are impaired. This results from direct injury to the muscles or (more commonly) because the neural impulses between the brain and these muscles are interrupted. However, an artificial respirator (also called a ventilator) can be used to compensate for the inability of the thoracic muscles to fill the lungs with air. Some of these machines use negative pressure to expand the chest wall (in which case they are called "iron lungs"); others use positive pressure to push air into the lungs. The respirators are equipped with devices to regulate the rate and depth of "breathing," which are normally controlled by the respiratory centers in the medulla. The machines cannot compensate entirely for the defective neural connections since they cannot regulate blood gas levels precisely. But, provided that the lungs themselves have not been ex-

Reprinted from President's Commission for the Study of Ethical Problems in Medicine and Biomedical and Behavioral Research, *Defining Death* (1981), pp. 13–20.

tensively damaged, gas exchange can continue and appropriate levels of oxygen and carbon dioxide can be maintained in the circulating blood.

Unlike the respiratory system, which depends on the neural impulses from the brain, the heart can pump blood without external control. Impulses from brain centers modulate the inherent rate and force of the heartbeat but are not required for the heart to contract at a level of function that is ordinarily adequate. Thus, when artificial respiration provides adequate oxygenation and associated medical treatments regulate essential plasma components and blood pressure, an intact heart will continue to beat, despite loss of brain functions. At present, however, no machine can take over the functions of the heart except for a very limited time and in limited circumstances (e.g., a heart-lung machine used during surgery). Therefore, when a severe injury to the heart or major blood vessels prevents the circulation of the crucial blood supply to the brain, the loss of brain functioning is inevitable because no oxygen reaches the brain.

LOSS OF VARIOUS BRAIN FUNCTIONS

The most frequent causes of irreversible loss of functions of the whole brain are: (1) direct trauma to the head, such as from a motor vehicle accident or a gunshot wound, (2) massive spontaneous hemorrhage into the brain as a result of ruptured aneurysm or complications of high blood pressure, and (3) anoxic damage from cardiac or respiratory arrest or severely reduced blood pressure.

Many of these severe injuries to the brain cause an accumulation of fluid and swelling in the brain tissue, a condition called cerebral edema. In severe cases of edema, the pressure within the closed cavity increases until it exceeds the systolic blood pressure, resulting in a total loss of blood flow to both the upper and lower portions of the brain. If deprived of blood flow for at least 10–15 minutes, the brain, including the brainstem, will completely cease functioning. Other pathophysiologic mechanisms also result in a progressive and, ultimately, complete cessation of intracranial circulation.

Once deprived of adequate supplies of oxygen and glucose, brain neurons will irreversibly lose all

activity and ability to function. In adults, oxygen and/or glucose deprivation for more than a few minutes causes some neuron loss. Thus, even in the absence of direct trauma and edema, brain functions can be lost if circulation to the brain is impaired. If blood flow is cut off, brain tissues completely self-digest (autolyze) over the ensuing days.

When the brain lacks all functions, consciousness is, of course, lost. While some spinal reflexes often persist in such bodies (since circulation to the spine is separate from that of the brain), all reflexes controlled by the brainstem as well as cognitive, affective and integrating functions are absent. Respiration and circulation in these bodies may be generated by a ventilator together with intensive medical management. In adults who have experienced irreversible cessation of the functions of the entire brain, this mechanically generated functioning can continue only a limited time because the heart usually stops beating within two to ten days. (An infant or small child who has lost all brain functions will typically suffer cardiac arrest within several weeks, although respiration and heartbeat can sometimes be maintained even longer.)

Less severe injury to the brain can cause mild to profound damage to the cortex, lower cerebral structures, cerebellum, brainstem, or some combination thereof. The cerebrum, especially the cerebral cortex, is more easily injured by loss of blood flow or oxygen than is the brainstem. A 4 to 6 minute loss of blood flow—caused by, for example, cardiac arrest—typically damages the cerebral cortex permanently, while the relatively more resistant brainstem may continue to function.

When brainstem functions remain, but the major components of the cerebrum are irreversibly destroyed, the patient is in what is usually called a "persistent vegetative state" or "persistent noncognitive state." Such persons may exhibit spontaneous, involuntary movements such as yawns or facial grimaces, their eyes may be open and they may be capable of breathing without assistance. Without higher brain functions, however, any apparent wakefulness does not represent awareness of self or environment (thus, the condition is often described as "awake but unaware"). The case of Karen Ann Quinlan has made this condition familiar to the general public. With necessary medical and nursing care—including feeding through intravenous or nasogastric tubes, and antibiotics for recurrent pulmonary infections—such patients can survive months or years, often without a respirator. (The longest survival exceeded 37 years.)

CONCLUSION: THE NEED FOR RELIABLE POLICY

Medical interventions can often provide great benefit in avoiding *irreversible* harm to a patient's injured heart, lungs, or brain by carrying a patient through a period of acute need. These techniques have, however, thrown new light on the interrelationship of these crucial organ systems. This has created complex issues for public policy as well.

For medical and legal purposes, partial brain impairment must be distinguished from complete and irreversible loss of brain functions or "whole brain death." The President's Commission, as subsequent chapters explain more fully, regards the cessation of the vital functions of the entire brain—and not merely portions thereof, such as those responsible for cognitive functions—as the only proper neurologic basis for declaring death. This conclusion accords with the overwhelming consensus of medical and legal experts and the public.

Present attention to the "definition" of death is part of a process of development in social attitudes and legal rules stimulated by the unfolding of biomedical knowledge. In the nineteenth century increasing knowledge and practical skill made the public confident that death could be diagnosed reliably using cardiopulmonary criteria. The question now is whether, when medical intervention may be responsible for a patient's respiration and circulation, there are other equally reliable ways to diagnose death. . . .

THE DEFINITION AND CRITERION OF DEATH
Charles M. Culver and Bernard Gert

Culver and Gert consider it essential to distinguish among the *definition* of death, the *criterion* of death, and the *tests* of death. In discussing the definition of death, they begin by giving reasons why death must be considered an event rather than a process. They define death as the permanent cessation of functioning of the *organism as a whole,* and they argue against a competing definition, according to which the permanent loss of consciousness and cognition is sufficient for death. In their view, patients who are in a chronic (permanent) vegetative state are alive but are no longer persons, and it is morally justifiable to allow them to die by discontinuing even "ordinary and routine care." With regard to the *criterion* of death, Culver and Gert maintain that the correct criterion is the permanent loss of functioning of the entire brain, not the permanent loss of cardiopulmonary function. They conclude with a brief discussion of the appropriate *tests* of death.

Much of the confusion arising from the current brain death controversy is due to the failure to distinguish three distinct elements: (1) the definition of death; (2) the medical criterion for determining that death

has occurred; and (3) the tests to prove that the criterion has been satisfied. We shall first define death in a way which makes its ordinary meaning explicit, then provide a criterion of death which fulfills this definition, and finally, indicate which tests have demonstrated perfect validity in determining that the criterion of death is satisfied.[1]

The definitions of death which appear in legal dictionaries and the new statutory definitions of death do not say what the layman actually means by death but merely set out the criteria by which physicians legally determine when death has occurred. *Death,* however, is not a technical term but a common term in everyday use. We believe that a proper understanding of the ordinary meaning of this word or concept must be developed before a medical criterion is chosen. We must decide what is ordinarily meant by death before physicians can decide how to measure it.

Agreement on the definition and criterion of death is literally a life-and-death matter. Whether a spontaneously breathing patient in a chronic vegetative state is classified as dead or alive depends on our understanding of the definition of death. Even given the definition, the status of a patient with a totally and permanently non-functioning brain who is being maintained on a ventilator depends on the criterion of death employed. Defining death is primarily a philosophical task; providing the criterion of death is primarily medical; and choosing the tests to prove that the criterion is satisfied is solely a medical matter.

THE DEFINITION OF DEATH

Death as a Process or an Event It has been claimed that death is a process rather than an event (Morison, 1971). This claim is supported by the fact that a standard series of degenerative and destructive changes occurs in the tissues of an organism, usually following but sometimes preceding the irreversible cessation of spontaneous ventilation and circulation. These changes include: necrosis of brain cells, necrosis of other vital organ cells, cooling, rigor mortis, dependent lividity, and putrefaction. This process actually persists for years, even centuries, until the skeletal remains have disintegrated, and could even be viewed as beginning with the failure of certain organ systems during life. Because these changes occur in a fairly regular and ineluctable fashion, it is claimed that the stipulation of any particular point in this process as the moment of death is arbitrary.

The following argument, however, shows the theoretical inadequacy of any definition which makes death a process. If we regard death as a process, then either (1) the process starts when the person is still living, which confuses the process of death with the process of dying, for we all regard someone who is dying as not yet dead, or (2) the process of death starts when the person is no longer alive, which confuses the process of death with the process of disintegration. Death should be viewed not as a process but as the event that separates the process of dying from the process of disintegration.

On a practical level, regarding death as a process makes it impossible to declare the time of death with any precision. This is not a trivial issue. There are pressing medical, legal, social, and religious reasons to declare the time of death with some precision, including the interpretation of wills, burial times and procedures, mourning times, and decisions regarding the aggressiveness of medical support. There are no countervailing practical or theoretical reasons for regarding death as a process rather than an event in formulating a definition of death. We shall say that death occurs at some definite time, although this time may not always be specifiable with complete precision.

Choices for a Definition of Death The definition of death must capture our ordinary use of the term, for *death,* as noted earlier, is a word used by everyone and is not primarily a medical or legal term. In this ordinary use, certain facts are assumed, and we shall assume them as well. Therefore we shall not apply our analysis to science fiction speculations, for example, about brains continuing to function independently of the rest of the organism (Gert, 1967, 1971). Thus we shall assume that all and only living organisms can die, that the living can be distinguished from the dead with very good reliability, and that the moment when an organism leaves the former state and enters the latter can be determined with a fairly high degree of precision. We shall regard death as permanent. We know that some people claim to have been dead for several minutes and then to have returned to life, but we regard this as only a dramatic way of saying that consciousness was temporarily lost (for example, because of a brief episode of cardiac arrest).

Although there are religious theories that death involves the soul leaving the body, we know that religious persons and secularists do not disagree in their ordinary application of the term *dead.* We acknowledge that the body can remain physically intact for some time after death and that some isolated parts of the organism may continue to function (for example, it is commonly believed that hair and nails continue to grow after death). We shall now present our definition of death and contrast it to a proposed alternative.

We define death as the permanent cessation of functioning of the organism as a whole. By the organism as a whole, we do not mean the whole organism, that is, the sum of its tissue and organ parts, but rather the highly complex interaction of its organ subsystems. The organism need not be whole or complete—it may have lost a limb or an organ (such as the spleen)—but it still remains an organism.

By the functioning of the organism as a whole, we mean the spontaneous and innate activities of integration of all or most subsystems (for example, neuroendocrine control) and at least limited response to the environment (for example, temperature change). However, it is not necessary that all of the subsystems be integrated. Individual subsystems may be replaced (for example, by pacemakers, ventilators, or pressors) without changing the status of the organism as a whole.

It is possible for individual subsystems to function for a time after the organism as a whole has permanently ceased to function. Spontaneous ventilation ceases either immediately after or just before the permanent cessation of functioning of the organism as a whole, but spontaneous circulation, with artificial ventilation, may persist for up to two weeks after the organism as a whole has ceased to function.

An example of an activity of the organism as a whole is temperature regulation. The control of this complex process is located in the hypothalamus and is important for normal maintenance of all cellular processes. It is lost when the organism as a whole has ceased to function.

Consciousness and cognition are sufficient to show the functioning of the organism as a whole in higher animals, but they are not necessary. Lower organisms never have consciousness and even when a higher organism is comatose, evidence of the functioning of the organism as a whole may still be evident, for example, in temperature regulation.

We believe that the permanent cessation of the functioning of the organism as a whole is what has traditionally been meant by death. This definition retains death as a biological occurrence which is not unique to human beings; the same definition applies to other higher animals. We believe that death is a biological phenomenon and should apply equally to related species. When we talk of the death of a human being, we mean the same thing as we do when we talk of the death of a dog or a cat. This is supported by our ordinary use of the term *death,* and by law and tradition. It is also in accord with social and religious practices and is not likely to be affected by future changes in technology.

An alternative definition of death as the irreversible loss of that which is essentially significant to the nature of man has been proposed by Veatch (1976). Though this definition initially seems very attractive, it does not state what we ordinarily mean when we speak of death. It is not regarded as self-contradictory to say that a person has lost that which is essentially significant to the nature of man, but is still alive. For example, we all acknowledge that permanently comatose patients in chronic vegetative states are sufficiently brain-damaged that they have irreversibly lost all that is essentially significant to the nature of man but we still consider them to be living (for example, Karen Ann Quinlan; see Beresford, 1977).

The patients described by Brierley and associates (1971) are also in this category. These patients had complete neocortical destruction with preservation of the brainstem and diencephalic (posterior brain) structures. They had isoelectric (flat) electroencephalograms (EEGs) (indicating neocortical death) and were permanently comatose, although they had normal spontaneous breathing and brainstem reflexes; they were essentially in a permanent, severe, chronic vegetative state (Jennett and Plum, 1972). They retained many of the vital functions of the organism as a whole, including neuroendocrine control (that is, homeostatic inter-relationships between the brain and various hormonal glands) and spontaneous circulation and breathing.

This alternative definition actually states what it means to cease to be a person rather than what it means for that person to die. *Person* is not a biological concept but rather a concept defined in terms of certain kinds of abilities and qualities of awareness. It is inherently vague. Death is a biological concept. Thus in a literal sense, death can be applied directly only to biological organisms and not to persons. We do not object to the phrase "death of a person," but the phrase in common usage actually means the death of the organism which was the person. For example, one might overhear in the hospital wards, "The person in room 612 died last night." In this common usage, one is referring to the death of the organism which was a person. By our analysis, Veatch (1976) and others have used the phrase "death of a person" metaphorically, applying it to an organism which has ceased to be a person but has not died.

Without question, consciousness and cognition are essential human attributes. If they are lost, life has lost its meaning. A patient in a chronic vegetative state is usually regarded as living in only the most basic biological sense. But it is just this basic biological sense that we want to capture in our definition of death. We must not confuse the death of an organism which was a person with an organism's ceasing to be a person. We are immediately aware of the loss of personhood in these patients and are repulsed by the idea of continuing to treat them as if they were persons. But were we to consider these chronic vegetative patients as actually dead, serious problems would arise. First, a slippery slope condition would be introduced wherein the question could be asked: How much neocortical damage is necessary before we declare a patient dead? Surely patients in a chronic vegetative state, although usually not totally satisfying the tests for neocortical destruction, have permanently lost their consciousness and cognition. Then what about the somewhat less severely brain-damaged patient?

By considering permanent loss of consciousness and cognition as a criterion for ceasing to be a person and not for death of the organism as a whole, the slippery slope phenomenon is put where it belongs: not in the definition of death, but in the determination of possible grounds for nonvoluntary euthanasia, that is, providing possible grounds for killing the organism, or allowing it to die, in those instances in which the organism is no longer a person. The justification of nonvoluntary euthanasia

must be kept strictly separate from the definition of death. Most of us would like our organism to die when we cease to be persons, but this should not be accomplished by blurring the distinctions between biological death and the loss of personhood.

When an organism ceases to be a person, that is, when it permanently loses all consciousness and cognition, then practical problems arise. How are we to treat this organism? (1) Should we treat it just as we treat a person, making every effort to keep it alive? (2) Should we cease caring for it, either in part or at all, and allow it to die? (3) Should we kill it?

In our view, an organism that is no longer a person has no claim to be treated as a person. But just as one treats a corpse with respect, even more so would one expect that such a living organism be treated with respect. This does not mean, however, that one should strive to keep the organism alive. No one benefits by doing this; on the contrary, given the care needed to keep such an organism alive, it seems an extravagant waste of both economic and human resources to attempt to do so. On the other hand, it seems unjustified to require anyone to actively kill it. Even though the organism is no longer a person, it still looks like a person, and unless there are overwhelming reasons for killing it, it seems best not to do anything that might weaken the prohibition against killing. This leaves the second alternative, discontinuing all care and allowing the patient to die. This can take either of two forms: discontinuing medical treatment or discontinuing all ordinary and routine care. The latter is the position we favor.

It is important to note that the patient will not suffer from lack of care, for since the patient is no longer a person this means that it has permanently lost all consciousness and cognition. Any patient who retains even the slightest capacity to suffer pain or discomfort of any kind remains a person and must be treated as such. We make this point to emphasize our position that only patients who have completely and permanently lost all consciousness and cognition should have all care discontinued. We believe that discontinuing all care and allowing the patient who is no longer a person to die is the preferred alternative, and the one that should be recommended to the legal guardian or next of kin as the course of action to be followed.

THE CRITERION OF DEATH

We have argued that the correct definition of death is permanent cessation of functioning of the organism as a whole. We will now inspect the two competing criteria of death: (1) the permanent loss of cardiopulmonary functioning and (2) the total and irreversible loss of functioning of the whole brain.

Characteristics of Optimum Criteria and Tests

Given that death is the permanent cessation of functioning of the organism as a whole, a criterion will yield a false-positive if it is satisfied, and yet it would still be possible for that organism to function as a whole. By far the most important requirement for a criterion of death is that it yield no false-positives.

A criterion of death, however, cannot have any exceptions; this is what enables it to serve as a legal definition of death. It is not sufficient that the criterion be correct 99.99 percent of the time. This means that not only can the criterion yield no false-positives, it can also yield no false-negatives. A criterion of death yields a false-negative if it is not satisfied and yet the organism as a whole has irreversibly ceased to function. Of course, one may sometimes determine death without using the criterion, but it can never be that the criterion is satisfied and yet the person is not dead, or that the criterion is not satisfied and the person is dead. This is why it is so easy to mistake a criterion for an ordinary definition; it is rather a kind of operational definition, and serves as part of the legal definition, but the real operational definition is provided by the tests which show whether or not the criterion is satisfied.

Permanent Loss of Cardiopulmonary Functioning

Permanent termination of heart and lung function has been used as a criterion of death throughout history. The ancients observed that all other bodily functions ceased shortly after cessation of these vital functions, and the irreversible process of bodily disintegration inevitably followed. Thus permanent loss of spontaneous cardiopulmonary function was found to predict permanent nonfunctioning of the organism as a whole. Further, if there were no permanent loss of spontaneous cardiopulmonary function, then the organism as a whole continued to function. Therefore permanent loss of cardiopulmonary function served as an adequate criterion of death.

Because of current ventilation/circulation technology, permanent loss of spontaneous cardiopulmonary functioning is no longer necessarily predictive of permanent nonfunctioning of the organism as a whole. Consider a conscious, talking patient who is unable to breathe because of suffering from poliomyelitis and who requires an iron lung (thus having permanent loss of spontaneous pulmonary function), who has also developed asystole (loss of spontaneous heartbeat) requiring a permanent pacemaker (thus having permanent loss of spontaneous cardiac function). It would be absurd to regard such a person as dead.

It might be proposed that it is not the permanent loss of *spontaneous* cardiopulmonary function that is the criterion of death, but rather the permanent loss of all cardiopulmonary function, whether spontaneous or artificially supported. But now that ventilation and circulation can be mechanically maintained, an organism with permanent loss of whole brain functioning can have permanently ceased to function as a whole days to weeks before the heart and lungs cease to function with artificial support. Thus this supposed criterion would not be satisfied, yet the person would be dead. The heart and lungs now seem to have no unique relationship to the functioning of the organism as a whole. Continued artificially supported cardiopulmonary function is no longer perfectly correlated with life, and permanent loss of spontaneous cardiopulmonary functioning is no longer perfectly correlated with death.

Total and Irreversible Loss of Whole Brain Functioning

The criterion for the cessation of functioning of the organism as a whole is the permanent loss of functioning of the entire brain. This criterion is perfectly correlated with the permanent cessation of functioning of the organism as a whole because it is the brain that is necessary for the functioning of the organism as a whole. It integrates, generates, interrelates, and controls complex bodily activities. A patient on a ventilator with a totally destroyed brain is merely a preparation of artificially maintained subsystems since the organism as a whole has ceased to function.

The brain generates the signal for breathing through brainstem ventilatory centers and aids in the control of circulation through brainstem blood pressure control centers. Destruction of the brain produces apnea (inability to breathe) and generalized vasodilatation (opening of the peripheral blood vessels); in all cases, despite the most aggressive support, the adult heart stops within a week and that of the child within two weeks (Ingvar et al., 1978). Thus when the organism as a whole has ceased to function, the artificially supported vital subsystems quickly fail. Many other functions of the organism as a whole, including neuroendocrine control, temperature control, food-searching behaviors, and sexual activity, reside in the more primitive regions (hypothalamus, brainstem) of the brain. Thus total and irreversible loss of functioning of the whole brain and not merely the neocortex is required as the criterion for the permanent loss of the functioning of the organism as a whole.

Using permanent loss of functioning of the whole brain as the criterion for death of the organism as a whole is also consistent with tradition. Throughout history, whenever a physician was called to ascertain the occurrence of death, his examination included the following important signs indicative of permanent loss of functioning of the whole brain: unresponsivity, lack of spontaneous movements including breathing; and absence of pupillary light response. Only one important sign, lack of heartbeat, was not directly indicative of whole brain destruction. But since the heartbeat stops within several minutes of apnea, permanent absence of the vital signs is an important sign of permanent loss of whole brain functioning. Thus, in an important sense, permanent loss of whole brain functioning has always been the underlying criterion of death.

THE TESTS OF DEATH

Given the definition of death as the permanent cessation of functioning of the organism as a whole, and the criterion of death as the total and irreversible cessation of functioning of the whole brain, the next step is the examination of the available tests of death. The tests must be such that they will never yield a false-positive result. Of secondary importance, they should produce few and relatively brief false-negatives.

Cessation of Heartbeat and Ventilation The physical findings of permanent absence of heartbeat and respiration are the traditional tests of death. In the vast majority of deaths not complicated by artificial ventilation, these classic tests are still applicable. They show that the criterion of death has been satisfied since they always quickly produce permanent loss of functioning of the whole brain. However, when mechanical ventilation is being used, these tests lose most of their utility due to the production of numerous false-negatives for as long a time as one to two weeks, that is, death of the organism as a whole with still intact circulatory-ventilatory subsystems. Thus though the circulation-ventilation tests will suffice in most instances of death, if there is artificial maintenance of circulation or ventilation the special tests for permanent cessation of whole brain functioning will be needed.

Irreversible Cessation of Whole Brain Functioning Numerous formalized sets of tests have been established to determine that the criterion of permanent loss of whole brain functioning has been met. These include, among others, tests described by the Harvard Medical School Ad Hoc Committee (Beecher, 1968) and the National Institutes of Health Collaborative Study of Cerebral Survival (1977). They have all been recently reviewed (Black, 1978; Molinari, 1978). What we call tests have sometimes been called "criteria," but it is important to distinguish these second-level criteria from the first-level criteria. While the first-level criteria must be for the death of the organism and must be understandable by the layman, the second-level criteria (tests) determine the permanent loss of functioning of the whole brain and need not be understandable by anyone except qualified clinicians. To avoid confusion, we prefer to use the designation "tests" for the second-level criteria.

All the proposed tests require total and permanent absence of all functioning of the brainstem and both hemispheres. They vary slightly from one set to another, but all require unresponsivity (deep coma), absent pupillary light reflexes, apnea (inability to breathe), and absent brainstem reflexes. They also require the absence of drug intoxication and low body temperature, and the newer sets require the demonstration that a lesion of the brain exists. Isoelectric (flat) EEGs are generally required, and tests disclosing the absence of cerebral blood flow are of confirmatory value (NIH Collaborative Study, 1977). All tests require the given loss of function to be present for a particular time interval, which in the case of the absence of cerebral blood flow may be as short as thirty minutes.

Current tests of irreversible loss of whole brain function may produce many false-negatives of a sort during the thirty-minute to twenty-four-hour interval between the successive neurologic examinations which the tests require. Certain sets of tests, particularly those requiring electrocerebral silence by EEG, may produce false-negatives if an EEG artifact is present and cannot confidently be distinguished from brain wave activity. Generally, a few brief false-negatives are tolerable and even inevitable, since tests must be delineated conservatively in order to eliminate any possibility of false-positives.

There are many studies which show perfect correlation between the loss of whole brain function tests of the Ad Hoc Committee of the Harvard Medical School and total brain necrosis at postmortem examination. Veith et al. (1977a) conclude that "the validity of the criteria [tests] must be considered to be established with as much certainty as is possible in biology or medicine" (p. 1652). Thus, when a physician ascertains that a patient satisfies the validated loss of whole brain function tests, he can be confident that the loss of whole brain functioning is permanent. Physicians should apply only tests which have been completely validated. . . .

NOTE

1 This [article] is adapted in part from Bernat, Culver, and Gert (1981).

REFERENCES

American Bar Association. House of Delegates redefines death, urges redefinition of rape, and undoes the Houston amendments. *American Bar Association Journal,* 1975, *61,* 463–464.

Beecher, Henry K. A definition of irreversible coma: report of the Ad Hoc Committee of the Harvard Medical School to examine the definition of brain death. *Journal of the American Medical Association,* 1968, *205,* 337–340.

Beresford, H. Richard. The Quinlan decision: problems and legislative alternatives. *Annals of Neurology,* 1977, *2,* 74–81.

Bernat, James L., Culver, Charles M., and Gert, Bernard. On the definition and criterion of death. *Annals of Internal Medicine,* 1981, *94,* 389–394.

Black, Peter M. Brain death. *New England Journal of Medicine,* 1978, *299,* 338–344, 393–401.

Brierley, J. B., Adams, J. H., Graham, D. I., and Simpson, J. A. Neocortical death after cardiac arrest. *Lancet,* 1971, *2,* 560–565.

Capron, Alexander M., and Kass, Leon R. A statutory definition of the standards for determining human death: an appraisal and a proposal. *University of Pennsylvania Law Review,* 1972, *121,* 87–118.

Gert, Bernard. Can the brain have a pain? *Philosophy and Phenomenological Research,* 1967, *27,* 432–436.

Gert, Bernard. Personal identity and the body. *Dialogue,* 1971, *10,* 458–478.

Hastings Center Task Force on Death and Dying. Refinements in criteria for the determination of death: an appraisal. *Journal of the American Medical Association,* 1972, *221,* 48–53.

Ingvar, David H., Brun, Arne, Johansson, Lars, and Sammuelsson, Sven M. Survival after severe cerebral anoxia with destruction of the cerebral cortex: the apallic syndrome. *Annals of the New York Academy of Science,* 1978, *315,* 184–214.

Jennett, B., and Plum, F. Persistent vegetative state after brain damage. A syndrome in search of a name. *Lancet,* 1972, *1,* 734–737.

Jonas, Hans. *Philosophical Essays: From Ancient Creed to Technological Man.* Englewood Cliffs, N.J.: Prentice-Hall, 1974, pp. 134–140.

Law Reform Commission of Canada. *Criteria for the Determination of Death.* Ottawa: Law Reform Commission of Canada, 1979.

Molinari, Gaetano F. Review of clinical criteria of brain death. *Annals of the New York Academy of Science,* 1978, *315,* 62–69.

Morison, Robert S. Death: process or event? *Science,* 1971, *173,* 694–698.

NIH Collaborative Study of Cerebral Survival. An appraisal of the criteria of cerebral death: a summary statement. *Journal of the American Medical Association,* 1977, *237,* 982–986.

President's Commission for the Study of Ethical Problems in
    Medicine and Biomedical and Behavioral Research.
    *"Defining Death," a Report on the Medical, Legal and
    Ethical Issues in the Determination of Death.* Washington,
    D.C., 1981.
Veatch, Robert M. *Death, Dying and the Biological Revolution:
    Our Last Quest for Responsibility.* New Haven, Conn.: Yale
    University Press, 1976.

Veith, Frank J., Fein, Jack M., Tendler, Moses D., Veatch,
    Robert M., Kleiman, Marc A., and Kalkines, George. Brain
    death I. A status report of medical and ethical
    considerations. *Journal of the American Medical
    Association,* 1977a, *238,* 1651–1655.
Veith, Frank J., Fein, Jack M., Tendler, Moses D., Veatch,
    Robert M., Kleiman, Marc A., and Kalkines, George. Brain
    death II. A status report of legal considerations. *Journal of
    the American Medical Association,* 1977b, *238,* 1744–1748.

PRAGMATISM AND THE DETERMINATION OF DEATH

Martin Benjamin

Benjamin clarifies various aspects of the debate over the determination of death, engaging the issue from the vantage point of American pragmatism. (He believes it is misleading to phrase the issue in terms of the *definition* of death.) Benjamin ultimately argues that death should be determined on the basis of "higher-brain" criteria rather than "whole-brain" criteria. Thus, he contends that both anencephalic infants and patients in a permanent vegetative state should be pronounced dead. Benjamin identifies the underlying philosophical issue as follows: "Exactly what is it that ceases to exist when we say someone like you or me is dead?" In his view, there are compelling pragmatic reasons to understand the underlying entity as a person rather than as a biological organism.

The individual has a stock of old opinions already, but he meets a new experience that puts them to a strain. . . . The result is an inward trouble to which his mind till then had been a stranger, and from which he seeks to escape by modifying his previous mass of opinions. He saves as much of it as he can, for in this matter of belief we are all extreme conservatives.
    William James[1]

What serious men not engaged in the professional business of philosophy most want to know is what modifications and abandonments of intellectual inheritance are required by the newer industrial, political, and scientific movements. They want to know what these newer movements mean when translated into general ideas. Unless professional philosophy can mobilize itself sufficiently to assist in this clarification and redirection of men's thoughts, it is likely to get more and more sidetracked from the main currents of contemporary life.
    John Dewey[2]

Reprinted with permission of the publisher from *Pragmatic Bioethics,* 2d
ed., edited by Glenn McGee (Cambridge: The MIT Press), pp. 193–206.
© 1999, 2003 Glenn McGee.

Recent debates over the determination of death illustrate these observations by James and Dewey. From about 1850 to the 1960s there was general agreement about the determination of death. An individual was pronounced dead when breathing and heartbeat had permanently ceased. In the mid-1960s, however, advances in medical knowledge and technology were enabling physicians to maintain respiration and circulation in patients with total loss of brain function. This new experience, in James's words, together with the development of organ transplantation, was placing considerable strain on our old opinions about the determination of death. The result was an inward trouble of mind from which physicians sought to escape by modifying our previous mass of opinions. This modification—declaring patients with heartbeat and respiration but total loss of brain function dead—saved as much of the previous mass of opinions as possible, confirming James's observation that "in this matter of belief we are all extreme conservatives."

Yet the change has not remained stable. Debate over the so-called definition of death continues to this day. An explanation is suggested by the passage from Dewey. Adopting new criteria for death required certain modifications and abandonments of intellectual inheritance that were not at the time adequately considered. Those in the forefront of change gave insufficient attention to the philosophical question of what these modifications and abandonments meant when translated into general ideas. This question ranged beyond the more-or-less immediate practical concerns of physicians. Therefore, to adapt Dewey's words, *until* serious men (and women) not engaged in the professional business of philosophy attend fully to the philosophical dimensions of the determination of death—and *until* professional philosophers adequately assist in this clarification and redirection of their thoughts—the debate is likely to continue.

In what follows, I develop this suggestion. I begin by explaining the controversy over the determination of death. Then I identify the general ideas—the possible modifications and abandonments of intellectual inheritance—at stake in the debate. I conclude by proposing a clarification and redirection of our understanding of the determination of death and defend it on pragmatic grounds.

BACKGROUND

In the not-so-distant past, respiration and circulation were considered the principal signs of human life, and their cessation was considered the mark of death. Individuals were pronounced dead when they had permanently stopped breathing or their hearts had stopped beating. In the mid-1960s, however, developments in mechanical respiration (together with related supportive measures) gave physicians the capacity to maintain respiration and circulation in patients who had undergone total and permanent loss of

brain function. Such patients—patients who were totally and permanently unconscious—were, according to the prevailing criteria, living human beings.

In 1968 a landmark article published by an ad hoc committee of the Harvard Medical School identified reliable clinical criteria for identifying respirator-dependent patients who have lost *all* brain functions, including primitive brain stem reflexes.[3] Patients satisfying these criteria, the committee said, were in "irreversible coma." The committee then proposed that patients in irreversible coma be declared dead and removed from the respirator. The publication of this article gave currency to the misleading term *brain death.*

Brain death, in the first and most literal sense, means the death of an organ, the brain. But death of an organ is one thing, and death of the organism of which it is a part quite another. Yet the term soon came to be used to refer to the latter as well. That is, a patient pronounced dead by use of the so-called Harvard criteria for irreversible coma was often said to be brain dead. The result was a misleading impression that there were now two kinds of death—ordinary (heart-lung) death and brain death.

The confusion may be avoided by scrupulously restricting the expression *brain death* to the death of the brain and using the term *brain criteria* to refer to the criteria for pronouncing a respirator-dependent patient with absolutely no brain function dead. Such a patient should be considered dead in the same way—and for the same reasons—as a patient whose heartbeat and respiration have permanently ceased. This important clarification, however, required taking account of certain philosophical considerations that in the late 1960s were given insufficient attention.

The motivation for the Harvard ad hoc committee's recommendation that irreversible coma (or the death of the brain) be accepted as a criterion for determining the death of the patient was clinical, not philosophical. First, the increasing number of respirator-dependent patients who met the Harvard criteria was becoming a burden on limited medical, technological, and financial resources. This seemed wasteful insofar as physicians believed such patients could no longer benefit from treatment. Second, the development of organ transplantation was increasing the demand for kidneys, hearts, and other organs.

Transplant surgeons wanted permission to remove healthy organs from irreversibly comatose respirator-dependent patients without being accused of murder. And third, waiting to pronounce such patients dead according to traditional heart-lung criteria prolonged the limbolike status—and related emotional costs—of friends and family members awaiting the inevitable.

After publication of the Harvard criteria, states began reconsidering their statutes on death. By 1980 twenty-four states had incorporated brain criteria. Then in 1981 a presidential commission undertook a comprehensive review of the "medical, legal, and ethical issues in the determination of death." The commission eventually endorsed brain criteria and, together with the American Medical Association and the American Bar Association, recommended adoption by all states of a model statute, the Uniform Determination of Death Act (UDDA):

> An individual who has sustained either (1) irreversible cessation of circulatory and respiratory functions or (2) irreversible cessation of all functions of the entire brain, including the brain stem, is dead. A determination of death must be made in accordance with accepted medical standards.[4]

Brain criteria for the determination of death have now been incorporated into the law of most states. Health professionals, lawyers, legislators, and the public generally agree that a patient who has lost all brain function is, despite respirator-assisted breathing and heartbeat, dead.

CONTINUING CONTROVERSY

Yet the debate has not ended. As specified by the UDDA, the new criteria require "irreversible cessation of *all* functions of the *entire* brain, *including the brain stem*"(my emphasis). But beginning with the case of Karen Ann Quinlan in 1976, the condition now dubbed a persistent vegetative state (PVS) has become both more prevalent and widely known. Patients in a vegetative state are unconscious because the parts of the brain necessary for thought and consciousness are no longer functioning. The state becomes permanent when it becomes irreversible.[5]

Such patients are totally and permanently unconscious. Yet they do not satisfy the current criteria for death; they have not lost *all* brain function. Because their brain stems continue to function and because the brain stem can regulate respiration, blood pressure, and a number of other vegetative functions, in the absence of cerebral function patients in a persistent vegetative state are often able to breathe and maintain their heartbeat without the assistance of a respirator.

Are such patients living or dead? According to the law, they are alive. The general criteria for death proposed by the Harvard ad hoc committee, endorsed by the president's commission, and adopted by the states explicitly require the permanent loss of *all* function of the brain, *including the brain stem*—and patients in a permanent vegetative state have functioning brain stems. But a number of bioethicists have recommended that such patients be pronounced dead.[6] Total and permanent loss of consciousness—and not total and permanent loss of *all* brain function, these bioethicists maintain—is what marks the line between human life and death.

The controversy is usually characterized as a debate over the definition of death. Defenders of the status quo are said to accept a "whole-brain" definition of death, while their opponents propose we adopt a "higher-brain" definition. This characterization is, however, misleading. The disagreement does not center on definition, but rather on what Dewey described as the "general ideas" underlying the "modifications and abandonments of intellectual inheritance" required by a "new scientific movement." The new scientific movement is, in this instance, the capacity to diagnose total and permanent loss of consciousness in patients for whom respiration and heartbeat may be medically maintained (in some cases, for over thirty years). The underlying general idea is whether being alive is, for the likes of you and me, solely a matter of biology or whether it also involves consciousness (or the potential for consciousness). This is a philosophical question, not simply a matter of definition.

THE MAIN QUESTION

We have no trouble understanding what people mean when they speak or write of the death of a human embryo, a lawn, a dog, a language, or an entire culture. In each case the entity to which the word *dead* (or one of its cognates) is applied has ceased to exist as a thing *of that kind.* The conditions of existence and death of any entity—be it a human embryo, a lawn, a dog, a language, or a culture—are determined by the kind of thing that it is. "Death" is the cessation of life, a ceasing to be. When we are puzzled over what it means to say, "Karen Anne Quinlan is dead," the problem centers not on the meaning of *dead,* but rather on the entity to which we refer; exactly what *kind* of entity is it, and what are the conditions of its existence? Are we referring only to a human biological organism, or are we referring to something else, something whose conditions of existence include consciousness or at least the potential for consciousness?

The so-called definition-of-death debate, then, is really a debate over how we should conceive the individual subject to which the words *is dead* are applied. Exactly what is it that ceases to exist when we say someone like you or me is dead? This is the difficult, unavoidable philosophical question generated by the capacity of modern medicine to sustain respiration and heartbeat in patients who are totally and permanently unconscious.

We owe the misplaced emphasis on definition, I suspect, to the fact that the terms of the problem were set by those who first encountered and addressed it—members of the medical community. Clinicians are understandably more comfortable talking about definitions than they are about opposing philosophical conceptions of the human individual. But the philosophical questions are now unavoidable. What exactly is it that has lost life or ceased to be when we say that someone like you or me is dead? What is so important about whatever has been lost when we pronounce death to justify the enormous difference between our treatment of the living and the dead? These are not, on reflection, easy questions. And there may be no single answer to them that ought, at this time, to be embraced by all of us, insofar as we are informed and rational. Still, we will not reach closure on the determination of death until we can satisfactorily address them.

DEATH OF THE ORGANISM AS A WHOLE

Though the Harvard ad hoc committee did not address these questions, eleven years later the president's commission did. Essential to human life, the commission argued, is the integrated functioning of the circulatory system, the respiratory system, and the central nervous system:

> Three organs—the heart, lungs, and brain—assume special significance . . . because their interrelationship is very close and the irreversible cessation of any one very quickly stops the other two and consequently halts the integrated functioning of the organism as a whole. Because they were easily measured, circulation and respiration were traditionally the basic "vital signs." But breathing and heartbeat are not life itself. They are simply used as signs—as one window for viewing a deeper and more complex reality: a triangle of interrelated systems with the brain at its apex.[7]

The subject of life and death is, then, the organism as a whole. The organism as a whole is alive when there is the integrated functioning of the circulatory, respiratory, and central nervous systems. The organism dies when the integrated functioning of these three systems is permanently disrupted. Permanent loss of any corner of the "triangle" soon leads to permanent loss of the other two.

According to the president's commission, then, adoption of brain criteria does not require a change in philosophical understanding. The subject of life and death has always been the organism as a whole, conceived as the integrating functioning of the circulatory, respiratory, and central nervous systems. Each set of criteria—heart-lung and brain—represents a different "window" for viewing the same state, death of the organism as a whole. "On this view," the commission wrote, "death is that moment at which the body's physiological system ceases to constitute an integrated whole. Even if life continues in individual cells or organs, life of the organism as a whole requires complex integration and without the latter, a person cannot properly be regarded as alive." The commission considered and explicitly rejected "higher-brain" criteria because, among other things, even if it could be shown that "higher" brain function is necessary for consciousness, the cessation of higher brain function "often cannot be assessed with the certainty that would be required in applying a statutory definition [of death]."[8]

Finally, the commission acknowledged with some pride that its proposal was "deliberately conservative." The UDDA incorporates legal recognition of a new way to diagnose death, but it does not put forth a new philosophical conception of death. Brain criteria identify the very same thing heart-lung criteria have traditionally identified—death of the organism as a whole. Therefore, in modifying our "old opinions" to accommodate a "new experience that put them to a strain," the commission sought to save as much of our "previous mass of opinions" as it could. "For in this matter of belief," as James put it, "we are all extreme conservatives."

DEATH OF THE PERSON

But, proponents of higher-brain criteria contend, the capacity to sustain biological life long after an individual becomes totally and permanently unconscious requires more extensive revision of our previous mass of opinions than the president's commission was willing to acknowledge. A "person"—where the word *person* designates the kind of being whose continued existence is generally of the utmost importance to us—may be dead even though the organism as a whole is alive.[9] What really matters to us, when we consider our own lives and the lives of others, is continued existence as persons, not continued existence as personless organisms.

Consider, for example, the following situation. In one part of a large urban hospital, infant Andrew is born with anencephaly. Anencephaly is a rare congenital condition marked by absence of a major portion of the brain, skull, and scalp. Anencephalic infants have functioning brain stems, but because they lack functioning cerebral hemispheres, they do not and never will experience any degree of consciousness. Andrew, though "alive" by current criteria, is totally and permanently unconscious. Without highly aggressive care, Andrew is likely to satisfy

the UDDA's criteria for death within a few days, if not hours. Even with aggressive care, he is unlikely to live for more than a week or two.

In a nearby hospital lies infant Helen. Helen has hypoplastic left heart syndrome, a congenital malformation very likely to lead to an early death. Apart from her seriously defective heart, Helen is healthy. Though his brain is seriously defective, Andrew has a healthy heart. Suppose, as may in reality be the case, it is surgically possible to replace Helen's defective heart with Andrew's healthy one. Such an operation is likely to significantly extend Helen's life. The surgeon cannot, however, wait until Andrew is pronounced dead. By the time Andrew satisfies the current criteria for death, his heart will have seriously deteriorated. So the question is whether, if both Helen's and Andrew's parents give their informed consent, it would be wrong for a surgeon to remove Andrew's heart and transplant it to Helen.

If by "wrong" we mean illegal, the answer is clear. Under current law, removing Andrew's heart would be an act of murder. Andrew is a living human being, and the cause of death would be the surgeon's cutting into his chest and removing his heart. But is removing Andrew's heart to save Helen's life a significant moral wrong? Indeed, might it not be wrong not to do the operation—wrong not only for Helen and her parents, but also for Andrew's parents? How, if Andrew is totally and permanently unconscious, would he be wronged by removing his heart? Removing his heart will not cause him pain or suffering, nor will it deprive him of a valuable future. As far as pain or prospects for future experience go, Andrew is no different than any cadaver organ donor. Why, then, should it be okay to save a life by transplanting the heart of a patient who satisfies whole-brain criteria for death, but wrong to save a life by transplanting Andrew's heart?

The Council on Ethical and Judicial Affairs of the American Medical Association reports: "In a survey of leading medical experts in ethics, two thirds of those surveyed stated that they consider the use of organs from anencephalic infants 'intrinsically moral,' and more than half stated their support for a change in the law to permit such use."[10] I am inclined to agree; and when I ask why the law should be changed, the answer that springs to mind is that there is an important sense in which Andrew is already dead. Though Andrew is certainly a living human organism, something central to my understanding of the wrongness of killing is missing in this and similar cases.

Exactly what this is comes into sharper focus when we shift our consideration from an infant with anencephaly to a patient in a permanent vegetative state. Both anencephalic infants and patients in a permanent vegetative state are totally and permanently unconscious. The main difference is that total and permanent unconsciousness is congenital in the former and acquired in the latter. Therefore, if anencephalic infants are to be pronounced dead because they are totally and permanently unconscious, we shall have to do the same with patients in a permanent vegetative state. Is there good reason to consider these patients dead?

Imagine you have just been diagnosed with a terrible disease that will soon ravage your body and end your life. A surgeon then comes along who offers the possibility of a dramatic new operation guaranteed to stop the disease in its tracks. There is, however, one very serious side effect. The operation is very long and the anesthetic very powerful. One of the consequences is that, although the disease will be cured, you will emerge from the operation in a permanent vegetative state. But, the surgeon cheerfully emphasizes, at least you will be alive! The operation will cure the disease, and your life will be saved. Finally, let us suppose, the operation is very expensive. To cover its costs you will have to use up your entire life savings and sell all your possessions. The question, now, is, will you agree to undergo the operation?

When I put this question to myself, the answer is clear. Whether or not I have the operation, it seems to me that *I* will be dead. That is, *I*—the being whose motivation for having the operation is to live to meet my grandchildren, watch them grow, finish the book I am working on, enjoy conversation and travel with my wife, and see the Chicago Cubs win the World Series—will not survive in either case. Whether I have the operation or forego it, *I*—whatever exactly *I* refers to here—will be dead. Though my body will survive the operation, *I*—the person whose body it

is—will not. The only difference from my perspective is whether the doctors will get my money or it will go to my family. And there is no question that I want it to go to my family.

The same general point can be made from a third-person perspective. Suppose someone develops a "permanent vegetative state drug"—a tasteless chemical compound that makes anyone who imbibes it totally and permanently unconscious. Then someone deliberately places this drug in the drink of one of your dearest friends or relatives. Soon after drinking it, your friend or relative becomes totally and permanently unconscious. The heinous perpetrator is then caught. How should he or she be charged? Should the charge be murder? If you (not unreasonably) answer yes, is it not because you believe that your friend or relative (the person you loved, whose well-being and future you valued, and whose company you cherished) is now dead? How persuaded would you be by a defense attorney arguing for a lesser charge by pointing out that your friend or family member still enjoys integrated functioning of the circulatory, respiratory, and central nervous systems and, on no less authority than that of a presidential commission, is alive?

As these examples suggest, there may be an important difference between a living human biological organism and whatever it is we regard as the subject of life and death when we say of ourselves or some other human being, *X,* "X is alive" or "X is dead." What, then, is the subject of the predicates *alive* and *dead* when applied to beings like you and me? Is it a biological organism (the class of which includes you and me, together with anencephalic infants and permanently vegetative patients) or, as my examples suggest, is it what I am calling a person? And can, in a small number of cases, the organism as a whole survive the death of the person? There will be no closure on the determination of death until there is closure on these fundamental questions.

Before considering a philosophically pragmatic response, we must consider an important objection to the personhood conception. Whether a person is in a permanent vegetative state, the objection correctly maintains, cannot be assessed by all physicians with the same degree of certainty as the death of the organism as a whole. But ease of application and a very high degree of certainty are necessary for criteria for death to be incorporated into the law. Therefore, the personhood conception must be rejected.[11]

The objection is, however, overstated. In the vast majority of cases, defenders of the personhood conception can point out, it is as easy to diagnose death under the personhood conception as it is under the biological conception because the two conceptions employ the same criteria for death. A person is dead if he or she sustains either: (1) irreversible cessation of circulatory and respiratory functions or (2) irreversible cessation of all functions of the entire brain, including the brain stem. Either the first criterion or the second is sufficient for total and permanent loss of consciousness. Indeed, it is the death of the person that provides the most plausible rationale for use of these criteria.

At the same time, the personhood conception explains why these conditions, although sufficient for pronouncing death, may not be necessary. Individuals in a permanent vegetative state are also totally and permanently unconscious (even though they have not undergone either irreversible cessation of respiration and circulation or total and irreversible cessation of all brain functions). If the most plausible rationale for the use of heart-lung and "whole-brain" criteria is that they give us a way to identify total and permanent loss of consciousness, anencephalic infants and others in a permanent vegetative state must also be regarded as dead, for they too are totally and permanently unconscious.

Therefore, even if we have doubts about our capacity to clearly and definitively diagnose a permanent vegetative state, the personhood conception may provide a more plausible rationale for our current criteria for death than does the "death of the organism as a whole" conception. Second, if we are willing to defer to neurologists, we will, after various periods of testing and observation, be able to identify with a high degree of certainty many cases of permanent vegetative state. Third, it is quite possible that more specific and reliable criteria for diagnosing a permanent vegetative state will emerge from further studies of large patient populations or the development of more refined technology (such as positron-emission tomographic [PET] scanners,

which can detect decreases in cerebral cortical metabolism consistent with unconsciousness and deep anesthesia).[12]

PRAGMATISM AND THE SUBJECT OF LIFE AND DEATH

How, then, should we conceive the subject of human life and death? Is it a biological organism, or is it a person? Whatever the answer to this question, pragmatists would say, it will not be discovered in a fixed, external reality, independent of and prior to our efforts to live and make sense of our lives in a complex, dynamic, social and natural world. "The trail of the human serpent," as James once put it, "is over everything."[13] Our conception of human death turns on our conception of the conditions of existence for beings like ourselves; and our conception of these conditions turns in part on a wide variety of factors, including human biology, our scientific and technological capacities, our beliefs about the world, and our reasonable aspirations, given our full set of values and principles. None of these elements is fixed or independent of the others. Significant changes in one will often occasion revisions in the others. There is, moreover, no way for us to show that any particular stage in this evolving web of reflective action and active belief is the last or final stage.

Which conception of the human individual—and its related conditions for existence—best coheres with the complex network of actions and beliefs giving shape and meaning to our lives? Is it principally a biological conception, centering on the integrated functioning of the organism as a whole? Or is it a social-psychological conception, centering on consciousness?

To fix this question pragmatically—to bring it "down to earth," as it were—we must ask ourselves such questions as, What really matters to us with respect to questions of life and death? Are we, when push comes to shove, deeply concerned with the continued existence of the integrated functioning of the circulatory, respiratory, and central nervous systems, independent of its contribution to consciousness? How willing are we to sacrifice other important values and principles—not to mention economic and social resources—to sustain the integrated functioning of a human organism as a whole? What conception of the subject of life and death provides the most practical and unified approach to the largest number of bioethical issues? And, most generally, what conception best coheres with the largest number of things that we are, on reflection, strongly inclined to do and believe? Though detailed and complete answers to these and related questions are beyond the scope of this [essay], my hunch is that conceiving the subject of life and death in terms of personhood will provide a more satisfactory answer to this family of questions than conceiving it in terms of biology alone.

First, when we ask what really matters to us with regard to human life and death—why, for example, we believe murder is so very wrong (and a physician's prima facie obligation to save life so very right)—the most plausible answer, it seems to me, turns on what Donald Marquis identifies as the "loss of a valuable future": "The loss of one's life is one of the greatest losses one can suffer. The loss of one's life deprives one of all the experience, activities, projects, and enjoyments that would otherwise have constituted one's future. Therefore, killing someone is wrong, primarily because the killing inflicts (one of) the greatest possible losses on the victim."[14]

But neither anencephalic infants nor those in a permanent vegetative state can be deprived of all of the experience, activities, projects, and enjoyments that would otherwise have constituted their future because they are, due to the absence or permanent loss of cerebral functioning, incapable of experiencing, doing, planning, or enjoying anything. If the loss of all possible experience, action, projects, or enjoyment is what makes killing prima facie wrong and the prospect of such experience, action, projects, or enjoyment what makes saving life prima facie right, both murder victims and patients are best conceived as biological persons, not simply as biological organisms.

Second, acceptance of the UDDA has not entirely eliminated the "inward trouble" of mind to which the Harvard criteria and the UDDA were a response. Many of us are, for example, troubled by the prohibition against transplanting hearts from anencephalic infants like Andrew in order to save the lives of infants with hypoplastic left heart syndrome like Helen. Moreover, we question spending over a billion dollars per year for an increasing number of permanently vegetative patients while millions of Americans are denied access to health care because of an inability to pay.

We are also disturbed by the fact that each year hundreds of persons in need of new hearts or livers die on waiting lists while the hearts and livers of patients in permanent vegetative states keep on going until they satisfy the UDDA, at which time their organs are no longer biologically suitable for transplantation. To what extent should we be willing to trade off the lives of infants like Helen, the resources used to maintain permanently vegetative patients, and the life-saving potential of their organs for the sake of the integrated functioning of various sets of circulatory, respiratory, and central nervous systems?

Finally, a shift from a mainly biological conception of human life and death to a more social-psychological conception may lead to plausible and coherent resolutions to a wide range of bioethical issues—from abortion and embryo research on the one hand to euthanasia and assisted suicide on the other. Exploring the ramifications of such a change—its overall human and economic costs, benefits, implications, and so on—may also lead to a better overall understanding of ourselves and of the value of our lives.

Whatever the results of such an inquiry (and I do not expect that it will soon be completed), it addresses one of the most basic, far-reaching philosophical questions of our time. Unless "professional philosophy can mobilize itself sufficiently to assist" in clarifying and redirecting our thoughts about these and related issues, it runs the risk, as foreseen by Dewey, of becoming "more and more sidetracked from the main currents of contemporary life."

NOTES

1 William James, *Pragmatism* (Indianapolis, Hackett, 1981), 31.
2 John Dewey, "The Need for a Recovery of Philosophy," in *John Dewey: The Middle Works, 1899–1924*, ed. Jo Ann Boydston, vol. 10 (Carbondale: Southern Illinois University Press, 1980), 4.
3 Ad Hoc Committee of the Harvard Medical School to Examine the Definition of Death, "A Definition of Irreversible Coma," *Journal of the American Medical Association* 205 (1968): 337–40.

4 President's Commission for the Study of Ethical Problems in Medicine and Biomedical and Behavioral Research, *Defining Death* (Washington: U.S. Government Printing Office, 1981), 73.

5 Multi-Society Task Force on PVS (American Academy of Neurology, Child Neurology Society, American Neurological Association, American Association of Neurological Surgeons, American Academy of Pediatrics), "Medical Aspects of the Persistent Vegetative State," *New England Journal of Medicine* 330 (1994): 1499–1508, 1572–79.

6 See, for example, Karen Gervais, *Redefining Death* (New Haven: Yale University Press, 1986); Gina Kolata, "Ethicists Debating a New Definition of Death," *New York Times,* 21 April 1992.

7 President's Commission, *Defining Death,* 33.

8 Ibid., 40.

9 For an illuminating analysis of complexities that I cannot explore here, see Jeff McMahan, "The Metaphysics of Brain Death," *Bioethics* 9 (1995): 91–126.

10 Council on Ethical and Judicial Affairs, American Medical Association, "The Use of Anencephalic Neonates as Organ Donors," *Journal of the American Medical Association* 273 (1995): 1614. The council, though supporting use of anencephalics as sources of organs, does not consider them dead.

11 President's Commission, *Defining Death,* 41–42.

12 Multi-Society Task Force on PVS, "Medical Aspects of the Persistent Vegetative State," 1578.

13 James, *Pragmatism,* 33.

14 Don Marquis, "Why Abortion Is Immoral," *Journal of Philosophy* 86 (1989): 189. Though I agree with Marquis's general point about what makes killing wrong, I disagree with his extending it to fetuses. If a fetus cannot plausibly be said to have a personal interest in its future, the loss of such a future cannot be a loss to the fetus (though, of course, it may be a loss to others with an interest in the fetus's future).

COMPETENT ADULTS AND THE REFUSAL OF LIFE-SUSTAINING TREATMENT

WITHHOLDING AND WITHDRAWING LIFE-SUSTAINING TREATMENT

Council on Ethical and Judicial Affairs, American Medical Association

In this brief excerpt from a much longer report, the AMA Council on Ethical and Judicial Affairs presents a series of clarifications related to the right of a competent patient to forgo life-sustaining treatment. In conjunction with a consideration of the traditional distinction between ordinary and extraordinary treatments, the council rejects the idea that it is never permissible to forgo artificial nutrition and hydration. Also rejected is the view that there is an ethically significant distinction between *withholding* and *withdrawing* life-sustaining treatment.

The principle of patient autonomy requires that physicians respect a competent patient's decision to forgo any medical treatment. This principle is not altered when the likely result of withholding or withdrawing a treatment is the patient's death.[1] The right of competent patients to forgo life-sustaining treatment has been upheld in the courts (for example, *In re Brooks Estate,* 32 Ill2d 361, 205 NE2d 435 [1965]; *In re Osborne,* 294 A2d 372 [1972]) and is generally accepted by medical ethicists.[1]

Reprinted with permission of the AMA from "Decisions Near the End of Life," *JAMA,* vol. 267, no. 16 (April 22/29, 1992), pp. 2229–2233.

Decisions that so profoundly affect a patient's well-being cannot be made independent of a patient's subjective preferences and values.[2] Many types of life-sustaining treatments are burdensome and invasive, so that the choice for the patient is not simply a choice between life and death.[3] When a patient is dying of cancer, for example, a decision may have to be made whether to use a regimen of chemotherapy that might prolong life for several additional months but also would likely be painful, nauseating, and debilitating. Similarly, when a patient is dying, there may be a choice between returning home to a natural death, or remaining in the hospital, attached to machinery, where the patient's life might be prolonged a few more days or weeks. In both cases, individuals might weigh differently the value of additional life vs the burden of additional treatment.

The withdrawing or withholding of life-sustaining treatment is not inherently contrary to the principles of beneficence and nonmaleficence. The physician is obligated only to offer sound medical treatment and to refrain from providing treatments that are detrimental, on balance, to the patient's well-being. When a physician withholds or withdraws a treatment on the request of a patient, he or she has fulfilled the obligation to offer sound treatment to the patient. The obligation to offer treatment does not include an obligation to impose treatment on an unwilling patient. In addition, the physician is not providing a harmful treatment. Withdrawing or withholding is not a treatment, but the forgoing of a treatment.

Some commentators argue that if a physician has a strong moral objection to withdrawing or withholding life-sustaining treatment, the physician may transfer the patient to another physician who is willing to comply with the patient's wishes.[1] It is true that a physician does not have to provide a treatment, such as an abortion, that is contrary to his or her moral values. However, if a physician objects to withholding or withdrawing the treatment and forces unwanted treatment on a patient, the patient's autonomy will be inappropriately violated even if it will take only a short time for the patient to be transferred to another physician.

Withdrawing or withholding some life-sustaining treatments may seem less acceptable than others. The distinction between "ordinary" vs "extraordinary" treatments has been used to differentiate ethically obligatory vs ethically optional treatments.[4] In other words, ordinary treatments must be provided, while extraordinary treatment may be withheld or withdrawn. Varying criteria have been proposed to distinguish ordinary from extraordinary treatment. Such criteria include customariness, naturalness, complexity, expense, invasiveness, and balance of likely benefits vs burdens of the particular treatment.[4,5] The ethical significance of all these criteria essentially are subsumed by the last criterion—the balance of likely benefits vs the burdens of the treatment.[4]

When a patient is competent, this balancing must ultimately be made by the patient. As stated earlier, the evaluation of whether life-sustaining treatment should be initiated, maintained, or forgone depends on the values and preferences of the patient. Therefore, treatments are not objectively ordinary or extraordinary. For example, artificial nutrition and hydration have frequently been cited as an objectively ordinary treatment which, therefore, must never be forgone. However, artificial nutrition and hydration can be very burdensome to patients. Artificial nutrition and hydration immobilize the patient to a large degree, can be extremely uncomfortable (restraints are sometimes used to prevent patients from removing nasogastric tubes), and can entail serious risks (for example, surgical risks from insertion of a gastrostomy tube and the risk of aspiration pneumonia with a nasogastric tube).

Aside from the ordinary vs extraordinary argument, the right to refuse artificial nutrition and hydration has also been contested by some because the provision of food and water has a symbolic significance as an expression of care and compassion.[6] These commentators argue that withdrawing or withholding food and water is a form of abandonment and will cause the patient to die of starvation and/or thirst. However, it is far from evident that providing nutrients through a nasogastric tube to a patient for whom it is unwanted is comparable to the typical human ways of feeding those who are hungry.[5] In addition, discomforting symptoms can be palliated so that a death that occurs after forgoing artificial nutrition and/or hydration is not marked by substantial suffering.[7,8] Such care requires constant attention to the patient's needs. Therefore, when comfort care is maintained, respecting a patient's decision to forgo artificial nutrition and hydration will not constitute an abandonment of the patient, symbolic or otherwise.

There is also no ethical distinction between withdrawing and withholding life-sustaining treatment.[1,4,9] Withdrawing life support may be emotionally more difficult than withholding life support because the physician performs an action that hastens death. When life-sustaining treatment is withheld, on the other hand, death occurs because of an omission rather than an action. However, as most bioethicists now recognize, such a distinction lacks ethical significance.[1,4,9] First, the distinction is often meaningless. For example, if a physician fails to provide a tube feeding at the scheduled time, would it be a withholding or a withdrawing of treatment? Second, ethical relevance does not lie with the distinction between acts and omissions, but with other factors such as the motivation and professional obligations of the physician. For example, refusing to initiate ventilator support despite the patient's need and request because the physician has been promised a share of the patient's inheritance is clearly ethically more objectionable than stopping a ventilator for a patient who has competently decided to forgo it. Third, prohibiting the withdrawal of life support would inappropriately affect a patient's decision to initiate such treatment. If treatment cannot be stopped once it is initiated, patients and physicians may be more reluctant to begin treatment when there is a possibility that the patient may later want the treatment withdrawn.[1]

While the principle of autonomy requires that physicians respect competent patients' requests to forgo life-sustaining treatments, there are potential negative consequences of such a policy. First, deaths may occur as a result of uninformed decisions or from pain and suffering that could be relieved with measures that will not cause the patient's death. Further, subtle or overt pressures from family, physicians, or society to forgo life-sustaining treatment may render the patient's choice less than free. These pressures could revolve around beliefs that such patients' lives no longer possess social worth and are an unjustifiable drain of limited health resources.

The physician must ensure that the patient has the capacity to make medical decisions before carrying out the patient's decision to forgo (or receive) life-sustaining treatment. In particular, physicians must be aware that the patient's decision-making capacity can be diminished by a misunderstanding of the medical prognosis and options or by a treatable state of depression. It is also essential that all efforts be made to maximize the comfort and dignity of patients who are dependent on life-sustaining treatment and that patients be assured of these efforts. With such assurances, patients will be less likely to forgo life support because of suffering or anticipated suffering that could be palliated.

The potential pressures on patients to forgo life-sustaining treatments are an important concern. The Council believes that the medical profession must be vigilant against such tendencies, but that the greater policy risk is of undermining patient autonomy.

REFERENCES

1 *Deciding to Forego Life-Sustaining Treatment: A Report on the Ethical, Medical, and Legal Issues in Treatment Decisions.* Washington, DC: President's Commission for the Study of Ethical Problems in Medicine and Biomedical and Behavioral Research; 1987.

2 Brock D. W. Death and dying. In: Veatch R. M, ed. *Medical Ethics.* Boston, Mass: Jones & Bartlett Publishing Inc; 1989.

3 Office of Technology Assessment Task Force. *Life-Sustaining Technologies and the Elderly.* Philadelphia, Pa: Science Information Resource Center; 1988.

4 Beauchamp T. L, Childress J. F. *Principles of Biomedical Ethics.* 3rd ed. New York, NY: Oxford University Press; 1989.

5 Lynn J., Childress J. F. Must patients always be given food and water? *Hastings Cent Rep.* October 1983: 17–21.

6 Ramsey P. *The Patient as Person.* New Haven, Conn: Yale University Press; 1970: 113–129.

7 Schmitz P., O'Brien M. Observations on nutrition and hydration in dying patients. In: Lynn J., ed. *By No Extraordinary Means: The Choice to Forgo Life-Sustaining Food and Water.* Bloomington, Ind: Indiana University Press; 1986.

8 Billings J. A. Comfort measures for the terminally ill: is dehydration painful? *J Am Geriatr Soc.* 1985; 33:808–810.

9 *Guidelines on the Termination of Life-Sustaining Treatment and the Care of the Dying: A Report by the Hastings Center.* Briarcliff Manor, NY: Hastings Center; 1987.

REFUSING LIFE-SUSTAINING TREATMENT AFTER CATASTROPHIC INJURY: ETHICAL IMPLICATIONS

Tia Powell and Bruce Lowenstein

Powell and Lowenstein present and discuss a case in which a severely disabled patient decided to refuse life-sustaining treatment (nutrition and hydration) in order to bring about her death. The authors compare and contrast this case with the more widely known case of Elizabeth Bouvia. They then express reservations about the suggestion that patient autonomy should be suspended for an extensive period of time as a patient undergoes rehabilitation in response to catastrophic injury. Powell and Lowenstein ultimately endorse the right of a competent disabled patient to refuse life-sustaining treatment, "no matter how much we may lament such a choice."

In theory, a competent patient may refuse any and all treatments, even those that sustain life. The problem with this theory, confidently and frequently asserted, is that the circumstances of real patients may so confound us with their complexity as to shake our confident assumptions to their core.

For instance, it is not the case that one may always and easily know which patients are competent. Indeed, evaluation of decision-making capacity is notoriously difficult. Not only may reasonable and experienced evaluators, say a judge and a psychiatrist, disagree, but also a person's capacity may change from hour to hour and may extend to some decisions yet not to others. And yet it is on this subtle art of capacity evaluation that life and death decisions often turn, especially when patients decline life-sustaining treatment.

An evaluation of capacity may consider the impact of serious medical or psychiatric illness, as well as the patient's life circumstances. A number of authors have addressed decision-making capacity in the setting of depression, fatal illness, and end-of-life treatment decisions.[1] Less commonly, these factors have been examined in the context of competent patients with chronic disability, rather than terminal illness.[2] In the world of rehabilitation medicine and disability, which is so strikingly different from acute

Journal of Law, Medicine & Ethics, vol. 24 (Spring 1996), pp. 54–61. © 1996. Reprinted with permission of the authors and the American Society of Law, Medicine & Ethics. All rights reserved.

medicine in other ways, assumptions about decision-making capacity may also differ. These different assumptions may lead to a crisis when chronically disabled (but not dying) patients refuse life-sustaining treatments. This crisis, in turn, forces a reexamination of the concept of decisional capacity in the rehabilitation context. In particular, the impact of catastrophic trauma on decisional capacity is judged differently in acute intensive care settings than in rehabilitation settings.

We review a complex case that highlights the difficulty in evaluating capacity to refuse life-sustaining treatments in the rehabilitation setting. As we shall see, the determination of this patient's capacity hinges on diverse factors, including depression, physician countertransference, and the ethos of disability and rehabilitation medicine. Although factors specific to the context of disability deserve careful examination in evaluations of capacity, we do not think, in this case or in general, that disabled patients should be held to a different standard of capacity than other patients.

CASE PRESENTATION: BB

BB was a thirty-seven-year-old woman, in good health, employed, and pursuing a marital separation. Without warning, she suffered a brain stem stroke in November 1993, resulting in the diagnosis of locked-in syndrome. She was left fully alert mentally, although quadriplegic and unable to speak; she preserved limited voluntary head movement, vertical gaze, blinking, and minimal voluntary movement of her left arm.

Before her stroke, BB had a history of major depression with psychotic features, with one previous psychiatric hospitalization ten years earlier. Over the past decade, her symptoms were well controlled with weekly psychotherapy and medications. She was an effective and skilled professional in a competitive technical field.

Roughly ten weeks after her injury, BB was transferred to a rehabilitation facility for possible weaning from a ventilator and for assistance with communication and mobility devices. She began to learn to communicate by means of an elaborate state-of-the-art computer system; she also had an appropriately modified power wheelchair.

BB expressed great eagerness to proceed with ventilatory weaning. After some difficulty, she succeeded in breathing without the ventilator. However, her success disappointed her, to the surprise of the staff. In this fashion, the medical team learned of BB's wish to die.

Although engaged in psychotherapy since her admission to the rehabilitation facility, BB had not confided in her therapists her desire to die. Indeed, although she exuded feelings of tension, anger, and anguish, she had kept psychotherapeutic contacts generally superficial. Now, the focus of psychotherapy shifted toward exploring the reasons why BB wanted to die. She described great suffering, which was primarily psychological rather than physical. She did not believe that she could ever accept life with her extreme physical limitations.

BB's treatment team encouraged her to reconsider. They informed BB that many persons who suffer catastrophic injury have suicidal ideas early in their rehabilitation, yet, after two or more years, may regain their desire to live. Thus, a decision to forgo life-sustaining treatment should wait until then.[3] On the basis of this information, BB promised to postpone for at least six months her wish to die.

However, three weeks later, BB changed her mind. She took three days to write a letter, using her specially adapted computer communication system. She cogently and forcefully described her reasons for wanting to die, and to do so by stopping all nutrition, hydration, and medications, except for mor-

phine as needed to control pain. She further stated that she wished to die at the rehabilitation hospital.

This new stance prompted formal evaluation of BB's capacity to make medical decisions, and specifically to forgo life-sustaining treatment. BB's attending psychologist and psychiatrist carefully reviewed the issue of her capacity to make this irrevocable medical decision. Her cognition clearly allowed her to understand her prognosis and to participate in everyday decisions. She had no formal thought disorder and no current evidence of disabling depression. However, BB had manifested significant fluctuations of mood since admission, as well as waxing and waning of her interest in her care, in a fashion consistent with early reaction to catastrophic injury. Because of these symptoms, the staff feared BB might indeed lack capacity, and engaged a forensic psychiatrist to evaluate her. This evaluation confirmed BB's capacity, as judged from the standpoint of an expert who was not involved in her daily care.

BB's family participated in discussions about her prognosis and wishes. They appreciated the enormity of BB's suffering, but fervently hoped that she would postpone her decision to die. They also supported her right to make her own decision.

Distress was great for many members of the staff who had worked with BB. In particular, members of her team felt extreme discomfort with the timing of BB's request. Were she to wait two years, a number of staff members said that they would still regret her decision to die, but that they would feel that her choice would be more truly the product of informed consent.

Meanwhile, BB's attending physician felt he could not continue to act as her doctor if she wanted to terminate food and fluid. The physician himself had recently been given a potentially fatal diagnosis. His determination to fight his own illness by every possible means stood in direct contrast to BB's choice. Physician and patient, both facing life and death decisions, chose opposite courses. Perhaps, for this reason, or others, the physician described to BB his idea of the suffering she would endure as she died of starvation and dehydration. He would not offer her pain medication, for to do so, in his opinion, would hasten her death, in violation of his ethical and personal beliefs.

At this point, BB and her doctor parted ways. After intense discussions among the staff, another physician—reluctantly and courageously—accepted BB as a patient.

The staff investigated various alternative discharge plans for BB. Of note, local hospices refused to accept BB, arguing that her request constituted assisted suicide. They would only accept a patient whose *illness,* and not whose choice, was leading to an imminent death. BB's disability made the option of dying at home an impossibility, as she would need significant assistance to manage pain, possible seizures, and routine care.

The staff requested an ethics consultation, but BB refused to meet with the ethicist, noting correctly that she had already been examined by an extraordinary number of health professionals. In addition, communication for her was physically arduous and time-consuming. The ethicist, however, did meet with the staff and the administration several times. These meetings focused on the process by which BB's decisions had evolved, rather than on the outcome. Initially, many staff members objected to carrying out a plan that they could not condone, just because the law permitted, indeed required, that they do so. The ethicist presented a different point of view. Staff members who believed that they could not ethically carry out BB's wishes could withdraw from her care. However, the ethicist urged them not to view their obligation as first and foremost a legal one, but rather as an ethical response to their competent yet suffering patient, who stated so movingly that caring for her as she died was the only way to care for her at all. In the ethicist's opinion, it is not always up to the health professional to determine how or when a patient dies, either because of medical limitations or because of legal power; yet this fact does not relieve caregivers from their obligation to care for the dying patient to the best of their ability.

The staff continued to work closely with BB, acknowledging her right to cease food and fluid, but encouraging her to wait or reconsider. BB wrote letters of thanks and farewell to many who had cared for her. Then, on August 15, 1994, she stopped receiving food and fluid. Over a period of about two weeks, she became gradually unresponsive, and ultimately fell into a coma. She denied significant amounts of pain, and required only minimal analgesics. During the first week of September, BB died.

RELEVANT CASES: DISABILITY AND REFUSAL OF LIFE-SUSTAINING TREATMENT

The most widely known—and quite controversial—case of a conscious patient who wished to die by refusing food and fluid while hospitalized is that of Elizabeth Bouvia.[4] Ms. Bouvia was a twenty-eight-year-old woman with cerebral palsy, a life-long, progressively degenerative neuromuscular disorder. Ms. Bouvia was quadriplegic, had significant chronic pain, and depended on a gastrostomy tube for nutrition. She had, disability notwithstanding, graduated from college, attended graduate school in social work, married, and suffered a miscarriage. Bouvia gained notoriety through a protracted and ultimately successful legal battle to secure the right to be cared for in a hospital while she died from starvation and dehydration. (Ms. Bouvia has not yet exercised that right.)

Bouvia's case is similar to BB's in a number of ways. First, both cases call into question the traditional distinction between refusing treatment, which may inadvertently lead to death, and actively seeking death. For instance, when a patient refuses a treatment like chemotherapy because the procedure itself is invasive, painful, or otherwise burdensome, that refusal may result in death. However, we accept this refusal more readily because we can say that the illness kills the patient, who has merely let nature take its course. The point for both Bouvia and BB was not simply to avoid an onerous or invasive treatment that *might* prolong life. They explicitly wanted to die. In order to die, they rejected a treatment—food and fluid—that had nothing in particular to do with illness, but is necessary to sustain life in all persons. Thus, Bouvia and BB did not first object to a treatment, and then reluctantly accept that their refusal might lead to death. They first and primarily objected to life with their disability, and then seized on treatment refusal as a means to end life.

For both Bouvia and BB, the overt wish to die led to evaluations of their capacity to make medical decisions. In both cases, the notion that a desire to die was in itself proof of incapacity was raised and rejected. Further, the Bouvia case helped establish, along with the case of Nancy Cruzan,[5] that nutrition and hydration are medical treatments, and are not inherently different from other life-sustaining measures, such as ventilatory support.

But Bouvia and BB are not alike in all respects. When Bouvia attempted to die by starvation, she had lived with cerebral palsy for her entire twenty-eight years. The duration of her disability sets her radically apart from individuals who have recently suffered catastrophic illness or injury, such as stroke, traumatic quadriplegia, or severe Guillain-Barre syndrome. In these persons, the onset of impairment is sudden and unexpected; the symptoms and inabilities are foreign and frightening. The dependency that ensues is often complete, following fast on a life with no knowledge of physical limitation. The sense of loss may be overwhelming.

Recently, a number of competent patients with severe permanent paralysis have fought for and won the right to stop life-sustaining treatments. These cases are more similar to BB's case than to Bouvia's in the onset and timing of their disability. Included in this group are patients with amyotrophic lateral sclerosis, locked in syndrome,[6] and spinal cord injury (SCI).[7]

Two of these cases bear closer examination. First, an eighteen-year-old male athlete suffered a C1 lesion with quadriplegia and ventilatory dependence after a diving accident.[8] He developed severe, painful spasticity of the head and face, which was unresponsive to medication. Two months post-injury, he told his parents that he wanted to die. They urged him to postpone his decision until he could complete rehabilitation efforts. He acquired a motorized wheelchair and advanced communication technology, and returned home to live with his family. This young man persisted in his wish to die. He requested legal proceedings to document his competency and to protect his parents. A judge acceded to his request that his parents remove him from the ventilator. He died twenty-five months after sustaining his injury.

Second, Ridley[9] presents the case of a twenty-three-year-old man with a high cervical injury sustained in a diving accident while he was intoxicated. This patient had a complex history of psychiatric disturbance, including substance abuse and multiple hospitalizations. After asking to die, he was evaluated by a psychiatrist, found competent and removed from the respirator.

Thus, in a number of cases, patients with catastrophic injuries have proved competent and exercised the right to refuse life-sustaining treatment. However, these cases are controversial, and not all ethicists or health care professionals support such decisions.[10]

CHALLENGES TO AUTONOMY

Because of legal precedents and their own ethical principles, the Ethics Committee of the American Academy of Neurology has published a position statement strongly defending the right of competent but profoundly paralyzed patients to cease all treatments.[11]

However, professionals who focus on rehabilitation medicine may not endorse such a position. Indeed, these professionals, at least in the initial phase of patients' recovery from traumatic injury, suggest that in some cases physicians override patient autonomy, particularly in regard to refusing life-sustaining treatment. For instance, Caplan, Callahan, and Haas suggest that because newly disabled patients have limited experience with disability and lack information about their options and outcomes, some level of paternalism may be justified in their early care and rehabilitation.[12] Caplan, Callahan, and Haas offer three reasons why the competence of patients with recent traumatic injuries may be questioned. They suggest that, first, such patients may not be able adequately to evaluate the risks and benefits of rehabilitation, the results of which may take months or years to appreciate. Second, they argue that it takes time—of an unspecified amount—to cope with the threat to self-identity posed by catastrophic injury. Third, they believe that surrogates may also have impaired judgment because they suffer, as do the patients, from the first two problems. Thus, Caplan, Callahan, and Haas opt for a kind of temporary suspension of patient autonomy, during which significant decision-making authority will accrue to the health care team, which may "initially ignore or override patient and family choice." However,

Caplan, Callahan, and Haas also impose on rehabilitation providers a duty to maximize autonomy and to return decision-making authority to patients once they have had an "opportunity to accommodate to the realities of their functional impairments."[13]

Some aspects of this model closely resemble ordinary standards for decision making in emergency care. In the immediate aftermath of significant trauma, patients often cannot make informed refusals of treatment, either because the patient's mental status is unclear or because physicians may not yet have made a reliable estimate of damage and prognosis. The difficulty with Caplan, Callahan, and Haas's proposal does not arise, therefore, from the idea of a temporary abridgment of autonomy, but from the related questions of how long to accept such an infringement on patients' rights, and how to determine what constitutes a sufficient opportunity to appreciate disability. Caplan, Callahan, and Haas do not offer specific answers to either of these questions, and this reticence leaves severely disabled patients in jeopardy. Are they suggesting that we suspend patients' rights to refuse treatment for the six months to two years that clinical lore suggests are necessary to reintegrate identity after catastrophic trauma? We would not support such a lengthy extension of emergency decision-making power for health care providers. We do favor extremely careful evaluations of capacity, along with maximal efforts to teach patients about options for rehabilitation, and to offer the best possible treatments. However, we would reserve for competent disabled patients the right to refuse life-saving care, no matter how much we may lament such a choice. . . .

REFERENCES

1 T. E. Quill, "Death and Dignity—A Case of Individualized Decision Making," *N. Engl. J. Med.,* 324 (1991): 691–94; S. Block and A. Billings, "Patient Requests for Euthanasia and Assisted Suicide in Terminal Illness," *Psychosomatics,* 36 (1995): 445–57; H. M. Chochinov et al., "Desire for Death in the Terminally Ill," *American Journal of Psychiatry,* 152 (1995): 1185–91; and M. Sullivan and S. Youngner, "Depression, Competence, and the Right to Refuse Lifesaving Treatment," *American Journal of Psychiatry,* 151 (1994): 971–78.

2 J. Shapiro, "No Less Worthy a Life," in J. Shapiro, *No Pity: People with Disabilities Forging a New Civil Rights Movement* (New York: Times Books, 1993): ch. 9; V. Michel, "Suicide by Persons with Disabilities Disguised as the Refusal of Life-Sustaining Treatment," *HEC Forum,* 7 (1995): 122–31; and B. Ridley, "Tom's Story: A Quadriplegic Who Refused Rehabilitation," *Rehabilitation Nursing,* 14 (1989): 250–53.

3 D. Patterson et al., "When Life Support Is Questioned Early in the Care of Patients with Cervical-Level Quadriplegia," *N. Engl. J. Med.,* 238 (1993): 506–09.

4 For further discussion of Bouvia, see: G. Annas, "When Suicide Prevention Becomes Brutality: The Case of Elizabeth Bouvia," *Hastings Center Report,* 14, no. 2 (1984): 20–21; G. Annas, "Elizabeth Bouvia: Whose Space Is This Anyway?," *Hastings Center Report,* 16, no. 2 (1986): 24–25; and F. Kane, "Keeping Elizabeth Bouvia Alive for the Public Good," *Hastings Center Report,* 15, no. 6 (1985): 5–8.

5 *Cruzan v. Director, Missouri Dep't of Health,* 497 U.S. 261 (1990).

6 *Satz v. Perlmutter,* 362 So. 2d 160 (Fla. App. Ct. 1978), *aff'd,* 379 So. 2d 359 (Fla. 1980); and *In re Requena,* No. P-326-86E (N.J. Super. Ct. Ch. Div. Sept. 24. 1986), *aff'd per curiam,* No. A-442-86T5 (N.J. Super. Ct. App. Div. Oct. 6, 1986). For amyotrophic lateral sclerosis, see *In re Farrell,* 108 N.J. 335, 529 A.2d 404 (N.J. 1987). For locked in syndrome, see *In re Rodas,* No. 86PR139 (Colo. Dist. Ct. Jan. 22, 1987), *modified,* (Colo. Dist. Ct. Apr. 3. 1987). All above cases are cited in J. Bernat et al., "Competent Patients with Advanced States of Permanent Paralysis Have the Right to Forgo Life-Sustaining Therapy," *Neurology,* 43 (1993): 224–25.

7 F. Maynard and A. Muth, "The Choice to End Life as a Ventilator-Dependent Quadriplegic," *Archives of Physical Medicine and Rehabilitation,* 68 (1987): 862–64.

8 *Id.* A C1 lesion is an injury sustained to the upper part of the spinal cord. The injury results in quadriplegia and ventilatory dependence.

9 Ridley, *supra* note 2.

10 J. R. Thobaben, "The Case of Mr. Sims," *HEC Forum,* 7 (1995): 94–109.

11 Report of the Ethics and Humanities Subcommittee of the American Academy of Neurology, "Position Statement: Certain Aspects of the Care and Management of Profoundly and Irreversibly Paralyzed Patients with Retained Consciousness and Cognition," *Neurology,* 43 (1993): 222–23.

12 A. Caplan, D. Callahan, and J. Haas, "Ethical and Policy Issues in Rehabilitation Medicine," *Hastings Center Report,* 17, no. 4 (1987): S1–S20.

13 *Id.* at 12.

SUICIDE BY PERSONS WITH DISABILITIES DISGUISED AS THE REFUSAL OF LIFE-SUSTAINING TREATMENT

Vicki Michel

Michel focuses attention on a series of court cases in which a disabled person who is not terminally ill has sought to refuse life-sustaining treatment in order to end his or her life. She believes that such cases are most accurately described as cases in which a person with disabilities has chosen suicide. Courts typically hold in these cases that a competent adult cannot be forced to accept life-sustaining treatment, but Michel—giving voice to a disability-rights perspective—is critical of the attitude toward disability often found in the thinking of the courts. In her view, the courts are far too ready to conclude that life as a dependent person is meaningless; thus, she charges them with discrimination on the basis of disability. She insists that courts have a responsibility to consider the context of a person's life and, in particular, to remember how the eradication of social barriers to a meaningful life can create life possibilities for a person with disabilities.

Cases involving the refusal of life-sustaining treatment by competent persons arise in three basic forms. First, there are those involving a terminally ill person who refuses the burden of continued treatment with the result that death comes somewhat sooner (by weeks or months) than it would have if treatment had been continued. These situations can be fairly described as involving "the process of dying" and courts and ethicists have agreed that no other interests should override the patient's choice about treatment during that process.

Second are those cases involving religious objections to treatment. These usually involve refusals of blood transfusions by Jehovah's Witnesses, and physicians find them particularly difficult because the medical prognosis is often one of return to health and normal functioning if the blood transfusion is given and death if it is not. Because Jehovah's Witnesses generally accept other medical treatment it is not reasonable to argue that this particular treatment refusal constitutes a suicide attempt; from a legal perspective the general right to make treatment decisions is strengthened by the First Amendment right to free exercise of religion. As a result, the dominant

view has been to uphold the right to refuse treatment in this context.

The third group of cases is the one I am going to address in this article. The cases in this group have been analyzed by the courts as cases about refusal of life-sustaining treatment. They involve nonterminally ill people with disabilities who ask to stop eating or to have ventilator support withdrawn in order that they may end their lives. It is clear from the facts of these cases that the person both intends and wants to die, unlike the situations in the first two categories of cases. Despite the clarity of the intention courts uniformly have refused to analyze these situations as involving suicide. This was demonstrated most recently in the case of *Thor v. Superior Court*[1], a decision by the California Supreme Court involving a quadriplegic prisoner who was refusing food and medical treatment. Like the *Bergstedt, Rodas, Rivlin, McAfee* and *Bouvia* cases before it, this case would be more accurately described as a case about a person with disabilities choosing suicide rather than simply another case about a competent patient refusing life-sustaining treatment.

Descriptively naming these cases matters because calling them treatment refusal cases masks the courts' judgments about the quality of life of persons with disabilities. By focusing on a person's right to make choices about life and death, courts act and

Reprinted with permission of the author and the publisher from *HEC Forum*, vol. 7, nos. 2-3 (1995), pp. 122–131. © 1995 Kluwer Academic Publishers.

speak as if disability is not an issue and in particular ignore the social conditions that may cause persons with disabilities to want to be dead rather than continue to struggle against social prejudice and discrimination. To the extent that this occurs, the respect for persons that is supposed to underlie the priority given to the value of personal autonomy is undermined in these court decisions. At the same time, to insist that a disability perspective is essential to understanding these cases creates the danger that in attempting to advocate for people with disabilities we risk imposing our view of their lives on them—that is, we may find ourselves telling people they *should* want to continue the struggle rather than give in to the social barriers to a meaningful life that they experience.

The tension between these concerns has been evident since Elizabeth Bouvia first asked Riverside County Hospital psychiatric ward, over ten year ago, to care for her while she starved herself to death. The February–March 1984 issue of *The Disability Rag* (an advocacy publication for the community of people with disabilities) was primarily devoted to articles about the case of Elizabeth Bouvia. In 1983, Elizabeth Bouvia was a 26-year-old woman with cerebral palsy who used a wheelchair, was married, and was in graduate school in social work. That year Ms. Bouvia suffered a series of losses that included a miscarriage, the breakup of her marriage, and being told that she would never be employable. Before long, Ms. Bouvia, whose life was of course much more complex than this description captures, became the focal point of a vehement dispute between civil libertarians and disability activists, a dispute which has not yet really cooled down and which has had a series of subsequent cases to fuel it over the years. The dispute is about whether a person with disabilities has a "right to die" that encompasses a right to refuse to eat and drink and then to refuse any medical means of nutrition and hydration necessitated by the refusal to take food and fluids by mouth. The physicians at Riverside said no—they were not willing to participate in a suicide, which is how they defined what Ms. Bouvia was up to. Ms. Bouvia's lawyer on the other hand tried to define it as a refusal of medical treatment, and although Elizabeth Bouvia failed to get the agreement of the Riverside trial

court, she was eventually able to establish through a California Second District Court of Appeal decision in 1986 that physicians could not legally administer nutrition and hydration over her objection even if her refusal to eat hastened her death.

Some members of the disability community objected. Paul Longmore, Ph.D., at that time a program specialist with the Program on the Study of Disability and Society at the University of Southern California, said the courts have appropriated disability rights to support the right to suicide. "It isn't a right to die case at all. It's disability case. When society has given us the right to live with dignity, then we will talk about the right to die. Not before"[2] (p. 5).

Subsequent cases have adopted the analytic structure established in *Bouvia*. A competent person cannot be forced to accept life-sustaining treatment over his or her objection. My argument is not with this statement as a general matter but rather with the attitude toward disability revealed in the decisions, an attitude which suggests that the court would have treated the case differently if the central character had not had a severe disability. The court in *Bouvia* said, "All decisions permitting cessation of. . .life-support procedures to some degree hastened the arrival of death. In part, at least, this was permitted because the quality of life during the time remaining in those cases had been terribly diminished. In Elizabeth Bouvia's view the quality of her life has been diminished to the point of hopelessness, uselessness, unenjoyability and frustration. She, as the patient, lying helplessly in bed, unable to care for herself, may consider her existence meaningless. She cannot be faulted for so concluding"[3] (p. 304).

Would a court ever make such a statement about a person without disabilities? Judicial comments like this simply reflect the societal view that not only is dependency the worse thing that can befall a person, but that life as a dependent person is a meaningless existence. Thus, it should have come as no surprise that the four mental health experts who spoke with Elizabeth Bouvia during her stay in Riverside concluded that her decision to end her life was reasonable. This despite the fact that when a person without disabilities voices a desire to die, he or she is first assumed to be clinically depressed and an appropriate candidate for psychiatric treatment.

Kenneth Bergstedt became a quadriplegic as the result of a swimming accident at age ten. His father cared for him and he lived what seemed to be a satisfactory life until he was thirty-one and his father was terminally ill. At that point Mr. Bergstedt asked the court to affirm that he had a right to die by refusing further ventilator support. The Nevada Supreme Court did so, denying that what Mr. Bergstedt wanted was to commit suicide. "If a competent adult is beset with an irreversible condition such as quadriplegia, where life must be sustained artificially and under circumstances of total dependence, the adult's attitude or motive may be presumed not to be suicidal"[4] (p. 627). The court also said that "the State has no overriding interest in interfering with the natural process of dying among citizens whose lives are irreparably devastated by injury or illness to the point where life may be sustained only by contrivance or radical intervention"[4] (p. 626). But does this make sense as a description of Kenneth Bergstedt's twenty-one years of life using ventilator support after his accident? Interestingly the court elsewhere in its opinion acknowledged that Kenneth led a meaningful life and noted that "it appeared to us that Kenneth needed some type of assurance that society would not cast him adrift in a sea of indifference after his father's passing"[4] (p. 628). To the point, the court said, "It is beyond cavil in one sense, that Kenneth was taking affirmative measures to hasten his own death. It is equally clear that *if Kenneth had enjoyed sound physical health but had viewed life as unbearably miserable because of his mental state, his liberty interest would provide no basis for asserting a right to terminate his life with or without the assistance of other persons. Our societal regard for the value of an individual life. . .would never countenance an assertion of liberty over life under such circumstances*"[4] (p. 625). (emphasis added)

In other words only if a person has serious disability does his or her liberty interest in being able to choose to die take precedence over the social interest in preserving individual lives! This is a shocking statement, but it and statements like it in other similar cases go unaddressed in the literature except in journals like *The Disability Rag* and *Issues in Law and Medicine* which tend to be dismissed as publications committed to advocacy.

Concerns about attitudes toward disability sometimes get tangled up with the concerns that arise from a right-to-life perspective. The right-to-life perspective makes life itself the ultimate value, leading to a view that killing, suicide, and letting die are all moral wrongs whether the person involved is competent, senile, or permanently unconscious. Personal autonomy in this view will generally be trumped by the value of life itself. The mainstream bioethics literature, on the other hand, has made autonomy the value that generally trumps anything else. Consistent with this view, the ACLU as counsel for Elizabeth Bouvia took the position that persons with disabilities have the same right to choose death by refusal of life-sustaining treatment as persons without disabilities. As a statement of a general principle this may not be objectionable but such a statement does not take account of the context of people's lives and in each of the cases that have reached the courts context has been both critical and unaccounted for in the legal proceedings. Kenneth Bergstedt was facing the impending loss of his care taker, his father. Elizabeth Bouvia had been told she would never be employable and was dealing with a miscarriage and a failing marriage as mentioned earlier.

The case of Larry McAfee in Georgia demonstrates the dramatic change in intention which can occur when the context changes through the opening up of life opportunities for a person with disabilities. McAfee was a quadriplegic, as a result of a motorcycle accident, who seemed likely to do well at rehabilitation in the years following the accident despite the devastating loss of his relationship with grandparents who were very important to him. But when insurance money ran out he had only Medicaid funding which was not sufficient to support living at home with attendants. McAfee went to court to get permission to end his ventilator support and die, but his case got the attention of disability activists who eventually energized both him and his parents; this led to opportunities to use his engineering talents and to get home care rather than state institutional care. McAfee no longer wanted to die although he made clear he would kill himself if forced to return to an institution[5] (ch. 9).

The point made by the disability community is that it is not the disability itself that makes life so unbearable that suicide seems a reasonable solution, but rather the conditions that people with disabilities have to contend with, including both social attitudes and the lack of accommodation and opportunity. When a person with disabilities says he or she wants to die it is outrageously discriminatory to *assume* this is a reasonable choice whereas someone without those disabilities would be referred for suicide prevention services. It should be shocking to hear a person's lawyer say, as Elizabeth Bouvia's lawyer did, that people with disabilities can't work and that "For Elizabeth Bouvia a natural death is the sanctuary from an existence so painful and degrading that its intentional infliction would be shunned as cruel, inhumane and repugnant."[6]

In 1983, disability activists wanted to talk to Elizabeth Bouvia. They hoped to convince her that she had other options. She rejected their efforts. In December 1983 she made a public statement including the following: "I appreciate the concern of disabled persons and the disabled community but would ask them to express their support for me by agreeing that my choice, as a competent individual, is mine to make, however much any other person disagrees with that choice"[2] (p. 5). Here is the tension between the civil libertarian and disability advocacy positions.

But the court opinions don't reflect the tension or the complexity. Instead they deny the reality of suicide by calling it treatment refusal and they say explicitly that they would treat the case differently if it involved someone who was not disabled. These sentiments merit critical analysis regardless of whether one agrees with the courts' ultimate holdings because they amount to discrimination on the basis of disability. These cases say that if you are not disabled and you are suicidal the state has an interest in making sure your decision is not due to mental disorder, and to promote that interest can insist on psychiatric evaluation and involuntary hospitalization for diagnosis and sometimes treatment. But if you are a person with disabilities your desire to end your life is presumed reasonable. In addition, if you want to accomplish your demise by refusing to eat, even if you are capable of taking food by mouth, your refusal will be considered a refusal of medical treatment despite the fact that you didn't need medical treatment to get nourishment until you refused to eat.

The most recent decision of this kind, the California Supreme Court decision in the *Thor* case mentioned earlier, illustrates this analytic structure perfectly.[1,7]

Howard Andrews was an inmate serving a life sentence. In 1991, he jumped off a wall in prison and sustained injuries causing him to become quadriplegic. There seems to be agreement that Andrews was depressed both prior to and after this incident. Subsequently, he refused spoon feeding, which was an effective way for him to receive nutrition as long as he cooperated. He also refused treatment for medical problems. Dr. Thor, the prison physician, went to court for permission to place a gastrostomy tube to feed Andrews over his objection. The trial and appellate courts held that Andrews had a right to refuse life-sustaining treatment and the California Supreme Court affirmed their decision.

In one sense the decision is unremarkable. It can be viewed as simply consistent with other California opinions (*Bartling, Bouvia,* etc.) which have said that competent, non-terminally ill persons' rights to refuse life-sustaining treatment outweigh any asserted state interests in keeping them alive. But it is worth looking at Andrews' situation more closely. When we do, the case looks more like a *real* "right to die" case than like a treatment refusal case. Andrews, after all, apparently attempted suicide by jumping off a wall prior to his becoming quadriplegic. He is refusing spoon feeding, not artificial nutrition and hydration, and no one has yet asserted that spoon feeding is medical treatment. In this case, the need for feeding as medical treatment arises only from the refusal of spoon feeding, not from the patient's inability to tolerate spoon feeding, as is typical in most other artificial feeding cases.

Thus this case seems to be about a suicide attempt, not a treatment refusal. The amicus brief from the California Medical Association (CMA) is the only brief in the case that acknowledges this. The brief asserts that it doesn't matter whether Andrews is attempting suicide; he has a right to refuse an unwanted medical intervention no matter what caused his underlying medical condition. This is a defensible position. It does not pretend that refusing life-sustaining treatment is never attempted suicide and it suggests that the state interest in preventing suicide is not very compelling.

What is disturbing about the court's opinion? The court notes that "with respect to the prevention of suicide, the state has expressed a limited interest at best," and goes on to say, "a necessary distinction exists between a person suffering from a serious life-threatening disease or debilitating injury who rejects medical intervention that only prolongs but never cures the affliction and an individual who deliberately sets in motion a course of events aimed at his or her own demise and attempts to enlist the assistance of others."[1] Howard Andrews seems to be in the latter category, but the court inexplicably places him in the former.

Noting that Andrews has a "profoundly disabling" condition that causes him to be totally dependent on others, the court accepts the Nevada Supreme Court's view in *Bergstedt* that, "as the quality of life diminishes because of physical deterioration, the State's interest in preserving life may correspondingly decrease." In other words, the court believes it is Andrews' disability that causes the state to have little interest in preserving his life. This analysis is reinforced by footnote 16 of the opinion which says, "Under the facts of this case we have no occasion to address and therefore do not decide any related issues that might arise in the event an otherwise healthy inmate with no underlying affliction engages in a course of conduct for nonmedical reasons, such as a hunger strike, that subsequently necessitates therapeutic intervention to prevent death."[1] Howard Andrews was such a healthy inmate who jumped off a wall presumably for "nonmedical" reasons and then refused spoon feeding, also for nonmedical reasons, thus "necessitat[ing] therapeutic intervention."

This is not to suggest that the state should force feed quadriplegic inmates who have decided that death is a better alternative than life in prison in that condition. But it is disturbing to find that the court treats an inmate with disabilities differently from one without disabilities, who similarly decides to choose death over life in prison and to accomplish this refuses to eat. The court gives every indication that the state's interest in preserving the life of a person without disabilities would be viewed as more substantial.

The fact that Andrews was in prison added a factor that should have helped the court see the relevance of context in considering an "autonomous" decision to die. The CMA in its amicus brief was again the only participant to raise ethical concerns stemming from the inherently coercive character of incarceration. The CMA brief suggested that, because the prison environment puts the voluntariness of inmate decisions into question, there should be judicial involvement before accepting a decision to refuse life-sustaining treatment. CMA raises the question of whether a disabled prisoner has had access to rehabilitative services that meet the community care standards, to a physician of his choosing, to visitors, to a social support system, and so on. The ironic thing about this very valid point is that it is the very lack of access to these things *outside* of prisons that can lead to despair and the desire to die on the part of people with disabilities.

The difficult question is how courts are to take context into account. The Nevada Supreme Court in the *Bergstedt* decision made an attempt in this direction despite also buying into the questionable analytic structure discussed above. The court created a new state interest that must be considered in cases where a competent person who is not terminally ill wants to reject life-sustaining treatment. This is the "state's interest in encouraging the charitable and humane care of afflicted persons"[4] (p. 628). The court noted that efforts to improve the lives of people with disabilities "are indicative of the highest social character—a society attuned to the worth of an individual irrespective of physical or mental handicap."[4] (p. 628)

Although the tone here sounds somewhat patronizing of people with disabilities and also seems to view opportunities for them as a matter of charity rather than entitlement, the court is still moving in the right direction. At least a court with a case like Larry McAfee's would have to explore his life circumstances and consider whether he was aware of all his options. And under the Nevada decision each of these cases would *have* to be reviewed by a judge.

The cases described here are certainly just the tip of the iceberg. They are not likely to have had major impact on the lives of people with disabilities generally compared to the years of activist struggle that led to both local victories and ultimately to the passage of the Americans with Disabilities Act. But it is worth wondering why the bioethics literature includes so little from a disability rights perspective and why in both these "right to die" cases and in the cases about treatment decisions for newborns with disabilities so little weight is given to that perspective. Perhaps it is unrealistic to expect this literature to reflect a more constructive and contextual understanding of difference than others. I hope not. Martha Minow has given the question of difference thoughtful consideration in her book, *Making All the Difference.*[8] In a chapter titled "Dying and Living" she makes a point that will serve well as my conclusion and as something ethics committees and courts would do well to keep in mind. "Preserving life in a doubtful case may be the only way to guard against underestimations of the potential life experience of the disabled person. Once we recognize the extent to which social attitudes construct the meaning of disabilities—that disabilities are critically relational in their social meaning and their actual impact on peo-ple's lives—we may work for changes in institutional arrangements to benefit those who have been labeled handicapped. The historical record cautions against underestimating and stigmatizing those whose prospects may well change with medical advances and changes in social attitudes. Hence, the fact of life alone—and the possibilities for change that it implies—may supply the core meaning to its quality"[8] (p. 321).

REFERENCES

1 *Thor v. Superior Court* 21 Cal Rptr. 2d.357 (1993).
2 *The Disability Rag.* Feb/Mar; 1984.
3 *Bouvia v. Superior Court* 225 Cal Rpt. 297 (Cal. App 2d Dist 1986).
4 *McKay v. Bergstedt* 801 P2d 617 (Nev. 1990).
5 Shapiro P. *No Pity.* New York, N.Y.: New York Times Books; 1993.
6 Memorandum of Points and Authorities in Support of Application for TRO and injunctions in the Bouvia case, Nov. 1, 1983.
7 The following discussion of the *Thor* case is adapted from *Ethical Currents* #35; September 1993.
8 Minow M. *Making All the Difference.* Ithaca, N.Y.: Cornell University Press; 1993.

DNR ORDERS AND MEDICAL FUTILITY

ETHICS AND COMMUNICATION IN DO-NOT-RESUSCITATE ORDERS
Tom Tomlinson and Howard Brody

Tomlinson and Brody emphasize the importance of distinguishing among three distinct rationales for DNR orders: (1) CPR would be futile and thus offer no medical benefit; (2) there would be an unacceptable quality of life *after* CPR; (3) there is presently—*before* CPR—an unacceptable quality of life. In their view, whereas the first rationale involves a purely medical judgment, the second and third involve judgments that are properly made by the patient or the patient's family. Also, whereas the first and second do not imply that other forms of life-prolonging treatment are inappropriate, the third does have such an implication. The authors analyze the proper purposes of physician communication with patients and families by reference to the underlying rationale of a DNR order. They also argue that failure to make clear the underlying rationale of a DNR order is a potent source of confusion among professional staff.

Despite the extensive literature devoted to do-not-resuscitate (DNR) orders, they continue to raise vexing problems for physicians, house staff, nurses, and policy makers. The difficulties include physicians' ambivalence about who should be consulted before a DNR order is written, the frustration of house officers and nurses who are asked to continue complicated or invasive treatments of a patient for whom a DNR order has been written, and hospital administrators' uncertainty and confusion over what their DNR policies should be.

Many of these problems arise from the failure to distinguish among three distinct rationales for DNR orders and to appreciate their differing implications. Although some commentators, notably Annas,[1] have insisted that different justifications for a DNR order should be explicitly distinguished, the majority view has lumped them all together uncritically:

> A decision not to resuscitate is considered for a variety of reasons: a request by a patient or family; advanced age of the patient; poor prognosis; severe brain damage; extreme suffering or disability in a chronically or terminally ill patient; and in some instances, the enormous cost and personnel commitment as opposed to the low probability of patient recovery.[2]

Each of the reasons listed may be good in one circumstance or another. But this shopping-list approach hides important differences among three distinct rationales that need to be better articulated and understood.

THREE RATIONALES FOR DNR

No Medical Benefit A commonly accepted ethical principle is that physicians have no obligation to provide, and patients and families have no right to demand, medical treatment that is of no demonstrable benefit.[3] Patients or families may wrongly imagine that a futile treatment would be beneficial, but this imagined benefit does not generate a right to receive treatment; otherwise, patients would be enti-

tled to demand and receive laetrile and other quack therapies from their physicians.[4]

Although published data on survival after cardiopulmonary resuscitation (CPR) will not always be decisive in individual cases,[5,6] we believe there are circumstances when a DNR order is justified because resuscitation would almost certainly not be successful, and so would be of no benefit to the patient. This rationale for DNR orders has been discussed by Blackhall.[7]

Poor Quality of Life After CPR A second reason for withholding CPR is that the quality of life that would result after the cardiac arrest and the subsequent CPR effort is unacceptable, even though survival might be prolonged. The life that would remain might be of little or no benefit to the patient (as with permanent loss of consciousness), or the benefits might be far outweighed by likely burdens. For example, a patient who is physically disabled after a previous arrest may still have a life whose quality is acceptable to him or his family; but it can be predicted that if he should have another arrest, he would almost certainly deteriorate further into a condition he would consider unacceptable. The crucial feature of this rationale is that the arrest, the resuscitation effort, or both threaten a change in the patient's quality of life, from one that is at least minimally acceptable to one that is unacceptable.

Poor Quality of Life Before CPR The third rationale also involves a judgment about the quality of life, but here the judgment concerns the patient's current quality of life—before any anticipated arrest and resuscitation. Although the patient may survive the resuscitation, his current quality of life is judged to be unacceptable, either to him or to his family if he is incompetent. This rationale might be applied to a patient who was severely incapacitated, mentally or physically, or who suffered intolerably from a terminal or chronic disease. The crucial difference between this and the second rationale is that the judgment here concerns the patient's current quality of life, not merely the quality of life after an arrest.

With these distinctions in hand, it becomes apparent how vague many previous recommendations

Reprinted with permission of the publisher from the *New England Journal of Medicine,* vol. 318, no. 1 (January 7, 1988), pp. 43–46.

have been concerning the proper use of resuscitation. An example is the maxim advocated by the National Council on Cardiopulmonary Resuscitation and Emergency Cardiac Care, and often quoted with approval: "The purpose of CPR is the prevention of sudden, unexpected death. CPR is not indicated in certain situations, such as in cases of terminal irreversible illness where death is not unexpected."[1,8] "Cases of terminal irreversible illness" do not unequivocally exemplify just one kind of rationale for DNR orders, as this principle would suggest. A terminally ill patient may reasonably be given a DNR order for any of the three reasons just described, depending on the facts of the case. There could even be cases of terminal irreversible illness in which a DNR order would *not* be justified, because the resuscitation would not be futile and the patient would judge the quality of life both before and after the arrest to be acceptable.

This last possibility suggests the ethical danger of applying a single rule for the use of CPR unambiguously to all terminally ill patients, and also the ethical importance of the distinctions we have made. In what follows, we will substantiate the claim that these are distinctions that make a difference—for the ethics of DNR decisions, for communication with patients and families, for communication among health professionals, and for hospital policies. In these discussions, we will refer to two important contrasts among the three rationales.

CONTRASTS AMONG THE THREE RATIONALES

Relevance of Patient's Values The first important difference among the rationales concerns the relevance of the patient's or family's values to the justification for the DNR decision. When the decision is based on there being no medical benefit in resuscitation, then the value that the patient or the patient's family might place on the patient's life after an arrest is irrelevant: resuscitation would not provide any meaningful prolongation of the patient's life and so could not provide anything that the patient or his family could reasonably value. Consequently, when resuscitation offers no medical benefit, the physician can make a reasoned determination that a DNR

order should be written without any knowledge of the patient's values in the matter. The decision that CPR is unjustified because it is futile is a judgment that falls entirely within the physician's technical expertise.

By contrast, when the rationale depends on an assessment of the patient's quality of life, either before or after CPR, it requires the application of a set of values that determine whether the benefit of continued life outweighs any associated harm such as pain or disability. Since the physician's values may well differ from those of the patient or the patient's family acting as proxy, and since the patient has both a legal and a moral right to accept or refuse treatment in accordance with his or her values, the values used to make these quality-of-life determinations are properly the patient's. Therefore, the justification of a DNR order on the basis of either one of the quality-of-life rationales described above is not purely a matter for expert judgment: it requires that the decision be based on the values of the individual patient.

Generalizability to Other Treatments The other important area of contrast among the three rationales concerns their specificity to the event of an arrest and subsequent resuscitation, and the generalizations they allow about the appropriateness of treatment options besides CPR.

Both "no medical benefit" and "poor quality of life after CPR" are rationales that limit the scope of their judgments to resuscitation. A decision that resuscitation will be futile concerns that treatment alone and does not imply futility for other life-prolonging treatments. So too, the judgment that an arrest and subsequent resuscitation would result in an unacceptable quality of life for the patient pertains to the undesirable consequences of those specific events; it implies nothing about the consequences of other life-threatening events and their related treatments.

On the other hand, a DNR order based on the unacceptable quality of a patient's current life, before an anticipated or possible arrest, does not involve a judgment tied exclusively to the arrest and to CPR. Instead, it is a judgment that death would be preferable to continued survival, because of the burdens imposed either by disease or by necessary

TABLE 1   Contrasts Among Rationales for DNR Orders

Rationale	Patient's values relevant?	Implications for other treatments?
No medical benefit	No	No
Poor quality of life after CPR	Yes	No
Poor quality of life before CPR	Yes	Yes

life-prolonging treatment. Therefore, the same logic that supports the DNR order also supports the withholding or withdrawing of other life-prolonging measures, other things being equal.

These contrasts are summarized in Table 1.

COMMUNICATION WITH PATIENTS AND FAMILIES

The differences we have described among the three rationales have implications for the proper purposes of communicating with patients and families about DNR decisions. They also provide a basis for evaluating some of the published research in this area.

When the absence of medical benefit is the rationale for a DNR order, communication with the patient or family should aim at securing an understanding of the decision the physician has already made. Eliciting the patient's values or involving the family in the decision is not required because the decision is based on medical expertise. Rather, the discussion should inform them of the medical realities and attempt to persuade them of the reasonableness of the DNR order. (This is not to say that the physician should callously override or ignore the wishes of a patient or family that insists on resuscitation.)

When one of the quality-of-life rationales is involved, discussions with the patient or family have a different objective. Contemplating a DNR order justified by a quality-of-life rationale, a physician needs the patient's or family's permission (as an exercise of their rights), not merely their understanding (out of concern for their welfare). In such cases, it is inappropriate for the physician to begin by trying to persuade the patient or family to agree to the DNR order. It is presumptuous for the physician to believe that a DNR order is justified before he or she has knowledge of the only set of values—the patient's—that is relevant to a quality-of-life decision.

If we are correct on these points, then the President's Commission is wrong in claiming, with regard to all resuscitation decisions, that "the great weight accorded to competent patients' self-determination means that attending physicians have a duty to ascertain patients' preferences."[8] The right of self-determination, as well as the patient's preferences, is irrelevant to the determination that resuscitation would be of no medical benefit. When this is the rationale for a DNR decision, the physician has no duty to ascertain the patient's preferences.

Charlson et al. err on the other side by suggesting that DNR decisions should be discussed only with "patients whose hospital course is characterized by a slow, progressive deterioration," because statistically such patients account for the lowest post-CPR success and survival rates.[6] But these facts support their recommendation only on the false assumption that the sole valid reason for giving a DNR order is that CPR would be of no medical benefit.

Several recent studies of doctor-patient communication in DNR decisions are unhelpful when they do not distinguish among rationales. What, for example, should be made of the study[9] that indicated that one third of the DNR orders documented no discussion with either patient or family? We don't know how many of these cases involved DNR decisions based on the lack of medical benefit. In such cases, there would be no need for discussion, since the justification for the order would not rest on information about the patient's values or preferences. Other data showing a higher rate of communication[10] cannot be applauded until we know whether the communication had the proper objectives, pursuing understanding or permission only when each was appropriate. Future empirical studies in this area need to account explicitly for the ethical differences among the three rationales.

COMMUNICATION AMONG PHYSICIANS AND STAFF

In our experience, DNR orders can be potent sources of misunderstanding, dissension, and anger among the professional staff. These problems arise at least partly from uncertainty about which of the three rationales is being applied in a particular case.

An example is the case, described by Stuart Youngner,[11] of an elderly woman who had had a series of strokes but remained mentally alert. Both she and her family requested that if she should have a cardiac arrest, no resuscitative efforts should be made. Accordingly, she was given a DNR order. When she had a cardiac arrhythmia, however, she was successfully defibrillated. Both the patient and the family were very upset at what they considered a violation of their directive. Some physicians agreed; others did not consider the arrhythmia an arrest and so disagreed that the patient's wishes had been violated.

Youngner uses this case simply to illustrate that there can be disagreement over what constitutes a cardiac arrest. But this way of framing the problem makes the dispute seem semantic and legalistic, when it is more than that. The question of whether defibrillation fell under the scope of the DNR order is better answered by looking to the rationale behind the request of the patient and family and their physician's agreement. Was the order made because resuscitation was thought to be of no medical benefit? If so, defibrillation might not be covered under that rationale, if it were the physician's judgment that a fibrillation could be treated more successfully than another arrest mechanism, such as a complete heart block. Was the issue worry about the quality of life after an arrest? Again, it might be thought that damage after a successful resuscitation from fibrillation would be less severe than that after other forms of arrest. Only if the original order were grounded in concern for the patient's quality of life before CPR would its interpretation be unambiguous. In that case, no life-prolonging treatment for any form of cardiac arrest would be acceptable, because the life to be prolonged had been judged as unacceptable by the patient, independently of any further facts about the mechanism of the arrest or the characteristics of the resuscitation.

As this example illustrates, proper understanding or interpretation of a DNR order is impossible without knowing the rationale behind it. Unfortunately, one study reports that for almost half of DNR orders there is no written explanation or justification to serve as a guide.[9] Another study revealed that physicians writing DNR orders invariably intended the order to include other interventions besides CPR—antibiotics, blood transfusions, antiarrhythmic drugs. Nevertheless, 43 percent of the patients' charts failed to mention these other interventions.[12] Lipton found that in "60 percent of the cases physicians did not specify the intent or philosophy of the overall treatment plan subsequent to DNR designation" and that in only 35 percent of the cases was there any mention of other specific types of care to be either continued or withdrawn.[13]

In practice, clearly, the terms "DNR" or "no code" are left both ambiguous and vague. The ambiguity arises from the existence of two meanings—the explicit "no CPR" and the often inferred "no extraordinary measures." The vagueness arises under both meanings because the other treatments to be withheld, if any, can only be guessed at when the rationale for the order is missing. It is therefore not surprising that if three staff members hear that a patient has been assigned a "no code," they will each construct an idea of what the patient's true management plan is, and the three imagined plans may be radically different.

HOSPITAL POLICY

Some proposed DNR policies have tried to avoid both ambiguity and vagueness by insisting that a DNR order should have no implication for the continuation of other treatments besides CPR.[2,8] As the data show, this has simply not worked, for an obvious reason. One of the three rationales for DNR—indeed, the one that may be used most frequently—does have implications for other modes of treatment. If it does not, the DNR order is illogical or unfounded. Thus, hospital staff members who continue to believe that at least some DNR orders imply conclusions about other management options are correct, formal hospital policies notwithstanding. We therefore reject this principle as invalid for guiding hospital DNR policies.

DNR forms that simply include options for withholding other types of treatment besides CPR[12] are also inadequate. When they offer options independently of the overall rationale for the DNR order, the forms invite the automatic withholding of other treatments whenever a DNR decision is made, even when the rationale for that decision may not readily generalize to other life-prolonging treatments.

Finally, our analysis also suggests difficulties with DNR policies that combine categories of patient care with resuscitation status. A typical scheme divides patients into groups assigned to receive "full support, including CPR," "full support, excluding CPR," or "modified support, excluding CPR."[14] The trouble with such schemes is that they do not connect the use of the no-CPR categories to the rationale for the decision not to use CPR, which leads to incoherent treatment plans or unjustified generalization from the patient's no-CPR status. Thus, a patient whose no-CPR order was based on an unacceptable quality of life before CPR could be placed in the category requiring full support, excluding CPR. This would require nursing and medical staff to continue other treatments that were also unjustified, leading to the miscommunication and anger we have mentioned. Also, a patient could be assigned to the "modified support, excluding CPR" category merely on the basis of his or her no-CPR status, when such a generalization was unjustified by the rationale for the resuscitation decision.

REFERENCES

1 Annas GJ. CPR: when the beat should stop. Hastings Cent Rep 1982; 12(5):30–1.
2 Miles SH, Cranford R, Schultz AL. The do-not-resuscitate order in a teaching hospital: considerations and a suggested policy. Ann Intern Med 1982; 96:660–4.
3 President's Commission for the Study of Ethical Problems in Medicine and Biomedical and Behavioral Research. Making health care decisions: a report on the ethical and legal implications of informed consent in the patient-practitioner relationship. Vol. 1. Washington, D.C.: Government Printing Office, 1982:43–4. (Publication no. 0-383-515/8673.)
4 Brett A. S., McCullough L. B. When patients request specific interventions: defining the limits of the physician's obligation. N Engl J Med 1986; 315:1347–51.
5 Bedell S. E., Delbanco T. L., Cook E. F., Epstein F. H. Survival after cardiopulmonary resuscitation in the hospital. N Engl J Med 1983; 309:569–76.
6 Charlson M. E., Sax F. L, MacKenzie C. R., Fields SD., Braham R. L., Douglas R. G. Jr. Resuscitation: How do we decide? A prospective study of physicians' preferences and the clinical course of hospitalized patients. JAMA 1986; 255:1316–22.
7 Blackhall L. J. Must we always use CPR? N Engl J Med 1987; 317:1281–5.
8 President's Commission for the Study of Ethical Problems in Medicine and Biomedical and Behavioral Research. Deciding to forego life-sustaining treatment. Washington, D.C.: Government Printing Office, 1983. (Publication no. 0-402-884.)
9 Youngner S. J., Lewandowski W., McClish D. K., Juknialis B. W., Coulton C, Bartlett E. T. 'Do not resuscitate' orders: incidence and implications in a medical intensive care unit. JAMA 1985; 253:54–7.
10 Bedell S. E., Pelle D, Maher P. L., Cleary P. D. Do-not-resuscitate orders for critically ill patients in the hospital: How are they used and what is their impact? JAMA 1986; 256:233–7.
11 Youngner S. J. Do-not-resuscitate orders: no longer secret, but still a problem. Hastings Cent Rep 1987; 17(1):24–33.
12 Uhlmann R. E., Cassel C. K., McDonald W. J. Some treatment-withholding implications of no-code orders in an academic hospital. Crit Care Med 1984; 12:879–81.
13 Lipton H. L. Do-not-resuscitate decisions in a community hospital: incidence, implications, and outcomes. JAMA 1986; 256:1164–9.
14 Daila F., Boisaubin E. V, Sears D. A. Patient care categories: an approach to do-not-resuscitate decisions in a public teaching hospital. Crit Care Med 1986; 14:1066–7.

MEDICAL FUTILITY: A CONCEPTUAL AND ETHICAL ANALYSIS
Mark R. Wicclair

Wicclair explores some of the difficulties associated with the view that judgments of futility can provide a justification for the refusal of physicians to make certain treatments available to patients. His analysis is developed by reference to three senses of futility: (1) physiological futility; (2) futility in relation to the patient's goals; and

(3) futility in relation to standards of professional integrity. In Wicclair's view, judgments of futility almost always involve a reference to evaluative standards. Thus, since he believes that the language of futility tends to communicate a false sense of scientific objectivity, he ultimately recommends that physicians not use such language in expressing their opposition to providing certain treatments.

There is a growing consensus that patients who possess decision-making capacity have an ethical and legal right to accept or refuse medical interventions, including life-sustaining treatment.[1] Advance directives enable persons to express their wishes before losing decision-making capacity, and when patients who lack decision-making capacity have not executed advance directives with unambiguous instructions, surrogates can accept or refuse medical interventions on their behalf. However, a right to accept or refuse treatments *if they are offered* by physicians does not entail a right to demand or receive treatments that physicians are unwilling to offer. In fact, there is increasing support for the position that physicians are not obligated to give patients or their surrogates an opportunity to accept or refuse *medically futile* treatments.[2]

It might be thought that physicians are uniquely qualified to make determinations of medical futility because such judgments are based on knowledge and expertise that physicians possess and patients and surrogates lack. But is this belief correct? To answer this question, it is necessary to distinguish three senses of "futility": (1) Physiological futility: A medical intervention is futile if there is no reasonable chance that it will achieve its direct physiological (medical) objective.[3] For example, CPR is futile in this sense if there is no reasonable chance that it will succeed in restoring cardiopulmonary function; dialysis is futile if there is no reasonable chance that it will succeed in cleansing the patient's blood of toxins; and tube feeding is futile if there is no reasonable chance that it will succeed in providing the patient with life-sustaining nutrition. (2) Futility in relation to the patient's goals: A medical intervention is futile if there is no reasonable chance that it will achieve the patient's goals. For example, if the

patient's goal is to survive to leave the hospital, CPR is futile in this sense if there is no reasonable chance that it will enable the patient to do so. (3) Futility in relation to standards of professional integrity: A medical intervention is futile if there is no reasonable chance that it will achieve any goals that are compatible with norms of professional integrity.[4]

1. PHYSIOLOGICAL FUTILITY

Judgments of futility in the first sense (i.e., physiological futility) appear to be based on expertise that physicians possess and patients and surrogates typically lack. Physicians have scientific and clinical expertise that enables them to ascertain the likely physiological effects of medical interventions, and most patients and surrogates lack this ability. Consequently, if anyone is capable of determining that a medical intervention (e.g., CPR, chemotherapy, or dialysis) is unlikely to have a specified physiological effect in a particular case, it is the physician and not the patient or the patient's surrogate. However, there are still two reasons for doubting that the scientific and clinical expertise of physicians uniquely qualifies them to make futility judgments in this sense.

First, although their scientific and clinical expertise enables physicians to determine whether, in relation to a particular standard of reasonableness, there is a reasonable chance that a specified physiological outcome will occur, setting the standard of reasonableness involves a value judgment that goes beyond such expertise. Suppose a 79-year-old severely demented man is hospitalized with pneumonia. He appears to be responding to intravenous antibiotics. His physician believes that it is important to decide whether CPR should be initiated in the event of a cardiopulmonary arrest. The physician's scientific and clinical expertise uniquely qualifies her to determine whether the chance of restoring cardiopulmonary function is greater than X percent. However, unless X equals zero, that expertise does not uniquely qualify her to determine whether the chance of restoring cardiopulmonary function is reasonable or worthwhile only if it is greater than X percent.

Second, although the scientific and clinical expertise of physicians enables them to determine whether a medical intervention is likely to achieve a specified outcome, determining whether a particular outcome is an appropriate objective for a medical intervention involves value judgments that go beyond that expertise. Suppose a physician concludes that it would be futile to amputate the leg of a terminally ill cancer patient because an amputation would neither prevent the spread of the cancer nor significantly reduce pain. But the patient wants an amputation because he is disgusted by the thought of having a cancerous leg. Insofar as an amputation would achieve the patient's objective of removing a source of disgust and extreme displeasure, it would not be futile to the patient. The scientific and clinical expertise of the physician uniquely qualifies her to determine whether an amputation is likely to prevent the spread of the cancer or significantly reduce pain. However, that expertise does not uniquely qualify her to evaluate the patient's goal and to determine that the amputation is futile (inappropriate) even if there is a reasonable chance of achieving the patient's goal.

If a patient or surrogate wants a medical intervention that the physician deems to be futile because she concludes that there is no reasonable chance that the intervention will achieve its direct physiological (medical) objective, the physician can attempt to justify not offering it by citing standards of professional integrity. For example, the physician can claim that it is incompatible with those norms either (1) to attempt resuscitation when there is less than an X percent chance that it will restore cardiopulmonary function or (2) to amputate a limb because it disgusts a patient. However, the physician's decision not to offer a treatment would then involve a judgment of futility in the third sense (which will be considered later).

2. FUTILITY IN RELATION TO THE PATIENT'S GOALS

A medical intervention is futile in the second sense if there is no reasonable chance that it will achieve the patient's goals. Patients and surrogates may require assistance in identifying and clarifying goals,

and physicians can sometimes provide such assistance. However, ordinarily physicians are not uniquely qualified to identify a patient's goals.

Even when patients or their surrogates and physicians agree on goals, there are two possible sources of disagreement about whether a treatment is futile in relation to those goals. First, the patient or surrogate and the physician might disagree about the *probability* of achieving the patient's goals by means of the treatment. Suppose that the patient's primary goal is to survive to leave the hospital. The physician concludes that the chance of achieving this goal by means of CPR if the patient were to experience cardiac arrest is close to nil. The patient agrees that CPR would be futile if the physician were right, but the patient refuses to accept the physician's conclusion. Instead, he insists that there is a very good chance that he would survive to leave the hospital if he were to receive CPR after experiencing cardiac arrest. In such cases, the disputed judgments call for scientific and clinical expertise that physicians have and patients and surrogates typically lack. Consequently, in situations of this kind, the expertise of physicians appears to uniquely qualify them to make futility determinations.

Second, even if a patient or surrogate and the physician agree on the probability of achieving the patient's goals, they might disagree about whether the probability is high enough to warrant treatment. Whereas a physician might conclude that treatment is futile because of the low probability of achieving the patient's goals, the patient or surrogate might believe that despite the poor odds, it is still worth a try. As it is sometimes put, "there is always a chance for a miracle," and the patient or surrogate may not want to foreclose whatever slim chance there is. This disagreement between the physician and the patient or surrogate concerns the standard for determining whether the probability of achieving a specified outcome is "reasonable." To recall what was said in relation to the first sense of futility, although the scientific and clinical expertise of physicians enables them to determine whether, in relation to a particular standard of reasonableness, a chance of producing a specified outcome is reasonable, setting that standard involves a value judgment that goes beyond such expertise. Again, the physician can attempt to justify a particular standard of reasonableness by citing standards of professional integrity. However, the physician's decision to not offer treatment would then involve a judgment of futility in the third sense.

3. FUTILITY IN RELATION TO STANDARDS OF PROFESSIONAL INTEGRITY

The reasoning underlying the claim that physicians are uniquely qualified to make determinations of futility in the third sense is as follows. Since the best treatment choice for patients is a function of their individual preferences and values, the scientific and clinical expertise of physicians ordinarily does not uniquely qualify them to make treatment decisions for patients. However, as practitioners of medicine, physicians have a special responsibility to uphold standards of professional integrity. These are standards for the medical profession, and not merely personal standards of individual physicians. For example, performing abortions or withdrawing life support might be contrary to the personal standards of a particular physician, but she might not hold that it is improper for *any* physician to perform an abortion or withdraw life support. That is, she need not believe that it is wrong to perform such actions *as a physician.*

Among other things, standards of professional integrity identify the proper goals of medicine and the appropriate objectives and uses of medical interventions. These standards provide a basis for claiming, say, that whereas certain surgical procedures (e.g., surgically altering the size and shape of a person's nose) are properly used for cosmetic purposes, others (e.g., an amputation of a healthy leg or arm) are not.

Of more relevance to futility determinations, standards of professional integrity might provide a basis for a principle such as the following: A medical intervention is futile if the probability of achieving any appropriate treatment goal by means of that intervention is too low. Suppose a physician recommends a Do Not Resuscitate (DNR) order to a patient with widely metastasized liver cancer. The patient responds that she *wants* CPR if she suffers cardiopulmonary arrest. The physician carefully explains the burdens of CPR and states that it is futile because the patient is within a group that has less than a 1 percent chance of surviving to leave the hospital. The patient responds that any chance of extending her life, even if

it will be spent in the hospital, is worthwhile to her, and clearly outweighs the burdens of CPR. The physician can still maintain that CPR is futile because resuscitative efforts would be incompatible with norms of professional integrity. In effect, the physician would be claiming that the use of CPR in this case would constitute a *misuse* of that medical procedure.

It is important to recognize that this account of futility decisions is not based on the presumed special scientific and clinical expertise of physicians. Rather, it is based on norms associated with standards of professional integrity and the alleged special responsibility of physicians to uphold those norms. The term "standards of professional integrity" is ambiguous. It can be used descriptively or prescriptively (in an evaluative sense). Descriptively, "standards of professional integrity" can refer to: (1) an individual physician's standards (i.e., the physician's conception of the proper goals of medicine, the appropriate objectives and uses of medical interventions, and so forth), or (2) customary or currently accepted standards relating to the proper goals of medicine, the appropriate objectives and uses of medical interventions, and so forth. On some questions (e.g., whether Laetrile is an appropriate treatment for cancer) there may be enough agreement among members of the medical profession to warrant referring to "customary or currently accepted standards." However, on other questions (e.g., whether tube feeding is appropriate for patients who have been in a persistent vegetative state for over a month), there may be insufficient agreement. Prescriptively, "standards of professional integrity" refers to *valid* or *legitimate* standards. Such standards are valid if and only if their content is *worthy* of being adopted and maintained by members of the medical profession.[5]

If determinations that medical interventions are futile in the third sense can justify decisions to deny patients or their surrogates an opportunity to accept or refuse treatments, it can only be when futility judgments are based on *valid* standards of professional integrity.[6] Suppose Ms. P is a 76-year-old patient with lung cancer who suffers renal failure. Her physician is Dr. Q, and dialyzing patients under these circumstances is contrary to Dr. Q's conception of the appropriate objectives and uses of dialysis. Suppose it is not contrary to valid standards of professional integrity to dialyze Ms. P. If Dr. Q offers to refer Ms. P or her surrogate to a nephrologist who would be willing to dialyze Ms. P, then Dr. Q might justifiably assert that *he* is not obligated to dialyze her. However, Dr. Q cannot justifiably claim that Ms. P or her surrogate should be denied an opportunity to accept or refuse dialysis because dialyzing Ms. P would violate *his* and/or *customary* standards of professional integrity.

CONCLUSION

It is beyond the scope of this essay to provide criteria for identifying valid standards of professional integrity. By way of a modest conclusion about determinations of medical futility, however, I will suggest the following. The statement that a medical intervention is futile communicates a sense of scientific objectivity and finality and tends to suggest that clinical data alone can decisively demonstrate that it is justified to deny patients or surrogates an opportunity to accept or refuse the treatment. However, standards of professional integrity almost always are an essential component of judgments of futility in every sense, and these standards are *evaluative*. Whereas a medical intervention may be futile in relation to one conception of the proper goals of medicine and the appropriate objectives and uses of that intervention, it may not be futile in relation to another conception. For example, according to one conception of the proper objectives and uses of mechanical ventilation, it may be futile for patients with advanced Alzheimer's disease; and according to another conception, ventilatory support may not be futile for such patients. Similarly, according to one conception of the proper objectives and uses of CPR, resuscitative efforts can be futile if the probability of survival until discharge is less than 2 percent; and according to another conception, resuscitative efforts may not be futile in the same circumstances. A key issue, then, is whether or not the medical intervention is *appropriate* from the perspective of valid standards of professional integrity.

Since the term "futility" tends to communicate a false sense of scientific objectivity and finality and to obscure the evaluative nature of the corresponding judgments, it is recommended that physicians avoid using the term to justify not offering medical interventions. Instead of saying, "life-extending treatment is not an option because it is futile," it is recommended that physicians explain the specific grounds for concluding that life-support generally, or a particular life-sustaining measure, is inappropriate in the circumstances. Whereas the statement that life-sustaining treatment is futile tends to discourage discussion, explaining the grounds for concluding that (some or all) life-extending interventions are inappropriate in the circumstances tends to invite discussion and point it in the right direction.

NOTES

1 See Alan Meisel, "The Legal Consensus About Forgoing Life-Sustaining Treatment: Its Status and Prospects," *Kennedy Institute of Ethics Journal*, Vol. 2, No. 4 (December 1992), pp. 309–45.

2 See, for example, Tom Tomlinson and Howard Brody, "Futility and the Ethics of Resuscitation," *Journal of the American Medical Association*, Vol. 264, No. 10 (Sept. 12, 1990), pp. 1276–1280; Lawrence J. Schneiderman, Nancy S. Jecker, and Albert R. Jonsen, "Medical Futility: Its Meaning and Ethical Implications," *Annals of Internal Medicine*, Vol. 112, No. 12 (June 15, 1990), pp. 949–954; and Steven H. Miles, "Medical Futility," *Law, Medicine & Health Care*, Vol. 20, No. 4 (Winter 1992), pp. 310–15.

3 This sense of futility might be further identified as *"specific physiological futility"* to distinguish it from *"general physiological futility."* A medical intervention is futile in the latter sense if there is no reasonable chance that it will have *any* physiological effect. However, it is rarely, if ever, the case that a medical intervention is unlikely to have *any* physiological effect. For example, although a blood transfusion or chemotherapy may not extend a patient's life, each is likely to produce some physiological changes (e.g., an alteration in blood count).

4 See Tomlinson and Brody, "Futility and the Ethics of Resuscitation."

5 Alternatively, validity can be understood as a *procedural* concept. For example, it might be said standards are valid if: (1) they were adopted through a fair democratic process open to physicians and the general public, or (2) they would be adopted if such a process were followed.

6 Even if physicians are not obligated to *offer* medically futile treatments to patients or their surrogates, it may still be appropriate to *discuss* treatment goals and plans with patients or their surrogates before implementing a decision to forgo such treatments. As Youngner puts it, "Don't offer, perhaps, but please discuss." Stuart J. Youngner, "Futility in Context," *Journal of the American Medical Association*, Vol. 264, No. 10 (Sept. 12, 1990), p. 1296.

ADVANCE DIRECTIVES AND TREATMENT DECISIONS FOR INCOMPETENT ADULTS

SOME REFLECTIONS ON ADVANCE DIRECTIVES
Thomas A. Mappes

Mappes discusses some of the problems associated with the construction and implementation of advance directives. He argues that standard-form living wills typically fail
to address adequately the problem posed by the prospect of existence in a severely
debilitated but nonterminal condition, and he further argues that this problem is not
easily solved, even if a person resolves to craft a more customized instructional directive. Mappes also provides a discussion of the relative importance of proxy and instructional directives. Next, he argues that although advance directives have a very
weighty moral authority, physicians are sometimes justified in refusing to honor the instructional directives of patients. Finally, he briefly considers both "the past wishes versus present interests problem" and the "problem of incompetent revocation."

There is no doubt in my mind that advance directives
can be a valuable and important tool for many of us,
but it has become increasingly clear that these instruments (especially living wills) are more problematic than originally anticipated.[1] In calling
attention to some of the problems associated with
the construction and implementation of advance directives, I do not really mean to suggest that advance
directives are unworthy of enthusiasm, but I do want
to insist that our enthusiasm needs to be somewhat
tempered by an awareness of various limitations and
problems.

There are two basic types of advance directives.
In executing an *instructional* directive, a competent
person specifies instructions about his or her care in
the event that decision-making capacity is lost. An
instructional directive, especially when it deals
specifically with a person's wishes regarding life-
sustaining treatment in various possible circumstances, is commonly called "a living will." In
executing a *proxy* directive, a competent person
specifies a substitute decision maker (i.e., a health-
care agent) to make health-care decisions for him or
her in the event that decision-making capacity is
lost. The legal mechanism for executing a proxy di-

rective is often called a "durable power of attorney
for health care."

It is helpful at this point to remind ourselves of
the sense behind a living will. Most of us can easily
imagine medical circumstances in which the continuation of our lives would be of no value to us. I
would certainly say, in the event that I should fall
into a persistent vegetative state (PVS), that the continuation of my life would have no value for me. [All
references to PVS in this paper assume that the vegetative state is reasonably believed to be irreversible (i.e., permanent).] Moreover, in some cases, I—and
I think many others—would want to say something
even stronger—not just that the continuation of my
life has *no* value for me, but that it has *negative*
value. If I were terminally ill and undermined by
pain, constraint, and/or indignity, with no reasonable
prospect of relief, I would be inclined to say that I
am better off dead; that is, it is in my best interests
for my life not to continue. Now, if I am competent
(i.e., if I retain decision-making capacity) at this
point, I can refuse life-sustaining treatment. But, as
we all know, the rigors of incurable illness and the
dying process frequently deprive previously competent agents of their decision-making capacity. A living will is a device that allows me to exercise some
measure of control over the circumstances of my
death. In a living will, I express my personal wishes
with regard to life-sustaining treatment in various

Reprinted with permission of the American Philosophical Association
from *Newsletter on Philosophy and Medicine,* in *APA Newsletters,* vol.
98, no. 1, Fall 1998, pp. 106–111.

possible circumstances. At its core, then, the living will is an expression of patient autonomy; the principal value that is being expressed is the value of self-determination. I am presently incompetent and cannot make decisions about life-sustaining treatment, but the living will has allowed me to make such decisions *prospectively*. I make decisions—while I am still competent—about how I want to be treated if I become incompetent, and the living will is the instrument that confers authority on these decisions and renders them efficacious.

A COMMON SHORTCOMING IN STANDARD-FORM LIVING WILLS: THE CIRCUMSTANCES TYPICALLY REQUIRED FOR ACTIVATION OF A LIVING WILL ARE TOO RESTRICTIVE

In speaking now of standard-form living wills, I have in mind principally the various forms that have emerged in conjunction with state statutes. In my judgment, most of these standard forms share a central shortcoming, to this effect, the circumstances typically required for activation of a living will are *too restrictive*. The problem I have in mind here was more extreme in the first generation of living wills but is still cause for concern in many states, including my own (Maryland).

The core of the problem is the way in which activation of a living will is so frequently tied to the presence of "terminal illness" or a "terminal condition"—categories that have usually been interpreted to exclude both a patient in a persistent vegetative state and one who is mired in a severely compromised state, for example, as a result of stroke or Alzheimer's disease. Although the definition of a "terminal condition" is itself a notoriously problematic issue, a terminal condition is often understood as a condition that is incurable and irreversible and, regardless of medical intervention, will lead to death in some suitably short period of time. Thus, a PVS patient is not necessarily terminally ill. Although irreversibly unconscious and hopelessly compromised, the patient might be sustained in this state for 10, 20, 30, 40 or more years. Similarly, a desparately compromised stroke victim might be in a relatively stable state and thus not qualify as terminally ill. And the Alzheimer's patient, despite the fact that he

or she is significantly debilitated and on a progressively worsening trajectory, also fails to qualify as terminally ill.

Many states (including my own) have by now effectively acted to deal with the first aspect of the problem that I am worried about; they have simply revised their standard-form living wills to ensure that the existence of PVS is an independent basis upon which to activate a living will. Although I find this development with regard to PVS an entirely welcome one, I am convinced that the other aspect of the overall problem remains largely unsolved. Even if the PVS issue has been effectively resolved in second generation standard-form living wills, it still remains the case that the circumstances typically required for activation of a living will are too restrictive.

Many of us, I believe, are deeply concerned about the prospect of existence in a *severely debilitated but nonterminal condition,* and we would like our living will to somehow address this concern. Would I, for example, want to be sustained as an Alzheimer's patient if I no longer had any idea who my friends and family were? Would I want antibiotics for my pneumonia in such a state? Would I even want nutrition and hydration in such a state? But with the emergence of such questions things get much more complicated. In fact, we are now faced with a whole new layer of complexity.

ANOTHER LAYER OF COMPLEXITY: DESIGNING AN INSTRUCTIONAL DIRECTIVE RESPONSIVE TO THE PROSPECT OF EXISTENCE IN A SEVERELY DEBILITATED BUT NONTERMINAL CONDITION

I am ruminating for a moment in terms of my own value system, recognizing of course that diverse personal and cultural values will lead different individuals to very different points of view on the issues at stake in this new layer of complexity. For one thing, I am not a religious person, so my attitudes and beliefs do not take account of any doctrinal authority or tradition. Obviously, many others will want to ensure that anything they say at this point would be in accord with the religious tradition they have embraced.

Certain general phrases come to my mind. I would not want life-sustaining treatment for myself in the event that I no longer have, and there is no reasonable possibility that I will regain, a "meaningful quality of life." That phrase certainly captures part of what I want to say, but were I to put it (or something like it) in an instructional directive, what would I really accomplish? Unless I go on to specify in some detail what counts *for me* as a *meaningful* quality of life, my instructional directive will be hopelessly vague. Other ideas are floating around in my mind. I certainly do not want to be condemned to an existence that I (as a presently competent person) would consider—here are the words—"demeaning" or "degrading" or "undignified." Perhaps I should add something like the following to my instructional directive: I do not want life-sustaining treatment if there is no reasonable prospect that I will recover from an *undignified* state of existence. Once again, we encounter the problem of vagueness. Unless I go on to specify in some detail what counts *for me* as an *undignified* state of existence, I will have provided very little effective guidance in my instructional directive.

Here is one other concern that I would consider very central to any instructional directive that I might want to prepare. I do not wish for my continued existence in a severely compromised state to be a burden—either an emotional or a financial burden—on those with whom I have shared my life—that is, my family and friends. I'm not at all sure exactly how to phrase what I want to say on this score; I only know that I am very strongly invested in this consideration, and I think many other people are as well. Perhaps I want to say something like this: Even if my life in a severely compromised state seems on balance to provide more benefits than burdens *for me,* I would not want my life to be sustained if the *collective burdens* to me, my family and friends are significant enough to outweigh the *collective benefits* to me, my family, and friends. At any rate, I think I have the prerogative as a presently competent person to stipulate that I do not want decisions about the continuation of my life in a severely compromised state to be made without regard for the impact of these decisions on my family and friends.

In focusing attention on some phrases that I resonate with, here is where I wind up. I don't want my life in a severely compromised state to be sustained if I no longer have a "meaningful" quality of life or if I am mired in an "undignified" state or if my continued existence constitutes a "significant burden" for those who love me. Now, on the one hand, I am interested in incorporating such phrases into an instructional directive that is more comprehensive than standard-form living wills. But, on the other hand, I recognize that numerous problems of interpretation are likely to arise unless I more effectively specify the meaning of these various phrases. Although this task is not an insurmountable one, I believe it is a very difficult one, even for those of us who have already thought a good bit about the issues at stake. One natural alternative is simply to include such phrases in an instructional directive and concurrently execute a proxy directive with the intention of having one's health-care agent resolve any problems of interpretation. If this strategy is chosen, of course, it would certainly be important for a person to discuss these matters in some detail with one's health-care agent.

THE RELATIVE VALUE OF ADVANCE DIRECTIVES

Should everyone have advance directives? It is very doubtful that an affirmative answer to this question could be sustained, but it does seem to me that there are very good reasons for many people to have at least some type of advance directive. Perhaps the best way to think about this is simply to say that, depending on individual circumstances, and depending on the type of advance directive we have in mind, there are more powerful reasons for some people to have advance directives than for other people to have them.

Let's focus attention first on the relative importance of a proxy directive. In many states, there is now established an explicit hierarchy for the identification of a surrogate decision maker for an incompetent person who has not executed a proxy directive. In Maryland, for example, the hierarchy looks like this:

- court-appointed guardian
- spouse
- adult child

- parent
- adult sibling
- close friend or other relative

I am reflecting, once again, in terms of the circumstances of my own life. There is no doubt in my mind that were I to lose decision-making capacity, I would want my spouse to make health-care decisions for me. But in Maryland, she will be empowered to do so even if I never execute a proxy directive appointing her as my health-care agent. So, in a way, it seems like I don't have a very compelling incentive to execute a proxy directive. But now I reflect further: What would happen if, for whatever reason, my spouse could not function as my surrogate? According to the established Maryland hierarchy, my parents are next in line, but they are approaching 80 and I would not want this responsibility to fall on them. So I reach this point in my deliberations: It makes sense for me to have a proxy directive in which I appoint my spouse as my health-care agent and, taking account of the possibility that she might ultimately be unable to function as my health-care agent, I name one of my three sisters as my backup health-care agent. And yet, since my first choice for a health-care decision maker is in accord with the state hierarchy, it may not seem like I have a really powerful incentive to have a proxy directive in place.

Suppose on the other hand that I were a gay male in a long-term relationship with my male partner. I would certainly execute a proxy directive naming my male partner as my health-care agent, because the more traditional logic of the state hierarchy is not about to lead to the identification of my partner as my surrogate decision maker. And similarly, anyone whose first choice for a surrogate decision maker does not accord with the reigning hierarchy has a very powerful motive for establishing a proxy directive. Suppose a person looks at the relevant state hierarchy and says: "You mean it's my brother who would make health-care decisions for me? My brother's a space cadet! I wouldn't trust him to take out the garbage." The person who says that is a person who has a very powerful incentive to execute a proxy directive.

Now, there is another consideration in all of this and, for me, it turns out to be a consideration of decisive importance. In Maryland, the health-care agent—that is, the person formally named in a proxy directive—has broader powers with regard to end-of-life decision making than does a surrogate identified in terms of the state hierarchy. A surrogate is authorized to reject life-sustaining treatment *only if* the patient is in a terminal condition, is in a so-called end-stage condition, or is in a persistent vegetative state; a health-care agent is not restricted to these three circumstances. Thus, for me, taking account of the fact that I would very much like to guard against the possibility of a prolonged existence in a severely compromised state, it would be very imprudent not to execute a proxy directive.

A more remote possibility also enters my mind. What if I were tragically injured and hospitalized in a state such as New York, where at present a surrogate (as contrasted with a designated health-care agent or proxy) essentially has no legal right to refuse life-sustaining treatment for a patient who has lost decision-making capacity? As a resident of Maryland, I already have a very strong reason to establish a proxy directive. When I consider that I am also a potential visitor to a state such as New York, I realize that the overall case for my having a proxy directive is at least slightly stronger. Of course, if I were a resident of New York, I would conclude that my need for a proxy directive (especially in the absence of a very explicit living will) was truly compelling.

Let's shift our focus now to the relative importance of instructional directives. I think I want to say, other things being equal, that the older a person is, the more compelling is the reason to think seriously about executing a living will. Do we really want to suggest that it is important for (healthy) young adults to have a living will? In teaching biomedical ethics to undergraduate students, I find that I do not so much want to encourage young adults to execute a living will at this point in their life as to educate them so that they will have the understanding necessary to think seriously about the possibility of doing so in due time.

A related consideration seems more or less obvious to me. Other things being equal, the more endangered a person's health, the more compelling is the reason to think seriously about the possibility of executing a living will. Further, in this vein, once a person is identified as a "heart" patient, or a "kidney" patient, or an ALS patient, it becomes possible to forsee with greater concreteness what sort of decline and dying process might lie ahead. And then, with appropriate education and support from both health-care professionals and family, it becomes more realistic to think through exactly what one might want in terms of life-sustaining treatment. Thus it becomes more feasible to craft a customized instructional directive, and I think there is often very good sense in doing so.

Instructional directives might well be of special value for individuals whose treatment preferences are unusual or at odds with what family members might be expected to favor. Instructional directives might also be of special value for those who would like to insulate their loved ones from the perceived burdens of end-of-life decision making, those who do not consider any likely surrogate or possible health-care agent sufficiently trustworthy or otherwise adequate to the task, and those who are essentially devoid of close personal ties. Of course, living wills originally evolved as a form of protection against overtreatment, and for most of us, that concern—despite a competing concern that cost controls now operative in the health-care system create a significant risk of undertreatment—may still provide a fairly strong incentive for establishing a living will, regardless of our age, degree of health, or special circumstances.

Let's ask then why so few people do in fact have living wills. One reason is obvious. On any given day, if I have a choice between working on my living will and working in the garden (or some such thing), I will probably decide to work in the garden. Thinking about my death is a rather unpleasant task; designing a new garden plot is a much more engaging activity. Moreover, the cultural and religious attitudes of many people are in various ways at odds with the whole idea of planning for death.[2] Closely related is the fact that some people are simply repelled by the thought that their choices could actually be implicated in the moment and manner of their death. However, I also want to suggest that the issues and concerns that can arise in drafting a living will can be very intimidating. I do not say that I am typical in the following regard, but I also do not think I am alone in saying that I have never seen a standard-form living will that did not make me nervous in some way, and often nervous in four or five

different ways at once. On the other hand, how many of us are prepared to strike out on our own and craft our own document?[3] Better perhaps to share our thoughts and concerns with our health-care agent and trust his or her judgment.

Joanne Lynn develops a related line of thought in an article entitled, "Why I Don't Have a Living Will." Lynn registers a host of complaints against standard-form living wills but, in the end, simply prefers a model of family decision making. She writes:

> I believe I have a trustworthy family and a supportive circle of friends. I would prefer to endure the outcome if they "err" in predicting my preferences, or even if they choose to ignore my preferences other than the preference for family decision-making, rather than to remove from them the opportunity and the burden of making the choices. I do not want anyone else presuming to impose what are taken to be my desires as expressed elsewhere upon that family.[4]

Many people, I believe, do not have living wills essentially because they feel secure within the fabric of family life. If difficult end-of-life decisions must be made for a family member who has lost decision-making capacity, then so be it; the decision-making resources of the family will be adequate to the task. Thus, from this point of view, there is simply no compelling need for living wills.

JUSTIFIED VERSUS UNJUSTIFIED REFUSALS TO HONOR ADVANCE DIRECTIVES

When patients have in fact gone to the trouble of establishing advance directives—and here I am thinking primarily of instructional directives—do physicians typically pay sufficient attention to them? There is perhaps good reason to believe the answer to this question is no, but rather than directly exploring worries that might arise on this score, I will briefly consider a closely related and more fundamental question: Is it ever justified for physicians to refuse to honor the advance directives of patients?[5]

Surely the value of patient autonomy is sufficient to ground a very strong moral presumption that advance directives should be followed, but a moral presumption is one thing and an unconditional moral requirement is something else. Advance directives must be accorded a very weighty moral authority, but I believe it is just wrongheaded to say that refusals to honor them can never be justified.

Suppose a person has explicitly written the following into an instructional directive: "Never put me on a ventilator." At face value, this instruction is as plain as anything could possibly be. It says, "*never* put me on a ventilator." But suppose further that this person, otherwise in good health, has been injured, is presently incompetent, and needs the temporary assistance of a ventilator in order to recover. The family of the patient insists that this instruction should be disregarded. The patient's daughter speaks for the family: "Look, Mom didn't really mean she wouldn't want a ventilator in this instance. She wrote that instruction after watching granddad's tortured existence on a ventilator in his last days. Mom only meant that she did not want her dying process to be prolonged on a ventilator." In this sort of case I think it would be morally perverse to "honor" a patient's advance directive. Surely we do not show respect for patient autonomy by slavishly following a written instruction when there is compelling reason to believe the written instruction does not convey what the patient really meant to say.

Here is a similar case that once arose at a hospital in my community. An ALS patient essentially decided that he would not want his life to be prolonged past the point at which he had lost all awareness, and he wanted to write an instructional directive to this effect. He explained what he wanted to say to a lawyer, who responded, very wrongly, "oh, you mean brain death." So the patient wound up with an instructional directive saying that he wanted life-prolonging treatment until he was brain dead, but this instruction was clearly not the one he meant to give. Now, I would say, in such a case, to the extent that there is clear evidence—based on the testimony of family and friends—that a written instruction does not in fact represent the actual wishes of a formerly competent patient, that a refusal to follow this instruction is morally permissible and perhaps even morally required.

I will briefly mention one other consideration relevant to the claim that the refusal to honor the provisions of an instructional directive might sometimes be justified. There is certainly an important difference in an instructional directive between a patient's *refusing* and *requesting* certain forms of

treatment. If a patient's instructional directive requests an experimental and very expensive form of treatment, and there is no mechanism in terms of which the treatment can be funded, there is certainly no obligation to provide it. Similarly, if a patient's instructional directive requests a so-called "medically ineffective" or "futile" treatment, there may well be no obligation to provide it.

TWO REMAINING PROBLEMS

Two final problems are sufficiently important to warrant explicit mention. The first can be identified as the "past wishes versus present interests problem." The second can be identified as the "problem of incompetent revocation."

The past-wishes-versus-present-interests problem is associated with the following kind of case. Someone has unambiguously stipulated in an advance directive that life-sustaining treatment should not be provided if she becomes seriously mentally debilitated; this patient is now severely mentally debilitated but is "pleasantly senile" and does not appear to be suffering. The problem is that life-sustaining treatment, although clearly incompatible with her *past wishes,* appears to be in her *present interests.* And there is a body of opinion that insists that the patient's present interests should take priority over the patient's past wishes.[6] A related issue involves the concept of personal identity. If mental deterioration is so severe that there is good reason to doubt that the present patient is essentially the "same person" as the one who executed the instructional directive, then what is the moral authority of the one to determine what happens to the other?[7]

My own view on the past-wishes-versus-present-interests problem is that the patient's past wishes should ultimately take priority over the patient's present interests, but I think this is a very difficult problem and I have constructed a more developed case to help us feel its force.

Albert H is a 77-year-old man who lives in a nursing home. His wife is deceased but their only child, a son, visits his father at least three times a week. Albert H began to exhibit the first signs of senility in his late sixties and his condition rapidly deteriorated. At this point he is categorized as severely but "pleasantly" demented. Albert H needs constant supervision and assistance with basic tasks but seems undisturbed by his situation. He loves to watch TV and smoke cigars. He seldom recognizes his son but talks enthusiastically with him and anyone else who will listen. He tells the same stories over and over again; in fact, he often tells the same story to a person 4 or 5 times in a row, forgetting that he has just told the story. Almost all of his stories derive from memories of childhood; he seems to have virtually no memories of his adult life. Apart from his mental deterioration, Albert H has no notable health problems.

When Albert H was in his early sixties, he had executed a formal advance directive. Among other things, he had clearly specified that, were he to become seriously mentally impaired, he should not be given life-sustaining treatments, including antibiotics. The problem now is that Albert H has contracted pneumonia, and this disease will probably be fatal unless it is countered with an antibiotic. Although Albert H's son is aware of his father's advance directive, he nevertheless believes that an antiobiotic should be provided. He argues that his father presently has no conception of the "indignity" of his existence. Since his life, however compromised, clearly has value to him (i.e., to Albert H), his son contends, it is in his best interest that the antiobiotic be provided.

Should Albert H's advance directive be overridden in this case? Is Albert H presently the same person as the person who wrote the advance directive? If not, does that former person have the right to dictate what happens to Albert H?[8]

Our final problem—a closely related one—is the problem of incompetent revocation.[9] A previously competent patient has unambiguously rejected some form of life-sustaining treatment in his or her living will. But now the patient, presently incompetent, confused and perhaps scared, insists on the treatment. The conflict here is between the *past* wishes of the previously competent patient and the *present* wishes of the now incompetent patient. Which should have priority? To my knowledge, state living-will statutes ordinarily provide for a patient—whether competent or incompetent—to revoke a living will at any time. Thus the system essentially gives priority to the present wishes of the incompetent patient over the past wishes of the pre-

viously competent patient. But one might feel that this is not a satisfactory resolution of the issue, and some people have attempted to deal with this contingency by incorporating something like the following provision into their living wills: "And if I ever say, while incompetent, that I *do* want treatment, I hereby instruct you to disregard what I say."

CONCLUSION

I think we must say that difficult and unresolved problems attend the construction and implementation of advance directives, especially living wills. At the same time, these documents can be immensely valuable within the context of many people's lives. We should acknowledge the valuable role that advance directives can play; we should not lose sight of the associated problems.

NOTES

1 For one avenue of approach to the many problems associated with advance directives, see the series of articles in Special Supplement, "Advance Care Planning: Priorities for Ethical and Empirical Research," *Hastings Center Report,* 24:6 (1994), pp. S1–S36.

2 See, for example, Sheila T. Murphy et al., "Ethnicity and Advance Care Directives," *Journal of Law, Medicine & Ethics,* 24 (1996), pp. 108–117.

3 Norman Cantor presents one example of a very sophisticated, fully individualized document in "My Annotated Living Will," *Law, Medicine & Health Care,* 18:1–2 (1990), pp. 114–122.

4 Joanne Lynn, "Why I Don't Have a Living Will," *Law, Medicine, & Health Care,* 19:1–2 (1991), p. 104.

5 For one approach to this issue, see Dan W. Brock, "Trumping Advance Directives," Special Supplement, *Hastings Center Report,* 21:5 (1991), pp. S5–S6.

6 See, for example, Rebecca S. Dresser and John A. Robertson, "Quality of Life and Non-Treatment Decisions for Incompetent Patients: A Critique of the Orthodox Approach," *Law, Medicine, & Health Care,* 17 (1989), pp. 234–244.

7 For an extensive discussion of this issue, see Allen E. Buchanan and Dan W. Brock, *Deciding for Others: The Ethics of Surrogate Decision Making* (New York: Cambridge University Press, 1989), Chapter 3, "Advance Directives, Personhood, and Personal Identity."

8 This case originally appeared in Thomas A. Mappes and David DeGrazia, eds., *Biomedical Ethics,* 4th ed. (New York: McGraw-Hill, 1996), pp. 637–638.

9 Nancy M.P. King discusses this problem in *Making Sense of Advance Directives,* rev. ed. (Wash., D.C.: Georgetown University Press, 1996), pp. 204–213.

MY ANNOTATED LIVING WILL
Norman L. Cantor

Cantor provides an example of a highly personalized living will. Regarding the desirability of medical treatment in the event of a fatal condition, he presents a systematic account of the relative significance of various factors in a determination of his best interests. The factors he discusses are physical pain, indignity, mental deterioration, physical disability, economic considerations, and the interests of others. One of Cantor's principal concerns is to avoid life-preserving treatments should he be reduced to an existence that he (as a presently competent person) would consider clearly demeaning (degrading, undignified). This underlying concern is apparent in the specific instructions he gives with regard to permanent unconsciousness, progressive degenerative disease, and senility.

. . . The following personal "living will" is offered for publication for two reasons. First, by addressing various medical conditions and issues, it may encourage other people to consider a full spectrum of situations in advance and thus to provide better guidance than is currently offered in the abbreviated living will forms often used.[1] Further, to the extent that persons adopt positions identical or close to the instructions given here, they will be reinforcing one conception of what constitutes "humane" treatment for a previously vigorous adult who faces a life-threatening illness or condition. The annotations—the explanatory comments provided in brackets and boldface print—are unabashedly aimed at recruiting converts to the substantive provisions presented in the document.

Reprinted with permission of the author and the American Society of Law, Medicine & Ethics from *Law, Medicine & Health Care,* vol. 18, nos. 1–2 (1990), pp. 115–119.

MY LIVING WILL

I. INTRODUCTION

I hereby make this declaration before _____ witnesses in accordance with my state's living will legislation (or natural death act). Nonetheless, I understand that my instructions may extend beyond the classes of situations covered in such legislation. **[Conformity with the relevant state legislation—as to which each person should consult with a lawyer—helps reinforce the instructions. A living will statute usually provides some form of explicit legal sanction for medical failure to implement the patient's instructions, as well as explicit legal protection for physicians' good faith implementation of these instructions. Compliance with the formal statutory format (witnesses, etc.) assures** **that these elements will apply to the particular living will being drafted. Nonetheless, particular state statutes may provide constraints which do not fit the wishes of persons like myself. For example, a statute may authorize discontinuance of life-preserving treatment only when death is imminent, or a statute may not include refusal of artificial nutrition within its range of rejectable medical interventions. My instructions are not drawn according to the substantive (as opposed to the procedural) bounds of the state legislation. My effort to fully describe my wishes, regardless of the ostensibly limited scope of a living will statute, is designed to invoke judicially developed, common law rights of self-determination** and bodily integrity. **Living Will Statutes generally preserve judicially developed rights of dying patients. Thus, even in a jurisdiction with a living will statute of limited scope, there is hope that medical care providers will adhere to the prior instructions of a currently incompetent patient even though those instructions appear to go beyond the statute's bounds.]**

I hereby designate _____ as my surrogate for purposes of implementing this document. I hereby authorize _____ [the designated surrogate] to act on my behalf with regard to all decisions regarding medical care after I have lost mental capacity to make my own medical decisions. This authorization includes, but is not limited to, authority to accept or refuse life-preserving measures, to hire and fire attending personnel, to admit and remove me from institutions, to gain access to relevant information, and to undertake litigation on my behalf. I have consulted with _____ [the designated surrogate] and I have confidence that (s)he will implement my instructions with devotion to their letter and spirit. In the event that _____ [the designated surrogate] is not available to make determinations at the relevant moment, I request that my attending physician and any guardian involved in determining my care adhere to the contents of this document. **[In the absence of a designated agent or representative of an incompetent patient, the attending physician(s) would customarily consult with the patient's spouse or next of kin or other close relative willing to assume responsibility for medical decision-making. This may be a satisfactory arrangement, depending on the individual situation. I prefer to designate in advance a particularly trusted person who has expressed understanding of, and sympathy with, the instructions presented in this living will document. My hope and expectation is that my designated representative will be able to implement my instructions in a clear-headed fashion without the excessive emotional involvement which might affect some in my family. It may be advisable to designate an alternative surrogate who would function if the primary designated representative is unavailable at the appropriate time. Note also that in some states, legislation**

prescribes certain formalities for the appointment of such a representative, and care should be taken to adhere to those requirements.]

This document applies to medical decisions on my behalf after I have become legally incompetent to make such decisions myself. **[Legal incompetence simply means that a patient no longer understands the nature and consequences of the particular medical decision in question. This is a judgment to be made by attending medical personnel in conjunction with the patient's representative(s). No formal process is ordinarily required in order to determine that decision-making competence is not present. My expectation is that my surrogate will strive to ensure that no premature determination of my incompetence is made, in addition to seeing that, once competence is lost, all medical decisions conform to my preferences as expressed in this document.]**

Before I turn to instructions relating to particular types of conditions, I mention certain guidelines which apply to all post-competence decisions on my behalf. First, while my instructions call for withholding of life-preserving medical care in various situations, palliative care is always to be provided. That is, pain relievers or sedatives should be provided to relieve intractable pain or extreme emotional upset insofar as the need for such palliative agents can be discerned. Also, I would always expect to be maintained in a clean, sheltered, and comfortable environment. Nursing care aimed at providing a clean and dignified environment should therefore always be furnished.

Second, the general criterion to be applied to decision-making on my behalf is my "best interests." In this document, I define various elements or factors to be considered in determining my best interests. According to these elements, it will sometimes be in my best interests to withhold life-preserving medical intervention and to permit me to die. In line with my normal preference and respect for life, any such terminal decision should be made only when that decision is clearly in my best interests.

Third, life-preserving medical treatment refers to all forms of medical intervention whether complex, like respirators, or simplistic, like blood transfusions or antibiotics. Different treatments may entail different consequences and side effects (e.g., the long term dependence on a dialysis machine), so that differentiations among types of treatment may have to be made in the course of actual decision-making. Yet there is no intention here to categorize certain treatments as ordinary and others as extraordinary for purposes of shaping my medical future. Best interests will have to be assessed on a case by case basis with regard to my specific condition and various proposed treatments.

II. SUBSTANTIVE INSTRUCTIONS ACCORDING TO HEALTH CONDITION

A. Permanent Unconsciousness In the event that my capacity for sentient existence—consciousness or awareness of my environment—is permanently lost, I request that all life-extending medical intervention be ended. An existence devoid of all awareness is to my mind a demeaning state for a human being, and I don't wish to be maintained in such a status. I realize that the status of permanent unconsciousness can sometimes be artificially prolonged for long periods. This knowledge that death is not necessarily imminent merely reinforces my conviction to reject all life-extending medical intervention in such an instance. I request only that the medical assessment of permanent unconsciousness be carefully made in accord with good medical practice and after consultation with a skilled neurologist other than the attending physician.

My rejection of medical intervention in the face of permanent unconsciousness is intended to be complete. It includes simplistic procedures such as blood transfusions, CPR, antibiotics, or other medicines, as well as more complicated procedures such as respirators or dialysis machines. In the event that my medical condition in the permanently unconscious state includes damage to the alimentary processes (inability to swallow or digest food), I request that artificial means of nutrition not be initiated or maintained. **[There are instances when a patient in permanent coma retains a swallowing reflex and can be fed manually. Some persons may desire to instruct that this feeding be ceased in order to permit the permanently unconscious being to expire. However, the legal status of such**

a request is uncertain. A patient is acknowledged to have a right to decline medical treatment, which has been understood by the courts to include artificial nutrition. There is no assurance that manual feeding will be included within declinable medical treatment. Moreover, there is some question whether medical ethics would permit personnel to cooperate with such a request.]

B. A Fatal Organ Deficiency At some point after I have become incompetent, disease or trauma will produce a fatal condition. By this I mean major dysfunction of a critical organ (such as the heart or kidneys) or an illness (such as cancer or pneumonia) which by its nature is life threatening. In the event that such a condition occurs, it is my desire that medical intervention be guided by my best interests as determined in accord with the following considerations.

1. Physical Pain. To the extent that analgesics still leave significant physical pain or produce prolonged stupor, this should be deemed a significant factor adverse to my best interests.

2. Indignity. There are certain conditions which for me, an independent person who has been extremely active in both intellectual and physical pursuits, would be demeaning and degrading. I understand that in my incompetent state I may not feel or sense the humiliation or degradation with which I am concerned. Nonetheless, it is important to me as a currently autonomous being to shape my medical future in accord with my conception of indignity. It is important to me to be remembered as a person possessing certain characteristics, whose absence I consider undignified or demeaning. I direct that medical intervention in the face of a fatal organ deficiency be guided by my conception of personal dignity described herein. In other words, my best interests as an incompetent person should be judged with the following elements of indignity in mind.

A major element of indignity for me is helplessness. If, for example, I permanently lose the capacity to feed myself, this is a significant blow to my dignity. Inability to dress or bathe myself should also be considered a distasteful blow to my dignity. Similarly, if I lose control of my bodily evacuations, so that I must be diapered or otherwise attended, this constitutes a significant blow to my dignity.

Another aspect of helplessness is physical restraint. It may be that in my incompetence I will physically resist administration of medical treatment or otherwise act out so as to necessitate physical restraint in order to protect myself or others. Such conduct may be purely instinctive without any awareness or reason behind the actions. Nonetheless, it is demeaning to be trussed up or physically restrained for significant periods. If prolonged or repeated restraint (or, alternatively, prolonged or repeated sedation reducing me to a stupor) is necessary, this involuntary restraint is to be considered a significant blow to my dignity. . . .

3. Mental Deterioration. By definition, this living will is relevant only when I have lost competence to make my own medical decisions. While it is difficult for me to conceive of life without such mental capacity, I understand that persons lacking such capacity can still derive enjoyment and benefit from their existences. Therefore, while the prospect of mental incompetence is troubling to me, that fact, by itself, should not be deemed a basis for withholding or withdrawing medical treatment.

At the same time, there is a level of severe mental dysfunction which for me is demeaning and degrading. For example, permanent inability to recognize and/or interact with my relatives or friends would, by itself, constitute an undesirable, degrading status. Along these lines, total incapacity to read and understand a newspaper or magazine would reflect a level of dysfunction demeaning to me. If I am permanently reduced to such a level of dysfunction, this would at least constitute a significant blow to my dignity.

[Some persons might question my moral right to dictate an end to life-preserving care for my future self—particularly in a situation where that future self is not actually suffering from the undignified state reached. Is this incompetent future self a different persona who deserves to be preserved unless shown to be suffering irremediably? My response is that my right to self-determination includes the prerogative of shaping my dying process even after competence has been lost.[2] Just as I have a legitimate right to shape

handling of my future corpse, or to dispose of my property after death, I think I have a right to dictate my post-competence medical fate. In dictating the precise course to be followed, I have tried to be sensitive to how I am actually likely to feel (or not feel) in an advanced debilitated state.

My preferences expressed in this document represent no disrespect for the mentally handicapped population. I understand that mentally handicapped individuals still deserve society's solicitous attention and care. I am simply defining my own preferences, as a mentally acute person, with regard to my own future incapacities and the personal indignity involved therein (see the section below relating to senility and organic brain syndrome).]

4. Physical Disability. I have always been a vigorous person who loves participating in athletics and hiking. Thus, it is hard to imagine existence without capacity to engage in such pursuits. Nonetheless, I consider myself resilient enough and life-affirming enough to adjust to a significant degree of physical disability, including even blindness or inability to walk. Consequently, physical incapacity by itself should not be regarded in my case as a demeaning or degrading state. (This last statement is of course subject to the conditions which I have described above as depriving me of dignity—such as incontinence or inability to feed myself. I reiterate that such extreme debilities should be considered as significant blows to my dignity.)

My degree of actual or prospective physical disability should be considered in conjunction with my level of mental dysfunction. That is, if my mental deterioration deprives me of the ability to cope with whatever physical disabilities are involved, that fact should be included in calculating my best interests. While severe physical disabilities would not by themselves be a basis for ending life-preserving care, such disabilities in combination with extreme mental deterioration might well prompt a determination that my best interests dictate the cessation of medical intervention in the face of a fatal organ deficiency.

5. Economic Considerations. In general, my best interests ought to be determined without reference to the costs attributable to my care. So long as it is in my best interests to be medically maintained, I would expect care to continue. This is said with awareness that my assets are sufficient to cover even expensive medical care, and that I have no dependents whose economic well-being is threatened by the exhaustion of my estate. **[Were the financial situation otherwise, my instructions might well be different. If I were the head of a family of dependents, I would specify that the expense of prospective medical care be a factor to be considered in decision-making. I would instruct that if the decision regarding best interests is borderline, the extreme expense of prospective care should be considered as a factor weighing against initiation or continuation of the treatment. In addition, I would mention that financial dependence on loved ones would constitute a significant blow to my dignity. This means that if a decision regarding my best interests is otherwise borderline, financial dependence of this sort should be considered a significant factor dictating against further medical intervention.]**

6. Interests of Others. In general, my best interests ought to be determined without reference to the discomfort, inconvenience, anguish, or frustration of those surrounding me during the dying process. This is so whether those affected be medical staff or family and friends. It is not that I am indifferent to the interests of such persons. Rather, I have attempted in this document to design a dying process which would not be prolonged beyond the point where I am no longer reaping some net benefit from existence. My assumption is that my instructions foreclose a protracted dying process in which I have declined to a level of indignity which would exact a serious toll upon those around me.

C. Progressive Degenerative Disease I am aware that there are a number of incurable diseases which gradually and insidiously cause physical and/or mental deterioration over a prolonged period, before eventually leading to death. Alzheimer's disease and ALS (Lou Gehrig's disease) provide two examples known to me. If my incompetence coincides with such an affliction, I direct that medical intervention be shaped in accord with the best interests formula outlined above. This directive means, *inter alia,* that when irreversible deterioration has reached a point

which can be defined as clearly demeaning, life-preserving medical care should not be continued. I understand that as a consequence death may be permitted much earlier than it would ensue if medical intervention were maintained until the most advanced stages of the disease process. My wish is to avoid those stages of the dying process in which my existence has clearly become degrading according to the standards described in this document.

A point may come in the degenerative disease process when my condition is clearly degrading, and medical intervention is either already in place or is being contemplated because the disease process has impacted on critical bodily systems. At that point, my wish is that life-preserving medical treatment be withheld or withdrawn. Again, this applies to all forms of treatment whether simplistic or complex, and includes artificial nutrition where normal alimentary processes have been incapacitated (whether by the underlying degenerative disease or any other pathology which has developed).

[The term "point" is used in this document advisedly. There will normally not be one magic moment (except perhaps for a lapse into permanent unconsciousness) when a degrading status is suddenly reached. Deterioration will more likely be gradual, both in physical and mental terms. Nonetheless, a stage will be reached when good faith application of the criteria presented here will prompt a conclusion that the patient's status is clearly degrading. The judgment of my representative (or other decision-maker in the absence of my chosen surrogate) will determine when that stage has been reached.]

D. Senility and Organic Brain Syndrome I understand that my mental faculties may become debilitated by these common afflictions of old age. There are obviously various degrees of mental incapacity connected with senility, and the condition may or may not be accompanied by serious physical afflictions. I address here senility serious enough so that competence to make important medical decisions has been lost. If a fatal organ deficiency or serious malignant disease coincides with senility or organic brain syndrome, I dictate that medical decisions be made according to the criteria listed above under "Fatal Organ Deficiencies." This means that my deteriorated mental status will be considered in accord with the approach described in the section on "mental deterioration."

A few words with regard to senility. As I have outlined in the section on "mental deterioration," the fact of mental incompetence is not in itself to be deemed degrading or undignified so as to prompt withholding of life-preserving medical intervention. There is such a thing as "pleasantly senile," where an individual can still enjoy existence despite the loss of some mental faculties. Even though this persona is not the way I relish being remembered, I do not instruct that medical care be withheld solely because of this level of mental dysfunction. At the same time, the dysfunction may become so acute that my condition is clearly demeaning or degrading as I have defined it above. (For example, when I am in such a stupor that I no longer can recognize or relate to friends or relatives.) At that stage, my best interests would dictate release from this demeaning status by withholding or withdrawing life-prolonging medical intervention.

The hardest issue for me in drafting this living will is how to deal with preventive or curative medical care once severe mental deterioration has set in, yet I am still physically healthy. I am referring to having reached a mental status that is clearly demeaning, yet my physical status entails no fatal organ deficiency or serious disease. I am concerned about treatment of pathological conditions which by themselves are not fatal, but which if not treated will develop into fatal conditions, such as minor infections which are treatable with antibiotics, or minor organ dysfunctions which are curable but which will lead to fatal dysfunctions if not treated. Should preventive and curative measures be withheld in order to facilitate onset of a dying process which will liberate me from my demeaning state?

My personal resolution of this issue is to say that such conditions should be treated during my incompetency up until the point when my mental status can be deemed clearly and permanently degrading under the criteria listed above. For example, existence in a semiconscious stupor, or existence without any recognition of relatives or friends, would trigger this instruction. Once such a status has been reached, even medical intervention for curable conditions should be withheld. Infections should not be treated with antibiotics unless the prospective pain and discomfort and indignity accompanying the ensuing dying process would outweigh the relief which death might offer from the currently degrading status. The same approach should be applied to minor kidney, heart, or other organ problems which would not normally be deemed fatal organ deficiencies. In short, once a clearly demeaning mental status has irreversibly set in, even minor medical problems should not be treated (except palliatively) unless the consequent dying process carries with it negative consequences for me which make continued maintenance in an albeit demeaning state consistent with my best interests.

There may be tension here between my preferences regarding preventive and curative care and the conscientious positions of some medical personnel. While I have no desire to force medical personnel to violate their conscientious scruples, I do want to have my instructions implemented. In the event that attending medical personnel (or the institutional host) cannot in good conscience honor my preferences, my representative(s) are instructed to seek alternative personnel who can, in good conscience, cooperate. Or, I should be transferred to another facility in which cooperation is available. . . .

REFERENCES

1 For another effort to assist in drafting medical directives, see L. Emmanuel & E. Emmanuel, "The Medical Directive," 261 *J.A.M.A.* 3288 (1989).

2 See Dworkin, "Autonomy and the Demented Self," 64:2 *Millbank Quarterly* (1986), pp. 4–16.

THE CONSCIOUS INCOMPETENT PATIENT

Rebecca Dresser

Dresser provides a brief account of the *Wendland* case, in which the California Supreme Court refused to authorize the cessation of nutrition and hydration for a conscious but seriously brain-damaged man. In such cases (i.e., in cases involving conscious incompetent patients who are not terminally ill, in explicit contrast to cases involving permanently unconscious patients and cases involving terminally ill patients), Dresser points out, there seems to be an emerging legal consensus on the appropriateness of a very high evidentiary standard—the "clear and convincing evidence" standard. One especially notable result of this legal consensus is the following: in the absence of formal advance directives, prior statements by a patient indicating a "general aversion" to being maintained in a compromised state do not provide "clear and convincing evidence."

In 1995, the Michigan Supreme Court decided one of the landmark cases in end of life decisionmaking. *In re Martin* involved a man who had suffered severe brain damage in a car accident.[1] He was seriously debilitated and unable to make decisions, but he retained some awareness of his surroundings. Though he had no advance directive, before the accident he had said that he would not want to live if he became "dependent on people and machines." His wife wanted the feeding tube removed, but his mother and sister opposed this action. The Michigan court refused to permit withdrawal of the patient's feeding tube.

Six years later, faced with a strikingly similar set of facts, the California Supreme Court issued a similar ruling. In *Wendland v. Wendland*,[2] the court unanimously refused to authorize cessation of a severely brain-damaged patient's medical nutrition and hydration. The patient, Robert Wendland, had been injured in a car accident. He was conscious and able to engage in "clear, though inconsistent, interaction with his environment in response to simple commands." It was unclear whether Wendland understood these commands. He was paralyzed, incontinent, and dependent on a gastrostomy tube for nutrition and hydration. Physicians believed that there would be no further improvement in his condition.

Robert Wendland had no advance directive, but his wife, brother, and daughter all said that before the accident he had expressed strong views about life-sustaining treatment. When his father-in-law was close to death and being maintained on a respirator, Robert Wendland told his wife, Rose, "I would never want to live like that, and I wouldn't want my children to see me like that." When his brother worried that drinking and driving could leave Wendland "like a vegetable," Wendland responded, "whatever you do, don't let that happen." His daughter reported that he had said, "if he could not be a provider for his family, if he could not do all the things that he enjoyed doing, . . . just basic things, feeding himself, talking, communicating, if he could not do those things, he would not want to live."

When Rose Wendland told the hospital that she wanted Robert's tube feeding stopped, the hospital ethics committee supported her request. Wendland's mother and sister disagreed, however, and obtained a restraining order preventing removal of the tube. The trial judge appointed Rose Wendland as Robert's conservator and later appointed an independent attorney as Robert's legal representative. The attorney eventually supported Rose Wendland's position. But the trial court ruled against them because the conservator had

Reprinted with permission of the author and the publisher from *Hastings Center Report,* vol. 32 (May–June 2002), pp. 9–10. Copyright © 2002 by The Hastings Center.

failed to supply clear and convincing evidence that Wendland, who was "not in a persistent vegetative state nor suffering from a terminal illness would, under the circumstances, want to die." Nor had she demonstrated by clear and convincing evidence that removing the tube would be in the patient's best interest.

Rose Wendland appealed the ruling and the intermediate appellate court reversed, based on its view that California law required physicians to implement whatever treatment decision the conservator thought would be in the patient's best interest, as long as that judgment was made in good faith. The California Supreme Court ruled against this interpretation of state law, however, and instead held that the relevant statutes required conservators to "make health care decisions for the conservatee in accordance with the conservatee's individual health care instructions, if any, and other wishes to the extent known to the conservator." The court also said that if evidence regarding the patient's prior preferences is inadequate or unavailable, the conservator must decide in accordance with the patient's best interest.

Besides setting forth the substantive standards governing treatment decisions by conservators, the California Supreme Court established a high standard of proof for cases like *Wendland*. The court declared that a decision based on the patient's prior wishes or best interest must be supported by clear and convincing evidence, rather than the less demanding preponderance of the evidence. The court determined that the latter standard was acceptable when applied to terminally ill or permanently unconscious patients, but that the stricter standard should govern when conservators seek to forgo nutrition and hydration from conscious patients still able to perceive the discomfort and other symptoms that dehydration and starvation could produce. According to the court, applying a lower standard of proof to cases involving conscious patients could be unconstitutional because it would give inadequate protection to the patient's right to life and the state's interest in preserving life.

AN EMERGING CONSENSUS?

The California court cited as support for its ruling three other state supreme court decisions holding that clear and relatively precise evidence of a con-

scious, non-terminally ill, incompetent patient's prior wishes is necessary before nutrition and hydration may be forgone.[3] In response to Rose Wendland's argument that such a demanding evidentiary standard would improperly burden the individual's right to control future treatment, the court declared its agreement with the U.S. Supreme Court's statement in *Cruzan:* "The differences between the choice made *by* a competent person to refuse medical treatment, and the choice made *for* an incompetent person by someone else to refuse medical treatment, are so obviously different that the State is warranted in establishing rigorous procedures for the latter class of cases."[4] Moreover, the California court noted, the stringent evidentiary standard would be required only in cases involving conscious but incompetent patients who have no terminal illness and who failed to name a health care agent or complete a formal advance directive. Thus the impact of the clear and convincing evidence requirement on end of life decisions would be limited.

Robert Wendland died of pneumonia shortly before the California Supreme Court issued its opinion. If he had lived, however, the court would not have permitted clinicians to remove his feeding tube. According to the court, the evidence in the case failed to satisfy the clear and convincing standard. Robert Wendland's prior remarks were too general to indicate his clear desire to refuse treatment in his present circumstances. The judges refused "to define the extreme factual predicates that, if proved by clear and convincing evidence, might support a conservator's decision that withdrawing life support would be in the best interest of a conscious conservatee." Nevertheless, they were certain that the evidence in *Wendland* was insufficient to support the claim that the patient's quality of life was low enough to make withdrawing treatment in his best interest.

Wendland may signal a developing legal consensus. The class of patients described in *Wendland*—conscious incompetent patients—includes not only patients with brain injuries, but a much larger population of people with Alzheimer's disease and other forms of dementia. As the court observed, other state supreme courts considering end of life treatment for such patients have issued decisions resembling *Wendland*. In essence, the courts have refused to authorize cessation of treatment based on evidence of an individual's former general aversion to being maintained in a vegetative or other dependent state.

In *Wendland,* the California Supreme Court also focused on the experiential interests retained by conscious incompetent patients. According to the court, such patients have a stronger interest in avoiding a possibly burdensome non-treatment decision than do unconscious patients. To override this interest, at least one of two conditions must be met. There must be evidence that patients felt strongly enough about their nontreatment preferences to make a formal advance directive or to leave other specific instructions that they would not want treatment in their current situation. Alternatively, there must be persuasive evidence that maintaining life would impose pain or other serious experiential burdens that outweigh any positive experiences patients could gain from having their lives prolonged.

UNRESOLVED QUESTIONS

Since the 1970s, most ethicists and policymakers have regarded the competent individual's prior treatment preferences as the most defensible guide to decisionmaking for incompetent patients. This view gave rise to legislation and court decisions authorizing the cessation of treatment based on a person's general desire not to be maintained in a compromised state. But this legal approach was formulated in response to treatment questions involving patients in the persistent vegetative state or with illnesses expected to produce death in a relatively short time. *Wendland* and the other state supreme court decisions indicate that courts will demand greater justi-

fication to authorize nontreatment for conscious incompetent patients who are not terminally ill.

What remains uncertain is how courts will handle cases in which there is stronger evidence of a conscious incompetent patient's prior preferences for, or current interests in, having treatment stopped. For example, what if Robert Wendland had made a formal advance directive naming his wife as his treatment decisionmaker? Would the court have approved Rose Wendland's request to have the feeding tube removed? What if Robert Wendland had made a directive refusing all forms of life support if he could not talk or feed himself? Would the court have authorized the treatment withdrawal? And what balance of burdens and benefits would satisfy the California Supreme Court's formulation of the best interest standard? What is the "extreme" fact situation that would make forgoing treatment in a conscious patient's best interest?

These will be the hard treatment questions facing courts, legislatures, and policymakers in the new century. With an increasing number of dementia patients and aging Baby Boomers seeking control over their future care, cases presenting such questions will inevitably arise. Morally defensible resolutions will demand a refined and expanded analysis of decisionmaking for these patients.

NOTES

1 *In re Martin,* 538 N.W.2d 399 (Mich. 1995).
2 *Wendland v. Wendland,* 110 Cal. Rptr. 2d 412 (Cal. 2001).
3 *In re Martin; In re Edna M. F.,* 563 N.W.2d 485 (Wis. 1997); *In re Conroy,* 486 A.2d 1209 (N.J. 1985).
4 *Cruzan v. Harmon,* 110 S. Ct. 2841, 2856 (1990).

THE TREATMENT OF IMPAIRED INFANTS

INVOLUNTARY EUTHANASIA OF DEFECTIVE NEWBORNS

John A. Robertson

Robertson denies that the undesirable consequences of treating a severely impaired (defective) newborn can morally justify nontreatment. The consequentialist argument directly under attack by Robertson has two versions. One version is based on the suffering of the severely impaired newborn, whereas the other version is based on the suffering of others (principally the family but also health professionals and society as a whole). The first version of the consequentialist argument, identified by Robertson as the "quality-of-life argument," maintains that withholding treatment is morally justified because the severely impaired newborn is better off dead. Although Robertson insists that it is often false that death is a better fate than continued life for the severely impaired newborn, his fundamental objection to the quality-of-life argument stems from his reluctance to accept proxy assessments of quality of life. The second version of the consequentialist argument holds that withholding treatment is morally justified because of the emotional and financial burden falling on those who would have to provide the continued care for a severely impaired child. Robertson's central objection to this version of the consequentialist argument has to do with its utilitarian spirit, but he also argues that it is seldom plausible to think that the suffering of others is so grave as to outweigh the impaired newborn's interest in life.

One of the most perplexing dilemmas of modern medicine concerns whether "ordinary"[1] medical care justifiably can be withheld from defective newborns. Infants with malformations of the central nervous system[2] such as anencephaly,[3] hydrocephaly,[4] Down's syndrome,[5] spina bifida,[6] and myelomeningocele[7] often require routine surgical or medical attention[8] merely to stay alive. Until recent developments in surgery and pediatrics, these infants would have died of natural causes. Today with treatment many will survive for long periods, although some will be severely handicapped and limited in their potential for human satisfaction and interaction. Because in the case of some defective newborns, the chances are often slim that they will ever lead normal human lives, it is now common practice for parents to request, and for physicians to agree, not to treat such infants. Without treatment the infant usually dies. . . .

If we reject the argument that defective newborns are not persons, the question remains whether circumstances exist in which the consequences of treatment as compared with nontreatment are so undesirable that the omission of care is justified. . . .

. . . Many parents and physicians deeply committed to the loving care of the newborn think that treating severely defective infants causes more harm

than good, thereby justifying the withholding of ordinary care. In their view the suffering and diminished quality of the child's life do not justify the social and economic costs of treatment. This claim has a growing commonsense appeal, but it assumes that the utility or quality of one's life can be measured and compared with other lives, and that health resources may legitimately be allocated to produce the greatest personal utility. This argument will now be analyzed from the perspective of the defective patient and others affected by his care.

A. THE QUALITY OF THE DEFECTIVE INFANT'S LIFE

Comparisons of relative worth among persons, or between persons and other interests, raise moral and methodological issues that make any argument that relies on such comparisons extremely vulnerable. Thus the strongest claim for not treating the defective newborn is that treatment seriously harms the infant's own interests, whatever may be the effects on others. When maintaining his life involves great physical and psychosocial suffering for the patient, a reasonable person might conclude that such a life is not worth living. Presumably the patient, if fully informed and able to communicate, would agree. One then would be morally justified in withholding lifesaving treatment if such action served to advance the best interests of the patient.

Congenital malformations impair development in several ways that lead to the judgment that deformed retarded infants are "a burden to them-selves."[9] One is the severe physical pain, much of it resulting from repeated surgery that defective infants will suffer. Defective children also are likely to de-velop other pathological features, leading to repeated fractures, dislocations, surgery, malfunctions, and other sources of pain. The shunt, for example, in-serted to relieve hydrocephalus, a common problem in defective children, often becomes clogged, neces-sitating frequent surgical interventions.

Pain, however, may be intermittent and man-ageable with analgesics. Since many infants and adults experience great pain, and many defective in-fants do not, pain alone, if not totally unmanageable, does not sufficiently show that a life is so worthless that death is preferable. More important are the psy-chosocial deficits resulting from the child's handi-caps. Many defective children never can walk even with prosthesis, never interact with normal children, never appreciate growth, adolescence, or the fulfill-ment of education and employment, and seldom are even able to care for themselves. In cases of severe retardation, they may be left with a vegetative exis-tence in a crib, incapable of choice or the most min-imal response to stimuli. Parents or others may reject them, and much of their time will be spent in hospitals, in surgery, or fighting the many illnesses that beset them. Can it be said that such a life is worth living?

There are two possible responses to the quality-of-life argument. One is to accept its premises but to question the degree of suffering in particular cases, and thus restrict the justification for death to the most extreme cases. The absence of opportunities for schooling, career, and interaction may be the fault of social attitudes and the failings of healthy persons, rather than a necessary result of congenital malformations. Psychosocial suffering occurs be-cause healthy, normal persons reject or refuse to re-late to the defective, or hurry them to poorly funded institutions. Most nonambulatory, mentally re-tarded persons can be trained for satisfying roles. One cannot assume that a nonproductive existence is necessarily unhappy: even social rejection and nonacceptance can be mitigated. Moreover, the psy-chosocial ills of the handicapped often do not differ in kind from those experienced by many persons.

With training and care, growth, development, and a full range of experiences are possible for most peo-ple with physical and mental handicaps. Thus, the claim that death is a far better fate than life cannot in most cases be sustained.

This response, however, avoids meeting the quality-of-life argument on its strongest grounds. Even if many defective infants can experience growth, interaction, and most human satisfactions if nurtured, treated, and trained, some infants are so severely retarded or grossly deformed that their re-sponse to love and care, in fact their capacity to be conscious, is always minimal. Although mongoloid and nonambulatory spina bifida children may expe-rience an existence we would hesitate to adjudge worse than death, the profoundly retarded, nonam-bulatory, blind, deaf infant who will spend his few years in the back-ward cribs of a state institution is clearly a different matter.

To repudiate the quality-of-life argument, there-fore, requires a defense of treatment in even these extreme cases. Such a defense would question the validity of any surrogate or proxy judgments of the worth or quality of life when the wishes of the per-son in question cannot be ascertained. The essence of the quality-of-life argument is a proxy's judgment that no reasonable person can prefer the pain, suf-fering, and loneliness of, for example, life in a crib at an IQ level of 20, to an immediate, painless death.

But in what sense can the proxy validly con-clude that a person with different wants, needs, and interests, if able to speak, would agree that such a life were worse than death? At the start one must be skeptical of the proxy's claim to objective disinter-estedness. If the proxy is also the parent or physi-cian, as has been the case in pediatric euthanasia, the impact of treatment on the proxy's interests, rather than solely on those of the child, may influence his assessment. But even if the proxy were truly neutral and committed only to caring for the child, the prob-lem of egocentricity and knowing another's mind re-mains. Compared with the situation and life prospects of a "reasonable man," the child's poten-tial quality of life indeed appears dim. Yet a standard based on healthy, ordinary development may be en-tirely inappropriate to this situation. One who has never known the pleasures of mental operation, ambulation, and social interaction surely does not suffer from their loss as much as one who has. While one who has known these capacities may prefer death to a life without them, we have no assurance that the handicapped person, with no point of comparison, would agree. Life, and life alone, whatever its limitations, might be of sufficient worth to him.

One should also be hesitant to accept proxy assessments of quality of life because the margin of error in such predictions may be very great. For instance, while one expert argues that by a purely clinical assessment he can accurately forecast the minimum degree of future handicap an individual will experience, such forecasting is not infallible, and risks denying care to infants whose disability might otherwise permit a reasonably acceptable quality of life. Thus given the problems in ascertaining another's wishes, the proxy's bias to personal or culturally relative interests, and the unreliability of predictive criteria, the quality of life argument is open to serious question. Its strongest appeal arises in the case of a grossly deformed, retarded, institutionalized child, or one with incessant unmanageable pain, where continued life is itself torture. But these cases are few, and cast doubt on the utility of any such judgment. Even if the judgment occasionally may be defensible, the potential danger of quality-of-life assessments may be a compelling reason for rejecting this rationale for withholding treatment.

B. THE SUFFERING OF OTHERS

In addition to the infant's own suffering, one who argues that the harm of treatment justifies violation of the defective infant's right to life usually relies on the psychological, social, and economic costs of maintaining his existence to family and society. In their view the minimal benefit of treatment to persons incapable of full social and physical development does not justify the burdens that care of the defective infant imposes on parents, siblings, health professionals, and other patients. Matson, a noted pediatric neurosurgeon, states:

> [I]t is the doctor's and the community's responsibility to provide [custodial] care and to minimize suffering; but, at the same time, it is also their responsibility not to prolong such individual, famil-

ial, and community suffering unnecessarily, and not to carry out multiple procedures and prolonged, expensive, acute hospitalization in an infant whose chance for acceptable growth and development is negligible.[10]

Such a frankly utilitarian argument raises problems. It assumes that because of the greatly curtailed orbit of his existence, the costs or suffering of others is greater than the benefit of life to the child. This judgment, however, requires a coherent way of measuring and comparing interpersonal utilities, a logical-practical problem that utilitarianism has never surmounted. But even if such comparisons could reliably show a net loss from treatment, the fact remains that the child must sacrifice his life to benefit others. If the life of one individual, however useless, may be sacrificed for the benefit of any person, however useful, or for the benefit of any number of persons, then we have acknowledged the principle that rational utility may justify any outcome. As many philosophers have demonstrated, utilitarianism can always permit the sacrifice of one life for other interests, given the appropriate arrangement of utilities on the balance sheet. In the absence of principled grounds for such a decision, the social equation involved in mandating direct, involuntary euthanasia becomes a difference of degree, not kind, and we reach the point where protection of life depends solely on social judgments of utility.

These objections may well be determinative. But if we temporarily bracket them and examine the extent to which care of the defective infant subjects others to suffering, the claim that inordinate suffering outweighs the infant's interest in life is rarely plausible. In this regard we must examine the impact of caring for defective infants on the family, health professions, and society-at-large.

The Family The psychological impact and crisis created by birth of a defective infant is devastating. Not only is the mother denied the normal tension release from the stresses of pregnancy, but both parents feel a crushing blow to their dignity, self-esteem, and self-confidence. In a very short time, they feel grief for the loss of the normal expected child, anger at fate, numbness, disgust, waves of helplessness, and disbelief. Most feel personal blame for the defect, or blame their spouse. Adding to the shock is fear that social position and mobility are permanently endangered. The transformation of a "joyously awaited experience into one of catastrophe and profound psychological threat"[11] often will reactivate unresolved maturational conflicts. The chances for social pathology—divorce, somatic complaints, nervous and mental disorders—increase and hard-won adjustment patterns may be permanently damaged.

The initial reactions of guilt, grief, anger, and loss, however, cannot be the true measure of family suffering caused by care of a defective infant, because these costs are present whether or not the parents choose treatment. Rather, the question is to what degree treatment imposes psychic and other costs greater than would occur if the child were not treated. The claim that care is more costly rests largely on the view that parents and family suffer inordinately from nurturing such a child.

Indeed, if the child is treated and accepted at home, difficult and demanding adjustments must be made. Parents must learn how to care for a disabled child, confront financial and psychological uncertainty, meet the needs of other siblings, and work through their own conflicting feelings. Mothering demands are greater than with a normal child, particularly if medical care and hospitalization are frequently required. Counseling or professional support may be nonexistent or difficult to obtain. Younger siblings may react with hostility and guilt, older with shame and anger. Often the normal feedback of child growth that renders the turmoil of childrearing worthwhile develops more slowly or not at all. Family resources can be depleted (especially if medical care is needed), consumption patterns altered, or standards of living modified. Housing may have to be found closer to a hospital, and plans for further children changed. Finally, the anxieties, guilt, and grief present at birth may threaten to recur or become chronic.

Yet, although we must recognize the burdens and frustrations of raising a defective infant, it does not necessarily follow that these costs require nontreatment, or even institutionalization. Individual and group counseling can substantially alleviate anxiety, guilt, and frustration, and enable parents to cope with underlying conflicts triggered by the birth and the adaptations required. Counseling also can reduce psychological pressures on siblings, who can be taught to recognize and accept their own possibly hostile feelings and the difficult position of their parents. They may even be taught to help their parents care for the child.

The impact of increased financial costs also may vary. In families with high income or adequate health insurance, the financial costs are manageable. In others, state assistance may be available. If severe financial problems arise or pathological adjustments are likely, institutionalization, although undesirable for the child, remains an option. Finally, in many cases, the experience of living through a crisis is a deepening and enriching one, accelerating personality maturation, and giving one a new sensitivity to the needs of spouse, siblings, and others. As one parent of a defective child states: "In the last months I have come closer to people and can understand them more. I have met them more deeply. I did not know there were so many people with troubles in the world."[12]

Thus, while social attitudes regard the handicapped child as an unmitigated disaster, in reality the problem may not be insurmountable, and often may not differ from life's other vicissitudes. Suffering there is, but seldom is it so overwhelming or so imminent that the only alternative is death of the child.

Health Professionals Physicians and nurses also suffer when parents give birth to a defective child, although, of course, not to the degree of the parents. To the obstetrician or general practitioner the defective birth may be a blow to his professional identity. He has the difficult task of informing the parents of the defects, explaining their causes, and dealing with the parents' resulting emotional shock. Often he feels guilty for failing to produce a normal baby. In addition, the parents may project anger or hostility on the physician, questioning his professional competence or seeking the services of other doctors. The physician also may feel that his expertise and training are misused when employed to maintain the life of an infant whose chances for a productive existence are so diminished. By neglecting other patients, he may feel that he is prolonging rather than alleviating suffering.

Nurses, too, suffer role strain from care of the defective newborn. Intensive-care-unit nurses may work with only one or two babies at a time. They face the daily ordeals of care—the progress and relapses—and often must deal with anxious parents who are themselves grieving or ambivalent toward the child. The situation may trigger a nurse's own ambivalence about death and mothering, in a context in which she is actively working to keep alive a child whose life prospects seem minimal.

Thus, the effects of care on physicians and nurses are not trivial, and must be intelligently confronted in medical education or in management of a pediatric unit. Yet to state them is to make clear that they can but weigh lightly in the decision of whether to treat a defective newborn. Compared with the situation of the parents, these burdens seem insignificant, are short term, and most likely do not evoke such profound emotions. In any case, these difficulties are hazards of the profession—caring for the sick and dying will always produce strain. Hence, on these grounds alone it is difficult to argue that a defective person may be denied the right to life.

Society Care of the defective newborn also imposes societal costs, the utility of which is questioned when the infant's expected quality of life is so poor. Medical resources that can be used by infants with a better prognosis, or throughout the health-care system generally, are consumed in providing expensive surgical and intensive-care services to infants who may be severely retarded, never lead active lives, and die in a few months or years. Institutionalization imposes costs on taxpayers and reduces the resources available for those who might better benefit from it, while reducing further the quality of life experienced by the institutionalized defective.

One answer to these concerns is to question the impact of the costs of caring for defective newborns. Precise data showing the costs to taxpayers or the trade-offs with health and other expenditures do not exist. Nor would ceasing to care for the defective necessarily lead to a reallocation within the health budget that would produce net savings in suffering or life; in fact, the released resources might not be reallocated for health at all. In any case, the trade-

offs within the health budget may well be small. With advances in prenatal diagnosis of genetic disorders many deformed infants who would formerly require care will be aborted beforehand. Then, too, it is not clear that the most technical and expensive procedures always constitute the best treatment for certain malformations. When compared with the almost seven percent of the GNP now spent on health, the money in the defense budget, or tax revenues generally, the public resources required to keep defective newborns alive seem marginal, and arguably worth the commitment to life that such expenditures reinforce. Moreover, as the Supreme Court recently recognized,[13] conservation of the taxpayer's purse does not justify serious infringement of fundamental rights. Given legal and ethical norms against sacrificing the lives of nonconsenting others, and the imprecisions in diagnosis and prediction concerning the eventual outcomes of medical care, the social cost argument does not compel nontreatment of defective newborns. . . .

NOTES

1 Few persons would argue that "extraordinary" care must be provided a defective newborn, or indeed, to any person. The difficult question, however, is to distinguish "ordinary" from "extraordinary" care. . . . In this article "ordinary" care refers to those medical and surgical procedures that would normally be applied in situations not involving physically or mentally handicapped persons.

2 The need for ordinary treatment will also arise with noncentral nervous system malformations such as malformations of the cardiovascular, respiratory, orogastrointestinal, urogenital, muscular and skeletal systems, as well as deformities of the eye, ear, face, endocrine glands, and skin. *See generally* J. Warkany, CONGENITAL MALFORMATIONS (1971). Often these defects will accompany central nervous system malformations. The medical-ethical dilemma discussed in this article has arisen chiefly with regard to central nervous system problems, perhaps because the presence of such defects seriously affects intelligence, social interaction, and the potential for development and growth, and will be discussed only in the context of the major central nervous system malformations. Parents of physically deformed infants with normal intelligence might face the same choice, but because of the child's capacity for development, pressure to withhold ordinary treatment will be less severe.

3 Anencephaly is partial or total absence of the brain. J. Warkany, *supra* note 2, at 189–99.

4 Hydrocephaly is characterized by an increase of free fluid in the cranial cavity which results in a marked enlargement of the head. *Id.* at 217. It is a symptom of many diverse

disorders, and is associated with hereditary and chromo-somal syndromes. *Id.* at 217–18. Warkany describes the symptoms as follows: "Bulging of the forehead, protrusion of the parietal areas and extension of the occipital region are characteristic changes. . . . The skin of the scalp is thin and stretched and its veins are dilated. . . . The head cannot be held up, and walking and talking are delayed. The legs are spastic, the tendon reflexes increased and convulsions may occur. Anorexia, vomiting and emaciation complicate severe cases. As a rule, hydrocephalic children are dull and lethargic. Blindness can develop, but hearing and the auditory memory may be good. Physical and mental devel-opment depend on several factors, such as rapidity of onset, intracranial pressure, compensatory growth of the head, nature of the basic malformations and progress or arrest of the process. Such variability makes the prognosis and evalu-ation of therapeutic measures difficult. Pressure on the hypothalamic area can cause obesity or precocious puberty in exceptional cases." *Id.* at 226–27.

5 Down's syndrome or mongolism is a chromosomal disorder producing mental retardation caused by the presence of 47 rather than 46 chromosomes in a patient's cells, and marked by a distinctively shaped head, neck, trunk, and abdomen. *Id.* at 311–12, 324. For summary of clinical and pathological characteristics, *see id.* at 324–31.

6 Spina bifida refers generally to midline defects of the osseous spine. The defect usually appears in the posterior aspects of the vertebral canal, and may be marked by an external saccular protrusion (spina bifida cystica). *Id.* at 272. Spina bifida is often seriously involved with urinary tract deficiency, hydrocephaly, and may involve paralysis of the lower extremities. *Id.* at 286–88. While there are important differences between spina bifida, meningoceles, and

myelomeningocele, the terms will be used interchangeably in discussing and evaluating the duty to treat.

7 The saccular enlargements of spina bifida cystica protruding through osseous defects of the vertebral column that contain anomalous meninges and spinal fluid but do not have neural elements affixed to their walls are called meningoceles. If the spinal cord or nerves are included in the formation of the sac, the anomaly is called myelomeningocele. *Id.* at 272. As with spina bifida, myelomeningocele may substantially interfere with locomotion, sphincter and bladder control, and may be accompanied by kyphoscoliosis and hydrocephaly leading to mental retardation. For a description of symptoms and treatment alternatives, *see* Lorber, *Results of Treatment of Myelomeningocele,* 13 DEVELOP. MED. & CHILD NEUROL. 279–303 (1971).

8 The infant might suffer from duodenal atresia and need surgery to connect the stomach to the intestine; or need an appendectomy; or antibiotics to fight pneumonia; or suffer from Respirator Distress Syndrome and need breathing assistance. In some cases the question is whether to begin or continue feeding.

9 Smith & Smith, *Selection for Treatment in Spina Bifida Cystica,* 4 BRIT. MED. J. 189, 195 (1973).

10 Matson, *Surgical Treatment of Myelomeningocele,* 42 PEDIATRICS 225, 226 (1968).

11 Goodman, *Continuing Treatment of Parents with Congenitally Defective Infants,* SOCIAL WORK, Vol. 9, No. I, at 92 (1964).

12 *Quoted in* Johns, *Family Reactions to the Birth of a Child with a Congenital Abnormality,* 26 OBSTET. GYNECOL. SURVEY 635, 637 (1971).

13 *Memorial Hosp. v. Maricopa County,* 415 U.S. 250 (1974).

STANDARDS OF JUDGMENT FOR TREATMENT OF IMPERILED NEWBORNS

Members of The Hastings Center Research Project on the Care of Imperiled Newborns

In this brief excerpt from a much longer report, the project group members address the problem of selective nontreatment. They first reject two distinctive sanctity-of-life positions—"vitalism" and "the medical indications policy." They then endorse the use of quality-of-life standards, with the provision that quality must be measured by reference to the infant's own well-being and not in terms of social utility. In their view, two distinctive quality-of-life standards are relevant to the problem of selective nontreatment. In most cases, the relevant standard is the best interest of the infant, which would allow (and, in fact, mandate) nontreatment only when continued life would be worse for the infant than an early death. In some cases, however, the rel-evant standard is that of "relational potential," which would make treatment optional for an infant who lacks the potential for human relationships.

As parents and clinicians evaluate specific strategies for responding to uncertainty, it is essential to ask how they should determine whether treatment is *ethically right* for a particular infant. The ethical questions can only be resolved by establishing reasonable standards of judgment against which to measure strategies and procedures.

"SANCTITY OF LIFE" STANDARDS

Many critics of the practice of selective nontreatment argue that we must concentrate on the *sanctity* of life. But what does it mean to base our decisions on the sanctity of each child's life? Does it mean that caregivers may *never* forgo treatment, or that they may do so only for the most catastrophically afflicted newborns? Without further specification, the "sanctity of life" standard remains a vague slogan, rather than a meaningful guide to decisionmaking.

Vitalism The most extreme sanctity of life position would hold that "where there is life, there is hope," and that so long as a child continues to cling to life, he or she must be treated. According to this view, which we shall call "vitalism," the mere presence of a heartbeat, respiration, or brain activity is a compelling reason to sustain all efforts to save the child's life. Only the moment of death relieves caregivers of their duty to treat. An adherent of this vitalist philosophy would accordingly hold that, except in cases where the child has been declared dead, all withholding and withdrawal of treatment is ethically wrong.

This most extreme sanctity of life position has few advocates. Its major flaw is that it would insist upon aggressive treatments even for those children who are deemed to be in the process of dying. If responsible physicians have concluded that a particular child cannot be saved, that he will soon die, then it seems pointless and cruel to continue to treat the child with medical interventions that are by no means benign. By insisting on treatment even in such hopeless cases, the vitalist can justly be accused of worshipping an abstraction, "life," rather than focusing on the concrete good of the patient. As theologian Paul Ramsey has cogently argued, the

appropriate response to a dying patient is not the futile imposition of painful medical treatments, but rather kind and respectful *care* designed to ease the child's passing.

The Medical Indications Policy A more reasonable sanctity of life position has been proposed by Paul Ramsey and adopted (with some modifications) in various versions of the Department of Health and Human Services so-called "Baby Doe Rules." According to this standard, each child possesses equal dignity and intrinsic worth (i.e. "sanctity") and therefore no child should be denied life-sustaining medical treatments simply on the basis of his or her "handicap" or future quality of life. Such treatments must be provided to all infants, except (1) when the infant is judged to be in the process of dying, or (2) when the contemplated treatment is itself deemed to be "medically contraindicated." As Ramsey puts it, *treatments* may be compared in order to see which will be medically beneficial for a child, but abnormal *children* may not be compared with normal children in order to determine who shall live.

This policy is supported by two complementary ethical principles. First, the "nondiscrimination principle" states that children with impairments may not be selected for nontreatment solely on the basis of their "handicapping condition." If an otherwise normal child would receive a certain treatment—for example, surgery to repair an intestinal blockage—then a child with an abnormality must receive like treatment. Failure to do so discriminates unfairly against the child with impairments.

Second, the "medical benefit principle" states that caregivers are obliged to provide any and all treatments deemed, according to "reasonable medical judgment," to be "medically beneficial" to the patient. This means that if a certain medical or surgical procedure would be likely to bring about its intended result of avoiding infection or some other fatal consequence, then it must be provided to the child.

Although this medical indications policy was obviously well intended, insofar as it attempted to prevent instances of *unjust* discrimination against newborns with impairments, we believe that it is an overly rigid and inappropriate guide to decisionmaking. The first problem is that the nondiscrimina-

Reprinted with permission of the publisher from *Hastings Center Report*, vol. 17 (December 1987), pp. 13–16.

tion principle would have decisionmakers ignore, not just relatively mild handicaps of the sort encountered in most children with spina bifida and Down syndrome, but also impairments that are genuinely catastrophic.

Consider, for example, the child suffering from severe birth asphyxia who also happens to have a grave heart defect. Although surgeons would be willing to operate to fix the heart of an otherwise normal infant, the fact that this particular infant will never be sufficiently conscious to interact with his environment would appear to be a factor that the child's caretakers might permissibly take into consideration. Should the child be subjected to major and painful cardiac surgery only so that he might subsist in a permanently unconscious state? Even though treatment might be withheld from such a grievously afflicted infant "solely on the basis of his handicap," such a decision would in no way count as *unjust* discrimination precisely because the child's handicap is so severe that he can no longer meaningfully be compared to an "otherwise normal" infant.

The second problem with the medical indications policy lies in its "medical benefit" principle. Although this principle works well in many cases—for example, mild to moderate spina bifida—it does so because we think that the treatment confers a benefit, not merely upon the child's spine, but rather upon the whole child.

QUALITY OF LIFE STANDARDS

Although we conclude that quality of life judgments are ethically proper, and indeed inevitable, a great deal of care must be given to specifying why quality of life matters and what qualitative conditions might justify the denial of treatment. Merely invoking the phrase "quality of life" will get us no farther than invocations of the "sanctity of life."

The phrase "quality of life," as used in medical contexts, is ambiguous and frequently misunderstood. It is sometimes used to denote the social worth of an individual, the value that individual has for society. According to this interpretation, a person's quality of life is determined by utilitarian criteria, measured by balancing the burdens and benefits to others, especially family members. It is this meaning of the phrase that gives rise to the

greatest worries about undertreatment of newborns with impairments.

This interpretation of quality of life has been defended on the grounds that external circumstances are crucially important in the outlook for certain newborns and because of the increased stress families undergo in raising children with disabilities. Despite the recognition that these external factors play a role in parental attitudes toward treatment, the consensus of this report is that "quality of life" should refer to the present or future characteristics of the infant, judged by standards of the infant's own well-being and not in terms of social utility.

Another way of understanding "quality of life" is as measured against a norm of "acceptable" life. Yet it is often noted that what would not be acceptable to some people, for themselves, is clearly acceptable to others. A danger lies in drawing the line too high, thereby ruling as "unacceptable" the life of a person with multiple handicaps or with mild-to-moderate mental retardation. When quality of life assessments are made for newborns with impairments, caution must be exercised to avoid this pitfall.

An example of drawing the line of "acceptable" life too high is "the ability to work or marry," a factor cited by the British pediatrician, John Lorber. An example of a very low standard is permanent coma, a criterion appearing in the 1984 Child Abuse Amendments. This threshold is so low as to be non-controversial.

A subset of the quality of life standard and an alternative to a medical indications policy is the standard known as the "best interest of the child." Traditionally, this standard has been employed by courts in making child custody determinations and other decisions involving placement of an infant or child.

Unlike the medical indications policy, the "best interest" standard does incorporate quality of life considerations. This standard holds that infants should be treated with life-sustaining therapy except when (1) the infant is dying, (2) treatment is medically contraindicated (the two exceptions built into the medical indications policy), and (3) continued life would be worse for the infant than an early death. The third condition opens the door to quality of life considerations, but requires that such considerations be viewed from the infant's point of view.

That is, certain states of being, marked by severe and intractable pain and suffering, can be viewed as worse than death. Thus, according to the best interest standard, there is room to consider the possibility that an infant's best interest can lie in withholding or withdrawing medical treatments, resulting in death.

Care must be taken, however, not to employ a standard based on the sensibilities of unimpaired adults; for example, one in which adult decisionmakers judge, from their own perspective, that they would not want to live a life with mental or physical disabilities. An infant-centered quality of life standard should be as objective as possible, in an attempt to determine whether continued life would be a benefit, from the child's point of view. An impaired child does not have the luxury of comparing his life to a "normal" existence; for such a child, it is a question of life with impairments versus no life at all.

The greatest merit of the best interest standard lies precisely in its child-centeredness. This focus on the individual child will aid decisionmakers in avoiding the twin evils of overtreatment, sanctioned by the medical indications policy, and undertreatment, which might result from allowing negative consequences for the family or society to determine what treatment is appropriate for the infant.

Although we believe the best interest of the infant should remain the primary standard for decisionmaking on behalf of newborns with impairments, it has limits. In addition to the undeniable problem of vagueness, there is the further question of the applicability of this standard to some of the most troubling dilemmas in the neonatal nursery. As one critic has noted about the standard suggested in the President's Commission report, *Deciding to Forgo Life-Sustaining Treatment:*

> The fact that the child-based best-interest standard would mandate treatment even in the face of a prognosis bereft of any distinctly human potentiality reveals a feature of that standard that has so far gone unnoticed. In such extreme cases, the best-interest standard tends to view the absence of pain as the only morally relevant consideration. No matter that the infant is doomed to a life of very short duration, and lacks the capacity for any distinctively human development or activity; so long as the child does not experience any severe burdens, interpreted from her

point of view, the fact that she can anticipate no distinctly human benefits is of no moral consequence.

In an article published in 1974, Father Richard McCormick explained and defended a quality of life viewpoint that differs from the best interest standard. Noting that modern medicine can keep almost anyone alive, he posed the question: "Granted that we can easily save the life, what kind of life are we saving?" McCormick admits this is a quality of life judgment, and holds that we must face the possibility of answering this question when it arises.

McCormick's guideline is "the potential for human relationships associated with the infant's condition." Translated into the language of "best interests," an individual who lacks any present capacity or future potential for human relationships can be said to have no interests at all, except perhaps to be free from pain and discomfort.

Our conclusion is that there is a need for two different standards embodying relational potential considerations. The prevailing "best interest" notion presupposes that all infants have interests, but for some, the burdens of continued life can outweigh the benefits. The alternative "relational potential" standard focuses on the potential of the individual for human relationships, and presumes that some severely neurologically impaired children cannot be said to have interests to which a best interest standard might apply. In employing these two standards, decisionmakers should first determine whether the best interest standard applies to the case at hand. For the large majority of infants this standard is applicable, and should be used to determine whether life-sustaining treatment should be administered. However, if an infant is so severely neurologically impaired as to render the best interest standard inapplicable, then the alternative standard, lack of potential for human relationships, becomes the relevant criterion, placing decisionmaking within the realm of parental discretion.

When the best interest standard is applicable, because the infant's best interest can be determined, decisionmakers are obligated either to institute or to forgo life-sustaining treatment. In contrast, the relational potential standard is nonobligatory: it permits the withholding or withdrawing of therapy from infants who lack the potential for human relationships, but it does not require that treatment be forgone. Continued treatment would not benefit such infants, but neither would it harm them. An example might be an infant born with trisomy 13. Most such infants do not survive beyond the first year of life, are severely or profoundly mentally retarded, and have multiple malformations. Their chances of being able to experience human interactions are minimal. Unlike the best interest standard, which is infant-centered, the relational potential standard allows the interests of others—e.g., family or society—to weigh in the decision about whether to treat. . . .

ANNOTATED BIBLIOGRAPHY

Bernat, James L.: "A Defense of the Whole-Brain Concept of Death," *Hastings Center Report* 28 (March–April 1998), pp. 14–23. Bernat answers a collection of arguments directed against the whole-brain approach to the definition of death.

Cantor, Norman L.: "Twenty-Five Years After *Quinlan:* A Review of the Jurisprudence of Death and Dying," *Journal of Law, Medicine & Ethics* 29 (Summer 2001), pp. 182–196. In the first part of this wide-ranging review article, Cantor clarifies the options that are legally available to a competent patient vis-à-vis the dying process. In the second part, he clarifies the end-of-life options legally available to surrogates acting on behalf of formerly competent patients.

Caplan, Arthur L., Robert H. Blank, and Janna C. Merrick, eds.: *Compelling Compassion: Government Intervention in the Treatment of Critically Ill Newborns* (Totowa, NJ: Humana Press, 1992). This book provides an extensive collection of material on the federal "Baby Doe" legislation.

Celesia, Gastone G.: "Persistent Vegetative State: Clinical and Ethical Issues," *Theoretical Medicine* 18 (1997), pp. 221–236. Celesia clarifies the clinical diagnosis of persistent vegetative state (PVS) and identifies relevant factors in predicting outcomes for PVS patients. He also distinguishes five subgroups of PVS patients and makes suggestions about the level of treatment appropriate for members of each subgroup.

DeGrazia, David: "Persons, Organisms, and Death: A Philosophical Critique of the Higher-Brain Approach," *Southern Journal of Philosophy* 37 (1999), pp. 419–440. Endorsing an "organismic" definition of death, DeGrazia counters various philosophical arguments that have been advanced in support of a higher-brain approach.

Dresser, Rebecca S., and John A. Robertson: "Quality of Life and Non-Treatment Decisions for Incompetent Patients: A Critique of the Orthodox Approach," *Law, Medicine & Health Care* 17 (Fall 1989), pp. 234–244. The authors argue against the orthodox approach to surrogate decision making, which emphasizes the desirability of advance directives and the priority of the substituted-judgment standard. Their principal complaint is that the orthodox approach allows an incompetent patient's past wishes to take priority over his or her present interests.

Fagerlin, Angela, and Carl E. Schneider: "Enough: The Failure of the Living Will," *Hastings Center Report* 34 (March–April 2004), pp. 30–42. Drawing extensively on empirical studies, Fagerlin and Schneider argue that policies designed to promote living wills are indefensible. They believe that several insoluble problems confront living wills.

Guidelines on the Termination of Life-Sustaining Treatment and the Care of the Dying: A Report by the Hastings Center (Bloomington: Indiana University Press, 1988). This document presents general guidelines on the decision-making process and other guidelines relevant to specific treatment modalities. Also included are guidelines on advance directives and the declaration of death.

Journal of the American Geriatrics Society 42 (August 1994). This issue features a collection of articles under the heading "Futility in Clinical Practice." Various aspects of the contemporary debate over medical futility are explored.

King, Nancy M. P.: *Making Sense of Advance Directives,* rev. ed. (Washington, DC: Georgetown University Press, 1996). In this useful book, King provides a comprehensive discussion of advance directives and the many issues associated with them.

Lynn, Joanne, ed.: *By No Extraordinary Means: The Choice to Forgo Life-Sustaining Food and Water* (Bloomington: Indiana University Press, 1986). This anthology provides a wide range of material on the issue of forgoing artificial nutrition and hydration.

Olick, Robert S.: *Taking Advance Directives Seriously: Prospective Autonomy and Decisions Near the End of Life* (Washington, DC: Georgetown University Press, 2001). Olick considers a number of challenges to advance directives and constructs an overall defense of their moral and legal weight.

Paris, John J., Jeffrey Ferranti, and Frank Reardon: "From the Johns Hopkins Baby to Baby Miller: What Have We Learned from Four Decades of Reflection on Neonatal Cases?" *Journal of Clinical Ethics* 12 (Fall 2001), pp. 207–214. The authors provide commentary on a series of prominent cases involving nontreatment decisions for severely impaired infants.

President's Commission for the Study of Ethical Problems in Medicine and Biomedical and Behavioral Research: *Deciding to Forego Life-Sustaining Treatment* (1983). Chapter 4 of this valuable document provides material on the determination of incapacity (incompetence), surrogate decision making, and advance directives. Chapter 5 deals with patients who have permanently lost consciousness but are not "brain-dead." Chapter 6 considers seriously ill newborns, and Chapter 7 is concerned with resuscitation decisions.

———: *Defining Death* (1981). In this document, the commission provides an overall account of its deliberations leading to the recommendation that the Uniform Determination of Death Act be adopted in all states.

Schneiderman, Lawrence J., Nancy S. Jecker, and Albert R. Jonsen: "Medical Futility: Its Meaning and Ethical Implications," *Annals of Internal Medicine* 112 (June 15, 1990), pp. 949–954. The authors distinguish between a quantitative and a qualitative sense of futility, and they assign an operational meaning to each sense. In a subsequent article—"Medical Futility: Response to Critiques," *Annals of Internal Medicine* 125 (October 15, 1996), pp. 669–674—the authors clarify and modify their original proposal and respond to several lines of criticism.

Stone, Jim: "Advance Directives, Autonomy and Unintended Death," *Bioethics* 8 (July 1994), pp. 223–246. Stone argues that living wills are typically confused and dangerous documents: Not only do they often fail to culminate in the avoidance of unwanted medical treatments, but they also create a substantial risk that patients' lives will be ended in ways that were never intended. He also argues that health-care professionals often fail to distinguish living wills from DNR orders.

Veatch, Robert M.: "The Impending Collapse of the Whole-Brain Definition of Death," *Hastings Center Report* 23 (July-August 1993), pp. 18–24. Favoring a higher-brain approach to the definition of death, Veatch presents objections to the whole-brain approach and responds to a set of arguments commonly made against the higher-brain approach. He also argues for the incorporation of a "conscience clause" in definition-of-death statutes.

Weir, Robert F.: *Selective Nontreatment of Handicapped Newborns: Moral Dilemmas in Neonatal Medicine* (New York: Oxford University Press, 1984). Weir surveys and critically analyzes a wide range of views (advanced by various pediatricians, attorneys, and ethicists) on the subject of selective nontreatment. He then presents and defends on overall policy for the guidance of decision making in this area.

Youngner, Stuart J.: "Do-Not-Resuscitate Orders: No Longer Secret, but Still a Problem," *Hastings Center Report* 17 (February 1987), pp. 24–33. Youngner argues for the importance of (1) the improved documentation and specification of DNR orders; (2) the involvement of patient, family, and staff (including nurses) in DNR decisions; and (3) the regular (at least daily) review of a patient's DNR status. He also insists that DNR status does not entail medical or psychological abandonment.

Youngner, Stuart J., Robert M. Arnold, and Renie Schapiro, eds.: *The Definition of Death: Contemporary Controversies* (Baltimore, MD: Johns Hopkins University Press, 1999). The articles in this useful collection address a wide range of issues associated with the definition and determination of death.

CHAPTER 6

SUICIDE, PHYSICIAN-ASSISTED SUICIDE, AND ACTIVE EUTHANASIA

INTRODUCTION

The mercy killing of patients, whether called "active euthanasia" (as it is here) or simply "euthanasia," is a topic of long-standing controversy in biomedical ethics. Can active euthanasia—especially in response to the request of a competent patient—be morally justified? Should it be legalized? Parallel questions can be raised about physician-assisted suicide, a closely related topic that has also generated intense discussion. This chapter is designed in large part to deal with ethical questions about active euthanasia and physician-assisted suicide. Its point of departure, however, is a consideration of the morality of suicide, an issue whose relevance is not restricted to a medical context.

WHAT IS SUICIDE?

Clarity in discussions of the morality of suicide can be greatly enhanced by paying some attention to the concept of suicide. Consider two people, one saying that suicide is always immoral and the other saying that suicide is sometimes morally acceptable. It is possible that these two people are in substantive moral agreement and differ only with regard to an operating definition of *suicide*. One of them may hold that suicide is systematically immoral but say that a certain action is not suicide and is therefore morally acceptable, whereas the other may consider the same action suicide but consider it a morally acceptable form of suicide. The following cases and the accompanying analysis are presented in order to shed some measure of light on the concept of suicide.

(1) A woman, having despaired of achieving a satisfying life, leaps to her death from the top of a city skyscraper. (2) An elderly man dies from a massive overdose of sleeping pills, leaving behind a note explaining that he is not bitter but that life seems to have passed him by. He has outlived his friends, he has no employment, he finds no enjoyment in his pastimes, and so forth. Both of these cases provide us with clear instances of suicide. In accordance with what might be called the standard definition of *suicide,* each of these cases is a suicide precisely because it features the *intentional termination of one's own life.* Consider a third case. (3) In time of war, a soldier is captured and subjected to torture. Feeling unable to resist any longer, but determined not to yield any information that would endanger the lives of his comrades, he hangs himself. This third case is noteworthy, in contrast to the first two, in that it features an other-directed rather than a self-directed motivation. Still, it seems to be a clear case of the intentional termination of one's own life. It is sometimes said that the self-killing in such cases is sacrificial rather than suicidal, but to deny that case 3 is a case of suicide is surely to abandon the standard definition of the term.

(4) A truck driver, foreseeing his own death, nevertheless steers his runaway truck into a concrete abutment to avoid hitting a schoolbus that has stopped on the roadway to discharge children. (5) In a somewhat similar and much discussed actual case, a certain Captain Oates fell ill and found himself physically unable to continue on with a party of explorers in the Antarctic. The explorers were struggling to find their way out of a blizzard. Captain Oates, determined to avoid further endangering his colleagues by hindering their progress, but unable to convince them to leave him to die, simply walked off to meet his death in the blizzard. One may feel some puzzlement as to whether cases 4 and 5 are to be identified as cases of suicide. As in case 3, the notion of sacrificial death may come to mind. Presumably, neither the truck driver nor Captain Oates wanted to die; each sacrificed his own life so that the lives of others might be protected. In contrast to case 3, however, it is plausible to say, in accordance with the standard definition, that cases 4 and 5 are not cases of suicide. In this view, it would be said that neither the truck driver nor Captain Oates *intentionally terminated* his life. While each initiated a chain of events that was foreseen as leading to his own death, neither initiated the chain of events because he desired to die; quite the contrary, he desired to attain some other objective—that is, the protection of others. Thus, the primary intention of the basic action (redirecting the truck, walking away from camp) was to protect others; one's own death, it is said, is foreseen but not intended.[1] Still, many would insist, contrary to the line of thought just developed, that both the truck driver and Captain Oates did intentionally terminate their lives. It was in their power to avoid their deaths, but they chose, seemingly in noble fashion, not to do so.

Consider one final case. (6) A Jehovah's Witness, as a matter of religious principle, refuses to consent to a blood transfusion and dies. Is this a case of suicide? This judgment turns, as does our judgment regarding cases 4 and 5, on the interpretation of the phrase *intentional termination.* The Jehovah's Witness, in many ways similar to the traditional Christian martyr, refuses to sacrifice religious principle and thereby brings about his or her own death. Those who say that case 6 is not a case of suicide point out that the Jehovah's Witness typically does not want to die. The Jehovah's Witness foresees but does not intend his or her own death. Those who say that case 6 is a case of suicide point out that, in effect, the avoidance of death is within the power of the Jehovah's Witness. Thus, in their view, choosing to refuse the blood transfusion constitutes an intentional termination of life.

Notice that, in certain circumstances, the refusal of life-sustaining treatment is undeniably suicide. Suppose a person in good health is accidentally injured and needs a routine surgical procedure in order to live (and fully recover). Suppose further that this person refuses medical intervention simply because he or she wants to die. In such a case, refusing life-sustaining treatment is simply a convenient way of committing suicide. The phrase *intentional termination,* however it is to be finally analyzed, clearly incorporates passive as well as active means. A person can commit suicide just as effectively by (passively) refusing to eat as by (actively) taking an overdose of drugs.

Ordinarily, the refusal of life-sustaining treatment by a terminally ill patient is not considered suicide—at least if the patient's death is reasonably imminent. Perhaps this is the case because the refusal of life-sustaining treatment in such cases is so naturally understood as a decision not to extend the dying process. On the other hand, consider a patient (not terminally ill) who is dissatisfied with the quality of life that has resulted from some incurable medical condition (e.g., paralysis) and refuses life-sustaining treatment for a treatable medical condition (e.g., pneumonia) that happens to arise. Is this not suicide?[2]

THE MORALITY OF SUICIDE

Under what conditions, if at all, is suicide morally acceptable? Classical literature on the morality of suicide provides a number of sources who issue a strong moral condemnation of suicide. St. Augustine, St. Thomas Aquinas, and Immanuel Kant are prominent examples. Augustine's arguments are dominantly theological in character, but Aquinas and Kant advance philosophical as well as religiously based arguments against suicide. According to Aquinas, suicide is to be condemned, not only because it violates our duty to God but also because it violates the natural law and, moreover, because it injures the community. Kant, in the first selection of this chapter, argues that suicide degrades human worth and is therefore always immoral. R. B. Brandt, in a very different vein, critically analyzes the most influential of the classical arguments against suicide and vigorously defends the view that suicide is not always immoral. This more liberal viewpoint, it is important to note, is not unprecedented in the classical literature on suicide. The Roman Stoic Seneca and the eighteenth-century Scottish philosopher David Hume are quite notable in their articulation and defense of such a view.

The more liberal view on the morality of suicide might be explicated in general terms as follows. Suicide is morally acceptable to the extent that it does no substantial damage to the interests of other individuals. Moreover, even in cases where suicide has some significant negative impact on others, no person is morally obliged to undergo extreme distress to prevent others from undergoing some smaller measure of discomfort, sadness, and so forth.

In his discussion, Brandt considers not only the morality of suicide but also the rationality of suicide. It is sometimes asserted that a suicidal intention is necessarily irrational and thus a symptom of mental illness and incompetence. In other words, it is impossible for a competent adult to have a suicidal intention. Although this point seems to be built into some psychiatric theories, many philosophers—and, today, many psychiatrists as well—consider it an implausible contention. Brandt, in particular, insists that suicide can be a rational choice, although he warns of the distorting effects that depression can exercise over human judgment.

THE MORALITY OF ACTIVE EUTHANASIA

There is both a narrow and a broad sense of *euthanasia.* The difference between the two is best understood by reference to the categories of killing and allowing to die, although the distinction between killing and allowing to die is itself a controversial one. Understood in the narrow sense, the category of euthanasia is limited to mercy *killing*. Thus, if a physician believes a terminally ill patient is better off dead and for that reason (mercifully) administers a lethal dose of a drug to the patient, this act is a paradigm of euthanasia. On the other hand, if a physician *allows a patient to die* (e.g., by withholding or withdrawing a respirator), this does not count as euthanasia. Although the narrow sense of euthanasia is becoming increasingly common, many writers still use the word *euthanasia* in the broad sense. Understood in the broad sense, the category of euthanasia encompasses both killing and allowing to die (on grounds of mercy). Of course, the underlying assumption in conceptualizing the withholding or withdrawal of treatment under the heading of euthanasia is that the physician withholds or withdraws life-sustaining treatment (mercifully) for the precise purpose of bringing about the patient's death. Those who use the broad sense of euthanasia typically distinguish between *active* euthanasia (i.e., killing) and *passive* euthanasia (i.e., allowing to die).

One other distinction is of central importance in discussions of euthanasia. *Voluntary* euthanasia proceeds in response to the (informed) request of a competent patient. *Nonvoluntary* euthanasia involves an individual who is incompetent to give consent. The possibility of nonvoluntary euthanasia might arise with regard to adults who have for any number of reasons (e.g., Alzheimer's disease) lost their decision-making capacity, and it might arise with regard to newborn infants or children. Both voluntary and nonvoluntary euthanasia may be further distinguished from *involuntary* euthanasia, which entails acting against the will or, at any rate, without the permission of a competent person. It is important to note, however, that some writers in biomedical ethics use the phrase *involuntary euthanasia* in referring to what has been identified here as nonvoluntary euthanasia.

If the voluntary/nonvoluntary distinction is combined with the active/passive distinction, four types of euthanasia can be distinguished: (1) voluntary active euthanasia, (2) nonvoluntary active euthanasia, (3) voluntary passive euthanasia, and (4) nonvoluntary passive euthanasia. Contemporary debate, however, focuses on the moral legitimacy of active euthanasia, especially voluntary active euthanasia. There is far less controversy about the moral legitimacy of passive euthanasia, whether voluntary or nonvoluntary. At any rate, the idea that it can be morally appropriate to withhold or withdraw life-sustaining treatment is firmly established, at least in the United States. This is not to say, of course, that there are no issues related to the specific conditions that must be satisfied in order for the withholding or withdrawal of life-sustaining treatment to be morally appropriate. (See Chapter 5 in this regard.)

James Rachels argues, in this chapter, for the moral legitimacy of active euthanasia. One of his central claims is that there is no morally significant distinction between killing and allowing to die. Daniel Callahan, by way of contrast, defends the coherence and moral importance of the distinction between killing and allowing to die. Callahan is opposed to active euthanasia and argues that killing patients is incompatible with the role of the physician in society. In his view, the power of the physician must be used "only to cure or comfort, never to kill." Dan W. Brock, in turn, rejects the idea that active euthanasia is incompatible with the fundamental professional commitments of a physician. Furthermore, in stating a case for the moral legitimacy of voluntary active euthanasia, Brock appeals to the centrality of two fundamental values—patient autonomy and patient well-being.

Those, like Rachels, who argue for the moral legitimacy of active euthanasia usually emphasize considerations of humaneness. When the intent is to provide an overall defense of voluntary active euthanasia, the humanitarian appeal is typically conjoined with an appeal to the primacy of individual autonomy. Thus, the overall case for the moral legitimacy of voluntary active euthanasia incorporates two basic arguments: (1) It is cruel and inhumane to refuse the plea of a terminally ill person for his or her life to be mercifully ended in order to avoid future suffering and/or indignity. (2) Autonomous choice should be respected to the extent that it does not result in harm to others. Since no one is harmed—at least in typical cases—by terminally ill patients' undergoing active euthanasia, a decision to have one's life ended in this fashion should be respected.

Those who argue against the moral legitimacy of active euthanasia typically rest their case on one or all of the following claims: (1) Killing an innocent person is inherently wrong. (2) Killing is incompatible with the professional responsibilities of the physician. (3) Any systematic acceptance of active euthanasia would lead to detrimental social consequences (e.g., via a lessening of respect for human life). This third line of argument is the one that is typically most emphasized in discussions concerning the legalization of active euthanasia.

PHYSICIAN-ASSISTED SUICIDE

Arguments for and against the moral legitimacy of physician-assisted suicide largely parallel the standard arguments for and against the moral legitimacy of voluntary active euthanasia, and one might wonder if there is a morally significant difference between these two practices. Physician-assisted suicide typically involves a physician in one or both of the following roles: (1) providing *information* to a patient about how to commit suicide in an effective manner and (2) providing the *means* necessary for an effective suicide (most commonly, by writing a prescription for a lethal amount of medication). Other modes of physician assistance in suicide might include providing moral support for the patient's decision, "supervising" the actual suicide, and helping the patient carry out the necessary physical actions. For example, a very frail patient might need a certain amount of physical assistance just to take pills.

In both physician-assisted suicide and voluntary active euthanasia, a physician plays an active role in bringing about the death of a patient. However, at face value, there is a difference between the two: In voluntary active euthanasia the physician ultimately kills the patient, whereas in physician-assisted suicide the patient ultimately kills himself or herself, albeit with the assistance of the physician. It is a controversial issue whether this difference in terms of ultimate causal agency can serve as a basis for the claim that there is a morally significant difference between physician-assisted suicide and voluntary active euthanasia.

An important development in the public debate over physician-assisted suicide took place in 1997, when the U.S. Supreme Court unanimously upheld the constitutionality of state statutes prohibiting physician-assisted suicide. In *Washington v. Glucksberg,* the Court rejected the claim that the Due Process Clause of the Fourteenth Amendment encompasses a fundamental right to physician-assisted suicide. In the companion case *Vacco v. Quill,* the Court rejected the claim that the Equal Protection Clause of the Fourteenth Amendment is violated by a state prohibiting physician-assisted suicide while at the same time permitting the withdrawal of life-sustaining treatment. In resolving this second case, the Court explicitly committed itself to the legitimacy and importance of drawing a distinction between assisting suicide and withdrawing life-sustaining treatment.

Each of the physician-assisted suicide cases was decided by a 9–0 vote, but the Court is not nearly so unified on the construction of the underlying issues as these unanimous votes might suggest. The Court's underlying fragmentation of viewpoint is reflected in a host of concurring opinions generated by the cases. Chief Justice William H. Rehnquist wrote the "Opinion of the Court" in each of the cases, but only four other justices actually concurred in these opinions, and one of these four, Justice Sandra Day O'Connor, also crafted a concurring opinion. Both of Chief Justice Rehnquist's opinions are reprinted in this chapter, as is the concurring opinion of Justice O'Connor. In another of this chapter's selections, David Orentlicher provides a commentary on the Supreme Court opinions on physician-assisted suicide. Orentlicher's analysis focuses on the Court's endorsement of the practice of *terminal sedation.*

The idea of terminal sedation naturally arises in those (presumably few) cases in which the severe pain or suffering of a terminally ill patient is resistant to established palliative techniques and can be alleviated only by *sedation into unconsciousness.* A frequent concomitant of terminal sedation, as actually practiced, is the withholding of nutrition and hydration. Thus, a patient who undergoes terminal sedation eventually dies either (1) as a result of the underlying disease or (2) from dehydration or starvation. Discussions of the ethics of terminal sedation frequently involve reference to the so-called Principle of Double Effect.[3] In accordance with this complex principle, a physician may never *intend* the death of a patient but may sometimes perform actions that *foreseeably* result in death. The principle is frequently cited as the underlying justification for providing a terminally ill patient with an adequate level of pain medication, even if the amount necessary to relieve pain is likely to hasten the patient's death (e.g., by depressing respiration).[4] In such a case, it is said, death can be understood as a foreseen but unintended consequence of providing the pain medication. Of course, those who are sympathetic to the tradition bound up with the Principle of Double Effect ordinarily reject physician-assisted suicide and active euthanasia on the grounds that these practices necessarily involve a physician in the intentional termination of a patient's life. But terminal sedation, it can be argued, is a morally acceptable practice precisely because the physician in sedating the patient to unconsciousness need intend only the relief of suffering, not the death of the patient. Orentlicher points out, however, that the Principle of Double Effect can justify only the sedation itself, not the withholding of nutrition and hydration.

PHYSICIAN-ASSISTED SUICIDE, ACTIVE EUTHANASIA, AND SOCIAL POLICY

Should active euthanasia be legalized? If so, in what form or forms and with what safeguards? Although active euthanasia is presently illegal in all 50 states and the District of Columbia, proposals for its legalization have been recurrently advanced. Most commonly, those proposals call for the legalization of *voluntary* active euthanasia.

There are some who consider active euthanasia in any form intrinsically immoral (sometimes on overtly religious grounds) and, for this reason, oppose the legalization of voluntary active euthanasia. Others are opposed to legalization because of their conviction that physicians in particular should not kill. Still others do not necessarily object to individual acts of voluntary active euthanasia but nevertheless stand opposed to any social policy that would permit its practice. The concern here is with the adverse social consequences of legalization. In this vein, it is alleged that vulnerable persons would be subject to abuse, that a disincentive for the availability of supportive services for the dying would be created, and that public trust and confidence in physicians would be undermined. Another consequentialist concern is embodied in a frequently made "slippery-slope" argument: the legalization of voluntary active euthanasia would lead us down a slippery slope to the legalization of nonvoluntary (and perhaps involuntary) euthanasia. Those who support the legalization of voluntary active euthanasia recognize that some unfortunate consequences may result from legalization. However, they typically seek to establish that potential dangers are either overstated or can be minimized with appropriate safeguards.

Although arguments advanced against the legalization of physician-assisted suicide largely parallel those advanced against the legalization of voluntary active euthanasia, it is frequently argued that there is far less risk of abuse involved in the legalization of physician-assisted suicide. This point of view is embraced by Timothy E. Quill, Christine K. Cassel, and Diane E. Meier in one of this chapter's readings. In this particular reading, the three physicians recommend the legalization of physician-assisted suicide in accordance with a set of conditions they present.

A concrete model for the legalization of physician-assisted suicide has emerged in Oregon, where physician-assisted suicide is now legal. In November 1994, voters in Oregon approved by a margin of 51 to 49 percent a ballot initiative known as the Oregon Death with Dignity Act. This law survived constitutional challenges and ultimately went into effect on October 27, 1997; it also survived a second referendum in November 1997 in which Oregon voters opposed repeal by a margin of 60 to 40 percent. The law permits physicians in Oregon to prescribe lethal drugs for competent, terminally ill adult patients who want to end their own lives. One of the most important and distinctive features of the Oregon model is a mandatory "waiting period." In Oregon, a physician cannot provide a patient with a prescription for a lethal dose of medication until 15 days after the patient's initial request. The Oregon Death with Dignity Act is reprinted in this chapter in the form originally approved by Oregon voters.[5]

Consider, for a moment, some of the issues that might arise in specifying appropriate limits for the practice of physician-assisted suicide and/or voluntary active euthanasia. Would we want to restrict availability to patients who are terminally ill (according to some definition), to patients who are experiencing unbearable suffering (according to some definition), or to patients who are *both* terminally ill and experiencing unbearable suffering?[6] And if voluntary active euthanasia is at issue, would we want to insist that a patient be competent at the time he or she undergoes active euthanasia, or would we also want to allow for the possibility of active euthanasia in accordance with an advance directive?

Voluntary active euthanasia is a well-established practice in The Netherlands (see Appendix, Case 32). One of the interesting aspects of the Dutch system is its requirement that active euthanasia be available only if the patient is experiencing unbearable suffering (with no prospect of improvement), but there is no requirement that the patient be terminally ill. Another interesting feature of the Dutch system is its explicit acceptance of an advance-directive principle. That is, active euthanasia may be provided for patients who have become incompetent but who had clearly expressed their request for active euthanasia in a written declaration while competent.

In one of this chapter's readings, Franklin G. Miller et al. call for the legalization of both voluntary active euthanasia and physician-assisted suicide in accordance with a suggested regulatory scheme.[7] John Arras, in turn, argues strongly against the legalization of any form of physician-assisted death, a category that includes both voluntary active euthanasia and physician-assisted suicide. Arras's opposition to legalization is based on the strong likelihood of detrimental social consequences, especially a negative impact on vulnerable patients; in this regard he develops a two-pronged slippery-slope argument. According to another important point of view, since terminally ill patients are already free to refuse hydration and nutrition and thereby bring about death, there is no compelling need to legalize either voluntary active euthanasia or physician-assisted suicide. James L. Bernat, Bernard Gert, and R. Peter Mogielnicki give articulate voice to this viewpoint in the final reading of this chapter.

T.A.M.

NOTES

1 The phrase "foreseen but not intended" derives from application of the Principle of Double Effect. This principle is explicitly discussed later in this Introduction.
2 See the Chapter 6 reading by Vicki Michel, "Suicide by Persons with Disabilities Disguised as the Refusal of Life-Sustaining Treatment."
3 For one useful articulation and critique of the Principle of Double Effect, see Timothy E. Quill, Rebecca Dresser, and Dan W. Brock, "The Rule of Double Effect—a Critique of Its Role in End-of-Life Decision Making," *New England Journal of Medicine* 337 (December 11, 1997), pp. 1768–1771.
4 Some commentators refer to the practice at issue here as *double-effect euthanasia.*
5 Further clarifications and small changes have subsequently been introduced in the language of the Oregon Death with Dignity Act. Current language can be accessed under "Legislative Statute" on the Oregon Department of Human Services home page (http://www.dhs.state.or.us/publichealth/chs/pas/pas.cfm). Also available on this site are annual statistical reports about the provision of physician-assisted suicide in Oregon. In 2003, 42 patients in Oregon used physician-assisted suicide to end their lives, compared to 38 who did so in 2002. On average, there are 31,000 deaths each year in Oregon.
6 For an argument to restrict availability (at least at the present time) to those who are terminally ill, see Martin Gunderson and David J. Mayo, "Restricting Physician-Assisted Death to the Terminally Ill," *Hastings Center Report* 30 (November–December 2000), pp. 17–23.
7 Miller's coauthors in this 1994 piece include Quill and Meier, whose views can be seen to have evolved from their 1992 article with Cassel. In this earlier article, Quill and Meier endorse the legalization of physician-assisted suicide but reject the legalization of voluntary active euthanasia.

THE MORALITY OF SUICIDE

SUICIDE

Immanuel Kant

Kant issues a blanket moral condemnation of suicide: "Suicide is in no circumstances permissible." In his view, suicide is characterized by the intention to destroy oneself. Thus, neither the "victim of fate" nor the person whose intemperance leads to a shortened life is guilty of suicide. Kant insists that suicide is self-contradictory, in the sense that the power of free will is used for its own destruction. In a related consideration, suicide is said to be a moral abomination because it degrades human worth. Kant also claims that suicide is rightly condemned on religious grounds.

DUTIES TOWARDS THE BODY IN REGARD TO LIFE

What are our powers of disposal over our life? Have we any authority of disposal over it in any shape or form? How far is it incumbent upon us to take care of it? These are questions which fall to be considered in connexion with our duties towards the body in regard to life. We must, however, by way of introduction, make the following observations. If the body were related to life not as a condition but as an accident or circumstance so that we could at will divest ourselves of it; if we could slip out of it and slip into another just as we leave one country for another, then the body would be subject to our free will and we could rightly have the disposal of it. This, however, would not imply that we could similarly dispose of our life, but only of our circumstances, of the movable goods, the furniture of life. In fact, however, our life is entirely conditioned by our body, so that we cannot conceive of a life not mediated by the body and we cannot make use of our freedom except through the body. It is, therefore, obvious that the body constitutes a part of ourselves. If a man destroys his body, and so his life, he does it by the use of his will, which is itself destroyed in the process. But to use the power of a free will for its own destruction is self-contradictory. If freedom is the condition of life it cannot be employed to abolish life and so to destroy and abolish itself. To use life for its own destruction, to use life for producing lifelessness, is self-contradictory. These preliminary remarks are sufficient to show that man cannot rightly have any power of disposal in regard to himself and his life, but only in regard to his circumstances. His body gives man power over his life; were he a spirit he could not destroy his life; life in the absolute has been invested by nature with indestructibility and is an end in itself; hence it follows that man cannot have the power to dispose of his life.

From Immanuel Kant, *Lectures on Ethics,* translated by Louis Infield (New York: Harper & Row, 1963), pp. 147–154. Reprinted by permission of Taylor & Francis Books Ltd.

SUICIDE

Suicide can be regarded in various lights; it might be held to be reprehensible, or permissible, or even heroic. In the first place we have the specious view that suicide can be allowed and tolerated. Its advocates argue thus. So long as he does not violate the proprietary rights of others, man is a free agent. With regard to his body there are various things he can properly do; he can have a boil lanced or a limb amputated, and disregard a scar; he is, in fact, free to do whatever he may consider useful and advisable. If then he comes to the conclusion that the most useful and advisable thing that he can do is to put an end to his life, why should he not be entitled to do so? Why not, if he sees that he can no longer go on living and that he will be ridding himself of misfortune, torment and disgrace? To be sure he robs himself of a full life, but he escapes once and for all from calamity and misfortune. The argument sounds most plausible. But let us, leaving aside religious considerations, examine the act itself. We may treat our body as we please, provided our motives are those of self-preservation. If, for instance, his foot is a hindrance to life, a man might have it amputated. To preserve his person he has the right of disposal over his body. But in taking his life he does not preserve his person; he disposes of his person and not of its attendant circumstances; he robs himself of his person. This is contrary to the highest duty we have towards ourselves, for it annuls the condition of all other duties; it goes beyond the limits of the use of free will, for this use is possible only through the existence of the Subject.

There is another set of considerations which make suicide seem plausible. A man might find himself so placed that he can continue living only under circumstances which deprive life of all value; in which he can no longer live conformably to virtue and prudence, so that he must from noble motives put an end to his life. The advocates of this view quote in support of it the example of Cato. Cato knew that the entire Roman nation relied upon him in their resistance to Caesar, but he found that he could not prevent himself from falling into Caesar's hands. What was he to do? If he, the champion of freedom, submitted, every one would say, "If Cato himself submits, what else can we do?" If, on the other hand, he killed himself, his death might spur on the Romans to fight to the bitter end in defence of their freedom. So he killed himself. He thought that it was necessary for him to die. He thought that if he could not go on living as Cato, he could not go on living at all. It must certainly be admitted that in a case such as this, where suicide is a virtue, appearances are in its favour. But this is the only example which has given the world the opportunity of defending suicide. It is the only example of its kind and there has been no similar case since. Lucretia also killed herself, but on grounds of modesty and in a fury of vengeance. It is obviously our duty to preserve our honour, particularly in relation to the opposite sex, for whom it is a merit; but we must endeavour to save our honour only to this extent, that we ought not to surrender it for selfish and lustful purposes. To do what Lucretia did is to adopt a remedy which is not at our disposal; it would have been better had she defended her honour unto death; that would not have been suicide and would have been right; for it is no suicide to risk one's life against one's enemies, and even to sacrifice it, in order to observe one's duties towards oneself.

No one under the sun can bind me to commit suicide; no sovereign can do so. The sovereign can call upon his subjects to fight to the death for their country, and those who fall on the field of battle are not suicides, but the victims of fate. Not only is this not suicide, but the opposite; a faint heart and fear of the death which threatens by the necessity of fate, is no true self-preservation; for he who runs away to save his own life, and leaves his comrades in the lurch, is a coward; but he who defends himself and his fellows even unto death is no suicide, but noble and high-minded; for life is not to be highly regarded for its own sake. I should endeavor to preserve my own life only so far as I am worthy to live. We must draw a distinction between the suicide and the victim of fate. A man who shortens his life by intemperance is guilty of imprudence and indirectly of his own death; but his guilt is not direct; he did not intend to kill himself; his death was not premeditated. For all our offences are either *culpa* or *dolus*. There is certainly no *dolus* here, but there is *culpa;* and we

can say of such a man that he was guilty of his own death, but we cannot say of him that he is a suicide. What constitutes suicide is the intention to destroy oneself. Intemperance and excess which shorten life ought not, therefore, to be called suicide; for if we raise intemperance to the level of suicide, we lower suicide to the level of intemperance. Imprudence, which does not imply a desire to cease to live, must, therefore, be distinguished from the intention to murder oneself. Serious violations of our duty towards ourselves produce an aversion accompanied either by horror or by disgust; suicide is of the horrible kind, *crimina carnis* of the disgusting. We shrink in horror from suicide because all nature seeks its own preservation; an injured tree, a living body, an animal does so; how then could man make of his freedom, which is the acme of life and constitutes its worth, a principle for his own destruction? Nothing more terrible can be imagined; for if man were on every occasion master of his own life, he would be master of the lives of others; and being ready to sacrifice his life at any and every time rather than be captured, he could perpetrate every conceivable crime and vice. We are, therefore, horrified at the very thought of suicide; by it man sinks lower than the beasts; we look upon a suicide as carrion, whilst our sympathy goes forth to the victim of fate.

Those who advocate suicide seek to give the widest interpretation to freedom. There is something flattering in the thought that we can take our own life if we are so minded; and so we find even right-thinking persons defining suicide in this respect. There are many circumstances under which life ought to be sacrificed. If I cannot preserve my life except by violating my duties towards myself, I am bound to sacrifice my life rather than violate these duties. But suicide is in no circumstances permissible. Humanity in one's own person is something inviolable; it is a holy trust; man is master of all else, but he must not lay hands upon himself. A being who existed of his own necessity could not possibly destroy himself; a being whose existence is not necessary must regard life as the condition of everything else, and in the consciousness that life is a trust reposed in him, such a being recoils at the thought of committing a breach of his holy trust by turning his life against himself. Man can only dispose over things; beasts are things in this sense; but man is not a thing, not a beast. If he disposes over himself, he treats his value as that of a beast. He who so behaves, who has no respect for human nature and makes a thing of himself, becomes for everyone an Object of freewill. We are free to treat him as a beast, as a thing, and to use him for our sport as we do a horse or a dog, for he is no longer a human being; he has made a thing of himself, and, having himself discarded his humanity, he cannot expect that others should respect humanity in him. Yet humanity is worthy of esteem. Even when a man is a bad man, humanity in his person is worthy of esteem. Suicide is not abominable and inadmissible because life should be highly prized; were it so, we could each have our own opinion of how highly we should prize it, and the rule of prudence would often indicate suicide as the best means. But the rule of morality does not admit of it under any condition because it degrades human nature below the level of animal nature and so destroys it. Yet there is much in the world far more important than life. To observe morality is far more important. It is better to sacrifice one's life than one's morality. To live is not a necessity; but to live honourably while life lasts is a necessity. We can at all times go on living and doing our duty towards ourselves without having to do violence to ourselves. But he who is prepared to take his own life is no longer worthy to live at all. The pragmatic ground of impulse to live is happiness. Can I then take my own life because I cannot live happily? No! It is not necessary that whilst I live I should live happily; but it is necessary that so long as I live I should live honourably. Misery gives no right to any man to take his own life, for then we should all be entitled to take our lives for lack of pleasure. All our duties towards ourselves would then be directed towards pleasure; but the fulfillment of those duties may demand that we should even sacrifice our life.

Is suicide heroic or cowardly? Sophistication, even though well meant, is not a good thing. It is not good to defend either virtue or vice by splitting hairs. Even right-thinking people declaim against suicide on wrong lines. They say that it is arrant cowardice. But instances of suicide of great heroism exist. We cannot, for example, regard the suicides of Cato and Atticus as cowardly. Rage, passion and insanity are the most frequent causes of suicide, and that is why persons who attempt suicide and are saved from it are so terrified at their own act that they do not dare to repeat the attempt. There was a time in Roman and in Greek history when suicide was regarded as honourable, so much so that the Romans forbade their slaves to commit suicide because they did not belong to themselves but to their masters and so were regarded as things, like all other animals. The Stoics said that suicide is the sage's peaceful death; he leaves the world as he might leave a smoky room for another, because it no longer pleases him; he leaves the world, not because he is no longer happy in it, but because he disdains it. It has already been mentioned that man is greatly flattered by the idea that he is free to remove himself from this world, if he so wishes. He may not make use of this freedom, but the thought of possessing it pleases him. It seems even to have a moral aspect, for if man is capable of removing himself from the world at his own will, he need not submit to any one; he can retain his independence and tell the rudest truths to the cruellest of tyrants. Torture cannot bring him to heel, because he can leave the world at a moment's notice as a free man can leave the country, if and when he wills it. But this semblance of morality vanishes as soon as we see that man's freedom cannot subsist except on a condition which is immutable. This condition is that man may not use his freedom against himself to his own destruction, but that, on the contrary, he should allow nothing external to limit it. Freedom thus conditioned is noble. No chance or misfortune ought to make us afraid to live; we ought to go on living as long as we can do so as human beings and honourably. To bewail one's fate and misfortune is in itself dishonourable. Had Cato faced any torments which Caesar might have inflicted upon him with a resolute mind and remained steadfast, it would have been noble of him; to violate himself was not so. Those who advocate suicide and teach that there is authority for it necessarily do much harm in a republic of free men. Let us imagine a state in which men held as a general opinion that they were entitled to commit suicide, and that there was even merit and honour in so doing. How dreadful everyone would find them. For he who does not respect his life even in principle cannot be restrained from the most dreadful vices; he recks neither king nor torments.

But as soon as we examine suicide from the standpoint of religion we immediately see it in its true light. We have been placed in this world under certain conditions and for specific purposes. But a suicide opposes the purpose of his Creator; he arrives in the other world as one who has deserted his post; he must be looked upon as a rebel against God. So long as we remember the truth that it is God's intention to preserve life, we are bound to regulate our activities in conformity with it. We have no right to offer violence to our nature's powers of self-preservation and to upset the wisdom of her arrangements. This duty is upon us until the time comes when God expressly commands us to leave this life. Human be-

ings are sentinels on earth and may not leave their posts until relieved by another beneficent hand. God is our owner; we are His property; His providence works for our good. A bondman in the care of a beneficent master deserves punishment if he opposes his master's wishes.

But suicide is not inadmissible and abominable because God has forbidden it; God has forbidden it because it is abominable in that it degrades man's inner worth below that of the animal creation. Moral philosophers must, therefore, first and foremost show that suicide is abominable. We find, as a rule, that those who labour for their happiness are more liable to suicide; having tasted the refinements of pleasure, and being deprived of them, they give way to grief, sorrow, and melancholy.

THE MORALITY AND RATIONALITY OF SUICIDE
R. B. Brandt

Operating on the assumption that suicide is to be understood as the intentional termination of one's own life, Brandt sets himself firmly against the view that suicide is always immoral. He critically analyzes, and finds wanting, various classes of arguments that have been advanced to support the alleged immorality of suicide: (1) theological arguments, (2) arguments from natural law, and (3) arguments to the effect that suicide necessarily harms other persons or society in general. Brandt does acknowledge that there is some obligation to refrain from committing suicide when that act would be injurious to others, but he insists that this obligation may often be overridden by other morally relevant considerations. Clearly, for Brandt, suicide is sometimes morally acceptable. He also insists that a person's decision to commit suicide may be quite rational, although he is careful to warn of potential errors in judgment. He concludes by analyzing the various factors that are relevant in establishing the moral obligation of other persons toward those who are contemplating suicide.

THE MORAL REASONS FOR AND AGAINST SUICIDE

[Assuming that there is suicide if and only if there is intentional termination of one's own life,] persons who say suicide is morally wrong must be

asked which of two positions they are affirming: Are they saying that *every* act of suicide is wrong, *everything considered;* or are they merely saying that there is always *some* moral obligation—doubtless of serious weight—not to commit suicide, so that very often suicide is wrong, although it is possible that there are *countervailing considerations* which in particular situations make it right or even a moral duty? It is quite evident that the first position is absurd; only the second has a chance of being defensible.

In order to make clear what is wrong with the first view, we may begin with an example. Suppose an army pilot's single-seater plane goes out of control over a heavily populated area; he has the choice of staying in the plane and bringing it down where it will do little damage but at the cost of certain death for himself, and of bailing out and letting the plane fall where it will, very possibly killing a good many civilians. Suppose he chooses to do the former, and so, by our definition, commits suicide. Does anyone want to say that his action is morally wrong? Even Immanuel Kant, who opposed suicide in all circumstances, apparently would not wish to say that it is; he would, in fact, judge that this act is not one of suicide, for he says, "It is no suicide to risk one's life against one's enemies, and even to sacrifice it, in order to preserve one's duties toward oneself."[1] St. Thomas Aquinas, in his discussion of suicide, may seem to take the position that such an act would be wrong, for he says, "It is altogether unlawful to kill oneself," admitting as an exception only the case of being under special command of God. But I believe St. Thomas would, in fact, have concluded that the act is right because the basic intention of the pilot was to save the lives of civilians, and whether an act is right or wrong is a matter of basic intention.[2]

In general, we have to admit that there are things with some moral obligation to avoid which, on account of other morally relevant considerations, it is sometimes right or even morally obligatory to do. There may be some obligation to tell the truth on every occasion, but surely in many cases the consequences of telling the truth would be so dire that one is obligated to lie. The same goes for promises. There is some moral obligation to do what one has promised (with a few exceptions); but, if one can keep a trivial promise only at serious cost to another person (i.e., keep an appointment only by failing to give aid to someone injured in an accident), it is surely obligatory to break the promise.

The most that the moral critic of suicide could hold, then, is that there is *some* moral obligation not to do what one knows will cause one's death; but he surely cannot deny that circumstances exist in which there are obligations to do things which, in fact, will result in one's death. If so, then in principle it would

be possible to argue, for instance, that in order to meet my obligation to my family, it might be right for me to take my own life as the only way to avoid catastrophic hospital expenses in a terminal illness. Possibly the main point that critics of suicide on moral grounds would wish to make is that it is never right to take one's own life *for reasons of one's own personal welfare,* of any kind whatsoever. Some of the arguments used to support the immorality of suicide, however, are so framed that if they were supportable at all, they would prove that suicide is *never* moral.

One well-known type of argument against suicide may be classified as *theological.* St. Augustine and others urged that the Sixth Commandment ("Thou shalt not kill") prohibits suicide, and that we are bound to obey a divine commandment. To this reasoning one might first reply that it is arbitrary exegesis of the Sixth Commandment to assert that it was intended to prohibit suicide. The second reply is that if there is not some consideration which shows on the merits of the case that suicide is morally wrong, God had no business prohibiting it. It is true that some will object to this point, and I must refer them elsewhere for my detailed comments on the divine-will theory of morality.[3]

Another theological argument with wide support was accepted by John Locke, who wrote: ". . . Men being all the workmanship of one omnipotent and infinitely wise Maker; all the servants of one sovereign Master, sent into the world by His order and about His business; they are His property, whose workmanship they are made to last during His, not one another's pleasure . . . Every one . . . is bound to preserve himself, and not to quit his station wilfully. . . ."[4] And Kant: "We have been placed in this world under certain conditions and for specific purposes. But a suicide opposes the purpose of his Creator; he arrives in the other world as one who has deserted his post; he must be looked upon as a rebel against God. So long as we remember the truth that it is God's intention to preserve life, we are bound to regulate our activities in conformity with it. This duty is upon us until the time comes when God expressly commands us to leave this life. Human beings are sentinels on earth and may not leave their posts until relieved by another beneficent hand."[5] Unfortunately, however, even if we grant that it is the duty of human beings to do what God commands or intends them to do, more argument is required to show that God does *not* permit human beings to quit this life when their own personal welfare would be maximized by so doing. How does one draw the requisite inference about the intentions of God? The difficulties and contradictions in arguments to reach such a conclusion are discussed at length and perspicaciously by David Hume in his essay "On Suicide," and in view of the unlikelihood that readers will need to be persuaded about these, I shall merely refer those interested to that essay.[6]

A second group of arguments may be classed as arguments *from natural law.* St. Thomas says: "It is altogether unlawful to kill oneself, for three reasons. First, because everything naturally loves itself, the result being that everything naturally keeps itself in being, and resists corruptions so far as it can. Wherefore suicide is contrary to the inclination of nature, and to charity whereby every man should love himself. Hence suicide is always a mortal sin, as being contrary to the natural law and to charity."[7] Here St. Thomas ignores two obvious points. First, it is not obvious why a human being is morally bound to do what he or she has some inclination to do. (St. Thomas did not criticize chastity.) Second, while it is true that most human beings do feel a strong urge to live, the human being who commits suicide obviously feels a stronger inclination to do something else. It is as natural for a human being to dislike, and to take steps to avoid, say, great pain, as it is to cling to life.

A somewhat similar argument by Immanuel Kant may seem better. In a famous passage Kant writes that the maxim of a person who commits suicide is "From self-love I make it my principle to shorten my life if its continuance threatens more evil than it promises pleasure. The only further question to ask is whether this principle of self-love can become a universal law of nature. It is then seen at once that a system of nature by whose law the very same feeling whose function is to stimulate the furtherance of life should actually destroy life would contradict itself and consequently could not subsist as a system of nature. Hence this maxim cannot possibly hold as a universal law of nature and is therefore entirely opposed to the supreme principle of all duty."[8] What Kant finds contradictory is that the motive of

self-love (interest in one's own long-range welfare) should sometimes lead one to struggle to preserve one's life, but at other times to end it. But where is the contradiction? One's circumstances change, and, if the argument of the following section in this [paper] is correct, one sometimes maximizes one's own long-range welfare by trying to stay alive, but at other times by bringing about one's demise.

A third group of arguments, a form of which goes back at least to Aristotle, has a more modern and convincing ring. These are arguments to show that, in one way or another, a suicide necessarily does harm to other persons, or to society at large. Aristotle says that the suicide treats the *state* unjustly.[9] Partly following Aristotle, St. Thomas says: "Every man is part of the community, and so, as such, he belongs to the community. Hence by killing himself he injures the community."[10] Blackstone held that a suicide is an offense against the king "who hath an interest in the preservation of all his subjects," perhaps following Judge Brown in 1563, who argued that suicide cost the king a subject—"he being the head has lost one of his mystical members."[11] The premise of such arguments is, as Hume pointed out, obviously mistaken in many instances. It is true that Freud would perhaps have injured society had he, instead of finishing his last book, committed suicide to escape the pain of throat cancer. But surely there have been many suicides whose demise was not a noticeable loss to society; an honest man could only say that in some instances society was better off without them.

It need not be denied that suicide is often injurious to other persons, especially the family of a suicide. Clearly it sometimes is. But, we should notice what this fact establishes. Suppose we admit, as generally would be done, that there is some obligation not to perform any action which will probably or certainly be injurious to other people, the strength of the obligation being dependent on various factors, notably the seriousness of the expected injury. Then there is *some* obligation not to commit suicide, when that act would probably or certainly be injurious to other people. But, as we have already seen, many cases of *some* obligation to do something nevertheless are *not* cases of a duty to do that thing, *everything considered.* So it could sometimes be morally justified to commit suicide, even if the act will harm someone. Must a man with a terminal illness undergo excruciating pain because his death will cause his wife sorrow—when she will be caused sorrow a month later anyway, when he is dead of natural causes? Moreover, to repeat, the fact that an individual has some obligation not to commit suicide when that act will probably injure other persons does not imply that, everything considered, it is wrong for him to do it, namely, that in all circumstances suicide *as such* is something there is some obligation to avoid.

Is there any sound argument, convincing to the modern mind, to establish that there is (or is not) *some moral obligation* to avoid suicide *as such,* an obligation, of course, which might be overridden by other obligations in some or many cases? (Captain Oates may have had a moral obligation not to commit suicide as such, but his obligation not to stand in the way of his comrades getting to safety might have been so strong that, everything considered, he was justified in leaving the polar camp and allowing himself to freeze to death.)

To present all the arguments necessary to answer this question convincingly would take a great deal of space. I shall, therefore, simply state one answer to it which seems plausible to some contemporary philosophers. Suppose it could be shown that it would maximize the long-run welfare of everybody affected if people were taught that there is a moral obligation to avoid suicide—so that people would be motivated to avoid suicide just because they thought it wrong (would have anticipatory guilt feelings at the very idea), and so that other people would be inclined to disapprove of persons who commit suicide unless there were some excuse. . . . One might ask: how could it maximize utility to mold the conceptual and motivational structure of persons in this way? To which the answer might be: feeling in this way might make persons who are impulsively inclined to commit suicide in a bad mood, or a fit of anger or jealousy, take more time to deliberate; hence, some suicides that have bad effects generally might be prevented. In other words, it might be a good thing in its effects for people to feel about suicide in the way they feel about breach of promise or injuring others, just as it might be a good thing for people to

feel a moral obligation not to smoke, or to wear seat belts. However, it might be that negative moral feelings about suicide as such would stand in the way of action by those persons whose welfare really is best served by suicide and whose suicide is the best thing for everybody concerned.

WHEN A DECISION TO COMMIT SUICIDE IS RATIONAL FROM THE PERSON'S POINT OF VIEW

The person who is contemplating suicide is obviously making a choice between future world-courses; the world-course that includes his demise, say, an hour from now, and several possible ones that contain his demise at a later point. One cannot have precise knowledge about many features of the latter group of world-courses, but it is certain that they will all end with death some (possibly short) finite time from now.

Why do I say the choice is between *world-courses* and not just a choice between future life-courses of the prospective suicide, the one shorter than the other? The reason is that one's suicide has some impact on the world (and one's continued life has some impact on the world), and that conditions in the rest of the world will often make a difference in one's evaluation of the possibilities. One *is* interested in things in the world other than just oneself and one's own happiness.

The basic question a person must answer, in order to determine which world-course is best or rational for him to choose, is which he *would* choose under conditions of optimal use of information, when *all* of his desires are taken into account. It is not just a question of what we prefer *now,* with some clarification of all the possibilities being considered. Our preferences change, and the preferences of tomorrow (assuming we can know something about them) are just as legitimately taken into account in deciding what to do now as the preferences of today. Since any reason that can be given today for weighting heavily today's preference can be given tomorrow for weighting heavily tomorrow's preference, the preferences of any time-stretch have a rational claim to an equal vote. Now the importance of that fact is this: we often know quite well that our desires, aversions, and preferences may change after a short while. When a person is in a state of despair—perhaps brought about by a rejection in love or discharge from a long-held position—nothing but the thing he cannot have seems desirable; everything else is turned to ashes. Yet we know quite well that the passage of time is likely to reverse all this; replacements may be found or other types of things that are available to us may begin to look attractive. So, if we were to act on the preferences of today alone, when the emotion of despair seems more than we can stand, we might find death preferable to life; but, if we allow for the preferences of the weeks and years ahead, when many goals will be enjoyable and attractive, we might find life much preferable to death. So, if a choice of what is best is to be determined by what we want not only now but later (and later desires on an equal basis with the present ones)—as it should be—then what is the best or preferable world-course will often be quite different from what it would be if the choice, or what is best for one, were fixed by one's desires and preferences now.

Of course, if one commits suicide there are no future desires or aversions that may be compared with present ones and that should be allowed an equal vote in deciding what is best. In that respect the course of action that results in death is different from any other course of action we may undertake. I do not wish to suggest the rosy possibility that it is often or always reasonable to believe that next week "I shall be more interested in living than I am today, if today I take a dim view of continued existence." On the contrary, when a person is seriously ill, for instance, he may have no reason to think that the preference-order will be reversed—it may be that tomorrow he will prefer death to life more strongly.

The argument is often used that one can never be *certain* what is going to happen, and hence one is never rationally justified in doing anything as drastic as committing suicide. But we always have to live by probabilities and make our estimates as best we can. As soon as it is clear beyond reasonable doubt not only that death is now preferable to life, but also that it will be every day from now until the end, the rational thing is to act promptly.

Let us not pursue the question of whether it is rational for a person with a painful terminal illness to commit suicide; it is. However, the issue seldom

arises, and few terminally ill patients do commit suicide. With such patients matters usually get worse slowly so that no particular time seems to call for action. They are often so heavily sedated that it is impossible for the mental processes of decision leading to action to occur; or else they are incapacitated in a hospital and the very physical possibility of ending their lives is not available. Let us leave this grim topic and turn to a practically more important problem: whether it is rational for persons to commit suicide for some reason other than painful terminal physical illness. Most persons who commit suicide do so, apparently, because they face a nonphysical problem that depresses them beyond their ability to bear.

Among the problems that have been regarded as good and sufficient reasons for ending life, we find (in addition to serious illness) the following: some event that has made a person feel ashamed or lose his prestige and status; reduction from affluence to poverty; the loss of a limb or of physical beauty; the loss of sexual capacity; some event that makes it seem impossible to achieve things by which one sets store; loss of a loved one; disappointment in love; the infirmities of increasing age. It is not to be denied that such things can be serious blows to a person's prospects of happiness.

Whatever the nature of an individual's problem, there are various plain errors to be avoided—errors to which a person is especially prone when he is depressed—in deciding whether, everything considered, he prefers a world-course containing his early demise to one in which his life continues to its natural terminus. Let us forget for a moment the relevance to the decision of preferences that he may have tomorrow, and concentrate on some errors that may infect his preference as of today, and for which correction or allowance must be made.

In the first place, depression, like any severe emotional experience, tends to primitivize one's intellectual processes. It restricts the range of one's survey of the possibilities. One thing that a rational person would do is compare the world-course containing his suicide with his *best* alternative. But his best alternative is precisely a possibility he may overlook if, in a depressed mood, he thinks only of how badly off he is and cannot imagine any way of improving his situation. If a person is disappointed in love, it is possible to adopt a vigorous plan of action that carries a good chance of acquainting him with someone he likes at least as well; and if old age prevents a person from continuing the tennis game with his favorite partner, it is possible to learn some other game that provides the joys of competition without the physical demands.

Depression has another insidious influence on one's planning; it seriously affects one's judgment about probabilities. A person disappointed in love is very likely to take a dim view of himself, his prospects, and his attractiveness; he thinks that because he has been rejected by one person he will probably be rejected by anyone who looks desirable to him. In a less gloomy frame of mind he would make different estimates. Part of the reason for such gloomy probability estimates is that depression tends to repress one's memory of evidence that supports a nongloomy prediction. Thus, a rejected lover tends to forget any cases in which he has elicited enthusiastic response from ladies in relation to whom he has been the one who has done the rejecting. Thus his pessimistic self-image is based upon a highly selected, and pessimistically selected, set of data. Even when he is reminded of the data, moreover, he is apt to resist an optimistic inference.

Another kind of distortion of the look of future prospects is not a result of depression, but is quite normal. Events distant in the future feel small, just as objects distant in space look small. Their prospect does not have the effect on motivational processes that it would have if it were of an event in the immediate future. Psychologists call this the "goal-gradient" phenomenon; a rat, for instance, will run faster toward a perceived food box than a distant unseen one. In the case of a person who has suffered some misfortune, and whose situation now is an unpleasant one, this reduction of the motivational influence of events distant in time has the effect that present unpleasant states weigh far more heavily than probable future pleasant ones in any choice of world-courses.

If we are trying to determine whether we now prefer, or shall later prefer, the outcome of one world-course to that of another (and this is leaving aside the questions of the weight of the votes of preferences at a later date), we must take into account

these and other infirmities of our "sensing" machinery. Since knowing that the machinery is out of order will not tell us what results it would give if it were working, the best recourse might be to refrain from making any decision in a stressful frame of mind. If decisions have to be made, one must recall past reactions, in a normal frame of mind, to outcomes like those under assessment. But many suicides seem to occur in moments of despair. What should be clear from the above is that a moment of despair, if one is seriously contemplating suicide, ought to be a moment of reassessment of one's goals and values, a reassessment which the individual must realize is very difficult to make objectively, because of the very quality of his depressed frame of mind.

A decision to commit suicide may in certain circumstances be a rational one. But a person who wants to act rationally must take into account the various possible "errors" and make appropriate rectification of his initial evaluations.

THE ROLE OF OTHER PERSONS

What is the moral obligation of other persons toward those who are contemplating suicide? The question of their moral blameworthiness may be ignored and what is rational for them to do from the point of view of personal welfare may be considered as being of secondary concern. Laws make it dangerous to aid or encourage a suicide. The risk of running afoul of the law may partly determine moral obligation, since moral obligation to do something may be reduced by the fact that it is personally dangerous.

The moral obligation of other persons toward one who is contemplating suicide is an instance of a general obligation to render aid to those in serious distress, at least when this can be done at no great cost to one's self. I do not think this general principle is seriously questioned by anyone, whatever his moral theory; so I feel free to assume it as a premise. Obviously the person contemplating suicide is in great distress of some sort; if he were not, he would not be seriously considering terminating his life.

How great a person's obligation is to one in distress depends on a number of factors. Obviously family and friends have special obligations to devote time to helping the prospective suicide— which others do not have. But anyone in this kind of distress has a moral claim on the time of any person who knows the situation (unless there are others more responsible who are already doing what should be done).

What is the obligation? It depends, of course, on the situation, and how much the second person knows about the situation. If the individual has decided to terminate his life if he can, and it is clear that he is right in this decision, then, if he needs help in executing the decision, there is a moral obligation to give him help. On this matter a patient's physician has a special obligation, from which any talk about the Hippocratic oath does not absolve him. It is true that there are some damages one cannot be expected to absorb, and some risks which one cannot be expected to take, on account of the obligation to render aid.

On the other hand, if it is clear that the individual should not commit suicide, from the point of view of his own welfare, or if there is a presumption that he should not (when the only evidence is that a person is discovered unconscious, with the gas turned on), it would seem to be the individual's obligation to intervene, prevent the successful execution of the decision, and see to the availability of competent psychiatric advice and temporary hospitalization, if necessary. Whether one has a right to take such steps when a clearly sane person, after careful reflection over a period of time, comes to the conclusion that an end to his life is what is best for him and what he wants, is very doubtful, even when one thinks his conclusion a mistaken one; it would seem that a man's own considered decision about whether he wants to live must command respect, although one must concede that this could be debated.

The more interesting role in which a person may be cast, however, is that of adviser. It is often important to one who is contemplating suicide to go over his thinking with another, and to feel that a conclusion, one way or the other, has the support of a respected mind. One thing one can obviously do, in rendering the service of advice, is to discuss with the person the various types of issues discussed above, made more specific by the concrete circumstances of his case, and help him find whether, in view, say, of the damage his suicide would do to others, he has a moral obligation to refrain, and whether it is rational or best for him, from the point of view of his own welfare, to take this step or adopt some other plan instead.

To get a person to see what is the rational thing to do is no small job. Even to get a person, in a frame of mind when he is seriously contemplating (or perhaps has already unsuccessfully attempted) suicide, to recognize a plain truth of fact may be a major operation. If a man insists, "I am a complete failure," when it is obvious that by any reasonable standard he is far from that, it may be tremendously difficult to get him to see the fact. But there is another job beyond that of getting a person to see what is the rational thing to do; that is to help him *act* rationally, or *be* rational, when he has conceded what would be the rational thing.

How either of these tasks may be accomplished effectively may be discussed more competently by an experienced psychiatrist than by a philosopher. Loneliness and the absence of human affection are states which exacerbate any other problems; disappointment, reduction to poverty, and so forth, seem less impossible to bear in the presence of the affection of another. Hence simply to be a friend, or to find someone a friend, may be the largest contribution one can make either to helping a person be rational or see clearly what is rational for him to do; this service may make one who was contemplating suicide feel that there is a future for him which it is possible to face.

NOTES

1 Immanuel Kant, *Lectures on Ethics,* New York: Harper Torchbook (1963), p. 150.

2 See St. Thomas Aquinas, *Summa Theologica,* Second Part of the Second Part, Q. 64, Art. 5. In Article 7, he says: "Nothing hinders one act from having two effects, only one of which is intended, while the other is beside the intention. Now moral acts take their species according to what is intended, and not according to what is beside the intention, since this is accidental as explained above" (Q. 43, Art. 3: I–II, Q. 1, Art. 3, as 3). Mr. Norman St. John-Stevas, the most articulate contemporary defender of the Catholic view, writes as follows: "Christian thought allows certain exceptions to its general condemnation of suicide. That covered by a particular divine inspiration has already been noted. Another exception arises where suicide is the method

imposed by the state for the execution of a just death penalty. A third exception is *altruistic* suicide, of which the best known example is Captain Oates. Such suicides are justified by invoking the principles of double effect. The act from which death results must be good or at least morally indifferent; some other good effect must result: The death must not be directly intended or the real means to the good effect, and a grave reason must exist for adopting the course of action" [*Life, Death and the Law,* Bloomington, Ind.: Indiana University Press (1961), pp. 250–51]. Presumably the Catholic doctrine is intended to allow suicide when this is required for meeting strong moral obligations; whether it can do so consistently depends partly on the interpretation given to "real means to the good effect." Readers interested in pursuing further the Catholic doctrine of double effect and its implications for our problem should read Philippa Foot, "The Problem of Abortion and the Doctrine of Double Effect," *The Oxford Review,* 5:5–15 (Trinity 1967).

3 R. B. Brandt, *Ethical Theory,* Englewood Cliffs, N.J.: Prentice-Hall (1959), pp. 61–82.
4 John Locke, *Two Treatises of Government,* Ch. 2.
5 Kant, *Lectures on Ethics,* p. 154.
6 This essay appears in collections of Hume's works.
7 For an argument similar to Kant's, see also St. Thomas Aquinas, *Summa Theologica,* II, II, Q. 64, Art. 5.
8 Immanuel Kant, *The Fundamental Principles of the Metaphysic of Morals,* trans. H. J. Paton, London: The Hutchinson Group (1948), Ch. 2.
9 Aristotle, *Nicomachaean Ethics,* Bk. 5, Ch. 10, p. 1138a.
10 St. Thomas Aquinas, *Summa Theologica,* II, II, Q. 64, Art. 5.
11 Sir William Blackstone, *Commentaries,* 4:189; Brown in *Hales v. Petit,* I Plow. 253, 75 E.R. 387 (C. B. 1563). Both cited by Norman St. John-Stevas, *Life, Death and the Law,* p. 235.

THE MORALITY OF ACTIVE EUTHANASIA

ACTIVE AND PASSIVE EUTHANASIA
James Rachels

In this classic article, Rachels identifies the "conventional doctrine" on the morality of euthanasia as the doctrine that allows passive euthanasia but does not allow active euthanasia. He then argues that the conventional doctrine may be challenged for four reasons. First, active euthanasia is in many cases more humane than passive euthanasia. Second, the conventional doctrine leads to decisions concerning life and death on irrelevant grounds. Third, the doctrine rests on a distinction between killing and letting die that itself has no moral importance. Fourth, the most common argument in favor of the doctrine is invalid.

The distinction between active and passive euthanasia is thought to be crucial for medical ethics. The idea is that it is permissible, at least in some cases, to withhold treatment and allow a patient to die, but it is never permissible to take any direct action designed to kill the patient. This doctrine seems to be accepted by most doctors, and it is endorsed in a statement adopted by the House of Delegates of the American Medical Association on December 4, 1973:

The intentional termination of the life of one human being by another—mercy killing—is contrary

Reprinted by permission from the *New England Journal of Medicine,* vol. 292, no. 2 (January 9, 1975), pp. 78–80.

to that for which the medical profession stands and is contrary to the policy of the American Medical Association.

The cessation of the employment of extraordinary means to prolong the life of the body when there is irrefutable evidence that biological death is imminent is the decision of the patient and/or his immediate family. The advice and judgment of the physician should be freely available to the patient and/or his immediate family.

However, a strong case can be made against this doctrine. In what follows I will set out some of the relevant arguments, and urge doctors to reconsider their views on this matter.

To begin with a familiar type of situation, a patient who is dying of incurable cancer of the throat is in terrible pain, which can no longer be satisfactorily alleviated. He is certain to die within a few days, even if present treatment is continued, but he does not want to go on living for those days since the pain is unbearable. So he asks the doctor for an end to it, and his family joins in the request.

Suppose the doctor agrees to withhold treatment, as the conventional doctrine says he may. The justification for his doing so is that the patient is in terrible agony, and since he is going to die anyway, it would be wrong to prolong his suffering needlessly. But now notice this. If one simply withholds treatment, it may take the patient longer to die, and so he may suffer more than he would if more direct action were taken and a lethal injection given. This fact provides strong reason for thinking that, once the initial decision not to prolong his agony has been made, active euthanasia is actually preferable to passive euthanasia, rather than the reverse. To say otherwise is to endorse the option that leads to more suffering rather than less, and is contrary to the humanitarian impulse that prompts the decision not to prolong his life in the first place.

Part of my point is that the process of being "allowed to die" can be relatively slow and painful, whereas being given a lethal injection is relatively quick and painless. Let me give a different sort of example. In the United States about one in 600 babies is born with Down's syndrome. Most of these babies are otherwise healthy—that is, with only the usual pediatric care, they will proceed to an otherwise normal infancy. Some, however, are born with congenital defects such as intestinal obstructions that require operations if they are to live. Sometimes, the parents and the doctor will decide not to operate, and let the infant die. Anthony Shaw describes what happens then:

> . . . When surgery is denied [the doctor] must try to keep the infant from suffering while natural forces sap the baby's life away. As a surgeon whose natural inclination is to use the scalpel to fight off death, standing by and watching a salvageable baby die is the most emotionally exhausting experience I know. It is easy at a conference, in a theoretical discussion, to decide that such infants should be allowed to die. It is altogether different to stand by in the nursery and watch as dehydration and infection wither a tiny being over hours and days. This is a terrible ordeal for me and the hospital staff—much more so than for the parents who never set foot in the nursery.[1]

I can understand why some people are opposed to all euthanasia, and insist that such infants must be allowed to live. I think I can also understand why other people favor destroying these babies quickly and painlessly. But why should anyone favor letting "dehydration and infection wither a tiny being over hours and days"? The doctrine that says that a baby may be allowed to dehydrate and wither, but may not be given an injection that would end its life without suffering, seems so patently cruel as to require no further refutation. The strong language is not intended to offend, but only to put the point in the clearest possible way.

My second argument is that the conventional doctrine leads to decisions concerning life and death made on irrelevant grounds.

Consider again the case of the infants with Down's syndrome who need operations for congenital defects unrelated to the syndrome to live. Sometimes, there is no operation, and the baby dies, but when there is no such defect, the baby lives on. Now, an operation such as that to remove an intestinal obstruction is not prohibitively difficult. The reason why such operations are not performed in these cases is, clearly, that the child has Down's syndrome and the parents and doctor judge that because of that fact it is better for the child to die.

But notice that this situation is absurd, no matter what view one takes of the lives and potentials of such babies. If the life of such an infant is worth preserving, what does it matter if it needs a simple operation? Or, if one thinks it better that such a baby should not live on, what difference does it make that it happens to have an unobstructed intestinal tract? In either case, the matter of life and death is being decided on irrelevant grounds. It is the Down's syndrome, and not the intestines, that is the issue. The matter should be decided, if at all, on that basis, and not be allowed to depend on the essentially irrelevant question of whether the intestinal tract is blocked.

What makes this situation possible, of course, is the idea that when there is an intestinal blockage, one can "let the baby die," but when there is no such defect there is nothing that can be done, for one must not "kill" it. The fact that this idea leads to such results as deciding life or death on irrelevant grounds is another good reason why the doctrine should be rejected.

One reason why so many people think that there is an important moral difference between active and passive euthanasia is that they think killing someone is morally worse than letting someone die. But is it? Is killing, in itself, worse than letting die? To investigate this issue, two cases may be considered that are exactly alike except that one involves killing whereas the other involves letting someone die. Then, it can be asked whether this difference makes any difference to the moral assessments. It is important that the cases be exactly alike, except for this one difference, since otherwise one cannot be confident that it is this difference and not some other that accounts for any variation in the assessments of the two cases. So, let us consider this pair of cases:

In the first, Smith stands to gain a large inheritance if anything should happen to his six-year-old cousin. One evening while the child is taking his bath, Smith sneaks into the bathroom and drowns the child, and then arranges things so that it will look like an accident.

In the second, Jones also stands to gain if anything should happen to his six-year-old cousin. Like Smith, Jones sneaks in planning to drown the child in his bath. However, just as he enters the bathroom Jones sees the child slip and hit his head, and fall face down in the water. Jones is delighted; he stands by, ready to push the child's head back under if it is necessary, but it is not necessary. With only a little thrashing about, the child drowns all by himself, "accidentally," as Jones watches and does nothing.

Now Smith killed the child, whereas Jones "merely" let the child die. That is the only difference between them. Did either man behave better, from a moral point of view? If the difference between killing and letting die were in itself a morally important matter, one should say that Jones's behavior was less reprehensible than Smith's. But does one really want to say that? I think not. In the first place,

both men acted from the same motive, personal gain, and both had exactly the same end in view when they acted. It may be inferred from Smith's conduct that he is a bad man, although that judgment may be withdrawn or modified if certain further facts are learned about him—for example, that he is mentally deranged. But would not the very same thing be inferred about Jones from his conduct? And would not the same further considerations also be relevant to any modification of this judgment? Moreover, suppose Jones pleaded, in his own defense, "After all, I didn't do anything except just stand there and watch the child drown. I didn't kill him; I only let him die." Again, if letting die were in itself less bad than killing, this defense should have at least some weight. But it does not. Such a "defense" can only be regarded as a grotesque perversion of moral reasoning. Morally speaking, it is no defense at all.

Now, it may be pointed out, quite properly, that the cases of euthanasia with which doctors are concerned are not like this at all. They do not involve personal gain or the destruction of normal, healthy children. Doctors are concerned only with cases in which the patient's life is of no further use to him, or in which the patient's life has become or will soon become a terrible burden. However, the point is the same in these cases: the bare difference between killing and letting die does not, in itself, make a moral difference. If a doctor lets a patient die, for humane reasons, he is in the same moral position as if he had given the patient a lethal injection for humane reasons. If his decision was wrong—if, for example, the patient's illness was in fact curable—the decision would be equally regrettable no matter which method was used to carry it out. And if the doctor's decision was the right one, the method used is not in itself important.

The AMA policy statement isolates the crucial issue very well; the crucial issue is "the intentional termination of the life of one human being by another." But after identifying this issue, and forbidding "mercy killing," the statement goes on to deny that the cessation of treatment is the intentional termination of life. This is where the mistake comes in, for what is the cessation of treatment, in these circumstances, if it is not "the intentional termination of the life of one human being by another"? Of course it is exactly that, and if it were not, there would be no point to it.

Many people will find this judgment hard to accept. One reason, I think, is that it is very easy to conflate the question of whether killing is, in itself, worse than letting die, with the very different question of whether most actual cases of killing are more reprehensible than most actual cases of letting die. Most actual cases of killing are clearly terrible (think, for example, of all the murders reported in the newspapers), and one hears of such cases every day. On the other hand, one hardly ever hears of a case of letting die, except for the actions of doctors who are motivated by humanitarian reasons. So one learns to think of killing in a much worse light than of letting die. But this does not mean that there is something about killing that makes it in itself worse than letting die, for it is not the bare difference between killing and letting die that makes the difference in these cases. Rather, the other factors—the murderer's motive of personal gain, for example, contrasted with the doctor's humanitarian motivation—account for different reactions to the different cases.

I have argued that killing is not in itself any worse than letting die; if my contention is right, it follows that active euthanasia is not any worse than passive euthanasia. What arguments can be given on the other side? The most common, I believe, is the following:

> "The important difference between active and passive euthanasia is that, in passive euthanasia, the doctor does not do anything to bring about the patient's death. The doctor does nothing, and the patient dies of whatever ills already afflict him. In active euthanasia, however, the doctor does something to bring about the patient's death: he kills him. The doctor who gives the patient with cancer a lethal injection has himself caused his patient's death; whereas if he merely ceases treatment, the cancer is the cause of the death."

A number of points need to be made here. The first is that it is not exactly correct to say that in passive euthanasia the doctor does nothing, for he does do one thing that is very important: he lets the patient die. "Letting someone die" is certainly different, in some respects, from other types of action—mainly in

that it is a kind of action that one may perform by way of not performing certain other actions. For example, one may let a patient die by way of not giving medication, just as one may insult someone by way of not shaking his hand. But for any purpose of moral assessment, it is a type of action nonetheless. The decision to let a patient die is subject to moral appraisal in the same way that a decision to kill him would be subject to moral appraisal: it may be assessed as wise or unwise, compassionate or sadistic, right or wrong. If a doctor deliberately let a patient die who was suffering from a routinely curable illness, the doctor would certainly be to blame for what he had done, just as he would be to blame if he had needlessly killed the patient. Charges against him would then be appropriate. If so, it would be no defense at all for him to insist that he didn't "do anything." He would have done something very serious indeed, for he let his patient die.

Fixing the cause of death may be very important from a legal point of view, for it may determine whether criminal charges are brought against the doctor. But I do not think that this notion can be used to show a moral difference between active and passive euthanasia. The reason why it is considered bad to be the cause of someone's death is that death is regarded as a great evil—and so it is. However, if it has been decided that euthanasia—even passive euthanasia—is desirable in a given case, it has also been decided that in this instance death is no greater an evil than the patient's continued existence. And if this is true, the usual reason for not wanting to be the cause of someone's death simply does not apply.

Finally, doctors may think that all of this is only of academic interest—the sort of thing that philosophers may worry about but that has no practical bearing on their own work. After all, doctors must be concerned about the legal consequences of what they do, and active euthanasia is clearly forbidden by the law. But even so, doctors should also be concerned with the fact that the law is forcing upon them a moral doctrine that may well be indefensible, and has a considerable effect on their practices. Of course, most doctors are not now in the position of being coerced in this matter, for they do not regard themselves as merely going along with what the law requires. Rather, in statements such as the AMA policy statement that I have quoted, they are endorsing this doctrine as a central point of medical ethics. In that statement, active euthanasia is condemned not merely as illegal but as "contrary to that for which the medical profession stands," whereas passive euthanasia is approved. However, the preceding considerations suggest that there is really no moral difference between the two, considered in themselves (there may be important moral differences in some cases in their *consequences,* but, as I pointed out, these differences may make active euthanasia,

and not passive euthanasia, the morally preferable option). So, whereas doctors may have to discriminate between active and passive euthanasia to satisfy the law, they should not do any more than that. In particular, they should not give the distinction any added authority and weight by writing it into official statements of medical ethics.

NOTE

1 Shaw A.: "Doctor, Do We Have a Choice?" *The New York Times Magazine,* January 30, 1972, p. 54.

KILLING AND ALLOWING TO DIE

Daniel Callahan

Callahan maintains that there is a valid distinction between killing and allowing to die, and he defends the distinction by reference to three overlapping perspectives—metaphysical, moral, and medical. In terms of a metaphysical perspective, Callahan emphasizes that the external world is distinct from the self and has its own causal dynamism. In terms of a moral perspective, he emphasizes the difference between *physical causality* and *moral culpability.* In conjunction with a medical perspective, he insists that killing patients is incompatible with the role of the physician in society.

. . . No valid distinction, many now argue, can be made between killing and allowing to die, or between an act of commission and one of omission. The standard distinction being challenged rests on the commonplace observation that lives can come to an end as the result of: (a) the direct action of another who becomes the cause of death (as in shooting a person), and (b) the result of impersonal forces where no human agent has acted (death by lightning, or by disease). The purpose of the distinction has been to separate those deaths caused by human action, and those caused by nonhuman events. It is, as a distinction, meant to say something about human beings and their relationship to the world. It is a way of articulating the difference between those actions

for which human beings can be held rightly responsible, or blamed, and those of which they are innocent. At issue is the difference between physical causality, the realm of impersonal events, and moral culpability, the realm of human responsibility.

The challenges encompass two points. The first is that people can become equally dead by our omissions as well as our commissions. We can refrain from saving them when it is possible to do so, and they will be just as dead as if we shot them. It is our decision itself that is the reason for their death, not necessarily how we effectuate that decision. That fact establishes the basis of the second point: if we *intend* their death, it can be brought about as well by omitted acts as by those we commit. The crucial moral point is not how they die, but our intention about their death. We can, then, be responsible for the death of another by intending that they die and accomplish that end by standing aside and allowing them to die.

Despite these criticisms—resting upon ambiguities that can readily be acknowledged—the distinction between killing and allowing to die remains, I contend, perfectly valid. It not only has a logical validity but, no less importantly, a social validity whose place must be central in moral judgments. As a way of putting the distinction into perspective, I want to suggest that it is best understood as expressing three different, though overlapping, perspectives on nature and human action. I will call them the metaphysical, the moral, and the medical perspectives.

METAPHYSICAL

The first and most fundamental premise of the distinction between killing and allowing to die is that there is a sharp difference between the self and the external world. Unlike the childish fantasy that the world is nothing more than a projection of the self, or the neurotic person's fear that he or she is responsible for everything that goes wrong, the distinction is meant to uphold a simple notion: there is a world external to the self that has its own, and independent, causal dynamism. The mistake behind a conflation of killing and allowing to die is to assume that the self has become master of everything within and outside of the self. It is as if the conceit that modern man might ultimately control nature has been internalized: that, if the self might be able to influence nature by its actions, then the self and nature must be one.

Of course that is a fantasy. The fact that we can intervene in nature, and cure or control many diseases, does not erase the difference between the self and the external world. It is as "out there" as ever, even if more under our sway. That sway, however great, is always limited. We can cure disease, but not always the chronic illness that comes with the cure. We can forestall death with modern medicine, but death always wins in the long run because of the innate limitations of the body, inherently and stubbornly beyond final human control. And we can distinguish between a diseased body and an aging body, but in the end if we wait long enough they always become one and the same body. To attempt to deny the distinction between killing and allowing to die is, then, mistakenly to impute more power to human action than it actually has and to accept the conceit that nature has now fallen wholly within the realm of human control. Not so.

MORAL

At the center of the distinction between killing and allowing to die is the difference between physical causality and moral culpability. To bring the life of another to an end by an injection kills the other directly; our action is the physical cause of the death. To allow someone to die from a disease we cannot cure (and that we did not cause) is to permit the disease to act as the cause of death. The notion of physical causality in both cases rests on the difference between human agency and the action of external nature. The ambiguity arises precisely because we can be morally culpable for killing someone (if we have no moral right to do so, as we would in self-defense) and no less culpable for allowing someone to die (if we have both the possibility and the obligation of keeping that person alive). Thus there are cases where, morally speaking, it makes no difference whether we killed or allowed to die; we are equally responsible. In those instances, the lines of physical causality and moral culpability happen to cross. Yet the fact that they can cross in some cases in no way shows that they are always, or even usually, one and the same. We can normally find the difference in all but the most obscure cases. We should not, then, use the ambiguity of such cases to do away altogether with the distinction between killing and allowing to die. The ambiguity may obscure, but does not erase, the line between the two.

There is one group of ambiguous cases that is especially troublesome. Even if we grant the ordinary validity between killing and allowing to die, what about those cases that combine (a) an illness that renders a patient unable to carry out an ordinary biological function (to breathe or eat on his own, for example), and (b) our turning off a respirator or removing an artificial feeding tube? On the level of physical causality, have we killed the patient or allowed him to die? In one sense, it is our action that shortens his life, and yet in another sense his underlying disease brings his life to an end. I believe it reasonable to say that, since his life was being sustained by artificial means (respirator or feeding tube) made necessary because of the fact that he had an incapacitating disease, his disease is the ultimate reality behind his death. But for its reality, there would be no need for artificial sustenance in the first place and no moral issue at all. To lose sight of the paramount reality of the disease is to lose sight of the difference between our selves and the outer world.

I quickly add, and underscore, a moral point: the person who, without good moral reason, turns off a respirator or pulls a feeding tube, can be morally culpable; that the patient has been allowed to die of his underlying condition does not morally excuse him. The moral question is whether we are obliged to continue treating a life that is being artificially sustained. To cease treatment may or may not be morally acceptable; but it should be understood, in either case, that the physical cause of death was the underlying disease.

MEDICAL

An important social purpose of the distinction between killing and allowing to die has been that of protecting the historical role of the physician as one who tries to cure or comfort patients rather than to kill patients. Physicians have been given special knowledge about the body, knowledge that can be used to kill or to cure. They are also given great privileges in making use of that knowledge. It is thus all the more important that physicians' social role and power be, and be seen to be, a limited power. It may be used only to cure or comfort, never to kill. They have not been given, nor should they be given, the power to use their knowledge and skills to bring life to an end. It would open the way for powerful misuse and, no less importantly, represent an intrinsic violation of what it has meant to be a physician.

Yet if it is possible for physicians to misuse their knowledge and power to kill people directly, are they thereby required to use that same knowledge always to keep people alive, always to resist a disease that can itself kill the patient? The traditional answer has been: not necessarily. For the physician's ultimate obligation is to the welfare of the patient, and excessive treatment can be as detrimental to that welfare as inadequate treatment. Put another way, the obligation to resist the lethal power of disease is limited—it ceases when the patient is unwilling to have it resisted, or where the resistance no longer serves the patient's welfare. Behind this moral premise is the recognition that disease (of some kind) ultimately triumphs and that death is both inevitable sooner or later and not, in any case, always the greatest human evil. To demand of the physician that he always struggle against disease, as if it was in his power always to conquer it, would be to fall into the same metaphysical trap mentioned above: that of assuming that no distinction can be drawn between natural and human agency.

A final word. I suggested [in an earlier discussion] that the most potent motive for active euthanasia and assisted suicide stems from a dread of the power of medicine. That power then seems to take on a drive of its own regardless of the welfare or wishes of patients. No one can easily say no—not physicians, not patients, not families. My guess is that happens because too many have already come to believe that it is their choice, and their choice alone, which brings about death; and they do not want to exercise that kind of authority. The solution is not to erase the distinction between killing and allowing to die, but to underscore its validity and importance. We can bring disease as a cause of death back into the care of the dying.

VOLUNTARY ACTIVE EUTHANASIA

Dan W. Brock

In this excerpt from a much longer article, Brock argues that two fundamental ethical values support the ethical permissibility of voluntary active euthanasia. These values are individual self-determination (autonomy) and individual well-being, the same two values that support the consensus view that patients have a right to make decisions about life-sustaining treatment. Brock also argues that allowing physicians to perform euthanasia is not incompatible with the "moral center" of medicine.

... The central ethical argument for [voluntary active] euthanasia is familiar. It is that the very same two fundamental ethical values supporting the consensus on patient's rights to decide about life-sustaining treatment also support the ethical permissibility of euthanasia. These values are individual self-determination or autonomy and individual well-being. By self-determination as it bears on euthanasia, I mean people's interest in making important decisions about their lives for themselves according to their own values or conceptions of a good life, and in being left free to act on those decisions. Self-determination is valuable because it permits people to form and live in accordance with their own conception of a good life, at least within the bounds of justice and consistent with others doing so as well. In exercising self-determination people take responsibility for their lives and for the kinds of persons they become. A central aspect of human dignity lies in people's capacity to direct their lives in this way. The value of exercising self-determination presupposes some minimum of decision-making capacities or competence, which thus limits the scope of euthanasia supported by self-determination; it cannot justifiably be administered, for example, in cases of serious dementia or treatable clinical depression.

Does the value of individual self-determination extend to the time and manner of one's death? Most people are very concerned about the nature of the last stage of their lives. This reflects not just a fear of experiencing substantial suffering when dying, but also a desire to retain dignity and control during this last period of life. Death is today increasingly preceded by a long period of significant physical and mental decline, due in part to the technological interventions of modern medicine. Many people adjust to these disabilities and find meaning and value in new activities and ways. Others find the impairments and burdens in the last stage of their lives at some point sufficiently great to make life no longer worth living. For many patients near death, maintaining the quality of one's life, avoiding great suffering, maintaining one's dignity, and ensuring that

Reprinted with permission of the author and the publisher from *Hastings Center Report*, vol. 22 (March/April 1992), pp. 11, 16. © The Hastings Center.

others remember us as we wish them to, become of paramount importance and outweigh merely extending one's life. But there is no single, objectively correct answer for everyone as to when, if at all, one's life becomes all things considered a burden and unwanted. If self-determination is a fundamental value, then the great variability among people on this question makes it especially important that individuals control the manner, circumstances, and timing of their dying and death.

The other main value that supports euthanasia is individual well-being. It might seem that individual well-being conflicts with a person's self-determination when the person requests euthanasia. Life itself is commonly taken to be a central good for persons, often valued for its own sake, as well as necessary for pursuit of all other goods within a life. But when a competent patient decides to forgo all further life-sustaining treatment then the patient, either explicitly or implicitly, commonly decides that the best life possible for him or her with treatment is of sufficiently poor quality that it is worse than no further life at all. Life is no longer considered a benefit by the patient, but has now become a burden. The same judgment underlies a request for euthanasia: continued life is seen by the patient as no longer a benefit, but now a burden. Especially in the often severely compromised and debilitated states of many critically ill or dying patients, there is no objective standard, but only the competent patient's judgment of whether continued life is no longer a benefit.

Of course, sometimes there are conditions, such as clinical depression, that call into question whether the patient has made a competent choice, either to forgo life-sustaining treatment or to seek euthanasia, and then the patient's choice need not be evidence that continued life is no longer a benefit for him or her. Just as with decisions about treatment, a determination of incompetence can warrant not honoring the patient's choice; in the case of treatment, we then transfer decisional authority to a surrogate, though in the case of voluntary active euthanasia a determination that the patient is incompetent means that choice is not possible.

The value or right of self-determination does not entitle patients to compel physicians to act contrary to their own moral or professional values.

Physicians are moral and professional agents whose own self-determination or integrity should be respected as well. If performing euthanasia became legally permissible, but conflicted with a particular physician's reasonable understanding of his or her moral or professional responsibilities, the care of a patient who requested euthanasia should be transferred to another. . . .

. . . Permitting physicians to perform euthanasia, it is said, would be incompatible with their fundamental moral and professional commitment as healers to care for patients and to protect life. Moreover, if euthanasia by physicians became common, patients would come to fear that a medication was intended not to treat or care, but instead to kill, and would thus lose trust in their physicians. This position was forcefully stated in a paper by Willard Gaylin and his colleagues:

> The very soul of medicine is on trial. . . . This issue touches medicine at its moral center; if this moral center collapses, if physicians become killers or are even licensed to kill, the profession—and, therewith, each physician—will never again be worthy of trust and respect as healer and comforter and protector of life in all its frailty.

These authors go on to make clear that, while they oppose permitting anyone to perform euthanasia, their special concern is with physicians doing so:

> We call on fellow physicians to say that they will not deliberately kill. We must also say to each of our fellow physicians that we will not tolerate killing of patients and that we shall take disciplinary action against doctors who kill. And we must say to the broader community that if it insists on tolerating or legalizing active euthanasia, it will have to find non-physicians to do its killing.[1]

If permitting physicians to kill would undermine the very "moral center" of medicine, then almost certainly physicians should not be permitted to perform euthanasia. But how persuasive is this claim? Patients should not fear, as a consequence of

permitting *voluntary* active euthanasia, that their physicians will substitute a lethal injection for what patients want and believe is part of their care. If active euthanasia is restricted to cases in which it is truly voluntary, then no patient should fear getting it unless she or he has voluntarily requested it. (The fear that we might in time also come to accept non-voluntary, or even involuntary, active euthanasia is a slippery slope worry I address [in a later section].) Patients' trust of their physicians could be increased, not eroded, by knowledge that physicians will provide aid in dying when patients seek it.

Might Gaylin and his colleagues nevertheless be correct in their claim that the moral center of medicine would collapse if physicians were to become killers? This question raises what at the deepest level should be the guiding aims of medicine, a question that obviously cannot be fully explored here. But I do want to say enough to indicate the direction that I believe an appropriate response to this challenge should take. In spelling out above what I called the positive argument for voluntary active euthanasia, I suggested that two principal values—respecting patients' self-determination and promoting their well-being—underlie the consensus that competent patients, or the surrogates of incompetent patients, are entitled to refuse any life-sustaining treatment and to choose from among available alternative treatments. It is the commitment to these two values in guiding physicians' actions as healers, comforters, and protectors of their patients' lives that should be at the "moral center" of medicine, and these two values support physicians' administering euthanasia when their patients make competent requests for it.

What should not be at that moral center is a commitment to preserving patients' lives as such, without regard to whether those patients want their lives preserved or judge their preservation a benefit to them. . . .

REFERENCE

1 Willard Gaylin, Leon R. Kass, Edmund D. Pellegrino, and Mark Siegler, "Doctors Must Not Kill," *JAMA* 259 (1988): 2139–40.

THE SUPREME COURT, PHYSICIAN-ASSISTED SUICIDE, AND TERMINAL SEDATION

OPINION OF THE COURT IN *WASHINGTON V. GLUCKSBERG*
Chief Justice William H. Rehnquist

At issue in this case is the constitutionality of the State of Washington's ban on assisted suicide—in particular, whether it violates the Due Process Clause of the Fourteenth Amendment. Although the Supreme Court unanimously upholds Washington's assisted-suicide ban, the fact that this case has produced five separate concurring opinions indicates that the Court remains fragmented on the most appropriate way of constructing the underlying issues. Chief Justice Rehnquist, in this opinion joined by four other justices, rejects the contention (asserted by the Ninth Circuit Court of Appeals) that a competent, terminally ill adult can claim a constitutionally protected right to physician assistance in suicide. On his analysis, no such liberty interest is protected by the Due Process Clause of the Fourteenth Amendment; thus, no basis exists for a fundamental-right claim. It follows, he argues, that the constitutionality of Washington's assisted-suicide ban can be established merely by showing that the ban is rationally related to legitimate government interests. In order to display how this requirement is clearly met, the Chief Justice identifies and discusses the relevant state interests.

The question presented in this case is whether Washington's prohibition against "caus[ing]" or "aid[ing]" a suicide offends the Fourteenth Amendment to the United States Constitution. We hold that it does not.

It has always been a crime to assist a suicide in the State of Washington. In 1854, Washington's first Territorial Legislature outlawed "assisting another in the commission of self-murder." Today, Washington law provides: "A person is guilty of promoting a suicide attempt when he knowingly causes or aids another person to attempt suicide." Wash. Rev. Code 9A.36.060(1) (1994). "Promoting a suicide attempt" is a felony, punishable by up to five years' imprisonment and up to a $10,000 fine. At the same time, Washington's Natural Death Act, enacted in 1979, states that the "withholding or withdrawal of life-sustaining treatment" at a patient's direction "shall not, for any purpose, constitute a suicide."

Petitioners in this case are the State of Washington and its Attorney General. Respondents Harold Glucksberg, M.D., Abigail Halperin, M.D., Thomas A. Preston, M.D., and Peter Shalit, M.D.,

United States Supreme Court. 521 U.S. 702 (1997).

are physicians who practice in Washington. These doctors occasionally treat terminally ill, suffering patients, and declare that they would assist these patients in ending their lives if not for Washington's assisted-suicide ban. In January 1994, respondents, along with three gravely ill, pseudonymous plaintiffs who have since died and Compassion in Dying, a nonprofit organization that counsels people considering physician-assisted suicide, sued in the United States District Court, seeking a declaration that Wash. Rev. Code 9A.36.060(1) (1994) is, on its face, unconstitutional. *Compassion in Dying v. Washington* (WD Wash. 1994).

The plaintiffs asserted "the existence of a liberty interest protected by the Fourteenth Amendment which extends to a personal choice by a mentally competent, terminally ill adult to commit physician-assisted suicide." Relying primarily on *Planned Parenthood v. Casey* (1992) and *Cruzan v. Director, Missouri Dept. of Health* (1990), the District Court agreed and concluded that Washington's assisted-suicide ban is unconstitutional because it "places an undue burden on the exercise of [that] constitutionally protected liberty interest." The District Court also decided that the Washington statute violated the Equal Protection Clause's requirement that "'all persons similarly situated . . . be treated alike.'"

A panel of the Court of Appeals for the Ninth Circuit reversed, emphasizing that "[i]n the two hundred and five years of our existence no constitutional right to aid in killing oneself has ever been asserted and upheld by a court of final jurisdiction." *Compassion in Dying v. Washington* (1995). The Ninth Circuit reheard the case en banc, reversed the panel's decision, and affirmed the District Court. *Compassion in Dying v. Washington* (1996). Like the District Court, the en banc Court of Appeals emphasized our *Casey* and *Cruzan* decisions. The court also discussed what is described as "historical" and "current societal attitudes" toward suicide and assisted suicide, and concluded that "the Constitution encompasses a due process liberty interest in controlling the time and manner of one's death—that there is, in short, a constitutionally-recognized 'right to die.'" After "[w]eighing and then balancing" this interest against Washington's various interests, the court held that the State's assisted-suicide ban was unconstitutional "as applied to terminally ill competent adults who wish to hasten their deaths with medication prescribed by their physicians." The court did not reach the District Court's equal-protection holding. We granted certiorari and now reverse.

I

We begin, as we do in all due-process cases, by examining our Nation's history, legal traditions, and practices. In almost every State—indeed, in almost every western democracy—it is a crime to assist a suicide. The States' assisted-suicide bans are not innovations. Rather, they are longstanding expressions of the States' commitment to the protection and preservation of all human life. Indeed, opposition to and condemnation of suicide—and, therefore, of assisting suicide—are consistent and enduring themes of our philosophical, legal, and cultural heritages.

More specifically, for over 700 years, the Anglo-American common-law tradition has punished or otherwise disapproved of both suicide and assisting suicide. . . .

For the most part, the early American colonies adopted the common-law approach. . . . [For example,] Virginia . . . required ignominious burial for suicides, and their estates were forfeit to the crown.

Over time, however, the American colonies abolished these harsh common-law penalties. . . . [H]owever, . . . the movement away from the common law's harsh sanctions did not represent an acceptance of suicide; rather, . . . this change reflected the growing consensus that it was unfair to punish the suicide's family for his wrongdoing. . . . [C]ourts continued to condemn [suicide] as a grave public wrong.

That suicide remained a grievous, though nonfelonious, wrong is confirmed by the fact that colonial and early state legislatures and courts did not retreat from prohibiting assisting suicide. . . . And the prohibitions against assisting suicide never contained exceptions for those who were near death. . . .

The earliest American statute explicitly to outlaw assisting suicide was enacted in New York in 1828. . . . By the time the Fourteenth Amendment was ratified, it was a crime in most States to assist a suicide. . . .

Though deeply rooted, the States' assisted-suicide bans have in recent years been reexamined and, generally, reaffirmed. Because of advances in medicine and technology, Americans today are increasingly likely to die in institutions, from chronic illnesses. Public concern and democratic action are therefore sharply focused on how best to protect dignity and independence at the end of life, with the result that there have been many significant changes in state laws and in the attitudes these laws reflect. Many States, for example, now permit "living wills," surrogate health-care decisionmaking, and the withdrawal or refusal of life-sustaining medical treatment. At the same time, however, voters and legislators continue for the most part to reaffirm their States' prohibitions on assisting suicide. . . .

. . . Against this backdrop of history, tradition, and practice, we now turn to respondents' constitutional claim.

II

The Due Process Clause guarantees more than fair process, and the "liberty" it protects includes more than the absence of physical restraint. The Clause also provides heightened protection against government interference with certain fundamental rights and liberty interests. In a long line of cases, we have held that, in addition to the specific freedoms protected by the Bill of Rights, the "liberty" specially protected by the Due Process Clause includes the rights to marry, to have children, to direct the education and upbringing of one's children, to marital privacy, to use contraception, to bodily integrity, and to abortion. We have also assumed, and strongly suggested, that the Due Process Clause protects the traditional right to refuse unwanted lifesaving medical treatment.

But we "ha[ve] always been reluctant to expand the concept of substantive due process because guideposts for responsible decisionmaking in this unchartered area are scarce and open-ended." By extending constitutional protection to an asserted right or liberty interest, we, to a great extent, place the matter outside the arena of public debate and legislative action. We must therefore "exercise the utmost care whenever we are asked to break new ground in this field," lest the liberty protected by the Due Process Clause be subtly transformed into the policy preferences of the members of this Court.

Our established method of substantive-due-process analysis has two primary features: First, we have regularly observed that the Due Process Clause specially protects those fundamental rights and liberties which are, objectively, "deeply rooted in this Nation's history and tradition" and "implicit in the concept of ordered liberty," such that "neither liberty nor justice would exist if they were sacrificed." Second, we have required in substantive-due-process cases a "careful description" of the asserted fundamental liberty interest. Our Nation's history, legal traditions, and practices thus provide the crucial "guideposts for responsible decisionmaking" that direct and restrain our exposition of the Due Process Clause. As we stated recently . . . , the Fourteenth Amendment "forbids the government to infringe . . . 'fundamental' liberty interests *at all,* no matter what process is provided, unless the infringement is narrowly tailored to serve a compelling state interest." . . .

Turning to the claim at issue here, the Court of Appeals stated that "[p]roperly analyzed, the first issue to be resolved is whether there is a liberty interest in determining the time and manner of one's death," or, in other words, "[i]s there a right to die?"

Similarly, respondents assert a "liberty to choose how to die" and a right to "control of one's final days," and describe the asserted liberty as "the right to choose a humane, dignified death" and "the liberty to shape death." As noted above, we have a tradition of carefully formulating the interest at stake in substantive-due-process cases. For example, although *Cruzan* is often described as a "right to die" case, we were, in fact, more precise: we assumed that the Constitution granted competent persons a "constitutionally protected right to refuse lifesaving hydration and nutrition." The Washington statute at issue in this case prohibits "aid[ing] another person to attempt suicide," Wash. Rev. Code §9A.36.060(1) (1994), and, thus, the question before us is whether the "liberty" specially protected by the Due Process Clause includes a right to commit suicide which itself includes a right to assistance in doing so.

We now inquire whether this asserted right has any place in our Nation's traditions. Here, as discussed above, we are confronted with a consistent and almost universal tradition that has long rejected the asserted right, and continues explicitly to reject it today, even for terminally ill, mentally competent adults. To hold for respondents, we would have to reverse centuries of legal doctrine and practice, and strike down the considered policy choice of almost every State.

Respondents contend, however, that the liberty interest they assert *is* consistent with this Court's substantive-due-process line of cases, if not with this Nation's history and practice. Pointing to *Casey* and *Cruzan,* respondents read our jurisprudence in this area as reflecting a general tradition of "self-sovereignty" and as teaching that the "liberty" protected by the Due Process Clause includes "basic and intimate exercises of personal autonomy." According to respondents, our liberty jurisprudence, and the broad, individualistic principles it reflects, protects the "liberty of competent, terminally ill adults to make end-of-life decisions free of undue government interference." The question presented in this case, however, is whether the protections of the Due Process Clause include a right to commit suicide with another's assistance. With this "careful description" of respondents' claim in mind, we turn to *Casey* and *Cruzan.*

In *Cruzan,* we considered whether Nancy Beth Cruzan, who had been severely injured in an automobile accident and was in a persistive vegetative state, "ha[d] a right under the United States Constitution which would require the hospital to withdraw life-sustaining treatment" at her parents' request. We began with the observation that "[a]t common law, even the touching of one person by another without consent and without legal justification was a battery." We then discussed the related rule that "informed consent is generally required for medical treatment." After reviewing a long line of relevant state cases, we concluded that "the common-law doctrine of informed consent is viewed as generally encompassing the right of a competent individual to refuse medical treatment." Next, we reviewed our own cases on the subject, and stated that "[t]he principle that a competent person has a constitutionally protected liberty interest in refusing unwanted medical treatment may be inferred from our prior decisions." Therefore, "for purposes of [that] case, we assume[d] that the United States Constitution would grant a competent person a constitutionally protected right to refuse lifesaving hydration and nutrition." We concluded that, notwithstanding this right, the Constitution permitted Missouri to require clear and convincing evidence of an incompetent patient's wishes concerning the withdrawal of life-sustaining treatment.

Respondents contend that in *Cruzan* we "acknowledged that competent, dying persons have the right to direct the removal of life-sustaining medical treatment and thus hasten death," and that "the constitutional principle behind recognizing the patient's liberty to direct the withdrawal of artificial life support applies at least as strongly to the choice to hasten impending death by consuming lethal medication." Similarly, the Court of Appeals concluded that "*Cruzan,* by recognizing a liberty interest that includes the refusal of artificial provision of life-sustaining food and water, necessarily recognize[d] a liberty interest in hastening one's own death."

The right assumed in *Cruzan,* however, was not simply deduced from abstract concepts of personal autonomy. Given the common-law rule that forced medication was a battery, and the long legal tradition protecting the decision to refuse unwanted medical treatment, our assumption was entirely consistent with this Nation's history and constitutional traditions. The decision to commit suicide with the assistance of another may be just as personal and profound as the decision to refuse unwanted medical treatment, but it has never enjoyed similar legal protection. Indeed, the two acts are widely and reasonably regarded as quite distinct. See *Quill v. Vacco* (1997). In *Cruzan* itself, we recognized that most States outlawed assisted suicide—and even more do today—and we certainly gave no intimation that the right to refuse unwanted medical treatment could be somehow transmuted into a right to assistance in committing suicide.

Respondents also rely on *Casey.* There, the Court's opinion concluded that "the essential holding of *Roe v. Wade* should be retained and once again reaffirmed." We held, first, that a woman has a right, before her fetus is viable, to an abortion "without undue interference from the State"; second, that States may restrict post-viability abortions, so long as exceptions are made to protect a woman's life and health; and third, that the State has legitimate interests throughout a pregnancy in protecting the health of the woman and the life of the unborn child. In reaching this conclusion, the opinion discussed in some detail this Court's substantive-due-process tradition of interpreting the Due Process Clause to protect certain fundamental rights and "personal decisions relating to marriage, procreation, contraception, family relationships, child rearing, and education," and noted that many of those rights and liberties "involv[e] the most intimate and personal choices a person may make in a lifetime."

The Court of Appeals, like the District Court, found *Casey* " 'highly instructive' " and " 'almost prescriptive' " for determining " 'what liberty interest may inhere in a terminally ill person's choice to commit suicide' ":

> Like the decision of whether or not to have an abortion, the decision how and when to die is one of "the most intimate and personal choices a person may make in a lifetime," a choice "central to personal dignity and autonomy."

. . . That many of the rights and liberties protected by the Due Process Clause sound in personal autonomy does not warrant the sweeping conclusion that any and all important, intimate, and personal decisions are so protected, and *Casey* did not suggest otherwise.

The history of the law's treatment of assisted suicide in this country has been and continues to be one of the rejection of nearly all efforts to permit it. That being the case, our decisions lead us to conclude that the asserted "right" to assistance in committing suicide is not a fundamental liberty interest protected by the Due Process Clause. The Constitution also requires, however, that Washington's assisted-suicide ban be rationally related to legitimate government interests. This requirement is unquestionably met here. As the court below recognized, Washington's assisted-suicide ban implicates a number of state interests.

First, Washington has an "unqualified interest in the preservation of human life." The State's prohibition on assisted suicide, like all homicide laws, both reflects and advances its commitment to this interest. This interest is symbolic and aspirational as well as practical:

> While suicide is no longer prohibited or penalized, the ban against assisted suicide and euthanasia shores up the notion of limits in human relationships. It reflects the gravity with which we view the decision to take one's own life or the life of another, and our reluctance to encourage or promote these decisions. New York State Task Force on Life and the Law, When Death is Sought: Assisted Suicide and Euthanasia in the Medical Context 131–132 (May 1994) (hereinafter New York Task Force).

Respondents admit that "[t]he State has a real interest in preserving the lives of those who can still contribute to society and enjoy life." The Court of Appeals also recognized Washington's interest in protecting life, but held that the "weight" of this interest depends on the "medical condition and the wishes of the person whose life is at stake." Washington, however, has rejected this sliding-scale approach and, through its assisted-suicide ban, insists that all persons' lives, from beginning to end, regardless of physical or mental condition, are under the full protection of the law. As we have previously

affirmed, the States "may properly decline to make judgments about the 'quality' of life that a particular individual may enjoy." This remains true, as *Cruzan* makes clear, even for those who are near death.

Relatedly, all admit that suicide is a serious public-health problem, especially among persons in otherwise vulnerable groups. The State has an interest in preventing suicide, and in studying, identifying, and treating its causes.

Those who attempt suicide—terminally ill or not—often suffer from depression or other mental disorders. See New York Task Force 13–22, 126–128 (more than 95% of those who commit suicide had a major psychiatric illness at the time of death; among the terminally ill, uncontrolled pain is a "risk factor" because it contributes to depression). Research indicates ... that many people who request physician-assisted suicide withdraw that request if their depression and pain are treated. The New York Task Force, however, expressed its concern that, because depression is difficult to diagnose, physicians and medical professionals often fail to respond adequately to seriously ill patients' needs. Thus, legal physician-assisted suicide could make it more difficult for the State to protect depressed or mentally ill persons, or those who are suffering from untreated pain, from suicidal impulses.

The State also has an interest in protecting the integrity and ethics of the medical profession. In contrast to the Court of Appeals' conclusion that "the integrity of the medical profession would [not] be threatened in any way by [physician-assisted suicide]," the American Medical Association, like many other medical and physicians' groups, has concluded that "[p]hysician-assisted suicide is fundamentally incompatible with the physician's role as healer." American Medical Association, Code of Ethics §2.211 (1994). And physician-assisted suicide could, it is argued, undermine the trust that is essential to the doctor-patient relationship by blurring the time-honored line between healing and harming.

Next, the State has an interest in protecting vulnerable groups—including the poor, the elderly, and disabled persons—from abuse, neglect, and mistakes. The Court of Appeals dismissed the State's concern that disadvantaged persons might be pressured into physician-assisted suicide as "ludicrous on its face." We have recognized, however, the real risk of subtle coercion and undue influence in end-of-life situations. Similarly, the New York Task Force warned that "[l]egalizing physician-assisted suicide would pose profound risks to many individuals who are ill and vulnerable. . . . The risk of harm is greatest for the many individuals in our society whose autonomy and well-being are already compromised by poverty, lack of access to good medical care, advanced age, or membership in a stigmatized social group." New York Task Force 120. If physician-assisted suicide were permitted, many might resort to it to spare their families the substantial financial burden of end-of-life health-care costs.

The State's interest here goes beyond protecting the vulnerable from coercion; it extends to protecting disabled and terminally ill people from prejudice, negative and inaccurate stereotypes, and "societal indifference." The State's assisted-suicide ban reflects and reinforces its policy that the lives of terminally ill, disabled, and elderly people must be no less valued than the lives of the young and healthy, and that a seriously disabled person's suicidal impulses should be interpreted and treated the same way as anyone else's.

Finally, the State may fear that permitting assisted suicide will start it down the path to voluntary and perhaps even involuntary euthanasia. The Court of Appeals struck down Washington's assisted-suicide ban only "as applied to competent, terminally ill adults who wish to hasten their deaths by obtaining medication prescribed by their doctors." Washington insists, however, that the impact of the court's decision will not and cannot be so limited. If suicide is protected as a matter of constitutional right, it is argued, "every man and woman in the United States must enjoy it." The Court of Appeals' decision, and its expansive reasoning, provide ample support for the State's concerns. The court noted, for example, that the "decision of a duly appointed surrogate decision maker is for all legal purposes the decision of the patient himself," that "in some instances, the patient may be unable to self-administer the drugs and . . . administration by the physician . . . may be the only way the patient may be able to receive them," and that not only physicians, but also family members and loved ones, will inevitably participate in assisting suicide. Thus, it turns out that what is couched as a limited right to "physician-assisted suicide" is likely, in effect, a much broader license, which could prove extremely difficult to police and contain. Washington's ban on assisting suicide prevents such erosion. . . .

We need not weigh exactly the relative strengths of these various interests. They are unquestionably important and legitimate, and Washington's ban on assisted suicide is at least reasonably related to their promotion and protection. We therefore hold that Wash. Rev. Code §9A.36.060(1) (1994) does not violate the Fourteenth Amendment, either on its face or "as applied to competent, terminally ill adults who wish to hasten their deaths by obtaining medication prescribed by their doctors."

Throughout the Nation, Americans are engaged in an earnest and profound debate about the morality, legality, and practicality of physician-assisted suicide. Our holding permits this debate to continue, as it should in a democratic society. The decision of the en banc Court of Appeals is reversed. . . .

OPINION OF THE COURT IN *VACCO V. QUILL*

Chief Justice William H. Rehnquist

The issue raised by this case is whether the State of New York's ban on assisted suicide violates the Equal Protection Clause of the Fourteenth Amendment. Although the Supreme Court unanimously holds that New York's assisted-suicide ban does not violate the Equal Protection Clause, the fact that this case—like its companion case, *Washington v. Glucksberg* (1997)—has spawned multiple concurring opinions indicates that the Court remains fragmented on the most appropriate way of constructing the underlying issues. Chief Justice Rehnquist, in this opinion joined by four other justices, insists that it is "both important and logical" to draw a distinction between assisting suicide and withdrawing life-sustaining treatment. Thus, in his view, there is no basis for the contention (asserted by the Second Circuit Court of Appeals) that New York law—by prohibiting assisted suicide yet allowing the withdrawal of life-sustaining treatment—fails to "treat equally all competent persons who are in the final stages of fatal illness and wish to hasten their own deaths."

In New York, as in most States, it is a crime to aid another to commit or attempt suicide, but patients may refuse even lifesaving medical treatment. The question presented by this case is whether New York's prohibition on assisting suicide therefore violates the Equal Protection Clause of the Fourteenth Amendment. We hold that it does not.

Petitioners are various New York public officials. Respondents Timothy E. Quill, Samuel C. Klagsbrun, and Howard A. Grossman are physicians who practice in New York. They assert that although it would be "consistent with the standards of [their] medical practice[s]" to prescribe lethal medication for "mentally competent, terminally ill patients" who are suffering great pain and desire a doctor's help in taking their own lives, they are deterred from doing so by New York's ban on assisting suicide. Respondents, and three gravely ill patients who have since died, sued the State's Attorney General in the United States District Court. They urged that because New York permits a competent person to refuse life-sustaining medical treatment, and because the refusal of such treatment is "essentially the same thing" as physician-assisted suicide, New York's assisted-suicide ban violates the Equal Protection Clause.

The District Court disagreed: "[I]t is hardly unreasonable or irrational for the State to recognize a difference between allowing nature to take its course, even in the most severe situations, and intentionally using an artificial death-producing device." The court noted New York's "obvious legitimate interests in preserving life, and in protecting vulnerable persons,"

United States Supreme Court. 521 U.S. 793 (1997).

and concluded that "[u]nder the United States Constitution and the federal system it establishes, the resolution of this issue is left to the normal democratic processes within the State."

The Court of Appeals for the Second Circuit reversed. The court determined that, despite the assisted-suicide ban's apparent general applicability, "New York law does not treat equally all competent persons who are in the final stages of fatal illness and wish to hasten their deaths," because "those in the final stages of terminal illness who are on life-support systems are allowed to hasten their deaths by directing the removal of such systems; but those who are similarly situated, except for the previous attachment of life-sustaining equipment, are not allowed to hasten death by self-administering prescribed drugs." In the court's view, "[t]he ending of life by [the withdrawal of life-support systems] is *nothing more nor less than assisted suicide*" (emphasis added). The Court of Appeals then examined whether this supposed unequal treatment was rationally related to any legitimate state interest, and concluded that "to the extent that [New York's statutes] prohibit a physician from prescribing medications to be self-administered by a mentally competent, terminally-ill person in the final stages of his terminal illness, they are not rationally related to any legitimate state interest." We granted certiorari and now reverse.

The Equal Protection Clause commands that no State shall "deny to any person within its jurisdiction the equal protection of the laws." This provision creates no substantive rights. Instead, it embodies a general rule that States must treat like cases alike but may treat unlike cases accordingly. If a legislative classification or distinction "neither burdens a fundamental right nor targets a suspect class, we will uphold [it] so long as it bears a rational relation to some legitimate end."

New York's statutes outlawing assisting suicide affect and address matters of profound significance to all New Yorkers alike. They neither infringe fundamental rights nor involve suspect classifications. These laws are therefore entitled to a "strong presumption of validity."

On their faces, neither New York's ban on assisting suicide nor its statutes permitting patients to refuse medical treatment treat anyone differently than anyone else or draw any distinctions between persons. *Everyone,* regardless of physical condition, is entitled, if competent, to refuse unwanted lifesaving medical treatment; *no one* is permitted to assist a suicide. Generally speaking, laws that apply even-handedly to all "unquestionably comply" with the Equal Protection Clause.

The Court of Appeals, however, concluded that some terminally ill people—those who are on life-support systems—are treated differently than those who are not, in that the former may "hasten death" by ending treatment, but the latter may not "hasten death" through physician-assisted suicide. This conclusion depends on the submission that ending or refusing lifesaving medical treatment "is nothing more nor less than assisted suicide." Unlike the Court of Appeals, we think the distinction between assisting suicide and withdrawing life-sustaining treatment, a distinction widely recognized and endorsed in the medical profession and in our legal traditions, is both important and logical; it is certainly rational. ("When the basic classification is rationally based, uneven effects upon particular groups within a class are ordinarily of no constitutional concern.")

The distinction comports with fundamental legal principles of causation and intent. First, when a patient refuses life-sustaining medical treatment, he dies from an underlying fatal disease or pathology; but if a patient ingests lethal medication prescribed by a physician, he is killed by that medication.

Furthermore, a physician who withdraws, or honors a patient's refusal to begin, life-sustaining medical treatment purposefully intends, or may so intend, only to respect his patient's wishes and "to cease doing useless and futile or degrading things to the patient when [the patient] no longer stands to benefit from them." Assisted Suicide in the United States, Hearing before the Subcommittee on the Constitution of the House Committee on the Judiciary, 104th Cong., 2d Sess., 368 (1996) (testimony of Dr. Leon R. Kass). The same is true when a doctor provides aggressive palliative care; in some cases, painkilling drugs may hasten a patient's death, but the physician's purpose and intent is, or may be, only to ease his patient's pain. A doctor who assists a suicide, however, "must, necessarily and indubitably, intend primarily that the patient be made dead." *Id.,* at 367. Similarly, a patient who commits suicide with a doctor's aid necessarily has the specific intent to end his or her own life, while a patient who refuses or discontinues treatment might not.

The law has long used actors' intent or purpose to distinguish between two acts that may have the same result. Put differently, the law distinguishes actions taken "because of" a given end from actions taken "in spite of" their unintended but foreseen consequences. ("When General Eisenhower ordered American soldiers onto the beaches of Normandy, he knew that he was sending many American soldiers to certain death. . . . His purpose, though, was to . . . liberate Europe from the Nazis.")

Given these general principles, it is not surprising that many courts, including New York courts, have carefully distinguished refusing life-sustaining treatment from suicide. . . .

Similarly, the overwhelming majority of state legislatures have drawn a clear line between assisting suicide and withdrawing or permitting the refusal of unwanted lifesaving medical treatment by prohibiting the former and permitting the latter. And "nearly all states expressly disapprove of suicide and assisted suicide either in statutes dealing with durable powers of attorney in health-care situations, or in 'living will' statutes." Thus, even as the States move to protect and promote patients' dignity at the end of life, they remain opposed to physician-assisted suicide.

New York is a case in point. The State enacted its current assisted-suicide statutes in 1965.[1] Since then, New York has acted several times to protect patients' common-law right to refuse treatment. In so doing, however, the State has neither endorsed a general right to "hasten death" nor approved physician-assisted suicide. Quite the opposite: The State has reaffirmed the line between "killing" and "letting die." More recently, the New York State Task Force on Life and the Law studied assisted suicide and euthanasia and, in 1994, unanimously recommended against legalization. When Death is Sought: Assisted Suicide and Euthanasia in the Medical Context vii (1994). In the Task Force's view, "allowing decisions to forego life-sustaining treatment and allowing assisted suicide or euthanasia have radically different consequences and meanings for public policy." *Id.,* at 146.

This Court has also recognized, at least implicitly, the distinction between letting a patient die and making that patient die. In *Cruzan v. Director, Mo. Dept. of Health* (1990), we concluded that "[t]he principle that a competent person has a constitutionally protected liberty interest in refusing unwanted medical treatment may be inferred from our prior decisions," and we assumed the existence of such a right for purposes of that case. But our assumption of a right to refuse treatment was grounded not, as the Court of Appeals supposed, on the proposition that patients have a general and abstract "right to hasten death," but on well established, traditional rights to bodily integrity and freedom from unwanted touching. In fact, we observed that "the majority of States in this country have laws imposing criminal penalties on one who assists another to commit suicide." *Cruzan* therefore provides no support for the notion that refusing life-sustaining medical treatment is "nothing more nor less than suicide."

For all these reasons, we disagree with respondents' claim that the distinction between refusing lifesaving medical treatment and assisted suicide is "arbitrary" and "irrational."[2] Granted, in some cases, the line between the two may not be clear, but certainty is not required, even were it possible. Logic and contemporary practice support New

York's judgment that the two acts are different, and New York may therefore, consistent with the Constitution, treat them differently. By permitting everyone to refuse unwanted medical treatment while prohibiting anyone from assisting a suicide, New York law follows a longstanding and rational distinction.

New York's reasons for recognizing and acting on this distinction—including prohibiting intentional killing and preserving life; preventing suicide; maintaining physicians' role as their patients' healers; protecting vulnerable people from indifference, prejudice, and psychological and financial pressure to end their lives; and avoiding a possible slide towards euthanasia—are discussed in greater detail in our opinion in *Glucksberg, ante.* These valid and important public interests easily satisfy the constitutional requirement that a legislative classification bear a rational relation to some legitimate end.

The judgment of the Court of Appeals is reversed. . . .

NOTES

1 It has always been a crime, either by statute or under the common law, to assist a suicide in New York.

2 Respondents also argue that the State irrationally distinguishes between physician-assisted suicide and "terminal sedation," a process respondents characterize as "induc[ing] barbiturate coma and then starv[ing] the person to death." Petitioners insist, however, that "'[a]lthough proponents of physician-assisted suicide and euthanasia contend that terminal sedation is covert physician-assisted suicide or euthanasia, the concept of sedating pharmacotherapy is based on informed consent and the principle of double effect.'" Reply Brief for Petitioners 12 (quoting P. Rousseau, Terminal Sedation in the Care of Dying Patients, 156 Archives Internal Med. 1785, 1785–1786 ([1996]). Just as a State may prohibit assisting suicide while permitting patients to refuse unwanted lifesaving treatment, it may permit palliative care related to that refusal, which may have the foreseen but unintended "double effect" of hastening the patient's death. See New York Task Force, "When Death is Sought," at 163 ("It is widely recognized that the provision of pain medication is ethically and professionally acceptable even when the treatment may hasten the patient's death, if the medication is intended to alleviate pain and severe discomfort, not to cause death").

CONCURRING OPINION IN *WASHINGTON V. GLUCKSBERG* AND *VACCO V. QUILL*

Justice Sandra Day O'Connor

In this concurring opinion, Justice O'Connor emphasizes that in both Washington and New York there are presently no legal barriers to terminally ill patients' obtaining adequate pain-relieving medication, "even to the point of causing unconsciousness and hastening death." If terminally ill patients did not, in fact, have access to such palliative care, she seems to suggest, there might be grounds for a different conclusion regarding physician-assisted suicide.

Death will be different for each of us. For many, the last days will be spent in physical pain and perhaps the despair that accompanies physical deterioration and a loss of control of basic bodily and mental functions. Some will seek medication to alleviate that pain and other symptoms.

The Court frames the issue in *Washington v. Glucksberg* as whether the Due Process Clause of the Constitution protects a "right to commit suicide which itself includes a right to assistance in doing so," and concludes that our Nation's history, legal traditions, and practices do not support the existence of such a right. I join the Court's opinions because I agree that there is no generalized right to "commit suicide." But respondents urge us to address the narrower question whether a mentally competent person who is experiencing great suffering has a constitutionally cognizable interest in controlling the circumstances of his or her imminent death. I see no need to reach that question in the context of the facial challenges to the New York and Washington laws at issue here. ("The Washington statute at issue in this case prohibits 'aid[ing] another person to attempt suicide,' . . . and, thus, the question before us is whether the 'liberty' specially protected by the Due Process Clause includes a right to commit suicide which itself includes a right to assistance in doing so"). The parties and *amici* agree that in these States a patient who is suffering from a terminal illness and who is experiencing great pain has no legal barriers to obtaining medication, from qualified physicians, to alleviate that suffering, even to the point of causing unconsciousness and hastening death. In this light, even assuming that we would recognize such an interest, I agree that the State's interests in protecting those who are not truly competent or facing imminent death, or those whose decisions to hasten death would not truly be voluntary, are sufficiently weighty to justify a prohibition against physician-assisted suicide.

Every one of us at some point may be affected by our own or a family member's terminal illness. There is no reason to think the democratic process will not strike the proper balance between the interests of terminally ill, mentally competent individuals who would seek to end their suffering and the State's interests in protecting those who might seek to end life mistakenly or under pressure. As the Court recognizes, States are presently undertaking extensive and serious evaluation of physician-assisted suicide and other related issues. In such circumstances, "the . . . challenging task of crafting appropriate procedures for safeguarding . . . liberty interests is entrusted to the 'laboratory' of the States . . . in the first instance."

In sum, there is no need to address the question whether suffering patients have a constitutionally cognizable interest in obtaining relief from the suffering that they may experience in the last days of their lives. There is no dispute that dying patients in Washington and New York can obtain palliative care, even when doing so would hasten their deaths. The difficulty in defining terminal illness and the risk that a dying patient's request for assistance in ending his or her life might not be truly voluntary justifies the prohibitions on assisted suicide we uphold here.

United States Supreme Court. 521 U.S. 702 (1997).

THE SUPREME COURT AND PHYSICIAN-ASSISTED SUICIDE: REJECTING ASSISTED SUICIDE BUT EMBRACING EUTHANASIA

David Orentlicher

Orentlicher analyzes the Supreme Court opinions on physician-assisted suicide in reference to the practice of *terminal sedation*. In Orentlicher's view, terminal sedation is often a form of euthanasia. Thus, he argues that the Court's acceptance of terminal sedation undermines the most important arguments against the legalization of assisted suicide. Moreover, Orentlicher contends, assisted suicide is ethically less problematic than terminal sedation.

In rejecting a constitutional right to physician-assisted suicide earlier this year,[1,2] the U.S. Supreme Court appeared to preserve the distinction between the withdrawal of life-sustaining treatment and assisted suicide or euthanasia. In fact, however, the Court undermined the distinction when it endorsed terminal sedation. Terminal sedation seems consistent with traditional medical care but often is a form of euthanasia. Moreover, it is a practice that is ethically more problematic than assisted suicide or voluntary euthanasia.

THE SUPREME COURT'S OPINIONS

In deciding against a right to assisted suicide, the Court faced the claim that such a right is necessary for some patients to ensure that they can avoid intolerable pain in their final days. Although physical pain is almost always treatable, some pain cannot be relieved by analgesia. In response to this concern, hospice providers and other medical professionals assured the Court that even the most severe suffering could be alleviated by sedating the patient into unconsciousness. According to the brief of the American Medical Association, for example,

> The pain of most terminally ill patients can be controlled throughout the dying process without heavy sedation or anesthesia. . . . For a very few patients, however, sedation to a sleep-like state may be necessary in the last days or weeks of life to prevent the patient from experiencing severe pain.[3]

Reprinted by permission of the publisher from *The New England Journal of Medicine,* vol. 337 (October 23, 1997), pp. 1236–1239. Copyright © 1997 Massachusetts Medical Society. All rights reserved.

With this assurance from the medical profession, Justices Sandra Day O'Connor, Stephen Breyer, and Ruth Bader Ginsburg wrote in their concurring opinions that the case for a right to assisted suicide had not been made. If a right to assisted suicide turned on the need to relieve the suffering of patients, the alternative of terminal sedation made such a right unnecessary.[1,2]

An important question, then, is whether terminal sedation really is a good alternative to assisted suicide.

TERMINAL SEDATION

At the end of life, terminally ill patients may have intolerable pain, shortness of breath, delirium, or persistent vomiting that is refractory to the usual therapies.[4-7] Intolerable pain may be caused by several conditions, including cancer that has metastasized to the spine, intestinal obstruction, and headache due to massive intracerebral edema.[4] Intolerable shortness of breath can result from several conditions, too, including lung and other cancers, chronic obstructive lung disease, and congestive heart failure.[8] In cases of intolerable and refractory suffering, adequate relief can be obtained only by sedating the patient, often deeply. Although the frequency of intolerable and refractory symptoms is uncertain, studies have found them in 15 to 50 percent of terminally ill patients referred for palliative care.[4,9] With terminal sedation, opioids, benzodiazepines, barbiturates, neuroleptic drugs, or combinations of these agents are used to sedate the patient.[4,10]

The sedation is maintained until the patient dies, usually within a few days, either from the underlying illness or from a second step that is typically part of terminal sedation—the withholding of nutrition and hydration. In most cases, terminal sedation shortens the patient's life by only hours to days, but it may shorten life by as much as several weeks.

At first glance, terminal sedation seems consistent with accepted practices. It is appropriate for physicians to treat the pain and other suffering of patients aggressively, even if doing so is likely to hasten death. On closer examination, however, terminal sedation at times is tantamount to euthanasia, or a kind of "slow euthanasia."[11]

TERMINAL SEDATION AS A FORM OF EUTHANASIA

In many cases, terminal sedation amounts to euthanasia because the sedated patient often dies from the combination of two intentional acts by the physician—the induction of stupor or unconsciousness and the withholding of food and water. Without these two acts, the patient would live longer before succumbing to illness.

It might be argued that death by terminal sedation is morally acceptable because death is due to the withdrawal of nutrition and hydration. As courts have consistently recognized,[12,13] it is ethically and legally permissible for patients to die because life-sustaining treatment has been discontinued.

Although death from dehydration or starvation during terminal sedation resembles death resulting from the withdrawal of treatment, it is in principle more like euthanasia. We permit the withdrawal of life-sustaining treatment while rejecting assisted suicide and euthanasia because, it is argued, the patient dies from the underlying disease, not from the active intervention of the physician.[1,13] A patient in a persistent vegetative state dies after the removal of a feeding tube because the patient's medical condition is responsible for the patient's inability to eat or drink. But this is not what happens in terminal sedation accompanied by the withholding of nutrition and hydration. In such cases, the patient dies from the induced stupor or coma. It is the physician-created state of diminished consciousness that renders the patient unable to eat, not the patient's underlying disease.

We might justify terminal sedation on the grounds that the patient's underlying disease creates the need for the sedation by causing the patient to ask for palliation. But that logic would also justify assisted suicide and euthanasia. In the case of assisted suicide or euthanasia, it is the patient's underlying disease that causes the patient to ask for a life-ending drug.

Proponents of terminal sedation might defend the practice by citing the principle of the double effect. According to that principle, physicians may take steps that might hasten the patient's death as long as the steps constitute a reasonable effort to treat the patient's suffering and the patient's death is not intended.[14] For example, it is permissible to give analgesics or sedatives to alleviate a patient's pain even if the drugs might halt the patient's breathing. However, the principle of the double effect justifies only the sedation that is part of terminal sedation. We cannot justify the withdrawal of food and water during terminal sedation, for that step does nothing to relieve the patient's suffering but only serves to bring about the patient's death. If it is argued that the withdrawal of food and water is a permissible act, then we are back to the previous response that it is permissible only because the patient's inability to eat or drink results from an underlying disease.

Terminal sedation is not only a type of euthanasia; it is also ethically more problematic than either assisted suicide or voluntary euthanasia. Terminal sedation poses the same risks of abuse as assisted suicide or euthanasia. At the same time, it serves fewer of the purposes of right-to-die law.

To see how terminal sedation carries the same risks as assisted suicide or euthanasia, we can consider a twist on the case of Janet Adkins, the woman with early Alzheimer's disease who became the first person to die with Dr. Jack Kevorkian's assistance. Let us assume that Ms. Adkins expressed her despair and her desire to consult Dr. Kevorkian to her personal physician. Suppose, further, that, in response, Ms. Adkins's physician suggested that she consider terminal sedation accompanied by the withholding of nutrition and hydration. If we are troubled by Ms. Adkins's suicide at the hands of Dr. Kevorkian, then we should be equally troubled if she had undergone terminal sedation at the hands of her personal physician. Like assisted suicide or euthanasia, terminal sedation can be provided to people whose illnesses are not yet serious or whose suffering results from a treatable depression. Moreover, like euthanasia, terminal sedation poses a risk of abuse that goes beyond the risks associated with assisted suicide. Assisted suicide requires the active participation of the patient[15]; terminal sedation, however, can be induced without the patient's consent or even the patient's knowledge. Accordingly, any incompetent patient could be terminally sedated.

Terminal sedation also serves fewer of the purposes of right-to-die law than assisted suicide or euthanasia. Although terminal sedation ensures a painless death, it forces patients to accept a dying process that is prolonged as compared with what it would be if assisted suicide or euthanasia were performed. Terminal sedation requires that patients linger in a state that may profoundly compromise their dignity and further distort the memory they leave behind. Terminal sedation also prevents patients from retaining some control over the timing and circumstances of their death, a control that may be critical to their psychological well-being.[16]

Because terminal sedation is often a type of euthanasia, the Court's acceptance of it undermines key objections to the legalization of assisted suicide. Many opponents of assisted suicide concede that it is morally acceptable in some circumstances, as when a person is suffering severe and intractable pain and will die shortly from metastatic cancer. However, these opponents argue, it will not be possible to limit assisted suicide to morally acceptable cases. Once we permit assisted suicide for some persons, we will have no principle that justifies denying it to other persons who claim great suffering.[17,18] Yet, if we can limit terminal sedation to appropriate cases, we can limit assisted suicide in the same way. By whatever criteria physicians use to decide when terminal sedation is appropriate therapy, they can also decide when assisted suicide is appropriate therapy.

The endorsement of terminal sedation undermines another key argument against legalizing assisted suicide. The distinction between the withdrawal of treatment and assisted suicide is often justified on the ground that, in the case of treatment withdrawal, the patient does not intend to die but intends only to be free of a burdensome medical treat-

ment.[2,13] In requesting assisted suicide, it is argued, the patient seeks relief from suffering by choosing a "treatment" that is uniformly fatal. Yet when a patient agrees to deep sedation accompanied by the withholding of nutrition and hydration, the patient also chooses a treatment that is uniformly fatal. If intent is not relevant to terminal sedation, it is also not relevant to assisted suicide.

TERMINAL SEDATION VERSUS ASSISTED SUICIDE

If terminal sedation is essentially euthanasia in many cases, why did three concurring Supreme Court justices endorse the practice, and why did the five-justice majority expressly reject the claim that terminal sedation "is covert physician-assisted suicide"?[2]

The Court's decision suggests that it cares as much about why a patient wishes to die as about how a patient dies. In approving terminal sedation despite the fact that it amounts to euthanasia at times, the Court is essentially saying that the right to die primarily reflects a moral sentiment: that people who are dying and suffering intolerably should be allowed to die even if they cannot do so simply by refusing life-sustaining treatment.[19]

In addition, a right to terminal sedation may be necessary to protect a patient's right to refuse life-sustaining treatment. Without a right to terminal sedation, physicians would have to tell terminally ill patients who are experiencing intolerable and refractory suffering that they could be sedated for relief but that, once sedated, they could no longer have nutrition and hydration withheld or withdrawn. These patients would be forced to choose between obtaining relief from their suffering and retaining their right to refuse life-sustaining treatment. That would be an unfair choice to put to dying patients.

Although we can explain why the Court accepted terminal sedation, we still need to explain why the Court rejected the ethically better alternative of assisted suicide. That decision appears to reflect considerations of symbolism. Although terminal sedation can effectively constitute euthanasia, it looks on the surface like a combination of the accepted practices of aggressive comfort care and withdrawal of treatment. Moreover, in practice, it appears to be limited to appropriate cases. No one is suggesting that physicians are administering terminal sedation to people who are not seriously ill or who really should be treated with psychological counseling and antidepressant drugs. In contrast, many suicides in this country are committed by people who are psychologically depressed but have no serious physical illness. The Court may have been concerned about the message it would send to these people if it permitted assisted suicide for terminally ill persons.

Nevertheless, the Court's deference to symbolic considerations creates its own problems of symbolism; assisted suicide is rejected only by embracing what is essentially euthanasia. Moreover, the symbolic benefits come at a substantial cost to patients. Patients who undergo terminal sedation are required to accept a form of death that may be less desirable for them and that is more vulnerable to abuse.

ACKNOWLEDGMENTS

I am indebted to Judy Failer, Ph.D., John Hansen-Flascben, M.D., and Timothy Quill, M.D., for their contributions.

REFERENCES

1 *Washington v. Glucksberg,* 117 S. Ct. 2258 (1997).
2 *Vacco v. Quill,* 117 S. Ct. 2293 (1997).
3 Brief of the American Medical Association, et al., as *amici curiae* in support of petitioners, at 6, *Washington v. Glucksberg,* 117 S. Ct. 2258 (1997) (No. 96–110).
4 Cherny N. I., Portenoy R. K. Sedation in the management of refractory symptoms: guidelines for evaluation and treatment. J Palliat Care 1994; 10(2):31–8.
5 Quill T. E., Brody R. V. 'You promised me I wouldn't die like this!': a bad death as a medical emergency. Arch Intern Med 1995; 155:1250–4.
6 Greene W. R., Davis W. H. Titrated intravenous barbiturates in the control of symptoms in patients with terminal cancer. South Med J 1991; 84:332–7.
7 Ramani S., Karnad A. B. Long-term subcutaneous infusion of midazolam for refractory delirium in terminal breast cancer. South Med J 1996; 89: 1101–3.
8 Reuben D. B., Mor V. Dyspnea in terminally ill cancer patients. Chest 1986;89:234–6.
9 Enck R. E. The medical care of terminally ill patients. Baltimore: Johns Hopkins University Press, 1994:166–72.
10 Truog R. D., Berde C. B., Mitchell C., Grier H. E. Barbiturates in the care of the terminally ill. N Engl J Med 1992; 327:1678–82.
11 Billings J. A, Block S. D. Slow euthanasia. J Palliat Care 1996; 12(4):21–30.
12 *Cruzan v. Director, Missouri Dept. of Health,* 497 U.S. 261 (1990).
13 *In re Conroy,* 486 A.2d 1209, 1224 (N.J. 1985).
14 Beauchamp T. L., Childress J. F. Principles of biomedical ethics. 4th ed. New York: Oxford University Press, 1994:206–11.
15 Angell M. The Supreme Court and physician-assisted suicide—the ultimate right. N Engl J Med 1997; 336:50–3.
16 Brock DW. Voluntary active euthanasia. Hastings Cent Rep 1992; 22(2):10–22.
17 Callahan D. When self-determination runs amok. Hastings Cent Rep 1992; 22(2):52–5.
18 Kamisar Y. Against assisted suicide—even a very limited form. Univ Detroit Mercy Law Rev 1995; 72:735–69.
19 Orentlicher D. The legalization of physician-assisted suicide. N Engl J Med 1996; 335:663–7.

PHYSICIAN-ASSISTED SUICIDE, ACTIVE EUTHANASIA, AND SOCIAL POLICY

CARE OF THE HOPELESSLY ILL: PROPOSED CLINICAL CRITERIA FOR PHYSICIAN-ASSISTED SUICIDE

Timothy E. Quill, Christine K. Cassel, and Diane E. Meier

The authors oppose the legalization of voluntary (active) euthanasia but endorse the legalization of physician-assisted suicide as "the policy best able to respond to patients' needs and to protect vulnerable people." In an effort to clarify the conditions under which physician-assisted suicide should be permitted, they introduce a set of relevant criteria. In their view, there are six conditions that must be satisfied, and there is also a documentation requirement.

... Although physician-assisted suicide and voluntary euthanasia both involve the active facilitation of a wished-for death, there are several important distinctions between them.[1] In assisted suicide, the final act is solely the patient's, and the risk of subtle coercion from doctors, family members, institutions, or other social forces is greatly reduced.[2] The balance of power between doctor and patient is more nearly equal in physician-assisted suicide than in euthanasia. The physician is counselor and witness and makes the means available, but ultimately the patient must be the one to act or not act. In voluntary euthanasia, the physician both provides the means and carries out the final act, with greatly amplified power over the patient and an increased risk of error, coercion, or abuse.

In view of these distinctions, we conclude that legalization of physician-assisted suicide, but not of voluntary euthanasia, is the policy best able to respond to patients' needs and to protect vulnerable people. From this perspective, physician-assisted suicide forms part of the continuum of options for comfort care, beginning with the forgoing of life-sustaining therapy, including more aggressive symptom-relieving measures, and permitting physician-assisted suicide only if all other alternatives have failed and all criteria have been met. Active voluntary euthanasia is excluded from this continuum because of the risk of abuse it presents. We recognize that this exclusion is made at a cost to competent, incurably ill patients who cannot swallow or move and who therefore cannot be helped to die by assisted suicide. Such persons, who meet agreed-on criteria in other respects, must not be abandoned to their suffering; a combination of decisions to forgo life-sustaining treatments (including food and fluids) with aggressive comfort measures (such as analgesics and sedatives) could be offered, along with a commitment to search for creative alternatives. We acknowledge that this solution is less than ideal, but we also recognize that in the United States access to medical care is currently too inequitable, and many doctor-patient relationships too impersonal, for us to tolerate the risks of permitting

active voluntary euthanasia. We must monitor any change in public policy in this domain to evaluate both its benefits and its burdens.

We propose the following clinical guidelines to contribute to serious discussion about physician-assisted suicide. Although we favor a reconsideration of the legal and professional prohibitions in the case of patients who meet carefully defined criteria, we do not wish to promote an easy or impersonal process.[3] If we are to consider allowing incurably ill patients more control over their deaths, it must be as an expression of our compassion and concern about their ultimate fate after all other alternatives have been exhausted. Such patients should not be held hostage to our reluctance or inability to forge policies in this difficult area.

PROPOSED CLINICAL CRITERIA FOR PHYSICIAN-ASSISTED SUICIDE

Because assisted suicide is extraordinary and irreversible treatment, the patient's primary physician must ensure that the following conditions are clearly satisfied before proceeding. First, the patient must have a condition that is incurable and associated with severe, unrelenting suffering. The patient must understand the condition, the prognosis, and the types of comfort care available as alternatives. Although most patients making this request will be near death, we acknowledge the inexactness of such prognostications[4-6] and do not want to exclude arbitrarily persons with incurable, but not imminently terminal, progressive illnesses, such as amyotrophic lateral sclerosis or multiple sclerosis. When there is considerable uncertainty about the patient's medical condition or prognosis, a second opinion or opinions should be sought and the uncertainty clarified as much as possible before a final decision about the patient's request is made.

Second, the physician must ensure that the patient's suffering and the request are not the result of inadequate comfort care. All reasonable comfort-oriented measures must at least have been considered, and preferably have been tried, before the means for a physician-assisted suicide are provided. Physician-assisted suicide must never be used to circumvent the struggle to provide comprehensive care or find acceptable alternatives. The physician's

Reprinted with permission of the publisher from the *New England Journal of Medicine*, vol. 327 (November 5, 1992), pp. 1381–1383.

prospective willingness to provide assisted suicide is a legitimate and important subject to discuss if the patient raises the question, since many patients will probably find the possibility of an escape from suffering more important than the reality.

Third, the patient must clearly and repeatedly, of his or her own free will and initiative, request to die rather than continue suffering. The physician should understand thoroughly what continued life means to the patient and why death appears preferable. A physician's too-ready acceptance of a patient's request could be perceived as encouragement to commit suicide, yet it is important not to force the patient to "beg" for assistance. Understanding the patient's desire to die and being certain that the request is serious are critical steps in evaluating the patient's rationality and ensuring that all alternative means of relieving suffering have been adequately explored. Any sign of ambivalence or uncertainty on the part of the patient should abort the process, because a clear, convincing, and continuous desire for an end of suffering through death is a strict requirement to proceed. Requests for assisted suicide made in an advance directive or by a health care surrogate should not be honored.

Fourth, the physician must be sure that the patient's judgment is not distorted. The patient must be capable of understanding the decision and its implications. The presence of depression is relevant if it is distorting rational decision making and is reversible in a way that would substantially alter the situation. Expert psychiatric evaluation should be sought when the primary physician is inexperienced in the diagnosis and treatment of depression, or when there is uncertainty about the rationality of the request or the presence of a reversible mental disorder the treatment of which would substantially change the patient's perception of his or her condition.[7]

Fifth, physician-assisted suicide should be carried out only in the context of a meaningful doctor-patient relationship. Ideally, the physician should have witnessed the patient's previous illness and suffering. There may not always be a preexisting relationship, but the physician must get to know the patient personally in order to understand fully the reasons for the request. The physician must understand why the patient considers death to be the best of a limited number of very unfortunate options. The primary physician must personally confirm that each of the criteria has been met. The patient should have no doubt that the physician is committed to finding alternative solutions if at any moment the patient's mind changes. Rather than create a new subspecialty focused on death,[8] assistance in suicide should be given by the same physician who has been struggling with the patient to provide comfort care, and who will stand by the patient and provide care until the time of death, no matter what path is taken.[3]

No physician should be forced to assist a patient in suicide if it violates the physician's fundamental values, although the patient's personal physician should think seriously before turning down such a request. Should a transfer of care be necessary, the personal physician should help the patient find another, more receptive primary physician.

Sixth, consultation with another experienced physician is required to ensure that the patient's request is voluntary and rational, the diagnosis and prognosis accurate, and the exploration of comfort-oriented alternatives thorough. The consulting physician should review the supporting materials and should interview and examine the patient.

Finally, clear documentation to support each condition is required. A system must be developed for reporting, reviewing, and studying such deaths and clearly distinguishing them from other forms of suicide. The patient, the primary physician, and the consultant must each sign a consent form. A physician-assisted suicide must neither invalidate insurance policies nor lead to an investigation by the medical examiner or an unwanted autopsy. The primary physician, the medical consultant, and the family must be assured that if the conditions agreed on are satisfied in good faith, they will be free from criminal prosecution for having assisted the patient to die.

Informing family members is strongly recommended, but whom to involve and inform should be left to the discretion and control of the patient. Similarly, spiritual counseling should be offered, depending on the patient's background and beliefs. Ideally, close family members should be an integral part of the decision-making process and should understand and support the patient's decision. If there is a major dispute between the family and the patient about how to proceed, it may require the involvement of an ethics committee or even of the courts. It is to be hoped, however, that most of these painful decisions can be worked through directly by the patient, the family, and health care providers. Under no circumstances should the family's wishes and requests override those of a competent patient.

THE METHOD

In physician-assisted suicide, a lethal amount of medication is usually prescribed that the patient then ingests. Since this process has been largely covert and unstudied, little is known about which methods are the most humane and effective. If there is a change in policy, there must be an open sharing of information within the profession, and a careful analysis of effectiveness. The methods selected should be reliable and should not add to the patient's suffering. We must also provide support and careful monitoring for the patients, physicians, and families affected, since the emotional and social effects are largely unknown but are undoubtedly far-reaching.

Assistance with suicide is one of the most profound and meaningful requests a patient can make of a physician. If the patient and the physician agree that there are no acceptable alternatives and that all the required conditions have been met, the lethal medication should ideally be taken in the physician's presence. Unless the patient specifically requests it, he or she should not be left alone at the time of death.

In addition to the personal physician, other health care providers and family members should be encouraged to be present, as the patient wishes. It is of the utmost importance not to abandon the patient at this critical moment. The time before a controlled death can provide an opportunity for a rich and meaningful goodbye between family members, health care providers, and the patient. For this reason, we must be sure that any policies and laws enacted to allow assisted suicide do not require that the patient be left alone at the moment of death in order for the assisters to be safe from prosecution. . . .

REFERENCES

1 Weir R. F. The morality of physician-assisted suicide. Law Med Health Care 1992; 20:116–26.
2 Glover J. Causing death and saving lives. New York: Penguin Books, 1977:182–9.
3 Jecker N. S. Giving death a hand: when the dying and the doctor stand in a special relationship. J Am Geriatr Soc 1991; 39:831–5.
4 Poses R. M., Bekes C, Copare F. J., Scott W. E. The answer to "What are my chances, doctor?" depends on whom is asked: prognostic disagreement and inaccuracy for critically ill patients. Crit Care Med 1989; 17:827–33.
5 Charlson M. E. Studies of prognosis: progress and pitfalls. J Gen Intern Med 1987; 2:359–61.
6 Schonwetter R. S., Teasdale T. A., Storey P., Luchi R. J. Estimation of survival time in terminal cancer patients: an impedance to hospice admissions? Hospice J 1990; 6:65–79.
7 Conwell Y., Caine E. D. Rational suicide and the right to die—reality and myth. N Engl J Med 1991; 325:1100–3.
8 Benrubi G. I. Euthanasia—the need for procedural safeguards. N Engl J Med 1992; 326:197–9.

THE OREGON DEATH WITH DIGNITY ACT

This Oregon law permits physicians to prescribe lethal drugs for Oregon adult residents who are terminally ill and who want to end their own lives. In order for a patient to be eligible for such assistance, the attending physician must determine that the patient has a terminal disease—a diagnosis entailing that the patient is expected to die within six months—and a consulting physician must confirm this diagnosis. Prominent among the other stipulated requirements are the following: (1) The patient must make an initial oral request; reiterate the oral request after 15 days have passed; and also submit a written request, supported by two witnesses. (2) Before writing the prescription, the attending physician must wait at least 15 days after the patient's initial request and at least 48 hours after the written request. (3) The attending physician must fully inform the patient about the diagnosis, prognosis, and feasible alternatives, including comfort care, hospice care, and pain control. (4) Both the attending physician and the consulting physician must certify that the patient is "capable" (i.e., has decision-making capacity), is acting voluntarily, and has made an informed choice. (5) If either physician believes that the patient's judgment might be impaired (e.g., by depression), the patient must be referred for counseling.

Section 1: General Provisions

1.01 Definitions

The following words and phrases, whenever used in this Act, shall have the following meanings:

(1) "Adult" means an individual who is 18 years of age or older.

(2) "Attending physician" means the physician who has primary responsibility for the care of the patient and treatment of the patient's terminal disease.

(3) "Consulting physician" means a physician who is qualified by specialty or experience to make a professional diagnosis and prognosis regarding the patient's disease.

(4) "Counseling" means a consultation between a state licensed psychiatrist or psychologist and a patient for the purpose of determining whether the patient is suffering from a psychiatric or psychological disorder, or depression causing impaired judgment.

(5) "Health care provider" means a person licensed, certified, or otherwise authorized or permitted by the law of this State to administer health care in the ordinary course of business or practice of a profession, and includes a health care facility.

(6) "Incapable" means that in the opinion of a court or in the opinion of the patient's attending physician or consulting physician, a patient lacks the ability to make and communicate health care decisions to health care providers, including communication through persons familiar with the patient's manner of communicating if those persons are available. Capable means not incapable.

(7) "Informed decision" means a decision by a qualified patient, to request and obtain a prescription to end his or her life in a humane and dignified manner, that is based on an appreciation of the relevant facts and after being fully informed by the attending physician of:

(a) his or her medical diagnosis;

(b) his or her prognosis;

(c) the potential risks associated with taking the medication to be prescribed;

(d) the probable result of taking the medication to be prescribed;

(e) the feasible alternatives, including, but not limited to, comfort care, hospice care and pain control.

(8) "Medically confirmed" means the medical opinion of the attending physician has been confirmed by a consulting physician who has examined the patient and the patient's relevant medical records.

(9) "Patient" means a person who is under the care of a physician.

(10) "Physician" means a doctor of medicine or osteopathy licensed to practice medicine by the Board of Medical Examiners for the State of Oregon.

(11) "Qualified patient" means a capable adult who is a resident of Oregon and has satisfied the requirements of this Act in order to obtain a prescription for medication to end his or her life in a humane and dignified manner.

(12) "Terminal disease" means an incurable and irreversible disease that has been medically confirmed and will, within reasonable medical judgment, produce death within six (6) months.

Section 2: Written Request for Medication to End One's Life in a Humane and Dignified Manner

2.01 Who may initiate a written request for medication

An adult who is capable, is a resident of Oregon, and has been determined by the attending physician and consulting physician to be suffering from a terminal disease, and who has voluntarily expressed his or her wish to die, may make a written request for medication for the purpose of ending his or her life in a humane and dignified manner in accordance with this Act.

2.02 Form of the written request

(1) A valid request for medication under this Act shall be in substantially the form described in Section 6 of this Act, signed and dated by the patient and witnessed by at least two individuals who, in the presence of the patient, attest that to the best of their knowledge and belief the patient is capable, acting voluntarily, and is not being coerced to sign the request.

(2) One of the witnesses shall be a person who is not:

    (a) A relative of the patient by blood, marriage or adoption;

    (b) A person who at the time the request is signed would be entitled to any portion of the estate of the qualified patient upon death under any will or by operation of law; or

    (c) An owner, operator or employee of a health care facility where the qualified patient is receiving medical treatment or is a resident.

(3) The patient's attending physician at the time the request is signed shall not be a witness.

(4) If the patient is a patient in a long term care facility at the time the written request is made, one of the witnesses shall be an individual designated by the facility and having the qualifications specified by the Department of Human Resources by rule.

Section 3: Safeguards

3.01 Attending physician responsibilities

The attending physician shall:

(1) Make the initial determination of whether a patient has a terminal disease, is capable, and has made the request voluntarily;

(2) Inform the patient of:

    (a) his or her medical diagnosis;

    (b) his or her prognosis;

    (c) the potential risks associated with taking the medication to be prescribed;

    (d) the probable result of taking the medication to be prescribed;

    (e) the feasible alternatives, including, but not limited to, comfort care, hospice care and pain control.

(3) Refer the patient to a consulting physician for medical confirmation of the diagnosis, and for determination that the patient is capable and acting voluntarily;

(4) Refer the patient for counseling if appropriate pursuant to Section 3.03;

(5) Request that the patient notify next of kin;

(6) Inform the patient that he or she has an opportunity to rescind the request at any time and in any manner, and offer the patient an opportunity to rescind at the end of the 15 day waiting period pursuant to Section 3.06;

(7) Verify, immediately prior to writing the prescription for medication under this Act, that the patient is making an informed decision;

(8) Fulfill the medical record documentation requirements of Section 3.09;

(9) Ensure that all appropriate steps are carried out in accordance with this Act prior to writing a prescription for medication to enable a qualified patient to end his or her life in a humane and dignified manner.

3.02 Consulting physician confirmation

Before a patient is qualified under this Act, a consulting physician shall examine the patient and his or her relevant medical records and confirm, in writing, the attending physician's diagnosis that the patient is suffering from a terminal disease, and verify that the patient is capable, is acting voluntarily and has made an informed decision.

3.03 Counseling referral

If in the opinion of the attending physician or the consulting physician a patient may be suffering from a psychiatric or psychological disorder, or depression causing impaired judgment, either physician shall refer the patient for counseling. No medication to end a patient's life in a humane and dignified manner shall be prescribed until the person performing the counseling determines that the person is not suffering from a psychiatric or psychological disorder, or depression causing impaired judgment.

3.04 Informed decision

No person shall receive a prescription for medication to end his or her life in a humane and dignified manner unless he or she has made an informed decision as defined in Section 1.01(7). Immediately prior to writing a prescription for medication under this Act, the attending physician shall verify that the patient is making an informed decision.

3.05 Family notification

The attending physician shall ask the patient to notify next of kin of his or her request for medication pursuant to this Act. A patient who declines or is unable to notify next of kin shall not have his or her request denied for that reason.

3.06 Written and oral requests

In order to receive a prescription for medication to end his or her life in a humane and dignified manner, a qualified patient shall have made an oral request and a written request, and reiterate the oral request to his or her attending physician no less than fifteen (15) days after making the initial oral request. At the time the qualified patient makes his or her second oral request, the attending physician shall offer the patient an opportunity to rescind the request.

3.07 Right to rescind request

A patient may rescind his or her request at any time and in any manner without regard to his or her mental state. No prescription for medication under this Act may be written without the attending physician offering the qualified patient an opportunity to rescind the request.

3.08 Waiting periods

No less than fifteen (15) days shall elapse between the patient's initial and oral request and the writing of a prescription under this Act. No less than 48 hours shall elapse between the patient's written request and the writing of a prescription under this Act.

3.09 Medical record documentation requirements

The following shall be documented or filed in the patient's medical record:

(1) All oral requests by a patient for medication to end his or her life in a humane and dignified manner;

(2) All written requests by a patient for medication to end his or her life in a humane and dignified manner;

(3) The attending physician's diagnosis and prognosis, determination that the patient is capa-

ble, acting voluntarily and has made an informed decision.

(4) The consulting physician's diagnosis and prognosis, and verification that the patient is capable, acting voluntarily and has made an informed decision;

(5) A report of the outcome and determinations made during counseling, if performed;

(6) The attending physician's offer to the patient to rescind his or her request at the time of the patient's second oral request pursuant to Section 3.06; and

(7) A note by the attending physician indicating that all requirements under this Act have been met and indicating the steps taken to carry out the request, including a notation of the medication prescribed.

3.10 Residency requirement

Only requests made by Oregon residents, under this Act, shall be granted.

3.11 Reporting requirements

(1) The Health Division shall annually review a sample of records maintained pursuant to this Act.

(2) The Health Division shall make rules to facilitate the collection of information regarding compliance with this Act. The information collected shall not be a public record and may not be made available for inspection by the public.

(3) The Health Division shall generate and make available to the public an annual statistical report of information collected under Section 3.11(2) of this Act.

3.12 Effect on construction of wills, contracts and statutes

(1) No provision in a contract, will or other agreement, whether written or oral, to the extent the provision would affect whether a person may make or rescind a request for medication to end his or her life in a humane and dignified manner, shall be valid.

(2) No obligation owing under any currently existing contract shall be conditioned or affected by the making or rescinding of a request, by a person, for medication to end his or her life in a humane and dignified manner.

3.13 Insurance or annuity policies

The sale, procurement, or issuance of any life, health, or accident insurance or annuity policy or the rate charged for any policy shall not be conditioned upon or affected by the making or rescinding of a request, by a person, for medication to end his or her life in a humane and dignified manner. Neither shall a qualified patient's act of ingesting medication to end his or her life in a humane and dignified manner have an effect upon a life, health, or accident insurance or annuity policy.

3.14 Construction of Act

Nothing in this Act shall be construed to authorize a physician or any other person to end a patient's life by lethal injection, mercy killing or active euthanasia. Actions taken in accordance with this Act shall not, for any purpose, constitute suicide, assisted suicide, mercy killing or homicide, under the law.

Section 4: Immunities and Liabilities

4.01 Immunities

Except as provided in Section 4.02:

(1) No person shall be subject to civil or criminal liability or professional disciplinary action for participating in good faith compliance with this Act. This includes being present when a qualified patient takes the prescribed medication to end his or her life in a humane and dignified manner.

(2) No professional organization or association, or health care provider, may subject a person to censure, discipline, suspension, loss of license, loss of privileges, loss of membership or other penalty for participating or refusing to participate in good faith compliance with this Act.

(3) No request by a patient for or provision by an attending physician of medication in good faith compliance with the provisions of this Act shall constitute neglect for any purpose of law or provide the sole basis for the appointment of a guardian or conservator.

(4) No health care provider shall be under any duty, whether by contract, by statute or by any other legal requirement to participate in the provision to a qualified patient of medication to end his or her life in a humane and dignified manner. If a health care provider is unable or unwilling to carry out a patient's request under this Act, and the patient transfers his or her care to a new health care provider, the prior health care provider shall transfer, upon request, a copy of the patient's relevant medical records to the new health care provider.

4.02 Liabilities

(1) A person who without authorization of the patient willfully alters or forges a request for medication or conceals or destroys a rescission of that request with the intent or effect of causing the patient's death shall be guilty of a Class A felony.

(2) A person who coerces or exerts undue influence on a patient to request medication for the purpose of ending the patient's life, or to destroy a rescission of such a request, shall be guilty of a Class A felony.

(3) Nothing in this Act limits further liability for civil damages resulting from other negligent conduct or intentional misconduct by any persons.

(4) The penalties in this Act do not preclude criminal penalties applicable under other law for conduct which is inconsistent with the provisions of this Act.

Section 5: Severability

5.01 Severability

Any section of this Act being held invalid as to any person or circumstance shall not affect the application of any other section of this Act which can be given full effect without the invalid section or application.

Section 6: Form of the Request

6.01 Form of the request

A request for a medication as authorized by this Act shall be in substantially the following form:

REQUEST FOR MEDICATION TO
END MY LIFE IN A HUMANE AND DIGNIFIED MANNER

I, _____, am an adult of sound mind.

I am suffering from _____, which my attending physician has determined is a terminal disease and which has been medically formed by a consulting physician.

I have been fully informed of my diagnosis, prognosis, the nature of medication to be prescribed and potential associated risks, the expected result, and the feasible alternatives, including comfort care, hospice care and pain control.

I request that my attending physician prescribe medication that will end my life in a humane and dignified manner.

INITIAL ONE:

_____ I have informed my family of my decision and taken their opinions into consideration.

_____ I have decided not to inform my family of my decision.

_____ I have no family to inform of my decision.

I understand that I have the right to rescind this request at any time.

I understand the full import of this request and I expect to die when I take the medication to be prescribed.

I make this request voluntarily and without reservation, and I accept full moral responsibility for my actions.

Signed: _____

Dated: _____

DECLARATION OF WITNESSES

We declare that the person signing this request:

(a) Is personally known to us or has provided proof of identity;

(b) Signed this request in our presence;

(c) Appears to be of sound mind and not under duress, fraud or undue influence;

(d) Is not a patient for whom either of us is attending physician.

_____ Witness 1/Date

_____ Witness 2/Date

NOTE: One witness shall not be a relative (by blood, marriage or adoption) of the person signing this request, shall not be entitled to any portion of the person's estate upon death and shall not own, operate or be employed at a health care facility where the person is a patient or resident. If the patient is an inpatient at a health care facility, one of the witnesses shall be an individual designated by the facility.

REGULATING PHYSICIAN-ASSISTED DEATH

Franklin G. Miller, Timothy E. Quill, Howard Brody, John C. Fletcher, Lawrence O. Gostin, and Diane E. Meier

The authors recommend legalization of physician-assisted death (a category that includes voluntary active euthanasia as well as physician-assisted suicide) in accordance with a regulatory scheme that they believe embodies adequate safeguards. In their view, physician-assisted death should be made available only to adults who retain decision-making capacity, but the practice should not be restricted solely to patients who are terminally ill; physician-assisted death should also be an available option for patients suffering from incurable, debilitating diseases. The authors insist that physician-assisted death must be considered a "treatment of last resort"—to be made available only if standard comfort-care measures fail to provide adequate relief from suffering. Certified palliative-care consultants, working in conjunction with regional palliative-care committees, are the cornerstone of the proposed regulatory scheme.

Public-opinion polls have consistently shown that approximately 60 percent of the American public favors legal reform allowing physician-assisted death as a last resort to end the suffering of competent patients.[1] Yet the voters in Washington State in 1991 and California in 1992 narrowly defeated referendums that would have permitted physicians to prescribe or administer lethal treatment to terminally ill patients. The lack of adequate safeguards to protect vulnerable patients and prevent abuse may have been an important factor in the rejection of these legislative proposals.[2] In this article we describe a policy of legalized physician-assisted death restricted to competent patients suffering from terminal illness or incurable, debilitating disease who voluntarily request to end their lives. Integral to this policy is a framework of regulation with safeguards that we believe are adequate to protect patients, preserve the professional integrity of physicians, and assure the public that voluntary physician-assisted death occurs only as a last resort.

Voluntary physician-assisted death serves the moral goals of relief of suffering and self-determination on the part of patients.[3–5] It becomes a permissible option when comfort care ceases to be effective for the terminally or incurably ill. ("Comfort care" refers to palliative and supportive treatment used in hospice programs and elsewhere.) Comfort care ought to be the standard medical treatment for patients who are suffering from a terminal illness or who have refused curative or life-sustaining treatment.[3] It is aimed at relieving symptoms, enhancing the quality and meaning of the patient's remaining life, and easing the process of dying. As a treatment of last resort, physician-assisted death becomes a legitimate option only after standard measures for comfort care have been found unsatisfactory by competent patients in the context of their own situation and values. Accordingly, the policy we recommend aims to promote comfort care and to permit voluntary physician-assisted death only in the relatively infrequent but troubling cases in which comfort care is inadequate. . . .

THE RATIONALE FOR REGULATION

Decisions about medical treatment are normally made in the privacy of the doctor-patient relationship.[6] Yet regulatory safeguards providing independent monitoring of medical decisions that involve physician-assisted death are necessary for two reasons. First, any treatment whose purpose is to cause death lies outside standard medical practice, which is defined here as medically indicated interventions aimed at promoting health and healing and

Reprinted by permission of the publisher from *The New England Journal of Medicine,* vol. 331 (July 14, 1994), pp. 119–123. Copyright © 1994 Massachusetts Medical Society. All rights reserved.

alleviating the suffering of patients. Currently accepted standards of comfort care allow for the use of aggressive palliative treatment that may indirectly and unintentionally contribute to a patient's death.[3] However, standards of comfort care stop short of permitting death to be caused intentionally as a means of ending unrelievable suffering.

We regard physician-assisted death as a nonstandard medical practice reserved for extraordinary circumstances, when it is requested voluntarily by a patient whose suffering has become intolerable and who has no other satisfactory options. Although we argue that physician-assisted death should be permitted as a treatment of last resort, we do not claim that patients have a right to physician-assisted death, as they do to standard medical care. Physicians must carefully assess patients' requests for assistance in dying and thoroughly explore alternatives for comfort care.[7] In addition, they must consider their own values and willingness to participate in physician-assisted death. Because of the nonstandard nature of physician-assisted death, even when patients and physicians agree that there are no acceptable alternatives, regulatory oversight should be required.

The second reason for regulating physician-assisted death is the risk of abuse of vulnerable patients. In addition to the highly publicized and problematic assisted suicides in which Jack Kevorkian has participated, there is evidence of a relatively widespread secret practice of physician-assisted death in the United States, which is completely unregulated.[8] Voluntary physician-assisted death has been widely practiced in the Netherlands in recent years, although it remains technically illegal.[9] Studies indicate that Dutch physicians have provided lethal treatment to some suffering incompetent patients who have made no request to die.[10–12] The Dutch practice of physician-assisted death is carried out mainly in the privacy of the doctor-patient relationship, subject to guidelines that are not independently monitored.

The risks of abuse in the absence of regulatory safeguards might be greater in the United States than in the Netherlands because of the pressures for cost containment in our health care system, the burdens imposed on family members by the responsibility of caring for dying patients, and our cultural penchant for seeking technological solutions to complex medical and social problems. Therefore, an acceptable policy of legalized physician-assisted death must include independent monitoring to ensure that it is used only as a treatment of last resort in response to the voluntary requests of competent patients who are suffering from terminal or incurable illnesses.

LEGISLATION AS AN APPROPRIATE VEHICLE FOR REFORM

We believe that state legislation is the most appropriate means of expanding the options of suffering patients while establishing adequate safeguards, and of achieving greater clarity and fairness in policies concerning physician-assisted death. Legislators are elected and demonstrably accountable for their decisions. They also have the opportunity for the careful consideration of policy decisions through public hearings and debate. Accordingly, they can thoughtfully design laws and regulatory procedures to guide professional practice and safeguard against abuse.

Several attempts to legalize physician-assisted death have come in the form of state referendums. Though referendums epitomize democracy, they can be inadequate mechanisms for the development of complex public policy. Votes on referendums are subject to substantial influence by interest groups that can afford to spend large amounts of money on advertising. More important, the electorate can only approve or disapprove the proposed legislation but cannot alter its language. As demonstrated in Washington and California, referendums often offer simple solutions without careful attention to clear criteria, rigorous procedures, and adequate safeguards.

A federal district court judge recently held that a Washington State law prohibiting assisted suicide unconstitutionally interferes with liberty and privacy interests protected by the Fourteenth Amendment.[13] This case raises the question of whether the judicial branch of government might provide the impetus for reform. It is conceivable that reasoning applied to treatment-refusal cases could also be applied to physician-assisted death.[14,15] The chief disadvantage of judicial activism in this area is the difficulty courts may have in specifying detailed criteria and procedures to protect vulnerable patients.

State legislatures are better positioned to design adequate safeguards for the appropriate use of physician-assisted death.

OBJECTIVES OF REGULATORY POLICY

We believe a policy regulating physician-assisted death should be designed with the following objectives: (1) to promote comfort care as standard treatment for dying patients; (2) to permit physician-assisted death only for competent patients suffering from terminal or incurable debilitating illnesses who voluntarily and repeatedly request to die; (3) to develop and promote practice guidelines for voluntary physician-assisted death aimed at making lethal treatment available only as a last resort for unrelievable suffering; (4) to provide independent and impartial oversight of decisions to pursue voluntary physician-assisted death without undue disruption of the doctor-patient relationship; (5) to provide a mechanism for prospective committee review of difficult or disputed cases; and (6) to ensure public accountability.

THE SCOPE OF LEGALIZED PHYSICIAN-ASSISTED DEATH

Our recommended policy reflects choices concerning two difficult issues: whether physician-assisted death should be limited to physician-assisted suicide, thus excluding voluntary, active euthanasia, and whether eligible patients must be only those for whom death is imminent or whether those who are not terminally ill but who suffer from incurable and debilitating conditions such as amyotrophic lateral sclerosis may also be considered eligible. We have opted for a liberal, inclusive policy with respect to these issues. To confine legalized physician-assisted death to assisted suicide unfairly discriminates against patients with unrelievable suffering who resolve to end their lives but are physically unable to do so. The method chosen is less important than the careful assessment that precedes assisted death. Limiting physician-assisted death to patients with terminal illness would deny this option of last resort to incurably, but not terminally, ill patients who make a rational decision to end their lives because of unremitting suffering. Physician-assisted death

would be appropriate only after thorough consideration of potential ways to improve the patient's quality of life. We believe that the regulatory safeguards described below would minimize the risks associated with the legalization of physician-assisted death for patients who are not terminally ill and with the possibility of voluntary, active euthanasia.

OVERVIEW OF POLICY

The general responsibility for regulating physician-assisted death would be lodged with regional palliative-care committees. Case-specific oversight of decisions to undertake physician-assisted death would be provided by physicians certified as palliative-care consultants, who would report to the palliative-care committees. Treating physicians would be prohibited from providing lethal treatment without prior consultation and review by an independent, certified palliative-care consultant. The palliative-care committee would be available for prospective review in difficult or disputed cases.

In order to ensure that physician-assisted death is voluntary, which is the inviolable cornerstone of this policy, only adults with decision-making capacity should be eligible for physician-assisted death. Written or witnessed oral consent by the patient must be obtained. No physician would be obligated to participate in physician-assisted death. Treating physicians would be required to report death by assisted suicide or the administration of lethal treatment to the proper public authority. Physicians who provided lethal treatment without compliance with the legal requirements would be liable to professional sanctions and criminal penalties.

PALLIATIVE-CARE CONSULTANTS

Independent and impartial oversight by a certified palliative-care consultant is a vital safeguard in this proposed policy of legalized physician-assisted death. Palliative-care consultants would be physicians with experience in treating dying patients, who were knowledgeable about and committed to comfort care, skilled in the assessment of the decision-making capacity of patients suffering from terminal or incurable conditions, and well educated about the ethics of end-of-life decision making. In order to institute effective consultation, new programs for the training and certification of palliative-care consultants would need to be developed and implemented. We do not envision the creation of a new medical specialty devoted to palliative-care consultation. Rather, certified consultants would be practicing physicians who routinely care for severely ill and dying patients and spend part of their time in the role of palliative-care consultant. It is essential that these consultants, who would oversee decisions to perform physician-assisted death, be aware firsthand of the clinical reality faced by suffering patients and their physicians.

The requirement for oversight by a member of an approved panel of palliative-care consultants goes beyond the guidelines in the Netherlands and the referendum questions in Washington and California, which merely stipulated consultation with a physician other than the treating physician.[16] The goal is to require a rigorous, independent second opinion by an accountable expert in the light of the objectives of the regulatory policy.

Review by an independent palliative-care consultant would be required whenever a patient and a physician, after thorough deliberation, agreed to pursue the option of physician-assisted death. This consultative oversight would include the examination of medical records and interviews with the treating physician, the patient, and interested members of the patient's family. The consultant would review the patient's diagnosis and prognosis and explore whether the treating physician and patient had considered carefully all reasonable alternatives.[17] The process of consultation might lead to improved pain management or the use of other means of comfort care. The consultant would assess the voluntariness of the patient's request to die and the strength of his or her resolve, paying careful attention to the possibility of distorted thinking or undue pressure by others who might be burdened with caring for the patient. The consultant could request additional expert advice if there was uncertainty about the patient's competence or medical condition or about the adequacy of palliative measures.

Certified palliative-care consultants would have the authority to override agreements by patients and physicians to undertake physician-assisted death. The

consultants would be required to prepare a reasoned and clearly articulated statement justifying their judgment that physician-assisted death was inappropriate. In addition, the patient and physician would have the right to appeal the consultant's judgment to the palliative-care committee. In all cases the palliative-care consultant would prepare a confidential written report that would be submitted to the palliative-care committee for retrospective monitoring. The palliative-care consultants would have the option of referring difficult or uncertain cases for prospective review to the palliative-care committees.

PALLIATIVE-CARE COMMITTEES

Regional palliative-care committees, made up of professional and lay members, would perform a variety of functions. The committees would develop, issue, and revise practice guidelines for physicians to supplement the legal requirements for physician-assisted death. For example, in order to avoid undue influence on vulnerable patients, the request for the consideration of lethal treatment must come from patients, and physicians should accede only after fully exploring the meaning of the patients' request to die and the available alternatives.[7]

The palliative-care committees would be responsible for educating clinicians and the public about methods of comfort care (including pain management), ethical standards of informed refusal and discontinuation of life-sustaining treatment, and the option of physician-assisted death. This educational activity would cover topics such as the law, practice guidelines, and the relevant regulations; how treating physicians should respond to requests by patients for the termination of life; methods of comfort care as an alternative to physician-assisted death; and effective methods of lethal treatment. The committees would engage in routine retrospective monitoring of cases of physician-assisted death, basing their review on reports filed by the palliative-care consultants. Finally, the committees would review prospectively difficult cases referred by palliative-care consultants and appeals from patients or their primary care physicians when their negotiated requests for physician-assisted death were disapproved by the palliative-care consultants.

BALANCING THE BENEFITS AND BURDENS OF REGULATION

The process of regulation should be aimed at striking a balance between competing imperatives. On the one hand, physician-assisted death should not be an easy way out for suffering patients and their physicians. On the other hand, oversight should not be so restrictive and onerous as to deprive patients of an adequate response to intolerable suffering.

It might be objected that the policy we recommend is unworkable because it is too cumbersome and intrusive. Such an objection might be justified in the case of a policy requiring mandatory prior committee review or a court hearing to authorize physician-assisted death. Review by a certified palliative-care consultant, however, seems comparable to other consultations by specialists. For a decision of this magnitude, an independent expert opinion is clearly desirable. Some patients and physicians might still feel burdened by such oversight, especially in difficult cases referred or appealed to the palliative-care committee. We believe that this is a price worth paying to protect vulnerable patients and to ensure public accountability. Critical to the success of this policy, however, would be the timely availability of palliative-care consultants, education that emphasized the sensitive nature of the oversight function, and scrupulous protection of confidentiality.

EVALUATIVE RESEARCH

Since there is no guarantee that the danger of abuse can be completely eliminated, a policy of regulating physician-assisted death should be viewed as experimental, and evaluative research should be built into any implementing legislation. Such research would be designed to determine and assess how physician-assisted death worked in practice, and to provide information helpful for modifying guidelines and procedures with the aim of improving the policy.

Two types of research would be desirable. First, to assess the effects of the policy, aggregate data should be collected and analyzed. These might include the number and disposition of cases reviewed by palliative-care consultants and palliative-care committees; the demographic characteristics and medical condition of patients requesting physician-assisted death; the location, methods, and circumstances of physician-assisted death; the attitudes of participating physicians and family members; the physicians' opinions of the regulatory process; and the long-term consequences for participants. Second, we recommend research into the personal and cultural meaning of physician-assisted death. In-depth interviews might be conducted with some patients, family members, treating physicians, and palliative-care consultants; researchers might witness the entire process of considering, reviewing, and providing physician-assisted death, subject to requirements of informed consent and confidentiality.

CONCLUSIONS

The ethical norms of relieving suffering and respecting patients' rights to self-determination support the permissibility of voluntary physician-assisted death as a last resort for terminally or incurably ill patients. The availability of the extraordinary option of lethal treatment, however, must be accompanied by careful regulation to minimize the risk of abuse. We recommend that physician-assisted death be legalized with adequate safeguards to protect vulnerable patients, preserve the professional integrity of physicians, and ensure accountability to the public. The policy we have outlined would ensure independent and impartial review of decisions to provide physician-assisted death in response to unrelievable suffering, without undue disruption of the doctor-patient relationship. We hope one or more states will decide democratically to expand the options for dying or incurably ill patients by implementing a policy that both promotes comfort care and permits voluntary physician-assisted death as a last resort.

REFERENCES

1 Blendon R. J., Szalay U. S., Knox R. A. Should physicians aid their patients in dying? The public perspective. JAMA 1992; 267:2658–62.
2 McGough P. M. Washington state initiative 119: the first public vote on legalizing physician-assisted death. Cambridge Q Healthcare Ethics 1993; 2: 63–7.
3 Quill T. E. Death and dignity. New York: W.W. Norton, 1993.
4 Brody H. Assisted death—a compassionate response to a medical failure. N Engl J Med 1992; 327:1384–8.
5 Miller F. G., Fletcher J. C. The case for legalized euthanasia. Perspect Biol Med 1993; 36:159–76.

6 Annas G. J., Glantz L. H., Mariner WK. The right of privacy protects the doctor-patient relationship. JAMA 1990; 263:858–61.

7 Quill T. E. Doctor, I want to die. Will you help me? JAMA 1993; 270:870–3.

8 Meier D. E. Doctors' attitudes and experiences with physician-assisted death: a review of the literature. In: Humber J. M., Almeder R. F., Kasting G. A., eds. Physician-assisted death. Totowa, N.J.: Humana Press, 1994:5–24.

9 van der Maas P. J., van Delden J. J. M., Pijnenborg L, Looman CWN. Euthanasia and other medical decisions concerning the end of life. Lancet 1991; 338:669–74.

10 Gomez C. F. Regulating death. New York: Free Press, 1991.

11 ten Have H. A., Welie J. V. Euthanasia: normal medical practice? Hastings Cent Rep 1992; 22:34–8.

12 Pijnenborg L., van der Maas P. J., van Delden J. J. M., Looman C. W. N. Life-terminating acts without explicit request of patient. Lancet 1993; 341:1196–9.

13 Egan T. Federal judge says ban on suicide aid is unconstitutional. New York Times. May 5, 1994:A1.

14 Note: physician-assisted suicide and the right to die with assistance. Harvard Law Rev 1992; 105:2021.

15 Gostin L., Weir R. F. Life and death choices after Cruzan: case law and standards of professional conduct, Milbank Q. 1991; 69:143–73.

16 A dozen caveats concerning the discussion of euthanasia in the Netherlands. In: Battin M. P. The least worst death. New York: Oxford University Press, 1994:130–44.

17 Quill T. E., Cassel C. K., Meier D. E. Care of the hopelessly ill—proposed clinical criteria for physician-assisted suicide. N Engl J Med 1992; 327: 1380–4.

ON THE SLIPPERY SLOPE IN THE EMPIRE STATE: THE NEW YORK STATE TASK FORCE ON PHYSICIAN-ASSISTED DEATH

John D. Arras

Arras provides an account of the considerations that led the New York State Task Force on Life and the Law to oppose legalization of both physician-assisted suicide and active euthanasia. Although some members of the task force also based their opposition to legalization on other arguments, the entire membership agreed that the likely social consequences of legalization are sufficiently problematic to warrant strong opposition. Arras constructs the argument from social consequences as a "slippery-slope" argument, and he essentially distinguishes two prongs—each somewhat complex—in the overall argument. The first prong, based on an analysis of the logic of justification for legalization, focuses concern on the likelihood that any initial narrowly drawn policy for the legalization of physician-assisted death would lead to an expansion of the original boundaries. The second prong of the slippery-slope argument focuses concern on the strong likelihood that any system providing criteria for the availability of physician-assisted death would be abused. Arras also provides a brief exposition of the task force's call for "a positive program of clinical and social reform," and he concludes by offering a critical response to the regulatory scheme proposed by Miller et al. in the previous selection.

THE TASK FORCE AND ITS CONCLUSIONS

Created by Governor Mario Cuomo in 1984, the New York State Task Force on Life and the Law has provided ethical analysis and policy recommenda-

Reprinted with permission of the American Philosophical Association from *Newsletter on Philosophy and Medicine,* in *APA Newsletters,* vol. 95, no. 2, Spring 1996, pp. 80–83.

tions to the people and legislature of New York on a host of important issues in bioethics, including brain death, organ transplantation, surrogate parenting, and forgoing life-sustaining treatment. The Task Force is composed of 25 members drawn from a wide variety of professional affiliations and geographical locations within the state. The membership includes clergy representing all four great New

York religions—i.e., Catholics, Jews, Protestants, and the ACLU—as well as physicians, nurses, social workers, attorneys, law professors, consumer advocates, and two philosopher/bioethicists (Professor Samuel Gorovitz of Syracuse University and, until recently, myself).

Although the Task Force had consistently displayed strong enthusiasm for the value of individual autonomy in its previous reports on DNR orders,[1] health care proxies,[2] and surrogate decision making,[3] it emphasized the limits of autonomy in its May 1994 report, *When Death Is Sought: Assisted Suicide and Euthanasia in the Medical Context.* In an extraordinary display of consensus within a nonpartisan and strongly pluralistic group, the Task Force had unanimously agreed to retain the present legal and policy barriers to physician-assisted suicide (PAS) and active euthanasia.

In spite of their agreement to uphold the ban on PAS and active euthanasia, the members disagreed sharply over the rationale for this conclusion. One faction strongly condemned both practices as inherently immoral, as violations of the moral rule against killing the innocent. Another faction primarily objected to the fact that physicians were being called upon to do the killing. While conceding that killing the terminally ill or assisting in their suicides might not always be morally wrong for others to do, this group maintained that the participation of physicians in such practices would undermine their role as healers and fatally compromise the physician-patient relationship. Finally, a third faction, the one to which I belonged during my tenure with the Task Force, readily conceded that neither PAS nor active euthanasia were always morally wrong, whether practiced by ordinary citizens or by physicians. On the contrary, we believed that in certain rare instances early release from a painful or intolerably degrading existence might constitute both a positive good and an important exercise of personal autonomy for the individual. Indeed, several of us conceded that should such a terrible fate befall us, we would hope to find a thoughtful, compassionate, and courageous physician (such as Dr. Timothy Quill) to release us from our misery. But in spite of these important concessions, these members shrank from endorsing or regulating PAS and active euthanasia due to fears bearing on the social consequences of liberalization.

Notwithstanding these internal disagreements, the entire membership of the Task Force agreed that the law should not be changed. We also unanimously endorsed the reasoning of the third faction bearing on the dangers of the slippery slope. Because this reasoning proved decisive within the deliberations of the Task Force, I shall devote the remainder of this brief commentary to a fuller exposition of the argument from social consequences. This complex argument is not only important for understanding the position of the Task Force, but it is also crucial for evaluating some recent proposals for legalization and regulation.

MORALITY VERSUS POLICY

Crucial to the Task Force's analysis was the distinction between the morality of individual acts and the wisdom of social policy. Much of the debate in the popular media is driven by the depiction of especially dramatic and poignant instances of suffering humanity, desperate for release from the painful thrall of terminal illness. Quite understandably, many if not most of us are prompted to respond, "Should such a terrible fate ever befall me, I would certainly not want to suffer interminably; I would want the option of an early exit and the help of my trusted physician in securing it." The problem, however, lies in getting from such compelling individual cases to social policy. The issue is not simply, "What would I want?", but rather what is the best social policy all things considered. The Task Force warns that we cannot make this jump from individual case to policy without endangering the autonomy and the very lives of others, many of whom are numbered among our most vulnerable citizens.

THE WISH TO DIE AND THE FAILURE OF MEDICINE

The Task Force recognized that many people advocate legalization because they fear a loss of control at the end of life. They fear falling victim to the technological imperative; they fear dying in chronic and uncontrolled pain; and they fear the psychological suffering attendant upon the relentless disintegration of the self. All of these fears, it so happens, are eminently justified. As the SUPPORT study recently demonstrated with such depressing clarity, physicians routinely ignore the documented wishes of patients and all-too-often allow patients to die with un-controlled pain.[4] Studies of cancer patients have shown that over 50% suffer from unrelieved pain. The Task Force found that uncontrolled pain, particularly when accompanied by feelings of hopelessness and untreated depression, is a significant contributing factor for suicide and suicidal ideation.

Clinical depression is another major factor. Depression accompanied by feelings of hopelessness is the strongest predictor of suicide for both individuals who are terminally ill and those who are not. Yet most doctors are not trained to notice depression, especially in complex cases such as the elderly suffering from terminal illness. And even when doctors succeed in diagnosing depression, they often do not successfully treat it with readily available medications in sufficient amounts.

The Task Force found that the vast majority of patients who request PAS or euthanasia are capable of being successfully treated both for their depression and their pain, and that when they receive adequate psychiatric and palliative care, their requests to die are usually withdrawn. In other words, patients given the requisite control over their lives and relief from depression and pain usually lose interest in PAS and euthanasia. This fact is of enormous importance for our evaluation of PAS and euthanasia as social policies, for if the root causes or motivations for assisted death can be successfully addressed for most patients through the delivery of technically competent and compassionate medicine, the case for changing the law loses much of its urgency.

But it does not, alas, lose all of its urgency. The Task Force recognized as well that a small percentage of patients suffer from conditions both physical and psychological that lie beyond the current reach of medicine and humane care. Some pain cannot be alleviated short of inducing a permanent state of unconsciousness in the patient; and some depression is unconquerable. For such unfortunate patients, the present law can represent an insuperable barrier to a dignified and decent death. While the Task Force expressed its compassion for the sufferings of such patients, its members were ultimately convinced that they could not be helped in a public way—i.e., be given publicly-sanctioned assistance in committing suicide—without endangering a far greater number of highly vulnerable patients.

In this sense, the Task Force members were painfully aware of the "tragic" nature of the choice confronting them. Whether they opted for a reaffirmation of the current legal restraints or for a policy of legitimation and regulation, there were bound to be victims. The victims of the current policy are easy to identify; they are on the news, the talk shows and the documentaries, and often on Dr. Kevorkian's roster of "patients." But who would be the victims of a more permissive policy? What exactly does the slippery slope argument amount to here?

AN "OPTION WITHOUT LIMITS"

The Task Force's first point is that a socially sanctioned practice of PAS would in all likelihood prove difficult, if not impossible, to cabin within its originally anticipated boundaries. The proponents of legalization usually begin with a wholesomely modest policy agenda, limiting their suggested reforms to a narrow and highly specified range of potential candidates and practices. "Give us PAS, not the more controversial practice of active euthanasia, for presently competent patients who are terminally ill and suffering unbearable pain." But the logic of the case for PAS, based as it is upon the twin pillars of patient autonomy and mercy, makes it highly unlikely that society could stop with this modest proposal once it had ventured out on the slope. As numerous other critics have pointed out, if autonomy is the prime consideration, then additional constraints based upon terminal illness and/or unbearable pain would appear hard to justify. Indeed, if autonomy is crucial, the requirement of unbearable suffering would appear to be entirely subjective. Who is to say—other than the patient herself—how much suffering is too much? Likewise, the requirement of terminal illness seems an arbitrary standard against which to judge patients' own subjective evaluation of their quality of life. If my life is no longer worth living, why should a terminally ill cancer patient be granted PAS but not me, merely because my suffering is due to my "non-terminal" ALS or intractable psychiatric disorder?

Alternatively, if pain and suffering are deemed crucial to the justification of legalization, it is hard to see how the proposed barrier of contemporaneous consent of competent patients could withstand serious erosion. If the logic of PAS is at all similar to that of forgoing life-sustaining treatments—and we have every reason to think it so— then it would seem almost inevitable that a case would soon be made to permit PAS for incompetent patients who had left advance directives, followed by a "substituted judgment" test for patients who "would have wanted" PAS, and finally an "objective" test for patients (including newborns) whose best interests would be served by PAS or active euthanasia even in the absence of any subjective intent.

In the same way, the joint justifications of autonomy and mercy would combine to undermine the plausibility of a line drawn between PAS and active euthanasia. As the authors of one highly publicized proposal have come to see, the logic of justification for active euthanasia is identical to that of PAS.[5] Legalizing PAS while continuing to ban active euthanasia, would serve only to discriminate unfairly against patients who are suffering and wish to end their lives, but cannot do so because of some physical impairment. Surely these patients, it will be said, are "the worst off group" and therefore the most in need of the assistance of others who will do for them what they can no longer accomplish on their own.

None of these initial slippery slope considerations, it must be conceded, constitute knock-down objections to further liberalization of our laws and practices. It is not obvious, after all, that each of these highly predictable shifts—e.g., from terminal to "merely" incurable, from contemporaneous consent to best interests, and from PAS to active euthanasia—are patently immoral and unjustifiable. Still, in pointing out this likely slippage, the Task Force is calling on society to think about the likely consequences of taking the first tentative step onto the slope. If all of the extended practices predicted above pose substantially greater risks for vulnerable patients than the more highly circumscribed initial liberalization proposals, then we need to factor in these additional risks even as we ponder those more modest proposals.[6]

THE LIKELIHOOD OF ABUSE

The second prong of the slippery slope argument deployed by the Task Force argues that whatever criteria for justifiable PAS and active euthanasia are

ultimately chosen, abuse of the system is highly likely to follow. In other words, patients who fall outside the ambit of our justifiable criteria will soon be candidates for death. This prong resembles what I have elsewhere called an "empirical slope"[7] argument, since it is based not on the close logical resemblance of concepts or justifications, but rather on an empirical prediction of what is likely to happen once we insert a particular social practice into our existing social system.

The Task Force made three assumptions about the requirements of any potentially justifiable social policy of PAS or active euthanasia. First, it would have to insist that all requests for death be voluntary; second, that all reasonable alternatives to PAS and active euthanasia must be explored before acceding to a patient's wishes; and third, a reliable system of reporting all cases must be established in order to effectively monitor these practices and respond to abuses. We argued that, given social reality as we know it, all three assumptions are problematic.

With regard to the voluntariness requirement, we contended that many requests would not be sufficiently voluntary. In addition to the subtly coercive influences of physicians and family members, perhaps the most slippery aspect of this slope is the highly predictable failure of most physicians reliably to diagnose and treat reversible clinical depression, especially in the elderly population. As one geriatric psychiatrist testified, we now live in the "golden age" of treating depression but the "lead age" of diagnosing it.[8] We have the tools, but physicians are not adequately trained and motivated to use them. So unless dramatic changes are effected in the practice of medicine, we can predict with confidence that many instances of PAS and active euthanasia will constitute abuses of the original criterion of voluntariness.

As to the second requirement, given the abysmal track record of physicians in responding adequately to pain and suffering, we can also confidently predict that in many cases all reasonable alternatives will not have been exhausted. Instead of vigorously addressing the pharmacologic and psycho-social needs of such patients, physicians will no doubt continue to ignore, undertreat, or treat them in an impersonal manner. The result will be more depression, desperation, and requests for physician-assisted death from patients who could have been successfully treated. The root causes of this predictable lapse are manifold, but include such factors as the inaccessibility of decent primary care to over 37 million Americans, the appalling lack of training in palliative care even among primary care physicians and cancer specialists, discrimination in the delivery of pain control (and other medical treatments) on the basis of race and economic status, various myths shared by both physicians and patients about the supposed ill effects of pain medications, and restrictive state laws on access to opioids.

Finally, the Task Force doubts that any reporting system would be sufficiently effective to adequately monitor these practices. A great deal depends here on the extent to which patients and practitioners will regard these practices as essentially *private* matters to be discussed and acted upon within the privacy of the doctor-patient relationship. As the Dutch experience has conclusively demonstrated, physicians will be extremely loath to report instances of PAS and active euthanasia to public authorities, largely for fear of bringing the harsh glare of publicity upon families at times when privacy is most needed. The likely result of this lack of oversight will be society's inability to respond appropriately to disturbing incidents and long-term trends. In other words, the practice will not be as amenable to regulation as the proponents contend.

A PRUDENTIAL CONCLUSION

The Task Force's argument can be summed up, then, as follows:

1. The number of "genuine cases" justifying PAS and/or active euthanasia will be relatively small. Patients who receive good personal care, good pain relief, treatment for depression, and adequate psychosocial supports tend not to persist in a desire to die.

2. The social risks of legalization are serious and highly predictable. They include the expansion of these practices to nonvoluntary cases and the widespread failure to pursue readily available alternatives to suicide motivated by pain, depression, and hopelessness.

3. Rather than propose a momentous and dangerous policy shift for a relatively small number of "genuine cases"—a shift, by the way, that would surely involve a great deal of persistent social division and strife analogous to that involved in the abortion controversy—we should instead attempt to redirect the public debate toward a goal on which we can and should all agree—viz., the manifest and urgent need to reform the way we die in America. Instead of launching a highly divisive and dangerous campaign for PAS, why not attack the problem at its root with an ambitious program of reform in the areas of access to primary care and the education of physicians in palliative care? At least as far as the "slippery slope faction" within the Task Force is concerned, we should thus first see to it that every person in this country has access to adequate, affordable, and nondiscriminatory primary and palliative care. At the end of this long and arduous process, when we finally have an equitable, effective, and compassionate health care system in place, we might well want to reopen the discussion of PAS and active euthanasia.

4. Finally, with regard to those few unfortunate patients who are truly beyond the pale of good palliative and psychiatric care, some Task Force members took limited solace from the fact that many such patients will still be able to find compassionate physicians who, like Dr. Quill, will ultimately be willing, albeit in fear and trembling, to "take small risks for patients [they] really care about." Such actions will continue to take place within the privacy of the patient-physician relationship, however, and will thus not threaten vulnerable patients and the social fabric to the extent that would result from full legalization and regulation. To be sure, this kind of continuing covert PAS will not be subject to regulation, but the mere threat of possible criminal sanctions and revocation of licensure will continue to serve as a powerful disincentive to abuse for the vast majority of

physicians. Moreover, as we have seen, it is highly unlikely that the proposals for legalization would result in truly effective oversight.

A POSITIVE AGENDA

Instead of conceiving this as a choice between legalization/regulation, with all of their attendant risks, and the abandonment of patients to their pain and suffering, the Task Force thus recommends a positive program of clinical and social reform. On the clinical level, physicians must learn how better to listen to their patients, to unflinchingly engage them in sensitive discussions of their needs and the meaning of their requests for assisted death, to deliver appropriate palliative care, to distinguish fact from fiction in the ethics and law of pain relief, to diagnose and treat clinical depression, and, finally, to ascertain and respect their patients' wishes for control regarding the forgoing of life-sustaining treatments. On the social level, the Task Force perceives a need for major initiatives in medical and public education regarding pain control, in the sensitization of insurance companies and licensing agencies to issues of the quality of dying, and in the reform of state laws that currently hinder access to pain relieving medications.

A RECENT CHALLENGE

The Task Force's slippery slope argument has recently been indirectly challenged by the authors of an interesting new legislative proposal for regulation.[9] Two points about this proposal are worth briefly mentioning here before closing. First, the authors concede what some of them had explicitly denied in a previous proposal, viz., that the logic of the matter cannot effectively distinguish between PAS and active euthanasia on the one hand, and between terminal illness and ("merely") incurable conditions like ALS on the other. They should thus be commended for forthrightly identifying the crucial parameters of the issue for public debate.

Second, the authors propose an additional safeguard designed to address most of our "empirical slope" objections: viz., a requirement of independent and impartial oversight by a certified palliative-care consultant within a national network of palliative-care committees. Before any choice for death arrived at by patient and physician could be sanctioned within this proposed system, a certified consultant would have to review the patient's diagnosis and prognosis, the possibility of available but untried alternatives for palliative care, the voluntariness and strength of the patient's wish to die, and so on. Consultants would presumably all be well versed in the techniques of palliative care, the nuances of competency, bioethics and law, and in the lived reality of dying patients. Should a patient and/or physician disagree with the verdict of a consultant, they could appeal the case to the consultant's regional committee.

To be sure, this part of the proposal marks a significant improvement over past proposals and legislative ballot initiatives. The requirements that voluntariness and competency be verified by a skilled diagnostician/clinician, and that either PAS or active euthanasia be permitted only after the failure of all other reasonable alternatives, would both go a long way toward providing serious safeguards and assuaging the Task Force's fears of an unalterably slippery slope. I for one, however, have a couple of reservations.

First, there is the lingering fear, expressed throughout the Task Force's report, that any legislative proposal would have to be implemented within the present context of deep and pervasive discrimination against the poor and members of minority groups. We have every reason to expect that a policy that worked tolerably well in an affluent community like Scarsdale might not work so well in a community like Bedford-Stuyvesant or Harlem. There is also reason to worry about any policy of PAS initiated within a growing system of managed care, capitation, and physician-incentives for delivering less care. Expert palliative care is no doubt an expensive and time-consuming proposition, requiring more rather than less time spent just talking with patients. It is highly doubtful that the context of physician-patient conversation within this new dispensation will be at all conducive to humane decisions untainted by subtle economic coercion.

Second, it must be noted that the impressive safeguards required by this proposal would entail significant costs in terms of privacy and autonomy for both patients and physicians. Even though these particular authors deny that their brief is based upon a "right to PAS"—which would itself be based upon the right to privacy in the same manner as abortion[10]; —they will have a hard time explaining this to patients whose appeals have been rejected by the palliative-care consultant and committee. Just as the elaborate paraphernalia of committee review of abortion decisions was swept aside by autonomy-driven judicial decisions in *Roe* v. *Wade* and *Doe* v. *Bolton* (1973), so here patients imbued with the rhetoric of autonomy will surely ask, "Who do these so-called 'consultants' and 'God-committees' think they are, passing judgment on the quality of my own very personal suffering?" And physicians, for their part, will surely be mightily offended by the implication that they cannot be trusted to handle these matters in a competent and sensitive way within the privacy of the physician-patient relationship without a new layer of intrusive and expensive bureaucracy. Indeed, to my mind, the biggest problem for the proponents of this plan would come, not from opponents of PAS on slippery slope grounds, but rather from patients and physicians eager, in the age of Newt, to cast off all remaining vestiges of state-sponsored bureaucracy. In short, the proposed regulations are plausible, at least in theory; but whether they could be sold to skeptical legislatures is a different and much more difficult question.

NOTES

1 *Do Not Resuscitate Orders,* April 1986.

2 *Life-Sustaining Treatment: Making Decisions and Appointing a Health Care Agent,* July 1987.

3 *When Others Must Choose: Deciding for Patients Without Capacity,* May 1992.

4 SUPPORT Principal Investigators, "A Controlled Trial to Improve Care for Seriously Ill Hospitalized Patients: The Study to Understand Prognoses and Preferences for Outcomes and Risks of Treatments (SUPPORT)," *JAMA* 274:20 (November 22/29): 1995. 1591–98.

5 See Timothy Quill, Christine Cassel, and Diane Meier, "Care of the Hopelessly Ill: Proposed Clinical Criteria for Physician-Assisted Suicide," *NEJM* 327:19 (Nov. 5, 1992): 1380–84, where the authors approve of PAS but disapprove of active euthanasia because it poses excessive social risks. Quill and Meier have subsequently conceded the untenability of this distinction in Franklin Miller et al., "Regulating Physician-Assisted Death," *NEJM* 331 (July 14, 1994): 119–123.

6 During the APA Eastern Division Session sponsored by the Committees on Philosophy and Medicine and Philosophy and Law (December 29, 1995) panel discussion, Professor Dan Brock echoed the Dutch view. He held that if one is really concerned with the slippery slope, then allowing surrogates to forgo life-sustaining treatments for incompetents poses far greater risks to autonomy than a policy of physician-assisted death solidly based upon a requirement of the contemporaneous informed consent of the ill person. While Brock may be correct that our current practices surrounding surrogate decision making are subject to abuse and need to be hedged in with further safeguards, I believe that he seriously underestimates the social risks involved with PAS and euthanasia. One crucial dissimilarity between our current practice of forgoing life-sustaining treatment and physician-assisted death is that allowing the latter practice would surely implicate many more people in a hospital. The second crucial difference is that abolishing the firmly entrenched practice of surrogate decision making would throw the health care system into chaos and impose undignified deaths on vast numbers of incompetent patients, whereas continuing to withhold official sanction for physician-assisted death would, at worst, merely continue the status quo.

7 John Arras, "The Right to Die on the Slippery Slope," *Social Theory and Practice,* 8:3 (Fall 1982): 285–328.

8 Dr. Gary Kennedy of the Division of Geriatrics, Montefiore Medical Center, Albert Einstein College of Medicine.

9 Franklin Miller, Timothy Quill, Howard Brody, John Fletcher, Lawrence Gostin, and Diane Meier, "Regulating Physician-Assisted Death," *NEJM* 331 (July 14, 1994): 119–123.

10 See Ronald Dworkin, *Life's Dominion* (New York: Knopf, 1993) for an elegant and powerful restatement of the view that in a pluralistic society individuals should have rights against governmental interference with deeply personal "private choices," such as abortion and euthanasia.

PATIENT REFUSAL OF HYDRATION AND NUTRITION: AN ALTERNATIVE TO PHYSICIAN-ASSISTED SUICIDE OR VOLUNTARY ACTIVE EUTHANASIA

James L. Bernat, Bernard Gert, and R. Peter Mogielnicki

Bernat, Gert, and Mogielnicki focus attention on patient refusal of hydration and nutrition as a means whereby competent patients can effectively bring about their own death. They argue, based on the existing consensus that physicians are morally and legally required to honor the rational refusal of treatment by competent patients, that there is no need to legalize physician-assisted suicide or voluntary active euthanasia. Their basic point is that patient refusal of hydration and nutrition already provides a feasible (and much less problematic) alternative for patients who desire to shorten the dying process. In the course of developing their overall argument, the authors address a series of conceptual issues related to the distinction between killing and letting die. They also emphasize that the feasibility of patient refusal of hydration and nutrition as an alternative to physician-assisted suicide and voluntary active euthanasia depends upon further confirmation of the factual claim "that lack of hydration and nutrition does not cause unmanageable suffering in terminally ill patients."

Public and scholarly debates on legalizing physician-assisted suicide (PAS) and voluntary active euthanasia (VAE) have increased dramatically in recent years.[1-5] These debates have highlighted a significant moral controversy between those who regard PAS and VAE as morally permissible and those who do not. Unfortunately, the adversarial nature of this controversy has led both sides to ignore an alternative that avoids moral controversy altogether and has fewer associated practical problems in its implementation. In this article, we suggest that educating chronically and terminally ill patients about the feasibility of patient refusal of hydration and nutrition (PRHN) can empower them to control their own destiny without requiring physicians to reject the taboos on PAS and VAE that have existed for millennia. To be feasible, this alternative requires confirmation of the preliminary scientific evidence that death by starvation and dehydration need not be accompanied by suffering.

Reprinted with permission of the publisher from *Archives of Internal Medicine,* vol. 153 (December 27, 1993), pp. 2723–2728. Copyright © 1993, American Medical Association.

DEFINITIONS

Before proceeding, we will define several terms. Patients are *competent* to make a decision about their health care if they have the capacity to understand and appreciate all the information necessary to make a rational decision. Patient competence, freedom from coercion, and the receipt of adequate information from the physician are the elements of valid (informed) consent or refusal of treatment.[6,7]

A decision is *rational* if it does not produce harm to the patient (eg, death, pain, or disability) without an adequate reason (eg, to avoid suffering an equal or greater harm). It is rational to rank harms in different ways. For example, it is rational to rank immediate death as worse than several months of suffering from a terminal disease; it is also rational to rank the suffering as worse than immediate death. We count as irrational only those rankings that result in the person suffering great harm and that would be rejected as irrational by almost everyone in the person's culture or subculture.[6,7]

Physician-assisted suicide occurs when the physician provides the necessary medical means for the patient to commit suicide, but death is not the direct result of the physician's act. In PAS, a physician accedes to the rational *request* of a competent patient to be provided with the necessary medical means for the patient to commit suicide. A suicide is *physician-assisted* if the physician's participation is a necessary but not sufficient component to the suicide. For example, a physician who complies with a dying patient's request to write a prescription for 100 pentobarbital tablets that the patient plans to swallow at a later time to commit suicide would be performing PAS.

Voluntary active euthanasia ("killing") occurs when a physician accedes to the rational *request* of a competent patient for some act by the physician to cause the death of the patient, which usually follows immediately on its completion. The physician's act in VAE is both necessary and sufficient to produce the patient's death. For example, a physician who complies with a dying patient's request to kill him mercifully with a lethal intravenous injection of pentobarbital sodium would be performing VAE.

Voluntary passive euthanasia ("letting die") occurs when a physician abides by the rational *refusal* of treatment by a competent patient with the knowledge that doing so will result in the patient dying sooner than if the physician had overruled the patient's refusal and had started or continued treatment. For example, when a physician complies with the refusal of a ventilator-dependent patient with motor neuron disease to receive further mechanical ventilatory support, and the patient dies as the result of extubation, this act is an example of voluntary passive euthanasia. Providing medical treatment to alleviate the pain and discomfort that normally accompanies extubation neither alters the fact that the physician is letting the patient die nor makes the act PAS. *Patient refusal of hydration and nutrition* is an example of voluntary passive euthanasia.

There are critical differences in the morality and legality of these acts. Physician-assisted suicide is legally prohibited in many jurisdictions, and there is a current controversy about whether it is moral. Voluntary active euthanasia is classified as criminal homicide and hence is strictly illegal in nearly every jurisdiction. Like PAS, its morality remains controversial. By contrast, there is no disagreement that physicians are morally and legally prohibited from overruling the rational refusal of therapy by a competent patient even when they know that death will result. There is also no disagreement that physicians are allowed to provide appropriate treatment for the pain and suffering that may accompany such refusals. In other words, physicians are morally and legally *required* to respect the competent patient's rational refusal of therapy, and they are morally and legally allowed to provide appropriate treatment for the pain and suffering involved. Physicians also are morally and legally required to abide by such refusals given as advance directives.[8]

CONFUSION CONCERNING KILLING VS LETTING DIE

Three areas of terminologic confusion that have clouded clear thinking about the morality of physician involvement in the care of the dying patient are (1) requests vs refusals by patients, (2) acts vs omissions by physicians, and (3) "natural" vs other causes of death.

PATIENTS' REQUESTS VS REFUSALS

Physicians are morally and legally required to honor a competent patient's rational *refusal* of therapy.[9–11] This requirement arises from the moral and legal prohibition against depriving a person of freedom and from the liberty-based right of a person to be left alone. In the medical context, it requires that the patient provide valid consent before any medical tests or treatments may be performed.

The moral and legal requirement to honor a refusal does not extend, however, to honoring a patient's *request* for specific therapy or other acts. Physicians should honor such requests or refuse to honor them on the basis of their professional judgment about the legal, moral, or medical appropriateness of doing so. A common example of the exercise of this freedom is physicians' refusal to prescribe requested narcotics in situations in which they judge narcotics to be inappropriate.

Confusion arises when the patient's refusal is framed misleadingly in terms resembling a request.[12] For example, a patient's "request" that no cardiopulmonary resuscitation be attempted is actually a refusal of permission for cardiopulmonary resuscitation. Similarly, written advance directives "requesting" the cessation or omission of other therapies are really refusals of treatment. Some writers have added to the confusion by simply talking of the patient's "choice" to forgo therapy as if there were no morally significant distinction between refusing and requesting.[12]

The distinction between requests and refusals has a critical importance in understanding the distinction between voluntary passive euthanasia (letting die) and VAE (killing). Patient *refusals* must be honored when they represent the rational decisions of competent patients even when physicians know death will result. There is no moral requirement to honor patient *requests* when physicians know death will result and there may be legal prohibitions against doing so.

PHYSICIANS' ACTS VS OMISSIONS

Some philosophers have misunderstood the definitions of VAE (killing) and passive euthanasia (letting die, including PRHN) and their moral significance by basing the distinction between killing and letting die on the distinction between acts and omissions.[13,14] In so doing, they have followed many physicians who have concentrated solely on what they themselves do (acts) or do not do (omissions) in distinguishing between killing and letting die. This way of distinguishing between killing and letting die creates a false moral distinction between a physician turning off intravenous feeding (act) and not replacing the intravenous solution container when it is empty (omission). When the distinction between killing and letting die is made in this way, it undermines legitimate medical and legal practice that permits allowing to die and does not permit killing.

This mistaken narrow focus on what the physician does or does not do without taking into account the larger context in which the physician acts or does not act can lead to the mistaken conclusion that PAS and VAE are really no different from voluntary passive euthanasia or "letting die." Recognition of the key role of whether or not the action is in response to the *patient's request* or the *patient's refusal* casts the issue in a clearer light.

As a matter of medical and legal practice, on the basis of a rational refusal of a competent patient, it is permitted either not to begin ventilatory therapy or to stop it; not to start treatment with antibiotics or to discontinue antibiotics; and not to start artificial hydration and nutrition or to cease them. All of these acts and omissions are morally and legally permitted when they result from a rational refusal by a competent patient. Indeed, it is misleading to say that these acts are morally and legally permitted, for they are morally and legally *required*. It is the rational refusal by a competent patient that is decisive here, not whether the physician acts or omits acting. It is the patient's refusal that makes the physician's acts and omissions "letting die" rather than "killing." Whether honoring this refusal requires the physician to act or omit acting is irrelevant. That is why those who base the distinction between killing and letting die on the distinction between acts and omissions mistakenly conclude that no morally relevant distinction exists.

'NATURAL' VS OTHER CAUSES OF DEATH

The term *natural,* as in "death by natural causes," has been another source of confusion. *Natural* is often used as a word of praise or, more generally, as a way of condoning something that otherwise would be considered unacceptable. Thus, voluntary passive euthanasia is often presented as acceptable because it allows the patient to "die a natural death." Because the death was caused by the disease process, no person is assigned responsibility for the death. The freedom from responsibility for the patient's death is psychologically helpful for the physician. To make some state laws authorizing advance directives more acceptable to the public, they even have been labeled "natural death acts."

When death results from lack of hydration and nutrition, however, it is less plausible to say that "the death was caused by the disease process." Thus, someone must be assigned responsibility for the patient's death, and physicians wish to avoid this responsibility. A partial explanation for the misuse of technology to prolong dying unjustifiably may be an attempt by physicians to avoid this psychological responsibility. Physicians who recognize that patients have the authority to refuse any treatment, including hydration and nutrition, are more likely to avoid unjustified feelings of responsibility for their deaths.

Just as it is erroneous to think that the distinction between acts and omissions has any moral relevance, so it is erroneous to think that anything morally significant turns on the use of the terms *natural* or *cause*. What is morally significant is that the terminally ill patient is competent and has made a rational decision to refuse further treatment. Indeed, it is not even important whether what the patient has refused counts as treatment. If the patient has refused, the physician has no moral or legal authority to overrule that refusal. It is morally and legally irrelevant whether or not the resulting death is considered natural.

PATIENT REFUSAL OF HYDRATION AND NUTRITION

We maintain that a preferable alternative to legalization of PAS and VAE is for physicians to educate patients that they may refuse hydration and nutrition and that physicians will help them do so in a way that minimizes suffering. Chronically or terminally ill patients who wish to gain more control over their deaths can then refuse to eat and drink and refuse enteral or parenteral feedings or hydration. The failure of the present debate to include this alternative may be the result of the confusion discussed above, an erroneous assumption that thirst and hunger remain strong drives in terminal illness, and a misconception that failure to satisfy these drives causes intractable suffering.

The stereotypic image of a parched person on a desert crawling toward a mirage of water, and narrative accounts of otherwise healthy shipwrecked victims adrift without water, have contributed to the general notion that life-threatening dehydration is unbearable.[15,16] Although this is true in the above circumstances, it is the consensus of experienced physicians and nurses that terminally ill patients dying of dehydration or lack of nutrition do not suffer if treated properly. In fact, maintaining physiologic hydration and adequate nutrition is difficult in most seriously ill patients because intrinsic thirst and hunger are usually diminished or absent.

Throughout the 1980s, many thinkers expressed serious reservations about allowing withdrawal of hydration and nutrition to become acceptable medical practice. These reservations, however, were not based on any information about the discomfort or suffering experienced by patients under these circumstances. Rather, caregivers experienced psychologic distress due in part to the failure to understand the distinction between killing and letting die, and the social implications of withdrawing or withholding food and fluids, particularly because of its symbolism as communicating lack of caring.[17,18]

However, if the distinction between killing and letting die is based as it should be on patients' requests vs patients' refusals, these latter considerations lose their force. Now the crucial consideration becomes the degree of suffering associated with lack of hydration and nutrition. If the associated suffering is trivial, PRHN clearly has major advantages over PAS or VAE. Only if this suffering is unmanageable does the choice become more difficult. Scientific studies and anecdotal reports both suggest that dehydration and starvation in the seriously ill do not cause significant suffering. Physicians and particularly nurses have written many observational pieces describing peaceful and apparently comfortable deaths by starvation and dehydration.[19–21] Lay observers have corroborated these reports.[22]

Surprisingly, the scientific literature is incomplete on this matter. Systematic studies of the symptoms preceding death are hard to find, and those that do exist commonly do not separate suffering attributable to the underlying disease from suffering attributable to dehydration.[23–25] During World War II, metabolic studies of starvation and of fluid deprivation noted incidentally that the thirst experienced by normal healthy volunteers was typically "not actually uncomfortable" and characteristically was "quenched by an amount of water much less than was lost."[26,27]

A handful of laboratory studies and clinical trials are consistent with these older observational comments, but the picture is far from complete. Starvation is known to produce increased levels of acetoacetate, β-hydroxybutyrate, and acetone.[28] Other ketones (methyl butyl ketone and methyl heptyl ketone) have been shown to have an anesthetic action on isolated squid axons.[29] Depriving male Wistar rats of water and food for periods ranging from 24 to 72 hours has been shown to increase the levels of some endogenous opioids in the hypothalamus, although levels elsewhere in the brain and other organs decrease.[30] Healthy elderly men (over 65 years old) have been demonstrated to experience reduced thirst and associated symptoms during a 24-hour period of water deprivation and, when given ad libitum access to water to correct their dehydration, do so much more slowly than young healthy men.[31]

Observational data on the experience of terminally ill patients dying of dehydration have been recorded most recently in the hospice literature. This evidence suggests that the overwhelming majority of hospice deaths resulting from lack of hydration and nutrition can be managed such that the patients remain comfortable.[19,32–35] In a 1990 survey of 826 members of the (US) Academy of Hospice Physicians, 89% of hospice nurses and 86% of hospice physicians reported that their terminal patients who died by cessation of hydration and nutrition had peaceful and comfortable deaths.[36]

Taken in toto, the anecdotal reports, laboratory studies, and the observations of nurses and physicians who care for terminally ill patients suggest that lack of hydration and nutrition does not cause unmanageable suffering in terminally ill patients and may even have an analgesic effect. Clinical experience with severely ill patients suggests that the major symptom of dry mouth can be relieved by ice chips, methyl cellulose, artificial saliva, or small sips of water insufficient to reverse progressive dehydration.

BENEFITS OF PRHN OVER PAS AND VAE

Unlike PAS and VAE, PRHN is recognized by all as consistent with current medical, moral, and legal practices. It does not compromise public confidence in the medical profession because it does not require physicians to assume any new role or responsibility that could alter their roles of healer, caregiver, and counselor. It places the proper emphasis on the duty of physicians to care for dying patients, because these patients need care and comfort measures during the dying period. It encourages physicians to engage in educational discussions with patients and families about dying and the desirability of formulating clear advance directives.

Legalization of PAS or VAE would likely create unintended and harmful social pressures and expectations. Many elderly or chronically ill patients could feel "the duty to die." They would request euthanasia not on the basis of personal choice but because they believed that their families considered them a burden and expected them to agree to be killed. Furthermore, patients might sense pressure from their physicians to consider VAE as an alternative and agree because the physicians must know what is best for them.[37] The meaning of "voluntary" euthanasia thus could become corrupted, causing the elderly and chronically ill to become victimized.

Unlike the "duty to die" resulting from legalizing PAS or VAE, it is unlikely that patients choosing to die by PRHN would feel as much social pressure or expectations from family members to die earlier because of the duration of the process and the opportunity therein for reconsideration and family interaction. Furthermore, it is much less likely that there would be pressure from physicians or other health professionals. Additionally, the several-day interval before unconsciousness ensues from PRHN would permit time for appropriate mourning and good-byes to family and friends.

Physicians may experience psychological stress about the patient's refusal of hydration and nutrition. Their moral and legal obligation to respect the treatment refusal should absolve some of the physician's discomfort. Physicians can seek no such solace in PAS or VAE because even if both were legalized, they would not be required. Physicians acceding to requests for PAS or VAE, even if it were legal, do so without legal or moral force compelling them to do so. This underscores the essential difference between passive euthanasia and PAS or VAE. It also lays bare the distress to be expected by physicians should they become involved with PAS and VAE in that they always will do so without an accompanying moral mandate.

Legalization of PAS or VAE would require the creation of a network of cumbersome legal safeguards to protect patients from abuse and misunderstanding or miscommunication. Despite such bureaucratic efforts, there would remain a risk that the practice of voluntary euthanasia would extend to involuntary cases, as has been alleged in the Dutch experience where VAE, although officially illegal, is permitted if physicians follow a series of judicial guidelines.[38,39] Furthermore, the safeguards would require the insinuation of courts, lawyers, and bureaucrats between the patient-family and the physician. The new legal requirements could have the effect of delaying the patient's death and generating unnecessary administrative complexity and expense.

Unlike PAS and VAE, PRHN is lawful already in most jurisdictions. Indeed, refusal of hydration and nutrition is listed as an option in commonly drafted advance directives in the United States. Communication errors, misunderstandings, and abuse are less likely with PRHN than with PAS or VAE and thus are less likely to result in an unwanted earlier death. The patient who refuses hydration and nutrition clearly demonstrates the seriousness and consistency of his or her desire to die. The several-day interval before the patient becomes unconscious provides time to reconsider the decision and for the family to accept that dying clearly represents the patient's wish. Furthermore, the process can begin immediately without first requiring legal approvals or other bureaucratic interventions. Thus, it may allow the patient to die faster than PAS or VAE, given the delays intrinsic to bureaucratic process.

THE PHYSICIAN'S ROLE IN PRHN

The current interest in legalizing PAS and VAE misplaces the emphasis of physicians' duties to their dying patients. Physicians should be more concerned about providing patients optimal terminal care than killing them or helping them kill themselves. Legalizing PAS would make it unnecessary for physicians to strive to maximize comfort measures in terminally ill patients and unnecessary for society to support research to improve the science of palliation.[12] By comparison, PRHN appropriately encourages the physician to attend to the medical treatment of dying patients.

The physician's traditional role has been summarized as "to cure sometimes, to relieve often, and to comfort always."[40] With PRHN, the physician can concentrate his or her energy on the last two of these three challenging tasks. In the modern era, this involves a number of important pragmatic matters worthy of review.

Terminal illness should be anticipated with all patients by education and offers of assistance in the design, completion, and implementation of advance directives for terminal care. Arrangements for appropriate home help and necessary nursing attendance must be addressed, as should appropriate means of avoiding well-intended but undesired resuscitation attempts by emergency medical technicians at the time of death. A pact should be made with the patient that the physician will do his or her best to minimize suffering during the dying process and will remain available to comfort the patient by physical presence as well as skillful treatment of symptoms, including pain, dyspnea, and dryness of the mouth.

Physicians caring for patients dying of PRHN have an important responsibility to provide adequate symptom control. Effective mouth care can relieve most of the unpleasant symptoms of thirst and mouth dryness. Physicians should be willing to prescribe narcotics and benzodiazepines in dosages sufficient to abate pain and other unpleasant sensations. They should not incorrectly limit the dosage of their prescriptions for fear of accelerating death; the intent should be to maintain adequate comfort during dying. The possibility of a hastened death as a complication of symptomatic treatment is an acceptable risk and does not count as PAS or VAE. There is evidence that adequate pain control in terminally ill cancer patients reduces the demand for PAS.[41] It is likely that adequate control of unpleasant symptoms during dying would also lessen demands for VAE.

There are several areas in PRHN where more work needs to be done. There remains a need for more systematic research on the phenomenology and pathophysiology of dying as a result of refusal of hydration and nutrition. Additional studies will help physicians understand the needs of dying patients and thereby ensure patient comfort throughout the dying process.

There needs to be societal acceptance that physicians have a moral duty to respect the rational wishes of competent, chronically ill but not terminally ill patients who wish to die by PRHN or other valid refusals of therapy. There is no reason why such patients should not have the same rights as the terminally ill to refuse life-sustaining therapies, including hydration and nutrition.[11] The American Academy of Neurology recently published a position statement asserting that chronically ill patients with severe paralysis and intact cognition, whether terminally ill or not, have the right to refuse life-sustaining therapy, including hydration and nutrition.[42,43]

The most pressing need is to dispel the myths about suffering caused by dehydration and to publicize as widely as possible to both physicians and their terminally ill patients the availability of PRHN as a means of shortening the dying process. Educational efforts should be directed to physicians, who are often ill-informed on this matter,[44] as well as to the general public. The emphasis on research and education on symptomatic treatments to relieve suffering during dying is fully compatible with the traditional and appropriate role of the physician as caregiver and comforter.

Since this manuscript was accepted for publication, other well-studied cases have been reported of comfortable deaths by patient refusal of hydration and nutrition.[45]

REFERENCES

1 Crigger B. J., ed. Dying well? a colloquy on euthanasia and assisted suicide. *Hastings Cent Rep.* 1992; 22:6–55.
2 Campbell C. S., Crigger B. J., eds. Mercy, murder, and morality: perspectives on euthanasia. *Hastings Cent Rep.* 1989; 19(suppl 1):1–32.
3 Pellegrino E. D. Doctors must not kill. *J Clin Ethics.* 1992; 3:95–102.
4 Quill T. E., Cassel C. K., Meier D. E. Care of the hopelessly ill: proposed clinical criteria for physician-assisted suicide. *N Engl J Med.* 1992; 327:1380–1384.
5 Brody H. Assisted death: a compassionate response to a medical failure. *N Engl J Med.* 1992; 327:1384–1388.
6 Culver C. M., Gert B. Basic ethical concepts in neurologic practice. *Semin Neurol.* 1984; 4:1–8.
7 Gert B., Culver C. M. Moral theory in neurologic practice. *Semin Neurol.* 1984; 4:9–14.
8 Gert B, Culver C. M. Distinguishing between active and passive euthanasia. *Clin Geriatr Med.* 1986; 2:29–36.
9 Culver C. M., Gert B. *Philosophy in Medicine: Conceptual and Ethical Issues in Medicine and Psychiatry.* New York, NY: Oxford University Press; 1982:20–64.
10 Gert B. *Morality: A New Justification of the Moral Rules.* New York, NY: Oxford University Press; 1988:282–303.
11 Meisel A. Legal myths about terminating life support. *Arch Intern Med.* 1991; 151:1497–1502.
12 Council on Ethical and Judicial Affairs, American Medical Association. Decisions near the end of life. *JAMA.* 1992; 267:2229–2233.
13 Rachels J. Active and passive euthanasia. *N Engl J Med.* 1975; 292:78–80.
14 Brock D. W. Voluntary active euthanasia. *Hastings Cent Rep.* 1992; 22:10–22.
15 Wolf A. V. *Thirst: Physiology of the Urge to Drink and Problems of Water Lack.* Springfield, Ill: Charles C Thomas Publisher; 1958:208–252, 375–463.
16 Critchley M. *Shipwreck Survivors: A Medical Study.* London, England: Churchill Ltd; 1943:24–40.
17 Derr P. G. Why food and fluids can never be denied. *Hastings Cent Rep.* 1986; 16:28–30.
18 Callahan D. On feeding the dying. *Hastings Cent Rep.* 1983; 13:22.
19 Andrews M., Levine A. Dehydration in the terminal patient: perception of hospice nurses. *Am J Hospice Care.* 1989; 3:31–34.
20 Zerwekh J. The dehydration question. *Nursing.* 1983; 13:47–51.
21 Printz L. A. Terminal dehydration, a compassionate treatment. *Arch Intern Med.* 1992; 152:697–700.
22 Nearing H. *Loving and Leaving the Good Life.* Post Mills, Vt: Chelsea Green Publishing Co; 1992.
23 Mogielnicki R. P., Nelson W. A., Dulac J. A study of the dying process in elderly hospitalized males. *J Cancer Educ.* 1990; 5:135–145.
24 Billings J. Comfort measures for the terminally ill: is dehydration painful? *J Am Geriatr Soc.* 1985; 33:808–810.
25 Morris J. N., Suissa S., Sherwood S., et al. Last days: a study of the quality of life of terminally ill cancer patients. *J Chronic Dis.* 1986; 39:47–62.
26 Winkler A. W., Danowski T. S., Elkinton J. R., Peters J. P. Electrolyte and fluid studies during water deprivation and starvation in human subjects and the effect of ingestion of fish, of carbohydrates, and of salt solutions. *J Clin Invest.* 1944; 23:807–811.
27 Black D. A. K., McCance R. A., Young W. F. A study of dehydration by means of balance experiments. *J Physiol.* 1944; 102:406–414.
28 Owen O., Caprio S., Reichard G., et al. Ketosis of starvation: a revisit and new perspectives. *Clin Endocrinol Metab.* 1983; 12:359–379.
29 Elliott J. R., Haydon D. A., Hendry B. M. Anaesthetic action of esters and ketones: evidence for an interaction with the sodium channel protein in squid axons. *J Physiol.* 1984; 354: 407–418.
30 Majeed N. H., Lason W., Prewlocka B., et al. Brain and peripheral opioid peptides after changes in ingestive behavior. *Neuroendocrinology.* 1986; 42:267–272.
31 Phillips P. A., Rolls B. J., Ledingham J. G. G., et al. Reduced thirst after water deprivation in healthy elderly men. *N Engl J Med.* 1984; 311: 753–759.
32 Miller R. J., Albright P. G. What is the role of nutritional support and hydration in terminal cancer patients? *Am J Hospice Care.* 1989; 6:33–38.
33 Cox S. S. Is dehydration painful? *Ethics Med.* 1987; 12:1–2.
34 Lichter I, Hunt E. The last 48 hours of life. *J Palliat Care.* 1990; 6:7–15.

35 Miller R. J. Hospice care as an alternative to euthanasia. *Law Med Health Care.* 1992; 20:127–132.

36 Miller R. J. Nutrition and hydration in terminal disease. *J Palliat Care.* In press.

37 Kamisar Y. Some non-religious views against proposed 'mercy-killing' legislation. *Minn Law Rev.* 1958; 42:969–1042.

38 Benrubi G. I. Euthanasia: the need for procedural safeguards. *N Engl J Med.* 1992; 326:197–199.

39 Van der Maas P. J., van Delden J. J. M., Pijnenborg L, Looman C. W. N. Euthanasia and other medical decisions concerning the end of life. *Lancet.* 1991; 338:669–674.

40 Strauss M. B, ed. *Familiar Medical Quotations.* Boston, Mass: Little Brown & Co; 1968:410.

41 Foley K. M. The relationship of pain and symptom management to patient requests for physician-assisted suicide. *J Pain Symptom Management* 1991; 6:289–297.

42 American Academy of Neurology. Position statement: certain aspects of the care and management of profoundly and irreversibly paralyzed patients with retained consciousness and cognition. *Neurology.* 1993; 53:222–223.

43 Bernat J. L, Cranford R. E, Kittredge F. I. Jr, Rosenberg RN. Competent patients with advanced states of permanent paralysis have the right to forgo life-sustaining therapy. *Neurology.* 1993; 43:224–225.

44 Ahronheim J. C., Gasner M. R. The sloganism of starvation. *Lancet.* 1990; 335:278–279.

45 Sullivan R. J. Accepting death without artificial nutrition or hydration. *J Gen Intern Med.* 1993; 8: 220–224.

ANNOTATED BIBLIOGRAPHY

Battin, Margaret Pabst: *Ethical Issues in Suicide* (Englewood Cliffs, NJ: Prentice Hall, 1995). In this useful book, Battin provides a comprehensive discussion of the traditional arguments concerning suicide. She also suggests an analysis of the concept of rational suicide, discusses suicide intervention as well as suicide facilitation, and considers the notion of suicide as a right. The book's final chapter provides a discussion of physician-assisted suicide.

Battin, M. Pabst, and David J. Mayo, eds.: *Suicide: The Philosophical Issues* (New York: St. Martin's Press, 1980). This valuable collection of articles includes material on the concept of suicide, the morality of suicide, and the rationality of suicide. There are also sections entitled "Suicide and Psychiatry" and "Suicide, Law, and Rights."

Battin, Margaret P., Rosamond Rhodes, and Anita Silvers, eds.: *Physician-Assisted Suicide: Expanding the Debate* (New York: Routledge, 1998). The essays in Part Two of this extensive collection debate the projected impact of physician-assisted suicide on vulnerable patients. Part Three considers physician-assisted suicide in reference to the practice of medicine, Part Four provides contrasting viewpoints on the issue of legalization, and Part Five presents religious perspectives.

Beauchamp, Tom L.: "Suicide." In Tom Regan, ed., *Matters of Life and Death,* 3rd ed. (New York: McGraw-Hill, 1993), pp. 69–120. In this long essay, Beauchamp provides both a conceptual analysis of suicide and an evaluation of various moral views. He also discusses suicide intervention and assisted suicide.

Beck, Robert N., and John B. Orr, eds.: *Ethical Choice: A Case Study Approach* (New York: Free Press, 1970). Section 2 of this work is entitled "Suicide" and conveniently reprints several classical sources on suicide: Seneca, St. Augustine, St. Thomas Aquinas, Hume, and Schopenhauer.

Coleman, Carl H., and Alan R. Fleischman: "Guidelines for Physician-Assisted Suicide: Can the Challenge Be Met?" *Journal of Law, Medicine & Ethics* 24 (Fall 1996), pp. 217–224. Coleman and Fleischman survey various proposals for regulating physician-assisted suicide and argue against legalization of the practice.

Gomez, Carlos F.: *Regulating Death: Euthanasia and the Case of The Netherlands* (New York: Free Press, 1991). Gomez describes and criticizes the practice of (active) euthanasia in The Netherlands. He argues that the Dutch system is plagued with inadequate controls.

Hastings Center Report 22 (March–April 1992). This issue provides a collection of articles under the heading "Dying Well? A Colloquy on Euthanasia and Assisted Suicide." Several of the articles deal specifically with the practice of (active) euthanasia in The Netherlands. Also, Dan W. Brock offers an extensive defense of voluntary active euthanasia, which Daniel Callahan opposes in "When Self-Determination Runs Amok."

Hedberg, Katrina, David Hopkins, and Melvin Kohn: "Five Years of Legal Physician-Assisted Suicide in Oregon," *New England Journal of Medicine* 348 (March 6, 2003), pp. 961–964. The authors, on behalf of Oregon Public Health Services, present statistical data on the practice of physician-assisted suicide in Oregon during the first five years (1998–2002) subsequent to legalization.

Legemaate, Johan: "The Dutch Euthanasia Act and Related Issues," *Journal of Law and Medicine* 11 (February 2004), pp. 312–323. Legemaate provides a discussion of the 2002 Dutch Termination of Life on Request and Assisted Suicide Act. He sets this legislation in historical context and considers international reactions to it. The full text of the act itself is included as an appendix to the article.

Mayo, David J., and Martin Gunderson: "Vitalism Revitalized: Vulnerable Populations, Prejudice, and Physician-Assisted Death," *Hastings Center Report* 32 (July–August 2002), pp. 14–21. Mayo and Gunderson reject the argument that physician-assisted death should not be legalized because people with disabilities (and members of other vulnerable populations) would be coerced into choosing physician-assisted death. The authors contend that this argument ultimately depends upon medical vitalism, the indefensible view that life should be prolonged whenever possible.

McStay, Rob: "Terminal Sedation: Palliative Care for Intractable Pain, post *Glucksberg* and *Quill,*" *American Journal of Law & Medicine* 29 (2003), pp. 45–76. McStay clarifies the legal basis of terminal sedation and describes how the debate about terminal sedation has played out among legal and medical commentators.

Miller, Franklin G., and Diane E. Meier: "Voluntary Death: A Comparison of Terminal Dehydration and Physician-Assisted Suicide," *Annals of Internal Medicine* 128 (April 1, 1998), pp. 559–562. Miller and Meier argue that terminal dehydration has some notable advantages over physician-assisted suicide.

Miller, Franklin G., Howard Brody, and Timothy E. Quill: "Can Physician-Assisted Suicide Be Regulated Effectively?" *Journal of Law, Medicine & Ethics* 24 (Fall 1996), pp. 225–232. The authors provide a further defense of their view that mandatory, independent palliative-care consultation is the key procedural safeguard necessary for the effective regulation of physician-assisted suicide.

Pellegrino, Edmund D.: "Doctors Must Not Kill," *Journal of Clinical Ethics* 3 (Summer 1992), pp. 95–102. Pellegrino contends (1) that the moral arguments in favor of (active) euthanasia are flawed, (2) that killing by physicians would seriously distort the healing relationship, and (3) that the social consequences of allowing such killing would be detrimental.

Prado, C. G.: *The Last Choice: Preemptive Suicide in Advanced Age,* 2nd ed. (Westport, CT: Praeger, 1998). Prado's basic claim is that it can be rational for an aging individual to commit suicide in order to avoid a demeaning decline. That is, he claims that suicide can be a rational choice even prior to the onset of unendurable mental or physical suffering.

Quill, Timothy E.: "Death and Dignity: A Case of Individualized Decision Making," *New England Journal of Medicine* 324 (March 7, 1991), pp. 691–694. Quill presents a brief account of a case, often referred to as "the case of Diane," in which he assisted in the suicide of one of his patients.

————, Bernard Lo, and Dan W. Brock: "Palliative Options of Last Resort: A Comparison of Voluntarily Stopping Eating and Drinking, Terminal Sedation, Physician-Assisted Suicide, and Voluntary Active Euthanasia," *JAMA* 278 (December 17, 1977), pp. 2099–2104. The authors compare and contrast the four identified practices. Both a clinical analysis and an ethical analysis are presented. Also provided is a brief discussion of appropriate safeguards for hastening death by any of the methods under discussion.

Rachels, James: "Euthanasia." In Tom Regan, ed., *Matters of Life and Death,* 3rd ed. (New York: McGraw-Hill, 1993), pp. 30–68. In this long essay, Rachels evaluates (1) arguments for and against the morality of active euthanasia and (2) arguments for and against legalizing it. He concludes that active euthanasia is morally acceptable and should be legalized.

Steinbock, Bonnie, and Alastair Norcross, eds.: *Killing and Letting Die,* 2nd ed. (New York: Fordham University Press, 1994). This anthology provides a wealth of material on the distinction between killing and letting die.

Wolf, Susan M.: "Gender, Feminism, and Death: Physician-Assisted Suicide and Euthanasia." In Susan M. Wolf, ed., *Feminism & Bioethics: Beyond Reproduction* (New York: Oxford University Press, 1996), pp. 282–317. Wolf provides an analysis of physician-assisted suicide and (active) euthanasia in reference to the category of gender. She also constructs feminist counterarguments to standard arguments in support of these practices, which she considers dangerous to women.

CHAPTER 7

ABORTION AND RESEARCH ON EMBRYONIC STEM CELLS

INTRODUCTION

The first object of concern in this chapter is the issue of the ethical (moral) acceptability of abortion. Some attention is then given to the social policy aspects of abortion, especially in conjunction with decisions made by the U.S. Supreme Court. Finally, attention is focused on the ethics of research on embryonic stem cells.

ABORTION: THE ETHICAL ISSUE

Discussions of the ethical acceptability of abortion often take for granted (1) an awareness of the various reasons that may be given for having an abortion and (2) a basic acquaintance with the biological development of a human fetus.

Reasons for Abortion Why would a woman have an abortion? The following catalog, not meant to provide an exhaustive survey, is sufficient to demonstrate the wide range of potential reasons for abortion. (1) In certain extreme cases, if the fetus is allowed to develop normally and come to term, the pregnant woman herself will die. (2) In other cases, it is not the woman's life but her health, physical or mental, that will be severely endangered if the pregnancy is allowed to continue. (3) There are also cases in which the pregnancy will probably, or surely, produce a severely impaired child,[1] and (4) there are others in which the pregnancy is the result of rape or incest.[2] (5) There are instances in which the pregnant woman is unmarried and faces the social stigma of illegitimacy. (6) In other instances, having a child, or having another child, will be an unbearable financial burden. (7) Certainly common, and perhaps most common of all, are those instances in which having a child will interfere with the happiness of the woman, the joint happiness of the couple, or even the combined happiness of a family unit that already includes children. There are almost endless possibilities in this final category. For example, the woman may desire a professional career, a couple may be content and happy together and feel their relationship would be damaged by the intrusion of a child, and parents may have older children and not feel up to raising another child.

The Biological Development of a Human Fetus During the course of a human pregnancy, in the nine-month period from conception to birth, the entity resulting from conception undergoes a continual process of change and development. *Conception* takes place when a male germ cell (the spermatazoon) combines with a female germ cell (the ovum), resulting in a single cell (the single-cell zygote), which embodies the full genetic code, twenty-three pairs of chromosomes. The single-cell zygote, also commonly identified as a newly formed *embryo,* soon begins a process of cellular division. While continuing to grow and beginning to take shape, the embryo moves through the fallopian tube and then undergoes gradual *implantation* at the uterine wall. The process of implantation is complete about eight to ten days after conception. The embryonic period continues until the end of the eighth week, and it is during this period—subsequent to implantation—that organ systems and other recognizably human characteristics begin to undergo noticeable development; in particular, rudimentary electrical activity in the brain may be detectable as early as the end of the sixth week. From the end of the eighth week until birth, the developing entity is formally designated a *fetus.* (The term *fetus,* however, is commonly used as a general term to designate the developing entity, whatever its stage of development.) Two other points in the development of the fetus are especially noteworthy as relevant to discussions of abortion, but these points are usually identified by reference to gestational age as calculated not from conception but from the first day of the woman's last menstrual period. Accordingly, somewhere around the sixteenth to the eighteenth week there usually occurs *quickening,* the point at which the woman begins to feel the movements of the fetus. And somewhere around the twenty-second week, *viability* becomes a realistic possibility. Viability is the point at which the fetus is capable of surviving outside the womb.

With the facts of fetal development in clear view, it may be helpful to describe the various abortion procedures. First-trimester abortions were at one time performed by *dilation and curettage (D&C),* but that procedure was essentially replaced in the 1970s by *vacuum aspiration,* often referred to as *suction abortion.* D&C involves the stretching (dilation) of the cervix and the scraping (curettage) of the inner walls of the uterus. In vacuum aspiration, the fetus is sucked out of the uterus by means of a tube connected to a suction pump. Although standard vacuum aspiration cannot effectively be performed prior to about two months after a pregnant woman's last period, a related technique—*manual vacuum aspiration (MVA)*—now provides the possibility of much earlier surgical abortion. In MVA, ultrasound is used to locate the tiny (smaller than a pea) gestational sac, which is then removed with a hand-held vacuum syringe. The use of RU-486, a chemical method for the termination of early pregnancies, is discussed later in this introduction.

Abortions beyond the first trimester require procedures such as *dilation and evacuation (D&E), induction techniques,* or *hysterotomy.* In D&E, which is the abortion procedure commonly used in the early stages of the second trimester, a forceps is used to dismember the fetus within the uterus; the fetal remains are then withdrawn through the cervix. In one notable induction technique, a saline solution injected into the amniotic cavity induces labor, thereby expelling the fetus. Another important induction technique employs prostaglandins (hormonelike substances) to induce labor. Hysterotomy—in essence, a miniature caesarean section—is a major surgical procedure and is uncommonly employed in the United States.

A brief discussion of fetal development, together with a cursory survey of various reasons for abortion, has prepared the way for a formulation of the ethical issue of abortion in its broadest terms. *Up to what point of fetal development, if any, and for what reasons, if any, is abortion ethically acceptable?* Some hold that abortion is *never* ethically acceptable, or at most that it is acceptable only when necessary to save the life of the pregnant woman. This view is frequently termed the *conservative* view on abortion. Others hold that abortion is *always* ethically acceptable—at any point of fetal development and for any of the standard reasons. This view is frequently termed the *liberal* view on abortion. Still others are anxious to defend perspectives that are termed *moderate* views, holding that abortion is ethically acceptable up to a certain point of fetal development and/or holding that some reasons provide a sufficient justification for abortion whereas others do not.

THE CONSERVATIVE VIEW AND THE LIBERAL VIEW

The *moral status* of the fetus has been a pivotal issue in discussions of the ethical acceptability of abortion. To say that the fetus has full moral status is to say that it is entitled to the same degree of moral consideration deserved by more fully developed human beings, such as the writer and the reader of these words. Assigning full moral status to the fetus entails, in particular, that the fetus has a right to life that must be taken as seriously as the right to life of any other human being. On the other hand, to say that the fetus has no significant moral status is to say that it has no rights worth mentioning. In particular, it does not possess a significant right to life. Conservatives typically claim that the fetus has full moral status, and liberals typically claim that the fetus has no significant moral status. (Some moderates argue that the fetus has a subsidiary or *partial* moral status.) Since the fetus has no significant moral status, the liberal is prone to argue, it has no more right to life than a piece of tissue, such as an appendix, and an abortion is no more morally objectionable than an appendectomy. Since the fetus has full moral status, the conservative is prone to argue, its right to life must be respected with the utmost seriousness, and an abortion, except perhaps to save the life of a pregnant woman, is as morally objectionable as any other murder.

Discussions of the moral status of the fetus often refer directly to the biological development of the fetus and pose the question: At what point in the continuous development of the fetus does a human life exist? In the context of such discussions, *human* implies full moral status, *nonhuman* implies no significant moral status, and any notion of partial moral status is systematically excluded. To distinguish the human from the nonhuman, to "draw the line," and to do so in a nonarbitrary way, is the central matter of concern. A conservative on abortion typically holds that the line must be drawn at conception. Usually the conservative argues that conception is the only point at which the line can be nonarbitrarily drawn. Against attempts to draw the line at points such as implantation, quickening, viability, or birth, considerations of continuity in the development of the fetus are pressed. The conservative argues that a line cannot be securely drawn anywhere along the path of fetal development. It is said that the line will inescapably slide back to the point of conception to find objective support—by reference to the fact that the full genetic code is present subsequent to conception, whereas it is not present prior to conception.

With regard to drawing the line, a liberal typically contends that the fetus remains nonhuman even in its most advanced stages of development. The liberal, of course, does not mean to deny that a fetus is biologically a human fetus. Rather, the claim is that the fetus is not human in any morally significant sense; that is, the fetus has no significant moral status. This point is often made in terms of the concept of personhood. Mary Anne Warren, who defends the liberal view on abortion in one of this chapter's selections, argues that the fetus is not a person. She also contends that the fetus bears so little resemblance to a person that it cannot be said to have a significant right to life. It is important to notice, as Warren analyzes the concept of personhood, that even a newborn baby is not a person. This conclusion, as might be expected, prompts Warren to a consideration of the moral justifiability of infanticide, an issue closely related to the problem of abortion.

Although the conservative view on abortion is most commonly predicated on the straightforward contention that the fetus is a person from conception, at least two other lines of argument have been advanced in its defense. One conservative, advancing what might be labeled "the presumption argument," writes:

> In being willing to kill the embryo, we accept responsibility for killing what we must admit *may* be a person. There is some reason to believe it is—namely the *fact* that it is a living, human individual and the inconclusiveness of arguments that try to exclude it from the protected circle of personhood.
>
> *To be willing to kill what for all we know could be a person is to be willing to kill it if it is a person.* And since we cannot absolutely settle if it is a person except by a metaphysical postulate, for all practical purposes we must hold that to be willing to kill the embryo is to be willing to kill a person.[3]

In accordance with this line of argument, although it may not be possible to show conclusively that the fetus is a person from conception, we must presume that it is. Another line of argument that has been advanced by some conservatives emphasizes the potential rather than the actual personhood of the fetus. Even if the fetus is not a person, it is said, there can be no doubt that it is a potential person. Accordingly, by virtue of its potential personhood, the fetus must be accorded a right to life. Warren, in response to this line of argument, argues that the potential personhood of the fetus provides no basis for the claim that it has a significant right to life.

The Roman Catholic church is a prominent proponent of the conservative view on abortion. In this chapter's first reading, Pope John Paul II gives voice to the Catholic tradition on the issue of abortion. In another reading in this chapter, Don Marquis argues for a conservative view on abortion, but he does not argue for what is commonly referred to as "the" conservative view on abortion. Whereas the standard conservative, such as John Paul II, is committed to a sanctity-of-life viewpoint, according to which the lives of all biologically human beings (assuming their moral innocence) are considered immune from attack, Marquis bases his opposition to abortion on a distinctive theory about the wrongness of killing. Although Marquis claims there is a strong moral presumption against abortion and although he clearly believes that the vast majority of abortions are seriously immoral, he is not committed to the standard conservative contention that the only possible exception is the case in which abortion is necessary to save the life of the pregnant woman.

MODERATE VIEWS

The conservative and liberal views, as explicated, constitute two extreme poles on the spectrum of ethical views on abortion. Each of the extreme views is marked by a formal simplicity. The conservative proclaims abortion to be immoral, irrespective of the stage of fetal development and irrespective of alleged justifying reasons. The one exception admitted by some conservatives is the case in which abortion is necessary to save the life of the pregnant woman.[4] The liberal proclaims abortion to be morally acceptable, irrespective of the stage of fetal development.[5] Moreover, there is no need to draw distinctions between those reasons that are sufficient to justify abortion and those that are not. No justification is needed. The moderate, in vivid contrast to both the conservative and the liberal, is unwilling either to condemn or to condone abortion in sweeping terms. Some abortions are morally justifiable; some are morally objectionable. In some moderate views, the stage of fetal development is a relevant factor in the assessment of the moral acceptability of abortion. In other moderate views, the alleged justifying reason is a relevant factor in the assessment of the moral acceptability of abortion. In still other moderate views, both the stage of fetal development and the alleged justifying reason are relevant factors in the assessment of the moral acceptability of abortion.

Moderate views have been developed in accordance with the following clearly identifiable strategies:

1. Moderation of the Conservative View   One strategy for generating a moderate view presumes the typical conservative contention that the fetus is a person (i.e., has full moral status) from conception. What is denied, however, is that we must conclude to the moral impermissibility of abortion in *all* or nearly all cases. In a widely discussed article reprinted in this chapter, Judith Jarvis Thomson attempts to moderate the conservative view in just this way. For Thomson, even if it is presumed that the fetus is a person from conception, abortion is morally justified in a significant range of cases.

2. Moderation of the Liberal View   A second strategy for generating a moderate view presumes the liberal contention that the fetus has no significant moral status, even in the latest stages of pregnancy. What is denied, however, is that we must conclude to the moral permissibility of abortion in *all* cases. It might be said, in accordance with this line of thought, that abortion, even though it does not violate the rights of the fetus (which is presumed to have no rights), remains ethically problematic to the extent that negative social consequences flow from its practice. Such an argument seems especially forceful in the later stages of pregnancy, when the fetus increasingly resembles a newborn infant. It is argued that very late abortions have a brutalizing effect on those involved and, in various ways, lead to the breakdown of attitudes associated with respect for human life. Thus, the conclusion is that very late abortions cannot be morally justified in the absence of weighty reasons.

3. Moderation in Drawing the Line   A third strategy for generating a moderate view—in fact, a whole range of moderate views—is associated with drawing-the-line discussions. Whereas the conservative typically draws the line between human (full moral status) and nonhuman (negligible moral status) at conception and the liberal typically draws that line at birth (or even somewhat later), a moderate view may be generated by drawing the line somewhere between these two extremes. For example, one might draw the line at implantation, at the point where brain activity begins, at quickening, at viability, and so forth.[6] Whereas drawing the line at implantation would tend to generate a rather conservative moderate view, drawing the line at viability would tend to generate a rather liberal moderate view. Wherever the line is drawn, it is the burden of any such moderate view to show that the point specified is a nonarbitrary one. Once such a point has been specified, however, it might be argued that abortion is ethically acceptable before that point and ethically unacceptable after that point. Of course, further stipulations may be added in accordance with strategies 1 and 2.

4. Moderation in the Assignment of Moral Status A fourth strategy for generating a moderate view is dependent upon assigning the fetus some sort of *partial moral status*.[7] It would seem that anyone who defends a moderate view based on the concept of partial moral status must first of all face the problem of explicating the nature of such partial moral status. Second, and closely related, is the problem of showing how the interests of those with partial moral status (or perhaps the claims that can be made on their behalf) are to be weighed against the interests and rights of those who have full moral status. In one of the readings in this chapter, Margaret Olivia Little presents a unique, nuanced discussion of the morality of abortion. Her overall analysis is calculated to be responsive to the particular identities, commitments, and personal ideals of individual women who face abortion decisions, but the point of departure for her analysis can be understood as the claim that the fetus has some sort of partial moral status.

ABORTION AND SOCIAL POLICY

In the United States, the Supreme Court's decision in *Roe v. Wade* (1973) has been the focal point of the social policy debate over abortion. This case had the effect, for all practical purposes, of legalizing "abortion on request." The Court held that it was unconstitutional for a state to have laws prohibiting the abortion of a previable fetus. According to the *Roe* Court, a woman has a constitutionally guaranteed right to terminate a pregnancy (prior to viability), although a state, for reasons related to maternal health, may restrict the manner and circumstances in which abortions are performed subsequent to the end of the first trimester. The reasoning underlying the Court's holding in *Roe* can be found in the majority opinion reprinted in this chapter.

Since the action of the Court in *Roe* had the practical effect of establishing a woman's legal right to choose whether or not to abort, it was enthusiastically received by "right-to-choose" forces. On the other hand, "right-to-life" forces, committed to the conservative view on the morality of abortion, vehemently denounced the Court for "legalizing murder." In response to *Roe,* right-to-life forces adopted a number of political strategies, several of which are discussed here.

Right-to-life forces originally worked for the enactment of a constitutional amendment directly overturning *Roe*. The proposed "human life amendment"—declaring the personhood of the fetus—was calculated to achieve the legal prohibition of abortion, allowing an exception only for abortions necessary to save the life of a pregnant woman. Right-to-life support also emerged for the idea of a constitutional amendment allowing Congress and/or each state to decide whether to restrict abortion. (If this sort of amendment were enacted, it would undoubtedly have the effect of prohibiting abortion or at least severely restricting it in a number of states.) Right-to-choose forces reacted in strong opposition to these proposed constitutional amendments. In their view, any effort to achieve the legal prohibition of abortion represents an illicit attempt by one group—conservatives on abortion—to impose their moral views on those who have different views.

In 1980, right-to-life forces were notably successful in working toward a more limited political aim, the cutoff of Medicaid funding for abortion. Medicaid is a social program designed to provide funds to pay for the medical care of impoverished people. At issue in *Harris v. McRae,* decided by the Supreme Court in 1980, was the constitutionality of the so-called Hyde amendment, legislation that had passed Congress with vigorous right-to-life support. The Hyde amendment, in the version considered by the Court, restricted federal Medicaid funding to (1) cases in which the pregnant woman's life is endangered and (2) cases of rape and incest. The Court, in a five-to-four decision, upheld the constitutionality of the Hyde amendment. According to the Court, a woman's right to an abortion does not entail *the right to have society fund the abortion.* However, if there is no constitutional obstacle to the cutoff of Medicaid funding for abortion, the question remains whether society's refusal to fund the abortions of poor women is an ethically sound social policy. Considerations of social justice are often pressed by those who argue that it is not.

With the decision of the Supreme Court in *Webster v. Reproductive Health Services* (1989), right-to-life forces celebrated a dramatic victory. Two crucial provisions of a Missouri statute were upheld. One provision bans the use of *public* facilities and *public* employees in the performance of abortions. Another requires physicians to perform tests to determine the viability of any fetus believed to be twenty weeks or older. From the perspective of right-to-life forces, the Court's holding in *Webster* represented the first benefits of a long-term strategy to undermine *Roe v. Wade* by controlling (through the political process) the appointment of new Supreme Court justices. More important than the actual holding of the case was the fact that the Court had apparently indicated its willingness to abandon *Roe.* In *Planned Parenthood of Southeastern Pennsylvania v. Casey, Governor of Pennsylvania* (1992), however, the Court once again reflected ongoing changes in its membership and reaffirmed the "essential holding" of *Roe.*

The emergence of RU-486 (mifepristone), a drug developed in France, has further complicated the social policy debate over abortion in the United States. RU-486 can be taken as an "abortion pill" and, in combination with a second drug taken to induce contractions, effectively terminates early pregnancies.[8] Throughout the 1990s, right-to-choose forces emphasized the importance of access to this private, nonsurgical form of abortion and worked to make RU-486 legally available in the United States. The drug first became legally available to pregnant women in the United States in September 2000, under a protocol approved by the Food and Drug Administration. Of course, right-to-life forces bitterly oppose the legal availability of RU-486. They refer to the drug as a "human pesticide" and denounce its use as "chemical warfare on the unborn."

Another dimension of the social policy debate over abortion in the United States involves the use of a rare, late-term abortion procedure known medically as *intact dilation and extraction* (intact D&X). Opponents of the procedure commonly refer to it as "partial-birth abortion." Intact D&X, which is sometimes used for late second-trimester abortions and for third-trimester abortions, can be understood as a variation on the D&E procedure discussed earlier. In one of its forms, intact D&X involves the partial, feet-first delivery of a fetus, followed by extraction of the brain in order to collapse the skull, so that the head can then pass through the cervix. Whereas D&E results in a dismembered fetus, intact D&X results in an "intact" fetus. The history of legislative efforts to ban "partial-birth abortion" is already complex, as is the history of constitutional challenges to such bans. In *Stenberg v. Carhart* (2000), the U.S. Supreme Court struck down Nebraska's ban on "partial-birth abortion." At the time this case was decided, similar bans existed in about thirty states. Subsequently, Congress passed the Partial Birth Abortion Ban Act of 2003. As of this writing (Fall 2004), the federal ban has been found unconstitutional by district court judges in San

Francisco, New York, and Lincoln, Nebraska, and further action in the courts is expected. In one of this chapter's readings, George J. Annas provides a rich account of the constitutional issues in *Stenberg* as they played out in the Supreme Court decision.

RESEARCH ON EMBRYONIC STEM CELLS

A human embryo reaches the so-called *blastocyst* stage of its development about five days after fertilization. At the blastocyst stage, the embryo contains both an inner cell mass that would normally develop into a fetus and an outer layer of cells that would normally become part of the placenta. The cells making up the inner cell mass of the blastocyst are capable of developing into virtually any type of human cell or tissue. If these cells are extracted, they are identified as embryonic stem cells. Such cells are believed to have great value for various research applications, especially in connection with hoped-for therapies for many diseases and conditions, including Alzheimer's disease, diabetes, and spinal cord injury. Of course, deriving stem cells from a human embryo at the blastocyst stage entails the destruction of that embryo. Hence, subsequent to reports in 1998 of the first successful derivation of embryonic stem cells from human embryos, a firestorm of controversy erupted around the possibility of research on embryonic stem cells. At the center of this controversy is the ethics of research on embryonic stem cells, although a related policy issue is also prominent in the overall societal debate—that is, whether and to what extent federal funding should be provided for research on embryonic stem cells. Discussion in this chapter is largely restricted to the ethics of research on embryonic stem cells and does not directly engage the funding issue.

Obviously, the issue of the moral status of the early embryo is crucially implicated in discussions of the ethics of research on embryonic stem cells. If full moral status is attributed to the early embryo, there would seem to be no ethical justification for the destruction of embryos necessary to derive embryonic stem cells for research purposes. On the other hand, if no significant moral status is attributed to the early embryo, there would seem to be no real problem with the derivation and use of embryonic stem cells for research purposes. But many commentators would attribute some sort of partial or intermediate moral status to the early embryo. In their view, an embryo is entitled to some measure of respect corresponding to its intermediate moral status. Advocates of this approach differ among themselves, however, regarding whether or not the respect due to the early embryo is compatible with the creation and destruction of embryos for research purposes. Bonnie Steinbock argues in this chapter that respect for embryos does not rule out the creation and destruction of embryos for research purposes. In her view, respect for embryos requires only that embryos not be used for unimportant or frivolous purposes. A contrasting view, given voice in this chapter by the President's Council on Bioethics, holds that if the early embryo is attributed an intermediate and developing moral status, this moral status will be the ground of a "special respect" for embryos, and this special respect must be understood as ruling out the creation of embryos solely for research applications that entail their very destruction. However, this view does not necessarily rule out the derivation of embryonic stem cells from already existing "spare" embryos—that is, embryos originally created for reproductive purposes but no longer needed.

In one of this chapter's readings, a document from the National Institutes of Health provides useful background information about so-called *pluripotent* stem cells and their potential therapeutic value. (Embryonic stem cells are the most prominent type of pluripotent stem cells.) The NIH document also provides background information on adult stem cells and their therapeutic potential. According to one important argument in the stem cell controversy, the potential therapeutic value of adult stem cells is so substantial that there is no compelling need for research on embryonic stem cells.

There is an important point at which the stem cell controversy intersects with the cloning controversy. The ethics of human reproductive cloning is fully discussed in Chapter 8, but it is essential at this time to explain the difference between *reproductive* cloning and *research* cloning. Both types of cloning involve somatic cell nuclear transfer (SCNT). In SCNT, the nucleus of a donor somatic cell is transferred into an egg cell whose nucleus has been extracted, and the overall result is the formation of a "cloned embryo." Reproductive cloning would involve the subsequent development of the cloned embryo, its implantation in the uterus of a woman, and the eventual birth of a human child, who would be a "clone" of the person who provided the original genetic material. Research cloning would involve the development of the embryo only to a certain stage, with the intention of studying its development or otherwise using it for research purposes.[9] One especially prominent possibility in this regard is allowing the cloned embryo to develop only to the blastocyst stage, then destroying it by extracting its stem cells. Thus, three important sources of embryonic stem cells can be identified: (1) "spare" embryos originally created for reproductive purposes by in vitro fertilization; (2) embryos expressly created for research purposes by in vitro fertilization; (3) cloned embryos expressly created for research purposes.

In *Human Cloning and Human Dignity: An Ethical Inquiry* (2002), the President's Council on Bioethics (PCB) considered both cloning to produce children (reproductive cloning) and cloning for biomedical research (research cloning).[10] Although members of the PCB unaminimously agreed on the moral impermissibility of reproductive cloning, the group found itself deeply divided on the ethics of research cloning. Reflecting this deep division, the PCB presented in its report both "the moral case for cloning-for-biomedical-research," expressing the views of one segment of the council, and "the moral case against cloning-for-biomedical-research," expressing the views of the other segment. Only the latter section of the report is reprinted in this chapter.[11] According to those members of the PCB morally opposed to research cloning, it is morally indefensible to create any embryo, whether by cloning or by in vitro fertilization, solely for research purposes. This part of their argument is explicitly based on underlying claims about the moral status of the early embryo, but there are also other dimensions in their overall argument against research cloning. In particular, it is argued that research cloning would "open the door" for reproductive cloning.

T.A.M.

NOTES

1 The first section of Chapter 8 provides an extensive discussion of prenatal diagnosis and selective abortion.

2 The expression *therapeutic abortion* suggests abortion for medical reasons. Accordingly, abortions corresponding to reasons 1, 2, and 3 are usually said to be therapeutic. More problematically, abortions corresponding to reason 4 have often been identified as therapeutic. Perhaps it is presumed that pregnancies resulting from rape or incest are traumatic and thus a threat to mental health. Alternatively, perhaps calling such an abortion "therapeutic" is just a way of indicating that it is thought to be justifiable.

3 Germain Grisez, *Abortion: The Myths, the Realities, and the Arguments* (New York: Corpus Books, 1970), p. 306.

4 In accordance with Roman Catholic moral teaching, the *direct* killing of innocent human life is forbidden. Hence, abortion is forbidden. Even if the pregnant woman's life is in danger, perhaps because her heart or

kidney function is inadequate, abortion is impermissible. In two special cases, however, procedures resulting in the death of the fetus are allowable. In the case of an ectopic pregnancy, where the developing fetus is lodged in the fallopian tube, the fallopian tube may be removed. In the case of a pregnant woman with a cancerous uterus, the cancerous uterus may be removed. In these cases, the death of the fetus is construed as *indirect* killing, the foreseen but unintended by-product of a surgical procedure designed to protect the life of the woman. If the distinction between direct and indirect killing is a defensible one (and this is a controversial issue), it might still be suggested that the distinction is not rightly applied in the Roman Catholic view of abortion. For example, some critics contend that abortion may be construed as indirect killing—indeed, an allowable form of indirect killing—in at least all cases in which it is necessary to save the life of the pregnant woman. For one helpful exposition and critical analysis of the Roman Catholic position on abortion, see Daniel Callahan, *Abortion: Law, Choice and Morality* (New York: Macmillan, 1970), Chapter 12, pp. 409–447.

5 In considering the liberal contention that abortions are morally acceptable irrespective of the stage of fetal development, we should take note of an ambiguity in the concept of abortion. Does *abortion* refer merely to the termination of a pregnancy in the sense of detaching the fetus from the pregnant woman, or does it entail the death of the fetus as well? Whereas the abortion of a previable fetus entails its death, the "abortion" of a viable fetus by means of hysterotomy (a miniature caesarean section) does not entail the death of the fetus and would seem to be tantamount to the birth of a baby. With regard to the "abortion" of a *viable* fetus, liberals can defend the woman's right to detach the fetus from her body without contending that the woman has the right to insist on the death of the child.

6 L.W. Sumner argues that the line should be drawn at the point at which the fetus becomes sentient, that is, capable of feeling pleasure and pain: "It is likely that a fetus is unable to feel pleasure or pain at the beginning of the second trimester and likely that it is able to do so at the end of that trimester. If this is so, then the threshold of sentience, and thus also the threshold of moral standing, occurs sometime during the second trimester." L.W. Sumner, "Abortion," in Donald Van DeVeer and Tom Regan, eds., *Health Care Ethics: An Introduction* (Philadelphia: Temple University Press, 1987), p. 179. Jeff McMahan also considers the problem of determining the onset of consciousness/sentience in the developing fetus. "Most neurologists accept that the earliest point at which consciousness is possible is around the twentieth week of pregnancy. . . . It is, however, unlikely that consciousness becomes possible until at least another month—that is, until around the sixth month." Jeff McMahan, *The Ethics of Killing* (New York: Oxford University Press, 2002), p. 267.

7 Callahan embraces this approach in *Abortion: Law, Choice and Morality*, pp. 493–501.

8 RU-486 is not to be confused with the "morning after" pill. RU-486 dislodges an embryo already implanted in the uterus; the "morning after" pill prevents implantation (although it may also prevent ovulation and fertilization).

9 Research cloning is sometimes called *therapeutic cloning* because the principal long-term aim underlying research on cloned embryos is the development of therapies for serious diseases and conditions.

10 This document is available on the council's website (www.bioethics.gov).

11 The corresponding section, located in Chapter 6 of the report, can be easily accessed at the council's website (see previous note).

THE MORALITY OF ABORTION

THE UNSPEAKABLE CRIME OF ABORTION
Pope John Paul II

Insisting that we must "call things by their proper name," Pope John Paul II identifies abortion as the *murder* of an innocent and defenseless human being. He considers some of the reasons ordinarily given to justify abortion and concludes that such reasons are never sufficient to justify the deliberate killing of an innocent human being. He then identifies several groups of people and claims that these groups, in various ways, share in the moral guilt associated with the practice of abortion. In the end, John Paul II argues that *from the moment of conception* a human being is a person or, at any rate, must be respected and treated as a person.

Among all the crimes which can be committed against life, procured abortion has characteristics making it particularly serious and deplorable. The Second Vatican Council defines abortion, together with infanticide, as an "unspeakable crime."[1]

But today, in many people's consciences, the perception of its gravity has become progressively obscured. The acceptance of abortion in the popular mind, in behaviour and even in law itself, is a telling sign of an extremely dangerous crisis of the moral sense, which is becoming more and more incapable of distinguishing between good and evil, even when the fundamental right to life is at stake. Given such a grave situation, we need now more than ever to have the courage to look the truth in the eye and to *call things by their proper name,* without yielding to convenient compromises or to the temptation of self-deception. In this regard the reproach of the Prophet is extremely straightforward: "Woe to those who call evil good and good evil, who put darkness for light and light for darkness" (*Is* 5:20). Especially in the case of abortion there is a widespread use of ambiguous terminology, such as "interruption of pregnancy," which tends to hide abortion's true nature and to attenuate its seriousness in public opinion. Perhaps this linguistic phenomenon is itself a symptom of an uneasiness of conscience. But no word has the power to change the reality of things: procured abortion is *the deliberate and direct killing, by whatever means it is carried out, of a human being in the initial phase of his or her existence, extending from conception to birth.*

The moral gravity of procured abortion is apparent in all its truth if we recognize that we are dealing with murder and, in particular, when we consider the specific elements involved. The one eliminated is a human being at the very beginning of life. No one more absolutely *innocent* could be imagined. In no way could this human being ever be considered an aggressor, much less an unjust aggressor! He or she is *weak,* defenseless, even to the point of lacking that minimal form of defence consisting in the poignant power of a newborn baby's cries and tears. The unborn child is *totally entrusted* to the protection and care of the woman carrying him or her in the womb. And yet sometimes it is precisely the mother herself who makes the decision and asks for the child to be eliminated, and who then goes about having it done.

It is true that the decision to have an abortion is often tragic and painful for the mother, insofar as the decision to rid herself of the fruit of conception is not made for purely selfish reasons or out of convenience, but out of a desire to protect certain important values such as her own health or a decent standard of living for the other members of the family. Sometimes it is feared that the child to be born would live in such conditions that it would be better if the birth did not take place. Nevertheless, these reasons and others like them, however serious and tragic, *can never justify the deliberate killing of an innocent human being.*

As well as the mother, there are often other people too who decide upon the death of the child in the womb. In the first place, the father of the child may be to blame, not only when he directly pressures the woman to have an abortion, but also when he indirectly encourages such a decision on her part by leaving her alone to face the problems of pregnancy:[2] in this way the family is thus mortally wounded and profaned in its nature as a community of love and in its vocation to be the "sanctuary of life." Nor can one overlook the pressures which sometimes come from the wider family circle and from friends. Sometimes the woman is subjected to such strong pressure that she feels psychologically forced to have an abortion: certainly in this case moral responsibility lies particularly with those who have directly or indirectly obliged her to have an abortion. Doctors and nurses are also responsible, when they place at the service of death skills which were acquired for promoting life.

But responsibility likewise falls on the legislators who have promoted and approved abortion laws, and, to the extent that they have a say in the matter, on the administrators of the health-care centres where abortions are performed. A general and no less serious responsibility lies with those who have encouraged the spread of an attitude of sexual permissiveness and a lack of esteem for motherhood, and with those who should have ensured—but did not—effective family and social policies in support

From *Evangelium Vitae,* encyclical letter of John Paul II, March 25, 1995. Reprinted with permission. © Libreria Editrice Vaticana, 00120 Città del Vaticano.

of families, especially larger families and those with particular financial and educational needs. Finally, one cannot overlook the network of complicity which reaches out to include international institutions, foundations and associations which systematically campaign for the legalization and spread of abortion in the world. In this sense abortion goes beyond the responsibility of individuals and beyond the harm done to them, and takes on a distinctly social dimension. It is a most serious *wound* inflicted on society and its culture by the very people who ought to be society's promoters and defenders. As I wrote in my *Letter to Families,* "we are facing an immense threat to life: not only to the life of individuals but also to that of civilization itself."[3] We are facing what can be called a *"structure of sin" which opposes human life not yet born.*

Some people try to justify abortion by claiming that the result of conception, at least up to a certain number of days, cannot yet be considered a personal human life. But in fact, "from the time that the ovum is fertilized, a life is begun which is neither that of the father nor the mother; it is rather the life of a new human being with his own growth. It would never be made human if it were not human already. This has always been clear, and . . . modern genetic science offers clear confirmation. It has demonstrated that from the first instant there is established the programme of what this living being will be: a person, this individual person with his characteristic aspects already well determined. Right from fertilization the adventure of a human life begins, and each of its capacities requires time—a rather lengthy time—to find its place and to be in a position to act."[4] Even if the presence of a spiritual soul cannot be ascertained by empirical data, the results themselves of scientific research on the human embryo provide "a valuable indication for discerning by the use of reason a personal presence at the moment of the first appearance of a human life: how could a human individual not be a human person?"[5]

Furthermore, what is at stake is so important that, from the standpoint of moral obligation, the mere probability that a human person is involved would suffice to justify an absolutely clear prohibition of any intervention aimed at killing a human embryo. Precisely for this reason, over and above all scientific debates and those philosophical affirmations to which the Magisterium has not expressly committed itself, the Church has always taught and continues to teach that the result of human procreation, from the first moment of its existence, must be guaranteed that unconditional respect which is morally due to the human being in his or her totality and unity as body and spirit: *"The human being is to be respected and treated as a person from the moment of conception;* and therefore from that same moment his rights as a person must be recognized, among which in the first place is the inviolable right of every innocent human being to life."[6] . . .

NOTES

1 Pastoral Constitution on the Church in the Modern World *Gaudium et Spes,* 51: "Abortus necnon infanticidium nefanda sunt crimina."

2 Cf. John Paul II, Apostolic Letter *Mulieris Dignitatem* (15 August 1988), 14: *AAS* 80 (1988), 1686.

3 No. 21: *AAS* 86 (1994), 920.

4 Congregation for the Doctrine of the Faith, *Declaration on Procured Abortion* (18 November 1974), Nos. 12–13: *AAS* 66 (1974), 738.

5 Congregation for the Doctrine of the Faith, Instruction on Respect for Human Life in Its Origin and on the Dignity of Procreation *Donum Vitae* (22 February 1987), I, No. 1: *AAS* 80 (1988), 78–79.

6 *Ibid., loc. cit.,* 79.

ON THE MORAL AND LEGAL STATUS OF ABORTION

Mary Anne Warren

Warren, defending the liberal view on abortion, promptly distinguishes two senses of the term *human:* (1) One is *human in the genetic sense* when one is a member of the biological species *Homo sapiens.* (2) One is *human in the moral sense* when one is a full-fledged member of the moral community. Warren attacks the presupposition underlying the standard conservative argument against abortion—that the fetus is human in the moral sense. She contends that the moral community, the set of beings with full and equal moral rights, consists of all and only people (persons). (Thus, she takes the concept of personhood to be equivalent to the concept of humanity in the moral sense.) After analyzing the concept of a person, she concludes that there is no stage of fetal development at which a fetus resembles a person enough to have a significant right to life. She also argues that the fetus's *potential* for being a person does not provide a basis for the claim that it has a significant right to life. It follows, in her view, that a woman's right to obtain an abortion is absolute. Abortion is morally justified at any stage of fetal development, and no legal restrictions should be placed on a woman's right to abort. In a concluding postscript, Warren briefly assesses the moral justifiability of infanticide.

The question which we must answer in order to produce a satisfactory solution to the problem of the moral status of abortion is this: How are we to define the moral community, the set of beings with full and equal moral rights, such that we can decide whether a human fetus is a member of this community or not? What sort of entity, exactly, has the inalienable rights to life, liberty, and the pursuit of happiness? Jefferson attributed these rights to all *men,* and it may or may not be fair to suggest that he intended to attribute them *only* to men. Perhaps he ought to have attributed them to all human beings. If so, then we arrive, first, at [John] Noonan's problem of defining what makes a being human, and, second, at the equally vital question which Noonan does not consider, namely, What reason is there for identifying the moral community with the set of all human beings, in whatever way we have chosen to define that term?

1 ON THE DEFINITION OF "HUMAN"

One reason why this vital second question is so frequently overlooked in the debate over the moral status of abortion is that the term 'human' has two distinct, but not often distinguished, senses. This fact results in a slide of meaning, which serves to conceal the fallaciousness of the traditional argument that since (1) it is wrong to kill innocent human

Reprinted by permission from vol. 57, no. 1, of *The Monist,* LaSalle, Illinois 61301. "Postscript on Infanticide" reprinted with permission of the author from *The Problem of Abortion,* second edition, edited by Joel Feinberg (Belmont, Calif.: Wadsworth, 1984).

beings, and (2) fetuses are innocent human beings, then (3) it is wrong to kill fetuses. For if 'human' is used in the same sense in both (1) and (2) then, whichever of the two senses is meant, one of these premises is question-begging. And if it is used in two different senses then of course the conclusion doesn't follow.

Thus, (1) is a self-evident moral truth,[1] and avoids begging the question about abortion, only if 'human being' is used to mean something like 'a full-fledged member of the moral community.' (It may or may not also be meant to refer exclusively to members of the species *Homo sapiens.*) We may call this the *moral* sense of 'human.' It is not to be confused with what we call the *genetic* sense, i.e., the sense in which *any* member of the species is a human being, and no member of any other species could be. If (1) is acceptable only if the moral sense is intended, (2) is non-question-begging only if what is intended is the genetic sense.

In "Deciding Who is Human," Noonan argues for the classification of fetuses with human beings by pointing to the presence of the full genetic code, and the potential capacity for rational thought.[2] It is clear that what he needs to show, for his version of the traditional argument to be valid, is that fetuses are human in the moral sense, the sense in which it is analytically true that all human beings have full moral rights. But, in the absence of any argument showing that whatever is genetically human is also morally human, and he gives none, nothing more than genetic humanity can be demonstrated by the presence of the human genetic code. And, as we will see, the *potential* capacity for rational thought can at most show that an entity has the potential for *becoming* human in the moral sense.

2 DEFINING THE MORAL COMMUNITY

Can it be established that genetic humanity is sufficient for moral humanity? I think that there are very good reasons for not defining the moral community in this way. I would like to suggest an alternative way of defining the moral community, which I will argue for only to the extent of explaining why it is, or should be, self-evident. The suggestion is simply that the moral community consists of all and only *people,* rather than all and only human beings,[3] and probably the best way of demonstrating its self-evidence is by considering the concept of personhood, to see what sorts of entity are and are not persons, and what the decision that a being is or is not a person implies about its moral rights.

What characteristics entitle an entity to be considered a person? This is obviously not the place to attempt a complete analysis of the concept of personhood, but we do not need such a fully adequate analysis just to determine whether and why a fetus is or isn't a person. All we need is a rough and approximate list of the most basic criteria of personhood, and some idea of which, or how many, of these an entity must satisfy in order to properly be considered a person.

In searching for such criteria, it is useful to look beyond the set of people with whom we are acquainted, and ask how we would decide whether a totally alien being was a person or not. (For we have no right to assume that genetic humanity is necessary for personhood.) Imagine a space traveler who lands on an unknown planet and encounters a race of beings utterly unlike any he has ever seen or heard of. If he wants to be sure of behaving morally toward these beings, he has to somehow decide whether they are people, and hence have full moral rights, or whether they are the sort of thing which he need not feel guilty about treating as, for example, a source of food.

How should he go about making this decision? If he has some anthropological background, he

might look for such things as religion, art, and the manufacturing of tools, weapons, or shelters, since these factors have been used to distinguish our human from our prehuman ancestors, in what seems to be closer to the moral than the genetic sense of 'human.' And no doubt he would be right to consider the presence of such factors as good evidence that the alien beings were people, and morally human. It would, however, be overly anthropocentric of him to take the absence of these things as adequate evidence that they were not, since we can imagine people who have progressed beyond, or evolved without ever developing, these cultural characteristics.

I suggest that the traits which are most central to the concept of personhood, or humanity in the moral sense, are, very roughly, the following:

1. Consciousness (of objects and events external and/or internal to the being), and in particular the capacity to feel pain;

2. Reasoning (the *developed* capacity to solve new and relatively complex problems);

3. Self-motivated activity (activity which is relatively independent of either genetic or direct external control);

4. The capacity to communicate, by whatever means, messages of an indefinite variety of types, that is, not just with an indefinite number of possible contents, but on indefinitely many possible topics;

5. The presence of self-concepts, and self-awareness, either individual or racial, or both.

Admittedly, there are apt to be a great many problems involved in formulating precise definitions of these criteria, let alone in developing universally valid behavioral criteria for deciding when they apply. But I will assume that both we and our explorer know approximately what (1)–(5) mean, and that he is also able to determine whether or not they apply. How, then, should he use his findings to decide whether or not the alien beings are people? We needn't suppose that an entity must have *all* of these attributes to be properly considered a person; (1) and (2) alone may well be sufficient for personhood, and quite probably (1)–(3) are sufficient. Neither do we need to insist that any one of these criteria is *necessary* for personhood, although once again (1) and (2) look like fairly good candidates for necessary conditions, as does (3), if 'activity' is construed so as to include the activity of reasoning.

All we need to claim, to demonstrate that a fetus is not a person, is that any being which satisfies *none* of (1)–(5) is certainly not a person. I consider this claim to be so obvious that I think anyone who denied it, and claimed that a being which satisfied none of (1)–(5) was a person all the same, would thereby demonstrate that he had no notion at all of what a person is—perhaps because he had confused the concept of a person with that of genetic humanity. If the opponents of abortion were to deny the appropriateness of these five criteria, I do not know what further arguments would convince them. We would probably have to admit that our conceptual schemes were indeed irreconcilably different, and that our dispute could not be settled objectively.

I do not expect this to happen, however, since I think that the concept of a person is one which is very nearly universal (to people), and that it is common to both proabortionists and antiabortionists, even though neither group has fully realized the relevance of this concept to the resolution of their dispute. Furthermore, I think that on reflection even the antiabortionists ought to agree not only that (1)–(5) are central to the concept of personhood, but also that it is a part of this concept that all and only people have full moral rights. The concept of a person is in part a moral concept; once we have admitted that *x* is a person we have recognized, even if we have not agreed to respect, *x*'s right to be treated as a member of the moral community. It is true that the claim that *x* is a *human being* is more commonly voiced as part of an appeal to treat *x* decently than is the claim that *x* is a person, but this is either because 'human being' is here used in the sense which implies personhood, or because the genetic and moral sense of 'human' have been confused.

Now if (1)–(5) are indeed the primary criteria of personhood, then it is clear that genetic humanity is neither necessary nor sufficient for establishing that an entity is a person. Some human beings are not people, and there may well be people who are not human beings. A man or woman whose conscious-

ness has been permanently obliterated but who remains alive is a human being which is no longer a person; defective human beings, with no appreciable mental capacity, are not and presumably never will be people; and a fetus is a human being which is not yet a person, and which therefore cannot coherently be said to have full moral rights. Citizens of the next century should be prepared to recognize highly advanced, self-aware robots or computers, should such be developed, and intelligent inhabitants of other worlds, should such be found, as people in the fullest sense, and to respect their moral rights. But to ascribe full moral rights to an entity which is not a person is as absurd as to ascribe moral obligations and responsibilities to such an entity.

3 FETAL DEVELOPMENT AND THE RIGHT TO LIFE

Two problems arise in the application of these suggestions for the definition of the moral community to the determination of the precise moral status of a human fetus. Given that the paradigm example of a person is a normal adult human being, then (1) How like this paradigm, in particular how far advanced since conception, does a human being need to be before it begins to have a right to life by virtue, not of being fully a person as of yet, but of being *like* a person? and (2) To what extent, if any, does the fact that a fetus has the *potential* for becoming a person endow it with some of the same rights? Each of these questions requires some comment.

In answering the first question, we need not attempt a detailed consideration of the moral rights of organisms which are not developed enough, aware enough, intelligent enough, etc., to be considered people, but which resemble people in some respects. It does seem reasonable to suggest that the more like a person, in the relevant respects, a being is, the stronger is the case for regarding it as having a right to life, and indeed the stronger its right to life is. Thus we ought to take seriously the suggestion that, insofar as "the human individual develops biologically in a continuous fashion . . . the rights of a human person might develop in the same way."[4] But we must keep in mind that the attributes which are relevant in determining whether or not an entity is enough like a person to be regarded as having some of the same moral rights are no different from those which are relevant to determining whether or not it is fully a person—i.e., are no different from (1)–(5)—and that being genetically human, or having recognizable human facial and other physical features, or detectable brain activity, or the capacity to survive outside the uterus, are simply not among these relevant attributes.

Thus it is clear that even though a seven- or eight-month fetus has features which make it apt to arouse in us almost the same powerful protective instinct as is commonly aroused by a small infant, nevertheless it is not significantly more personlike than is a very small embryo. It is *somewhat* more personlike; it can apparently feel and respond to pain, and it may even have a rudimentary form of consciousness, insofar as its brain is quite active. Nevertheless, it seems safe to say that it is not fully conscious, in the way that an infant of a few months is, and that it cannot reason, or communicate messages of indefinitely many sorts, does not engage in self-motivated activity, and has no self-awareness. Thus, in the *relevant* respects, a fetus, even a fully developed one, is considerably less personlike than is the average mature mammal, indeed the average fish. And I think that a rational person must conclude that if the right to life of a fetus is to be based upon its resemblance to a person, then it cannot be said to have any more right to life than, let us say, a newborn guppy (which also seems to be capable of feeling pain), and that a right of that magnitude could never override a woman's right to obtain an abortion, at any stage of her pregnancy.

There may, of course, be other arguments in favor of placing legal limits upon the stage of pregnancy in which an abortion may be performed. Given the relative safety of the new techniques of artificially inducing labor during the third trimester, the danger to the woman's life or health is no longer such an argument. Neither is the fact that people tend to respond to the thought of abortion in the later stages of pregnancy with emotional repulsion, since mere emotional responses cannot take the place of moral reasoning in determining what ought to be permitted. Nor, finally, is the frequently heard argument that legalizing abortion, especially late in the pregnancy, may erode the level of respect for human life, leading, perhaps, to an increase in unjustified euthanasia and other crimes. For this threat, if it is a threat, can be better met by educating people to the kinds of moral distinctions which we are making here than by limiting access to abortion (which limitation may, in its disregard for the rights of women, be just as damaging to the level of respect for human rights).

Thus, since the fact that even a fully developed fetus is not personlike enough to have any significant right to life on the basis of its personlikeness shows that no legal restrictions upon the stage of pregnancy in which an abortion may be performed can be justified on the grounds that we should protect the rights of the older fetus; and since there is no other apparent justification for such restrictions, we may conclude that they are entirely unjustified. Whether or not it would be *indecent* (whatever that means) for a woman in her seventh month to obtain an abortion just to avoid having to postpone a trip to Europe, it would not, in itself, be *immoral,* and therefore it ought to be permitted.

4 POTENTIAL PERSONHOOD AND THE RIGHT TO LIFE

We have seen that a fetus does not resemble a person in any way which can support the claim that it has even some of the same rights. But what about its *potential,* the fact that if nurtured and allowed to develop naturally it will very probably become a person? Doesn't that alone give it at least some right to life? It is hard to deny that the fact that an entity is a potential person is a strong prima facie reason for not destroying it; but we need not conclude from this that a potential person has a right to life, by virtue of that potential. It may be that our feeling that it is better, other things being equal, not to destroy a potential person is better explained by the fact that potential people are still (felt to be) an invaluable resource, not to be lightly squandered. Surely, if every speck of dust were a potential person, we would be much less apt to conclude that every potential person has a right to become actual.

Still, we do not need to insist that a potential person has no right to life whatever. There may well be something immoral, and not just imprudent, about wantonly destroying potential people, when doing so isn't necessary to protect anyone's rights. But even if a potential person does have some prima facie right to life, such a right could not possibly outweigh the right of a woman to obtain an abortion, since the rights of any actual person invariably outweigh those of any potential person, whenever the two conflict. Since this may not be immediately obvious in the case of a human fetus, let us look at another case.

Suppose that our space explorer falls into the hands of an alien culture, whose scientists decide to create a few hundred thousand or more human beings, by breaking his body into its component cells, and using these to create fully developed human beings, with, of course, his genetic code. We may imagine that each of these newly created men will have all of the original man's abilities, skills, knowledge, and so on, and also have an individual self-concept, in short that each of them will be a bona fide (though hardly unique) person. Imagine that the whole project will take only seconds, and that its chances of success are extremely high, and that our explorer knows all of this, and also knows that these people will be treated fairly. I maintain that in such a situation he would have every right to escape if he could, and thus to deprive all of these potential people of their potential lives; for his right to life outweighs all of theirs together, in spite of the fact that they are all genetically human, all innocent, and all have a very high probability of becoming people very soon, if only he refrains from acting.

Indeed, I think he would have a right to escape even if it were not his life which the alien scientists planned to take, but only a year of his freedom, or, indeed, only a day. Nor would he be obligated to stay if he had gotten captured (thus bringing all these people-potentials into existence) because of his own carelessness, or even if he had done so deliberately, knowing the consequences. Regardless of how he got captured, he is not morally obligated to remain in captivity for *any* period of time for the sake of permitting any number of potential people to come into actuality, so great is the margin by which one actual person's right to liberty outweighs whatever right to life even a hundred thousand potential people have. And it seems reasonable to conclude that the rights

of a woman will outweigh by a similar margin whatever right to life a fetus may have by virtue of its potential personhood.

Thus, neither a fetus's resemblance to a person, nor its potential for becoming a person provides any basis whatever for the claim that it has any significant right to life. Consequently, a woman's right to protect her health, happiness, freedom, and even her life,[5] by terminating an unwanted pregnancy, will always override whatever right to life it may be appropriate to ascribe to a fetus, even a fully developed one. And thus, in the absence of any overwhelming social need for every possible child, the laws which restrict the right to obtain an abortion, or limit the period of pregnancy during which an abortion may be performed, are a wholly unjustified violation of a woman's most basic moral and constitutional rights.[6]

POSTSCRIPT ON INFANTICIDE, FEBRUARY 26, 1982

One of the most troubling objections to the argument presented in this article is that it may appear to justify not only abortion but infanticide as well. A newborn infant is not a great deal more personlike than a nine-month fetus, and thus it might seem that if late-term abortion is sometimes justified, then infanticide must also be sometimes justified. Yet most people consider that infanticide is a form of murder, and thus never justified.

While it is important to appreciate the emotional force of this objection, its logical force is far less than it may seem at first glance. There are many reasons why infanticide is much more difficult to justify than abortion, even though if my argument is correct neither constitutes the killing of a person. In this country, and in this period of history, the deliberate killing of viable newborns is virtually never justified. This is in part because neonates are so very *close* to being persons that to kill them requires a very strong moral justification—as does the killing of dolphins, whales, chimpanzees, and other highly personlike creatures. It is certainly wrong to kill such beings just for the sake of convenience, or financial profit, or "sport."

Another reason why infanticide is usually wrong, in our society, is that if the newborn's parents do not want it, or are unable to care for it, there are (in most cases) people who are able and eager to adopt it and to provide a good home for it. Many people wait years for the opportunity to adopt a child, and some are unable to do so even though there is every reason to believe that they would be good parents. The needless destruction of a viable infant inevitably deprives some person or persons of a source of great pleasure and satisfaction, perhaps severely impoverishing their lives. Furthermore, even if an infant is considered to be unadoptable (e.g., because of some extremely severe mental or physical handicap) it is still wrong in most cases to kill it. For most of us value the lives of infants, and would prefer to pay taxes to support orphanages and state institutions for the handicapped rather than to allow unwanted infants to be killed. So long as most people feel this way, and so long as our society can afford to provide care for infants which are unwanted or which have special needs that preclude home care, it is wrong to destroy any infant which has a chance of living a reasonably satisfactory life.

If these arguments show that infanticide is wrong, at least in this society, then why don't they also show that late-term abortion is wrong? After all, third trimester fetuses are also highly person like, and many people value them and would much prefer that they be preserved; even at some cost to themselves. As a potential source of pleasure to some family, a viable fetus is just as valuable as a viable infant. But there is an obvious and crucial difference between the two cases: once the infant is born, its continued life cannot (except, perhaps, in very exceptional cases) pose any serious threat to the woman's life or health, since she is free to put it up for adoption, or, where this is impossible, to place it in a state-supported institution. While she might prefer that it die, rather than being raised by others, it is not clear that such a preference would constitute a right on her part. True, she may suffer greatly from the knowledge that her child will be thrown into the lottery of the adoption system, and that she will be unable to ensure its well-being, or even to know whether it is healthy, happy, doing well in school, etc.: for the law generally does not permit natural parents to remain in contact with their children, once they are adopted by another family. But there are surely better ways of dealing with these problems than by permitting infanticide in such cases. (It

might help, for instance, if the natural parents of adopted children could at least receive some information about their progress, without necessarily being informed of the identity of the adopting family.)

In contrast, a pregnant woman's right to protect her own life and health clearly outweighs other people's desire that the fetus be preserved—just as, when a person's life or limb is threatened by some wild animal, and when the threat cannot be removed without killing the animal, the person's right to self-protection outweighs the desires of those who would prefer that the animal not be harmed. Thus, while the moment of birth may not mark any sharp discontinuity in the degree to which an infant possesses a right to life, it does mark the end of the mother's absolute right to determine its fate. Indeed, if and when a late-term abortion could be safely performed without killing the fetus, she would have no absolute right to insist on its death (e.g., if others wish to adopt it or pay for its care), for the same reason that she does not have a right to insist that a viable infant be killed.

It remains true that according to my argument neither abortion nor the killing of neonates is properly considered a form of murder. Perhaps it is understandable that the law should classify infanticide as murder or homicide, since there is no other existing legal category which adequately or conveniently expresses the force of our society's disapproval of this action. But the moral distinction remains, and it has several important consequences.

In the first place, it implies that when an infant is born into a society which—unlike ours—is so impoverished that it simply cannot care for it adequately without endangering the survival of existing persons, killing it or allowing it to die is not necessarily wrong—provided that there is no *other* society which is willing and able to provide such care. Most human societies, from those at the hunting and gathering stage of economic development to the highly civilized Greeks and Romans, have permitted the practice of infanticide under such unfortunate circumstances, and I would argue that it shows a serious lack of understanding to condemn them as morally backward for this reason alone.

In the second place, the argument implies that when an infant is born with such severe physical anomalies that its life would predictably be a very short and/or very miserable one, even with the most heroic of medical treatment, and where its parents do not choose to bear the often crushing emotional, financial and other burdens attendant upon the artificial prolongation of such a tragic life, it is not morally wrong to cease or withhold treatment, thus allowing the infant a painless death. It is wrong (and sometimes a form of murder) to practice involuntary euthanasia on persons, since they have the right to decide for themselves whether or not they wish to continue to live. But terminally ill neonates cannot make this decision for themselves, and thus it is incumbent upon responsible persons to make the decision for them, as best they can. The mistaken belief that infanticide is always tantamount to murder is responsible for a great deal of unnecessary suffering, not just on the part of infants which are made to endure needlessly prolonged and painful deaths, but also on the part of parents, nurses, and other involved persons, who must watch infants suffering needlessly, helpless to end that suffering in the most humane way.

I am well aware that these conclusions, however modest and reasonable they may seem to some people, strike other people as morally monstrous, and that some people might even prefer to abandon their previous support for women's right to abortion rather than accept a theory which leads to such conclusions about infanticide. But all that these facts show is that abortion is not an isolated moral issue; to fully understand the moral status of abortion we may have to reconsider other moral issues as well,

issues not just about infanticide and euthanasia, but also about the moral rights of women and of non-human animals. It is a philosopher's task to criticize mistaken beliefs which stand in the way of moral understanding, even when—perhaps especially when—those beliefs are popular and widespread. The belief that moral strictures against killing should apply equally to *all* genetically human entities, and *only* to genetically human entities, is such an error. The overcoming of this error will undoubtedly require long and often painful struggle; but it must be done.

NOTES

1 Of course, the principle that it is (always) wrong to kill innocent human beings is in need of many other modifications, e.g., that it may be permissible to do so to save a greater number of other innocent human beings, but we may safely ignore these complications here.
2 John Noonan, "Deciding Who Is Human," *Natural Law Forum,* 13 (1968), 135.
3 From here on, we will use 'human' to mean genetically human, since the moral sense seems closely connected to, and perhaps derived from, the assumption that genetic humanity is sufficient for membership in the moral community.
4 Thomas L. Hayes, "A Biological View," *Commonweal,* 85 (March 17, 1967), 677–78; quoted by Daniel Callahan, in *Abortion: Law, Choice and Morality* (London: Macmillan & Co., 1970).
5 That is, insofar as the death rate, for the woman, is higher for childbirth than for early abortion.
6 My thanks to the following people, who were kind enough to read and criticize an earlier version of this paper: Herbert Gold, Gene Glass, Anne Lauterbach, Judith Thomson, Mary Mothersill, and Timothy Binkley.

WHY ABORTION IS IMMORAL
Don Marquis

Marquis argues that abortion, with rare exceptions, is seriously immoral. He bases this conclusion on a theory that he presents and defends about the wrongness of killing. In his view, killing another adult human being is wrong precisely because the victim is deprived of all the value—"activities, projects, experiences, and enjoyments"—of his or her future. Since abortion deprives a typical fetus of a "future like ours," he contends, the moral presumption against abortion is as strong as the presumption against killing another adult human being.

The view that abortion is, with rare exceptions, seriously immoral has received little support in the recent philosophical literature. No doubt most philosophers affiliated with secular institutions of higher education believe that the anti-abortion position is either a symptom of irrational religious dogma or a conclusion generated by seriously confused philosophical argument. The purpose of this essay is to undermine this general belief. This essay sets out an argument that purports to show, as well as any argument in ethics can show, that abortion is, except possibly in rare cases, seriously immoral, that it is in the same moral category as killing an innocent adult human being.

This argument is based on a major assumption: If fetuses are in the same category as adult human beings with respect to the moral value of their lives, then the *presumption* that any particular abortion is immoral is exceedingly strong. Such a presumption could be overridden only by considerations more compelling than a woman's right to privacy. The defense of this assumption is beyond the scope of this essay.[1]

Furthermore, this essay will neglect a discussion of whether there are any such compelling considerations and what they are. Plainly there are strong candidates: abortion before implantation, abortion when the life of a woman is threatened by a pregnancy or abortion after rape. The casuistry of these hard cases will not be explored in this essay. The purpose of this essay is to develop a general argument for the claim that, subject to the assumption above, the overwhelming majority of deliberate abortions are seriously immoral. . . .

. . . A necessary condition of resolving the abortion controversy is a . . . theoretical account of the wrongness of killing. After all, if we merely believe, but do not understand, why killing adult human beings such as ourselves is wrong, how could we conceivably show that abortion is either immoral or permissible? . . .

In order to develop such an account, we can start from the following unproblematic assumption concerning our own case: it is wrong to kill *us*. Why is it wrong? Some answers can be easily eliminated. It might be said that what makes killing us wrong is that a killing brutalizes the one who kills. But the brutalization consists of being inured to the performance of an act that is hideously immoral; hence, the brutalization does not explain the immorality. It might be said that what makes killing us wrong is the great loss others would experience due to our absence. Although such hubris is understandable, such an explanation does not account for the wrongness of killing hermits, or those whose lives are relatively independent and whose friends find it easy to make new friends.

A more obvious answer is better. What primarily makes killing wrong is neither its effect on the murderer nor its effect on the victim's friends and relatives, but its effect on the victim. The loss of one's life is one of the greatest losses one can suffer. The loss of one's life deprives one of all the experiences, activities, projects, and enjoyments that would otherwise have constituted one's future. Therefore, killing someone is wrong, primarily because the killing inflicts (one of) the greatest possible losses on the victim. To describe this as the loss of life can be misleading, however. The change in my biological state does not by itself make killing me wrong. The effect of the loss of my biological life is the loss to me of all those activities, projects, experiences, and enjoyments which would otherwise have constituted my future personal life. These activities, projects, experiences, and enjoyments are either valuable for their own sakes or are means to something else that is valuable for its own sake. Some parts of my future are not valued by me now, but will come to be valued by me as I grow older and as my values and capacities change. When I am killed, I am deprived both of what I now value which would have been part of my future personal life, but also what I would come to value. Therefore, when I die, I am deprived of all of the value of my future. Inflicting this loss on me is ultimately what makes killing me wrong. This being the case, it would seem that what makes killing *any* adult human being prima facie seriously wrong is the loss of his or her future.[2]

How should this rudimentary theory of the wrongness of killing be evaluated? It cannot be faulted for deriving an 'ought' from an 'is,' for it

Reprinted, as slightly modified by the author, with permission of the author and the publisher from the *Journal of Philosophy*, vol. 86 (April 1989).

does not. The analysis assumes that killing me (or you, reader) is prima facie seriously wrong. The point of the analysis is to establish which natural property ultimately explains the wrongness of the killing, given that it is wrong. A natural property will ultimately explain the wrongness of killing, only if (1) the explanation fits with our intuitions about the matter and (2) there is no other natural property that provides the basis for a better explanation of the wrongness of killing. This analysis rests on the intuition that what makes killing a particular human or animal wrong is what it does to that particular human or animal. What makes killing wrong is some natural effect or other of the killing. Some would deny this. For instance, a divine-command theorist in ethics would deny it. Surely this denial is, however, one of those features of divine-command theory which renders it so implausible.

The claim that what makes killing wrong is the loss of the victim's future is directly supported by two considerations. In the first place, this theory explains why we regard killing as one of the worst of crimes. Killing is especially wrong, because it deprives the victim of more than perhaps any other crime. In the second place, people with AIDS or cancer who know they are dying believe, of course, that dying is a very bad thing for them. They believe that the loss of a future to them that they would otherwise have experienced is what makes their premature death a very bad thing for them. A better theory of the wrongness of killing would require a different natural property associated with killing which better fits with the attitudes of the dying. What could it be?

The view that what makes killing wrong is the loss to the victim of the value of the victim's future gains additional support when some of its implications are examined. In the first place, it is incompatible with the view that it is wrong to kill only beings who are biologically human. It is possible that there exists a different species from another planet whose members have a future like ours. Since having a future like that is what makes killing someone wrong, this theory entails that it would be wrong to kill members of such a species. Hence, this theory is opposed to the claim that only life that is biologically human has great moral worth, a claim which many anti-abortionists have seemed to adopt. This opposi-

tion, which this theory has in common with personhood theories, seems to be a merit of the theory.

In the second place, the claim that the loss of one's future is the wrong-making feature of one's being killed entails the possibility that the futures of some actual nonhuman mammals on our own planet are sufficiently like ours that it is seriously wrong to kill them also. Whether some animals do have the same right to life as human beings depends on adding to the account of the wrongness of killing some additional account of just what it is about my future or the futures of other adult human beings which makes it wrong to kill us. No such additional account will be offered in this essay. Undoubtedly, the provision of such an account would be a very difficult matter. Undoubtedly, any such account would be quite controversial. Hence, it surely should not reflect badly on this sketch of an elementary theory of the wrongness of killing that it is indeterminate with respect to some very difficult issues regarding animal rights.

In the third place, the claim that the loss of one's future is the wrong-making feature of one's being killed does not entail, as sanctity of human life theories do, that active euthanasia is wrong. Persons who are severely and incurably ill, who face a future of pain and despair, and who wish to die will not have suffered a loss if they are killed. It is, strictly speaking, the value of a human's future which makes killing wrong in this theory. This being so, killing does not necessarily wrong some persons who are sick and dying. Of course, there may be other reasons for a prohibition of active euthanasia, but that is another matter. Sanctity-of-human-life theories seem to hold that active euthanasia is seriously wrong even in an individual case where there seems to be good reason for it independently of public policy considerations. This consequence is most implausible, and it is a plus for the claim that the loss of a future of value is what makes killing wrong that it does not share this consequence.

In the fourth place, the account of the wrongness of killing defended in this essay does straightforwardly entail that it is prima facie seriously wrong to kill children and infants, for we do presume that they have futures of value. Since we do believe that it is wrong to kill defenseless little babies, it is important that a theory of the wrongness of killing easily account for this. Personhood theories of the wrongness of killing, on the other hand, cannot straightforwardly account for the wrongness of killing infants and young children. Hence, such theories must add special ad hoc accounts of the wrongness of killing the young. The plausibility of such ad hoc theories seems to be a function of how desperately one wants such theories to work. The claim that the primary wrong-making feature of a killing is the loss to the victim of the value of its future accounts for the wrongness of killing young children and infants directly; it makes the wrongness of such acts as obvious as we actually think it is. This is a further merit of this theory. Accordingly, it seems that this value of a future-like-ours theory of the wrongness of killing shares strengths of both sanctity-of-life and personhood accounts while avoiding weaknesses of both. In addition, it meshes with a central intuition concerning what makes killing wrong.

The claim that the primary wrong-making feature of a killing is the loss to the victim of the value of its future has obvious consequences for the ethics of abortion. The future of a standard fetus includes a set of experiences, projects, activities, and such which are identical with the futures of adult human beings and are identical with the futures of young children. Since the reason that is sufficient to explain why it is wrong to kill human beings after the time of birth is a reason that also applies to fetuses, it follows that abortion is prima facie seriously morally wrong.

This argument does not rely on the invalid inference that, since it is wrong to kill persons, it is wrong to kill potential persons also. The category that is morally central to this analysis is the category of having a valuable future like ours; it is not the category of personhood. The argument to the conclusion that abortion is prima facie seriously morally wrong proceeded independently of the notion of person or potential person or any equivalent. Someone may wish to start with this analysis in terms of the value of a human future, conclude that abortion is, except perhaps in rare circumstances, seriously morally wrong, infer that fetuses have the right to life, and then call fetuses "persons" as a result of

their having the right to life. Clearly, in this case, the category of person is being used to state the *conclusion* of the analysis rather than to generate the *argument* of the analysis.

The structure of this anti-abortion argument can be both illuminated and defended by comparing it to what appears to be the best argument for the wrongness of the wanton infliction of pain on animals. This latter argument is based on the assumption that it is prima facie wrong to inflict pain on me (or you, reader). What is the natural property associated with the infliction of pain which makes such infliction wrong? The obvious answer seems to be that the infliction of pain causes suffering and that suffering is a misfortune. The suffering caused by the infliction of pain is what makes the wanton infliction of pain on me wrong. The wanton infliction of pain on other adult humans causes suffering. The wanton infliction of pain on animals causes suffering. Since causing suffering is what makes the wanton infliction of pain wrong and since the wanton infliction of pain on animals causes suffering, it follows that the wanton infliction of pain on animals is wrong.

This argument for the wrongness of the wanton infliction of pain on animals shares a number of structural features with the argument for the serious prima facie wrongness of abortion. Both arguments start with an obvious assumption concerning what it is wrong to do to me (or you, reader). Both then look for the characteristic or the consequence of the wrong action which makes the action wrong. Both recognize that the wrong-making feature of these immoral actions is a property of actions sometimes directed at individuals other than postnatal human beings. If the structure of the argument for the wrongness of the wanton infliction of pain on animals is sound, then the structure of the argument for the prima facie serious wrongness of abortion is also sound, for the structure of the two arguments is the same. The structure common to both is the key to the explanation of how the wrongness of abortion can be demonstrated without recourse to the category of person. In neither argument is that category crucial. . . .

Of course, this value of a future-like-ours argument, if sound, shows only that abortion is prima facie wrong, not that it is wrong in any and all circumstances. Since the loss of the future to a standard fetus, if killed, is, however, at least as great a loss as the loss of the future to a standard adult human being who is killed, abortion, like ordinary killing, could be justified only by the most compelling reasons. The loss of one's life is almost the greatest misfortune that can happen to one. Presumably abortion could be justified in some circumstances, only if the loss consequent on failing to abort would be at least as great. Accordingly, morally permissible abortions will be rare indeed unless, perhaps, they occur so early in pregnancy that a fetus is not yet definitely an individual. Hence, this argument should be taken as showing that abortion is presumptively very seriously wrong, where the presumption is very strong—as strong as the presumption that killing another adult human being is wrong. . . .

In this essay, it has been argued that the correct ethic of the wrongness of killing can be extended to fetal life and used to show that there is a strong presumption that any abortion is morally impermissible. If the ethic of killing adopted here entails, however, that contraception is also seriously immoral, then there would appear to be a difficulty with the analysis of this essay.

But this analysis does not entail that contraception is wrong. Of course, contraception prevents the actualization of a possible future of value. Hence, it follows from the claim that futures of value should be maximized that contraception is prima facie immoral. This obligation to maximize does not exist, however; furthermore, nothing in the ethics of killing in this paper entails that it does. The ethics of killing in this essay would entail that contraception is wrong only if something were denied a human future of value by contraception. Nothing at all is denied such a future by contraception, however.

Candidates for a subject of harm by contraception fall into four categories: (1) some sperm or other, (2) some ovum or other, (3) a sperm and an ovum separately, and (4) a sperm and an ovum together. Assigning the harm to some sperm is utterly arbitrary, for no reason can be given for making a sperm the subject of harm rather than an ovum. Assigning the harm to some ovum is utterly arbitrary, for no reason can be given for making an ovum the

subject of harm rather than a sperm. One might attempt to avoid these problems by insisting that contraception deprives both the sperm and the ovum separately of a valuable future like ours. On this alternative, too many futures are lost. Contraception was supposed to be wrong, because it deprived us of one future of value, not two. One might attempt to avoid this problem by holding that contraception deprives the combination of sperm and ovum of a valuable future like ours. But here the definite article misleads. At the time of contraception, there are hundreds of millions of sperm, one (released) ovum and millions of possible combinations of all of these. There is no actual combination at all. Is the subject of the loss to be a merely possible combination? Which one? This alternative does not yield an actual subject of harm either. Accordingly, the immorality of contraception is not entailed by the loss of a future-like-ours argument simply because there is no nonarbitrarily identifiable subject of the loss in the case of contraception. . . .

The purpose of this essay has been to set out an argument for the serious presumptive wrongness of abortion subject to the assumption that the moral permissibility of abortion stands or falls on the moral status of the fetus. Since a fetus possesses a property, the possession of which in adult human beings is sufficient to make killing an adult human being wrong, abortion is wrong. This way of dealing with the problem of abortion seems superior to other approaches to the ethics of abortion, because it rests on an ethics of killing which is close to self-evident, because the crucial morally relevant property clearly applies to fetuses, and because the argument avoids the usual equivocations on 'human life,' 'human being,' or 'person.' The argument rests neither on religious claims nor on Papal dogma. It is not subject to the objection of "speciesism." Its soundness is compatible with the moral permissibility of euthanasia and contraception. It deals with our intuitions concerning young children.

Finally, this analysis can be viewed as resolving a standard problem—indeed, *the* standard problem—concerning the ethics of abortion. Clearly, it is wrong to kill adult human beings. Clearly, it is not wrong to end the life of some arbitrarily chosen single human cell. Fetuses seem to be like arbitrarily chosen human cells in some respects and like adult humans in other respects. The problem of the ethics of abortion is the problem of determining the fetal property that settles this moral controversy. The thesis of this essay is that the problem of the ethics of abortion, so understood, is solvable.

NOTES

1 Judith Jarvis Thomson has rejected this assumption in a famous essay, "A Defense of Abortion," *Philosophy and Public Affairs* 1, #1 (1971), 47–66.

2 I have been most influenced on this matter by Jonathan Glover, *Causing Death and Saving Lives* (New York: Penguin, 1977), ch. 3; and Robert Young, "What Is So Wrong with Killing People?" *Philosophy*, LIV, 210 (1979): 515–528.

A DEFENSE OF ABORTION[1]

Judith Jarvis Thomson

In an effort to moderate the conservative view, Thomson argues that the standard conservative claim about the moral impermissibility of abortion cannot be sustained even if (for the sake of argument) it is presumed that the fetus is a person from conception. Her central point is that the moral impermissibility of abortion does not follow simply from the admission that the fetus (as a person) has a right to life. In her view, the right to life is to be understood as the right not to be killed unjustly and does not entail the right to use another person's body. In cases where the pregnant woman has not extended to the fetus the right to use her body, most prominently in the case of rape, Thomson holds that abortion is not unjust killing and thus does not violate the fetus's right to life. Thomson acknowledges that there may be cases in which the fetus (presumed to be a person) has a right to the use of the pregnant woman's body and, thus, some cases where abortion would be unjust killing. She proceeds to distinguish between the moral demands of justice and the moral demands of decency. In some cases, she maintains, an abortion does no injustice (to the fetus) yet may be subject to moral criticism on the grounds that minimal standards of moral decency are transgressed.

Most opposition to abortion relies on the premise that the fetus is a human being, a person, from the moment of conception. The premise is argued for, but, as I think, not well. Take, for example, the most common argument. We are asked to notice that the development of a human being from conception through birth into childhood is continuous; then it is said that to draw a line, to choose a point in this development and say "before this point the thing is not a person, after this point it is a person" is to make an arbitrary choice, a choice for which in the nature of things no good reason can be given. It is concluded that the fetus is, or anyway that we had better say it is, a person from the moment of conception. But this conclusion does not follow. Similar things might be said about the development of an acorn into an oak tree, and it does not follow that acorns are oak trees, or that we had better say they are. Arguments of this form are sometimes called "slippery slope arguments"—the phrase is perhaps self-explanatory—and it is dismaying that opponents of abortion rely on them so heavily and uncritically.

Philosophy and Public Affairs, vol. 1, no. 1 (1971), pp. 47–50, 54–66.
© 1971 by Princeton University Press. Reprinted by permission of Blackwell Publishing Ltd.

I am inclined to agree, however, that the prospects for "drawing a line" in the development of the fetus look dim. I am inclined to think also that we shall probably have to agree that the fetus has already become a human person well before birth. Indeed, it comes as a surprise when one first learns how early in its life it begins to acquire human characteristics. By the tenth week, for example, it already has a face, arms and legs, fingers and toes; it has internal organs, and brain activity is detectable.[2] On the other hand, I think that the premise is false, that the fetus is not a person from the moment of conception. A newly fertilized ovum, a newly implanted clump of cells, is no more a person than an acorn is an oak tree. But I shall not discuss any of this. For it seems to me to be of great interest to ask what happens if, for the sake of argument, we allow the premise. How, precisely, are we supposed to get from there to the conclusion that abortion is morally impermissible? Opponents of abortion commonly spend most of their time establishing that the fetus is a person, and hardly any time explaining the step from there to the impermissibility of abortion. Perhaps they think the step too simple and obvious to require much comment. Or perhaps instead they are simply being economical in argument. Many of those who defend abortion rely on the premise that the fetus is not a person, but only a bit of tissue that will become a person at birth; and why pay out more arguments than you have to? Whatever the explanation, I suggest that the step they take is neither easy nor obvious, that it calls for closer examination than it is commonly given, and that when we do give it this closer examination we shall feel inclined to reject it.

I propose, then, that we grant that the fetus is a person from the moment of conception. How does the argument go from here? Something like this, I take it. Every person has a right to life. So the fetus has a right to life. No doubt the mother has a right to decide what shall happen in and to her body; everyone would grant that. But surely a person's right to life is stronger and more stringent than the mother's right to decide what happens in and to her body, and so outweighs it. So the fetus may not be killed; an abortion may not be performed.

It sounds plausible. But now let me ask you to imagine this. You wake up in the morning and find yourself back to back in bed with an unconscious violinist. A famous unconscious violinist. He has been found to have a fatal kidney ailment, and the Society of Music Lovers has canvassed all the available medical records and found that you alone have the right blood type to help. They have therefore kidnapped you, and last night the violinist's circulatory system was plugged into yours, so that your kidneys can be used to extract poisons from his blood as well as your own. The director of the hospital now tells you, "Look, we're sorry the Society of Music Lovers did this to you—we would never have permitted it if we had known. But still, they did it, and the violinist now is plugged into you. To unplug you would be to kill him. But never mind, it's only for nine months. By then he will have recovered from his ailment, and can safely be unplugged from you." Is it morally incumbent on you to accede to this situation? No doubt it would be very nice of you if you did, a great kindness. But do you *have* to accede to it? What if it were not nine months, but nine years? Or longer still? What if the director of the hospital says, "Tough luck, I agree, but you've now got to stay in bed, with the violinist plugged into you, for the rest of your life. Because remember this. All persons have a right to life, and violinists are persons. Granted you have a right to decide what happens in and to your body, but a person's right to life outweighs your right to decide what happens in and to your body. So you cannot ever be unplugged from him." I imagine you would regard this as outrageous, which suggests that something really is wrong with that plausible-sounding argument I mentioned a moment ago.

In this case, of course, you were kidnapped; you didn't volunteer for the operation that plugged the violinist into your kidneys. Can those who oppose abortion on the ground I mentioned make an exception for a pregnancy due to rape? Certainly. They can say that persons have a right to life only if they didn't come into existence because of rape; or they can say that all persons have a right to life, but that some have less of a right to life than others, in particular, that those who came into existence because of rape have less. But these statements have a rather unpleasant sound. Surely the question of whether you have a right to life at all, or how much of it you have, shouldn't turn on the question of whether or not you are the product of a rape. And in fact the people who oppose abortion on the ground I mentioned do not make this distinction, and hence do not make an exception in case of rape.

Nor do they make an exception for a case in which the mother has to spend the nine months of her pregnancy in bed. They would agree that would be a great pity, and hard on the mother; but all the same, all persons have a right to life, the fetus is a person, and so on. I suspect, in fact, that they would not make an exception for a case in which, miraculously enough, the pregnancy went on for nine years, or even the rest of the mother's life.

Some won't even make an exception for a case in which continuation of the pregnancy is likely to shorten the mother's life; they regard abortion as impermissible even to save the mother's life. Such cases are nowadays very rare, and many opponents of abortion do not accept this extreme view. . . .

[1] Where the mother's life is not at stake, the argument I mentioned at the outset seems to have a much stronger pull. "Everyone has a right to life, so the unborn person has a right to life." And isn't the child's right to life weightier than anything other than the mother's own right to life, which she might put forward as ground for an abortion?

This argument treats the right to life as if it were unproblematic. It is not, and this seems to me to be precisely the source of the mistake.

For we should now, at long last, ask what it comes to, to have a right to life. In some views having a right to life includes having a right to be given at least the bare minimum one needs for continued life. But suppose that what in fact *is* the bare minimum a man needs for continued life is something he has no right at all to be given? If I am sick unto death, and the only thing that will save my life is the touch of Henry Fonda's cool hand on my fevered brow, then all the same, I have no right to be given the touch of Henry Fonda's cool hand on my fevered brow. It would be frightfully nice of him to fly in from the West Coast to provide it. It would be less nice, though no doubt well meant, if my friends flew out to the West Coast and carried Henry Fonda back with them. But I have no right at all against anybody that he should do this for me. Or again, to return to the story I told earlier, the fact that for continued life that violinist needs the continued use of your kidneys does not establish that he has a right to be given the continued use of your kidneys. He certainly has no right against you that *you* should give him continued use of your kidneys. For nobody has any right to use your kidneys unless you give him such a right; and nobody has the right against you that you shall give him this right—if you do allow him to go on using your kidneys, this is a kindness on your part, and not something he can claim from you as his due. Nor has he any right against anybody else that *they* should give him continued use of your kidneys. Certainly he had no right against the Society of Music Lovers that they should plug him into you in the first place. And if you now start to unplug yourself, having learned that you will otherwise have to spend nine years in bed with him, there is nobody in the world who must try to prevent you, in order to see to it that he is given something he has a right to be given.

Some people are rather stricter about the right to life. In their view, it does not include the right to be given anything, but amounts to, and only to, the right not to be killed by anybody. But here a related difficulty arises. If everybody is to refrain from killing that violinist, then everybody must refrain from doing a great many different sorts of things. Everybody must refrain from slitting his throat, everybody must refrain from shooting him—and everybody must refrain from unplugging you from him. But does he have a right against everybody that they shall refrain from unplugging you from him? To refrain from doing this is to allow him to continue to use your kidneys. It could be argued that he has a right against us that *we* should allow him to continue to use your kidneys. That is, while he had no right against us that we should give him the use of your kidneys, it might be argued that he anyway has a right against us that we shall not now intervene and deprive him of the use of your kidneys. I shall come back to third-party interventions later. But certainly the violinist has no right against you that *you* shall allow him to continue to use your kidneys. As I said, if you do allow him to use them, it is a kindness on your part, and not something you owe him.

The difficulty I point to here is not peculiar to the right to life. It reappears in connection with all the other natural rights; and it is something which an adequate account of rights must deal with. For present purposes it is enough just to draw attention to it. But I would stress that I am not arguing that people do not have a right to life—quite to the contrary, it seems to me that the primary control we must place on the acceptability of an account of rights is that it should turn out in that account to be a truth that all persons have a right to life. I am arguing only that having a right to life does not guarantee having either a right to be given the use of or a right to be allowed continued use of another person's body—even if one needs it for life itself. So the right to life will not serve the opponents of abortion in the very simple and clear way in which they seem to have thought it would.

[2] There is another way to bring out the difficulty. In the most ordinary sort of case, to deprive someone of what he has a right to is to treat him unjustly. Suppose a boy and his small brother are jointly given a box of chocolates for Christmas. If the older boy takes the box and refuses to give his brother any of the chocolates, he is unjust to him, for the brother has been given a right to half of them. But suppose that, having learned that otherwise it means nine years in bed with that violinist, you unplug yourself from him. You surely are not being unjust to him, for you gave him no right to use your kidneys, and no one else can have given him any such right. But we have to notice that in unplugging yourself, you are killing him; and violinists, like everybody else, have a right to life, and thus in the view we were considering just now, the right not to be killed. So here you do what he supposedly has a right you shall not do, but you do not act unjustly to him in doing it.

The emendation which may be made at this point is this: the right to life consists not in the right not to be killed, but rather in the right not to be killed unjustly. This runs a risk of circularity, but never mind: it would enable us to square the fact that the violinist has a right to life with the fact that you do not act unjustly toward him in unplugging yourself, thereby killing him. For if you do not kill him unjustly, you do not violate his right to life, and so it is no wonder you do him no injustice.

But if this emendation is accepted, the gap in the argument against abortion stares us plainly in the face: it is by no means enough to show that the fetus is a person, and to remind us that all persons have a right to life—we need to be shown also that killing the fetus violates its right to life, i.e., that abortion is unjust killing. And is it?

I suppose we may take it as a datum that in a case of pregnancy due to rape the mother has not given the unborn person a right to the use of her body for food and shelter. Indeed, in what pregnancy could it be supposed that the mother has given the unborn person such a right? It is not as if there were unborn persons drifting about the world, to whom a woman who wants a child says "I invite you in."

But it might be argued that there are other ways one can have acquired a right to the use of another person's body than by having been invited to use it by that person. Suppose a woman voluntarily indulges in intercourse, knowing of the chance it will issue in pregnancy, and then she does become pregnant; is she not in part responsible for the presence, in fact the very existence, of the unborn person inside her? No doubt she did not invite it in. But doesn't her partial responsibility for its being there itself give it a right to the use of her body?[3] If so, then her aborting it would be more like the boy's taking away the chocolates, and less like your unplugging yourself from the violinist—doing so would be depriving it of what it does have a right to, and thus would be doing it an injustice.

And then, too, it might be asked whether or not she can kill it even to save her own life: If she voluntarily called it into existence, how can she now kill it, even in self-defense?

The first thing to be said about this is that it is something new. Opponents of abortion have been so concerned to make out the independence of the fetus, in order to establish that it has a right to life, just as its mother does, that they have tended to overlook the possible support they might gain from making out that the fetus is *dependent* on the mother, in order to establish that she has a special kind of responsibility for it, a responsibility that gives it rights against her which are not possessed by any independent person—such as an ailing violinist who is a stranger to her.

On the other hand, this argument would give the unborn person a right to its mother's body only if her pregnancy resulted from a voluntary act, undertaken in full knowledge of the chance a pregnancy might result from it. It would leave out entirely the unborn person whose existence is due to rape. Pending the availability of some further argument, then, we would be left with the conclusion that unborn persons whose existence is due to rape have no right to the use of their mothers' bodies, and thus that aborting them is not depriving them of anything they have a right to and hence is not unjust killing.

And we should also notice that it is not at all plain that this argument really does go even as far as it purports to. For there are cases and cases, and the details make a difference. If the room is stuffy, and I therefore open a window to air it, and a burglar climbs in, it would be absurd to say, "Ah, now he can stay, she's given him a right to the use of her house—for she is partially responsible for his presence there, having voluntarily done what enabled him to get in, in full knowledge that there are such things as burglars, and that burglars burgle." It would be still more absurd to say this if I had had bars installed outside my windows, precisely to prevent burglars from getting in, and a burglar got in only because of a defect in the bars. It remains equally absurd if we imagine it is not a burglar who climbs in, but an innocent person who blunders or falls in. Again, suppose it were like this: people-seeds drift about in the air like pollen, and if you open your windows, one may drift in and take root in your carpets or upholstery. You don't want children, so you fix up your windows with fine mesh screens, the very best you can buy. As can happen, however, and on very, very rare occasions does happen, one of the screens is defective; and a seed drifts in and takes root. Does the person-plant who now develops have a right to the use of your house? Surely not—despite the fact that you voluntarily opened your windows, you knowingly kept carpets and upholstered furniture, and you knew that screens were sometimes defective. Someone may argue that you are responsible for its rooting, that it does have a right to your house, because after all you *could* have lived out your life with bare floors and furniture, or with sealed windows and doors. But this won't do—for by the same token anyone can avoid a pregnancy due to rape by having a hysterectomy, or anyway by never leaving home without a (reliable!) army.

It seems to me that the argument we are looking at can establish at most that there are *some* cases in which the unborn person has a right to the use of its mother's body, and therefore *some* cases in which abortion is unjust killing. There is room for much discussion and argument as to precisely which, if any. But I think we should sidestep this issue and leave it open, for at any rate the argument certainly does not establish that all abortion is unjust killing.

[3] There is room for yet another argument here, however. We surely must all grant that there may be cases in which it would be morally indecent to detach a person from your body at the cost of his life. Suppose you learn that what the violinist needs is not nine years of your life, but only one hour: all you need do to save his life is to spend one hour in that bed with him. Suppose also that letting him use your kidneys for that one hour would not affect your health in the slightest. Admittedly you were kidnapped. Admittedly you did not give anyone permission to plug him into you. Nevertheless it seems to me plain you *ought* to allow him to use your kidneys for that hour—it would be indecent to refuse.

Again, suppose pregnancy lasted only an hour, and constituted no threat to life or health. And suppose that a woman becomes pregnant as a result of rape. Admittedly she did not voluntarily do anything to bring about the existence of a child. Admittedly she did nothing at all which would give the unborn person a right to the use of her body. All the same it might well be said, as in the newly emended violinist story, that she *ought* to allow it to remain for that hour—that it would be indecent in her to refuse.

Now some people are inclined to use the term "right" in such a way that it follows from the fact that you ought to allow a person to use your body for the hour he needs, that he has a right to use your body for the hour he needs, even though he has not been given that right by any person or act. They may say that it follows also that if you refuse, you act unjustly toward him. This use of the term is perhaps so common that it cannot be called wrong; nevertheless it seems to me to be an unfortunate loosening of what we would do better to keep a tight rein on. Suppose that box of chocolates I mentioned earlier had not been given to both boys jointly, but was given only to the older boy. There he sits, stolidly eating his way through the box, his small brother watching enviously. Here we are likely to say "You ought not to be so mean. You ought to give your brother some of those chocolates." My own view is that it just does not follow from the truth of this that the brother has any right to any of the chocolates. If the boy refuses to give his brother any, he is greedy, stingy, callous—but not unjust. I suppose that the people I have in mind will say it does follow that the brother has a right to some of the chocolates, and thus that the boy does act unjustly if he refuses to give his brother any. But the effect of saying this is to obscure what we should keep distinct, namely the difference between the boy's refusal in this case and the boy's refusal in the earlier case, in which the box was given to both boys jointly, and in which the small brother thus had what was from any point of view clear title to half.

A further objection to so using the term "right" that from the fact that A ought to do a thing for B, it follows that B has a right against A that A do it for him, is that it is going to make the question of whether or not a man has a right to a thing turn on how easy it is to provide him with it; and this seems not merely unfortunate, but morally unacceptable. Take the case of Henry Fonda again. I said earlier that I had no right to the touch of his cool hand on my fevered brow, even though I needed it to save my life. I said it would be frightfully nice of him to fly in from the West Coast to provide me with it, but that I had no right against him that he should do so. But suppose he isn't on the West Coast. Suppose he has only to walk across the room, place a hand briefly on my brow—and lo, my life is saved. Then surely he ought to do it, it would be indecent to refuse. Is it to be said "Ah, well, it follows that in this case she has a right to the touch of his hand on her brow, and so it would be an injustice in him to refuse"? So that I have a right to it when it is easy for him to provide it, though no right when it's hard? It's rather a shocking idea that anyone's rights should fade away and disappear as it gets harder and harder to accord them to him.

So my own view is that even though you ought to let the violinist use your kidneys for the one hour he needs, we should not conclude that he has a right to do so—we would say that if you refuse, you are,

like the boy who owns all the chocolates and will give none away, self-centered and callous, indecent in fact, but not unjust. And similarly, that even supposing a case in which a woman pregnant due to rape ought to allow the unborn person to use her body for the hour he needs, we should not conclude that he has a right to do so; we should conclude that she is self-centered, callous, indecent, but not unjust, if she refuses. The complaints are no less grave; they are just different. However, there is no need to insist on this point. If anyone does wish to deduce "he has a right" from "you ought," then all the same he must surely grant that there are cases in which it is not morally required of you that you allow that violinist to use your kidneys, and in which he does not have a right to use them, and in which you do not do him an injustice if you refuse. And so also for mother and unborn child. Except in such cases as the unborn person has a right to demand it—and we were leaving open the possibility that there may be such cases—nobody is morally *required* to make large sacrifices, of health, of all other interests and concerns, of all other duties and commitments, for nine years, or even for nine months, in order to keep another person alive.

[4] We have in fact to distinguish between two kinds of Samaritan: the Good Samaritan and what we might call the Minimally Decent Samaritan. The story of the Good Samaritan, you will remember, goes like this:

> A certain man went down from Jerusalem to Jericho, and fell among thieves, which stripped him of his raiment, and wounded him, and departed, leaving him half dead.
>
> And by chance there came down a certain priest that way; and when he saw him, he passed by on the other side.
>
> And likewise a Levite, when he was at the place, came and looked on him, and passed by on the other side.
>
> But a certain Samaritan, as he journeyed, came where he was; and when he saw him he had compassion on him.
>
> And went to him, and bound up his wounds, pouring in oil and wine, and set him on his own beast, and brought him to an inn, and took care of him.
>
> And on the morrow, when he departed, he took out two pence, and gave them to the host, and said

unto him, "Take care of him; and whatsoever thou spendest more, when I come again, I will repay thee."

(Luke 10:30–35)

The Good Samaritan went out of his way, at some cost to himself, to help one in need of it. We are not told what the options were, that is, whether or not the priest and the Levite could have helped by doing less than the Good Samaritan did, but assuming they could have, then the fact they did nothing at all shows they were not even Minimally Decent Samaritans, not because they were not Samaritans, but because they were not even minimally decent.

These things are a matter of degree, of course, but there is a difference, and it comes out perhaps most clearly in the story of Kitty Genovese, who, as you will remember, was murdered while thirty-eight people watched or listened, and did nothing at all to help her. A Good Samaritan would have rushed out to give direct assistance against the murderer. Or perhaps we had better allow that it would have been a Splendid Samaritan who did this, on the ground that it would have involved a risk of death for himself. But the thirty-eight not only did not do this, they did not even trouble to pick up a phone to call the police. Minimally Decent Samaritanism would call for doing at least that, and their not having done it was monstrous.

After telling the story of the Good Samaritan, Jesus said "Go, and do thou likewise." Perhaps he meant that we are morally required to act as the Good Samaritan did. Perhaps he was urging people to do more than is morally required of them. At all events it seems plain that it was not morally required of any of the thirty-eight that he rush out to give direct assistance at the risk of his own life, and that it is not morally required of anyone that he give long stretches of his life—nine years or nine months—to sustaining the life of a person who has no special right (we were leaving open the possibility of this) to demand it.

Indeed, with one rather striking class of exceptions, no one in any country in the world is *legally* required to do anywhere near as much as this for anyone else. The class of exceptions is obvious. My main concern here is not the state of the law in re-

spect to abortion, but it is worth drawing attention to the fact that in no state in this country is any man compelled by law to be even a Minimally Decent Samaritan to any person; there is no law under which charges could be brought against the thirty-eight who stood by while Kitty Genovese died. By contrast, in most states in this country women are compelled by law to be not merely Minimally Decent Samaritans, but Good Samaritans to unborn persons inside them. This doesn't by itself settle anything one way or the other, because it may well be argued that there should be laws in this country—as there are in many European countries—compelling at least Minimally Decent Samaritanism.[4] But it does show that there is a gross injustice in the existing state of the law. And it shows also that the groups currently working against liberalization of abortion laws, in fact working toward having it declared unconstitutional for a state to permit abortion, had better start working for the adoption of Good Samaritan laws generally, or earn the charge that they are acting in bad faith.

I should think, myself, that Minimally Decent Samaritan laws would be one thing, Good Samaritan laws quite another, and in fact highly improper. But we are not here concerned with the law. What we should ask is not whether anybody should be compelled by law to be a Good Samaritan, but whether we must accede to a situation in which somebody is being compelled—by nature, perhaps—to be a Good Samaritan. We have, in other words, to look now at third-party interventions. I have been arguing that no person is morally required to make large sacrifices to sustain the life of another who has no right to demand them, and this even where the sacrifices do not include life itself; we are not morally required to be Good Samaritans or anyway Very Good Samaritans to one another. But what if a man cannot extricate himself from such a situation? What if he appeals to us to extricate him? It seems to me plain that there are cases in which we can, cases in which a Good Samaritan would extricate him. There you are, you were kidnapped, and nine years in bed with that violinist lie ahead of you. You have your own life to lead. You are sorry, but you simply cannot see giving up so much of your life to the sustaining of his. You cannot extricate yourself, and ask us to do so. I should have thought that—in light of his having no right to the use of your body—it was obvious that we do not have to accede to your being forced to give up so much. We can do what you ask. There is no injustice to the violinist in our doing so.

[5] Following the lead of the opponents of abortion, I have throughout been speaking of the fetus merely as a person, and what I have been asking is whether or not the argument we began with, which proceeds only from the fetus' being a person, really does establish its conclusion. I have argued that it does not.

But of course there are arguments and arguments, and it may be said that I have simply fastened on the wrong one. It may be said that what is important is not merely the fact that the fetus is a person, but that it is a person for whom the woman has a special kind of responsibility issuing from the fact that she is its mother. And it might be argued that all my analogies are therefore irrelevant—for you do not have that special kind of responsibility for that violinist, Henry Fonda does not have that special kind of responsibility for me. And our attention might be drawn to the fact that men and women both *are* compelled by law to provide support for their children.

I have in effect dealt (briefly) with this argument in section [2] above; but a (still briefer) recapitulation now may be in order. Surely we do not have any such "special responsibility" for a person unless we have assumed it, explicitly or implicitly. If a set of parents do not try to prevent pregnancy, do not obtain an abortion, and then at the time of birth of the child do not put it out for adoption, but rather take it home with them, then they have assumed responsibility for it, they have given it rights, and they cannot *now* withdraw support from it at the cost of its life because they now find it difficult to go on providing for it. But if they have taken all reasonable precautions against having a child, they do not simply by virtue of their biological relationship to the child who comes into existence have a special responsibility for it. They may wish to assume responsibility for it, or they may not wish to. And I am suggesting that if assuming responsibility for it would require large sacrifices, then they may refuse. A Good Samaritan would not refuse—or anyway, a Splendid Samaritan, if the sacrifices that had to be made were enormous.

But then so would a Good Samaritan assume responsibility for that violinist; so would Henry Fonda, if he is a Good Samaritan, fly in from the West Coast and assume responsibility for me.

[6] My argument will be found unsatisfactory on two counts by many of those who want to regard abortion as morally permissible. First, while I do argue that abortion is not impermissible, I do not argue that it is always permissible. There may well be cases in which carrying the child to term requires only Minimally Decent Samaritanism of the mother, and this is a standard we must not fall below. I am inclined to think it a merit of my account precisely that it does *not* give a general yes or a general no. It allows for and supports our sense that, for example, a sick and desperately frightened fourteen-year-old schoolgirl, pregnant due to rape, may *of course* choose abortion, and that any law which rules this out is an insane law. And it also allows for and supports our sense that in other cases resort to abortion is even positively indecent. It would be indecent in the woman to request an abortion, and indecent in a doctor to perform it, if she is in her seventh month, and wants the abortion just to avoid the nuisance of postponing a trip abroad. The very fact that the arguments I have been drawing attention to treat all cases of abortion, or even all cases of abortion in which the mother's life is not at stake, as morally on a par ought to have made them suspect at the outset.

Secondly, while I am arguing for the permissibility of abortion in some cases, I am not arguing for the right to secure the death of the unborn child. It is easy to confuse these two things in that up to a certain point in the life of the fetus it is not able to survive outside the mother's body; hence removing it from her body guarantees its death. But they are importantly different. I have argued that you are not morally required to spend nine months in bed, sustaining the life of that violinist; but to say this is by no means to say that if, when you unplug yourself, there is a miracle and he survives, you then have a right to turn round and slit his throat. You may detach yourself even if this costs him his life; you have no right to be guaranteed his death, by some other means, if unplugging yourself does not kill him. There are some people who will feel dissatisfied by this feature of my argument. A woman may be utterly devastated by the thought of a child, a bit of herself, put out for adoption and never seen or heard of again. She may therefore want not merely that the child be detached from her, but more, that it die. Some opponents of abortion are inclined to regard this as beneath contempt—thereby showing insensitivity to what is surely a powerful source of despair. All the same, I agree that the desire for the child's death is not one which anybody may gratify, should it turn out to be possible to detach the child alive.

At this place, however, it should be remembered that we have only been pretending throughout that the fetus is a human being from the moment of conception. A very early abortion is surely not the killing of a person, and so is not dealt with by anything I have said here.

NOTES

1 I am very much indebted to James Thomson for discussion, criticism, and many helpful suggestions.

2 Daniel Callahan, *Abortion: Law, Choice and Morality* (New York, 1970), p. 373. This book gives a fascinating survey of the available information on abortion. The Jewish tradition is surveyed in David M. Feldman, *Birth Control in Jewish Law* (New York, 1968), Part 5, the Catholic tradition in John T. Noonan, Jr., "An Almost Absolute Value in History," in *The Morality of Abortion*, ed. John T. Noonan, Jr. (Cambridge, Mass., 1970).

3 The need for a discussion of this argument was brought home to me by members of the Society for Ethical and Legal Philosophy, to whom this paper was originally presented.

4 For a discussion of the difficulties involved, and a survey of the European experience with such laws, see *The Good Samaritan and the Law*, ed. James M. Ratcliffe (New York, 1966).

THE MORALITY OF ABORTION
Margaret Olivia Little

Little argues that abortion is a morally weighty matter even if we put aside the claim that the fetus is a person. In her view, "burgeoning human life" matters morally; it has some degree of value (moral status) and, thus, to that extent is worthy of respect. From this general starting point, Little explores the morality of abortion, paying special attention to two themes—motherhood and respect for creation—that often play a role in the thinking of women struggling with a decision to continue or end pregnancy. She explains how each of these themes adds a layer of complexity to a woman's decision to continue or end pregnancy, and she ultimately argues that personal decisions about the morality of abortion depend in part on the unique way in which individual women construct their fundamental identities, commitments, and personal ideals.

. . . Just as we cannot assume that abortion is monstrous if fetuses are persons, so too we cannot assume that abortion is empty of moral import if they are not. Given all the ink that has been spilt on arbitrating the question of fetal personhood, one might be forgiven for having thought so: on some accounts, decisions about whether to continue or end a

Reprinted with permission of the publisher from *A Companion to Applied Ethics* (2003), edited by R. G. Frey and Christopher Heath Wellman, pp. 319–324. © 2003 by Blackwell Publishing Ltd.

pregnancy really are, from a moral point of view, just like decisions about whether to cut one's hair.

But as Ronald Dworkin (1993) has urged, to think abortion morally weighty does not require supposition that the fetus is a person, or even a creature with interests in continued life. Destruction of a Da Vinci painting, he points out, is not bad *for the painting*—the painting has no interests. Instead, it is regrettable because of the deep value it has. So, too, one of the reasons we might regard abortion as morally weighty does not have to do with its being bad *for the fetus*—a setback to its interests—for it may not satisfy the criteria of having interests. Abortion may be weighty, instead, because there is something precious and significant about germinating human life that deserves our deep respect. This, as Dworkin puts it, locates issues of abortion in a different neighborhood of our moral commitments: namely, the accommodation we owe to things of value. That an organism is a potential person may not make it a claims-bearer, but it does mean it has a kind of stature that is worthy of respect.

This intuition, dismissed by some as mere sentimentality, is, I think, both important and broadly held. Very few people regard abortion as the moral equivalent of contraception. Most think a society better morally—not just by public health measures—if it regards abortion as a back-up to failed contraception rather than as routine birth control. Reasons adequate for contraception do not translate transparently as reasons adequate for abortion. Indeed, there is a telling shift in presumption: for most people, it takes no reason at all to justify contracepting; it takes *some* reason to justify ending a pregnancy. That a human life has now begun matters morally.

Burgeoning human life, we might put it, is *respect-worthy*. This is why we care not just whether, but how, abortion is done—while crass jokes are made or with solemnity—and why we care how the fetal remains are treated. It is why the thought of someone aborting for genuinely trivial reasons—to fit into a favorite party dress, say—makes us morally queasy. Perhaps, most basically, it is why the thought of someone aborting with casual indifference fills us with misgiving. Abortion involves loss. Not just loss of the hope that various parties might have invested, but loss of something valuable in its own right. To respect something is to appreciate fully the value it has and the claims it presents to us; someone who aborts but never gives it a second thought has not exhibited genuine appreciation of the value and moral status of that which is now gone.

But if many share the intuition that early human life has a value deserving of respect, there is considerable disagreement about what that respect looks like. There is considerable conflict, that is, over what accommodation we owe to burgeoning human life.

In part, of course, this is due to disagreement over the *degree* of value such life should be accorded: those for whom it is thoroughly modest will have very different views on issues, from abortion to stem-cell research, from those for whom it is transcendent. But this is only part of the story. Obscured by analogies to Da Vinci paintings, some of the most important sources of conflict, especially for the vast middle rank of moderates, ride atop rough agreement on "degree" of fetal value. If we listen to women's own struggles about when it is morally decent to end pregnancy, what we hear are themes about *motherhood* and *respect for creation*. These themes are enormously complex, I want to argue, for they enter stories on both sides of the ledger: for some women, as reasons to continue pregnancy, and, for others, as reasons to end it. Let me start with motherhood.

For many women who contemplate abortion, the desire to end pregnancy is not, or not centrally, a desire to avoid the nine months of pregnancy; it is to avoid what lies on the far side of those months—namely, motherhood. If gestation were simply a matter of rendering, say, somewhat risky assistance to help a burgeoning human life they have come across—if they could somehow render that assistance without thereby adding a member to their family—the decision faced would be a far different one. But gestation does not just allow cells to become a person; it turns one into a mother.

One of the most common reasons women give for wanting to abort is that they do not want to become a mother—now, ever, again, with this partner, or no reliable partner, with these few resources, or these many that are now, after so many years of mothering, slated finally to another cause (Hursthouse, 1987: ch. 8.4). Nor does adoption represent a universal solution. To give up a child would be for some a life-long trauma; others occupy fortunate circumstances that would, by their own lights, make it unjustified to give over a child for others to rear. Or again—and most frequently—she does not want to raise a child just now but knows that if she *does* carry the pregnancy to term, she will not *want* to give up the child for adoption. Gestation, she knows, is likely to reshape her heart and soul, transforming her into a mother emotionally, not just officially; and it is precisely that transformation she does not want to undergo. It is because continuing pregnancy brings with it this new identity and, likely, relationship, then, that many feel it legitimate to decline.

But pregnancy's connection to motherhood also enters the phenomenology of abortion in just the opposite direction. For some women, that it would be her child is precisely why she feels she must continue the pregnancy, even if motherhood is not what she desired. To be pregnant is to have one's potential child knocking at one's door: to abort is to turn one's back on it, a decision, many women say, that would haunt them forever. On this view, the desire to avoid motherhood, so compelling as a reason to use contraception, is uneasy grounds to abort: for once an embryo is on the scene, it is not about rejecting motherhood, it is about rejecting one's *child*. Not literally, of course, since there is no child yet extant to stand as the object of rejection. But the stance one should take to pregnancy, sought or not, is one of *acceptance:* when a potential family member is knocking at the door, one should move over, make room, and welcome her in.

These two intuitive stances represent just profoundly different ways of *gestalting* the situation of ending pregnancy. On the first view, abortion is closer to contraception: hardly equivalent, because it means the demise of something of value. But the desire to avoid the enterprise and identity of motherhood is an understandable and honorable basis for deciding to end a pregnancy. Given that there is no child yet on the scene, one does not owe special openness to the relationship that stands at the end of pregnancy's trajectory. On the second view, abortion is closer to exiting a parental relationship: hardly equivalent, for one of the key relata is not yet fully present. But one's decision about whether to continue the pregnancy already feels specially constrained; that one would be related to the resulting person exerts now some moral force. It would take especially grave reasons to refuse assistance here, for the norms of parenthood already have toehold. Assessing the moral status of abortion, it turns out, then, is not just about assessing the contours of generic respect owed to burgeoning human life, it is about assessing the salience of *impending relationship*. And this is an issue that functions in different

ways for different women—and, sometimes, in one and the same woman.

In my own view, until the fetus is a person, we should recognize a moral prerogative to decline parenthood and end the pregnancy. Not because motherhood is necessarily a burden (though it can be), but because it so thoroughly changes what we might call one's fundamental *practical identity*. The enterprise of mothering restructures the self—changing the shape of one's heart, the primary commitments by which one lives one's life, the terms by which one judges one's life a success or a failure. If the enterprise is eschewed and one decides to give the child over to another, the identity of mother still changes the normative facts that are true of one, as there is now someone by whom one does well or poorly (see Ross, 1982). And either way—whether one rears the child or lets it go—to continue a pregnancy means that a piece of one's heart, as the saying goes, will forever walk outside one's body. As profound as the respect we should have for burgeoning human life, we should acknowledge moral prerogatives over identity-constituting commitments and enterprises as profound as motherhood.

Whether one agrees with this view or not, there is at any rate another layer of the moral story here. If women find themselves with different ways of *gestalting* the prospective relationship involved in pregnancy, it is in part because they have different identities, commitments, and ideals that such a prospect intersects with, commitments which, while permissibly idiosyncratic, are morally authoritative for *them*. If one woman feels already duty-bound by the norms of parenthood to nurture this creature, for example, it may be for the very good reason that, in an important personal sense, she already *is* its mother. She finds herself (perhaps to her surprise) with a maternal commitment to this creature. But taking on the identity of mother toward something just *is* to take on certain imperatives about its well-being as categorical. Her job is thus clear: it is to help this creature reach its fullest potential. For another woman, on the other hand, the identity of mother is yet to be taken on; it is tried on, perhaps accepted, but perhaps declined—in which case respect is owed, but love is saved, or confirmed, for others—other relationships, other projects, other passions.

And, again, if one woman feels she owes a stance of welcome to burgeoning human life that comes her way, it may be, not because she thinks such a stance authoritative for all, but because of the virtues around which her practical identity is now oriented: receptivity to life's agenda, for instance, or responsiveness to that which is most vulnerable. For another woman, the virtues to be exercised may tug in just the other direction: loyalty to treasured life plans, a commitment that it be she, not the chances of biology, that should determine her life's course, bolstering self-direction after a life too long ruled by serendipity and fate.

Deciding when it is morally decent to end a pregnancy, it turns out, is an admixture of settling impersonally or universally authoritative moral requirements, and of discovering and arbitrating—sometimes after agonizing deliberation, sometimes in a decision no less deep for its immediacy—one's own commitments, identity, and defining virtues.

A similarly complex story appears when we turn to the second theme. Another thread that appears in many women's stories in the face of unsought pregnancy is respect for the weighty responsibility involved in creating human life. Once again, it is a theme that pulls and tugs in different directions.

In its most familiar direction, it shows up in many stories of why an unsought pregnancy is continued. Many people believe that one's responsibility to nurture new life is importantly amplified if one is responsible for bringing about its existence in the first place. Just what it takes to count as responsible here is a point on which individuals diverge (whether voluntary intercourse with contraception is different from intercourse without use of birth control, and again from intentionally deciding to become pregnant at the IVF clinic). But triggering the relevant standard of responsibility for creation, it is felt, brings with it a heightened responsibility to nurture: it is disrespectful to create human life only to allow it to wither. Put more rigorously, one who is responsible for bringing about a creature that has intrinsic value in virtue of its potential to become a person has a special responsibility to enable it to reach that end state.

But the idea of respect for creation is also, if less frequently acknowledged, sometimes the reason why women are moved to *end* pregnancies. As Bar-

bara Katz Rothman (1989) puts it, decisions to abort often represent, not a decision to destroy, but a refusal to create. Many people have deeply felt convictions about the circumstances under which they feel it right for them to bring a child into the world. Can it be brought into a decent world, an intact family, a society that can minimally respect its agency? These considerations may persist even after conception has taken place; for while the *embryo* has already been created, a person has not. Some women decide to abort, that is, not because they do not *want* the resulting child—indeed, they may yearn for nothing more, and desperately wish that their circumstances were otherwise—but because they do not think bringing a child into the world the right thing for them to do.

These are abortions marked by moral language. A woman wants to abort because she knows she could not give up a child for adoption but feels she could not give the child the sort of life, or be the sort of parent, she thinks a child *deserves;* a woman who would have to give up the child thinks it would be *unfair* to bring a child into existence already burdened by rejection, however well grounded its reasons; a woman living in a country marked by poverty and gender apartheid wants to abort because she decides it would be *wrong* for her to bear a daughter whose life, like hers, would be filled with so much injustice and hardship.

Some have thought that such decisions betray a simple fallacy: unless the child's life were literally going to be worse than non-existence, how can one abort out of concern for the future child? But the worry here is not that one would be imposing a *harm* on the child by bringing it into existence (as though children who are in the situations mentioned have lives that are not worth living). The claim is that bringing about a person's life in these circumstances would do violence to her ideals of creating and parenthood. She does not want to bring into existence a daughter she cannot love and care for, she does not want to bring into existence a person whose life will be marked by disrespect or rejection.

Nor does the claim imply judgment on women who *do* continue pregnancies in similar circumstances—as though there were here an obligation to abort. For the norms in question, once again, need not be impersonally authoritative moral claims. Like ideals of good parenting, they mark out considerations all should be sensitive to, perhaps, but equally reasonable people may adhere to different variations and weightings. Still, they are normative for those who do have them; far from expressing mere matters of taste, the ideals one does accept carry an important kind of categoricity, issuing imperatives whose authority is not reducible to mere desire. These are, at root, issues about *integrity,* and the importance of maintaining integrity over one's participation in this enterprise precisely because it is so normatively weighty.

What is usually emphasized in the morality of abortion is the ethics of destruction, but there is a balancing ethics of creation. And for many people, conflict about abortion is a conflict *within* that ethics. On the one hand, we now have on hand an entity that has a measure of sanctity: that it has begun is reason to help it continue, perhaps especially if one has had a role in its procreation, which is why even early abortion is not normatively equivalent to contraception. On the other hand, not to end a pregnancy *is* to do something else, namely, to continue creating a person, and, for some women, pregnancy strikes in circumstances in which they cannot countenance that enterprise. For some, the sanctity of developing human life will be strong enough to tip the balance toward continuing the pregnancy; for others, their norms of respectful creation will hold sway. For those who believe that the norms governing creation of a person are mild relative to the normative telos of embryonic life, being a responsible

creator means continuing to gestate, and doing the best one can to bring about the conditions under which that creation will be more respectful. For others, though, the normativity of fetal telos is mild and their standards of respectful creation high, and the lesson goes in just the other direction: it is a sign of respect not to continue creating when certain background conditions, such as a loving family or adequate resources, are not in place.

However one thinks these issues settle out, they will not be resolved by austere contemplation of the value of human life. They require wrestling with the rich meanings of creation, responsibility, and kinship. And these issues, I have suggested, are just as much issues about one's integrity as they are about one's integrity as they are about what is impersonally obligatory. On many treatments of abortion, considerations about whether or not to continue a pregnancy are exhausted by preferences, on the one hand, and universally authoritative moral demands, on the other; but some of the most important terrain lies in between.

REFERENCES

Dworkin, R. (1993) *Life's Dominion: An Argument About Abortion, Euthanasia, and Individual Freedom.* New York: Alfred A. Knopf.

Hursthouse, R. (1987) *Beginning Lives.* Oxford: Open University Press.

Ross, S. L. (1982) Abortion and the death of the fetus. *Philosophy and Public Affairs,* 11:232–45.

Rothman, B. K. (1989) *Recreating Motherhood: Ideology and Technology in a Patriarchal Society.* New York: Norton.

ABORTION AND SOCIAL POLICY

MAJORITY OPINION IN *ROE V. WADE*
Justice Harry Blackmun

In this case, a pregnant single woman, suing under the fictitious name of Jane Roe, challenged the constitutionality of the existing Texas criminal abortion law. According to the Texas Penal Code, the performance of an abortion, except to save the life of the pregnant woman, constituted a crime that was punishable by a prison sentence of two to five years. At the time this case was finally resolved by the Supreme Court, abortion legislation varied widely from state to state. Some states, principally

New York, had already legalized abortion on demand. Most other states, however, had legalized various forms of therapeutic abortion but had retained some measure of restrictive abortion legislation.

Justice Blackmun, writing an opinion concurred in by six other justices, argues that a woman's decision to terminate a pregnancy is encompassed by a *right to privacy*—but only up to a certain point in the development of the fetus. As the right to privacy is not an absolute right, it must yield at some point to the state's legitimate interests. Justice Blackmun contends that the state has a legitimate interest in protecting the health of the mother and that this interest becomes compelling at approximately the end of the first trimester in the development of the fetus. He also contends that the state has a legitimate interest in protecting potential life and that this interest becomes compelling at the point of viability.

It is . . . apparent that at common law, at the time of the adoption of our Constitution, and throughout the major portion of the 19th century, abortion was viewed with less disfavor than under most American statutes currently in effect. Phrasing it another way, a woman enjoyed a substantially broader right to terminate a pregnancy than she does in most States today. At least with respect to the early stage of pregnancy, and very possibly without such a limitation, the opportunity to make this choice was present in this country well into the 19th century. Even later, the law continued for some time to treat less punitively an abortion procured in early pregnancy. . . .

Three reasons have been advanced to explain historically the enactment of criminal abortion laws in the 19th century and to justify their continued existence.

It has been argued occasionally that these laws were the product of a Victorian social concern to discourage illicit sexual conduct. Texas, however, does not advance this justification in the present case, and it appears that no court or commentator has taken the argument seriously. . . .

A second reason is concerned with abortion as a medical procedure. When most criminal abortion laws were first enacted, the procedure was a hazardous one for the woman. This was particularly true prior to the development of antisepsis. Antiseptic techniques, of course, were based on discoveries by Lister, Pasteur, and others first announced in 1867, but were not generally accepted and employed until

United States Supreme Court; January 22, 1973. 410 U.S. 113, 93 S.Ct. 705.

about the turn of the century. Abortion mortality was high. Even after 1900, and perhaps until as late as the development of antibiotics in the 1940s, standard modern techniques such as dilation and curettage were not nearly so safe as they are today. Thus it has been argued that a State's real concern in enacting a criminal abortion law was to protect the pregnant woman, that is, to restrain her from submitting to a procedure that placed her life in serious jeopardy.

Modern medical techniques have altered this situation. Appellants and various *amici* refer to medical data indicating that abortion in early pregnancy, that is, prior to the end of first trimester, although not without its risk, is now relatively safe. Mortality rates for women undergoing early abortions, where the procedure is legal, appear to be as low as or lower than the rates for normal childbirth. Consequently, any interest of the State in protecting the woman from an inherently hazardous procedure, except when it would be equally dangerous for her to forego it, has largely disappeared. Of course, important state interests in the area of health and medical standards do remain. The State has a legitimate interest in seeing to it that abortion, like any other medical procedure, is performed under circumstances that insure maximum safety for the patient. This interest obviously extends at least to the performing physician and his staff, to the facilities involved, to the availability of after-care, and to adequate provision for any complication or emergency that might arise. The prevalence of high mortality rates at illegal "abortion mills" strengthens, rather than weakens, the State's interest in regulating the conditions under which abortions are performed.

Moreover, the risk to the woman increases as her pregnancy continues. Thus the State retains a definite interest in protecting the woman's own health and safety when an abortion is performed at a late stage of pregnancy.

The third reason is the State's interest—some phrase it in terms of duty—in protecting prenatal life. Some of the argument for this justification rests on the theory that a new human life is present from the moment of conception. The State's interest and general obligation to protect life then extends, it is argued, to prenatal life. Only when the life of the pregnant mother herself is at stake, balanced against the life she carries within her, should the interest of the embryo or fetus not prevail. Logically, of course, a legitimate state interest in this area need not stand or fall on acceptance of the belief that life begins at conception or at some other point prior to live birth. In assessing the State's interest, recognition may be given to the less rigid claim that as long as at least *potential* life is involved, the State may assert interests beyond the protection of the pregnant woman alone.

Parties challenging state abortion laws have sharply disputed in some courts the contention that a purpose of these laws, when enacted, was to protect prenatal life. Pointing to the absence of legislative history to support the contention, they claim that most state laws were designed solely to protect the woman. Because medical advances have lessened this concern, at least with respect to abortion in early pregnancy, they argue that with respect to such abortions the laws can no longer be justified by any state interest. There is some scholarly support for this view of original purpose. The few state courts called upon to interpret their laws in the late 19th and early 20th centuries did focus on the State's interest in protecting the woman's health rather than in preserving the embryo and fetus. . . .

The Constitution does not explicitly mention any right of privacy. In a line of decisions, however, going back perhaps as far as *Union Pacific R. Co. v. Botsford* (1891), the Court has recognized that a right of personal privacy, or a guarantee of certain areas or zones of privacy, does exist under the constitution. In varying contexts the Court or individual Justices have indeed found at least the roots of that right in the First Amendment, . . . in the Fourth and Fifth Amendments . . . in the penumbras of the Bill of Rights . . . in the

Ninth Amendment . . . or in the concept of liberty guaranteed by the first section of the Fourteenth Amendment. . . . These decisions make it clear that only personal rights that can be deemed "fundamental" or "implicit in the concept of ordered liberty," . . . are included in this guarantee of personal privacy. They also make it clear that the right has some extension to activities relating to marriage, . . . procreation, . . . contraception, . . . family relationships, . . . and child rearing and education. . . .

This right of privacy, whether it be founded in the Fourteenth Amendment's concept of personal liberty and restrictions upon state action, as we feel it is, or, as the District Court determined, in the Ninth Amendment's reservation of rights to the people, is broad enough to encompass a woman's decision whether or not to terminate her pregnancy. . . .

. . . [A]ppellants and some *amici* argue that the woman's right is absolute and that she is entitled to terminate her pregnancy at whatever time, in whatever way, and for whatever reason she alone chooses. With this we do not agree. Appellants' arguments that Texas either has no valid interest at all in regulating the abortion decision, or no interest strong enough to support any limitation upon the woman's sole determination, is unpersuasive. The Court's decisions recognizing a right of privacy also acknowledges that some state regulation in areas protected by that right is appropriate. As noted above, a state may properly assert important interests in safe guarding health, in maintaining medical standards, and in protecting potential life. At some point in pregnancy, these respective interests become sufficiently compelling to sustain regulation of the factors that govern the abortion decision. The privacy right involved, therefore, cannot be said to be absolute. . . .

We therefore conclude that the right of personal privacy includes the abortion decision, but that this right is not unqualified and must be considered against important state interests in regulation.

We note that those federal and state courts that have recently considered abortion law challenges have reached the same conclusion. . . .

Although the results are divided, most of these courts have agreed that the right of privacy, however based, is broad enough to cover the abortion decision; that the right, nonetheless, is not absolute and is subject to some limitations; and that at some point the state interests as to protection of health, medical standards, and prenatal life, become dominant. We agree with this approach. . . .

The appellee and certain *amici* argue that the fetus is a "person" within the language and meaning of the Fourteenth Amendment. In support of this they outline at length and in detail the well-known facts of fetal development. If this suggestion of personhood is established, the appellant's case, of course, collapses, for the fetus' right to life is then guaranteed specifically by the Amendment. The appellant conceded as much on reargument. On the other hand, the appellee conceded on reargument that no case could be cited that holds that a fetus is a person within the meaning of the Fourteenth Amendment. . . .

All this, together with our observation, *supra,* that throughout the major portion of the 19th century prevailing legal abortion practices were far freer than they are today, persuades us that the word "person," as used in the Fourteenth Amendment, does not include the unborn. . . . Indeed, our decision in *United States v. Vuitch* (1971) inferentially is to the same effect, for we there would not have indulged in statutory interpretation favorable to abortion in specified circumstances if the necessary consequence was the termination of life entitled to Fourteenth Amendment protection.

. . . As we have intimated above, it is reasonable and appropriate for a State to decide that at some point in time another interest, that of health of the mother or that of potential human life, becomes significantly involved. The woman's privacy is no longer sole and any right of privacy she possesses must be measured accordingly.

Texas urges that, apart from the Fourteenth Amendment, life begins at conception and is present throughout pregnancy, and that, therefore, the State has a compelling interest in protecting that life from and after conception. We need not resolve the difficult question of when life begins. When those trained in the respective disciplines of medicine, philosophy, and theology are unable to arrive at any consensus, the judiciary, at this point in the development of man's knowledge, is not in a position to speculate as to the answer.

It should be sufficient to note briefly the wide divergence of thinking on this most sensitive and difficult question. There has always been strong support for the view that life does not begin until live birth. This was the belief of the Stoics. It appears to be the predominant, though not the unanimous, attitude of the Jewish faith. It may be taken to represent also the position of a large segment of the Protestant community, insofar as that can be ascertained; organized groups that have taken a formal position on the abortion issue have generally regarded abortion as a matter for the conscience of the individual and her family. As we have noted, the common law found greater significance in quickening. Physicians and their scientific colleagues have regarded that event with less interest and have tended to focus either upon conception or upon live birth or upon the interim point at which the fetus becomes "viable," that is, potentially able to live outside the mother's womb, albeit with artificial aid. Viability is usually placed at about seven months (28 weeks) but may occur earlier, even at 24 weeks. . . .

In areas other than criminal abortion the law has been reluctant to endorse any theory that life, as we recognize it, begins before live birth or to accord legal rights to the unborn except in narrowly defined situations and except when the rights are contingent upon live birth. . . . In short, the unborn have never been recognized in the law as persons in the whole sense.

In view of all this, we do not agree that, by adopting one theory of life, Texas may override the rights of the pregnant woman that are at stake. We repeat, however, that the State does have an important and legitimate interest in preserving and protecting the health of the pregnant woman, whether she be a resident of the State or a nonresident who seeks medical consultation and treatment there, and that it has still *another* important and legitimate interest in protecting the potentiality of human life. These interests are separate and distinct. Each grows in substantiality as the woman approaches term and, at a point during pregnancy, each becomes "compelling."

With respect to the State's important and legitimate interest in the health of the mother, the "compelling" point, in the light of present medical knowledge, is at approximately the end of the first trimester. This is so because of the now established medical fact ... that until the end of the first trimester mortality in abortion is less than mortality in normal childbirth. It follows that, from and after this point, a State may regulate the abortion procedure to the extent that the regulation reasonably relates to the preservation and protection of maternal health. Examples of permissible state regulation in this area are requirements as to the qualifications of the person who is to perform the abortion; as to the licensure of that person; as to the facility in which the procedure is to be performed, that is, whether it must be a hospital or may be a clinic or some other place of less-than-hospital status; as to the licensing of the facility; and the like.

This means, on the other hand, that, for the period of pregnancy prior to this "compelling" point, the attending physician, in consultation with his patient, is free to determine, without regulation by the State, that in his medical judgment the patient's pregnancy should be terminated. If that decision is reached, the judgment may be effectuated by an abortion free of interference by the State.

With respect to the State's important and legitimate interest in potential life, the "compelling" point is at viability. This is so because the fetus then presumably has the capability of meaningful life outside the mother's womb. State regulation protective of fetal life after viability thus has both logical and biological justifications. If the State is interested in protecting fetal life after viability, it may go so far as to proscribe abortion during that period except when it is necessary to preserve the life or health of the mother. . . .

To summarize and repeat:

1. A state criminal abortion statue of the current Texas type, that excepts from criminality only a life-saving procedure on behalf of the mother, without regard to pregnancy stage and without recognition of the other interests involved, is violative of the Due Process Clause of the Fourteenth Amendment.

    a. For the stage prior to approximately the end of the first trimester, the abortion decision and its effectuation must be left to the medical judgment of the pregnant woman's attending physician.

    b. For the stage subsequent to approximately the end of the first trimester, the State, in promoting its interest in the health of the mother, may, if it chooses, regulate the abortion procedure in ways that are reasonably related to maternal health.

    c. For the stage subsequent to viability the State, in promoting its interest in the potentiality of human life, may, if it chooses, regulate, and even proscribe, abortion except where it is necessary, in appropriate medical judgment, for the preservation of the life or health of the mother.

2. The State may define the term "physician," as it has been employed [here], to mean only a physician currently licensed by the State, and may proscribe any abortion by a person who is not a physician as so defined.

. . . The decision leaves the State free to place increasing restrictions on abortion as the period of pregnancy lengthens, so long as those restrictions are tailored to the recognized state interests. The decision vindicates the right of the physician to administer medical treatment according to his professional judgment up to the points where important state interests provide compelling justifications for intervention. Up to those points the abortion decision in all its aspects is inherently, and primarily, a medical decision, and basic responsibility for it must rest with the physician. If an individual practitioner abuses the privilege of exercising proper medical judgment, the usual remedies, judicial and intraprofessional, are available. . . .

"PARTIAL-BIRTH ABORTION" AND THE SUPREME COURT

George J. Annas

Annas reviews and interprets the issues at stake in the case of *Stenberg v. Carhart*, a case decided by the U.S. Supreme Court in 2000. In *Stenberg,* the Court declared unconstitutional a Nebraska law banning "partial-birth abortion" except when necessary to save the life of a pregnant woman. Annas explains Justice Breyer's reasoning in the majority opinion and provides a brief survey of the various concurring and dissenting opinions. He then offers some concluding commentary on the state of constitutional law regarding abortion.

Abortion has long been, and remains, the most politicized medical procedure in the United States. It has been the subject of more state and federal legislation than all other medical procedures combined. The U.S. Supreme Court, which almost never hears cases about medical procedures, has regularly heard cases over the past 25 years concerning the constitutionality of various state laws designed to limit abortion. Thus, it was only a matter of time before the Court would hear a case on the constitutionality of laws restricting so-called partial-birth abortion.[1] When the Court heard a challenge to Nebraska's law, statutes relating to partial-birth abortion had been enacted in 30 states, and two bills banning such abortions had been passed by Congress. All the appeals courts except one, the Seventh Circuit Court of Appeals, had found these laws unconstitutional, and the opinion of that court rested on an extremely narrow interpretation of the law.[2]

The controversies surrounding partial-birth abortion are over how to describe the procedure and whether physicians ever need to use it to protect the health of a pregnant woman. The Supreme Court confronted these issues in the case of *Stenberg* v. *Carhart* last summer [2000].[3]

THE NEBRASKA PARTIAL-BIRTH ABORTION LAW

The Nebraska law provides that "no partial birth abortion shall be performed in this state, unless such procedure is necessary to save the life of the mother

whose life is endangered by a physical disorder, physical illness, or physical injury, including a life-endangering physical condition caused by or arising from the pregnancy itself."[4] Like the federal acts twice passed by Congress and vetoed by President Bill Clinton, the Nebraska law defined partial-birth abortion as "an abortion in which the person performing the abortion partially delivers vaginally a living unborn child before killing the unborn child and completing the delivery." The law further defines the phrase "partially delivers vaginally a living unborn child before killing the unborn child" to mean "deliberately and intentionally delivering into the vagina a living unborn child, or a substantial portion thereof, for the purpose of performing a procedure that the person performing such procedure knows will kill the unborn child and does kill the unborn child."[4] Violation of the law is a felony that carries a prison term of up to 20 years, a fine of up to $25,000, and automatic revocation of a medical license.

Dr. Leroy Carhart, a Nebraska physician who performs abortions, sued in federal court to have the law declared unconstitutional. U.S. District Court judge Richard G. Kopf reviewed abortion procedures in detail, using a drawing of female pelvic anatomy as an attachment to his opinion, before holding that the statute was unconstitutional because it endangered women's lives and health and was void for vagueness because physicians could not know what conduct it proscribed.[5] The Court of Appeals for the Eighth Circuit affirmed the District Court ruling.[6] By a five-to-four vote, the Supreme Court ruled on June 28, 2000, that the Nebraska law and all other laws banning partial-birth abortion are unconstitutional.

THE MAJORITY DECISION

The opinion of the Court was written by Justice Stephen Breyer, one of only two current justices (the other is Ruth Bader Ginsburg) who had not previously expressed an opinion in a major decision about abortion. The opinion is best understood as a direct application to the Nebraska law of the principles articulated in the 1973 decision in *Roe* v. *Wade*[7] and the 1992 decision in *Planned Parenthood of Southeastern Pennsylvania* v. *Casey*.[8] In *Roe* the Court held that because a woman's right to privacy is "fundamental," states must demonstrate a "compelling interest" in order to restrict abortion, and they are unable to demonstrate such an interest before the time when the fetus becomes viable. Moreover, *Roe* made it clear that the state could not favor the life of the fetus over the life or health of the pregnant woman. The Court in *Casey* affirmed the core holding of *Roe,* that states cannot outlaw abortion before the time of fetal viability and can do so thereafter only if the woman's life and health are protected. States were permitted, however, to regulate abortions so long as any restriction did not impose an "undue burden" on the pregnant woman's liberty interest in terminating her pregnancy.

The Nebraska ban applies throughout pregnancy and has no exception to preserve a woman's health. Under *Roe* and *Casey,* the state of Nebraska had to demonstrate that the state had at least a legitimate interest in outlawing partial-birth abortions and that doing so would not place an undue burden on women. Because it is a criminal statute, the legislature had to be very clear about what exactly the statute prohibited. In order to determine exactly what was and was not prohibited, Justice Breyer, like the trial court judge, devoted nearly the entirety of his opinion to describing various abortion procedures and comparing them with the language of the Nebraska law.

HOW ABORTIONS ARE PERFORMED

Justice Breyer introduced his descriptions of abortion procedures by stating that they may seem "clinically cold or callous to some, perhaps horrifying to others," but that he saw no other way "to acquaint the reader with the technical distinctions among different abortion methods and related factual matters, upon which the outcome of this case depends." Breyer noted, among other facts, that 90 percent of abortions in the United States are performed before 12 weeks of gestation, and almost all the rest are performed between 12 and 24 weeks. Almost all second-trimester abortions are performed by means of dilation and evacuation, with variations depending on the stage of gestation. Breyer quoted a report from the American Medical Association (AMA) as saying that at 13 to 15 weeks of gestation, "D&E [dilation and evacuation] is similar to vacuum aspiration except that the cervix must be dilated more widely because surgical instruments are used to remove larger pieces of tissue." After 15 weeks, the AMA report continues, because of the increased size of the fetus and the rigidity of its bones, "dismemberment or other destructive procedures are more likely to be required . . . to remove fetal and placental tissue." And after 20 weeks, "some physicians use intrafetal potassium chloride or digoxin to induce fetal demise . . . to facilitate evacuation."[3]

Breyer then made a series of observations and factual conclusions that determined the outcome of the case. He found, first, that the various dilation-and-evacuation procedures have in common the dilation of the cervix, the removal of at least some fetal tissue with the use of surgical instruments, and (after the 15th week) the potential need for dismemberment of the fetus. When dismemberment does occur, it typically occurs "as the doctor pulls a portion of the fetus through the cervix into the birth canal." Breyer noted that a variation of dilation and evacuation, which the physicians who testified at the trial referred to as "intact D&E" or dilation and extraction, is used at 16 weeks at the earliest, when vacuum aspiration is ineffective and the fetal skull is too large to pass through the cervix. Dilation and extraction may proceed in two ways: if the fetus presents head first, the physician collapses the skull and then extracts the intact fetus through the cervix; if there is a breech presentation, the physician pulls the fetal body through the cervix, then collapses the skull, and then extracts the fetus.[3]

On the basis of information from medical textbooks and the position taken by the American College of Obstetricians and Gynecologists,[9] Breyer concluded that "intact D&E and D&X [dilation and extraction] are sufficiently similar for us [the Court] to use the terms interchangeably." There are no accurate statistics available on the number of dilation-and-extraction abortions performed in the United States, and Breyer cited estimates ranging from 640 to 5000 cases per year. He found that such abortions are performed for a variety of reasons, including reducing the danger caused by the passage of sharp bone fragments through the cervix, minimizing the number of surgical instruments used (and thereby decreasing the likelihood of uterine perforation), reducing the likelihood of infection, and helping to ensure the removal of all fetal tissue. Dilation and extraction is also the preferred method for fetuses with hydrocephaly and anomalies incompatible with fetal survival.[3]

All this was much more detail about a medical procedure than had ever appeared before in a Supreme Court opinion. The factual conclusions, however, were necessary to answering the two major constitutional questions posed by Nebraska's ban: Must a law prohibiting the use of a medical procedure for abortion contain an exception to protect the health of the pregnant woman as defined in *Roe?* And does the Nebraska law "unduly burden" a woman's right to choose to terminate her pregnancy as defined in *Casey?* Justice Breyer's answer to both of these questions was yes.

WOMEN'S HEALTH

Justice Breyer recited the rule, as stated in *Roe* v. *Wade,* that a state may outlaw abortion after the fetus is viable in order to promote its interest in protecting potential human life, "except where it is necessary, in appropriate medical judgment, for the preservation of the life or health of the mother." Breyer logically concluded that if *Roe* requires an exception for the mother's health after fetal viability, it must require one before viability, when the state has less of an interest in protecting fetal life.

Would the ban in fact adversely affect the health of pregnant women who want to terminate their pregnancies? Breyer concluded that it would, on the basis of the belief of "significant medical authority" that "in some circumstances, D&X would be the

safest procedure." Breyer found especially persuasive the brief to the Court in which the American College of Obstetricians and Gynecologists stated specifically that dilation and extraction "may be the best or most appropriate procedure in a particular circumstance to save the life or preserve the health of a woman."[3,9] Nebraska relied on a contrary statement of the AMA that "there does not appear to be any identified situation in which intact D&X is the only appropriate procedure to induce abortion."[3]

Breyer rejected the argument that the word "necessary," as used in the opinion *Planned Parenthood* v. *Casey*—"necessary, in appropriate medical judgment, for the preservation of the life or health of the mother"[8]—means an "absolute necessity" or requires "absolute proof." He concluded that the words "'appropriate medical judgment' must embody the judicial need to tolerate responsible differences of medical opinion." Breyer, who has special expertise in administrative law and risk assessment, went on to say that "the division of medical opinion about the matter at most means uncertainty, a factor that signals the presence of risk, not its absence." He concluded that "where substantial medical authority supports the proposition that banning a particular abortion procedure could endanger women's health, *Casey* requires the statute to include a health exception when the procedure is 'necessary, in appropriate medical judgment, for the preservation of the life or health of the mother.'"[3]

DISTINGUISHING BETWEEN DILATION AND EXTRACTION AND DILATION AND EVACUATION

The second constitutional issue was whether the statute imposed an "undue burden" on a woman's liberty to terminate her pregnancy before the fetus was viable. The answer to this question depended on whether the statute was precisely written so as to apply only to the rare dilation-and-extraction procedures and not to the more routine dilation-and-evacuation procedures as well. On the basis of the statute's descriptions of the procedure, Breyer concluded that its language "does not track the medical differences between D&E and D&X."

Breyer stated that it would have been a simple matter for the state legislature to provide an exception for dilation-and-evacuation procedures, but given the medical material he quoted in his opinion, it is difficult to see how this could be effectively done. The attorney general of Nebraska, for example, argued unpersuasively that the two procedures were actually distinguished by the words "substantial portion" of the fetus, which the attorney general interpreted as meaning "the child up to the head" and thus not including "a fetal arm or leg or anything less than the entire fetal body." Because of the vagueness of the statute, Justice Breyer concluded that the statute threatened physicians who would otherwise perform dilation-and-evacuation procedures, but who would not now perform them because they would "fear prosecution, conviction, and imprisonment." This results in placing "an undue burden on a woman's right to make an abortion decision."

THE CONCURRING OPINIONS

Justices John Paul Stevens, Sandra Day O'Connor, and Ruth Bader Ginsburg each wrote brief concurring opinions. Stevens emphasized that the extent of the rhetoric surrounding abortion often obscures the fact that, during the past 27 years, the core holding of *Roe* v. *Wade* "has been endorsed by all but 4 of the 17 justices who have addressed the issue." He also argued (persuasively, I think) that "the notion that either of these two equally gruesome procedures [dilation and extraction and dilation and evacuation after 15 weeks] performed at this late stage of gestation is more akin to infanticide than the other, or that the State furthers any legitimate interest by banning one but not the other, is simply irrational." Justice O'Connor agreed with Breyer but added that she thought "a ban on partial-birth abortion that only proscribed the D&X method of abortion and that included an exception to preserve the life and health of the mother would be constitutional." Justice Ginsburg emphasized that the Nebraska law would "not save any fetus from destruction" nor "protect the lives or health of pregnant women" and that therefore the state had no legitimate interest in enacting it.[3] She also cited Chief Judge Richard Posner, who had made this point in an extremely cogent dissent to the opinion of the Seventh Circuit Court. "These statutes," wrote Posner, "are not concerned with saving fetuses . . . [or] with protecting the health of

women. . . . They are concerned with making a statement in an ongoing war for public opinion. . . . The statement is that fetal life is more important than women's health."[2]

THE DISSENTING OPINIONS

There are four dissenting opinions, the two major ones written by Justices Anthony Kennedy and Clarence Thomas; Chief Justice William Rehnquist joined both of them, and Justice Antonin Scalia joined the Thomas dissent. Justice Kennedy objected to the majority's use of medical textbooks and terminology to describe abortion procedures, arguing that this technical language "views the procedures from the perspective of the abortionist, rather than from the perspective of a society shocked when confronted with a new method of ending human life . . . [and] may obscure matters for persons not trained in medical terminology." He did not refer to physicians as physicians, instead calling them "abortionists," and proceeded to describe the dilation-and-extraction procedure in lay terms. His version included such descriptions as the following: "with only the head of the fetus remaining in utero, the abortionist tears open the skull [using] . . . a pair of scissors."[3] Kennedy concluded that permitting an exception to preserve the health of the woman would be the equivalent of forbidding Nebraska to ban partial-birth abortion. In his words "A ban which depends on 'the appropriate medical judgment' of Dr. Carhart is no ban at all."[3]

Kennedy's central argument was that under *Casey,* states "have an interest in forbidding medical procedures which, in the State's reasonable determination, might cause the medical profession or society as a whole to become insensitive, even disdainful, to life, including life in the human fetus." But this argument could apply to all abortions, and it is not, in fact, what *Casey* held. Moreover, he argued that it is irrelevant that the majority of the justices cannot see the difference between dilation and evacuation and dilation and extraction. "The issue is not whether members of the judiciary can see a difference between the two procedures," Kennedy wrote. "It is whether Nebraska can." Regardless of whether physicians can distinguish between legal and illegal medical procedures, Kennedy argued that the state of Nebraska has a "right to declare a moral difference" between two medical procedures.

Kennedy also believes that there is a real difference, arguing, for instance, that "D&X perverts the natural birth process to a greater degree than D&E, commandeering the live birth process until the skull is pierced;" that the fetus is "killed outside of the womb;" and that dilation and extraction bears a "stronger resemblance to infanticide." Finding that the state has a legitimate interest in outlawing this abortion procedure, Kennedy then argued that the Court has no medical expertise sufficient to second-guess the Nebraska legislature on its determination that abortion by dilation and extraction is no safer than other methods of abortion and is therefore never medically necessary. In this view, outlawing dilation-and-extraction abortions (which Kennedy believes are the only type affected by the statute) would deprive no woman of access to a safe abortion, and thus cannot, under the terms set forth by *Casey,* place an undue burden on the pregnant woman.

Justice Thomas, like Kennedy, was upset by Breyer's "sanitized" medical descriptions, noting that since *Roe,* "this Court has never described the various methods of aborting a second- or third-trimester fetus." Thomas also argued that the statute's plain language can and should be interpreted as including only abortions by dilation and extraction, and not by dilation and evacuation. To the argument that "partial-birth abortion" is not a medical term, he replied simply and accurately, "There is, of course, no requirement that a legislature use terminology accepted by the medical community." Thomas disagreed that the state cannot second-guess physicians who believe use of a particular abortion method is necessary to preserve a woman's health. He argued that the majority opinion "eviscerates *Casey's* undue burden standard and imposes unfettered abortion on demand." In his view, the resolution of differences among physicians regarding the safety of abortion procedures should be left to the state legislatures.[3] The dissenters, in short, do not believe that physicians can be trusted to make good-faith decisions about the health of their patients.

CONSTITUTIONAL LAW AFTER *STENBERG*

The majority opinion in *Stenberg* demonstrates that five justices take *Roe* v. *Wade* and *Casey* seriously. By applying the basic principles of these decisions, the majority found the Nebraska statute unconstitutional for the following reasons: because it would place an undue burden on a woman's right to choose an abortion, as such a burden is defined in *Casey;* because it is so vague, in that it might be interpreted as applying to dilation and evacuation and might thus intimidate physicians, who might therefore not perform them; and because the statute provided no exception for protecting the health of the woman, as required by *Roe.* Thus, in this opinion, five justices strongly reaffirmed *Roe* and *Casey.*

The somewhat surprising vote, and the one that has caused pro-choice commentators the most concern, was that of Justice Kennedy, one of the three justices who wrote the joint opinion in *Casey* (the others are Sandra Day O'Connor and David Souter).[8,10] Kennedy stated that the Nebraska law did not impose an undue burden on women as defined by *Casey,* whereas O'Connor and Souter found that it did. Does this mean that Kennedy might change his mind about the *Casey* decision and vote to overrule it along with *Roe* v. *Wade* at some future time? No one can say for sure. But I do not believe that such a conclusion can be drawn from this case. In *Stenberg,* because five justices upheld *Roe* and *Casey,* Kennedy could express his own moral outrage at partial-birth abortion—and support Nebraska's right to express its moral outrage—without having his personal views change the outcome of the case or the constitutional status of either *Roe* or *Casey.*

The result in *Stenberg* was determined by *Roe* and *Casey.* Justice O'Connor may be correct in noting that it would be possible to craft a statute that meets constitutional requirements. But given the medical facts, such a statute would probably not apply to any patient in the real world. In my view, there is little likelihood that redrafted statutes will be the centerpiece of antiabortion activity at the state or federal level after this opinion. On the other hand, antiabortion forces will most likely renew their efforts to change the composition of the Court by lobbying for the appointment of justices with strong antiabortion stances.

Physicians should take comfort from the Court's strong protection of the application of medical judgment. In this regard, the opinion can be seen as reflecting *Roe* v. *Wade*'s strong endorsement of the privacy of the physician-patient relationship and the right of women and their physicians to make decisions about abortion.[11] The opinion reflects this endorsement by focusing much more attention on physicians and the medical techniques they use than it does on women and their lives and liberty. This focus was necessary because the statute under review aimed to restrict medical practice. *Casey,* on the other hand, dealt with restrictions of women's autonomy and therefore centered more on women, whose constitutional rights were directly at stake. The opinion's emphasis on physicians may also explain why Dr. Carhart entitled his presentation last October to an audience of Harvard medical students "Partial-Birth Abortion, the Supreme Court, and Physician Autonomy," as well as why he personally remains a target of antiabortion forces.[12]

MEDICINE AND ABORTION

A deeper discussion of the availability of safe abortions to protect women's lives and liberty may be too much to ask of the Supreme Court. Maybe, in the debate over abortion, we are all past the point at which facts and logic matter. As the decision in *Stenberg* underlines, the law can determine whether abortions

are permitted, but only physicians—with their patients—can determine how they may be performed safely. Ultimately, the central question regarding abortion remains who should make the decision: the state or women and their physicians together. The answer of the Supreme Court, as articulated in *Roe* v. *Wade* and its companion case, *Doe* v. *Bolton,*[13] and now strongly reinforced in *Stenberg,* is that the decision belongs to the woman and her physician together. In this respect, the Court has been remarkably consistent in all the abortion cases it has heard.

REFERENCES

1 Annas G. J. Partial-birth abortion, Congress, and the Constitution. N Engl J Med 1998; 339:279–83.
2 *The Hope Clinic v. Ryan,* 195 F.3d 857 (7th Cir. 1999) (Posner J, dissenting).
3 *Stenberg v. Carhart,* 530 U.S. 914 (2000).
4 Neb. Rev. Stat. Ann. sec. 28–328(1) (Supp. 1999).
5 *Carhart v. Stenberg,* 11 F. Supp.2d 1099 (Neb. 1998).
6 *Stenberg v. Carhart,* 192 F.3d 1142 (1999).
7 *Roe v. Wade,* 410 U.S. 113 (1973).
8 *Planned Parenthood of Southeastern Pennsylvania v. Casey,* 502 U.S. 1056 (1992).
9 Brief for American College of Obstetricians and Gynecologists et al. as Amici Curiae, 21–22.
10 Annas G. J. The Supreme Court, liberty, and abortion. N Engl J. Med 1992; 327:651–4.
11 Annas G. J., Glantz LH, Mariner WK. The right of privacy protects the doctor-patient relationship. JAMA 1990; 263:858–61.
12 Belluck P. After abortion victory, doctor's troubles persist. New York Times. November 7, 2000:A18.
13 *Doe v. Bolton,* 410 U.S. 179 (1973).

RESEARCH ON EMBRYONIC STEM CELLS

STEM CELLS: A PRIMER
National Institutes of Health

This NIH document is designed to provide a basic understanding of stem cells and their prospective therapeutic uses. So-called *pluripotent* stem cells can be derived either from fetal tissue or from human embryos at the blastocyst stage. (When pluripotent stem cells are derived from human embryos, they are commonly called *embryonic stem cells.*) Pluripotent stem cells seem to have great therapeutic potential, but significant technological problems must be overcome for this potential to be realized. Adult stem cells also seem to have significant therapeutic potential, but there is reason to believe that their therapeutic potential is more limited than that of pluripotent stem cells.

This primer presents background information on stem cells. It includes an explanation of what stem cells are; what pluripotent stem cells are; how pluripotent stem cells are derived; why pluripotent stem cells are important to science; why they hold such great promise for advances in health care; and what adult stem cells are.

Recent published reports on the isolation and successful culturing of the first human pluripotent stem cell lines have generated great excitement and have brought biomedical research to the edge of a new frontier. The development of these human pluripotent stem cell lines deserves close scientific examination, evaluation of the promise for new therapies, and prevention strategies, and open discussion of the ethical issues.

In order to understand the importance of this discovery as well as the related scientific, medical, and ethical issues, it is absolutely essential to first clarify the terms and definitions.

DEFINITIONS

DNA—abbreviation for deoxyribonucleic acid which makes up genes.
Gene—a functional unit of heredity which is a segment of DNA located in a specific site on a chromosome. A gene directs the formation of an enzyme or other protein.
Somatic cell—cell of the body other than egg or sperm.
Somatic cell nuclear transfer—the transfer of a cell nucleus from a somatic cell into an egg from which the nucleus has been removed.
Stem cells—cells that have the ability to divide for indefinite periods in culture and to give rise to specialized cells.
Pluripotent—capable of giving rise to most tissues of an organism.
Totipotent—having unlimited capability. Totipotent cells have the capacity to specialize into extraembryonic membranes and tissues, the embryo, and all postembryonic tissues and organs.

National Institutes of Health, May 2000.

WHAT IS A STEM CELL?

Stem cells have the ability to divide for indefinite periods in culture and to give rise to specialized cells. They are best described in the context of normal human development. Human development begins when a sperm fertilizes an egg and creates a single cell that has the potential to form an entire organism. This fertilized egg is *totipotent,* meaning that its potential is total. In the first hours after fertilization, this cell divides into identical totipotent cells. This means that either one of these cells, if placed into a woman's uterus, has the potential to develop into a fetus. In fact, identical twins develop when two totipotent cells separate and develop into two individual, genetically identical human beings. Approximately four days after fertilization and after several cycles of cell division, these totipotent cells begin to specialize, forming a hollow sphere of cells, called a blastocyst. The blastocyst has an outer layer of cells and inside the hollow sphere, there is a cluster of cells called the inner cell mass.

The outer layer of cells will go on to form the placenta and other supporting tissues needed for fetal development in the uterus. The inner cell mass cells will go on to form virtually all of the tissues of the human body. Although the inner cell mass cells can form virtually every type of cell found in the human body, they cannot form an organism because they are unable to give rise to the placenta and supporting tissues necessary for development in the human uterus. These inner cell mass cells are *pluripotent*—they can give rise to many types of cells but not all types of cells necessary for fetal development. Because their potential is not total, they are not totipotent and they are not embryos. In fact, if an inner cell mass cell were placed into a woman's uterus, it would not develop into a fetus.

The pluripotent stem cells undergo further specialization into stem cells that are committed to give rise to cells that have a particular function. Examples of this include blood stem cells which give rise to red blood cells, white blood cells, and platelets; and skin stem cells that give rise to the various types of skin cells. These more specialized stem cells are called *multipotent*.

While stem cells are extraordinarily important in early human development, multipotent stem cells are also found in children and adults. For example, consider one of the best understood stem cells, the blood stem cell. Blood stem cells reside in the bone marrow of every child and adult, and in fact, they can be found in very small numbers circulating in the blood stream. Blood stem cells perform the critical role of continually replenishing our supply of blood cells—red blood cells, white blood cells, and platelets—throughout life. A person cannot survive without blood stem cells.

HOW ARE PLURIPOTENT STEM CELLS DERIVED?

At present, human pluripotent cell lines have been developed from two sources[1] with methods previously developed in work with animal models.

(1) In the work done by Dr. [James] Thomson, pluripotent stem cells were isolated directly from the inner cell mass of human embryos at the blastocyst stage. Dr. Thomson received embryos from IVF (In Vitro Fertilization) clinics—these embryos were in excess of the clinical need for infertility treatment. The embryos were made for purposes of reproduction, not research. Informed consent was obtained from the donor couples. Dr. Thomson isolated the inner cell mass and cultured these cells producing a pluripotent stem cell line.

(2) In contrast, Dr. [John] Gearhart isolated pluripotent stem cells from fetal tissue obtained from terminated pregnancies. Informed consent was obtained from the donors after they had independently made the decision to terminate their pregnancy. Dr. Gearhart took cells from the region of the fetus that was destined to develop into the testes or the ovaries. Although the cells developed in Dr. Gearhart's lab and Dr. Thomson's lab were derived from different sources, they appear to be very similar.

The use of somatic cell nuclear transfer (SCNT) may be another way that pluripotent stem cells could be isolated. In studies with animals using SCNT, researchers take a normal animal egg cell and remove the nucleus (cell structure containing the chromosomes). The material left behind in the egg cell contains nutrients and other energy-producing materials that are essential for embryo development. Then, using carefully worked out laboratory conditions, a somatic cell—any cell other than an egg or a sperm cell—is placed next to the egg from which the nucleus had been removed, and the two are fused. The resulting fused cell, and its immediate descendants, are believed to have the full potential to develop into an entire animal, and hence are totipotent. As described these totipotent cells will soon form a blastocyst. Cells from the inner cell mass of this blastocyst could, in theory, be used to develop pluripotent stem cell lines. Indeed, any method by which a human blastocyst is formed could potentially serve as a source of human pluripotent stem cells.

POTENTIAL APPLICATIONS OF PLURIPOTENT STEM CELLS

There are several important reasons why the isolation of human pluripotent stem cells is important to science and to advances in health care. At the most fundamental level, pluripotent stem cells could help us to understand the complex events that occur during human development. A primary goal of this work would be the identification of the factors involved in the cellular decision-making process that results in cell specialization. We know that turning genes on and off is central to this process, but we do not know much about these "decision-making" genes or what turns them on or off. Some of our most serious medical conditions, such as cancer and birth defects, are due to abnormal cell specialization and cell division. A better understanding of normal cell processes will allow us to further delineate the fundamental errors that cause these often deadly illnesses.

Human pluripotent stem cell research could also dramatically change the way we develop drugs and test them for safety. For example, new medications could be initially tested using human cell lines. Cell lines are currently used in this way (for example, cancer cells). Pluripotent stem cells would allow testing in more cell types. This would not replace testing in whole animals and testing in human beings, but it would streamline the process of drug development. Only the drugs that are both safe and appear to have a beneficial effect in cell line testing would graduate to further testing in laboratory animals and human subjects.

Perhaps the most far-reaching potential application of human pluripotent stem cells is the generation of cells and tissue that could be used for so-called cell therapies. Many diseases and disorders result from disruption of cellular function or destruction of tissues of the body. Today, donated organs and tissues are often used to replace ailing or destroyed tissue. Unfortunately, the number of people suffering from these disorders far outstrips the number of organs available for transplantation. Pluripotent stem cells, stimulated to develop into specialized cells, offer the possibility of a renewable source of replacement cells and tissue to treat a myriad of diseases, conditions, and disabilities including Parkinson's and Alzheimer's diseases, spinal cord injury, stroke, burns, heart disease, diabetes, osteoarthritis, and rheumatoid arthritis. There is almost no realm of medicine that might not be touched by this innovation. Some details of two of these examples follow.

- Transplant of healthy heart muscle cells could provide new hope for patients with chronic heart disease whose hearts can no longer pump adequately. The hope is to develop heart muscle cells from human pluripotent stem cells and transplant them into the failing heart muscle in order to augment the function of the failing heart. Preliminary work in mice and other animals has demonstrated that healthy heart muscle cells transplanted into the heart successfully repopulate the heart tissue and work together with the host cells. These experiments show that this type of transplantation is feasible.
- In the many individuals who suffer from Type I diabetes, the production of insulin by specialized pancreatic cells, called islet cells, is disrupted. There is evidence that transplantation of either the entire pancreas or isolated islet cells could mitigate the need for insulin injections. Islet cell lines

derived from human pluripotent stem cells could be used for diabetes research and, ultimately, for transplantation.

While this research shows extraordinary promise, there is much to be done before we can realize these innovations. Technological challenges remain before these discoveries can be incorporated into clinical practice. These challenges, though significant, are not insurmountable.

First, we must do the basic research to understand the cellular events that lead to cell specialization in the human, so that we can direct these pluripotent stem cells to become the type(s) of tissue needed for transplantation.

Second, before we can use these cells for transplantation, we must overcome the well-known problem of immune rejection. Because human pluripotent stem cells derived from embryos or fetal tissue would be genetically different from the recipient, future research would need to focus on modifying human pluripotent stem cells to minimize tissue incompatibility or to create tissue banks with the most common tissue-type profiles.

The use of somatic cell nuclear transfer (SCNT) would be another way to overcome the problem of tissue incompatibility for some patients. For example, consider a person with progressive heart failure. Using SCNT, the nucleus of virtually any somatic cell from that patient could be fused with a donor egg cell from which the nucleus had been removed. With proper stimulation the cell would develop into a blastocyst: cells from the inner cell mass could be taken to create a culture of pluripotent cells. These cells could then be stimulated to develop into heart muscle cells. Because the vast majority of genetic information is contained in the nucleus, these cells would be essentially identical genetically to the person with the failing heart. When these heart muscle cells were transplanted back into the patient, there would likely be no rejection and no need to expose the patient to immune-suppressing drugs, which can have toxic effects.

ADULT STEM CELLS

As noted earlier, multipotent stem cells can be found in some types of adult tissue. In fact, stem cells are needed to replenish the supply cells in our body that normally wear out. An example, which was mentioned previously, is the blood stem cell.

Multipotent stem cells have not been found for all types of adult tissue, but discoveries in this area of research are increasing. For example, until recently, it was thought that stem cells were not present in the adult nervous system, but, in recent years, neuronal stem cells have been isolated from the rat and mouse nervous systems. The experience in humans is more limited. In humans, neuronal stem cells have been isolated from fetal tissue and a kind of cell that may be a neuronal stem cell has been isolated from adult brain tissue that was surgically removed for the treatment of epilepsy.

Do Adult Stem Cells Have the Same Potential as Pluripotent Stem Cells? Until recently, there was little evidence in mammals that multipotent cells such as blood stem cells could change course and produce skin cells, liver cells or any cell other than a blood stem cell or a specific type of blood cell; however, research in animals is leading scientists to question this view.

In animals, it has been shown that some adult stem cells previously thought to be committed to the development of one line of specialized cells are able to develop into other types of specialized cells. For example, recent experiments in mice suggest that when neural stem cells were placed into the bone marrow, they appeared to produce a variety of blood cell types. In addition, studies with rats have indicated that stem cells found in the bone marrow were able to produce liver cells. These exciting findings suggest that even after a stem cell has begun to specialize, the stem cell may, under certain conditions, be more flexible than first thought. At this time, demonstration of the flexibility of adult stem cells has been only observed in animals and limited to a few tissue types.

Why Not Just Pursue Research with Adult Stem Cells? Research on human adult stem cells suggests that these multipotent cells have great potential for use in both research and in the development of cell therapies. For example, there would be many advantages to using adult stem cells for transplantation. If we could isolate the adult stem cells from a patient,

coax them to divide and direct their specialization and then transplant them back into the patient, it is unlikely that such cells would be rejected. The use of adult stem cells for such cell therapies would certainly reduce or even avoid the practice of using stem cells that were derived from human embryos or human fetal tissue, sources that trouble many people on ethical grounds.

While adult stem cells hold real promise, there are some significant limitations to what we may or may not be able to accomplish with them. First of all, stem cells from adults have not been isolated for all tissues of the body. Although many different kinds of multipotent stem cells have been identified, adult stem cells for all cell and tissue types have not yet been found in the adult human. For example, we have not located adult cardiac stem cells or adult pancreatic islet stem cells in humans.

Second, adult stem cells are often present in only minute quantities, are difficult to isolate and purify, and their numbers may decrease with age. For example, brain cells from adults that may be neuronal stem cells have only been obtained by removing a portion of the brain of epileptics, not a trivial procedure.

Any attempt to use stem cells from a patient's own body for treatment would require that stem cells would first have to be isolated from the patient and then grown in culture in sufficient numbers to obtain adequate quantities for treatment. For some acute disorders, there may not be enough time to grow enough cells to use for treatment. In other disorders, caused by a genetic defect, the genetic error would likely be present in the patient's stem cells. Cells from such a patient may not be appropriate for transplantation. There is evidence that stem cells from adults may not have the same capacity to proliferate as younger cells do. In addition, adult stem cells may contain more DNA abnormalities, caused by exposure to daily living, including sunlight, toxins, and by expected errors made in DNA replication during the course of a lifetime. These potential weaknesses could limit the usefulness of adult stem cells.

Research on the early stages of cell specialization may not be possible with adult stem cells since they appear to be farther along the specialization pathway than pluripotent stem cells. In addition, one adult stem cell line may be able to form several, perhaps 3 or 4, tissue types, but there is no clear evidence that stem cells from adults, human or animal, are pluripotent. In fact, there is no evidence that adult stem cells have the broad potential characteristic of pluripotent stem cells. In order to determine the very best source of many of the specialized cells and tissues of the body for new treatments and even cures, it will be vitally important to study the developmental potential of adult stem cells and compare it to that of pluripotent stem cells.

SUMMARY

Given the enormous promise of stem cells to the development of new therapies for the most devastating diseases, it is important to simultaneously pursue all lines of research. Science and scientists need to search for the very best sources of these cells. When they are identified, regardless of their sources, researchers will use them to pursue the development of new cell therapies.

The development of stem cell lines, both pluripotent and multipotent, that may produce many tissues of the human body is an important scientific breakthrough. It is not too unrealistic to say that this research has the potential to revolutionize the practice of medicine and improve the quality and length of life.

NOTE

1 Michael Shamblott et al., "Derivation of Pluripotent Stem Cells from Cultured Human Primordial Germ Cells," *Proceedings of the National Academy of Sciences USA* 95 (1998): 13726–31; James Thomson et al., "Embryonic Stem Cell Lines Derived from Human Blastocysts," *Science* 282 (1998): 1145–47.

WHAT DOES "RESPECT FOR EMBRYOS" MEAN IN THE CONTEXT OF STEM CELL RESEARCH?
Bonnie Steinbock

Steinbock argues that research on embryonic stem cells is entirely compatible with respect for embryos. She rejects the view that research on adult stem cells should be aggressively pursued prior to conducting any research on embryonic stem cells. Distinguishing between respect for embryos and respect for persons, she argues that respect for embryos entails only that embryos not be used in unimportant or frivolous ways. Steinbock also argues that the use of embryos created by in vitro fertilization (IVF) solely for research purposes is as morally permissible as the use of "spare" embryos (i.e., those left over from IVF reproductive procedures).

Like abortion, embryo research polarizes those who believe that embryos have as much of a right to life as any born human being, and those who maintain that embryos are not the kinds of entities that can have rights, because rights are restricted either to persons or to sentient beings.[1] However, those who deny that embryos can be possessors of rights need not strip them of moral significance altogether. There is a "third alternative," which is that although human embryos do not have full moral status, or human moral status, they are a form of human life and, as such, deserving of respect. This is the view that virtually every commission considering the issue has taken, including the Human Embryo Research Panel of the National Institutes of Health (NIH)[2] and the Warnock Committee[3] in Great Britain. But what does "respect for embryos" mean? Is this simply an empty phrase, solemnly invoked by national commissions to soften or conceal the fact that they are endorsing killing embryos?

Reprinted with permission from *Women's Health Issues*, vol. 10, no. 3 (May/June 2000), pp. 127–130. Copyright © 2000 Jacobs Institute of Women's Health.

This was charged by Daniel Callahan,[4] who took the NIH Human Embryo Research Panel to task for failing to demonstrate (as opposed to merely asserting) that progress in scientific research depends on using human embryos. Callahan's point is not that respect for embryos entails that they never be destroyed or used in research. Rather, it is that the interests or goals to be accomplished by using human embryos in research must be shown to be compelling, and unreachable by other means. If less than compelling purposes can justify the destruction of embryos, or if compelling goals could be reached without destroying embryos, the idea that embryos are due profound respect rings hollow.

A similar view regarding embryonic stem (ES) cell research was expressed by Richard M. Doerflinger.[5] He cited advances in isolating and culturing adult stem (AS) cells and suggested that AS cells might be more clinically useful than embryonic cells because treatments based on a patient's own cells would avoid problems of tissue rejection[5]:

> No one can say with certainty at this time whether embryonic stem cells will have any clinical use that cannot equally well be addressed by other means. . . . At a minimum, an ethic that demands serious respect for human embryonic life will also demand that other, morally accepted alternatives be explored first. (p. 144)

The suggestion that other alternatives should be explored first makes sense only if there is some reason to believe that these alternatives are likely to yield comparable results. As a nonscientist, I cannot evaluate the research cited by Doerflinger. A recent article in *Science*[6] says, "Scientists are now speeding ahead with work on adult stem cells, hoping to discover whether their promise will rival that of embryonic stem (ES) cells." If that is so, it is possible that it will not be necessary to use ES cells for therapeutic purposes. At the same time, no one can accuse the National Bioethics Advisory Commission of simply assuming that there will be scientific benefits from embryonic stem cell research, or ignoring the possibility that AS could be used instead of ES cells. Its report, *Ethical Issues in Human Stem Cell Research,*[7] examines at great length the scientific evidence, and the possibility that AS cells can replace embryonic cells. It concludes that this is unlikely because ES cells have a property that AS cells do not: the ability to differentiate into all cell types. The report states[7]:

> . . . although much promising research currently is being conducted with stem cells obtained from adult organisms, studies in animals suggest that this approach will be scientifically and technically limited. . . . Moreover, because important biological differences exist between embryonic and adult stem cells, this source of stem cells should not be considered an alternative to ES and EG [embryonic germ] cell research. (p. ii)

This raises the intriguing question of how promising evidence for the utility of AS cells must be to pursue that line of research while delaying research using ES cells, out of respect for embryos. Certainly, if current research indicated that significant medical benefit was just as likely from research using AS, as opposed to ES, cells, respect for embryos would require us to use AS cells. However, no one is making this claim. Although no one can say for sure, the likelihood is that stopping research using ES cells and exploring instead the therapeutic possibilities of AS cells will result in the loss of significant medical benefits for people. A better alternative would be to conduct both kinds of research simultaneously. In any event, Doerflinger's reference to doing research with AS cells appears to be a red herring because it is clear from what he says in his Abstract that he rejects absolutely stem cell research that involves the destruction of human embryos. If such research is never morally acceptable, why go on about doing other research "first"? Doerflinger's views about embryo research derive from the right-to-life position on the moral status of the human embryo. They are unrelated to the "third alternative" which accords respect, but not full moral status, to the human embryo.

What, then, does respect for embryos require? It is important, first, to differentiate respect for embryos from respect for persons. Respect for persons means, as Kant instructs us, never treating persons as mere means to our ends, but always treating them as ends in themselves. This obscure phrase means that we must take seriously the ends—the projects, the goals—that other people have (at least if they are morally permissible ends). We cannot do this with embryos as they do not have ends of their own. Lacking the kinds of ends that persons have, embryos cannot be given the respect that is due to persons. Nevertheless, they have a significance and moral value that other bodily tissues do not have because they are "potent symbols of human life."[8] In this respect, embryos are like dead bodies, which also do not have interests.[9] Unlike dead bodies, embryos are potential human beings in the sense that, under certain conditions, embryos can develop into human persons. This potential gives them a significance and importance that does not belong to other cells of the body, and imposes restrictions on what it is permissible to do to embryos. We show respect for human embryos by not using them in unimportant or frivolous ways, say, to teach high school biology or to make cosmetics or jewelry. However, respect for embryos does not require refraining from research likely to have significant benefits, such as treating disease and prolonging life.

Embryonic stem cells can be derived from embryos remaining after infertility treatment (sometimes called "spare" embryos), or they can be derived from embryos made solely for research purposes using in vitro fertilization (IVF). Both involve the destruction of embryos. However, the NBAC report distinguished morally between the two. It recommended that an exception should be made to the present ban on federal funding of embryo research to permit funding of research using spare embryos, but it recommended that federal agencies should not fund research involving the derivation of human ES cells from embryos made solely for research purposes[7]:

> The primary objection to creating embryos specifically for research is that there is a morally relevant difference between generating an embryo for the sole purpose of creating a child and producing an embryo with no such goal. Those who object to creating embryos for research often appeal to arguments about

respecting human dignity by avoiding instrumental use of human embryos (i.e., using embryos merely as a means to some other goal does not treat them with appropriate respect or concern as a form of human life). (p. v)

Certainly, if one takes the right-to-life view of human embryos, it is morally wrong to create embryos and then destroy them, regardless of the purpose. However, according to the right-to-life view, it is also wrong to create more embryos than will be transferred for implantation; that is, it is wrong to create spare embryos and also wrong to use them in research. Because NBAC does not reject using spare embryos in research, but only creating embryos for the purpose of research, the question is, what justifies this distinction? Here is NBAC's argument[7]:

> Embryos that are discarded following the completion of IVF treatment were presumably created by individuals who had the primary intention of implanting them for reproductive purposes. . . . By contrast, research embryos are created for use in research and, in the case of stem cell research, their destruction in the process of research. Hence, one motivation that encourages serious consideration of the "discarded-created" distinction is a concern about instrumentalization—treating the embryo as a mere object—a practice that may increasingly lead us to think of embryos generally as means to our ends rather than as ends in themselves. (p. 56)

The first part of this paragraph simply reiterates the difference between spare and created embryos; it does not explain why there is a moral difference between the two. The last part attempts to provide a justification for a moral difference, but it relies on the view I have argued is conceptually confused: namely, that embryos should be treated as ends in themselves.

If we reject the view that embryos are ends in themselves, what follows? In my view, it makes no moral difference whether one creates an embryo for reproductive purposes but ends up using it in research, or whether one creates an embryo for the explicit purpose of research. Respect for embryos is demonstrated by restricting their use to important ends. Research that promises to cure disease and save lives clearly qualifies.

The acceptability of this view depends, of course, on one's view of the moral status of the embryo. If embryos are people, there is a moral difference between creating embryos for reproductive purposes and creating them for research purposes. Creating embryos for birth benefits the embryo, whereas creating them for research purposes harms (kills) the embryos to benefit others. But if you reject the idea that preimplantation embryos are the kinds of beings who can be benefited or harmed,[1] creating embryos for research purposes is just as acceptable as creating them for reproductive purposes. Both are valid; neither is frivolous. Therefore, neither contravenes the principle of respect for embryos as a form of human life.

REFERENCES

1 Steinbock B. Life before birth: The moral and legal status of embryos and fetuses. New York: Oxford University Press, 1992.

2 National Institutes of Health. Report of the human embryo research panel. Bethesda (MD): National Institutes of Health, 1994.

3 Warnock M. A question of life: The Warnock report on human fertilisation and embryology. New York: Basil Blackwell, 1985:63–4.

4 Callahan D. The puzzle of profound respect. Hastings Center Rep 1995;25:39–40.

5 Doerflinger R. The ethics of funding embryonic stem cell research: A Catholic viewpoint. Kennedy Inst Ethics J 1999; 9:137–50.

6 Vogel G. Capturing the promise of youth. Science 1999; 286:2238–9.

7 National Bioethics Advisory Commission. Ethical issues in human stem cell research, Vol. 1. Rockville (MD), 1999.

8 Robertson J. A. Symbolic issues in embryo research. Hastings Center Rep 1995; 2 5:37–8.

9 Feinberg J. The mistreatment of dead bodies. Hastings Center Rep 1985; 15:31–7.

THE MORAL CASE AGAINST CLONING-FOR-BIOMEDICAL-RESEARCH
President's Council on Bioethics

In this selection, the President's Council on Bioethics (PCB) presents an overall argument against "cloning-for-biomedical-research." (Because the council was deeply divided on the ethics of research cloning, the views expressed here must be understood as the views of only one segment of the council's membership.) The argument has obvious application, among other things, to the use of cloned embryos as a source of embryonic stem cells, but a central strand in the overall argument—"what we owe to the embryo"—also entails that it is wrong to create any embryo, whether by in vitro fertilization or by cloning, solely for the purpose of harvesting its stem cells. The extensive commentary presented herein on the issue of the moral status of the early embryo includes the claim that the embryo has either full moral status (is "one of us") or has the sort of intermediate and developing moral status that would ground "special respect." In either case, the argument goes, the moral status of the embryo rules out the creation of embryos solely for research applications that entail their very destruction. A second major strand in the overall argument against cloning-for-biomedical-research involves an appeal to "the moral well-being of society as a whole." In this regard, concerns are expressed about (1) crossing the boundary from sexual to asexual reproduction, (2) "the complete instrumentalization of nascent human life," and (3) opening the door to even greater moral hazards, such as cloning-to-produce-children.

. . . Those of us who maintain—for both principled and prudential reasons—that cloning-for-biomedical-research *should not* be pursued . . . begin by acknowledging that substantial human goods might be gained from this research. Although it would be wrong to speak in ways that encourage false hope in those who are ill, as if a cure were likely in the near future, we who oppose such research take seriously its potential for one day yielding substantial (and perhaps unique) medical benefits. Even apart from more distant possibilities for advances in regenerative medicine, there are more immediate possibilities for progress in basic research and for developing models to study different diseases. All of us whose lives benefit enormously from medical advances that began with basic research know how great is our collective stake in continued scientific investigations. Only for very serious reasons—to avoid moral wrongdoing, to avoid harm to society, and to avoid foolish or unnecessary risks—should progress toward increased knowledge and advances that might relieve suffering or cure disease be slowed.

We also observe, however, that the realization of these medical benefits—like all speculative research and all wagers about the future—remains uncertain. There are grounds for questioning whether the proposed benefits of cloning-for-biomedical-research will be realized. And there may be other morally unproblematic ways to achieve similar scientific results and medical benefits. For example, promising results in research with nonembryonic and adult stem cells suggest that scientists may be able to make progress in regenerative medicine without engaging in cloning-for-biomedical-research. We can move forward with other, more developed forms of human stem cell research and with animal cloning. We can explore other routes for solving the immune rejection problem or to finding valuable cellular models of human disease. Where such morally innocent alternatives exist, one could argue that the burden of persuasion lies on proponents to show not only that cloned embryo research is promising or desirable but that it is *necessary* to gain the sought-for

Reprinted from President's Council on Bioethics, *Human Cloning and Human Dignity: An Ethical Inquiry* (2002), pp. 150–165. Some notes omitted.

medical benefits. Indeed, the Nuremberg Code of research ethics enunciates precisely this principle—that experimentation should be "such as to yield fruitful results for the good of society, *unprocurable by other methods or means of study.*" Because of all the scientific uncertainties—and the many possible avenues of research—that burden cannot at present be met.

But, we readily concede, these same uncertainties mean that no one—not the scientists, not the moralists, and not the patients whose suffering we all hope to ameliorate—can know for certain which avenues of research will prove most successful. Research using cloned embryos may in fact, as we said above, yield knowledge and benefits unobtainable by any other means.

With such possible benefits in view, what reasons could we have for saying "no" to cloning-for-biomedical-research? Why not leave this possible avenue of medical progress open? Why not put the cup to our lips? In *The Winter's Tale,* Shakespeare has Leontes, King of Silicia, explain why one might not.[1]

> There may be in the cup
> A spider steep'd, and one may drink, depart,
> And yet partake no venom, for his knowledge
> Is not infected; but if one present
> The abhorr'd ingredient to his eye, make known
> How he hath drunk, he cracks his gorge, his sides
> With violent hefts. I have drunk, and seen the spider.

To discern the spider in the cup is to see the moral reality of cloning-for-biomedical-research differently. It is to move beyond questions of immediately evident benefits or harms alone toward deeper questions about what an ongoing program of cloning-for-biomedical-research would mean. In part, this approach compels us to think about embryo research generally, but cloning (even for research purposes alone) raises its own special concerns, since only cloned embryos could one day become cloned children. We need to consider and articulate the reasons why, despite the possibility of great benefits, society should nevertheless turn away and not drink from this cup, and why the reasons for "drinking with limits" . . . are finally not persuasive.

. . . We differ, among ourselves, on the relative importance of the various arguments presented below. But we all agree that *moral objections to the research itself* and *prudential considerations about where it is likely to lead* suggest that we should oppose cloning-for-biomedical-research, albeit with regret.

A. WHAT WE OWE TO THE EMBRYO

The embryo is, and perhaps will always be, something of a puzzle to us. In its rudimentary beginnings, it is so unlike the human beings we know and live with that it hardly seems to be one of us; yet, the fact of our own embryonic origin evokes in us respect for the wonder of emerging new human life. Even in the midst of much that is puzzling and uncertain, we would not want to lose that respect or ignore what we owe to the embryo.

The cell synthesized by somatic cell nuclear transfer, no less than the fertilized egg, is a human organism in its germinal stage. It is not just a "clump of cells" but an integrated, self-developing whole, capable (if all goes well) of the continued organic development characteristic of human beings. To be sure, the embryo does not yet have, except in potential, the full range of characteristics that distinguish the human species from others, but one need not have those characteristics in evidence in order to belong to the species. And of course human beings at some other stages of development—early in life, late in life, at any stage of life if severely disabled—do not forfeit their humanity simply for want of these distinguishing characteristics. We may observe different points in the life story of any human being— a beginning filled mostly with potential, a zenith at which the organism is in full flower, a decline in which only a residue remains of what is most distinctively human. But none of these points is itself the human being. That being is, rather, an organism with a continuous history. From zygote to irreversible coma, each human life is a single personal history.

But this fact still leaves unanswered the question of whether all stages of a human being's life have equal moral standing. Might there be sound biological or moral reasons for according the early-stage embryo only *partial* human worth or even none at all? If so, should such embryos be made available or even explicitly created for research that necessarily requires their destruction—especially if very real human good might come from it? Some of us who oppose cloning-for-biomedical-research hold that efforts to assign to the embryo a merely intermediate and developing moral status—that is, more humanly significant than other human cells, but less deserving of respect and protection than a human fetus or infant—are both biologically and morally unsustainable, and that the embryo is in fact fully "one of us": a human life in process, an equal member of the species *Homo sapiens* in the embryonic stage of his or her natural development. All of us who oppose going forward with cloning-for-biomedical-research believe that it is incoherent and self-contradictory for our colleagues . . . to claim that human embryos deserve "special respect" and to endorse nonetheless research that requires the creation, use, and destruction of these organisms, *especially when done routinely and on a large scale.*

The case for treating the early-stage embryo as simply the moral equivalent of all other human cells . . . is entirely unconvincing: it denies the continuous history of human individuals from zygote to fetus to infant to child; it misunderstands the meaning of potentiality—and, specifically, the difference between a "being-on-the-way" (such as a developing human embryo) and a "pile of raw materials," which has no definite potential and which might become anything at all; and it ignores the hazardous moral precedent that the routinized creation, use, and destruction of nascent human life would establish for other areas of scientific research and social life.

The more serious questions are raised—about individuality, potentiality, and "special respect"— by those who assign an intermediate and developing moral status to the human embryo, and who believe that cloned embryos can be used (and destroyed) for biomedical research while still according them special human worth. . . . But the arguments for this position—both biological and moral—are not convincing. For attempts to ground the special respect owed to a maturing embryo in certain of its developmental features do not succeed. And the invoking of a "special respect" owed to nascent human life seems to have little or no operative meaning once one sees what those who take this position are willing to countenance.

We are not persuaded by the argument that fourteen days marks a significant difference in moral status. Because the embryo's human and individual genetic identity is present from the start, nothing that happens later during the continuous development that follows—at fourteen days or any other time—is responsible for suddenly conferring a novel human individuality or identity. The scientific evidence suggests that the fourteen-day marker does not represent a biological event of moral significance; rather, changes that occur at fourteen days are merely the visibly evident culmination of more subtle changes that have taken place earlier and that are driving the organism toward maturity. Indeed, many advocates of cloning-for-biomedical-research implicitly recognize the arbitrariness of the fourteen-day line. The medical benefits to be gained by conducting research beyond the fourteen-day line are widely appreciated, and some people have already hinted that this supposed moral and biological boundary can be moved should the medical benefits warrant doing so. . . .

There are also problems with the claim that its capacity for "twinning" proves that the early embryo is not yet an individual or that the embryo's moral status is more significant after the capacity for twinning is gone. There is the obvious rejoinder that if one locus of moral status can become two, its moral standing does not thereby diminish but rather increases. More specifically, the possibility of twinning does not rebut the individuality of the early embryo from its beginning. The fact that where "John" alone once was there are now both "John" and "Jim" does not call into question the presence of "John" at the outset. Hence, we need not doubt that even the earliest cloned embryo is an individual human organism in its germinal stage. Its capacity for twinning may simply be one of the characteristic capacities of an individual human organism at that particular stage of development, just as the capacity for crawling, walking, and running, or cooing, babbling, and speaking are capacities that are also unique to particular stages of human development. Alternatively, from a developmental science perspective,

twinning may not turn out to be an intrinsic process within embryogenesis. Rather, it may be a response to a disruption of normal development from which the embryo recovers and then forms two. Twinning would thus be a testament to the resilience of self-regulation and compensatory repair within early life, not the lack of individuation in the early embryo. From this perspective, twinning is further testimony to the potency of the individual (in this case two) to fullness of form.

We are also not persuaded by the claim that in vitro embryos (whether created through IVF or cloning) have a lesser moral status than embryos that have been implanted into a woman's uterus, because they cannot develop without further human assistance. The suggestion that extra-corporeal embryos are not yet individual human organisms-on-the-way, but rather special human cells that acquire only through implantation the potential to become individual human organisms-on-the-way, rests on a misunderstanding of the meaning and significance of potentiality. An embryo is, by definition and by its nature, potentially a fully developed human person; its potential for maturation is a characteristic it *actually* has, and from the start. The fact that embryos have been created outside their natural environment—which is to say, outside the woman's body—and are therefore limited in their ability to realize their natural capacities, does not affect either the potential or the moral status of the beings themselves. A bird forced to live in a cage its entire life may never learn to fly. But this does not mean it is less of a bird, or that it lacks the immanent potentially to fly on feathered wings. It means only that a caged bird—like an in vitro human embryo—has been deprived of its proper environment. There may, of course, be good human reasons to create embryos outside their natural environments—most obviously, to aid infertile couples. But doing so does not obliterate the moral status of the embryos themselves.

As we have noted, many proponents of cloning-for-biomedical-research (and for embryo research more generally) do not deny that we owe the human embryo special moral respect. Indeed, they have wanted positively to affirm it. But we do not understand what it means to claim that one is treating cloned embryos with special respect when one decides to create them intentionally for research that necessarily leads to their destruction. This respect is allegedly demonstrated by limiting such research—and therefore limiting the numbers of embryos that may be created, used, and destroyed—to only the most serious purposes: namely, scientific investigations that hold out the potential for curing diseases or relieving suffering. But this self-limitation shows only that our purposes are steadfastly high-minded; it does not show that the *means* of pursuing these purposes are *respectful of the cloned embryos* that are necessarily violated, exploited, and destroyed in the process. To the contrary, a true respect for a being would nurture and encourage it toward its own flourishing.

It is, of course, possible to have reverence for a life that one kills. This is memorably displayed, for example, by the fisherman Santiago in Ernest Hemingway's *The Old Man and the Sea,* who wonders whether it is a sin to kill fish even if doing so would feed hungry people. But it seems difficult to claim—even in theory but especially in practice—the presence of reverence once we run a stockyard or raise calves for veal—that is, once we treat the animals we kill (as we often do) simply as resources or commodities. In a similar way, we find it difficult to imagine that biotechnology companies or scientists who routinely engaged in cloning-for-biomedical-research would evince solemn respect for human life each time a cloned embryo was used and destroyed. Things we exploit even occasionally tend to lose their special value. It seems scarcely possible to preserve a spirit of humility and solemnity while engaging in routinized (and in many cases corporately competitive) research that creates, uses, and destroys them.

The mystery that surrounds the human embryo is undeniable. But so is the fact that each human person began as an embryo, and that this embryo, once formed, had the unique potential to become a unique human person. This is the meaning of our embodied condition and the biology that describes it. If we add to this description a commitment to equal treatment—the moral principle that every human life deserves our equal respect—we begin to see how difficult it must be to suggest that a human

embryo, even in its most undeveloped and germinal stage, could simply be used for the good of others and then destroyed. Justifying our intention of using (and destroying) human embryos for the purpose of biomedical research would force us either to ignore the truth of our own continuing personal histories from their beginning in embryonic life or to weaken the commitment to human equality that has been so slowly and laboriously developed in our cultural history.

Equal treatment of human beings does not, of course, mean identical treatment, as all parents know who have more than one child. And from one perspective, the fact that the embryo seems to amount to so little—seems to be little more than a clump of cells—invites us to suppose that its claims upon us can also not amount to much. We are, many have noted, likely to grieve the death of an embryo less than the death of a newborn child. But, then, we are also likely to grieve the death of an eighty-five-year-old father less than the death of a forty-five-year-old father. Perhaps, even, we may grieve the death of a newborn child less than the death of a twelve-year-old. We might grieve differently at the death of a healthy eighty-year-old than at the death of a severely demented eighty-year-old. Put differently, we might note how even the researcher in the laboratory may react with excitement and anticipation as cell division begins. Thus, reproductive physiologist Robert Edwards, who, together with Dr. Patrick Steptoe, helped produce Louise Brown, the first "test-tube baby," said of her: "The last time I saw her, she was just eight cells in a test-tube. She was beautiful then, and she's still beautiful now."[2] The embryo seems to amount to little; yet it has the capacity to become what to all of us seems very much indeed. There is a trajectory to the life story of human beings, and it is inevitable—and appropriate—that our emotional responses should be different at different points in that trajectory. Nevertheless, these emotions, quite naturally and appropriately different, would be misused if we calibrated the degree of respect we owe each other on the basis of such responses. In fact, we are obligated to try to shape and form our emotional responses—and our moral sentiments—so that they are more in accord with the moral respect we owe to those whose capacities are least developed (or those whom society may have wrongly defined as "non-persons" or "nonentities").

In short, how we respond to the weakest among us, to those who are nowhere near the zenith of human flourishing, says much about our willingness to envision the boundaries of humanity expansively and inclusively. It challenges—in the face of what we can know and what we cannot know about the human embryo—the depth of our commitment to equality. If from one perspective the fact that the embryo seems to amount to little may invite a weakening of our respect, from another perspective its seeming insignificance should awaken in us a sense of shared humanity. This was once our own condition. From origins that seem so little came our kin, our friends, our fellow citizens, and all human beings, whether known to us or not. In fact, precisely because the embryo seems to amount to so little, our responsibility to respect and protect its life correspondingly increases. As Hans Jonas once remarked, a true humanism would recognize "the inflexible principle that utter helplessness demands utter protection."[3]

B. WHAT WE OWE TO SOCIETY

Having acknowledged all that, we would miss something if we stopped with what is owed to the embryo—with the language of respect, claims, or rights. An embryo may seem to amount to little or nothing, but that very insignificance tests not the embryo's humanity but our own. Even those who are uncertain about the precise moral status of the human embryo—indeed, even those who believe that it has only intermediate and developing status—have sound ethical-prudential reasons to refrain from using embryos for utilitarian purposes. Moreover, when the embryos to be used have been produced by cloning, there are additional moral dilemmas that go beyond the ethics of embryo research alone. There are principled reasons why people who *accept* research on leftover IVF embryos created initially for reproductive purposes should *oppose* the creation and use of cloned embryos explicitly for research. And there are powerful reasons to worry about where this research will lead us. All these objections have their ground not only in the embryo's character but also in our own, and in concern not only for the fate of nascent human life but for the moral well-being of society as a whole. *One need not believe the embryo is fully human to object vigorously to cloning-for-biomedical-research.*

We are concerned especially about three ways in which giving our moral approval to such research would harm the character of our common life and the way of life we want to transmit to future generations: (i) by crossing the boundary from sexual to asexual reproduction, in the process approving, whether recognized or not, genetic manipulation and control of nascent human life; (ii) by allowing and endorsing the complete instrumentalization of human embryos; and (iii) by opening the door to other—for some of us, far greater—moral hazards, such as cloning-to-produce-children or research on later-stage human embryos and fetuses.

1. Asexual Reproduction and the Genetic Manipulation of Embryos It is worth noting that human cloning—including cloning-for-biomedical-research itself and not simply cloning-to-produce-children— would cross a natural boundary between sexual and asexual reproduction, reducing the likelihood that we could either retrace our steps or keep from taking further steps. Cloning-for-biomedical-research and cloning-to-produce-children both begin with the same act of cloning: the production of a human embryo that is genetically virtually identical to its progenitor. The cloned embryo would therefore be the first human organism with a single genetic "parent" and, equally important, with a genetic constitution that is known and selected in advance. Both uses of cloning mark a significant leap in human power and human control over our genetic origins. Both involve deliberate genetic manipulation of nascent human life. It is, of course, precisely this genetic control that makes cloned embryos uniquely appealing and perhaps uniquely useful to those who seek to conduct research on them. But we should not be deceived about what we are agreeing to if we agree to start to clone: saying yes to cloned embryos in laboratories means saying yes *in principle* to an ever-expanding genetic mastery of one generation over the next.

2. The Complete Instrumentalization of Nascent Human Life

By approving the production of cloned embryos for the sole purpose of research, society would transgress yet another moral boundary: that separating the different ways in which embryos might become available for human experimentation. It is one thing, as some have argued, to conduct research on leftover embryos from IVF procedures, which were created in attempts to have a child and, once no longer needed or wanted, are "destined" for destruction in any case. It is quite another to create embryos *solely* for research that will unavoidably and necessarily destroy them. Thus, for example, the National Bioethics Advisory Commission (in its report on stem cell research) reasoned that in circumstances where embryos were going to be discarded anyway, it did not undermine the moral respect owed to them if they were destroyed in one way (through research) rather than another (by being discarded when no longer wanted for IVF).[4] By contrast, the Commission reasoned that it was much harder to embrace the language of respect for the embryo if it were produced solely for purposes of research and, having been used, then destroyed. This argument maintained the following moral and practical distinction: that embryos created for reproduction but no longer desired could, with proper consent, be used as research subjects, but that embryos ought not be produced solely in order to be used as research subjects. So long as we oppose morally and may perhaps one day prohibit legally the production of cloned children, it is in the very nature of the case that cloned human embryos will not be acquirable as "spare" embryos left over from attempts at reproduction. To the contrary, they will have to be produced solely and explicitly for the purpose of biomedical research, with no other end in view.

Some have argued that there is no significant moral difference between creating excess IVF embryos for reproduction *knowing in advance* that some will be discarded and creating cloned embryos for research *that leads necessarily* to their destruction. Because in both cases embryos are wittingly destroyed, there is, so the argument goes, no moral difference here.

When viewed simply in terms of the fates of embryos once they are created, the distinction between using leftover embryos and creating embryos solely for research may indeed be morally insignificant. But when viewed in terms of the different effects these two activities might have on the moral fabric of society—and the different moral dispositions of those who decide to produce embryos for these different purposes—the issue is more complex. In the eyes of those who create IVF embryos to produce a child, *every embryo,* at the moment of its creation, is *a potential child.* Even though more eggs are fertilized than will be transferred to a woman, each embryo is brought into being as an end in itself, not simply as a means to other ends. Precisely because one cannot tell which IVF embryo is going to reach the blastocyst stage, implant itself in the uterine wall, and develop into a child, the embryo "wastage" in IVF is more analogous to the embryo wastage in natural sexual intercourse practiced by a couple trying to get pregnant than it is to the creation and use of embryos that requires (without exception) their destruction.

Those who minimize or deny this distinction—between producing embryos hoping that one of them will become a child and producing embryos so that they can be used (and destroyed) in research—demonstrate the very problem we are worried about. Having become comfortable with seeing embryos as a means to noble ends (be it having a child or conducting biomedical research), they have lost sight of the fact that the embryos that we create as potential children are not means at all. Even those who remain agnostic about whether the human embryo is fully one of us should see the ways in which conducting such research would make us a different society: less humble toward that which we cannot fully understand, less willing to extend the boundaries of human respect ever outward, and more willing to transgress moral boundaries that we have, ourselves, so recently established, once it appears to be in our own interests to do so. We find it disquieting, even somewhat ignoble, to treat what are in fact seeds of the next generation as mere raw material for satisfying the needs of our own. Doing so would undermine the very prudence and humility to which defenders of limited embryo research often appeal:

the idea that, while a human embryo may not be fully one of us, it is not humanly nothing and therefore should not be treated as a resource alone. But that is precisely what cloning-for-biomedical-research would do.

3. Opening the Door to Other Moral Hazards

This leads directly to our third concern—that the cloning of human embryos for research will open the door to additional (and to some of us, far greater) moral hazards. Human suffering from horrible diseases never comes to an end, and, likewise, our willingness to use embryonic life in the cause of research, once permitted, is also unlikely to find any natural stopping point. To set foot on this slope is to tempt ourselves to become people for whom the use of nascent human life as research material becomes routinized and everyday. That much is inherent in the very logic of what we would do in cloning-for-biomedical-research.

In addition, the reasons justifying production of cloned embryos for research can be predicted to expand. Today, the demand is for stem cells; tomorrow it may be for embryonic and fetal organs. . . . Should this prove to be the case, pressure will increase to grow cloned human blastocysts to later stages—either in the uteruses of suitably prepared animal hosts or (eventually) using artificial placenta-like structures in the laboratory—in order to obtain the more useful tissues. . . .

We should not be self-deceived about our ability to set limits on the exploitation of nascent life. What disturbs us today we quickly or eventually get used to; yesterday's repugnance gives way to tomorrow's endorsement. A society that already tolerates the destruction of fetuses in the second and third trimesters will hardly be horrified by embryo and fetus farming (including in animal wombs), if this should turn out to be helpful in the cure of dreaded diseases. . . .

Finally, if we accept even limited uses of cloning-for-biomedical-research, we significantly increase the likelihood of cloning-to-produce-children. The technique will gradually be perfected and the cloned embryos will become available, and those who would be interested in producing cloned children will find it much easier to do so. The only way to prevent this from happening would be to prohibit, by law, the implantation of cloned embryos for the purpose of producing children. To do so, however, the government would find itself in the unsavory position of designating a class of embryos that it would be a felony not to destroy. It would *require,* not just permit, the destruction of cloned embryos—which seems to us the very opposite of showing such cloned embryos "special respect." . . .

NOTES

1 Brian Appleyard calls attention to this passage in his book, *Brave New Worlds: Staying Human in the Genetic Future* (New York: Viking, 1998).
2 Cited in Kass, L. "The Meaning of Life—in the Laboratory" *The Public Interest,* No. 146, pp. 45–46, Winter 2002.
3 Jonas, H. "Philosophical Reflections on Experimenting With Human Subjects" in *Readings on Ethical and Social Issues in Biomedicine,* ed. Richard W. Wertz (Prentice-Hall, 1973), p. 32.
4 National Bioethics Advisory Commission, *Ethical Issues in Human Stem Cell Research,* volume I, p. 53. Bethesda, MD: Government Printing Office, 1999.

ANNOTATED BIBLIOGRAPHY

Bolton, Martha Brandt: "Responsible Women and Abortion Decisions." In Onora O'Neill and William Ruddick, eds., *Having Children: Philosophical and Legal Reflections on Parenthood* (New York: Oxford University Press, 1979), pp. 40–51. In defending a moderate view on the morality of abortion, Bolton emphasizes the importance of contextual features in the life of a pregnant woman. She argues that the decision to bear a child must "fit" into a woman's life and make sense in terms of her responsibilities to her family and to the larger society.

Boonin, David: *A Defense of Abortion* (Cambridge: Cambridge University Press, 2003). Boonin contends (1) that the fetus does not acquire a right to life until the onset of organized cortical brain activity, which on his reading of the evidence occurs sometime between the 25th and 32nd week; and (2) that, even if the fetus had a right to life as early as conception, it would not follow from that fact that most abortions are morally impermissible.

Brody, Baruch: "On the Humanity of the Foetus." In Robert L. Perkins, ed., *Abortion: Pro and Con* (Cambridge, MA: Schenkman, 1974), pp. 69–90. Brody critically examines various proposals for "drawing the line" on the humanity of the fetus, ultimately suggesting that the most defensible view would draw the line at the point where fetal brain activity begins.

Dwyer, Susan, and Joel Feinberg, eds.: *The Problem of Abortion,* 3rd ed. (Belmont, CA: Wadsworth, 1997). This useful anthology features a wide range of articles on the moral justifiability of abortion. Also included is an extensive bibliography.

Engelhardt, H. Tristram, Jr.: "The Ontology of Abortion," *Ethics* 84 (April 1974), pp. 217–234. Engelhardt focuses attention on the issue of "whether or to what extent the fetus is a person." He argues that, strictly speaking, a human person is not present until the later stages of infancy. However, he finds the point of viability significant in that, with viability, an infant can play the social role of "child" and thus be treated "as if it were a person."

English, Jane: "Abortion and the Concept of a Person," *Canadian Journal of Philosophy* 5 (October 1975), pp. 233–243. English advances one line of argument calculated to moderate the conservative view on the morality of abortion and another line of argument calculated to moderate the liberal view.

Hansen, J-E. S.: "Embryonic Stem Cell Production Through Therapeutic Cloning Has Fewer Ethical Problems than Stem Cell Harvest from Surplus IVF Embryos," *Journal of Medical Ethics* 28 (April 2002), pp. 86–88. Hansen argues that an IVF embryo clearly lacks human moral status and a cloned embryo even more clearly lacks human moral status.

Langerak, Edward A.: "Abortion: Listening to the Middle," *Hastings Center Report* 9 (October 1979), pp. 24–28. Langerak suggests a theoretical framework for a moderate view that incorporates two "widely shared beliefs": (1) that there is something about the fetus *itself* that makes abortion morally problematic and (2) that late abortions are significantly more problematic than early abortions.

Noonan, John T., Jr.: "An Almost Absolute Value in History." In John T. Noonan, ed., *The Morality of Abortion: Legal and Historical Perspectives* (Cambridge, MA: Harvard University Press, 1970), pp. 51–59. In this well-known statement of the conservative view on the morality of abortion, Noonan argues that conception is the only objectively based and nonarbitrary point at which to "draw the line" between the nonhuman and the human.

Outka, Gene: "The Ethics of Human Stem Cell Research," *Kennedy Institute of Ethics Journal* 12 (June 2002), pp. 175–213. Outka surveys and analyzes various views on the ethics of human stem cell research. He ultimately argues that research on "excess" embryos can be justified by appeal to the "nothing is lost" principle, but the creation of embryos solely for research purposes cannot be justified.

Pojman, Louis P., and Francis J. Beckwith, eds.: *The Abortion Controversy: 25 Years After* Roe v. Wade: *A Reader,* 2nd ed. (Belmont, CA: Wadsworth, 1998). The articles in this long anthology are organized under eight headings, including "Evaluations of *Roe v. Wade,*" "Personhood Arguments on Abortion," and "Feminist Arguments on Abortion."

President's Council on Bioethics, *Monitoring Stem Cell Research* (2004). Chapter 2 of this report provides a description of "current federal law and policy." Chapter 3 presents an analysis of "recent developments in the ethical and policy debates," and Chapter 4 offers an account of "recent developments in stem cell research and therapy."

Ross, Steven L.: "Abortion and the Death of the Fetus," *Philosophy and Public Affairs* 11 (Summer 1982), pp. 232–245. Ross draws a distinction between abortion as the termination of pregnancy and abortion as the termination of the life of the fetus. He proceeds to defend abortion in the latter sense, insisting that it is justifiable for a woman to desire not only the termination of pregnancy but also the death of the fetus.

Ruse, Michael, and Christopher A. Pynes: *The Stem Cell Controversy: Debating the Issues* (Amherst, NY: Prometheus, 2003). This anthology offers sections on (1) the science of stem cells, (2) medical cures and promises, (3) moral issues, (4) religious issues, and (5) policy issues.

Sherwin, Susan: *No Longer Patient: Feminist Ethics and Health Care* (Philadelphia: Temple University Press, 1992). In Chapter 5 of this book (pp. 99–116), Sherwin presents an analysis of abortion that reflects her commitment to feminist ethics.

Steinbock, Bonnie: *Life Before Birth: The Moral and Legal Status of Embryos and Fetuses* (New York: Oxford University Press, 1992). Steinbock argues in Chapter 1 for "the interest view" of moral status—that is, the claim that "all and only beings who have interests have moral status." In Chapter 2, she provides an analysis of abortion.

Stone, Jim: "Why Potentiality Matters," *Canadian Journal of Philosophy* 17 (December 1987), pp. 815–830. Stone argues that a fetal right to life can be effectively grounded in the fact that a fetus is *potentially* an adult human being.

Strong, Carson: *Ethics in Reproductive and Perinatal Medicine: A New Framework* (New Haven, CT: Yale University Press, 1997). In Chapter 3, Strong argues for the view that the moral standing of the fetus progressively increases in strength as fetal development proceeds.

Tong, Rosemarie: *Feminist Approaches to Bioethics: Theoretical Reflections and Practical Applications* (Boulder, CO: Westview Press, 1997). In Chapter 6, Tong contrasts feminist and nonfeminist perspectives on abortion. She also distinguishes among various feminist approaches.

Tooley, Michael: *Abortion and Infanticide* (New York: Oxford University Press, 1983). In this long book, Tooley defends the liberal view on the morality of abortion. He insists that the question of the morality of abortion cannot be satisfactorily resolved "in isolation from the questions of the morality of infanticide and of the killing of nonhuman animals."

CHAPTER 8

GENETICS AND HUMAN REPRODUCTION

INTRODUCTION

With the rapid advance of knowledge and techniques in human genetics and the biology of human reproduction, a number of complex and troubling ethical issues have arisen. This chapter is designed to address some of the most important of these issues.

GENETIC DISEASE AND THE LANGUAGE OF GENETICS

Tay-Sachs disease is one prominent example of a genetic disease.[1] This disease, which most commonly affects Jewish children of Eastern European heritage, is characterized by progressive neurological degeneration and death in early childhood. Although a child afflicted with Tay-Sachs disease has the disease by virtue of his or her genetic inheritance, the child's parents do not have the disease. (Those afflicted with Tay-Sachs disease do not survive to reproduce.) The parents are *carriers*. Tay-Sachs carriers are those persons who have one normal gene and one variant, or defective, gene (the Tay-Sachs gene) at the same location on paired chromosomes. The Tay-Sachs gene is *recessive*. When it is paired with a normal gene, as is the case with the carrier, the normal gene is dominant. As a result, the carrier does not manifest the disease. However, if a child inherits the Tay-Sachs gene from both parents, then the child will be afflicted with Tay-Sachs disease.

Since Tay-Sachs disease is traceable to a recessive gene, it is said to be a recessive disease. Moreover, it is said to be an autosomal recessive disease; the word *autosomal* simply indicates that the defective genes are located on a pair of chromosomes other than the sex chromosomes. Furthermore, in the language of genetics, Tay-Sachs carriers are said to be in the *heterozygous* state, whereas a child afflicted with Tay-Sachs disease is said to be in the *homozygous* state, with regard to the Tay-Sachs gene. Carriers, having the Tay-Sachs gene paired with a different (normal) gene, are heterozygous with regard to the Tay-Sachs gene. The afflicted child, having two copies of the Tay-Sachs gene, is homozygous. The carrier is sometimes termed a "heterozygote"; the afflicted child, a "homozygote."

According to the (Mendelian) laws of heredity, when two carriers of a gene associated with an autosomal recessive disease produce offspring, there is one chance in four (25 percent) that their child will be afflicted with the genetic disease in question. There are two chances in four (50 percent) that their child will be, like them, a carrier. Finally, there is one chance in four (25 percent) that their child will be free both of the disease and of the carrier status.

Sickle-cell anemia is, like Tay-Sachs disease, a well-known autosomal recessive disease. Most commonly affecting people of African descent, sickle-cell anemia is characterized by acute episodes of pain (e.g., in the abdomen, chest, or joints) and exhibits a range of severity. There have been some notable treatment advances, but, at present, the average life expectancy for victims of sickle-cell anemia is less than 50. An estimated 10 percent of African Americans carry the sickle-cell gene.[2] As is characteristic of autosomal recessive diseases, if two carriers of the sickle-cell gene produce offspring, there is one chance in four (25 percent) that their child will be afflicted with sickle-cell anemia.

Cystic fibrosis provides one further example of an autosomal recessive disease. In the United States, since about 1 in 30 Caucasians carries the cystic fibrosis gene, about 1 in 900 Caucasian couples will be a carrier-carrier pairing and thus be at risk (one chance in four) of producing offspring with the disease. At present, although hopes are high for therapeutic advances, the median age of death for victims of cystic fibrosis is not much over 30. The disease is primarily characterized by a dysfunction of the exocrine glands. This dysfunction results in abnormal amounts of mucus, which can obstruct organ passages and produce intense pulmonary and digestive distress.

Huntington's disease provides a leading example of a genetic disease in the category of autosomal *dominant* diseases. Typically, the symptoms of Huntington's disease emerge only in the prime of life, between the ages of 35 and 50. It is characterized by mental and physical deterioration, leading to death within several years. The defective gene responsible for Huntington's disease is a dominant one. If a person has the defective gene, that person will eventually fall victim to the disease. Moreover, for any offspring of a person carrying the defective gene, there is one chance in two (50 percent) that the gene will be inherited.

In contrast to autosomal genetic diseases, some genetic diseases are linked to mutant genes located on the sex chromosomes. Prominent among the genetic diseases in this latter category are the so-called *X-linked diseases*. Hemophilia, a well-known disease characterized by uncontrollable bleeding, is a leading example of an X-linked disease. Of the 46 chromosomes that constitute the normal complement of genetic material in human beings, there are two sex chromosomes. A female has two X chromosomes, and a male has one X and one Y chromosome. In human reproduction, if the sperm fertilizing the egg provides an X chromosome, the child will be female. If the sperm fertilizing the egg provides a Y chromosome, the child will be male. (The egg always provides an X chromosome.) Hemophilia is a *recessive* X-linked disease. A female, therefore, will have the disease of hemophilia only if she has the mutant gene on both of her X chromosomes. If a female has one normal gene and one mutant gene, however, she will be a carrier. Since a male has only one X chromosome, if he has the mutant gene associated with hemophilia, he will have the disease. On the assumption that a female carrier mates with a male who is free of the disease, there is no risk that their female children will have the disease. Female children will inherit a normal gene from their father and thus themselves be free of the disease, although there is one chance in two (50 percent) that they will inherit their mother's mutant gene and be, like her, a carrier. In contrast, there is one chance in two (50 percent) that male children (of a female carrier and a disease-free male) will have the disease of hemophilia.

PRENATAL DIAGNOSIS AND SELECTIVE ABORTION

A number of techniques are presently employed for the detection of chromosomal abnormalities, many genetic diseases, and certain serious anatomical abnormalities in the fetus in utero. Among these techniques, amniocentesis and chorionic villi sampling (CVS) are the most prominent, although ultrasound is also of great importance. Ultrasound is a noninvasive technique that produces a visual representation of the developing fetus, thereby allowing the detection of many anatomical abnormalities.

In amniocentesis, a needle is inserted through a pregnant woman's abdomen, and a sample of the amniotic fluid surrounding the fetus is withdrawn. Diagnostic testing of fetal cells in the amniotic fluid makes it possible to detect the presence of various genetic diseases in the fetus. Also detectable, via chromosomal analysis, are conditions associated with an abnormal number of chromosomes or an abnormal arrangement of chromosomes. Down's syndrome, for example, is associated with the presence of an extra chromosome, namely, three instead of two number 21 chromosomes. Amniocentesis can also be employed for the detection of neural-tube defects (anencephaly and spina bifida). In this case, a positive diagnosis rests on the presence of increased levels of alphafetoprotein in the amniotic fluid.

Amniocentesis, first introduced in the late 1960s, has achieved wide acceptance among physicians as a relatively low-risk medical procedure. However, it is not ordinarily performed before the 15th or 16th week of gestation, and selective abortion must await the results of diagnostic testing, which may not be available until the 20th week or so. Since second-trimester abortions are more problematic (medically, psychologically, socially, and perhaps morally) than first-trimester abortions, a procedure capable of combining the prenatal diagnostic value of amniocentesis with the possibility of first-trimester abortion is much to be preferred, assuming, of course, that risk factors are within acceptable limits. Chorionic villi sampling (CVS), a procedure developed in Europe and first introduced in the United States in 1983, is now established as an alternative to amniocentesis in the detection of genetic diseases and chromosomal abnormalities. In CVS, a procedure that can be performed in the first trimester, usually around the 10th week, a small amount of tissue is extracted from the placenta, and the results of diagnostic testing on this tissue are typically available about seven days later. However, the risk of miscarriage is apparently somewhat greater for CVS than for amniocentesis.

Since prenatal diagnosis is ordinarily undertaken with an eye toward selective abortion, the practice of prenatal diagnosis clearly confronts us with one particular aspect of the more general problem of abortion, as discussed in Chapter 7. (There is also a close link with the problem of the treatment of impaired newborns, as discussed in Chapter 5.) Is the practice of selective abortion, on grounds of genetic defect, ethically acceptable? Leon R. Kass, in one of this chapter's selections, abstracts from the problem of abortion in general and argues specifically against the practice of selective (genetic) abortion. Kass's arguments resonate strongly with a viewpoint usually identified today as the *disability rights critique* of prenatal diagnosis and selective abortion.[3] Advocates of the disability rights critique claim, among other things, that the selection against disability embodied in selective abortion is a form of discrimination. Whether the disability rights critique of prenatal diagnosis and selective abortion can ultimately be sustained is a matter that continues to provoke intense debate.

MORALITY AND REPRODUCTIVE RISK

One important ethical issue associated with human genetics has to do with the morality of reproduction under circumstances of genetic risk. Laura M. Purdy argues, in this chapter, that it is morally wrong to reproduce when there is a high risk of serious genetic disease. In particular, she considers the case of Huntington's disease. If it is justifiable to maintain that there is a moral obligation of the sort that Purdy outlines, we may find ourselves once more faced with the problem of prenatal diagnosis and selective abortion. Clearly, in cases where prenatal diagnosis is available (e.g., Huntington's disease, Tay-Sachs disease, sickle-cell anemia, cystic fibrosis), selective abortion offers a means of sidestepping the risk of serious genetic disease.

Closely associated with the issue of the morality of reproduction under circumstances of genetic risk is another ethical issue, the justifiability of the use of coercive measures to achieve social control over individual reproductive decisions. It is one thing to say that certain reproductive choices are immoral and quite another to say that coercive measures for the control of reproductive choices are justified. Such coercive controls as compulsory sterilization and mandatory amniocentesis followed by forced abortion are widely rejected as invasive of fundamental rights. Mandatory screening programs for the identification of carriers, while surely less invasive than other coercive measures, are also viewed with suspicion by most commentators.

REPRODUCTIVE TECHNOLOGIES AND THE TREATMENT OF INFERTILITY

Human reproduction, as it naturally occurs, is characterized by sexual intercourse, tubal fertilization, implantation in the uterus, and subsequent in utero gestation. The expression *reproductive technologies* can be understood as applicable to an array of technical procedures that would replace the various steps in the natural process of reproduction, to a lesser or greater extent.[4]

Artificial insemination (also called assisted insemination) is a procedure that replaces sexual intercourse as a means of achieving tubal fertilization. Artificial insemination has long been available, primarily as a means of overcoming infertility on the part of a male, usually a husband. It is sometimes possible for a husband's infertility to be overcome by artificial insemination with the sperm of the *husband* (AIH). More often, at least in the past, a couple has found it necessary to turn to artificial insemination with the sperm of a *donor* (AID).[5] AID can also be employed when it has been established that the husband carries a mutant gene that would place a couple's offspring at genetic risk. Moreover, it has been suggested, most prominently in the work of the well-known geneticist Herman J. Muller, that AID be voluntarily employed as a way of achieving the aims of positive eugenics.[6] Muller recommended the formation of sperm banks that would collect and store the sperm of men judged to be "outstanding" in various ways. His idea was that any "enlightened" couple desiring a child would have recourse to one of these banks in order to arrange for the wife's artificial insemination. Another controversial use of AID is its use by unmarried women. Probably even more controversial is the use of artificial insemination within the context of a surrogacy arrangement. In the most typical case, a wife's infertility motivates a couple to seek out a so-called surrogate mother. The surrogate agrees to be artificially inseminated with the husband's sperm, in order to bear a child for the couple.

In vitro fertilization (IVF) literally means "fertilization in glass." The sperm of a husband (or a donor) is united, in a laboratory, with the ovum of a wife (or a donor). Whereas artificial insemination is a technically simple procedure, in vitro fertilization followed by embryo transfer (to the uterus for implantation) is a system of reproductive technology that features a high degree of technical sophistication. The first documented "test-tube baby," Louise Brown, was born in England in July 1978. Her birth was the culmination of years of collaboration between a gynecologist, Patrick Steptoe, and an embryologist, Robert Edwards. This pioneering team developed methods of obtaining mature eggs from a woman's ovaries (via a minor surgical procedure called a laparoscopy), effectively fertilizing eggs in the laboratory, cultivating them to the eight-cell stage, and then transferring a developing embryo to the uterus for implantation.

Reproductive centers throughout the United States now provide in vitro procedures for the treatment of infertility, although success rates continue to be somewhat disappointing. Since it is now possible, with the use of fertility drugs, to harvest a crop of mature eggs (perhaps ten or so) from a woman's ovaries, embryos are sometimes frozen (e.g., at the eight-cell stage) and then selectively thawed at appropriate times over a period of several months in an effort to achieve a successful implantation. Of course, the freezing of embryos may lead to other problems—for example, how to deal with frozen embryos no longer needed. However, the freezing of unfertilized eggs, which at face value may seem preferable to the freezing of embryos, has proven to be technically more difficult.

In vitro fertilization followed by embryo transfer is a system of reproductive technology that replaces not only sexual intercourse but also tubal fertilization in the natural process of reproduction. But consider also the future possibility of dispensing with implantation and in utero gestation as well. There seems to be no theoretical obstacle to totally artificial gestation, which would take place within the confines of an artificial womb. If *ectogenesis,* the process of artificial gestation, becomes a reality, then the combination of in vitro fertilization and ectogenesis would constitute a system of reproductive technology in which each element in the natural process of reproduction has been effectively replaced. At the present time, however, in vitro fertilization (accompanied by embryo transfer) is seen primarily as a means of overcoming certain forms of infertility—for example, infertility due to obstruction of the fallopian tubes.

One notable spinoff of IVF technology is a procedure called gamete intrafallopian transfer (GIFT). In this procedure, eggs are obtained as they would be for IVF, but instead of fertilization in vitro, the eggs are placed together with sperm in the fallopian tube (or tubes), where it is hoped that fertilization will take place in vivo (i.e., in the living situation). A closely related procedure is called zygote intrafallopian transfer (ZIFT). In ZIFT, a single-cell zygote, which is the product of in vitro fertilization, is transferred to the fallopian tube.

Intracytoplasmic sperm injection (ICSI), another spinoff of IVF technology, is a technique that was first developed in 1992. Now widely used in clinical practice, it was originally introduced to address problems of male infertility. In ICSI, a single sperm is injected into an egg to achieve fertilization in a laboratory dish. Even a man with a very low sperm count can become a biological father by the use of this technique, thereby allowing a couple to avoid the problems associated with the use of donor sperm in order to combat male infertility. At present, however, there are unresolved safety concerns about the use of ICSI, as there are about the use of IVF itself. These and related safety concerns are addressed in some detail by the President's Council on Bioethics in a selection reprinted in this chapter. In this selection, the council also presents a very useful account of state-of-the-art practice with regard to IVF and closely related procedures.

In contrast to a woman whose infertility can be traced to fallopian tube obstruction, consider a woman whose ovaries are either absent or nonfunctional. Since she has no ova, she cannot produce genetic offspring. If her uterus is functional, however, there is no biological obstacle to her bearing a child. Let us suppose that she wants to bear a child that is her husband's genetic offspring. Her problem can be addressed by some form of *egg donation*.[7] The most obvious possibility in this regard is in vitro fertilization of a donor egg with the husband's sperm, followed by embryo transfer to the wife.

In the case just discussed, a woman has a functional uterus but nonfunctional ovaries. Consider now the converse case—a woman has functional ovaries but a nonfunctional uterus. Perhaps she has had a hysterectomy. She is capable of becoming the *genetic* but not the *gestational* mother of a child. Now, suppose that she and her husband desire a child "of their own." This situation gives rise to the possibility of a surrogacy arrangement somewhat different from the kind predicated upon artificial insemination. In this case, in vitro fertilization could be employed to fertilize the wife's egg with the husband's sperm. The embryo could then be transferred to the uterus of a surrogate, who would agree to bear the child for the couple. The surrogate would then be the gestational but not the genetic mother of the child.

REPRODUCTIVE TECHNOLOGIES: ETHICAL CONCERNS

To what extent, if at all, is it ethically acceptable to employ the various reproductive technologies just described? Numerous ethical concerns have been expressed about these technologies, and a brief survey of the most prominent of these concerns should prove helpful.

Much of the ethical opposition to artificial insemination derives from religious views. AID especially has been attacked on the grounds that it illicitly separates procreation from the marriage relationship. Inasmuch as AID introduces a third party (the sperm donor) into a marriage relationship, it has been called a form of adultery. Even AIH, which cannot be accused of separating procreation from the marriage relationship, has not uniformly escaped attack. Some religious ethicists have gone so far as to contend that procreation is morally illicit whenever it is not the product of personal lovemaking. Although these sorts of objections frequently recur in discussions of egg donation, in vitro fertilization, and other reproductive technologies, they seem to have little force for those who do not share the basic worldview from which they proceed.

Some of the ethical opposition to in vitro fertilization (and related technologies) is based on the perceived "unnaturalness" of the procedure. Closely related is the charge that the procedure depersonalizes or dehumanizes procreation. Further, in this same vein, complaints are made against the "manufacture" and "commodification" of children. Another recurrent argument against in vitro fertilization is that its acceptance by society will lead to the acceptance of more and more objectionable developments in reproductive technology (e.g., ectogenesis).

In addition to arguments advanced in support of a wholesale rejection of in vitro fertilization, a number of concerns having a more limited scope can be identified. Some commentators have been quite willing to endorse the use of in vitro fertilization and embryo transfer within the framework of a marital relationship but object to any third-party involvement—that is, sperm or egg donation, embryo donation, and surrogate motherhood. Other critics object primarily to a frequent concomitant of in vitro procedures—the discarding of embryos considered unneeded or unsuitable for implantation. Those who consider even an early embryo a person (in the sense of having full moral status) are especially vocal on this score, and they also register a vigorous complaint against the use of surplus embryos for research purposes (see the stem cell discussion in Chapter 7), although they often endorse the idea of donating surplus embryos to another couple for attempted implantation. Of course, those who embrace a very different view of the moral status of the early embryo will typically argue that there is no ethical problem with either discarding surplus embryos or using them for research purposes.

Two readings in this chapter focus directly on the ethics of IVF.[8] Peter Singer provides a defense of IVF by countering many of the standard arguments against it. Susan Sherwin, in a very different spirit, works out a critique of IVF based on her commitment to feminist ethics. From a feminist point of view, she maintains, IVF is morally problematic for a number of closely related reasons. Although there is a diversity of views in the feminist community about the ethics of IVF, many feminists believe that the availability of IVF and other reproductive technologies is at best a mixed blessing for women.

In one of this chapter's readings, The New York State Task Force on Life and the Law presents an overall survey of ethical perspectives on reproductive technology. In another reading, Thomas H. Murray argues that the alternative reproductive practices made possible by contemporary technologies will not pass moral inspection if they fail to cohere with values at the core of family life. He is opposed in particular to the intrusion of marketplace values into the realm of family life. Thus, he is opposed to the *commercialization* of third-party involvement in reproduction, although he is not opposed to noncommercial third-party involvement. In Murray's view, payment for gamete donation (whether sperm or egg) is morally unsound, as is payment for the services of a surrogate mother.

Much of the ethical opposition to surrogate motherhood can be traced to (1) concerns about psychosocial problems likely to arise for the child who is born as a result of a surrogacy arrangement and (2) concerns that the practice will have a negative impact on family structure. However, as Murray's analysis makes clear, additional concerns can be raised about the practice of *commercial* surrogacy.

At present, the legal status of commercial surrogacy contracts varies from state to state, and legislatures have taken various approaches in attempting to deal with the social policy aspects of surrogacy. One option is for a state simply to recognize commercial surrogacy contracts as valid and legally enforceable. Another option is for the state to prohibit commercial surrogacy contracts altogether. Bonnie Steinbock argues, in this chapter, against the legal prohibition of surrogacy contracts, although she insists on the importance of state regulation. In her view, commercial surrogacy contracts should be permitted only if provision is made for a "waiting period" subsequent to birth. During this period, the surrogate would have the opportunity to change her mind about surrending her parental rights.

In the celebrated Baby M case (see Appendix, Case 41), the "surrogate" was both the genetic and gestational mother of a child. Other cases involve purely gestational surrogates—that is, women who have agreed to carry a child for a couple, each of whom is a genetic parent. Here the surrogate is the gestational but not the genetic mother of a child. If this type of surrogacy agreement breaks down, the following issue arises: Should we identify the genetic mother or the gestational mother as the child's legal mother?

HUMAN CLONING

With the announcement in February 1997 of the successful cloning of a sheep in Scotland, much attention has been focused on the prospect of human cloning.[9] Accordingly, the following sequence of events can be imagined. A mature human egg will be obtained from a woman and enucleated in a laboratory—that is, the nucleus of the egg cell will be removed. Meanwhile, a somatic cell from an adult human being (who might be anyone, including the woman who has provided the egg) will be obtained and enucleated. The extracted nucleus, which contains the donor's heretofore unique genotype (assuming the donor is not an identical twin), will then be inserted into the egg cell, and the renucleated egg will be activated, so that it will develop in the way that a newly fertilized egg ordinarily develops.[10] Embryo transfer (not necessarily into the uterus of the woman from whom the original egg was obtained) and subsequent in utero gestation will then lead to the birth of a human "clone." In contrast to offspring resulting from sexual reproduction, where the resultant genotype is the result of contributions by two parents, the clone will have the same genotype as his or her "parent."[11]

The type of cloning just described, somatic cell nuclear transfer (SCNT), is the focal point of concern in contemporary debates about the ethics of human cloning. Another important process, less dramatic than SCNT, is also considered by many commentators to be a type of cloning. This process involves the splitting of a very early embryo (e.g., at the eight-cell stage) and thus the formation of duplicate embryos. The embryo-splitting type of cloning is not technically difficult, and because it does not necessarily result in a "time lag" between identical twins in the way that SCNT does, many commentators consider it less problematic than SCNT. It may be important to realize, however, that embryo splitting followed by implantation of some embryos and freezing of others for later implantation would, in fact, lead to identical twins of different ages.

Many of the ethical concerns that can be raised about human cloning are continuous with concerns that have been raised about other reproductive technologies, but the prospect of human cloning also seems to confront us with some distinctive ethical concerns. In one of this chapter's selections, Leon R. Kass constructs four lines of argument against human cloning and maintains that it is deeply unethical. Also in this chapter, Thomas H. Murray expresses some serious reservations about human cloning. Robert Wachbroit presents a very different point of view on the ethics of human cloning. His arguments are calculated to defend human cloning in response to the various concerns raised by its critics.

Two presidential commissions have explicitly confronted the possibility of human (SCNT) cloning. In 1997, the National Bioethics Advisory Commission submitted its report *Cloning Human Beings*. In concluding that it is morally unacceptable "at this time" for anyone to attempt to create a child by cloning, the commission placed special emphasis on safety concerns. The commission's central recommendation was that federal legislation be enacted to prohibit anyone from attempting to create a child via cloning, although it also recommended incorporation of a sunset clause calculated to ensure that Congress would reconsider after three to five years whether a ban was still needed. No legislative action was forthcoming in response to commission recommendations. In 2002, the President's Council on Bioethics submitted its report *Human Cloning and Human Dignity: An Ethical Inquiry*.[12] The council considered both cloning-to-produce-children (reproductive cloning) and cloning-for-biomedical-research (research cloning). (The distinction between reproductive and research cloning is articulated in the Introduction to Chapter 7, in conjunction with the discussion of embryonic stem cells.) Members of the council unanimously agreed that reproductive cloning is morally unacceptable and unanimously recommended that Congress ban all attempts at reproductive cloning. The council also recommended a four-year national moratorium (that is, a temporary ban) on research cloning, although in this case only 10 of the 17 voting members of the council favored the moratorium. At the date of this writing (Fall 2004), political wrangling over the stem-cell issue has stymied any legislative action by Congress.

PREIMPLANTATION GENETIC DIAGNOSIS

Preimplantation genetic diagnosis (PGD) is a procedure that has emerged against the background of IVF technology. In PGD, embryos produced by IVF can be analyzed for chromosomal abnormalities and selected genetic diseases *before* implantation is attempted. The most common form of PGD involves extracting one or two cells from the preimplantation embryo, often around the eight-cell stage. Testing of these extracted cells allows affected embryos to be identified and discarded. Embryos that are unaffected are available for implantation. Couples at risk for the transmission of genetic disease sometimes choose IVF and PGD in order to avoid the problem of selective abortion that is associated with prenatal diagnosis during pregnancy. Some of the issues raised by the use of PGD to screen out embryos with chromosomal abnormality or genetic disease are continuous with issues raised by the practice of prenatal diagnosis and selective abortion. In particular, both practices feature a selection process against disability that advocates of the disability rights critique allege to be discriminatory. Of course, many commentators reject this claim of discrimination and argue for the ethical acceptability of both practices. Is PGD ethically preferable to prenatal diagnosis and selective abortion? The answer to this question surely depends in part on the issue of the moral status of the preimplantation embryo vis-à-vis the moral status of the developing fetus.

Although the standard medical use of PGD is to select against embryos with chromosomal or genetic disorders, other possible uses can be identified. In one of this chapter's readings, John A. Robertson surveys these various uses, both medical and nonmedical. Nonmedical uses of PGD are especially controversial. These uses include selecting embryos on the basis of gender (sex) and selecting embryos for desired traits (e.g., perfect pitch). In a closely related reading in this chapter, the President's Council on Bioethics considers whether it is likely that significant demand will emerge for PGD in order to select embryos for desired traits. In the course of its analysis, the council effectively clarifies a number of practical problems confronting this possible extension of PGD use.

GENETIC ENGINEERING, GENE THERAPY, AND ENHANCEMENT

Two important distinctions are involved in discussions of the ethics of genetic engineering (intervention, manipulation). *Therapeutic* genetic engineering, commonly called "gene therapy," involves interventions directed at the cure of disease. *Nontherapeutic* genetic engineering, often called "enhancement engineering," involves interventions directed at the enhancement of human traits (e.g., height) and capabilities (e.g., memory). *Somatic-cell* genetic interventions involve introducing modifications into nonreproductive cells (e.g., blood cells), so that the resultant changes are not passed on to future generations. *Germline* genetic interventions involve introducing modifications into sperm, ova, or preimplantion embryos, so that the resultant changes are passed on to future generations. By reference to these two distinctions, four categories of genetic engineering can be distinguished: (1) somatic-cell gene therapy, (2) germ-line gene therapy, (3) somatic-cell enhancement (nontherapeutic) engineering, and (4) germ-line enhancement (nontherapeutic) engineering.

It may be possible in the foreseeable future to cure a wide range of genetic diseases (e.g., cystic fibrosis and hemophilia) by the genetic manipulation of somatic cells. It is also hoped that somatic-cell gene therapy will eventually provide effective treatment for such diseases as cancer and cardiovascular disease. Despite the complaint that any use of genetic engineering places human beings in the role of "playing God," the continued development and use of somatic-cell gene therapy is widely endorsed and relatively uncontroversial— that is, in theory. In practice, progress in the development of somatic-cell gene therapy has been mostly disappointing, and numerous ethical and policy issues are associated with the conduct of clinical trials. Some of these issues are highlighted in this chapter by Sophia Kolehmainen, in conjunction with her discussion of the tragic case of Jesse Gelsinger, an eighteen-year-old male who died in 1999 as a result of his participation in a gene therapy clinical trial. In a closely related reading in this chapter, Marina Cavazzana-Calvo, Adrian Thrasher, and Fulvio Mavilio provide the valuable perspective of researchers in the field of genetic therapy. The point of departure for their analysis is the successful treatment of patients suffering from severe combined immunodeficiencies (SCIDs)—first reported in 2000 and widely celebrated as the first real success of gene therapy—followed by the unfortunate realization in 2002 that two of ten patients successfully treated had developed leukemia as a side-effect of the gene therapy.

There is extensive debate about the ethical acceptability of both germ-line gene therapy and enhancement engineering in any form. In one of this chapter's selections, LeRoy Walters and Julie Gage Palmer review the arguments commonly made for and against the use of germ-line gene therapy. Their analysis culminates in an endorsement of germ-line gene therapy, at least in principle. In another selection, Walter Glannon defends the treatment-enhancement distinction and argues that enhancement engineering (genetic enhancement) is morally objectionable. A contrasting view of the ethics of enhancement engineering is offered by Dan W. Brock.

T.A.M.

NOTES

1 Discussion of genetic disease in this section is limited to *Mendelian* diseases—that is, those produced by a single-gene defect. Polygenetic (or multigenetic) diseases are produced by the interaction of several genes, and many common diseases (e.g., cancer and cardiovascular disease) are the product of genetic predisposition (involving multiple genes) in combination with environmental factors.

2 A single copy of the sickle-cell gene is believed to make the carrier more resistant to malaria, an advantage especially in tropical climates.

3 For one helpful articulation of the disability rights critique of prenatal diagnosis and selective abortion, see Erik Parens and Adrienne Asch, "The Disability Rights Critique of Prenatal Genetic Testing: Reflections and Recommendations," in Erik Parens and Adrienne Asch, eds., *Prenatal Testing and Disability Rights* (Washington, DC: Georgetown University Press, 2000), pp. 3–43.

4 A broader conception of *reproductive technologies* would encompass other forms of technical assistance calculated to aid the process of reproduction—for example, the use of "fertility drugs" to stimulate ovulation.

5 More recently, the problem of male infertility has been effectively addressed by ICSI, a procedure discussed in a subsequent paragraph.

6 See, for example, Herman J. Muller, "Means and Aims in Human Genetic Betterment," in T. M., Sonneborn, ed., *The Control of Human Heredity and Evolution* (New York: Macmillan, 1965), pp. 100–122. Roughly, positive eugenics aims at enhancing the genetic heritage of the species, whereas negative eugenics aims at preventing deterioration of the gene pool. However, use of the word *eugenics* is frequently attended with

much confusion. So-called eugenics programs have usually featured elements of government coercion, but eugenics need not be understood as entailing coercion.

7 Egg donation might also be considered when a woman's own ova would place her offspring at risk for genetic disease.

8 In another reading already mentioned, "Assisted Reproduction," the President's Council on Bioethics contributes—at least indirectly—to an overall understanding of the ethics of IVF.

9 In this section, "human cloning" refers to *reproductive* cloning, not *research* cloning. (See the Introduction to Chapter 7.)

10 In the case of Dolly, the first cloned sheep, an entire somatic cell was fused with an enucleated egg by means of an electric current.

11 Strictly speaking, the clone's genotype will be almost identical to the genotype of the "parent." Mitochondrial DNA in the enucleated egg cell will also make a small contribution to the clone's genotype.

12 This valuable document is available on the council's website (http://www.bioethics.gov).

REPRODUCTIVE RISK, PRENATAL DIAGNOSIS, AND SELECTIVE ABORTION

IMPLICATIONS OF PRENATAL DIAGNOSIS FOR THE HUMAN RIGHT TO LIFE
Leon R. Kass

Setting aside a discussion of the moral problem of abortion in general, Kass focuses on some of the ethical difficulties associated with the abortion of fetuses known by amniocentesis to be genetically defective. He maintains that the practice of *genetic* abortion, inasmuch as it involves a qualitative assessment of fetuses, represents a threat to the "radical moral equality of all human beings." As a result of the practice of genetic abortion, Kass suggests, we will be inclined to take a more negative view of those who are genetically defective or otherwise "abnormal." Thus, we will be inclined to treat them in a second-class manner. Moreover, he contends, to commit ourselves to the practice of genetic abortion is to reflect acceptance of a very dangerous principle, that "defectives should not be born."

It is especially fitting on this occasion to begin by acknowledging how privileged I feel and how pleased I am to be a participant in this symposium. I suspect that I am not alone among the assembled in considering myself fortunate to be here. For I was conceived after antibiotics yet before amniocentesis, late enough to have benefited from medicine's ability to prevent and control fatal infectious diseases, yet early enough to have escaped from medicine's ability to prevent me from living to suffer from my genetic diseases. To be sure, my genetic vices are, as far as I know them, rather modest, taken individually—myopia, asthma and other allergies, bilateral

Reprinted by permission of the author and Kluwer Academic/Plenum Publishers from *Ethical Issues in Human Genetics,* edited by Bruce Hilton et al., 1973.

forefoot adduction, bowleggedness, loquaciousness, and pessimism, plus some four to eight as yet undiagnosed recessive lethal genes in the heterozygous condition—but, taken together, and if diagnosable prenatally, I might never have made it.

Just as I am happy to be here, so am I unhappy with what I shall have to say. Little did I realize when I first conceived the topic, "Implications of Prenatal Diagnosis for the Human Right to Life," what a painful and difficult labor it would lead to. More than once while this paper was gestating, I considered obtaining permission to abort it, on the grounds that, by prenatal diagnosis, I knew it to be defective. My lawyer told me that I was legally in the clear, but my conscience reminded me that I had made a commitment to deliver myself of this paper, flawed or not. Next time, I shall practice better contraception.

Any discussion of the ethical issues of genetic counseling and prenatal diagnosis is unavoidably haunted by a ghost called the morality of abortion. This ghost I shall not vex. More precisely, I shall not vex the reader by telling ghost stories. However, I would be neither surprised nor disappointed if my discussion of an admittedly related matter, the ethics of aborting the genetically defective, summons that hovering spirit to the reader's mind. For the morality of abortion is a matter not easily laid to rest, recent efforts to do so notwithstanding. A vote by the legislature of the State of New York can indeed legitimatize the disposal of fetuses, but not of the moral questions. But though the questions remain, there is likely to be little new that can be said about them, and certainly not by me.

Yet before leaving the general question of abortion, let me pause to drop some anchors for the discussion that follows. Despite great differences of opinion both as to what to think and how to reason about abortion, nearly everyone agrees that abortion is a moral issue.[1] What does this mean? Formally, it means that a woman seeking or refusing an abortion can expect to be asked to justify her action. And we can expect that she should be able to give reasons for her choice other than "I like it" or "I don't like it." Substantively, it means that, in the absence of good reasons for intervention, there is some presumption in favor of allowing the pregnancy to continue once it has begun. A common way of expressing this presumption is to say that "the fetus has a right to continued life."[2] In this context, disagreement concerning the moral permissibility of abortion concerns what rights (or interests or needs), and whose, override (take precedence over, or outweigh) this fetal "right." Even most of the "opponents" of abortion agree that the mother's right to live takes precedence, and that abortion to save her life is permissible, perhaps obligatory. Some believe that a woman's right to determine the number and spacing of her children takes precedence, while yet others argue that the need to curb population growth is, at least at this time, overriding.

Hopefully, this brief analysis of what it means to say that abortion is a moral issue is sufficient to establish two points. First, that the fetus is a living thing with some moral claim on us not to do it violence, and therefore, second, that justification must be given for destroying it.

Turning now from the general questions of the ethics of abortion, I wish to focus on the special ethical issues raised by the abortion of "defective" fetuses (so-called "abortion for fetal indications"). I shall consider only the cleanest cases, those cases where well-characterized genetic diseases are diagnosed with a high degree of certainty by means of amniocentesis, in order to side-step the added moral dilemmas posed when the diagnosis is suspected or possible, but unconfirmed. However, many of the questions I shall discuss could also be raised about cases where genetic analysis gives only a statistical prediction about the genotype of the fetus, and also about cases where the defect has an infectious or chemical rather than a genetic cause (e.g., rubella, thalidomide).

My first and possibly most difficult task is to show that there is anything left to discuss once we have agreed not to discuss the morality of abortion in general. There is a sense in which abortion for genetic defect is, after abortion to save the life of the mother, perhaps the most defensible kind of abortion. Certainly, it is a serious and not a frivolous reason for abortion, defended by its proponents in sober and rational speech—unlike justifications based upon the false notion that a fetus is a mere part of a woman's body, to be used and abused at her pleasure. Standing behind genetic abortion are serious and well-intentioned people, with reasonable ends in view: the prevention of genetic diseases, the elimination of suffering in families, the preservation of precious financial and medical resources, the protection of our genetic heritage. No profiteers, no sexploiters, no racists. No arguments about the connection of abortion with promiscuity and licentiousness, no perjured testimony about the mental health of the mother, no arguments about the seriousness of the population problem. In short, clear objective data, a worthy cause, decent men and women. If abortion, what better reason for it?

Yet if genetic abortion is but a happily wagging tail on the dog of abortion, it is simultaneously the nose of a camel protruding under a rather different tent. Precisely because the quality of the fetus is central to the decision to abort, the practice of genetic abortion has implications which go beyond those raised by abortion in general. What may be at stake here is the belief in the radical moral equality of all human beings, the belief that all human beings possess equally and independent of merit certain fundamental rights, one among which is, of course, the right to life.

To be sure, the belief that fundamental human rights belong equally to all human beings has been but an ideal, never realized, often ignored, sometimes shamelessly. Yet it has been perhaps the most powerful moral idea at work in the world for at least two centuries. It is this idea and ideal that animates most of the current political and social criticism around the globe. It is ironic that we should acquire the power to detect and eliminate the genetically unequal at a time when we have finally succeeded in removing much of the stigma and disgrace previously attached to victims of congenital illness, in providing them with improved care and support, and in preventing, by means of education, feelings of guilt on the part of their parents. One might even wonder whether the development of amniocentesis and prenatal diagnosis may represent a backlash against these same humanitarian and egalitarian tendencies in the practice of medicine, which, by helping to sustain to the age of reproduction persons with genetic disease has itself contributed to the increasing incidence of genetic disease, and with it, to increased pressures for genetic screening, genetic counseling, and genetic abortion.

No doubt our humanitatian and egalitarian principles and practices have caused us some new difficulties, but if we mean to weaken or turn our backs on them, we should do so consciously and thoughtfully. If, as I believe, the idea and practice of genetic abortion points in that direction, we should make ourselves aware of it. . . .

GENETIC ABORTION AND THE LIVING DEFECTIVE

The practice of abortion of the genetically defective will no doubt affect our view of and our behavior toward those abnormals who escape the net of detection and abortion. A child with Down's syndrome or with hemophilia or with muscular dystrophy born at a time when most of his (potential) fellow sufferers were destroyed prenatally is liable to be looked upon by the community as one unfit to be alive, as a second-class (or even lower) human type. He may be seen as a person who need not have been, and who would not have been, if only someone had gotten to him in time.

The parents of such children are also likely to treat them differently, especially if the mother would have wished but failed to get an amniocentesis because of ignorance, poverty, or distance from the testing station, or if the prenatal diagnosis was in error. In such cases, parents are especially likely to resent the child. They may be disinclined to give it the kind of care they might have before the advent of amniocentesis and genetic abortion, rationalizing that a second-class specimen is not entitled to first-class treatment. If pressed to do so, say by physicians, the parents might refuse, and the courts may become involved. This has already begun to happen.

In Maryland, parents of a child with Down syndrome refused permission to have the child operated on for an intestinal obstruction present at birth. The physicians and the hospital sought an injunction to require the parents to allow surgery. The judge ruled in favor of the parents, despite what I understand to be the weight of precedent to the contrary, on the grounds that the child was Mongoloid, that is, had the child been "normal," the decision would have gone the other way. Although the decision was not appealed to and hence not affirmed by a higher court, we can see through the prism of this case the possibility that the new powers of human genetics will strip the blindfold from the lady of justice and will make official the dangerous doctrine that some men are more equal than others.

The abnormal child may also feel resentful. A child with Down syndrome or Tay-Sachs disease will probably never know or care, but what about a child with hemophilia or with Turner's syndrome? In the past decade, with medical knowledge and power over the prenatal child increasing and with parental authority over the postnatal child decreasing, we have seen the appearance of a new type of legal action, suits for wrongful life. Children have brought suit against their parents (and others) seeking to recover damages for physical and social handicaps inextricably tied to their birth (e.g., congenital deformities, congenital syphilis, illegitimacy). In some of the American cases, the courts have recognized the justice of the child's claim (that he was injured due to parental negligence), although they have so far refused to award damages, due to policy considerations. In other countries, e.g., in Germany, judgments with compensation have gone for the plaintiffs. With the spread of amniocentesis and genetic abortion, we can only expect such cases to increase. And here it will be the soft-hearted rather than the hard-hearted judges who will establish the doctrine of second-class human beings, out of compassion for the mutants who escaped the traps set out for them.

It may be argued that I am dealing with a problem which, even if it is real, will affect very few people. It may be suggested that very few will escape the traps once we have set them properly and widely, once people are informed about amniocentesis, once the power to detect prenatally grows to its full capacity, and once our "superstitious" opposition to abortion dies out or is extirpated. But in order even to come close to this vision of success, amniocentesis will have to become part of every pregnancy—either by making it mandatory, like the test for syphilis, or by making it "routine medical practice," like the Pap smear. Leaving aside the other problems with universal amniocentesis, we could expect that the problem for the few who escape is likely to be even worse precisely because they will be few.

The point, however, should be generalized. How will we come to view and act toward the many "abnormals" that will remain among us—the retarded, the crippled, the senile, the deformed, and the true mutants—once we embark on a program to root out genetic abnormality? For it must be remembered that we shall always have abnormals—some who escape detection or whose disease is undetectable *in utero,* others as a result of new mutations, birth injuries, accidents, maltreatment, or disease—who will require our care and protection. The existence of "defectives" cannot be fully prevented, not even by totalitarian breeding and weeding programs. Is it not likely that our principle with respect to these people will change from "We try harder" to "Why

accept second best?" The idea of "the unwanted because abnormal child" may become a self-fulfilling prophecy, whose consequences may be worse than those of the abnormality itself.

GENETIC AND OTHER DEFECTIVES

The mention of other abnormals points to a second danger of the practice of genetic abortion. Genetic abortion may come to be seen not so much as the prevention of genetic disease, but as the prevention of birth of defective or abnormal children—and, in a way, understandably so. For in the case of what other diseases does preventive medicine consist in the elimination of the patient-at-risk? Moreover, the very language used to discuss genetic disease leads us to the easy but wrong conclusion that the afflicted fetus or person is rather than has a disease. True, one is partly defined by his genotype, but only partly. A person is more than his disease. And yet we slide easily from the language of possession to the language of identity, from "He has hemophilia" to "He is a hemophiliac," from "She has diabetes" through "She is diabetic" to "She is a diabetic," from "The fetus has Down syndrome" to "The fetus is a Down's." This way of speaking supports the belief that it is defective persons (or potential persons) that are being eliminated, rather than diseases.

If this is so, then it becomes simply accidental that the defect has a genetic cause. Surely, it is only because of the high regard for medicine and science, and for the accuracy of genetic diagnosis, that genotypic defectives are likely to be the first to go. But once the principle, "Defectives should not be born," is established, grounds other than cytological and biochemical may very well be sought. Even ignoring racialists and others equally misguided—of course, they cannot be ignored—we should know that there are social scientists, for example, who believe that one can predict with a high degree of accuracy how a child will turn out from a careful, systematic study of the socio-economic and psycho-dynamic environment into which he is born and in which he grows up. They might press for the prevention of socio-psychological disease, even of "criminality," by means of prenatal environmental diagnosis and abortion. I have heard rumor that a crude, unscientific form of eliminating potential "phenotypic defectives" is already being practiced in some cities, in that submission to abortion is allegedly being made a condition for the receipt of welfare payments. "Defectives should not be born" is a principle without limits. We can ill-afford to have it established.

Up to this point, I have been discussing the possible implications of the practice of genetic abortion for our belief in and adherence to the idea that, at least in fundamental human matters such as life and liberty, all men are to be considered as equals, that for these matters we should ignore as irrelevant the real qualitative differences amongst men, however important these differences may be for other purposes. Those who are concerned about abortion fear that the permissible time of eliminating the unwanted will be moved forward along the time continuum, against newborns, infants, and children. Similarly, I suggest that we should be concerned lest the attack on gross genetic inequality in fetuses be advanced along the continuum of quality and into the later stages of life.

I am not engaged in predicting the future; I am not saying that amniocentesis and genetic abortion will lead down the road to Nazi Germany. Rather, I am suggesting that the principles underlying genetic abortion simultaneously justify many further steps down that road. The point was very well made by Abraham Lincoln:

> If A can prove, however conclusively, that he may, of right, enslave B—Why may not B snatch the same argument and prove equally, that he may enslave A?
>
> You say A is white, and B is black. It is color, then; the lighter having the right to enslave the darker? Take care. By this rule, you are to be slave to the first man you meet with a fairer skin than your own.
>
> You do not mean color exactly? You mean the whites are intellectually the superiors of the blacks, and, therefore have the right to enslave them? Take care again. By this rule, you are to be slave to the first man you meet with an intellect superior to your own.

> But, say you, it is a question of interest; and, if you can make it your interest, you have the right to enslave another. Very well. And if he can make it his interest, he has the right to enslave you.[3]

Perhaps I have exaggerated the dangers; perhaps we will not abandon our inexplicable preference for generous humanitarianism over consistency. But we should indeed be cautious and move slowly as we give serious consideration to the question "What price the perfect baby?"[4] . . .

NOTES

1 This strikes me as by far the most important inference to be drawn from the fact that men in different times and cultures have answered the abortion question differently. Seen in this light, the differing and changing answers themselves suggest that it is a question not easily put under, at least not for very long.

2 Other ways include: one should not do violence to living or growing things; life is sacred; respect nature; fetal life has value; refrain from taking innocent life; protect and preserve life. As some have pointed out, the terms chosen are of different weight, and would require reasons of different weight to tip the balance in favor of abortion. My choice of the "rights" terminology is not meant to beg the questions of whether such rights really exist, or of where they come from. However, the notion of a "fetal right to life" presents only a little more difficulty in this regard than does the notion of a "human right to life," since the former does not depend on a claim that the human fetus is already "human." In my sense of terms "right" and "life," we might even say that a dog or fetal dog has a "right to life," and that it would be cruel and immoral for a man to go around performing abortions even on dogs for no good reason.

3 Lincoln, A. (1854). In *The Collected Works of Abraham Lincoln,* R. P. Basler, editor. New Brunswick, New Jersey, Rutgers University Press, Vol. II, p. 222.

4 For a discussion of the possible biological rather than moral price of attempts to prevent the birth of defective children see Motulsky, A. G., G. R. Fraser, and J. Felsenstein (1971). In Symposium on Intra-uterine Diagnosis, D. Bergsma, editor. *Birth Defects: Original Article Series,* Vol. 7, No. 5. Also see Neel, J. (1972). In *Early Diagnosis of Human Genetic Defects: Scientific and Ethical Considerations,* M. Harris, editor. Washington, D.C., U.S. Government Printing Office, pp. 366–380.

GENETICS AND REPRODUCTIVE RISK:
CAN HAVING CHILDREN BE IMMORAL?

Laura M. Purdy

Purdy argues that it can be morally wrong to reproduce in circumstances of genetic risk, most clearly in cases where there is a high risk of serious genetic disease. In developing her overall argument, she is committed to the view that we have a duty to try to provide a *minimally satisfying life* for our children. Much of Purdy's analysis focuses on Huntington's disease, and she emphasizes how the emergence of reliable genetic testing has opened up new possibilities for those at risk of passing on the disease.

Is it morally permissible for me to have children?[1] A decision to procreate is surely one of the most significant decisions a person can make. So it would seem that it ought not to be made without some moral soul-searching.

There are many reasons why one might hesitate to bring children into this world if one is concerned about their welfare. Some are rather general, like the deteriorating environment or the prospect of poverty. Others have a narrower focus, like continuing civil war in Ireland, or the lack of essential social support for child rearing persons in the United States. Still others may be relevant only to individuals at risk of passing harmful diseases to their offspring.

There are many causes of misery in this world, and most of them are unrelated to genetic disease. In the general scheme of things, human misery is most efficiently reduced by concentrating on noxious social and political arrangements. Nonetheless, we shouldn't ignore preventable harm just because it is confined to a relatively small corner of life. So the question arises: can it be wrong to have a child because of genetic risk factors?[2]

Unsurprisingly, most of the debate about this issue has focused on prenatal screening and abortion: much useful information about a given fetus can be made available by recourse to prenatal testing. This fact has meant that moral questions about reproduction have become entwined with abortion politics, to the detriment of both. The abortion connection has made it especially difficult to think about whether it is wrong to prevent a child from coming into being since doing so might involve what many people see as wrongful killing; yet there is no necessary link between the two. Clearly, the existence of genetically compromised children can be prevented not only by aborting already existing fetuses but also by preventing conception in the first place.

Worse yet, many discussions simply assume a particular view of abortion, without any recognition of other possible positions and the difference they make in how people understand the issues. For example, those who object to aborting fetuses with genetic problems often argue that doing so would undermine our conviction that all humans are in some important sense equal.[3] However, this position rests on the assumption that conception marks the point at which humans are endowed with a right to life. So aborting fetuses with genetic problems looks morally the same as killing "imperfect" people without their consent.

This position raises two separate issues. One pertains to the legitimacy of different views on abortion. Despite the conviction of many abortion activists to the contrary, I believe that ethically respectable views can be found on different sides of the debate, including one that sees fetuses as developing humans without any serious moral claim on continued life. There is no space here to address the details, and doing so would be once again to fall into the trap of letting the abortion question swallow up all others. Fortunately, this issue need not be resolved here. However, opponents of abortion need to face the fact that many thoughtful individuals do not *see* fetuses as moral persons. It follows that their reasoning process and hence the implications of their decisions are radically different from those envisioned by opponents of prenatal screening and abortion. So where the latter see genetic abortion as murdering people who just don't measure up, the former see it as a way to prevent the development of persons who are more likely to live miserable lives. This is consistent with a world view that values persons equally and holds that each deserves high quality life. Some of those who object to genetic abortion appear to be oblivious to these psychological and logical facts. It follows that the nightmare scenarios they paint for us are beside the point: many people simply do not share the assumptions that make them plausible.

How are these points relevant to my discussion? My primary concern here is to argue that conception can sometimes be morally wrong on grounds of genetic risk, although this judgment will not apply to those who accept the moral legitimacy of abortion and are willing to employ prenatal screening and selective abortion. If my case is solid, then those who oppose abortion must be especially careful not to conceive in certain cases, as they are, of course, free to follow their conscience about abortion. Those like myself who do not see abortion as murder have more ways to prevent birth.

HUNTINGTON'S DISEASE

There is always some possibility that reproduction will result in a child with a serious disease or handicap. Genetic counselors can help individuals determine whether they are at unusual risk and, as the Human Genome Project rolls on, their knowledge will increase by quantum leaps. As this knowledge becomes available, I believe we ought to use it to determine whether possible children are at risk *before* they are conceived.

I want in this paper to defend the thesis that it is morally wrong to reproduce when we know there is a high risk of transmitting a serious disease or defect. This thesis holds that some reproductive acts are wrong, and my argument puts the burden of proof on those who disagree with it to show why its

conclusions can be overridden. Hence it denies that people should be free to reproduce mindless of the consequences.[4] However, as moral argument, it should be taken as a proposal for further debate and discussion. It is not, by itself, an argument in favor of legal prohibitions of reproduction.[5]

There is a huge range of genetic diseases. Some are quickly lethal; others kill more slowly, if at all. Some are mainly physical, some mainly mental; others impair both kinds of function. Some interfere tremendously with normal functioning, others less. Some are painful, some are not. There seems to be considerable agreement that rapidly lethal diseases, especially those, like Tay-Sachs, accompanied by painful deterioration, should be prevented even at the cost of abortion. Conversely, there seems to be substantial agreement that relatively trivial problems, especially cosmetic ones, would not be legitimate grounds for abortion.[6] In short, there are cases ranging from low risk of mild disease or disability to high risk of serious disease or disability. Although it is difficult to decide where the duty to refrain from procreation becomes compelling, I believe that there are some clear cases. I have chosen to focus on Huntington's Disease to illustrate the kinds of concrete issues such decisions entail. However, the arguments presented here are also relevant to many other genetic diseases.[7]

The symptoms of Huntington's Disease usually begin between the ages of thirty and fifty. It happens this way:

> Onset is insidious. Personality changes (obstinacy, moodiness, lack of initiative) frequently antedate or accompany the involuntary choreic movements. These usually appear first in the face, neck, and arms, and are jerky, irregular, and stretching in character. Contractions of the facial muscles result in grimaces; those of the respiratory muscles, lips, and tongue lead to hesitating, explosive speech. Irregular movements of the trunk are present; the gait is shuffling and dancing. Tendon reflexes are increased. . . . Some patients display a fatuous euphoria; others are spiteful, irascible, destructive, and violent. Paranoid reactions are common. Poverty of thought and impairment of attention, memory, and judgment occur. As the disease progresses, walking becomes impossible, swallowing difficult, and dementia profound. Suicide is not uncommon.[8]

The illness lasts about fifteen years, terminating in death.

Huntington's Disease is an autosomal dominant disease, meaning that it is caused by a single defective gene located on a non-sex chromosome. It is passed from one generation to the next via affected individuals. Each child of such an affected person has a fifty percent risk of inheriting the gene and thus of eventually developing the disease, even if he or she was born before the parent's disease was evident.[9]

Until recently, Huntington's Disease was especially problematic because most affected individuals did not know whether they had the gene for the disease until well into their childbearing years. So they had to decide about childbearing before knowing whether they could transmit the disease or not. If, in time, they did not develop symptoms of the disease, then their children could know they were not at risk for the disease. If unfortunately they did develop symptoms, then each of their children could know there was a fifty percent chance that they, too, had inherited the gene. In both cases, the children faced a period of prolonged anxiety as to whether they would develop the disease. Then, in the 1980s, thanks in part to an energetic campaign by Nancy Wexler, a genetic marker was found that, in certain circumstances, could tell people with a relatively high degree of probability whether or not they had the gene for the disease.[10] Finally, in March 1993, the defective gene itself was discovered.[11] Now individuals can find out whether they carry the gene for the disease, and prenatal screening can tell us whether a given fetus has inherited it. These technological developments change the moral scene substantially.

How serious are the risks involved in Huntington's Disease? Geneticists often think a ten percent risk is high.[12] But risk assessment also depends on what is at stake: the worse the possible outcome the more undesirable an otherwise small risk seems. In medicine, as elsewhere, people may regard the same result quite differently. But for devastating diseases like Huntington's this part of the judgment should be unproblematic: no one wants a loved one to suffer in this way.[13]

There may still be considerable disagreement about the acceptability of a given risk. So it would be difficult in many circumstances to say how we should respond to a particular risk. Nevertheless, there are good grounds for a conservative approach, for it is reasonable to take special precautions to avoid very bad consequences, even if the risk is small. But the possible consequences here *are* very bad: a child who may inherit Huntington's Disease has a much greater than average chance of being subjected to severe and prolonged suffering. And it is one thing to risk one's own welfare, but quite another to do so for others and without their consent.

Is this judgment about Huntington's Disease really defensible? People appear to have quite different opinions. Optimists argue that a child born into a family afflicted with Huntington's Disease has a reasonable chance of living a satisfactory life. After all, even children born of an afflicted parent still have a fifty percent chance of escaping the disease. And even if afflicted themselves, such people will probably enjoy some thirty years of healthy life before symptoms appear. It is also possible, although not at all likely, that some might not mind the symptoms caused by the disease. Optimists can point to diseased persons who have lived fruitful lives, as well as those who seem genuinely glad to be alive. One is Rick Donohue, a sufferer from the Joseph family disease: "You know, if my mom hadn't had me, I wouldn't be here for the life I have had. So there is a good possibility I will have children."[14] Optimists therefore conclude that it would be a shame if these persons had not lived.

Pessimists concede some of these facts, but take a less sanguine view of them. They think a fifty percent risk of serious disease like Huntington's appallingly high. They suspect that many children born into afflicted families are liable to spend their youth in dreadful anticipation and fear of the disease. They expect that the disease, if it appears, will be perceived as a tragic and painful end to a blighted life. They point out that Rick Donohue is still young, and has not experienced the full horror of his sickness. It is also well-known that some young persons have such a dilated sense of time that they can hardly envision themselves at thirty or forty, so the prospect of pain at that age is unreal to them.[15]

More empirical research on the psychology and life history of sufferers and potential sufferers is clearly needed to decide whether optimists or pessimists have a more accurate picture of the experiences of individuals at risk. But given that some will surely realize pessimists' worst fears, it seems unfair to conclude that the pleasures of those who deal best with the situation simply cancel out the suffering of those others when that suffering could be avoided altogether.

I think that these points indicate that the morality of procreation in situations like this demands further investigation. I propose to do this by looking first at the position of the possible child, then at that of the potential parent.

POSSIBLE CHILDREN AND POTENTIAL PARENTS

The first task in treating the problem from the child's point of view is to find a way of referring to possible future offspring without seeming to confer some sort of morally significant existence upon them. I will follow the convention of calling children who might be born in the future but who are not now conceived "possible" children, offspring, individuals, or persons.

Now, what claims about children or possible children are relevant to the morality of childbearing in the circumstances being considered? Of primary importance is the judgment that we ought to try to provide every child with something like a minimally satisfying life. I am not altogether sure how best to formulate this standard but I want clearly to reject the view that it is morally permissible to conceive individuals so long as we do not expect them to be so miserable that they wish they were dead.[16] I believe that this kind of moral minimalism is thoroughly unsatisfactory and that not many people would really want to live in a world where it was the prevailing standard. Its lure is that it puts few demands on us, but its price is the scant attention it pays to human well-being.

How might the judgment that we have a duty to try to provide a minimally satisfying life for our children be justified? It could, I think, be derived fairly straightforwardly from either utilitarian or contractarian theories of justice, although there is no space here for discussion of the details. The net result of such analysis would be the conclusion that neglecting this duty would create unnecessary unhappiness or unfair disadvantage for some persons.

Of course, this line of reasoning confronts us with the need to spell out what is meant by "minimally satisfying" and what a standard based on this concept would require of us. Conceptions of a minimally satisfying life vary tremendously among societies and also within them. *De Rigueur* in some circles are private music lessons and trips to Europe, while in others providing eight years of schooling is a major accomplishment. But there is no need to consider this complication at length here since we are concerned only with health as a prerequisite for a minimally satisfying life. Thus, as we draw out what such a standard might require of us, it seems reasonable to retreat to the more limited claim that parents should try to ensure something like normal health for their children. It might be thought that even this moderate claim is unsatisfactory since in some places debilitating conditions are the norm, but one could circumvent this objection by saying that parents ought to try to provide for their children health normal for that culture, even though it may be inadequate if measured by some outside standard.[17] This conservative position would still justify efforts to avoid the birth of children at risk for Huntington's Disease and other serious genetic diseases in virtually all societies.[18]

This view is reinforced by the following considerations. Given that possible children do not presently exist as actual individuals, they do not have a right to be brought into existence, and hence no one is maltreated by measures to avoid the conception of a possible person. Therefore, the conservative course that avoids the conception of those who would not be expected to enjoy a minimally satisfying life is at present the only fair course of action. The alternative is a laissez-faire approach which brings into existence the lucky, but only at the expense of the unlucky. Notice that attempting to avoid the creation of the unlucky does not necessarily lead to *fewer* people being brought into being; the question boils down to taking steps to bring those with better prospects into existence, instead of those with worse ones.

I have so far argued that if people with Huntington's Disease are unlikely to live minimally satisfying lives, then those who might pass it on should not have genetically related children. This is consonant with the principle that the greater the danger of serious problems, the stronger the duty to avoid them. But this principle is in conflict with what people think of as the right to reproduce. How might one decide which should take precedence?

Expecting people to forego having genetically related children might seem to demand too great a sacrifice of them. But before reaching that conclusion we need to ask what is really at stake. One reason for wanting children is to experience family life, including love, companionship, watching kids grow, sharing their pains and triumphs, and helping to form members of the next generation. Other reasons emphasize the validation of parents as individuals within a continuous family line, children as a source of immortality, or perhaps even the gratification of producing partial replicas of oneself. Children may also be desired in an effort to prove that one is an adult, to try to cement a marriage or to benefit parents economically.

Are there alternative ways of satisfying these desires? Adoption or new reproductive technologies can fulfil many of them without passing on known genetic defects. Replacements for sperm have been available for many years via artificial insemination by donor. More recently, egg donation, sometimes in combination with contract pregnancy,[19] has been used to provide eggs for women who prefer not to use their own. Eventually it may be possible to clone individual humans, although that now seems a long way off. All of these approaches to avoiding the use of particular genetic material are controversial and have generated much debate. I believe that tenable moral versions of each do exist.[20]

None of these methods permits people to extend both genetic lines, or realize the desire for immortality or for children who resemble both parents; nor is it clear that such alternatives will necessarily succeed in proving that one is an adult, cementing a marriage, or providing economic benefits. Yet, many people feel these desires strongly. Now, I am sympathetic to William James's dictum regarding desires: "Take any demand, however slight, which any creature, however weak, may make. Ought it not, for its own sole sake be satisfied? If not, prove why not."[21] Thus a world where more desires are satisfied is generally better than one where fewer are. However, not all desires can be legitimately satisfied

since, as James suggests, there may be good reasons—such as the conflict of duty and desire—why some should be overruled.

Fortunately, further scrutiny of the situation reveals that there are good reasons why people should attempt—with appropriate social support—to talk themselves out of the desires in question or to consider novel ways of fulfilling them. Wanting to see the genetic line continued is not particularly rational when it brings a sinister legacy of illness and death. The desire for immortality cannot really be satisfied anyway, and people need to face the fact that what really matters is how they behave in their own lifetime. And finally, the desire for children who physically resemble one is understandable, but basically narcissistic, and its fulfillment cannot be guaranteed even by normal reproduction. There are other ways of proving one is an adult, and other ways of cementing marriages—and children don't necessarily do either. Children, especially prematurely ill children, may not provide the expected economic benefits anyway. Nongenetically related children may also provide benefits similar to those that would have been provided by genetically related ones, and expected economic benefit is, in many cases, a morally questionable reason for having children.

Before the advent of reliable genetic testing, the options of people in Huntington's families were cruelly limited. On the one hand, they could have children, but at the risk of eventual crippling illness and death for them. On the other, they could refrain from childbearing, sparing their possible children from significant risk of inheriting this disease, perhaps frustrating intense desires to procreate—only to discover, in some cases, that their sacrifice was unnecessary because they did not develop the disease. Or they could attempt to adopt or try new reproductive approaches.

Reliable genetic testing has opened up new possibilities. Those at risk who wish to have children can get tested. If they test positive, they know their possible children are at risk. Those who are opposed to abortion must be especially careful to avoid conception if they are to behave responsibly. Those not opposed to abortion can responsibly conceive children, but only if they are willing to test each fetus and abort those who carry the gene. If individuals at risk test negative, they are home free.

What about those who cannot face the test for themselves? They can do prenatal testing and abort fetuses who carry the defective gene. A clearly positive test also implies that the parent is affected, although negative tests do not rule out that possibility. Prenatal testing can thus bring knowledge that enables one to avoid passing the disease to others, but only, in some cases, at the cost of coming to know with certainty that one will indeed develop the disease. This situation raises with peculiar force the question of whether parental responsibility requires people to get tested.

Some people think that we should recognize a right "not to know." It seems to me that such a right could be defended only where ignorance does not put others at serious risk. So if people are prepared to forego genetically related children, they need not get tested. But if they want genetically related children then they must do whatever is necessary to ensure that affected babies are not the result. There is, after all, something inconsistent about the claim that one has a right to be shielded from the truth, even if the price is to risk inflicting on one's children the same dread disease one cannot even face in oneself.

In sum, until we can be assured that Huntington's Disease does not prevent people from living a minimally satisfying life, individuals at risk for the disease have a moral duty to try not to bring affected babies into this world. There are now enough options available so that this duty needn't frustrate their reasonable desires. Society has a corresponding duty to facilitate moral behavior on the part of individuals. Such support ranges from the narrow and concrete (like making sure that medical testing and counseling is available to all) to the more general social environment that guarantees that all pregnancies are voluntary, that pronatalism is eradicated, and that women are treated with respect regardless of the reproductive options they choose.

NOTES

1 This paper is loosely based on "Genetic Diseases: Can Having Children Be Immoral?" originally published in *Genetics Now,* ed. John L. Buckley (Washington, DC: University Press of America, 1978) and subsequently anthologized in a number of medical ethics texts. Thanks to Thomas Mappes and David DeGrazia for their helpful suggestions about updating the paper.

2 I focus on genetic considerations, although with the advent of AIDS the scope of the general question here could be expanded. There are two reasons for sticking to this relatively narrow formulation. One is that dealing with a smaller chunk of the problem may help us think more clearly, while realizing that some conclusions may nonetheless be relevant to the larger problem. The other is the peculiar capacity of some genetic problems to affect ever more individuals in the future.

3 For example, see Leon Kass, "Implications of Prenatal Diagnosis for the Human Right to Life," *Ethical Issues in Human Genetics,* eds. Bruce Hilton et al. (New York: Plenum Press, 1973).

4 This is, of course, a very broad thesis. I defend an even broader version in "Loving Future People," *Reproduction, Ethics and the Law,* ed. Joan Callahan (Bloomington: Indiana University Press, forthcoming).

5 Why would we want to resist legal enforcement of every moral conclusion? First, legal action has many costs, costs not necessarily worth paying in particular cases. Second, legal enforcement would tend to take the matter in question out of the realm of debate and treat it as settled. But in many cases, especially where mores or technology are rapidly evolving, we don't want that to happen. Third, legal enforcement would undermine individual freedom and decision-making capacity. In some cases, the ends envisioned are important enough to warrant putting up with these disadvantages, but that remains to be shown in each case.

6 Those who do not see fetuses as moral persons with a right to life may nonetheless hold that abortion is justifiable in these cases. I argue at some length elsewhere that lesser defects can cause great suffering. Once we are clear that there is nothing discriminatory about failing to conceive particular possible individuals, it makes sense, other things being equal, to avoid the prospect of such pain if we can. Naturally, other things rarely are equal. In the first place, many problems go undiscovered until a baby is born. Secondly, there are often substantial costs associated with screening programs. Thirdly, although women should be encouraged to consider the moral dimensions of routine pregnancy, we do not want it to be so fraught with tension that it becomes a miserable experience. (See "Loving Future People.")

7 It should be noted that failing to conceive a single individual can affect many lives: in 1916, nine hundred and sixty-two cases could be traced from six seventeenth-century arrivals in America. See Gordon Rattray Taylor, *The Biological Time Bomb* (New York, 1968), p. 176.

8 *The Merck Manual* (Rahway, NJ: Merck, 1972), pp. 1363, 1346. We now know that the age of onset and severity of the disease is related to the number of abnormal replications of the glutamine code on the abnormal gene. See Andrew Revkin, "Hunting Down Huntington's," *Discover,* December 1993, p. 108.

9 Hymie Gordon, "Genetic Counseling," *JAMA,* Vol. 217, n. 9 (August 30, 1971), p. 1346.

10 See Revkin, "Hunting Down Huntington's," pp. 99–108.

11 "Gene for Huntington's Disease Discovered," *Human Genome News,* Vol. 5, n. 1 (May 1993), p. 5.

12 Charles Smith, Susan Holloway, and Alan E. H. Emery, "Individuals at Risk in Families—Genetic Disease," *Journal of Medical Genetics,* Vol. 8 (1971), p. 453.

13 To try to separate the issue of the gravity of the disease from the existence of a given individual, compare this situation with how we would assess a parent who neglected to vaccinate an existing child against a hypothetical viral version of Huntington's.

14 *The New York Times,* September 30, 1975, p. 1, col. 6. The Joseph family disease is similar to Huntington's Disease except that symptoms start appearing in the twenties. Rick Donohue was in his early twenties at the time he made this statement.

15 I have talked to college students who believe that they will have lived fully and be ready to die at those ages. It is astonishing how one's perspective changes over time, and how ages that one once associated with senility and physical collapse come to seem the prime of human life.

16 The view I am rejecting has been forcefully articulated by Derek Parfit, *Reasons and Persons* (Oxford: Oxford University Press, 1984). For more discussion, see "Loving Future People."

17 I have some qualms about this response since I fear that some human groups are so badly off that it might still be wrong for them to procreate, even if that would mean great changes in their cultures. But this is a complicated issue that needs its own investigation.

18 Again, a troubling exception might be the isolated Venezuelan group Nancy Wexler found where, because of in-breeding, a large proportion of the population is affected by Huntington's. See Revkin, "Hunting Down Huntington's."

19 Or surrogacy, as it has been popularly known. I think that "contract pregnancy" is more accurate and more respectful of women. Eggs can be provided either by a woman who also gestates the fetus or by a third party.

20 The most powerful objections to new reproductive technologies and arrangements concern possible bad consequences for women. However, I do not think that the arguments against them on these grounds have yet shown the dangers to be as great as some believe. So although it is perhaps true that new reproductive technologies and arrangements shouldn't be used lightly, avoiding the conceptions discussed here is well worth the risk. For a series of viewpoints on this issue, including my own "Another Look at Contract Pregnancy," see Helen B. Holmes, *Issues in Reproductive Technology I: An Anthology* (New York: Garland Press, 1992).

21 *Essays in Pragmatism,* ed. A. Castell (New York, 1948), p. 73.

REPRODUCTIVE TECHNOLOGIES

IVF: THE SIMPLE CASE
Peter Singer

Singer identifies seven distinct objections that have been made to the use of in vitro fertilization (IVF) even in the "simple case"—a case in which a married couple is infertile, only eggs and sperm provided by the couple are involved, and all resulting embryos are transferred to the wife's uterus. He takes some of these objections more seriously than others but ultimately concludes that none should "count against going ahead" with IVF in the simple case.

The so-called simple case of IVF is that in which a married, infertile couple use an egg taken from the

From *Ethical Issues at the Outset of Life* (1987), edited by William B. Weil, Jr., and Martin Benjamin, pp. 44–49. Based on work done with Deane Wells and previously published in *Making Babies* (revised edition, 1985). Reprinted with the permission of Scribner, an imprint of Simon & Schuster Adult Publishing Group. Copyright © 1984, 1985 by Peter Singer and Deane Wells.

wife and sperm taken from the husband, and all embryos created are inserted into the womb of the wife. This case allows us to consider the ethics of IVF in itself, without the complications of the many other issues that can arise in different circumstances. Then we can go on to look at these complications separately.

THE TECHNIQUE

The technique itself is now well known and is fast becoming a routine part of infertility treatment in many countries. The infertile woman is given a hormone treatment to induce her ovaries to produce more than one egg in her next cycle. Her hormone levels are carefully monitored to detect the precise moment at which the eggs are ripening. At this time the eggs are removed. This is usually done by laparoscopy, a minor operation in which a fine tube is inserted into the woman's abdomen and the egg is sucked out up the tube. A laparoscope, a kind of periscope illuminated by fiber optics, is also inserted into the abdomen so that the surgeon can locate the place where the ripe egg is to be found. Instead of laparoscopy, some IVF teams are now using ultrasound techniques, which eliminate the need for a general anesthetic.

Once the eggs have been collected they are placed in culture in small glass dishes known as petri dishes, not in test tubes despite the popular label of "test-tube babies." Sperm is then obtained from the male partner by means of masturbation and placed with the egg. Fertilization follows in at least 80 percent of the ripe eggs. The resulting embryos are allowed to cleave once or twice and are usually transferred to the woman some 48 to 72 hours after fertilization. The actual transfer is done via the vagina and is a simple procedure.

It is after the transfer, when the embryo is back in the uterus and beyond the scrutiny of medical science, that things are most likely to go wrong. Even with the most experienced IVF teams, the majority of embryos transferred fail to implant in the uterus. One pregnancy for every five transfers is currently considered to be a good working average for a competent IVF team. Many of the newer teams fail to achieve anything like this rate. Nevertheless, there are so many units around the world now practicing IVF that thousands of babies have been produced as a result of the technique. IVF has ceased to be experimental and is now a routine, if still "last resort" method of treating some forms of infertility.

OBJECTIONS TO THE SIMPLE CASE

There is some opposition to IVF even in the simple case. The most frequently heard objections are as follows:

1. IVF is unnatural.
2. IVF is risky for the offspring.
3. IVF separates the procreative and the conjugal aspects of marriage and so damages the marital relationship.
4. IVF is illicit because it involves masturbation.
5. Adoption is a better solution to the problem of childlessness.
6. IVF is an expensive luxury and the resources would be better spent elsewhere.
7. IVF allows increased male control over reproduction and hence threatens the status of women in the community.

We can deal swiftly with the first four of these objections. If we were to reject medical advances on the grounds that they are "unnatural" we would be rejecting modern medicine as a whole, for the very purpose of the medical enterprise is to resist the ravages of nature which would otherwise shorten our lives and make them much less pleasant. If anything is in accordance with the nature of our species, it is the application of our intelligence to overcome adverse situations in which we find ourselves. The application of IVF to infertile couples is a classic example of this application of human intelligence.

The claim that IVF is risky for the offspring is one that was argued with great force before IVF became a widely used technique. It is sufficient to note that the results of IVF so far have happily refuted these fears. The most recent Australian figures, for example, based on 934 births, indicate that the rate of abnormality was 2.7%, which is very close to the national average of 1.5%. When we take into account the greater average age of women seeking IVF, as compared with the childbearing population as a whole, it does not seem that the *in vitro* technique itself adds to the risk of an abnormal offspring. This view is reinforced by the fact that the abnormalities were all ones that arise with the ordinary method of reproduction; there have been no new "monsters" produced by IVF (1). Perhaps we still cannot claim with statistical certainty that the risk of defect is no higher with IVF than with the more common method of conception; but if the risk is higher at all, it would appear to be only very slightly higher, and still within limits which may be considered acceptable.

The third and fourth objections have been urged by spokesmen for certain religious groups, but they are difficult to defend outside the confines of particular religions. Few infertile couples will take seriously the view that their marital relationship will be damaged if they use the technique which offers them the best chance of having their own child. It is in any case extraordinarily paternalistic for anyone else to tell a couple that they should not use IVF because it will harm their marriage. That, surely, is for them to decide.

The objection to masturbation comes from a similar source and can be even more swiftly dismissed. Religious prohibitions on masturbation are taboos from past times which even religious spokesmen are beginning to consider outdated. Moreover, even if one could defend a prohibition on masturbation for sexual pleasure—perhaps on the (very tenuous) ground that sexual activity is wrong unless it is directed either toward procreation or toward the strengthening of the bond between marriage partners—it would be absurd to extend a prohibition with that kind of rationale to a case in which masturbation is being used in the context of a marriage and precisely in order to make reproduction possible. (The fact that some religions do persist in regarding masturbation as wrong, even in these circumstances, is indicative of the folly of an ethical system based on absolute rules, irrespective of the circumstances in which those rules are being applied, or the consequences of their application.)

OVERPOPULATION AND THE ALLOCATION OF RESOURCES

The next two objections, however, deserve more careful consideration. In an overpopulated world in which there are so many children who cannot be properly fed and cared for, there is something incongruous about using all the ingenuity of modern medicine to create more children. And similarly, when there are so many deaths caused by preventable diseases, is there not something wrong with the priorities which lead us to develop expensive techniques for overcoming the relatively less serious problem of infertility?

These objections are sound to the following extent: in an ideal world we would find loving families for unwanted children before we created additional children; and in an ideal world we would clear up all the preventable ill-health and malnutrition-related diseases before we went on to tackle the problem of infertility. But is it appropriate to ask, of IVF alone, whether it can stand the test of measurement against what we would do in an ideal world? In an ideal world, none of us would consume more than our fair share of resources. We would not drive expensive cars while others die for the lack of drugs costing a few cents. We would not eat a diet rich in wastefully produced animal products while others cannot get enough to nourish their bodies. We cannot demand more of infertile couples than we are ready to demand of ourselves. If fertile couples are free to have large families of their own, rather than adopt destitute children from overseas, infertile couples must also be free to do what they can to have their own families. In both cases, overseas adoption, or perhaps the adoption of local children who are unwanted because of some impairment, should be considered; but if we are not going to make this compulsory in the former case, it should not be made compulsory in the latter.

There is a further question: to what extent do infertile couples have a right to assistance from community medical resources? Again, however, we must not single out IVF for harsher treatment than we give to other medical techniques. If tubal surgery is available and covered by one's health insurance, or is offered as part of a national health scheme, then why should IVF be treated any differently? And if infertile couples can get free or subsidized psychiatry to help them overcome the psychological problems of infertility, there is something absurd about denying them free or subsidized treatment which could overcome the root of the problem, rather than the symptoms. By today's standards, after all, IVF is not an inordinately expensive medical technique; and there is no country, as far as I know, which limits its provision of free or subsidized health care to those cases in which the patient's life is in danger. Once we extend medical care to cover cases of injury, incapacity, and psychological distress, IVF has a strong claim to be included among the range of free or subsidized treatments available.

THE EFFECT ON WOMEN

The final objection is one that has come from some feminists. In a recently published collection of essays by women titled *Test-Tube Women: What Future for Motherhood?,* several contributors are suspicious of the new reproductive technology. None is more hostile than Robyn Rowland, an Australian sociologist, who writes:

> Ultimately the new technology will be used for the benefit of men and to the detriment of women. Although technology itself is not always a negative development, the real question has always been—who controls it? Biological technology is in the hands of men (2).

And Rowland concludes with a warning as dire as any uttered by the most conservative opponents of IVF:

> What may be happening is the last battle in the long war of men against women. Women's position is most precarious . . . we may find ourselves without a product of any kind with which to bargain. For the history of "mankind" women have been seen in terms of their value as childbearers. We have to ask, if that last power is taken and controlled by men, what role is envisaged for women in the new world? Will women become obsolete? Will we be fighting to retain or reclaim the right to bear children—has patriarchy conned us once again? I urge you sisters to be vigilant. (2)

I can see little basis for such claims. For a start, women have figured quite prominently in the leading IVF teams in Britain, Australia, and the United States: Jean Purdy was an early colleague of Edwards and Steptoe in the research that led to the birth of Louise Brown; Linda Mohr has directed the development of embryo freezing at the Queen Victoria Medical Centre in Melbourne; and in the United States Georgeanna Jones and Joyce Vargyas have played leading roles in the groundbreaking clinics in Norfolk, Virginia, and at the University of Southern California, respectively. It seems odd for a feminist to neglect the contributions these women have made.

Even if one were to grant, however, that the technology remains predominantly in male hands, it has to be remembered that it was developed in response to the needs of infertile couples. From interviews I have conducted and meetings I have attended, my impression is that while both partners are often very concerned about their childlessness, in those cases in which one partner is more distressed than the other by this situation, that partner is usually the woman. Feminists usually accept that this is so, attributing it to the power of social conditioning in a patriarchal society; but the origin of the strong female desire for children is not really what is in question here. The question is: in what sense is the new technology an instrument of male domination over women? If it is true that the technology was developed at least as much in response to the needs of women as in response to the needs of men, then it is hard to see why a feminist should condemn it.

It might be objected that whatever the origins of IVF and no matter how benign it may be when used to help infertile couples, the further development of techniques such as ectogenesis—the growth of the embryo from conception totally outside the body, in an artificial womb—will reduce the status of women. Again, it is not easy to see why this should be so. Ectogenesis will, if it is ever successful, provide a choice for women. Shulamith Firestone argued several years ago in her influential feminist work *The Dialectic of Sex* (3) that this choice will remove the fundamental biological barrier to complete equality. Hence Firestone welcomed the prospect of ectogenesis and condemned the low priority given by our male-dominated society to research in this area.

Firestone's view is surely more in line with the drive to sexual equality than the position taken by Rowland. If we argue that to break the link between women and childbearing would be to undermine the status of women in our society, what are we saying about the ability of women to obtain true equality in other spheres of life? I am not so pessimistic about the abilities of women to achieve equality with men across the broad range of human endeavor. For that reason I think women will be helped, rather than harmed, by the development of a technology which makes it possible for them to have children without being pregnant. As Nancy Breeze, a very differently inclined contributor to the same collection of essays, puts it:

> Two thousand years of morning sickness and stretch marks have not resulted in liberation for women or

children. If you should run into a Petri dish, it could turn out to be your best friend. So rock it; don't knock it! (4)

So to sum up this discussion of the ethics of the simple case of IVF: the ethical objections urged against IVF under these conditions are not strong. They should not count against going ahead with IVF when it is the best way of overcoming infertility and when the infertile couple are not prepared to consider adoption as a means of overcoming their problem. There is, admittedly, a serious question about how much of the national health budget should be al-

located to this area. But then, there are serious questions about the allocation of resources in other areas of medicine as well.

REFERENCES

1 Abstract. Proceedings of the Fifth Scientific Meeting of the Fertility Society of Australia, Adelaide, Dec 2–6, 1986.
2 Rowland R. Reproductive technologies: The final solution to the woman question? In: Arditti R., Klein R. D., Minden S., eds., Test-tube women: What future for motherhood? London: Pandora, 1984.
3 Firestone S. The dialectic of sex. New York: Bantam, 1971.
4 Breeze N. Who is going to rock the petri dish? In: Arditti R., Klein R. D., Minden S., eds, Test-tube women: What future for motherhood? London: Pandora, 1984.

FEMINIST ETHICS AND IN VITRO FERTILIZATION
Susan Sherwin

Sherwin outlines the nature of feminist ethics and provides a feminist critique of in vitro fertilization (IVF). She maintains that IVF is morally problematic for a number of closely related reasons, including the following: (1) Although the desires of infertile couples for access to IVF are understandable and worthy of sympathetic regard, such desires themselves emerge from social arrangements and cultural values that are deeply oppressive to women; (2) IVF technology gives the appearance of providing women with increased reproductive freedom but in reality threatens women with a significant decrease of reproductive freedom. Sherwin also insists that those who find themselves in moral opposition to IVF have a responsibility to support medical and social developments that would reduce the perceived need of couples for IVF.

Many authors from all traditions consider it necessary to ask why it is that some couples seek [IVF] technology so desperately. Why is it so important to so many people to produce their 'own' child? On this question, theorists in the analytic tradition seem to shift to previously rejected ground and suggest that this is a natural, or at least a proper, desire. Englehardt, for example, says, 'The use of technology in the fashioning of children is integral to the goal of rendering the world congenial to persons.'[1] Bayles

Reprinted with permission of the author and the publisher from *Canadian Journal of Philosophy,* Supplementary Volume 13 (1987), pp. 276–284.

more cautiously observes that 'A desire to beget for its own sake . . . is probably irrational'; nonetheless, he immediately concludes, 'these techniques for fulfilling that desire have been found ethically permissible.'[2] R. G. Edwards and David Sharpe state the case most strongly: 'the desire to have children must be among the most basic of human instincts, and denying it can lead to considerable psychological and social difficulties.'[3] Interestingly, although the recent pronouncement of the Catholic Church assumes that 'the desire for a child is natural,'[4] it denies that a couple has a right to a child: 'The child is not an object to which one has a right.'[5]

Here, I believe, it becomes clear why we need a deeper sort of feminist analysis. We must look at the sort of social arrangements and cultural values that underlie the drive to assume such risks for the sake of biological parenthood. We find that the capitalism, racism, sexism, and elitism of our culture have combined to create a set of attitudes which views children as commodities whose value is derived from their possession of parental chromosomes. Children are valued as privatized commodities, reflecting the virility and heredity of their parents. They are also viewed as the responsibility of their parents and are not seen as the social treasure and burden that they are. Parents must tend their needs on pain of prosecution, and, in return, they get to keep complete control over them. Other adults are inhibited from having warm, stable interactions with the children of others—it is as suspect to try to hug and talk regularly with a child who is not one's own as it is to fondle and hang longingly about a car or a bicycle which belongs to someone else—so those who wish to know children well often find they must have their own.

Women are persuaded that their most important purpose in life is to bear and raise children; they are told repeatedly that their life is incomplete, that they are lacking in fulfillment if they do not have children. And, in fact, many women do face a barren existence without children. Few women have access to meaningful, satisfying jobs. Most do not find themselves in the centre of the romantic personal relationships which the culture pretends is the norm for heterosexual couples. And they have been socialized to be fearful of close friendships with others—they are taught to distrust other women, and to avoid the danger of friendship with men other than their husbands. Children remain the one hope for real intimacy and for the sense of accomplishment which comes from doing work one judges to be valuable.

To be sure, children can provide that sense of self-worth, although for many women (and probably for all mothers at some times) motherhood is not the romanticized satisfaction they are led to expect. But there is something very wrong with a culture where childrearing is the only outlet available to most women in which to pursue fulfillment. Moreover, there is something wrong with the ownership theory

of children that keeps other adults at a distance from children. There ought to be a variety of close relationships possible between children and adults so that we all recognize that we have a stake in the well-being of the young, and we all benefit from contact with their view of the world.

In such a world, it would not be necessary to spend the huge sums on designer children which IVF requires while millions of other children starve to death each year. Adults who enjoyed children could be involved in caring for them whether or not they produced them biologically. And, if the institution of marriage survives, women and men would marry because they wished to share their lives together, not because the men needed someone to produce heirs for them and women needed financial support for their children. That would be a world in which we might have reproductive freedom of choice. The world we now live in has so limited women's options and self-esteem, it is legitimate to question the freedom behind women's demand for this technology, for it may well be largely a reflection of constraining social perspectives.

Nonetheless, I must acknowledge that some couples today genuinely mourn their incapacity to produce children without IVF and there are very significant and unique joys which can be found in producing and raising one's own children which are not accessible to persons in infertile relationships. We must sympathize with these people. None of us shall live to see the implementation of the ideal cultural values outlined above which would make the demand for IVF less severe. It is with real concern that some feminists suggest that the personal wishes of couples with fertility difficulties may not be compatible with the overall interests of women and children.

Feminist thought, then, helps us to focus on different dimensions of the problem than do other sorts of approaches. But, with this perspective, we still have difficulty in reaching a final conclusion on whether to encourage, tolerate, modify, or restrict this sort of reproductive technology. I suggest that we turn to the developing theories of feminist ethics for guidance in resolving this question.[6]

In my view, a feminist ethics is a moral theory that focusses on relations among persons as well as on individuals. It has as a model an inter-connected social fabric, rather than the familiar one of isolated, independent atoms; and it gives primacy to bonds among people rather than to rights to independence. It is a theory that focuses on concrete situations and persons and not on free-floating abstract actions.[7] Although many details have yet to be worked out, we can see some of its implications in particular problem areas such as this.

It is a theory that is explicitly conscious of the social, political, and economic relations that exist among persons; in particular, as a feminist theory, it attends to the implications of actions or policies on the status of women. Hence, it is necessary to ask questions from the perspective of feminist ethics in addition to those which are normally asked from the perspective of mainstream ethical theories. We must view issues such as this one in the context of the social and political realities in which they arise, and resist the attempt to evaluate actions or practices in isolation (as traditional responses in biomedical ethics often do). Thus, we cannot just address the question of IVF per se without asking how IVF contributes to general patterns of women's oppression. As Kathryn Pyne Addelson has argued about abortion,[8] a feminist perspective raises questions that are inadmissible within the traditional ethical frameworks, and yet, for women in a patriarchal society, they are value questions of greater urgency. In particular, a feminist ethics, in contrast to other approaches in biomedical ethics, would take seriously the concerns just reviewed which are part of the debate in the feminist literature.

A feminist ethics would also include components of theories that have been developed as 'feminine ethics,' as sketched out by the empirical work of Carol Gilligan.[9] (The best example of such a theory is the work of Nel Noddings in her influential book *Caring*.)[10] In other words, it would be a theory that gives primacy to interpersonal relationships and woman-centered values such as nurturing, empathy, and co-operation. Hence, in the case of IVF, we must care for the women and men who are so despairing about their infertility as to want to spend the vast sums and risk the associated physical and emotional costs of the treatment, in pursuit of 'their own children.' That is, we should, in Noddings' terms, see

their reality as our own and address their very real sense of loss. In so doing, however, we must also consider the implications of this sort of solution to their difficulty. While meeting the perceived desires of some women—desires which are problematic in themselves, since they are so compatible with the values of a culture deeply oppressive to women— this technology threatens to further entrench those values which are responsible for that oppression. A larger vision suggests that the technology offered may, in reality, reduce women's freedom and, if so, it should be avoided.

A feminist ethics will not support a wholly negative response, however, for that would not address our obligation to care for those suffering from infertility; it is the responsibility of those who oppose further implementation of this technology to work towards the changes in the social arrangements that will lead to a reduction of the sense of need for this sort of solution. On the medical front, research and treatment ought to be stepped up to reduce the rates of peral sepsis and gonorrhea which often result in tubal blockage, more attention should be directed at the causes and possible cures for male infertility, and we should pursue techniques that will permit safe reversible sterilization providing women with better alternatives to tubal ligation as a means of fertility control; these sorts of technology would increase the control of many women over their own fertility and would be compatible with feminist objectives. On the social front, we must continue the social pressure to change the status of women and children in our society from that of breeder and possession respectively; hence, we must develop a vision of society as community where all participants are valued members, regardless of age or gender. And we must challenge the notion that having one's wife produce a child with his own genes is sufficient cause for the wives of men with low sperm counts to be expected to undergo the physical and emotional assault such technology involves.

Further, a feminist ethics will attend to the nature of the relationships among those concerned. Annette Baier has eloquently argued for the importance of developing an ethics of trust,[11] and I believe a feminist ethics must address the question of the degree of trust appropriate to the relationships involved. Feminists have noted that women have little reason to trust the medical specialists who offer to respond to their reproductive desires, for, commonly women's interests have not come first from the medical point of view.[12] In fact, it is accurate to perceive feminist attacks on reproductive technology as expressions of the lack of trust feminists have in those who control the technology. Few feminists object to reproductive technology per se; rather they express concern about who controls it and how it can be used to further exploit women. The problem with reproductive technology is that it concentrates power in reproductive matters in the hands of those who are not directly involved in the actual bearing and rearing of the child; i.e., in men who relate to their clients in a technical, professional, authoritarian manner. It is a further step in the medicalization of pregnancy and birth which, in North America, is marked by relationships between pregnant women and their doctors which are very different from the traditional relationships between pregnant women and midwives. The latter relationships fostered an atmosphere of mutual trust which is impossible to replicate in hospital deliveries today. In fact, current approaches to pregnancy, labour, and birth tend to view the mother as a threat to the fetus who must be coerced to comply with medical procedures designed to ensure delivery of healthy babies at whatever cost necessary to the mother. Frequently, the fetus-mother relationship is medically characterized as adversarial and the physicians choose to foster a sense of alienation and passivity in the role they permit the mother. However well IVF may serve the interests of the few women with access to it, it more clearly serves the interests (be they commercial, professional, scholarly, or purely patriarchal) of those who control it.

Questions such as these are a puzzle to those engaged in the traditional approaches to ethics, for they always urge us to separate the question of evaluating the morality of various forms of reproductive technology in themselves, from questions about particular uses of that technology. From the perspective of a feminist ethics, however, no such distinction can be meaningfully made. Reproductive technology is not an abstract activity, it is an activity done in particular contexts and it is those contexts which must be addressed.

Feminist concerns [make] clear the difficulties we have with some of our traditional ethical concepts; hence, feminist ethics directs us to rethink our basic ethical notions. Autonomy, or freedom of choice, is not a matter to be determined in isolated instances, as is commonly assumed in many approaches to applied ethics. Rather it is a matter that involves reflection on one's whole life situation. The freedom of choice feminists appeal to in the abortion situation is freedom to define one's status as childbearer, given the social, economic, and political significance of reproduction for women. A feminist perspective permits us to understand that reproductive freedom includes control of one's sexuality, protection against coerced sterilization (or iatrogenic sterilization, e.g., as caused by the Dalkon Shield), and the existence of a social and economic network of support for the children we may choose to bear. It is the freedom to redefine our roles in society according to our concerns and needs as women.

In contrast, the consumer freedom to purchase technology, allowed only to a few couples of the privileged classes (in traditionally approved relationships), seems to entrench further the patriarchal notions of woman's role as childbearer and of heterosexual monogamy as the only acceptable intimate relationship. In other words, this sort of choice does not seem to foster autonomy for women on the broad scale. IVF is a practice which seems to reinforce sexist, classist, and often racist assumptions of our culture; therefore, on our revised understanding of freedom, the contribution of this technology to the general autonomy of women is largely negative.

We can now see the advantage of a feminist ethics over mainstream ethical theories, for a feminist analysis explicitly accepts the need for a political component to our understanding of ethical issues. In this, it differs from traditional ethical theories and it also differs from a simply feminine ethics approach, such as the one Noddings offers, for Noddings seems to rely on individual relations exclusively and is deeply suspicious of political alliances as potential threats to the pure relation of caring. Yet, a full understanding of both the threat of IVF, and the alternative action necessary should we decide to reject IVF, is possible only if it includes a political dimension reflecting on the role of women in society.

From the point of view of feminist ethics, the primary question to consider is whether this and other forms of reproductive technology threaten to reinforce the lack of autonomy which women now experience in our culture—even as they appear, in the short run, to be increasing freedom. We must recognize that the interconnections among the social forces oppressive to women underlie feminists' mistrust of this technology which advertises itself as increasing women's autonomy.[13] The political perspective which directs us to look at how this technology fits in with general patterns of treatment for women is not readily accessible to traditional moral theories, for it involves categories of concern not accounted for in those theories—e.g., the complexity of issues which makes it inappropriate to study them in isolation from one another, the role of oppression in shaping individual desires, and potential differences in moral status which are connected with differences in treatment.

It is the set of connections constituting women's continued oppression in our society which inspires feminists to resurrect the old slippery slope arguments to warn against IVF. We must recognize that women's existing lack of control in reproductive matters begins the debate on a pretty steep incline. Technology with the potential to further remove control of reproduction from women makes the slope very slippery indeed. This new technology, though offered under the guise of increasing reproductive freedom, threatens to result, in fact, in a significant decrease in freedom, especially since it is a technology that will always include the active involvement of designated specialists and will not ever be a private matter for the couple or women concerned.

Ethics ought not to direct us to evaluate individual cases without also looking at the implications of our decisions from a wide perspective. My argument is that a theory of feminist ethics provides that wider perspective, for its different sort of methodology is sensitive to both the personal and the social dimensions of issues. For that reason, I believe it is the only ethical perspective suitable for evaluating issues of this sort.

NOTES

1 H. Tristram Englehardt, *The Foundations of Bioethics* (Oxford: Oxford University Press 1986), 239.
2 Michael Bayles, *Reproductive Ethics* (Englewood Cliffs, NJ: Prentice-Hall 1984) 31.
3 Robert G. Edwards and David J. Sharpe, 'Social Values and Research in Human Embryology,' *Nature* 231 (May 14, 1971), 87.
4 Joseph Card Ratzinger and Alberto Bovone, 'Instruction on Respect for Human Life in Its Origin and on the Dignity of Procreation: Replies to Certain Questions of the Day' (Vatican City: Vatican Polyglot Press 1987), 33.
5 Ibid., 34.
6 Many authors are now working on an understanding of what feminist ethics entail. Among the Canadian papers I am familiar with are Kathryn Morgan's 'Women and Moral Madness,' Sheila Mullett's 'Only Connect: The Place of Self-Knowledge in Ethics,' both in this volume, and Leslie Wilson's 'Is a Feminine Ethics Enough?' *Atlantis* (forthcoming).
7 Susan Sherwin, 'A Feminist Approach to Ethics,' *Dalhousie Review* 64, 4 (Winter 1984–85) 704–13.
8 Kathryn Pyne Addelson, 'Moral Revolution,' in Marilyn Pearsall, ed., *Women and Values* (Belmont, CA: Wadsworth 1986), 291–309.
9 Carol Gilligan, *In a Different Voice* (Cambridge, MA: Harvard University Press 1982).
10 Nel Noddings, *Caring* (Berkeley: University of California Press 1984).
11 Annette Baier, 'What Do Women Want in a Moral Theory?' *Nous* 19 (March 1985) 53–64, and 'Trust and Antitrust,' *Ethics* 96 (January 1986) 231–60.
12 Linda Williams presents this position particularly clearly in her invaluable work 'But What Will They Mean for Women? Feminist Concerns About the New Reproductive Technologies,' No. 6 in the *Feminist Perspective* Series, CRIAW.
13 Marilyn Frye vividly describes the phenomenon of interrelatedness which supports sexist oppression by appeal to the metaphor of a bird cage composed of thin wires, each relatively harmless in itself, but, collectively, the wires constitute an overwhelming barrier to the inhabitant of the cage. Marilyn Frye, *The Politics of Reality: Essays in Feminist Theory* (Trumansburg, NY: The Crossing Press 1983), 4–7.

ETHICAL DEBATES ABOUT INFERTILITY AND ITS TREATMENT

The New York State Task Force on Life and the Law

In this reading, a chapter reprinted from a much longer report on assisted reproductive technologies, the task force begins by clarifying the issues involved in debates about how to define *infertility*. The task force then organizes the contemporary debate about the use of assisted reproductive technologies by distinguishing among three groups of commentators. One group of commentators is opposed to any use of assisted reproductive technology. A second group, emphasizing the importance of autonomous choice, is committed to the claim that individuals have a right to use the entire range of assisted reproductive technologies. A third group argues that the right to use assisted reproductive technologies is sometimes outweighed by competing societal interests. The task force concludes its discussion by considering different perspectives on the question of whether children can be harmed by the very technologies that allow them to be born.

With an increasing number of physicians now providing assisted reproductive technologies (ARTs) and more infertile people opting for these services, many segments of society seem already to have concluded that assisted reproduction is a reasonable response to fertility problems. According to some commentators, this conclusion reflects an assumption that those who are infertile will, and perhaps should, want to find a way to create a child who is genetically, or at least gestationally, related to them. Yet, some have challenged the wisdom of this assumption, criticizing societal pressures on women to achieve biological motherhood at all costs and expressing concern about both the risks and the limited success rates of the technologies involved.

This chapter reviews the debate over the appropriateness of using assisted reproduction as a response to infertility. The ethical implications of particular aspects of the practice of assisted reproduction are discussed in Part II of this report.

DEFINING INFERTILITY

Discussions of the appropriateness of using assisted reproduction as a response to infertility often begin with debates about how to define infertility. Many

The New York State Task Force on Life and the Law, *Assisted Reproductive Technologies: Analysis and Recommendations for Public Policy* (April 1998), Chapter 3, pp. 95–104.

commentators, as well as advocacy organizations representing infertile individuals, characterize infertility as a disease. These commentators argue that "diseases are physical or mental conditions of an organism that result in deviations from normal species function,"[1] and, at least for those who desire biological children, infertility is a deviation from normal function.[2] Noting that infertility can be caused by a range of physical conditions, they define the disease of infertility as "the result of specific physical dysfunctions in the reproductive organs and/or other bodily systems, including such conditions as congenital malformations of the reproductive organs, endometriosis, hormonal imbalances, and immunologic factors."[3] Some commentators argue that because infertility "adversely affects a basic and important human capacity,"[4] and because some people experience it as distressing and limiting, it should be assigned "a relatively high priority with respect to other disease states."[5]

A number of feminist commentators object to the characterization of infertility as a disease requiring medical treatment. They believe that society's approach to infertility is distorted by viewing it as an illness to be solved, rather than as a physical difference that people may or may not wish to take steps to affect.[6] As one commentator observes, "Medicalizing subfertility with the help of procreative technologies sets up norms: bodily norms, behavioral norms, ethical norms."[7] Once infertility is viewed as a medical condition, this commentator argues, the infertile woman is expected to obtain treatment to "normalize her into pregnancy."[8] Other commentators are also critical of the societal emphasis on treatment for infertility, noting that infertility specialists expect their patients to "pursue all available treatments," not acknowledging any difference in kind among the treatments or the possibility that medical treatment may not be the most reasonable solution for a particular patient.[9]

These critics also argue that the term "treatment" misrepresents what actually happens in assisted reproduction. In their view, assisted reproduction does not treat infertility but, instead, bypasses it. In fact, they argue, many of the women who are "treated" by the use of assisted reproduction do not suffer from any physical difference of their own, but are being treated for "a rather unusual 'disease' "—sterility—"that exists in another person, a male partner."[10]

Other commentators maintain that there are many instances in medicine when treatment does not cure the condition or disease but instead "modifies its expression," enabling the patient to achieve a desired goal.[11] As one commentator argues, "The fact that [ARTs] do not correct infertility, but only allow a person to overcome the functional deficit of the disease does not mean that their use is not medical treatment for a disease. Many medical and rehabilitative treatments, including many that are standardly covered by health care insurance, do not correct the underlying condition, but only correct for its attendant disability."[12] For example, just as assisted reproduction enables an infertile person to reproduce without restoring that person's fertility, glasses enable a visually-impaired person to see, insulin enables a diabetic to live, and a hearing aid enables a hearing-impaired person to hear, all without correcting the underlying medical problem.

One commentator proposes that infertility should be described as a disability rather than a disease. This nomenclature acknowledges both the inherently social nature of the problem and the fact that medical treatment may be an appropriate response.[13] This commentator maintains that characterizing infertility as a disability rather than a disease broadens the types of responses one will consider. In the case of a disease, medical treatment is almost always viewed as the answer. In the case of a disability, medical treatment could cure or bypass the disability, but there are also "equally important non-medical ways of managing disability, ways that address the handicapping effects of the disability—like learning sign language, having wheelchair ramps, adopting babies."[14]

While the debate about how to define infertility may seem like a matter of semantics, commentators argue that the definition significantly affects both individual and societal responses. Some people note that unless infertility is viewed as a disease, it will be difficult to justify the provision of insurance coverage for assisted reproductive services, which could make these procedures accessible to many more infertile people.[15] Other people maintain that calling infertility a disease leads to the conclusion that medical treatment is the only proper response to the inability to conceive a child. In their view, this attitude reinforces society's expectation that all women will procreate and thus makes it more difficult for women to define themselves in other ways.[16] However, some commentators argue that the relevant question is not whether infertility is a disease, but whether particular responses to infertility are themselves appropriate. Even if infertility services "do not treat an illness or disease," these commentators maintain, they may be an appropriate use of medical services because they "relieve the misfortune of an impediment to the satisfaction of a desire for a 'good' in life not otherwise available."[17]

ASSISTED REPRODUCTION AS A RESPONSE TO INFERTILITY

Secular and religious commentators have expressed differing opinions on the appropriateness of using assisted reproduction as a response to infertility.[18] While some commentators oppose all ARTs, others defend the individual's right to use the entire range of available technologies. A third group supports the use of at least some of the technologies, but believes that in some cases their use must be limited to protect the interests of any children who might result and of society.

Opposition to Assisted Reproduction Some commentators reject assisted reproduction as a misguided solution to infertility. They maintain that making babies in a laboratory is a "degradation of parenthood."[19] One commentator, for example, argues that it is wrong to create a baby in a laboratory because it takes the creation of a child out of the marital relationship and inserts the practice of medicine and technology where it does not belong. He also argues that assisted reproduction is the "thin edge of the wedge," which will inevitably lead to the broader manipulation of genetic material in the laboratory and the utilization of science to create the perfect child.[20] According to this commentator, "Medical practice loses its way into an entirely different human activity—manufacture (which most wants to satisfy desires)—if it undertakes either to produce a child without curing infertility as a condition or to produce simply the desired sort of child."[21] Another commentator expresses a similar concern that assisted reproduction could lead to undesirable scientific advances. "The decisions we must now make," he notes, "may very well help to determine whether human beings will eventually be produced in laboratories. Once the genies let the babies into the bottle, it may be impossible to get them out again."[22]

Many of these commentators express particular concern about the impact of assisted reproduction on the way in which children are valued. They fear that "the child conceived through reproductive techniques becomes a means to an end of adult happiness, vanity, or obsession with genetic lineage."[23] Their concern is that the child will be viewed not as an invaluable and unique treasure but rather as a product valued for its cost and ostensible quality. Worried that children will be seen as just another product to be manufactured, bought, and sold, these commentators ask whether children are "more likely to flourish in a culture where making children is governed by the same rules that govern the making of automobiles or VCRs."[24]

Some commentators believe that the high cost of assisted reproduction will turn children into commodities from which parents will demand certain performance and perfection. The unattractive, slow, or disabled child will become unacceptable, in much the same way that a defective product is unacceptable and usually returned. These commentators are particularly concerned about the use of assisted reproduction to prevent the creation of children with undesirable traits. While most commentators do not object to pre-implantation genetic testing or sex selection to avoid the transmission of genetic diseases, many object to these practices when they are used for "morally frivolous reasons."[25]

Some feminists also oppose the use of assisted reproduction but for different reasons. Echoing their criticism of viewing infertility as a disease, they argue that assisted reproduction represents yet another attempt by male doctors to dominate women's bodies, and that it reinforces the view of women as primarily mothers. "Although [in vitro fertilization] appears to offer more choices and hence more freedom to women," states one commentator, "in fact it threatens to undermine women's freedom in the long run. It does this both by reinforcing sex-role stereotypes in which a woman's worth is dependent upon her reproductive capacity and also by reinforcing the power of men in the reproductive sphere."[26] These commentators argue that we live in a society in which "to choose to be childless is still socially disapproved and to be childless in fact is to be stigmatized as selfish and uncaring. In such a situation, to offer the hope of becoming a mother to a childless woman is a coercive offer."[27] They believe that the very existence of technology that allows some infertile women to give birth to a genetically, or at least gestationally, related child pushes all infertile women, and women with infertile partners, to continue trying to reproduce despite the odds, rather than coming to terms with their infertility.[28]

Other commentators have raised objections to ARTs because of concerns that they "reflect and reinforce the racial hierarchy in America."[29] As one commentator notes, although black women have higher infertility rates than white women,[30] "one of the most striking features of the new reproduction is that it is used almost exclusively by white people."[31] She maintains that, in addition to the high cost of infertility treatment, this racial disparity results from deliberate efforts by physicians to steer black women away from assisted reproduction.[32] She also argues that the desire among some white people to have a genetically related child reflects a long tradition of efforts "to preserve white racial purity."[33]

Assisted Reproduction: An Autonomous Right

At the other end of the spectrum are those who believe that decisions about the use of assisted reproduction should be left to the individuals involved, with the state playing only a limited regulatory role.[34] These commentators believe that all forms of assisted reproduction can be acceptable as long as the individuals utilizing them behave responsibly. As one notes, "In vitro fertilization and techniques that allow us to study and control human reproduction are morally neutral instruments for the realization of profoundly important human goals, which are bound up with the realization of the good of others: children for infertile parents and greater health for the children that will be born."[35] These commentators dispute the contention that children created through assisted reproduction will inevitably be treated as commodities, arguing that "the critical issue is not whether something involves monetary exchange as one of its aspects, but whether it is treated as reducible solely to its monetary features."[36]

The position of these commentators is based in large part on a determination that individuals have a right to procreate, and that this right includes a right to procreate non-coitally.[37] Although the Supreme Court has not explicitly recognized an affirmative constitutional right to procreate, as opposed to the more limited right to avoid procreation, most commentators assume that such a right exists, at least within marriage.[38] This assumption is based in part on a strong tradition in this country "of regarding questions of reproduction and family life as private matters."[39]

In the case of assisted reproduction, many commentators argue that this tradition of procreative liberty and privacy requires respect for autonomy as the guiding principle for all decision making. As such, they support the regulation of assisted reproduction only when its purpose is to protect autonomous choice and prevent coercion. In general, they conclude that the best way to achieve these goals is through the process of informed consent. For a patient considering assisted reproduction, commentators suggest that informed consent should include counseling that provides complete information about the likelihood of success, the risks and costs of the procedure, and medical and lifestyle alternatives available to the patient.[40] They also support state efforts to improve the quality of care available, as long as regulations "do not limit access to medically appropriate treatment."[41] In addition, they endorse regulations that provide uniform reporting of success rates of particular treatments and particular programs to protect the interests of patients as consumers.[42]

Some feminist commentators have adopted this autonomy-based view of assisted reproduction.[43] They believe that assisted reproduction increases women's reproductive freedom by expanding their choices about when to reproduce and allowing them to do so without a partner of the opposite sex.[44] They emphasize that with adequate informed consent women can be protected from exploitation by the commercial assisted reproduction market.[45] Some of these commentators believe that a technological solution to infertility is particularly appropriate in light of the fact that many women are infertile as a result of technological developments such as intrauterine devices and drugs such as diethylstilbestrol (DES). They conclude that "the drive to make use of the new reproductive technologies derives not simply from the fact of infertility, nor from its apparent increase, but from the social and medical circumstances under which infertility has been sustained."[46]

A Middle Ground In the middle are those commentators who believe that individuals have a right to choose assisted reproduction to enable them to create a family but that other interests may outweigh this right in certain circumstances. Commentators taking this position stress that procreative liberty, like other individual rights, is not an absolute and must always be balanced against the well-being of society and the best interests of existing children and the children who may be born as a result of ARTs.[47] They urge society to proceed cautiously, particularly when the technologies will have significant ramifications for people other than the individual or couple trying to reproduce.[48]

These commentators emphasize that the use of ARTs implicates important societal interests. Society has an interest in the impact of assisted reproduction on future generations, the effect on societal resources, and the implications for the value attached to human life. Society must also be concerned with the principle of beneficence, which emphasizes the impact of actions on others, in contrast to autonomy, which is concerned only with the protection of individual choice. As one commentator notes, "A commitment to the creation of a just society requires that an individual desire for genetically related children cannot be held up as an end commanding significant government resources and energy if as a 'good' it encourages the exploitation of vulnerable persons or fosters negative attitudes towards persons or groups of persons."[49]

Commentators taking this middle position recognize some of the concerns raised by opponents of assisted reproduction, particularly the risk that children will come to be viewed as commodities rather than individuals to be valued in their own right. In addition, many of these commentators express particular concern about third party participants in assisted reproduction, especially egg donors and surrogates, who may undergo significant medical risks without any possibility of direct benefit.[50] In general, however, these commentators conclude that the risks involved in assisted reproduction should be addressed by limiting or regulating particular practices rather than by prohibiting the use of the technologies entirely.

Some of these commentators emphasize the consequences of assisted reproduction for societal fairness or distributive justice. They ask whether substantial sums should be spent on assisted reproduction when there are children already born who need homes and infertile low-income women who cannot afford assisted reproduction but might benefit from money spent on preventive health measures or other forms of treatment.[51] These commentators maintain that concerted efforts to prevent infertility are at least as important, if not more so, than the continuing pursuit of new technological ways to bypass the infertile condition.[52]

Critics of the current emphasis on ARTs also note that while these technologies may be beneficial to a small, elite group of women who have the time and financial resources to pursue them, women as a social group would benefit much more if those resources were used to address breast cancer, AIDS, and the poverty that kills and maims many women and children. As one commentator notes, "The issue should not be increasing access to experimental, costly, and debilitating technologies but rather implementing priorities that prevent maternal morbidity and infant mortality as well as ensure basic access to nutrition, sanitation, prenatal care, and the prevention of disease."[53]

Harm to Children as the Critical Factor For many commentators, determining the best interests of children is the primary factor in assessing the appropriateness of particular types of ARTs.[54] The debate about the effect of assisted reproduction on the children who are created raises complex philosophical questions about whether children can be harmed by the technologies that allow them to be born.

Some commentators maintain that assisted reproduction can never harm the children who result because without assisted reproduction the children would not exist. As one commentator concludes, "Risking damage to offspring would not seem to wrong the offspring if it were not possible for them to be conceived or born without undergoing the risk of damage."[55] According to these commentators, this position is reflected in state court decisions refusing to recognize the tort of "wrongful life," which would allow an infant to recover damages from a physician who negligently failed to inform the infant's parents of fetal defects which, if known, might have prompted the parents to terminate the pregnancy that led to the infant's birth.[56]

Those who maintain that children can be harmed by the use of assisted reproduction respond that creating a child under certain circumstances can be wrong even if after birth the child would prefer life to nonexistence.[57] As one commentator notes, "Even if we cannot ascribe a preference for nonexistence to the child, surely we can say that this life is so awful that no one could possibly wish it for the child."[58] These commentators argue that "in deciding whether to have children, people should not only be concerned with their own interests in reproducing. They must think also, and perhaps primarily, of the welfare of the children they will bear. They should ask themselves, 'What kind of life is my child likely to have?'"[59]

According to several commentators, the claim that children cannot be harmed by assisted reproduction unless their life is worse than nonexistence reflects a failure to distinguish between the interests of existing children and those of children not yet conceived. One commentator argues that the view that children cannot be harmed by the technologies that allow them to exist "assumes that children with an interest in existing are waiting in a spectral world of nonexistence where their situation is less desirable than it would be were they released into this world."[60] This assumption is wrong, she argues, because unlike death, nonexistence before life is "neither good nor bad."[61] In comparison to such a state, a life of substantial suffering can indeed be harmful, even if a person already alive would prefer that life to no existence at all. Participants in a workshop on the ethics of reproductive medicine similarly concluded that "no one is ever harmed by not being born at all, by not being implanted into someone's uterus, but one can be very badly harmed if brought into the world with a lethal and terrible disease."[62]

Some commentators argue that it should not matter whether children can technically be "harmed" by the use of technologies that allow them to be born, because the use of those technologies can be "wrongful" even if they do not cause direct harm. One commentator, for example, maintains that when assisted reproduction leads to the birth of a child with a disease or disability that is serious but not so debilitating that the child would prefer never to have been born, it is possible to conclude that "the action is wrong, although the person who suffers the handicap is not harmed." Such "nonharmful wrongs," he concludes, might constitute "legitimate and possibly sufficient grounds for restricting procreative liberty."[63]

Those commentators who believe that children can be harmed by the use of assisted reproduction acknowledge the difficulty of determining the type of risks to a child that would make a decision to procreate ethically problematic. Noting the cultural variability of concepts of health, one commentator argues that such judgments must take into account "the nature of the disorder from which the child would suffer, the circumstances into which the child would be brought, and the ameliorative resources available for that child."[64] Ultimately, she argues, the question to be determined is whether the child will be born with an "inadequate opportunity for health."[65] Another commentator similarly argues that the relevant question is whether the child will be born "in circumstances where there is not a decent minimum opportunity for development."[66]

NOTES

1 D. W. Brock, "Funding New Reproductive Technologies: Should They Be Included in Health Insurance Benefit Packages?" in *New Ways of Making Babies: The Case of Egg Donation,* ed. C. B. Cohen (Bloomington: Indiana University Press, 1996), 213, 224.

2 Ibid., 225.

3 RESOLVE, *Ethical Issues Related to Medical Treatment of Infertility* (Somerville, MA: RESOLVE, 1995), 4.

4 A. L. Caplan, "The Ethics of In Vitro Fertilization," *Primary Care* 13 (1986): 241, 249–250.

5 Ibid., 250.

6 J. G. Raymond, *Women as Wombs* (San Francisco: Harper, 1993), 2.

7 H. L. Nelson, "Dethroning Choice: Analogy, Personhood, and the New Reproductive Technologies," *Journal of Law, Medicine and Ethics* 23 (1995): 129, 133.

8 Ibid.

9 P. Lauritzen, *Pursuing Parenthood: Ethical Issues in Assisted Reproduction* (Bloomington: Indiana University Press, 1993), xiv–xv.

10 Raymond, 2–3.

11 R. G. Edwards, "Fertilization of Human Eggs in Vitro: A Defense," in *The Ethics of Reproductive Technology,* ed. K. D. Alpern (New York: Oxford University Press, 1992), 75.

12 Brock, "Funding," 225.

13 B. K. Rothman, *Recreating Motherhood* (New York: Norton, 1989), 143.

14 Ibid., 144.

15 For a discussion of the ethical debates surrounding insurance coverage for assisted reproduction, see Chapter 17, pages 433–435. [The chapter citation here, as in subsequent notes, refers to the task force report *Assisted Reproductive Technologies* (April 1998).]

16 P. Lauritzen, "What Price Parenthood?" *Hastings Center Report* 20, no. 2 (1990): 40.

17 J. Spike and J. Greenlaw, "Case Study: Ethics Consultation," *Journal of Law, Medicine and Ethics* 22 (1994): 348.

18 For a discussion of religious perspectives on assisted reproduction, see Chapter 4.

19 L. R. Kass, "Making Babies—The New Biology and the Old Morality," *Public Interest* 26 (1972): 49.

20 P. Ramsey, "Shall We 'Reproduce'? II; Rejoinders and Future Forecast," *Journal of the American Medical Association* 220 (1972): 1481.

21 Ibid., 1482.

22 L. R. Kass, "The Meaning of Life—In the Laboratory," in *The Ethics of Reproductive Technology,* 108.

23 M. M. Schultz, "Reproductive Technology and Intent-Based Parenthood: An Opportunity for Gender Neutrality," *Wisconsin Law Review* (1990): 297, 334.

24 T. H. Murray, "New Reproductive Technologies and the Family," in *New Ways of Making Babies,* 62.

25 Schultz, 364. For further discussion of pre-implantation genetic testing and sex selection, see Chapter 7, pages 165–169.

26 K. Lebacqz, "Feminism and Bioethics: An Overview," *Second Opinion* 17, no. 2 (1991): 11.

27 Lauritzen, "What Price Parenthood?" 40 (describing feminist positions).

28 M. A. Warren, "IVF and Women's Interests: An Analysis of Feminist Concerns," *Bioethics* 2 (1988): 37, 45.

29 D. E. Roberts, "Race and the New Reproduction," *Hastings Law Journal* 47 (1996): 935, 937.

30 Ibid., 939.

31 Ibid., 937.

32 Ibid., 940.

33 Ibid., 943.

34 Ethics Committee of the American Fertility Society, "Ethical Considerations of Assisted Reproductive Technologies," *Fertility and Sterility* 62, Supplement 1 (1994): 13S.

35 H. T. Engelhardt, Jr., *The Foundations of Bioethics* (New York: Oxford University Press, 1986), 241.

36 Schultz, "Reproductive Technology," 336.

37 J. A. Robertson, "Embryos, Families, and Procreative Liberty: The Legal Structure of the New Reproduction," *Southern California Law Review* 59 (1986): 939, 960.

38 See Chapter 6, pages 135–137.

39 A. M. Capron, "The New Reproductive Possibilities: Seeking a Moral Basis for Concerted Action in a Pluralistic Society," *Law, Medicine and Health Care* (1984): 193.

40 J. A. Nisker, "A User-Friendly Framework for Exploration of Ethical Issues in Reproductive Medicine," *Assisted Reproduction Reviews* 5 (1995): 273.

41 RESOLVE, *Statements of Principle* (Somerville, MA: RESOLVE, 1995).

42 Ibid.

43 Warren, "IVF and Women's Interests," 41–42.

44 Brock, "Funding," 222.

45 Raymond, *Women as Wombs,* 88; Warren, 38–39.

46 J. H. Hollinger, "From Coitus to Commerce: Legal and Social Consequences of Noncoital Reproduction," *Journal of Law Reform* 18 (1985): 865, 876.

47 Lauritzen, *Pursuing Parenthood,* 66–67; C. B. Cohen, "Unmanaged Care: The Need to Regulate New Reproductive Technologies in the United States," *Bioethics* 11 (1997): 348, 360 ("The reproductive interests of those who are subfertile must be weighed against the harm and wrong that fulfilling those interests might do to the resulting children, to third party participants, to those persons themselves, and to society.").

48 Lauritzen, *Pursuing Parenthood,* 67.

49 M. A. Ryan, "The Argument for Unlimited Procreative Liberty: A Feminist Critique," *Hastings Center Report* 20, no. 4 (1990): 6, 12.

50 See Chapter 10, page 243.

51 Ryan, "A Feminist Critique," 12; Roberts, "Race," 948; E. Bartholet, *Family Bonds: Adoption and the Politics of Parenting* (Boston: Houghton Mifflin, 1993), 36–37.

52 Warren, "IVF and Women's Interests," 49.

53 Raymond, *Women as Wombs,* 137.

54 C. B. Cohen, "'Give Me Children or I Shall Die!' New Reproductive Technologies and Harm to Children," *Hastings Center Report* 26, no. 2 (1996): 19, 26.

55 Robertson, "Embryos," 988; see also J. A. Robertson, *Children of Choice: Freedom and the New Reproductive Technologies* (Princeton: Princeton University Press, 1994), 75–76.

56 See, e.g., *Becker v. Schwartz,* 46 N.Y.2d 401, 386 N.E.2d 807 (1978). A few courts have allowed such claims. See *Procanik v. Cillo,* 478 A.2d 722 (N.J. 1984); *Harbeson v. Parke-Davis,* 656 P.2d 483 (Wash. 1983); *Turpin v. Sortini,* 643 P.2d 954 (Cal. 1982).

57 B. Steinbock and R. McClamrock, "When Is Birth Unfair to the Child?" *Hastings Center Report* 24, no. 6 (1994): 15.

58 B. Steinbock, *Life Before Birth* (New York: Oxford University Press, 1992), 120.

59 Steinbock and McClamrock, 17.

60 Cohen, "Give Me Children," 21.

61 Ibid., 23.

62 B. Steinbock, "Workshop Summary: Ethics of Reproductive Medicine: Responsibilities and Challenges," *Assisted Reproduction Reviews* 7 (1997): 39.

63 D. W. Brock, "Book Review: *Children of Choice: Freedom and the New Reproductive Technologies,*" *Texas Law Review* 74 (1995): 187, 204–205.

64 Cohen, "Give Me Children," 25.

65 Ibid., 24.

66 C. Strong, *Ethics in Reproductive and Perinatal Medicine: A New Framework* (New Haven: Yale University Press, 1997), 92.

ASSISTED REPRODUCTION

President's Council on Bioethics

In this selection, the President's Council on Bioethics begins by providing a rich description of state-of-the-art practice in the field of "assisted reproduction," understanding by that phrase IVF and closely related procedures. Next, the council expresses concern about "the intersection of two key factors": (1) Technologies in the field of assisted reproduction are sometimes introduced into clinical practice without adequate testing; (2) The vulnerability of patients suffering from infertility may lead them to take undue risks. Finally, the council surveys the risk factors associated with assisted reproduction, first in reference to the children born as a result of these technologies, then in reference to the women who choose to use them.

I. TECHNIQUES AND PRACTICES

Most methods of assisted reproduction involve five discrete phases: (1) collection and preparation of gametes; (2) fertilization; (3) transfer of an embryo or multiple embryos to a woman's uterus; (4) pregnancy; and (5) delivery and birth. We will discuss each phase separately. . . .

A. Collection and Preparation of Gametes The precursors of human life are the gametes: sperm and ova. Parents seeking to conceive through assisted reproduction usually provide their own gametes. In the United States in the year 2001, 75.2 percent of the ART [assisted reproductive technology] cycles undertaken used never-frozen, nondonor ova or embryos and another 13.7 percent used frozen nondonor ova or embryos. Of the remaining 11.1 percent of cycles using donor embryos, the breakdown is as follows: 3.2 percent of the embryos were previously cryopreserved, and 8 percent were not.[1] . . .

Acquiring ova for use in artificial reproduction is significantly more onerous, painful, and risky than acquiring sperm (though its risks are still low in absolute terms). In the normal course of ovulation, one mature oocyte is produced per menstrual cycle. However in assisted reproduction—to increase the

probability of success—many more ova are typically retrieved and fertilized. Thus, the ova source (who is usually also the gestational mother) undergoes a drug-induced process intended to stimulate her ovaries to produce many mature oocytes in a single cycle. This procedure, commonly referred to as "superovulation," requires the daily injection of a synthetic gonadatropin analog, accompanied by frequent monitoring using blood tests and ultrasound examinations. This treatment begins midway through the previous menstrual cycle and continues until just before ova retrieval. The synthetic gonadatropin analogs give the clinician greater control over ovarian stimulation and prevent premature release of the ova. . . .

When blood testing and ultrasound monitoring suggest that the ova are sufficiently mature, the clinician attempts to harvest them. This is typically achieved by ultrasound-guided transvaginal aspiration. In this procedure, a needle guided by ultrasound is inserted through the vaginal wall and into the mature ovarian follicles. An ovum is withdrawn (along with some fluid) from each follicle. This is an outpatient procedure. Risks and complications are low, but may include accidental puncture of nearby organs such as the bowel, ureter, bladder, or blood vessels, as well as the typical risks accompanying outpatient surgery (for example, risks related to administration of anesthesia, infection, etc.).

Once sperm and ova have been collected, they are cultured and treated to maximize the probability of success. . . .

Reprinted from President's Council on Bioethics, *Reproduction & Responsibility: The Regulation of New Biotechnologies* (2004), Chapter 2. Many notes omitted.

B. Fertilization Once the ova and sperm have been properly prepared, the clinician attempts to induce fertilization—the union of sperm and ovum culminating in the fusion of their separate pronuclei and the initiation of a new, integrated, self-directing organism. It is common practice to attempt to fertilize all available ova.[2] Fertilization can be achieved through a number of means including (1) "classical" IVF, (2) gamete intrafallopian transfer (GIFT), (3) intracytoplasmic sperm injection (ICSI). . . .

IVF is the most common method of artificial fertilization. In 2001, it was used by 99 percent of ART patients. As noted previously, both sperm and ovum are cultured to maximize the probability of fertilization. The ova are examined and rated for maturity in an effort to calculate the optimal time for fertilization. They are usually placed in a tissue culture medium and left undisturbed for two to twenty-four hours. . . . Once the gametes are adequately prepared, thousands of tiny droplets of sperm are placed in the culture medium containing a single ovum. After 24 hours, each of the oocytes is examined to determine whether fertilization has occurred.

GIFT was introduced in 1984 as an alternative to standard IVF. Today, attempts at fertilization via GIFT are rare. In 2001, they accounted for less than 1 percent of all attempts at fertilization used by ART patients. As the name suggests, fertilization using GIFT occurs within the woman's body. Ovarian stimulation and retrieval are performed in the same manner as in IVF. In a single procedure, ova are retrieved, combined with the sperm outside the body, and then transferred back into the fallopian tube where it is hoped that fertilization itself will occur. . . .

A new and increasingly popular technique for fertilization is intracytoplasmic sperm injection. As the name implies, with ICSI, ovum-sperm fusion is accomplished not by chance, but by injecting a single sperm directly into an oocyte. . . . A single sperm is selected and drawn into a thin pipette from which it is injected into the cytoplasm of the ovum cell.

ICSI is indicated in cases of severe male-factor infertility, in which male patients have either malformed sperm or an abnormally low sperm count. ICSI is also ideal for patients whose sperm would

not otherwise penetrate the exterior of an oocyte. ICSI was used in 49.2 percent of all ART cycles in 2001. However, 42.2 percent of those ICSI cycles were undertaken by couples *without* male-factor infertility. The growing popularity of this technique most likely has to do with the wish to increase the control over, and success rates for, fertilization: ICSI, unlike standard IVF, guarantees the entrance of a single sperm directly into a single egg. . . .

Because in many cases not all embryos are transferred in each cycle, cryopreservation of embryos has become an integral part of ART.[3] . . . A recently reported study by the Society for Assisted Reproductive Technology and RAND estimates that 400,000 embryos are in cryostorage in the United States.[4]

Most ART patients do not receive cryopreserved embryos. In 2001, only 14 percent of all ART cycles involved transfer of frozen embryos. The rate of live births for cycles using cryopreserved embryos is significantly lower than it is for never-frozen embryos (23.4 percent versus 33.4 percent). Experts estimate that only 65 percent of frozen embryos survive the thawing process. There are, however, incentives for couples to use cryopreserved embryos; doing so eliminates the cost and effort of further oocyte retrieval. This can decrease the cost of a future cycle by roughly $6,000. . . . Cryopreservation also reduces pressure to implant all embryos at once, thus reducing the risk of high-order multiple pregnancies.

C. Transfer . . . Typically, the embryos are transferred on the second or third day after fertilization, at the four- to eight-cell stage. To maximize the probability of implantation, some clinicians cultivate embryos until the blastocyst stage (five days after fertilization) before transferring them to the uterus. . . .

Once the embryos have been selected and prepared, they are transferred into the uterus. The total number of embryos transferred per cycle varies, usually according to the age of the recipient. For women under 35, the average number of never-frozen embryos transplanted per transfer procedure was 2.8. For women 35 to 37, 38 to 40, and 41 to 42, the average numbers of never-frozen embryos transplanted per transfer procedure were, respectively, 3.1, 3.4, and 3.7. . . .

Typically embryos are transferred into the uterus using a catheter. The catheter is inserted through the woman's cervix and the embryos are injected into her uterus (along with some amount of the culture fluid). This procedure does not require anesthesia. Following injection, the patient must lie still for at least one hour. While the transfer procedure is regarded as simple, different practitioners tend to achieve different outcomes.

An alternative method of embryo transfer is zygote intrafallopian transfer (ZIFT). In ZIFT, the embryo is placed (via laparoscopy) directly into the fallopian tube, rather than into the uterus. In this way, it is similar to the transfer of gametes in GIFT. Some individuals opt for ZIFT on the theory that it enhances the likelihood of implantation, given that the embryo matures en route to the uterus, presumably as it would in natural conception and implantation. Additionally, many patients prefer ZIFT to GIFT because the process of fertilization and early development of the embryo may be monitored. However, ZIFT remains a rare choice, accounting for 0.8 percent of all ART cycles in 2001.

D. Pregnancy Successful implantation of an embryo in the uterine lining marks the beginning of pregnancy. In 2001, 32.8 percent of the ART cycles undertaken resulted in clinical pregnancy.[5] This number varied according to patient age. . . .

Multiple gestations are common among pregnancies facilitated by assisted reproductive technologies. The rate of multiple-fetus pregnancies from ART cycles using never-frozen, nondonor ova or embryos in 2001 was 36.7 percent. For the same time period, the multiple infant birth rate in the United States was 3 percent. The extraordinarily high rate of multiple pregnancies resulting from assisted reproduction is almost entirely attributable to the transfer of multiple embryos per cycle.

In an effort to reduce the risks of multiple pregnancy, practitioners sometimes employ a procedure termed "fetal reduction," the reduction in the number of fetuses in utero by selective abortion. Fetuses are selected for destruction based on size, position, and viability (in the clinician's judg-ment). The clinician, using ultrasound for guidance, inserts a needle through the mother's abdomen (transabdominal multifetal reduction) through the uterine wall. The clinician then administers a lethal injection to the heart of the selected fetus—typically potassium chloride. The dead fetus's body decomposes and is resorbed. To be effective, transabdominal multifetal reduction must be performed at ten to twelve weeks' gestation. In an alternative procedure, transvaginal multifetal reduction, a needle is inserted through the vagina. Transvaginal multifetal reduction must be performed between six and eight weeks gestation (eight weeks is recommended).

E. Delivery In 2001, for never-frozen nondonor ova or embryos, the overall rate of live births per cycle[6] was 27 percent (33.4 percent live births per transfer).[7] Among these pregnancies, 82.2 percent resulted in live births. Of these resulting 21,813 live births, 35.8 percent were multiple infant births (32 percent twins and 3.8 percent triplets or more). . . .

F. Disposition of Unused Embryos As mentioned above, in many cases of ART there are in vitro embryos that remain untransferred following a successful cycle. There are five possible outcomes for such an embryo: (1) it may remain in cryostorage until transferred into the mother's uterus in a future ART cycle; (2) it may be donated to another person or couple seeking to initiate a pregnancy; (3) it may be donated for purposes of research; (4) it may remain in cryostorage indefinitely; or (5) it may be thawed and destroyed. . . .

II. ETHICAL CONSIDERATIONS

The development and practice of assisted reproductive technologies have yielded great goods. They have relieved the suffering of many who are afflicted with infertility, helping them to conceive biologically related children. Yet these activities also raise a variety of ethical issues. Some concern the well-being of the participants in assisted reproduction. . . .

The intersection of two key factors—patient vulnerability and novel (in some cases untested) technology—defines much of the arena of concern.

First, assisted reproduction is generally practiced on patients who are experiencing great emotional strain. When it succeeds it can be a source of great joy—as it has been for tens of thousands of parents each year. But success is far from universal, especially for older patients; and even when it happens, the process and the circumstances surrounding it can be difficult to bear. Those suffering from infertility often come to practitioners of assisted reproduction after prolonged periods of failure and dismay. This vulnerability may lead some individuals to take undue risks (such as to insist on transferring an unduly large number of embryos). The occasional irresponsible clinician may even pressure patients to take such risks, for the sake of improving his reportable success rates.

Second, some assisted reproductive technologies have been used in clinical practice without prior rigorous testing in primates or studies of long-term outcomes. IVF itself was performed on at least 1,200 women before it was reported to have been performed on chimps, although it had been extensively investigated in rabbits, hamsters, and mice. The same is true for ICSI. The reproductive use of ICSI was first introduced by Belgian researchers in 1992. Two years later, relying on a two-study review of safety and efficacy, ASRM (The American Society for Reproductive Medicine) declared ICSI to be a "clinical" rather than "experimental" procedure. Yet the first nonhuman primate conceived by ICSI was born only in 1997 and the first successful ICSI procedure in mice was reported in 1995. Absent long-term studies of the children conceived using ICSI or other novel procedures, it is unclear to what extent these alterations in the ART process affect the health and development of the children so conceived. . . .

A. Well-Being of the Child The central figure in the process of assisted reproduction, directly affected by every action taken but incapable of consenting to such actions, is the child born with the aid of ART. Each intervention or stage in the ART process might affect this child's health and well-being: gamete retrieval and preparation, fertilization, embryo culture, embryo transfer, pregnancy, and of course birth. . . .

There have been very few comprehensive or long-term studies of the health and well-being of children born using ART, although more than 170,000 such children have been born in the United States. The fact that no major investigation or public study has yet been called for in this area might suggest that there is no discernible health crisis in assisted reproduction, as does the fact that demand for ART has grown substantially and continuously since its inception. At the same time, however, our ability to know this with certainty is limited, both because of the absence of major longitudinal studies of the well-being of children born using different assisted reproduction techniques, and because the oldest person conceived through ART is only in her mid-twenties.

Some recent studies have associated various birth defects and developmental difficulties with the uses of various technologies and practices of assisted reproduction. None of these studies provide a causal link between ART and the dysfunctions observed, and some commentators have taken issue with some of the methodologies used. Nevertheless, these findings have raised some concerns. One such study concluded that children conceived by assisted reproduction are twice as likely to suffer major birth defects as children conceived without such assistance.[8] Other recent studies have reached similar conclusions. Additional studies have associated the use of assisted reproduction technologies with a higher incidence of diseases and malformations, including Beckwith-Wiedemann syndrome (BWS),[9] . . .

While many are concerned about the increased risk to children suggested by these studies, the overall incidence of such harms is low enough that infertile couples have not been deterred in their efforts to conceive using IVF or ICSI. Indeed, ART clinicians (and in some cases the authors of these studies) advise their patients that such data should not dissuade them from pursuing infertility treatment.

ICSI has raised concerns among some observers largely for the very reasons that it has proven so successful as a means of fertilization: ICSI circumvents the ovum's natural barrier against sperm otherwise incapable of insemination. Some suspect that removing this barrier may permit a damaged sperm (for example, aneuploid or with damaged DNA) to fertilize an ovum, resulting in spontaneous abortion or harm to the resulting child. Some male ART patients have a gene mutation or a chromosomal deletion that renders them infertile. Yet, if a sperm can be retrieved from these patients, they may be able to conceive a child via ICSI, possibly passing along the genetic abnormality to the resulting child. . . .

It is a matter of concern that there have been few longitudinal studies analyzing the long-term effects of ICSI on the children born with its aid. The Belgian group that pioneered ICSI has collected a database that details neonatal outcome and congenital malformations in children conceived through ICSI. But there do not seem to be any ongoing or published studies of this kind investigating the long-term effects of ICSI beyond the neonatal stage. . . .

Multiple gestations, far more common in the context of assisted reproduction than in natural conception, have a higher incidence of adverse impacts on the health of the children born. Such pregnancies greatly increase the risk of prenatal death. Multiple pregnancies are also more likely to lead to premature birth; and prematurity is associated with myriad health problems including serious infection, respiratory distress syndrome, and heart defects. One in ten children born following high-order pregnancies dies before one year of age. Children born following a multiple pregnancy are at greater risk for such disabilities as blindness, respiratory dysfunction, and brain damage. Moreover, infants born following such a pregnancy tend to have an extremely low birthweight, which is itself associated with a number of health problems, including some that manifest themselves only later in life, such as hypertension, cardiac disease, stroke, and osteoporosis in middle age. Interestingly, the higher incidence of low birthweight may not be limited to infants born from multiple pregnancies. According to recent studies, singletons born with the aid of ART tend to have an abnormally high incidence of prematurity and low birthweight.

So-called "fetal reduction" aims to reduce the problems associated with multiple pregnancy. But fetal reduction is itself potentially associated with a number of adverse effects on the children who remain following the procedure. . . .

Taken together, the significance of these various studies is uncertain. They raise a broad range of concerns, but the scale of the research has been limited. In many cases, there are observed correlations between ART and a higher incidence of certain health problems in the resulting children. But in most studies, there is no demonstrable causal relationship between a particular facet of ART and the undesirable health effect. Infertile individuals seeking assisted reproduction may be disproportionately afflicted with heritable disorders, and these may in part account for the higher incidence of birth and developmental abnormalities in ART children compared to those conceived in vivo. The results are therefore still preliminary. The need seems clear for more data to determine what risks, if any, different assisted reproduction techniques present to the well-being of the future child. Moreover, in cases where ART is the only available means for individuals or couples to conceive a biologically related child, it is an important ethical and social question what level of increased risk can be privately justified by patients and doctors, and what level of increased risk should be publicly justified by society as a whole, especially should the society bear the costs of caring for any resulting health problems.

B. Well-Being of Women in the ART Process Another concern is for the well-being of the women who participate directly in the process of assisted reproduction.

Aside from the discomforts and burdens of ovarian stimulation and monitoring, there are also some risks attached to hormonal stimulation. One such risk is "ovarian hyperstimulation syndrome," characterized by dramatic enlargement of the ovaries and fluid imbalances that can be (in extreme cases) life threatening. Complications can include rupture of the ovaries, cysts, and cancers. The reported incidence of severe ovarian hyperstimulation syndrome is between 0.5 and 5.0 percent. Additionally, adverse side effects of the hormones administered during superovulation have included memory loss, neurological dysfunction, cardiac disorders, and even sudden death. There do not appear to be any studies on the incidence of such side effects. . . .

Multiple pregnancies are far more common following ART, owing especially to the practice of transferring multiple embryos but also to the higher incidence of spontaneous twinning with any single embryo. Multiple pregnancies pose greater risks to mothers than do singleton pregnancies. A woman carrying multiple fetuses has a greater chance of suffering from high blood pressure, anemia, or pre-eclampsia. Because multiple-gestation pregnancies are generally more taxing on the mother's body, they are likelier to aggravate pre-existing medical conditions. Moreover, such pregnancies expose the woman to higher risks of uterine rupture, placenta previa, or abruption. . . .

NOTES

1 Centers for Disease Control and Prevention (CDC), *2001 Assisted Reproductive Technology Success Rates, National Summary and Fertility Clinic Reports,* Atlanta, Georgia: Government Printing Office, 2003, p. 14. [Subsequent figures cited for 2001 also derive from this document.]

2 The number of ova collected depends on a number of variables, including the donor's age, health, and other factors. In some cases, ten or more ova are fertilized in a single cycle.

3 There is not yet a reliable method of freezing unfertilized ova. This is perhaps due to their large size and high water content. Additionally, it seems that freezing an ovum toughens the zona pellucida in a way that can inhibit sperm penetration.

4 Hoffman, D., et al., "Cryopreserved Embryos in the United States and Their Availability for Research," *Fertility and Sterility* 79: 1063–1069 (2003).

5 This statistic is for never-frozen, nondonor ova or embryos—the most common approach in 2001.

6 A "cycle" is initiated when a woman begins the process of superovulation and monitoring. (CDC Report, p. 4.) Not all cycles result in successful ova collection, fertilization, transfer, pregnancy, or birth.

7 There seems to be a negative association between cryopreservation and implantation. For all pregnancies initiated using frozen, nondonor embryos, the success rate was 20.3 percent live births per transfer. . . .

8 Hansen, M., et al., "The Risk of Major Birth Defects After Intracytoplasmic Sperm Injection and In Vitro Fertilization," *The New England Journal of Medicine* 346: 725 (2002). Specifically, among the children in the study conceived by IVF, 9 percent were diagnosed with a major birth defect or defects by the age of one year. Among children conceived using ICSI, the rate was 8.6 percent. The incidence of such abnormalities among children in the study who were conceived by natural means was 4.2 percent.

9 Researchers at Johns Hopkins University noted that among the patients listed in the 1994 Beckwith-Wiedemann registry, IVF conception was six times more common than in the general population. That is, 4.6 percent of the patients in the registry were conceived through IVF, as compared with 0.8 percent of the national population. Children with BWS have symptoms that can include an abnormally large tongue (which can cause respiratory difficulties), abdominal wall defects (including umbilical hernia and protrusion of intestine or other abdominal organs from the child's navel), low blood sugar, lethargy, poor feeding, seizures, and enlargement of organs and some tissues. BWS sufferers are predisposed to Wilms' tumor, hepatoblastoma, neuroblastoma, and other cancers. Despite their findings, JHU researchers suggested that parents should not alter their plans to use IVF. See, for example, DeBaun, M. R., et al., "Association of in vitro fertilization with Beckwith-Wiedemann syndrome and epigenetic alterations of LIT_1 and H_{19}," *American Journal of Human Genetics* 72: 156–160 (2003).

GAMETE DONATION AND SURROGACY

FAMILIES, THE MARKETPLACE, AND VALUES: NEW WAYS OF MAKING BABIES
Thomas H. Murray

Murray argues that alternative reproductive practices should be judged morally unacceptable to the extent that they fail to cohere with or threaten to undermine values at the core of family life. He argues explicitly against a competing framework of moral analysis, according to which reproductive liberty and marketplace values are of overriding significance. Indeed, Murray argues against any intrusion of marketplace values into the realm of family life. He is not opposed to third-party involvement in reproduction, but he is opposed to the *commercialization* of such involvement. Thus, he objects to commercial surrogacy, and he objects to the practice of paying men for providing their sperm and paying women for providing their ova.

... The values embedded in certain alternative reproductive practices form a constellation that aligns poorly with other values at the heart of family life. Two contrasting images of values and relationships within families illustrate the point.

The champion of procreative liberty celebrates control and choice and portrays decisions about whether and how to acquire children as similar to decisions to acquire other new entities, only more important than most. If choice is valued in selecting a new appliance, all the more should it be valued in selecting a new child. If we are permitted to make voluntary agreements to spend our money to obtain new objects, all the more important to allow us similar freedom of contract and commerce to obtain new children, with one caveat: the children should not be harmed.

The other image is harder to label. It sees a role for values like control and choice within families but insists that these are not the principal values for which we make families; it is aware of the tension between unbridled liberty and control, on the one hand, and the values at the core of family life, on the other. It is vigilant against the encroachment of marketplace values into the family sphere because it recognizes that in commercial relationships the goal is to purchase a good or service, not to deepen the relationship, whereas all that is most valuable in family life centers on nurturing relationships.[1] Potential ways of adding children to the family must be scrutinized to assure that they will not undermine the values sought in family life, now or in the long run.[2]

In a defense of cloning human embryos, John Robertson, an ardent exponent of reproductive liberty, argues that couples wishing to "adopt" (his word) an embryo that is a clone of already living children should know all they want to know about those children. He says, "The right of adoptive parents to receive as full information as possible about the children whom they seek to adopt is increasingly recognized. There is no reason why the same principle should not apply to embryo 'adoptions.' Even though the couple seeking the embryos will be

choosing embryos on the basis of expected characteristics, such a choice is neither invalid nor immoral."[3] A couple, that is, may exercise quality control through choice.

The emphasis here on control and choice does not fit well with our understanding of families. Good families are characterized more by acceptance than control. Furthermore, families are the preeminent realm of unchosen obligations. We may choose our spouses (although a persuasive argument could be made that for most of us this choice bears scarce resemblance to the model of rational, autonomous, carefully considered decision making). We may choose to have a child, but—unless we are "adopting" one of Robertson's cloned embryos—we do not choose to have this *particular* child, with its interests, moods, and manners. And as offspring, we certainly did not choose our parents. Yet most of us would agree that we do have moral obligations to our parents, as well as to our spouses and children. An interesting problem for an ethics that enshrines autonomous choice as the fundamental requirement for moral obligation is this: How do you explain the enormously powerful web of moral obligations that supports family life, despite the only partly chosen or wholly unchosen nature of those relationships?

Some of the new reproductive practices require enlisting third parties. Women or men supply gametes, couples provide embryos, and women gestate their own or someone else's fetus. Justifying the involvement of third parties usually builds on the values of choice and control and invokes liberty. The question immediately arises, Why would any third party agree to participate in another couple's effort to have a child? For many people the answer is obvious: money. Robertson states the case bluntly: "If collaborative reproduction is viewed positively, reproduction contracts become the instruments of reproductive freedom."[4] He acknowledges the implication of this view:

> Legal liberty allows persons to treat each other as means to reproductive ends, with their negotiating ability and other resources determining the fate of future offspring. The extracorporeal embryo, that potent symbol of human life, becomes subject to the vagaries of a market that drives people to buy or sell

reproductive factors and services. Yet such freedom also allows people to determine and satisfy their welfare more efficaciously than by government prescription. In liberal society, the invisible hand of procreative preference must be allowed to flourish, despite the qualms of those who think it debases our humanity.[5]

Freedom equals the right to make a contract, to welcome, in Robertson's memorable paraphrase of Adam Smith, "the invisible hand of procreative preference." The price we pay for that freedom, including a market for human embryos, is the necessary cost of liberty, or so Robertson argues. With admirable tenacity, Robertson leads us down the reproductive path paved by the values of the market—individual liberty, choice, personal preference, contract, and commercialization. We are now in a position to see where we have arrived—and what beautiful, perhaps fragile, shoots have been bulldozed in the rush to build this particular highway.

The difference between the two images is clearest in their responses to surrogate motherhood for pay. How does a paid surrogate childbearer explain to her other children what has happened? Does she say, "Mommy loves her children so much that she wants to give another woman a chance to have her own children to love"? Does she add, "Oh, by the way, it also lets us buy groceries/pay off the mortgage/go to Disney World/finish the third floor"? What do her children think about their own security? Their relationship with their parents? What have they learned about the nature of the parent-child relationship? Have they learned that it is subject to the same harsh rules of supply and demand as any other commodity? Will such doubts make them more secure, contribute to their emotional development?

What of the surrogate herself? David H. Smith observes that the surrogate contract signed by Mary Beth Whitehead, biological mother of the famous Baby M, gave striking power over Mrs. Whitehead to William Stern, her fetus's biological father. Indeed, the contract gave Mr. Stern "rights Whitehead's husband would not have had if he and Whitehead had engendered a child." Smith grants the appeal of such control to the Sterns, but he worries about the "status they impose upon the surrogate, whose entire life is subordinated to 'the delivery of a product' for another."[6] He considers the analogy of surrogacy to slavery, admitting that there are important dissimilarities but insisting that "surrogacy is like slavery in the absence of reciprocity, in the fact that one person becomes what Aristotle called an 'animated tool' of another, serving simply as a means to another's end."[7]

We need to think not only about the impact on those directly and immediately involved but also about the values, practices, and institutions that affect families now and in the future. Are children likely to flourish in a culture where making children is governed by the same rules that govern the making of automobiles or VCRs? Or is their flourishing more assured in a culture where making children, and matching children with nurturing adults, is treated as a sphere separate from the marketplace, a sphere governed by the ethics of gift and relationship, not contract and commerce?

My claim is not that a market in children, embryos, or gametes violates some abstract principle in the noumenal realm. Rather, it is that given the sort of creatures we humans are, our patterns of psychosocial development, our needs at different stages of our lives—given these facts, certain values, institutions, and practices support our mutual flourishing better than others. Specifically, the values of the marketplace are ill suited for nurturing the values, institutions, and practices that support the flourishing of children and adults within families.

A market in gametes, or even in offspring, might not be a moral and social problem for other sorts of creatures for whom rationality is preeminent. But such a market is a threat for us humans who need affection, trust, and, above all, intimate and enduring relationships in order to flourish.

Note that I did not say that those hypothetical beings for whom a reproductive market might be acceptable were more *rational*—only that for them rationality is preeminent. What would it take for us humans to be most rational in understanding the ethical and policy implications of alternative means of reproduction? It would make no sense whatsoever to ignore what sort of creatures we really are, what circumstances are most conducive to our mutual flourishing. No doubt, there is disagreement about just what institutions and practices are the most likely to support our flourishing. But responsible practical moral reasoning cannot wish such matters away. We cannot honestly pretend to resolve these questions with a strictly moral or legal argument—an appeal to individual autonomy or reproductive liberty, for example. We must take into account factual as well as moral considerations in our practical moral judgments.

Some reproductive alternatives are more troubling than others. For a variety of reasons, a man might produce some normal sperm but not be able to place enough of them in a good position to reach an ovum ready for fertilization. Artificially inseminating a woman with her husband's sperm, for example, strikes most people as eminently acceptable. (The Roman Catholic church is an exception to this general chorus of approval.) Using another man's sperm is more complicated morally.

The usual practice in the United States, known as artificial insemination by donor, or AID, is a misnomer. The "donor" is usually paid for his sperm, making him a sperm vendor. I think this is a serious confusion, not a minor semantic quibble. Calling the supplier of sperm a donor invokes the realm of gifts, and with it the sphere of family and friendship. In commercial sperm banks, the vendors are actually anonymous strangers, paid for their "product" and then sent away, with presumably no more interest in what happens to it subsequently than a seller of office supplies has with what happens to his or her Post-it notes. Some men who sell or donate sperm discover later that they care about what has happened to it.[8] This is evidence that the market is a poor description of what transpires when gametes are transferred from one party to another. Because the market fails as a description, it is unlikely to be a faithful guide to ethical understanding as well.

So far, discussions about the ethics of alternative reproduction in the United States have paid scant attention to the practice of paying for sperm. The prospect of a man sitting in a booth and ejaculating into a container is the source of many jokes. But if I am correct about the dangers of the values of the market intruding on the sphere of the family, then AIV—artificial insemination by vendor—should make us uneasy. Not because of any sexual

squeamishness, but because commerce in this realm may threaten what is genuinely valuable within it. Using gametes provided by another man raises other morally relevant difficulties.[9] Even if, as seems likely, those are outweighed by the good of creating new parent-child relationships, we should be concerned about the impact of commercializing the practice.

Suppose we stopped paying for sperm and instead asked men to be genuine donors. Would that create a shortage of sperm? There are reasons to believe that it would not. First, several countries find an adequate number of such volunteers.[10] Second, there is the analogy with blood. In the United States it used to be assumed that you could only obtain an adequate supply of whole blood by paying individuals for it, or by offering them some other advantage. That assumption was false. People give blood because they are convinced other persons need it and they do not have to undergo great inconvenience to make a donation.[11] Like donations of blood, donations of sperm can assuage an important form of human suffering.

Whatever moral difficulties we find in a market for sperm, they are magnified in the market for ova because of the much greater physical risks involved. There are fewer healthy ova available for treating infertility than there are women who want them. Getting healthy ova to use in in vitro fertilization (IVF) and related procedures is a much more elaborate and invasive procedure than what is required to obtain sperm. The woman who will be the source of these eggs typically takes hormones that stimulate her ovaries to ripen multiple eggs, which must then be removed by aspiration or laparoscopy. Why would a woman go through such an ordeal? In many instances, the woman is a genuine donor, providing an egg for a relative or a friend. In other cases, the woman receives money. Compensating the supplier is fine, according to the American Fertility Society's "Guidelines for Gamete Donation: 1993." The guidelines say that "donors should be compensated for the direct and indirect expenses associated with their participation, their inconvenience and time, and to some degree, for the risk and discomfort undertaken."[12] One proposal calculates that with all the interviewing, testing, examinations, the procedure itself, and a full day to recover, an egg donation takes fifty-six hours of a woman's time. Assuming that men are paid $25 an hour for sperm, the authors of this proposal conclude that a woman should "receive $1,400 for her time alone, exclusive of any compensation for travel, risk, or inconvenience."[13] They ask, "Since it is standard to compensate men for sperm donation, shouldn't the policy be equal pay for equal time?"[14] A survey of infertility programs found that women who were paid for their ova received an average of $1,548, with a range from $750 to $3,500.[15]

MARKET VALUES AND THE VALUES OF FAMILY LIFE

"Equal pay for equal work" sums it up well. Paying individuals for their biological products makes them vendors, not donors. And it places the interactions between the parties squarely in the marketplace. Markets are built on the premise that individuals are rational pursuers of their own satisfaction and that choice and control are preeminent values. Market enthusiasts claim that the more things we allow the market to distribute, the better off we are. In practice, most market proponents recognize that some things should not be bought and sold. But the moral logic of some market advocates encompasses even children.[16] Explanations of why we should not allow children to be bought and sold often rely on two kinds of arguments: either that children have intrinsic moral value or worth and that such things should never be bought, sold, or owned; or that the consequences for children will be bad. I want to suggest a different line of argument.

The key errors in market analyses of the sphere of the family are a faulty set of presuppositions coupled to a dry, shrunken conception of human flourishing. The presuppositions include the notion that people are best understood as rational, isolated individuals in selfish pursuit of their own satisfaction, with the values of choice and control preeminent. There are problems with each piece of this model of human life. The emphasis on the *rational* underestimates the importance of the emotional in human life. The emphasis on the *isolated individual* discounts the great significance of relationships for people's flourishing. The assumption that people's motiva-

tions are essentially *selfish* fails to comprehend the complexity of human motivation, especially in the sphere of family life. . . . The celebration of *control* and *choice* fails to acknowledge the very limited role these values play in family life, indeed that a disproportionate emphasis on either can destroy families.

If children flourish best in stable, loving families, then we harm them by promoting a view of human relationship that equates the decision to initiate such a relationship with the decision to buy a wide-screen television or a medium-priced car. If adults flourish best in enduring, warm relationships and if caring for children also contributes to the flourishing of adults, then we should encourage practices and policies that support such relationships. To the extent that the dry view of human flourishing implicit in marketplace values shrinks our perceptions and undermines our support for family life, it threatens not merely children but adults as well.

I am not arguing that marketplace values are linked in some tight logical or mechanistic way so that where one is present the others follow inexorably. Rather, I am claiming that they form a mutually supportive web of compatible considerations. The focus on rational individuals seeking the maximum of satisfaction for themselves supports choice and control as values. The same focus tends to evaluate all things—objects, entertainments, other people—according to how well they satisfy the individual's desires. I like crusty bread, so I chose a bread machine with that feature; you like hazel eyes and curly black hair, so should you choose your children by those characteristics?

WHAT DIFFERENCE DOES IT MAKE?

If we set aside the moral framework of contract and market in favor of one more in tune with what we value about families, how would we regard alternative methods of reproduction? Most significant would be a shift in how we frame the moral question. The currently fashionable way to think about such matters is to place individual liberty and choice on one side of the balance and the harms caused on the other side. Robertson uses this strategy frequently and skillfully. His analysis of surrogacy provides a typical example.[17] Robertson emphasizes the voluntary nature of the agreement between the paying couple and the paid surrogate. He looks at potential harms to the couple and the surrogate as unlikely, not that different from other things we already tolerate, and in any event a consequence of their own free choice.

The child-product of the surrogacy contract is a more difficult story. But not much more difficult. The prospect of harms to such children could be dismissed as implausible or unproved, or as not so different from other practices we tolerate anyway, especially adoption. The parallel with harms to the adults involved in surrogacy ends there. Robertson, like other defenders of commercial surrogacy, cannot use the child's fictitious "consent" to justify any harms that might come to it. But he has another strategy. The child, he argues, benefits because "but for the surrogacy contract, this child would not exist at all. . . . [E]ven if the child does suffer identity problems, as adopted children often do . . . this child has benefited, or at least has not been wronged, for without the surrogate arrangement, she would not have been born at all."[18]

Try now to imagine some novel method of bringing children into the world which this way of framing the issues would condemn, as long as the adults participating did so freely. Cloning human embryos? No problem. Cloning embryos, freezing some and thawing them out later for implantation in someone else? Still no problem. Implanting an aborted fetus's ovary, with its millions of yet-unripe eggs, into a woman's body, so that she might become pregnant with that fetus's ova? It is difficult to see how anyone who frames the argument as Robertson and other enthusiasts do could make a strong objection to the practice. Who is harmed? Not the woman who chose to abort the fetus and gave her consent to using its ovaries. Certainly not the woman or her spouse who wants this supply of healthy ova. As for any children born from these eggs, who could prove they would have been better off never existing?

Would it matter if the reason the woman desired the fetal ovary was her own infertility, or because she is thirty-five and wanted to avoid the increased risk of birth defects that comes from older eggs? Or that she and her spouse wanted children with blue eyes, or some other genetically linked characteristics? I doubt that Robertson or most other supporters of reproductive alternatives would embrace such bizarre practices. But, it is also hard to see how, given the way they structure the ethical balancing, they could argue persuasively against them. You would have to demonstrate harms of such magnitude and certainty to individuals who have not, by their own choice, accepted the risks, that they overwhelm the powerful presumption in favor of liberty. Robertson, for one, looks with favor on doing genetic screening on and then freezing embryos while a woman is young, "until education, career, or relationship goals are worked out. They can then be transferred to the woman when there is a lower risk of a handicapped birth than if fertilization occurred shortly before implantation."[19]

What of healthy fertile women, who want to have their own genetic child, but do not want to go through pregnancy? Robertson believes that "surrogacy for convenience . . . may turn out to be more acceptable if it proves to be an effective way for women to combine work and reproduction. . . . As long as surrogate interests are protected, an optimal situation for all might result from surrogacy for convenience, if one accepts the change in the concept of mother that it would appear to entail."[20] This is precisely the inexorable moral logic of the marketplace, a logic that sweeps everything before it, deterred only by compelling evidence of serious, direct harm to those who have not consented by virtue of their own participation. As for the children thus created, we would have to prove that they would have been better off never being born.

New York State's Task Force on Life and the Law argues that the way the question is framed essentially dictates the answer because it presupposes that the children in question already exist. The task force suggests an alternative framing: whether, given the disadvantages of commercial surrogacy for future children, the practice should be permitted in the first place.[21] We should extend the task force's question and ask if these alternative means of creating children support or interfere with what we value in family and parenthood. Would they, on balance, create not just individual parent-child relationships but the kind of relationships that foster mutuality, loyalty, and love; relationships that endure, that survive the inevitable occasions when the relationship is causing a great deal more pain than pleasure? Beyond individual relationships, would they help build social attitudes and institutions that support the flourishing of children and adults within families?

I am suspicious of practices such as paying gamete suppliers or surrogate childbearers that thrust the values of the market into the heart of the family. It would be ridiculous to argue that all children born of such arrangements are irreparably damaged, or their relationships with their rearing parents warped. But I do not think it is silly to worry about the effect such practices have on our intimate relationships more generally and on parent-child relationships in particular. Unreflective ideological commitments can and do lead us astray, away from what we genuinely and deeply value. The attitudes and institutions that provide the absolutely necessary cultural support for what we value can be eroded, so gradually that we scarcely notice.

I agree with Robertson and other proponents of new reproductive arrangements about the enormous importance of children in the lives of adults. We both want to promote social practices that match children with nurturing adults. But where he regards contract and commercialization as "the instruments of reproductive freedom," I view them as, at best, threats and, at worst, inimical to the values families are meant to promote. They should be our culture's last resort, if we allow resort to them at all. Cultural meanings are shared creations, and their protection, or change, a shared project.

There is enough reason for concern to throw the burden of proof back onto the shoulders of proponents of marketplace values in reproduction. Show us that the practices you advocate do not threaten what we value about family life and that reasonable alternatives are lacking. Artificial insemination by vendor, for example, would not be justifiable because a nonmarket alternative exists—genuine donors.

To protect the few against the tyranny of the majority, the law may have to permit in the name of liberty some practices that we believe are unwise. But our moral vision must remain clear. If commercializing reproductive practices threatens cultural meanings and institutions, then our respect for political liberty does not require us to welcome such prac-

tices. Some commentators argue that procreative liberty is a fundamental constitutional right. Under our constitution, the government must have a compelling purpose to justify interfering with a fundamental constitutional right. But other experts disagree with the claim that our reproductive rights encompass practices such as gestation for pay. Alex Capron and Margaret Radin conclude that the "claim that the right to privacy protects surrogacy may be more plausible for noncommercial than for commercial surrogacy; even if the Constitution should be understood as including a right to bear a child for someone else, it should not be interpreted as including a right to be paid for it."[22] They argue that there is no obstacle in the Constitution to prevent a community from banning commercial surrogacy agencies, brokers, or advertising. I believe that we should prohibit commercial surrogacy.

There is another kind of surrogacy—gift surrogacy. A woman who is willing to bear her sister's or best friend's child out of loyalty and affection is acting in harmony with the values we prize in families. I would urge caution on the part of everyone involved, but I see what she is doing as an act of generosity, an extraordinary gift. Despite the outward physiological similarity between surrogacy-for-love and surrogacy-for-pay, the meanings of the two acts could not be more different. The former builds on a relationship of affection to create new affectionate relationships. The latter transmutes the creation of a child into a commercial transaction—a sort of reverse alchemy, turning gold into dross. . . .

. . . The uncritical celebration of procreative liberty and other marketplace values in reproduction is indeed a threat to what we value about families. Reproductive alternatives need to be examined in the light of those same values.

NOTES

1 Even incursions of the market as simple as children's allowances must be handled carefully. See Viviana Zelizer, *Pricing the Priceless Child* (New York: Basic Books, 1985).

2 David H. Smith makes a related distinction. In a discussion of surrogacy, he describes alternative "ways of thinking about a woman's relationship to a child she bears and indeed to her own reproductive processes. In one of these perspectives the relationship between self and reproductive involvement is extrinsic and contingent. Pregnancy is

viewed externally and objectively as a temporary state one is in for any one of a number of reasons. The self calculates its reasons for pregnancy, mode and form of personal involvement. . . . Another perspective on body is also possible: I identify myself with my body. I not only control it, but I have to listen to it. . . . I have embodied involvements with others, involvements that are constitutive of me as a self. These constitutive, involving embodiments are clearest in our relations with our parents and our children." Smith, "Wombs for Rent, Selves for Sale?" *Journal of Contemporary Health Law and Policy* 4 (1988): 30–31.

3   John A. Robertson, "The Question of Human Cloning," *Hastings Center Report* (March 1994): 6–14.

4   Robertson, "Embryos, Families and Procreative Liberty: The Legal Structure of the New Reproduction," *Southern California Law Review* 59, no. 5 (1986): 1031. Robertson's commitment to reproductive liberty is clear in both the title and the text of his book, *Children of Choice: Freedom and the New Reproductive Technologies* (Princeton: Princeton University Press, 1994). In it he restates his guiding principle: "I propose that procreative liberty be given presumptive priority in all conflicts, with the burden on opponents of any particular technique to show that harmful effects from its use justify limiting procreative choice" (p. 16).

5   Ibid., 1040.

6   Smith, "Wombs for Rent, Selves for Sale?" 33.

7   Ibid, 34.

8   See K. R. Daniels, "Semen Donors: Their Motivations and Attitudes to Their Offspring," *Journal of Reproductive and Infant Psychology* 7 (1989): 121–127, and R. Rowland, "Attitudes and Opinions of Donors on an Artificial Insemination by Donor (AID) Programme," *Clinical Reproduction and Fertility* 2 (1983): 249–259.

9   Paul Lauritzen, *Pursuing Parenthood* (Bloomington: Indiana University Press, 1993).

10   Ken R. Daniels and Karyn Taylor, "Secrecy and Openness in Donor Insemination," *Politics and the Life Sciences* 12, no. 2 (1993): 155–170, confirm that Australia and New Zealand rely on genuine donors. In the same issue of the journal, Jacques Lansac affirms that France uses only sperm donors, not vendors ("One Father Only: Donor Insemination and CECOS in France," pp. 185–186).

11   Alvin W. Drake, Stan N. Finkelstein, and Harvey M. Sapolsky, *The American Blood Supply* (Cambridge: MIT Press, 1982).

12   American Fertility Society, "Guidelines for Gamete Donation: 1993," *Fertility and Sterility, Supplement 1* 59, no. 2 (1993): 5S–9S, 6S; sec. VI.A.

13   Machelle M. Seibel and Ann Kiessling, "Compensating Egg Donors: Equal Pay for Equal Time?" *New England Journal of Medicine* 328, no. 10 (1993): 737.

14   Ibid.

15   Andrea Mechanick Braverman, "Survey Results on the Current Practice of Ovum Donation," *Fertility and Sterility* 59, no. 6 (1993): 1216–1220.

16   In a famous article, Landes and Posner consider "some tentative and reversible steps toward a free baby market in order to determine experimentally the social costs and benefits of using the market in this area." "The Economics of the Baby Shortage," *Journal of Legal Studies,* 7, no. 2 (1978): 347.

17   John A. Robertson, "Surrogate Mothers: Not So Novel After All," *Hastings Center Report* 13, no. 5 (1983): 28–34.

18   Ibid., 29.

19   Robertson, "Embryos, Families and Procreative Liberty," 1030.

20   Ibid.

21   New York State Task Force on Life and the Law, *Surrogate Parenting: Analysis and Recommendations for Public Policy* (1988). The task force concluded unanimously that public policy ought to discourage surrogate parenting and proposed legislation to ban fees to surrogates or brokers and to void surrogacy contracts. Their response to the argument that children born under surrogacy arrangements are better off because otherwise they would not have been born at all is as follows:

> But this argument assumes the very factor under deliberation—the child's conception and birth. The assessment for public policy occurs prior to conception when the surrogate arrangements are made. The issue then is not whether a particular child should be denied life, but whether children should be conceived in circumstances that would place them at risk. The notion that children have an interest in being born prior to their conception and birth is not embraced in other public policies and should not be assumed in the debate on surrogate parenting. (p. 120)

I am grateful to John Arras for pointing out this argument to me.

22   Alexander M. Capron and Margaret J. Radin, "Choosing Family Law Over Contract Law as a Paradigm for Surrogate Motherhood," *Law, Medicine & Health Care* 16, nos. 1–2 (1988): 34, 40.

SURROGATE MOTHERHOOD AS PRENATAL ADOPTION
Bonnie Steinbock

Steinbock maintains that commercial surrogacy contracts should not be prohibited by the state. She argues that it is unjustifiably paternalistic for the state to ban surrogacy in an effort to protect the potential surrogate from a choice that may later be regretted. She also argues that concerns about a negative psychological impact on potential offspring are insufficient to warrant an outright ban. Moreover, in her view, commercial surrogacy is neither inherently exploitive nor inconsistent with human dignity. In dealing with the charge that commercial surrogacy amounts to baby selling, she insists that payment to the surrogate can be understood as compensation for "the risks, sacrifice, and discomfort the surrogate undergoes during pregnancy." Although Steinbock considers the legal prohibition of surrogacy contracts to be incompatible with a proper regard for the value of individual freedom, she believes that the practice of surrogacy should be regulated by the state. In particular, she would insist that surrogacy contracts be structured so as to allow the surrogate a postnatal waiting period, during which she would be free to change her mind and keep the child. (Steinbock makes several references to the Baby M case; for the facts of this case, see Appendix, Case 41.)

The recent case of "Baby M" has brought surrogate motherhood to the forefront of American attention. Ultimately, whether we permit or prohibit surrogacy depends on what we take to be good reasons for preventing people from acting as they wish. A growing number of people want to be, or hire, surrogates; are there legitimate reasons to prevent them? Apart from its intrinsic interest, the issue of surrogate motherhood provides us with an opportunity to examine different justifications for limiting individual freedom.

. . . I examine claims that surrogacy is ethically unacceptable because it is exploitive, inconsistent with human dignity, or harmful to the children born of such arrangements. I conclude that these reasons justify restrictions on surrogate contracts, rather than an outright ban. . . .

SHOULD SURROGACY BE PROHIBITED?

On June 27, 1988, Michigan became the first state to outlaw commercial contracts for women to bear children for others.[1] Yet making a practice illegal

From *Law, Medicine, and Health Care*, vol. 16 (Spring 1988). Reprinted with permission of the author and the publisher (American Society of Law, Medicine & Ethics).

does not necessarily make it go away: witness black-market adoption. The legitimate concerns that support a ban on surrogacy might be better served by careful regulation. However, some practices, such as slavery, are ethically unacceptable, regardless of how carefully regulated they are. Let us consider the arguments that surrogacy is intrinsically unacceptable.

Paternalistic Arguments These arguments against surrogacy take the form of protecting a potential surrogate from a choice she may later regret. As an argument for banning surrogacy, as opposed to providing safeguards to ensure that contracts are freely and knowledgeably undertaken, this is a form of paternalism.

At one time, the characterization of a prohibition as paternalistic was a sufficient reason to reject it. The pendulum has swung back, and many people are willing to accept at least some paternalistic restrictions on freedom. Gerald Dworkin points out that even Mill made one exception to his otherwise absolute rejection of paternalism: he thought that no one should be allowed to sell himself into slavery, because to do so would be to destroy his future autonomy.

This provides a narrow principle to justify some paternalistic interventions. To preserve freedom in the long run, we give up the freedom to make certain choices, those that have results that are "far-reaching, potentially dangerous and irreversible."[2] An example would be a ban on the sale of crack. Virtually everyone who uses crack becomes addicted and, once addicted, a slave to its use. We reasonably and willingly give up our freedom to buy the drug, to protect our ability to make free decisions in the future.

Can a Dworkinian argument be made to rule out surrogacy agreements? Admittedly, the decision to give up a child is permanent, and may have disastrous effects on the surrogate mother. However, many decisions may have long-term, disastrous effects (e.g., postponing childbirth for a career, having an abortion, giving a child up for adoption). Clearly we do not want the state to make decisions for us in all these matters. Dworkin's argument is rightly restricted to paternalistic interferences that protect the individual's autonomy or ability to make decisions in the future. Surrogacy does not involve giving up one's autonomy, which distinguishes it from both the crack and selling-oneself-into-slavery examples. Respect for individual freedom requires us to permit people to make choices they may later regret.

Moral Objections ... We must all agree that a practice that exploits people or violates human dignity is immoral. However, it is not clear that surrogacy is guilty on either count.

Exploitation The mere fact that pregnancy is *risky* does not make surrogate agreements exploitive, and therefore morally wrong. People often do risky things for money; why should the line be drawn at undergoing pregnancy? The usual response is to compare surrogacy and kidney-selling. The selling of organs is prohibited because of the potential for coercion and exploitation. But why should kidney-selling be viewed as intrinsically coercive? A possible explanation is that no one would do it, unless driven by poverty. The choice is both forced and dangerous, and hence coercive.

The situation is quite different in the case of the race-car driver or stuntman. We do not think that they are *forced* to perform risky activities for money:

they freely choose to do so. Unlike selling one's kidneys, these are activities that we can understand (intellectually, anyway) someone choosing to do. Movie stuntmen, for example, often enjoy their work, and derive satisfaction from doing it well. Of course they "do it for the money," in the sense that they would not do it without compensation; few people are willing to work "for free." The element of coercion is missing, however, because they enjoy the job, despite the risks, and could do something else if they chose.

The same is apparently true of most surrogates. "They choose the surrogate role primarily because the fee provides a better economic opportunity than alternative occupations, but also because they enjoy being pregnant and the respect and attention that it draws."[3] Some may derive a feeling of self-worth from an act they regard as highly altruistic: providing a couple with a child they could not otherwise have. If these motives are present, it is far from clear that the surrogate is being exploited. Indeed, it seems objectionally paternalistic to insist that she is.

Human Dignity It may be argued that even if womb-leasing is not necessarily exploitive, it should still be rejected as inconsistent with human dignity. But why? As John Harris points out, hair, blood, and other tissue is often donated or sold; what is so special about the uterus?[4]

Human dignity is more plausibly invoked in the strongest argument against surrogacy, namely, that it is the sale of a child. Children are not property, nor can they be bought or sold. It could be argued that surrogacy is wrong because it is analogous to slavery, and so is inconsistent with human dignity.

However, there are important differences between slavery and a surrogate agreement. The child born of a surrogate is not treated cruelly or deprived of freedom or resold; none of the things that make slavery so awful are part of surrogacy. Still, it may be thought that simply putting a market value on a child is wrong. Human life has intrinsic value; it is literally priceless. Arrangements that ignore this violate our deepest notions of the value of human life. It is profoundly disturbing to hear in a television documentary on surrogacy the boyfriend of a surrogate say, quite candidly, "We're in it for the money."

[The trial court judge in the Baby M case] accepted the premise that producing a child for money denigrates human dignity, but he denied that this happens in a surrogate agreement. Ms. Whitehead was not paid for the surrender of the child to the father: she was paid for her willingness to be impregnated and carry Mr. Stern's child to term. The child, once born, is his biological child. "He cannot purchase what is already his."[5]

This is misleading, and not merely because Baby M is as much Ms. Whitehead's child as Mr. Stern's. It is misleading because it glosses over the fact that the surrender of the child was part—indeed, the whole point—of the agreement. If the surrogate were paid merely for being willing to be impregnated and carrying the child to term, then she would fulfill the contract upon giving birth. She could take the money *and* the child. Mr. Stern did not agree to pay Ms. Whitehead merely to *have* his child, but to provide him with a child. The New Jersey Supreme Court held that this violated New Jersey's laws prohibiting the payment or acceptance of money in connection with adoption.

One way to remove the taint of baby-selling would be to limit payment to medical expenses associated with the birth or incurred by the surrogate during pregnancy (as is allowed in many jurisdictions, including New Jersey, in ordinary adoptions). Surrogacy could be seen, not as baby-selling, but as a form of adoption. Nowhere did the Supreme Court find any legal prohibition against surrogacy when there is no payment, and when the surrogate has the right to change her mind and keep the child. However, this solution effectively prohibits surrogacy, since few women would become surrogates solely for self-fulfillment or reasons of altruism.

The question, then, is whether we can reconcile paying the surrogate, beyond her medical expenses, with the idea of surrogacy as prenatal adoption. We can do this by separating the terms of the agreement, which include surrendering the infant at birth to the biological father, from the justification for payment. The payment should be seen as compensation for the risks, sacrifice, and discomfort the surrogate undergoes during pregnancy. This means that if, through no fault on the part of the surrogate, the baby is stillborn, she should still be paid in full, since she has

kept her part of the bargain. (By contrast, in the Stern-Whitehead agreement, Ms. Whitehead was to receive only $1,000 for a stillbirth).[6] If, on the other hand, the surrogate changes her mind and decides to keep the child, she would break the agreement, and would not be entitled to any fee or to compensation for expenses incurred during pregnancy. . . .

. . . There are sound moral and policy . . . reasons to provide a postnatal waiting period in surrogate agreements. As the Baby M case makes painfully clear, the surrogate may underestimate the bond created by gestation and the emotional trauma caused by relinquishing the baby. Compassion requires that we acknowledge these findings, and not deprive a woman of the baby she has carried because, before conception, she underestimated the strength of her feelings for it. Providing a waiting period, as in ordinary postnatal adoptions, will help protect women from making irrevocable mistakes, without banning the practice.

Some may object that this gives too little protection to the prospective adoptive parents. They cannot be sure that the baby is theirs until the waiting period is over. While this is hard on them, a similar burden is placed on other adoptive parents. If the absence of a guarantee serves to discourage people from entering surrogacy agreements, that is not necessarily a bad thing, given all the risks inherent in such contracts. In addition, this requirement would make stricter screening and counseling of surrogates essential, a desirable side-effect.

Harm to Others Paternalistic and moral objections to surrogacy do not seem to justify an outright ban. What about the effect on the offspring of such contracts? We do not yet have solid data on the effects of being a "surrogate child." Any claim that surrogacy creates psychological problems in the children is purely speculative. But what if we did discover that such children have deep feelings of worthlessness from learning that their natural mothers deliberately created them with the intention of giving them away? Might we ban surrogacy as posing an unacceptable risk of psychological harm to the resulting children?

Feelings of worthlessness are harmful. They can prevent people from living happy, fulfilling lives. However, a surrogate child, even one whose life is miserable because of these feelings, cannot claim to have been harmed by the surrogate agreement. Without the agreement, the child would never have existed. Unless she is willing to say that her life is not worth living because of these feelings, that she would be better off never having been born, she cannot claim to have been harmed by being born of a surrogate mother.

Elsewhere I have argued that children can be *wronged* by being brought into existence, even if they are not, strictly speaking, *harmed.*[7] They are wronged if they are deprived of the minimally decent existence to which all citizens are entitled. We owe it to our children to see that they are not born with such serious impairments that their most basic interests will be doomed in advance. If being born to a surrogate is a handicap of this magnitude, comparable to being born blind or deaf or severely mentally retarded, then surrogacy can be seen as wronging the offspring. This would be a strong reason against permitting such contracts. However, it does not seem likely. Probably the problems arising from surrogacy will be like those faced by adopted children and children whose parents divorce. Such problems are not trivial, but neither are they so serious that the child's very existence can be seen as wrongful.

If surrogate children are neither harmed nor wronged by surrogacy, it may seem that the argument for banning surrogacy on grounds of its harmfulness to the offspring evaporates. After all, if the children themselves have no cause for complaint, how can anyone else claim to reject it on their behalf? Yet it seems extremely counter-intuitive to suggest that the risk of emotional damage to the children born of such arrangements is not even relevant to our deliberations. It seems quite reasonable and proper—even morally obligatory—for policymakers to think about the possible detrimental effects of new reproductive technologies, and to reject those likely to create physically or emotionally damaged people. The explanation for this must involve the idea that it is wrong to bring people into the world in a harmful condition, even if they are not, strictly speaking, harmed by having been brought into existence. Should evidence emerge that surrogacy produces

children with serious psychological problems, that would be a strong reason for banning the practice.

There is some evidence on the effect of surrogacy on the other children of the surrogate mother. One woman reported that her daughter, now seventeen, who was eleven at the time of the surrogate birth, "is still having problems with what I did, and as a result she is still angry with me." She explains: "Nobody told me that a child could bond with a baby while you're still pregnant. I didn't realize then that all the times she listened to his heartbeat and felt his legs kick that she was becoming attached to him."[8]

A less sentimental explanation is possible. It seems likely that her daughter, seeing one child given away, was fearful that the same might be done to her. We can expect anxiety and resentment on the part of children whose mothers give away a brother or sister. The psychological harm to these children is clearly relevant to a determination of whether surrogacy is contrary to public policy. At the same time, it should be remembered that many things, including divorce, remarriage, and even moving to a new neighborhood, create anxiety and resentment in children. We should not use the effect on children as an excuse for banning a practice we find bizarre or offensive.

CONCLUSION

There are many reasons to be extremely cautious of surrogacy. I cannot imagine becoming a surrogate, nor would I advise anyone else to enter into a contract so fraught with peril. But the fact that a practice is risky, foolish, or even morally distasteful is not sufficient reason to outlaw it. It would be better for the state to regulate the practice, and minimize the potential for harm, without infringing on the liberty of citizens.

NOTES

1 *New York Times,* June 28, 1988, A20.
2 Gerald Dworkin, "Paternalism," in R. A. Wasserstrom, ed., *Morality and the Law* (Belmont, Cal.: Wadsworth, 1971); reprinted in J. Feinberg and H. Gross, eds., *Philosophy of Law,* 3d ed. (Belmont, Cal.: Wadsworth, 1986), 265.
3 John Robertson, "Surrogate Mothers: Not So Novel After All," *Hastings Center Report,* 13, no. 5 (1983): 29; citing P. Parker, "Surrogate Mother's Motivations: Initial Findings," *American Journal of Psychiatry,* 140 (1983): 1.

4 J. Harris, *The Value of Life* (London: Routledge & Kegan Paul, 1985), 144.

5 *In re Baby "M,"* 217 N.J. Super. 372, 525 A.2d 1157 (1987).

6 George Annas, "Baby M: Babies (and Justice) for Sale," *Hastings Center Report,* 17, no. 3 (1987): 14.

7 Bonnie Steinbock, "The Logical Case for 'Wrongful Life,'" *Hastings Center Report,* 16, no. 2 (1986): 15.

8 "Baby M Case Stirs Feelings of Surrogate Mothers," *New York Times,* March 2, 1987, B1.

HUMAN CLONING

CLONING OF HUMAN BEINGS
Leon R. Kass

In this testimony presented to the National Bioethics Advisory Commission (NBAC), Kass urges the commission to declare human cloning deeply unethical and to recommend a legal ban. Calling attention to the widespread sense of repugnance elicited by the prospect of human cloning, he advances four lines of argument against its use. These arguments are based on (1) considerations related to the ethics of experimentation, (2) concerns about identity and individuality, (3) the dangers of transforming procreation into manufacture, and (4) the negative impact upon our understanding of what it means to have children.

Mr. Chairman, Members of the Commission.

I am deeply grateful for the opportunity to present some of my thoughts about the ethics of human cloning, by which I mean precisely—the production of cloned human beings. This topic has occupied me off and on for over 30 years; it was the subject of one of my first publications in bioethics 25 years ago. Since that time, we have in some sense been softened up to the idea of human cloning—through movies, cartoons, jokes, and intermittent commentary in the mass media, occasionally serious, more often lighthearted. We have become accustomed to new practices in human reproduction—in vitro fertilization, embryo manipulation, and surrogate pregnancy—and, in animal biotechnology, to transgenic animals and a burgeoning science of genetic engineering. Changes in the broader culture make it now more difficult to express a common, respectful understanding of sexuality, procreation, nascent life, and the meaning of motherhood, fatherhood, and the links between the generations. In a world whose once-given natural boundaries are blurred by technological change and whose moral boundaries are seemingly up for grabs, it is, I believe, much more difficult than it once was to make persuasive the still compelling case against human cloning. As Raskolnikov put it, "Man gets used to everything—the beast!"

Therefore, the first thing of which I want to persuade you is not to be complacent about what is here at issue. Human cloning, though in some respects continuous with previous reproductive technologies, also represents something radically new, both in itself and in its easily foreseeable consequences. The stakes here are very high indeed. Let me exaggerate, but in the direction of the truth: You have been asked to give advice on nothing less than whether human procreation is going to remain human, whether children are going to be made rather than begotten, and whether it is a good thing, humanly speaking, to say yes to the road which leads (at best) to the dehumanized rationality of Brave New World. If I could persuade you of nothing else, it would be this: What we have here is not business as usual, to be fretted about for a while but finally to be given our seal of

Testimony presented to the National Bioethics Advisory Commission. March 14, 1997, Washington, D.C.

approval, not least because it appears to be inevitable. Rise to the occasion, address the subject in all its profundity, and advise as if the future of our humanity may hang in the balance.

"Offensive." "Grotesque." "Revolting." "Repugnant." "Repulsive." These are the words most commonly heard these days regarding the prospect of human cloning. Such reactions one hears both from the man or woman in the street and from the intellectuals, from believers and atheists, from humanists and scientists. Even Dolly's creator, Dr. Wilmot, has said he "would find it offensive" to clone a human being. People are repelled by many aspects of human cloning: The prospect of mass production of human beings, with large clones of look-alikes, compromised in their individuality; the idea of father-son or mother-daughter twins; the bizarre prospects of a woman giving birth to a genetic copy of herself, her spouse, or even her deceased father or mother; the creation of embryonic genetic duplicates of oneself, to be frozen away in case of later need for homologous organ transplantation; the narcissism of those who would clone themselves, the arrogance of others who think they know who deserves to be cloned or which genotype any child-to-be should be thrilled to receive; the Frankensteinian hubris to create human life and increasingly to control its destiny; man playing at being God. Almost no one sees any compelling reason for human cloning; almost everyone anticipates its possible misuses and abuses. Many feel oppressed by the sense that there is nothing we can do to prevent it from happening. This makes the prospect all the more revolting.

Revulsion is surely not an argument, and some of yesterday's repugnances are today calmly accepted. But in crucial cases, repugnance is often the emotional bearer of deep wisdom, beyond reason's power fully to articulate it. Can anyone really give an argument fully adequate to the horror which is father-daughter incest (even with consent) or having sex with animals or eating human flesh, or even just raping or murdering another human being? Would anyone's failure to give full rational justification for his revulsion at these practices make that revulsion ethically suspect? Not at all. In my view, our repugnance at human cloning belongs in this category. We are repelled by the prospect of cloning human beings not because of the strangeness or novelty of the undertaking, but because we intuit and feel, immediately and without argument, the violation of things we rightfully hold dear. I doubt very much whether I can give the proper rational voice to this horror, but in the remarks that follow I will try. But please consider seriously that this may be one of those instances about which the heart has its reasons that reason cannot adequately know.

I will raise four kinds of objections: the ethics of experimentation; identity and individuality; fabrication and manufacture; despotism and the violation of what it means to have children.

First, any attempt to clone a human being would constitute an unethical experiment upon the resulting child-to-be. As the animal experiments indicate, there is grave risk of mishaps and deformities. Moreover, one cannot presume a future cloned child's consent to be a clone, even a healthy one. Thus, we cannot ethically get to know even whether or not human cloning is feasible.

I understand, of course, the philosophical difficulty of trying to compare life with defects against non-existence. But common sense tells us that it is irrelevant. It is surely true that people can harm and even maim children in the very act of conceiving them, say, by paternal transmission of the HIV virus or maternal transmission of heroin dependence. To do so intentionally, or even negligently, is inexcusable and clearly unethical.

Second, cloning creates serious issues of identity and individuality. The cloned person may experience concerns about his distinctive identity not only because he will be in genotype and appearance identical to another human being, but, in this case, it will be to a twin who might be his "father" or "mother"—if one can still call them that. What would be the psychic burdens of being the "child" or "parent" of your twin? Moreover, the cloned individual will be saddled with a genotype that has already lived. He will not be fully a surprise to the world: people are likely always to compare his performances in life with that of his alter ego. True, his nurture and circumstance in life will be different; genotype is not exactly destiny. But one must also expect parental and other efforts to shape this new life after the original—or at least to view the child with the original version firmly in mind. For why else did they clone from the star basketball player, mathematician, and beauty queen—or even dear old Dad—in the first place?

Genetic distinctiveness not only symbolizes the uniqueness of each human life and the independence of its parents that each human child rightfully attains. It can also be an important support for living a worthy and dignified life. Such arguments apply with great force to any large-scale replication of human individuals. But they are, in my view, sufficient to rebut even the first attempts to clone a human being. One must never forget that these are human beings upon whom our eugenic or merely playful fantasies are to be enacted.

Third, human cloning would represent a giant step toward turning begetting into making, procreation into manufacture (literally, something "hand made"), a process already begun with in vitro fertilization and genetic testing of embryos. With cloning, not only is the process in hand, but the total genetic blueprint of the cloned individual is selected and determined by the human artisans. To be sure, subsequent development is still according to natural processes; and the resulting children will still be recognizably human. But we here would be taking a major step into making man himself simply another one of the man-made things. Human nature becomes merely the last part of nature to succumb to the technological project, which turns all of nature into raw material at human disposal, to be homogenized by our rationalized technique according to the subjective prejudices of the day.

How does begetting differ from making? In natural procreation, we two human beings come together, complementarily male and female, to give existence to another being who is formed, exactly as we were, by what we are—living, hence perishable, hence aspiringly erotic human beings. But in clonal reproduction, and in the more advanced forms of manufacture to which it leads, we give existence to a being not by what we are but by what we intend and design. As with any product of our making, no matter how excellent, the artificer stands above it, not as an equal but as a superior, transcending it by his will and creative prowess. Scientists who clone animals make it perfectly clear that they are engaged

in instrumental making; the animals are, from the start, designed as means to serve rational human purpose. In human cloning, scientists and prospective "parents" would be adopting the same technocratic mentality to human children: human children would be their artifacts. Such an arrangement is profoundly dehumanizing, no matter how good the product. Mass-scale cloning of the same individual makes the point vividly; but the violation of human equality, freedom, and dignity are present even in a single planned clone.

Finally, and perhaps most important, the practice of human cloning by nuclear transfer—like other anticipated forms of genetic engineering of the next generation—would enshrine and aggravate a profound and mischief-making misunderstanding of the meaning of having children and of the parent-child relationship. When a couple now chooses to procreate, the partners are saying yes to the emergence of new life in its novelty, are saying yes not only to having a child but also, tacitly, to having whatever child this child turns out to be. Whether we know it or not, we are thereby also saying yes to our own finitude and mortality, to the necessity of our replacement and the limits of our control. In this ubiquitous way of nature, to say yes to the future by procreating means precisely that we are relinquishing our grip, even as we thereby take up our own share in what we hope will be the immortality of human life and the human species. This means that our children are not our children: They are not our property, they are not our possessions. Neither are they supposed to live our lives for us, or anyone else's life but their own. To be sure, we seek to guide them on their way, imparting to them not just life but nurture, love, and a way of life; to be sure, they bear our hopes that they will surpass us in goodness and happiness, enabling us in small measure to transcend our own limitations. But their genetic distinctiveness and independence is the natural foreshadowing of the deep truth that they have their own and never-before-enacted life to live. Though sprung from a past, they take an uncharted course into the future.

Much mischief is already done by parents who try to live vicariously through their children; children are sometimes compelled to fulfill the broken dreams of unhappy parents; John Doe, Jr. or the III is under the burden of having to live up to his fore-bear's name. But in cloning, such overbearing parents take at the start a decisive step which contradicts the entire meaning of the open and forward-looking nature of parent-child relations. The child is given a genotype that has already lived, with full expectation that this blueprint of a past life ought to be controlling of the life that is to come. Cloning is inherently despotic, for it seeks to make one's children or someone else's children after one's own image (or an image of one's choosing) and their future according to one's will. In some cases, the despotism may be mild and benevolent, in others, mischievous and downright tyrannical. But despotism—the control of another through one's will—it will unavoidably be.

What then should we do? We should declare human cloning deeply unethical in itself and dangerous in its likely consequences. In so doing, we shall have the backing of the overwhelming majority not only of our fellow Americans, but of the human race—including, I believe, most practicing scientists. Next, we should do all that we can to prevent human cloning from happening, by an international legal ban if possible, by a unilateral national ban, at a minimum. Scientists can, of course, secretly undertake to violate such a law, but they will at least be deterred by not being able to stand up proudly to claim the credit for their technological bravado and success. Such a ban on human cloning will not harm the progress of basic genetic science and technology; on the contrary, it will reassure the public that scientists are happy to proceed without violating the deep ethical norms and intuitions of the human community.

The President has given this Commission a glorious opportunity. In a truly unprecedented way, you can strike a blow for the human control of the technological project, for wisdom, prudence, and human dignity. The prospect of human cloning, so repulsive to contemplate, in fact provides the occasion—as well as the urgent necessity—of deciding whether we shall be slaves of unregulated progress, and ultimately its artifacts, or whether we shall remain free human beings who guide our technique toward the enhancement of human dignity. To seize the occasion, we—you—must, as the late Paul Ramsey said, "raise the ethical questions with a serious and not a frivolous conscience. A man of frivolous conscience announces that there are ethical quandaries ahead that we must urgently consider before the future catches up with us. By this he often means that we need to devise a new ethics that will provide the rationalization for doing in the future what men are bound to do because of new actions and interventions science will have made possible. In contrast a man of serious conscience means to say in raising urgent ethical questions that there may be some things that men should never do. The good things that men do can be made complete only by the things they refuse to do."

EVEN IF IT WORKED, CLONING WOULDN'T BRING HER BACK
Thomas H. Murray

> Murray argues that we must face several "hard truths" about human cloning. One of these hard truths is that cloning—at least at this stage of technological development—does not produce healthy, normal offspring. The other hard truths he identifies are asserted in opposition to the idea that if cloning did produce healthy offspring, parents could sensibly use it to replace a dead child.

Eleven days ago, as I awaited my turn to testify at a congressional hearing on human reproductive clon-

Reprinted with permission of the author from *The Washington Post,* April 8, 2001.

ing, one of five scientists on the witness list took the microphone. Brigitte Boisselier, a chemist working with couples who want to use cloning techniques to create babies, read aloud a letter from "a father,

(Dada)." The writer, who had unexpectedly become a parent in his late thirties, describes his despair over his 11-month-old son's death after heart surgery and 17 days of "misery and struggle." The room was quiet as Boisselier read the man's words: "I decided then and there that I would never give up on my child. I would never stop until I could give his DNA—his genetic make-up—a chance."

I listened to the letter writer's refusal to accept the finality of death, to his wish to allow his son another opportunity at life through cloning, and I was struck by the futility and danger of such thinking. I had been asked to testify as someone who has been writing and teaching about ethical issues in medicine and science for more than 20 years; but I am also a grieving parent. My 20-year-old daughter's murder, just five months ago, has agonizingly reinforced what I have for years argued as an ethicist: Cloning can neither change the fact of death nor deflect the pain of grief.

Only four years have passed since the birth of the first cloned mammal—Dolly the sheep—was announced and the possibility of human cloning became real. Once a staple of science fiction, cloning was now the stuff of scientific research. A presidential commission [the National Bioethics Advisory Commission], of which I am a member, began to deliberate the ethics of human cloning; scientists disavowed any interest in trying to clone people; and Congress held hearings but passed no laws. A moratorium took hold, stable except for the occasional eruption of self-proclaimed would-be cloners such as Chicago-based physicist Richard Seed and a group led by a man named Rael who claims that we are all clones of alien ancestors.

Recently, Boisselier, Rael's chief scientist, and Panos Zavos, an infertility specialist in Kentucky, won overnight attention when they proclaimed that they would indeed create a human clone in the near future. The prospect that renegade scientists might try to clone humans reignited the concern of lawmakers, which led to the recent hearings before the House Energy and Commerce subcommittee on oversight and investigations.

Cloning advocates have had a difficult time coming up with persuasive ethical arguments. Indulging narcissism—so that someone can create many Mini-Me's—fails to generate much support

for their cause. Others make the case that adults should have the right to use any means possible to have the child they want. Their liberty trumps everything else; the child's welfare barely registers, except to avoid a life that would be worse than never being born, a standard akin to dividing by zero—no meaningful answer is possible. The strategy that has been the most effective has been to play the sympathy card—and who evokes more sympathy than someone who has lost a child?

Sadly, I'm in a position to correct some of these misunderstandings. I'm not suggesting that my situation is the same as that of the letter's author. Not better. Not worse. Simply different. His son was with him for less than a year, our daughter for 20; his son died of disease in a hospital; Emily, daughter to Cynthia and me, sister to Kate and Matt, Nicky and Pete, was reported missing from her college campus in early November. Her body was found more than five weeks later. She had been abducted and shot.

As I write those words, I still want to believe they are about someone else, a story on the 11 o'clock news. Cynthia and I often ask each other, how can this be our life? But it is our life and Emily, as a physical, exuberant, loving presence, is not in the same way a part of it anymore. Death changes things and, I suspect, the death of a child causes more wrenching grief than any other death. So I am told; so my experience confirms.

I want to speak, then, to the author of that letter, father to father, grieving parent to grieving parent; and to anyone clinging to unfounded hope that cloning can somehow repair the arbitrariness of disease, unhappiness and death. I have nothing to sell you, I don't want your money, and I certainly don't want to be cruel. But there are hard truths here that some people, whether through ignorance or self-interest, are obscuring.

The first truth is that cloning does not result in healthy, normal offspring. The two scientific experts on animal cloning who shared the panel with Boisslier reported the results of the cattle, mice and other mammals cloned thus far: They have suffered staggering rates of abnormalities and death; some of the females bearing them have been injured and some have died. Rudolf Jaenisch, an expert on mouse cloning at MIT's Whitehead Institute for Biomedical Research, told the subcommittee that he did not believe there was a single healthy cloned mammal in existence—not even Dolly, the sheep that started it all, who is abnormally obese.

Scientists do not know why cloning fails so miserably. One plausible explanation begins with what we already know—that as the cells of an embryo divide and begin to transform into the many varieties of tissue that make up our bodies, most of the genes in each cell are shut down, leaving active only those that the cell needs to perform its specific role. A pancreatic islet cell, for example, needs working versions of the genes that recognize when a person needs the hormone insulin, then cobble it together and shunt it into the bloodstream. All of that individual's other genetic information is in that islet cell, but most of it is chemically locked, like an illegally parked car immobilized by a tire boot.

To make a healthy clone, scientists need to unlock every last one of those tire boots in the cell that is to be cloned. It is not enough to have the genes for islet cells; every gene will be needed sometime, somewhere. Unless and until scientists puzzle out how to restore all the genes to their original state, we will continue to see dead, dying and deformed clones.

You do not need to be a professional bioethicist, then, to see that trying to make a child by cloning, at this stage in the technology, would be a gross violation of international standards protecting people from overreaching scientists, a blatant example of immoral human experimentation.

Some scientists claim they can avoid these problems. Zavos, who spoke at the hearing, has promised to screen embryos and implant only healthy ones. But Zavos failed to give a single plausible reason to believe that he can distinguish healthy from unhealthy cloned embryos.

Now for the second truth: Even if cloning produced a healthy embryo, the result would not be the same person as the one whose genetic material was used. Each of us is a complex amalgam of luck, experience and heredity. Where in the womb an embryo burrows, what its mother eats or drinks, what stresses she endures, her age—all these factors shape the developing fetus. The genes themselves conduct an intricately choreographed dance, turning on and off, instructing other genes to do the same in response to their interior rhythms and to the pulses of the world outside. How we become who we are remains a mystery.

About the only thing we can be certain of is that we are much more than the sum of our genes. As I said in my testimony, perhaps the best way to extinguish the enthusiasm for human cloning would be to clone Michael Jordan. Michael II might well have no interest in playing basketball but instead long to become an accountant. What makes Michael I great is not merely his physical gifts, but his competitive fire, his determination, his fierce will to win.

Yet another hard truth: Creating a child to stand in for another—dead—child is unfair. No child should have to bear the oppressive expectation that he or she will live out the life denied to his or her idealized genetic avatar. Parents may joke about their specific plans for their children; I suspect their children find such plans less amusing. Of course, we should have expectations for our children: that they be considerate, honest, diligent, fair and more. But we cannot dictate their temperament, talents or interests. Cloning a child to be a reincarnation of someone else is a grotesque, fun-house mirror distortion of parental expectations.

Which brings me to the final hard truth: There is no real escape from grief.

Cynthia and I have fantasized about time running backward so that we could undo Emily's murder. We would give our limbs, our organs, our lives to bring her back, to give her the opportunity to live out her dream of becoming an Episcopal priest, of retiring as a mesmerizing old woman sitting on her porch on Cape Cod, surrounded by her grandchildren and poodles.

But trying to recreate Emily from her DNA would be chasing an illusion. Massive waves of sorrow knock us down, breathless; we must learn to live with them. When our strength returns we stagger to our feet, summon whatever will we can, and do what needs to be done. Most of all we try to hold each other up. We can no more wish our grief away than King Canute could stem the ocean's tide.

So I find myself wanting to say to the letter writer, and to the scientists who offer him and other sorrowing families false hope: There are no technological fixes for grief; cloning your dear dead son will not repair the jagged hole ripped out of the tapestry of your life. Your letter fills me with sadness for you and you wife, not just for the loss of your child but also for the fruitless quest to quench your grief in a genetic replica of the son you lost. It would be fruitless even—especially—if you succeeded in creating a healthy biological duplicate. But there is little chance of that.

Emily lived until a few months shy of her 21st birthday. In those years our lives became interwoven in ways so intricate that I struggle for words to describe how Cynthia and I now feel. We were fortunate to have her with us long enough to see her become her own person, to love her whole-heartedly and to know beyond question that she loved us. Her

loss changes us forever. Life flows in one direction; science cannot reverse the stream or reincarnate the dead.

The Emily we knew and loved would want us to continue to do what matters in our lives, to love each other, to do good work, to find meaning. Not to forget her, ever: We are incapable of that. Why would we want to? She was a luminous presence in our family, an extraordinary friend, a promising young philosopher. And we honor her by keeping her memory vibrant, not by trying to manufacture a genetic facsimile. And that thought makes me address the letter's author once more: I have to think that your son, were he able to tell you, would wish for you the same.

GENETIC ENCORES: THE ETHICS OF HUMAN CLONING
Robert Wachbroit

Wachbroit constructs a series of arguments in response to the various concerns raised by critics of human cloning. First of all, because Wachbroit believes that many such concerns are based on false beliefs about genetic influence, he argues directly against the view identified as genetic determinism. He then addresses concerns raised about the interests and rights of human clones; his conclusion is that concerns about the negative impact of cloning on those produced by this process are not sufficient to sustain a moral objection to cloning. Next, in attempting to minimize concerns about the social consequences of the cloning process, Wachbroit compares cloning with two closely related technologies—assisted reproductive technologies and genetic engineering—and he concludes that in some ways cloning is actually less problematic than these other two technologies. Finally, Wachbroit considers the reasons that might motivate the use of cloning to create a child, and he responds to the argument that a permissive social policy regarding cloning essentially constitutes an endorsement of a narcissitic motivation for having children.

The successful cloning of an adult sheep, announced in Scotland this past February [1997], is one of the most dramatic recent examples of a scientific discovery becoming a public issue. During the last few months, various commentators—scientists and theologians, physicians and legal experts, talk-radio hosts and editorial writers—have been busily responding to the news, some calming fears, others raising alarms about the prospect of cloning a human being. At the request of the President, the National Bioethics Advisory Commission (NBAC) held hearings and prepared a report on the religious, ethical, and legal issues surrounding human cloning. While

Reprinted with permission of the publisher from *Report from the Institute for Philosophy & Public Policy,* vol. 17, no. 4, Fall 1997, pp. 1–7.

declining to call for a permanent ban on the practice, the Commission recommended a moratorium on efforts to clone human beings, and emphasized the importance of further public deliberation on the subject.

An interesting tension is at work in the NBAC report. Commission members were well aware of "the widespread public discomfort, even revulsion, about cloning human beings." Perhaps recalling the images of Dolly the ewe that were featured on the covers of national news magazines, they noted that "the impact of these most recent developments on our national psyche has been quite remarkable." Accordingly, they felt that one of their tasks was to articulate, as fully and sympathetically as possible, the range of concerns that the prospect of human cloning had elicited.

Yet it seems clear that some of these concerns, at least, are based on false beliefs about genetic influence and the nature of the individuals that would be produced through cloning. Consider, for instance, the fear that a clone would not be an "individual" but merely a "carbon copy" of someone else—an automaton of the sort familiar from science fiction. As many scientists have pointed out, a clone would not in fact be an identical *copy,* but more like a delayed identical *twin.* And just as identical twins are two separate people—biologically, psychologically, morally and legally, though not genetically—so, too, a clone would be a separate person from her noncontemporaneous twin. To think otherwise is to embrace a belief in genetic determinism—the view that genes determine everything about us, and that environmental factors or the random events in human development are insignificant.

The overwhelming scientific consensus is that genetic determinism is false. In coming to understand the ways in which genes operate, biologists have also become aware of the myriad ways in which the environment affects their "expression." The genetic contribution to the simplest physical traits, such as height and hair color, is significantly mediated by environmental factors (and possibly by stochastic events as well). And the genetic contribution to the traits we value most deeply, from intelligence to compassion, is conceded by even the most enthusiastic genetic researchers to be limited and indirect.

It is difficult to gauge the extent to which "repugnance" toward cloning generally rests on a belief in genetic determinism. Hoping to account for the fact that people "instinctively recoil" from the prospect of cloning, James Q. Wilson wrote, "There is a natural sentiment that is offended by the mental picture of identical babies being produced in some biological factory." Which raises the question: once people learn that this picture is mere science fiction, does the offense that cloning presents to "natural sentiment" attenuate, or even disappear? Jean Bethke Elshtain cited the nightmare scenarios of "the man and woman on the street," who imagine a future populated by "a veritable army of Hitlers, ruthless and remorseless bigots who kept reproducing themselves until they had finished what the historic Hitler failed to do: annihilate us." What happens, though, to the "pity and terror" evoked by the topic of cloning when such scenarios are deprived (as they deserve to be) of all credibility?

Richard Lewontin has argued that the critics' fears—or at least, those fears that merit consideration in formulating public policy—dissolve once genetic determinism is refuted. He criticizes the NBAC report for excessive deference to opponents of human cloning, and calls for greater public education on the scientific issues. (The Commission in fact makes the same recommendation, but Lewontin seems unimpressed.) Yet even if a public education campaign succeeded in eliminating the most egregious misconceptions about genetic influence, that wouldn't settle the matter. People might continue to express concerns about the interests and rights of human clones, about the social and moral consequences of the cloning process, and about the possible motivations for creating children in this way.

INTERESTS AND RIGHTS

One set of ethical concerns about human clones involves the risks and uncertainties associated with the current state of cloning technology. This technology has not yet been tested with human subjects, and scientists cannot rule out the possibility of mutation or other biological damage. Accordingly, the NBAC report concluded that "at this time, it is morally unacceptable for anyone in the public or private sector, whether in a research or clinical setting, to attempt to create a child using somatic cell nuclear transfer cloning." Such efforts, it said, would pose "unacceptable risks to the fetus and/or potential child."

The ethical issues of greatest importance in the cloning debate, however, do not involve possible failures of cloning technology, but rather the consequences of its success. Assuming that scientists were able to clone human beings without incurring the risks mentioned above, what concerns might there be about the welfare of clones?

Some opponents of cloning believe that such individuals would be wronged in morally significant ways. Many of these wrongs involve the denial of what Joel Feinberg has called "the right to an open future." For example, a child might be constantly compared to the adult from whom he was cloned, and thereby burdened with oppressive expectations. Even worse, the parents might actually limit the child's opportunities for growth and development: a child cloned from a basketball player, for instance, might be denied any educational opportunities that were not in line with a career in basketball. Finally, regardless of his parents' conduct or attitudes, a child might be burdened by the *thought* that he is a copy and not an "original." The child's sense of self-worth or individuality or dignity, so some have argued, would thus be difficult to sustain.

How should we respond to these concerns? On the one hand, the existence of a right to an open future has a strong intuitive appeal. We are troubled by parents who radically constrict their children's possibilities for growth and development. Obviously, we would condemn a cloning parent for crushing a child with oppressive expectations, just as we might condemn fundamentalist parents for utterly isolating their children from the modern world, or the parents of twins for inflicting matching wardrobes and rhyming names. But this is not enough to sustain an objection to cloning itself. Unless the claim is that cloned parents cannot help but be oppressive, we would have cause to say they had wronged their children only because of their subsequent, and avoidable, sins of bad parenting—not because they had chosen to create the child in the first place. (The possible reasons for making this choice will be discussed below.)

We must also remember that children are often born in the midst of all sorts of hopes and expectations; the idea that there is a special burden associated with the thought "There is someone who is genetically just like me" is necessarily speculative. Moreover, given the falsity of genetic determinism, any conclusions a child might draw from observing the person from whom he was cloned would be uncertain at best. His knowledge of his future would differ only in degree from what many children already know once they begin to learn parts of their family's (medical) history. Some of us knew that we would be bald, or to what diseases we might be susceptible. To be sure, the cloned individual might know more about what he or she could become. But because our knowledge of the effect of environment on development is so incomplete, the clone would certainly be in for some surprises.

Finally, even if we were convinced that clones are likely to suffer particular burdens, that would not be enough to show that it is wrong to create them. The child of a poor family can be expected to suffer specific hardships and burdens, but we don't thereby conclude that such children shouldn't be born. Despite the hardships, poor children can experience parental love and many of the joys of being alive: the deprivations of poverty, however painful, are not decisive. More generally, no one's life is entirely free of some difficulties or burdens. In order for these considerations to have decisive weight, we have to be able to say that life doesn't offer any compensating benefits. Concerns expressed about the welfare of human clones do not appear to justify such a bleak assessment. Most such children can be expected to have lives well worth living; many of the imagined harms are no worse than those faced by children acceptably produced by more conventional means. If there is something deeply objectionable about cloning, it is more likely to be found by examining implications of the cloning process itself, or the reasons people might have for availing themselves of it.

CONCERNS ABOUT PROCESS

Human cloning falls conceptually between two other technologies. At one end we have the assisted reproductive technologies, such as in vitro fertilization, whose primary purpose is to enable couples to produce a child with whom they have a biological connection. At the other end we have the emerging technologies of genetic engineering—specifically, gene transplantation technologies—whose primary purpose is to produce a child that has certain traits. Many proponents of cloning see it as part of the first technology: cloning is just another way of providing a couple with a biological child they might otherwise be unable to have. Since this goal and these other technologies are acceptable, cloning should be acceptable as well. On the other hand, many opponents of cloning see it as part of the second technology: even though cloning is a transplantation of an entire nucleus and not of specific genes, it is nevertheless an attempt to produce a child with certain traits. The deep misgivings we may have about the genetic manipulation of offspring should apply to cloning as well.

The debate cannot be resolved, however, simply by determining which technology to assimilate cloning to. For example, some opponents of human cloning see it as continuous with assisted reproductive technologies; but since they find those technologies objectionable as well, the assimilation does not indicate approval. Rather than argue for grouping cloning with one technology or another, I wish to suggest that we can best understand the significance of the cloning process by comparing it with these other technologies, and thus broadening the debate.

To see what can be learned from such a comparative approach, let us consider a central argument that has been made against cloning—that it undermines the structure of the family by making identities and lineages unclear. On the one hand, the relationship between an adult and the child cloned from her could be described as that between a parent and offspring. Indeed, some commentators have called cloning "asexual reproduction," which clearly suggests that cloning is a way of generating *descendants*. The clone, on this view, has only one biological parent. On the other hand, from the point of view of genetics, the clone is a *sibling,* so that cloning is more accurately described as "delayed twinning" rather than as asexual reproduction. The clone, on this view, has two biological parents, not one—they are the same parents as those of the person from whom that individual was cloned.

Cloning thus results in ambiguities. Is the clone an offspring or a sibling? Does the clone have one biological parent or two? The moral significance of these ambiguities lies in the fact that in many societies, including our own, lineage identifies responsibilities. Typically, the parent, not the sibling, is responsible for the child. But if no one is unambiguously the parent, so the worry might go, who is responsible for the clone? Insofar as social identity is based on biological ties, won't this identity be blurred or confounded?

Some assisted reproductive technologies have raised similar questions about lineage and identity. An anonymous sperm donor is thought to have no parental obligations towards his biological child. A surrogate mother may be required to relinquish all parental claims to the child she bears. In these cases, the social and legal determination of "who is the parent" may appear to proceed in defiance of profound biological facts, and to subvert attachments that we as a society are ordinarily committed to upholding. Thus, while the *aim* of assisted reproductive technologies is to allow people to produce or raise a child to whom they are biologically connected, such technologies may also involve the creation of social ties that are permitted to override biological ones.

In the case of cloning, however, ambiguous lineages would seem to be less problematic, precisely because no one is being asked to relinquish a claim on a child to whom he or she might otherwise acknowledge a biological connection. What, then, are the critics afraid of? It does not seem plausible that someone would have herself cloned and then hand the child over to her parents, saying, "You take care of her! She's *your* daughter!" Nor is it likely that, if the cloned individual did raise the child, she would suddenly refuse to pay for college on the grounds that this was not a sister's responsibility. Of course, policymakers should address any confusion in the social or legal assignment of responsibility resulting from cloning. But there are reasons to think that this would be *less* difficult than in the case of other reproductive technologies.

Similarly, when we compare cloning with genetic engineering, cloning may prove to be the less troubling of the two technologies. This is true even though the dark futures to which they are often alleged to lead are broadly alike. For example, a recent *Washington Post* article examined fears that the development of genetic enhancement technologies might "create a market in preferred physical traits." The reporter asked, "Might it lead to a society of DNA haves and have-nots, and the creation of a new underclass of people unable to keep up with the genetically fortified Joneses?" Similarly, a member of the National Bioethics Advisory Commission expressed concern that cloning might become "almost a preferred practice," taking its place "on the continuum of providing the best for your child." As a consequence, parents who chose to "play the lottery of old-fashioned reproduction would be considered irresponsible."

Such fears, however, seem more warranted with respect to genetic engineering than to cloning. By offering some people—in all probability, members of the upper classes—the opportunity to acquire desired traits through genetic manipulation, genetic engineering could bring about a biological reinforcement (or accentuation) of existing social divisions. It is hard enough already for disadvantaged children to compete with their more affluent counterparts, given the material resources and intellectual opportunities that are often available only to children of privilege. This unfairness would almost certainly be compounded if genetic manipulation came into the picture. In contrast, cloning does not bring about "improvements" in the genome: it is, rather, a way of *duplicating* the genome—with all its imperfections. It wouldn't enable certain groups of people to keep getting better and better along some valued dimension.

To some critics, admittedly, this difference will not seem terribly important. Theologian Gilbert Meilaender, Jr., objects to cloning on the grounds that children created through this technology would be "designed as a product" rather than "welcomed as a gift." The fact that the design process would be more selective and nuanced in the case of genetic engineering would, from this perspective, have no moral significance. To the extent that this objection reflects a concern about the commodification of human life, we can address it in part when we consider people's reasons for engaging in cloning.

REASONS FOR CLONING

This final area of contention in the cloning debate is as much psychological as it is scientific or philosophical. If human cloning technology were safe and widely available, what use would people make of it? What reasons would they have to engage in cloning?

In its report to the President, the Commission imagined a few situations in which people might avail themselves of cloning. In one scenario, a husband and wife who wish to have children are both carriers of a lethal recessive gene:

> Rather than risk the one in four chance of conceiving a child who will suffer a short and painful existence, the couple considers the alternatives: to forgo rearing children; to adopt; to use prenatal diagnosis and selective abortion; to use donor gametes free of the recessive trait; or to use the cells of one of the adults and attempt to clone a child. To avoid donor gametes and selective abortion, while maintaining a genetic tie to their child, they opt for cloning.

In another scenario, the parents of a terminally ill child are told that only a bone marrow transplant can save the child's life. "With no other donor available, the parents attempt to clone a human being from the cells of the dying child. If successful, the new child will be a perfect match for bone marrow transplant, and can be used as a donor without significant risk or discomfort. The net result: two healthy children, loved by their parents, who happen [sic] to be identical twins of different ages."

The Commission was particularly impressed by the second example. That scenario, said the NBAC report, "makes what is probably the strongest possible case for cloning a human being, as it demonstrates how this technology could be used for lifesaving purposes." Indeed, the report suggests that it would be a "tragedy" to allow "the sick child to die because of a moral or political objection to such cloning." Nevertheless, we should note that many people would be morally uneasy about the use of a minor as a donor, regardless of whether the child were a result of cloning. Even if this unease is justifiably overridden by other concerns, the "transplant scenario" may not present a more compelling case for cloning than that of the infertile couple desperately seeking a biological child.

Most critics, in fact, decline to engage the specifics of such tragic (and presumably rare) situations. Instead, they bolster their case by imagining very different scenarios. Potential users of the technology, they suggest, are narcissists or control freaks—people who will regard their children not as free, original selves but as products intended to meet more or less rigid specifications. Even if such people are not genetic determinists, their recourse to cloning will indicate a desire to exert all possible influence over what "kind" of child they produce.

The critics' alarm at this prospect has in part to do, as we have seen, with concerns about the psychological burdens such a desire would impose on the clone. But it also reflects a broader concern about the values expressed, and promoted, by a society's reproductive policies. Critics argue that a society that enables people to clone themselves thereby endorses the most narcissistic reason for having children—to perpetuate oneself through a genetic encore. The demonstrable falsity of genetic determinism may detract little, if at all, from the strength of this motive. Whether or not clones will have a grievance against their parents for producing them with this motivation, the societal indulgence of that motivation is improper and harmful.

It can be argued, however, that the critics have simply misunderstood the social meaning of a policy that would permit people to clone themselves even in the absence of the heartrending exigencies described in the NBAC report. This country has developed a strong commitment to reproductive autonomy. (This commitment emerged in response to the dismal history of eugenics—the very history that is sometimes invoked to support restrictions on cloning.) With the exception of practices that risk coercion and exploitation—notably baby-selling and commercial surrogacy—we do not interfere with people's freedom to create and acquire children by almost any means, for almost any reason. This policy does not reflect a dogmatic libertarianism. Rather, it recognizes the extraordinary personal importance and private character of reproductive decisions, even those with significant social repercussions.

Our willingness to sustain such a policy also reflects a recognition of the moral complexities of parenting. For example, we know that the motives people have for bringing a child into the world do not necessarily determine the manner in which they raise him. Even when parents start out as narcissists, the experience of childrearing will sometimes transform their initial impulses, making them caring, respectful, and even self-sacrificing. Seeing their child grow and develop, they learn that she is not merely an extension of themselves. Of course, some parents never make this discovery; others, having done so, never forgive their children for it. The pace and extent of moral development among parents (no less than among children) is infinitely variable. Still, we are justified in saying that those who engage in cloning will not, by virtue of this fact, be immune to the transformative effects of parenthood—even if it is the case (and it won't always be) that they begin with more problematic motives than those of parents who engage in the "genetic lottery."

Moreover, the nature of parental motivation is itself more complex than the critics often allow. Though we can agree that narcissism is a vice not to be encouraged, we lack a clear notion of where pride in one's children ends and narcissism begins. When, for example, is it unseemly to bask in the reflected glory of a child's achievements? Imagine a champion gymnast who takes delight in her daughter's athletic prowess. Now imagine that the child was actually cloned from one of the gymnast's somatic cells. Would we have to revise our moral assessment of her pleasure in her daughter's success? Or suppose a man wanted to be cloned and to give his child opportunities he himself had never enjoyed. And suppose that, rightly or wrongly, the man took the child's success as a measure of his own untapped potential—an indication of the flourishing life he might have had. Is *this* sentiment blamable? And is it all that different from what many natural parents feel?

CONCLUSION

Until recently, there were few ethical, social, or legal discussions about human cloning via nuclear transplantation, since the scientific consensus was that such a procedure was not biologically possible. With the appearance of Dolly, the situation has changed. But although it now seems more likely that human cloning will become feasible, we may doubt that the practice will come into widespread use.

I suspect it will not, but my reasons will not offer much comfort to the critics of cloning. While the technology for nuclear transplantation advances, other technologies—notably the technology of genetic engineering—will be progressing as well. Human genetic engineering will be applicable to a wide variety of traits; it will be more powerful than cloning, and hence more attractive to more people. It will also, as I have suggested, raise more troubling questions than the prospect of cloning has thus far.

SOURCES

National Bioethics Advisory Commission, "Cloning Human Beings: Report and Recommendations" (June 9, 1997).

James Q. Wilson, "The Paradox of Cloning," *Weekly Standard* (May 26, 1997).

Jean Bethke Elshtain, "Ewegenics," *New Republic* (March 31, 1997).

R. C. Lewontin, "The Confusion Over Cloning," *New York Review of Books* (October 23, 1997).

Leon Kass, "The Wisdom of Repugnance," *New Republic* (June 2, 1997).

Susan Cohen, "What Is a Baby? Inside America's Unresolved Debate About the Ethics of Cloning," *Washington Post Magazine* (October 12, 1997).

Rick Weiss, "Genetic Enhancements' Thorny Ethical Traits," *Washington Post* (October 12, 1997).

PREIMPLANTATION GENETIC DIAGNOSIS

EXTENDING PREIMPLANTATION GENETIC DIAGNOSIS: MEDICAL AND NON-MEDICAL USES

John A. Robertson

Robertson surveys the established, emerging, and prospective uses of preimplantation genetic diagnosis (PGD), emphasizing the distinction between medical and non-medical uses. PGD has principally been used to screen out embryos with aneuploidy (i.e., chromosomal abnormality) and Mendelian disease (i.e., genetic disease produced by a single-gene defect). As Robertson explains, newer medical uses include screening embryos for cancer susceptibility and late onset disorders, as well as HLA matching for existing children. He considers all of these medical uses of PGD to be ethically acceptable. Turning his attention to possible nonmedical uses of PGD, he identifies a series of factors that he considers relevant to their ethical assessment. Robertson applies his suggested ethical scheme in some detail to two nonmedical uses of PGD: (1) selection on the basis of gender and (2) selection for a perfect-pitch gene, should such a gene exist and be identified. He argues that the case against PGD for gender (sex) selection of a first child is much stronger than the case against gender selection for subsequent children in order to achieve gender "balance" in the family. His analysis also suggests that the case for allowing couples to use PGD to select for perfect pitch is fairly strong.

Debate about new reproductive technologies often cites preimplantation genetic diagnosis (PGD)—the technique by which early human embryos are genetically screened for selection for transfer to the uterus—as a practice that needs close ethical, legal, and social scrutiny. The use of PGD is growing, as are the indications for it. This article describes medical and non-medical extensions of PGD, and discusses the ethical, legal, and policy issues which they raise.

Reprinted with permission of the publisher from *Journal of Medical Ethics*, vol. 29 (August 2003), pp. 213–216. © 2003 BMJ Publishing Group & Institute of Medical Ethics.

PGD AND ITS PREVALENCE

PGD has been available since 1990 for testing of aneuploidy in low prognosis in vitro fertilisation (IVF) patients, and for single gene and X linked diseases in at risk couples. One cell (blastomere) is removed from a cleaving embryo and tested for the genetic or chromosomal condition of concern. Some programmes analyse polar bodies extruded from oocytes during meiosis, rather than blastomeres.[1] Cells are then either karyotyped to identify chromosomal abnormalities, or analysed for single gene mutations and linked markers.

Physicians have performed more than 3000 clinical cycles of PGD since 1990, with more than 700 children born as a result. The overall pregnancy rate of 24% is comparable to assisted reproductive practices which do not involve embryo or polar body biopsy.[1] Four centres (Chicago, Livingston (New Jersey), Bologna, and Brussels) accounted for nearly all the reported cases. More than 40 centres worldwide offer the procedure, however, including other centres in the United States and Europe, four centres in London and centres in the eastern Mediterranean, Southeast Asia, and Australia.

More than two thirds of PGD has occurred to screen out embryos with chromosomal abnormalities in older IVF patients and in patients with a history of miscarriage. About 1000 cycles have involved single gene mutational analysis.[1] Mutational analysis requires additional skills beyond karyotyping for aneuploidies, including the ability to conduct the multiplex polymerase chain reaction (PCR) of the gene of interest and related markers.

Several new indications for PGD single gene mutational analysis have recently been reported. New uses include PGD to detect mutations for susceptibility to cancer and for late onset disorders such as Alzheimer's disease.[2,3] In addition, parents with children needing hematopoietic stem cell transplants have used PGD to ensure that their next child is free of disease and a good tissue match for an existing child.[4] Some persons are also requesting PGD for gender selection for both first and later born children, and others have speculated that selection of embryos for a variety of non-medical traits is likely in the future.

PGD is ethically controversial because it involves the screening and likely destruction of embryos, and the selection of offspring on the basis of expected traits. While persons holding right to life views will probably object to PGD for any reason, those who view the early embryo as too rudimentary in development to have rights or interests see no principled objection to all PGD. They may disagree, however, over whether particular reasons for PGD show sufficient respect for embryos and potential offspring to justify intentional creation and selection of embryos. Donation of unwanted embryos to infertile couples reduces this problem somewhat, but there are too few such couples to accept all unwanted embryos, and in any event, the issue of selecting offspring traits remains.

Although ethical commentary frequently mentions PGD as a harbinger of a reproductive future of widespread genetic selection and alteration of prospective offspring, its actual impact is likely to be quite limited.[5,6] Even with increasing use the penetrance of PGD into reproductive practice is likely to remain a very small percentage of the 150 000 plus cycles of IVF performed annually throughout the world. Screening for susceptibility and late onset diseases is limited by the few diseases for which single gene predispositions are known. Relatively few parents will face the need to conceive another child to provide an existing child with matched stem cells. Nor are nonmedical uses of PGD, other than for gender, likely to be practically feasible for at least a decade or more. Despite the limited reach of PGD, the ethical, legal, and policy issues that new uses raise, deserve attention.

NEW MEDICAL USES

New uses of PGD may be grouped into medical and non-medical categories. New medical uses include not only screening for rare Mendelian diseases, but also for susceptibility conditions, late onset diseases, and HLA matching for existing children.

Embryo screening for susceptibility and late onset conditions are logical extensions of screening for serious Mendelian diseases. For example, using PGD to screen out embryos carrying the p53 or BRCA1&2 mutations prevent the birth of children who would face a greatly increased lifetime risk of cancer, and hence require close monitoring, prophylactic surgery, or other preventive measures. PGD for highly penetrant adult disorders such as Alzheimer's or Huntington's disease prevents the birth of a child who will be healthy for many years, but who in her late thirties or early forties will experience the onset of progressive neurological disease leading to an early death.

Although these indications do not involve diseases that manifest themselves in infancy or childhood, the conditions in question lead to substantial health problems for offspring in their thirties or forties.[7] Avoiding the birth of children with those conditions thus reflects the desire of parents to have offspring with good prospects for an average life span. If PGD is accepted to exclude offspring with early onset genetic diseases, it should be accepted for later onset conditions as well.

PGD for adult onset disorders does mean that a healthy child might then be born to a person with those conditions who is likely to die or become incompetent while the child is dependent on her.[8] But that risk has been tolerated in other cases of assisted reproduction, such as intrauterine insemination with sperm of a man who is HIV positive, IVF for women with cystic fibrosis, and use of gametes stored prior to cancer therapy. As long as competent caregivers will be available for the child, the likely death or disability of a parent does not justify condemning or stopping this use, anymore than that reproduction by men going off to war should be discouraged.

A third new medical indication—HLA matching to an existing child—enables a couple to have their next child serve as a matched hematopoietic stem cell donor for an existing sick child. It may also ensure that the new child does not also suffer from that same disease. The availability of PGD, however, should not hinge on that fact, as the Human Fertilisation and Embryology Authority, in the UK, now requires.[9] A couple that would coitally conceive a child to be a tissue donor should be free to use PGD to make sure that that child will be a suitable match, regardless of whether that child is also at risk for genetic disease. Parents who choose PGD for this purpose are likely to value the new child for its own

sake, and not only for the stem cells that it will make available. They do not use the new child as a "mere means" simply because they have selected HLA matched embryos for transfer.[10, 11]

NON-MEDICAL USES OF PGD

More ethically troubling has been the prospect of using PGD to screen embryos for genes that do not relate to the health of resulting children or others in the family. Many popular accounts of PGD assume that it will eventually be used to select for such non-medical traits as intelligence, height, sexual orientation, beauty, hair and eye colour, memory, and other factors.[5, 6] Because the genetic basis of those traits is unknown, and in any case is likely to involve many different genes, they may not be subject to easy mutational analysis, as Mendelian disease or susceptibility conditions are. Aside from gender, which is identifiable through karyotyping, it is unrealistic to think that non-medical screening for other traits, with the possible exception of perfect pitch, will occur anytime soon.

Still, it is useful to consider the methodology that ethical assessment of non-medical uses of PGD, if available, should follow. The relevant questions would be whether the proposed use serves valid reproductive or rearing interests; whether those interests are sufficient to justify creating and destroying embryos; whether selecting for a trait will harm resulting children; whether it will stigmatise existing persons, and whether it will create other social harms.

To analyse how these factors interact, I discuss PGD for sex selection and for children with perfect pitch. Similar issues would arise with PGD for sexual orientation, for hair and eye color, and for intelligence, size, and memory.

PGD for Gender Selection The use of medical technology to select the sex of offspring is highly controversial because of the bias against females which it usually reflects or expresses, and the resulting social disruptions which it might cause. PGD for gender selection faces the additional problem of appearing to be a relatively weak reason for creating and selecting embryos for discard or transfer.

The greatest social effects of gender selection arise when the gender of the first child is chosen. Selection for first children will overwhelmingly favour males, particularly if one child per family population policies apply. If carried out on a large scale, it could lead to great disparities in the sex ratio of the population, as has occurred in China and India through the use of ultrasound screening and abortion.[12, 13] PGD, however, is too expensive and inaccessible to be used on a wide scale for sex selection purposes. Allowing it to be used for the first child is only marginally likely to contribute to societal sex ratio imbalances. But its use is likely to reflect cultural notions of male privilege and may reinforce entrenched sexism toward women.

The use of PGD to choose a gender opposite to that of an existing child or children is much less susceptible to a charge of sexism. Here a couple seeks variety or "balance" in the gender of offspring because of the different rearing experiences that come with rearing children of different genders. Psychologists now recognise many biologically based differences between male and female children, including different patterns of aggression, learning, and spatial recognition, as well as hormonal differences.[14, 15] It may not be sexist in itself to wish to have a child or children of each gender, particularly if one has two or more children of the same gender.

Some feminists, however, would argue that any attention to the gender of offspring is inherently sexist, particularly when social attitudes and expectations play such an important role in constructing sex role expectations and behaviours.[16] Other feminists find the choice of a child with a gender different from existing children to be morally defensible as long as "the intention and consequences of the practice are not sexist," which is plausibly the case when gender variety in children is sought.[17] Desiring the different rearing experiences with boys and girls does not mean that the parents, who have already had children of one gender, are sexists or likely to value unfairly one or the other gender.[18]

Based on this analysis the case is weak for allowing PGD for the first child, but may be acceptable for gender variety in a family. With regard to the first child, facilitating preferences for male firstborns carries a high risk of promoting sexist social mores. It may also strike many persons as too trivial a concern to meet shared notions of the special respect due pre-implantation embryos. A proponent of gender selection, however, might argue that cultural preferences for firstborn males should be tolerated, unless a clearer case of harm has been shown. If PGD is not permitted, pregnancy and abortion might occur instead.

The case for PGD for gender variety is stronger because the risk of sexism is lessened. A couple would be selecting the gender of a second or subsequent children for variety in rearing experiences, and not out of a belief that one gender is privileged over another. Gender selection in that case would occur without running the risks of fostering sexism and hurting women.[18]

The question still arises whether the desire for gender variety in children, even if not sexist, is a strong enough reason to justify creating and discarding embryos. The answer depends on how strong an interest that is. No one has yet marshalled the evidence showing that the need or desire for gender variety in children is substantial and important, or whether many parents would refrain from having another child if PGD for gender variety were not possible. More evidence of the strength and prevalence of this need would help in reaching a conclusion. If that case is made, then PGD for gender variety might be acceptable as well.[19]

The ethics committee of the American Society of Reproductive Medicine (ASRM) has struggled with these issues in a series of recent opinions. It initially addressed the issue of PGD for gender selection generally, and found that it "should be discouraged" for couples not going through IVF, and "not encouraged" for couples who were, but made no distinction between PGD for gender selection of first and later children.[20] Subsequently, it found that *preconception* gender selection would be acceptable for purposes of gender variety but not for the first child.[18]

Perceiving these two positions to be inconsistent, a doctor who wanted to offer PGD for gender selection inquired of the ethics committee why preconception methods for gender variety, which lacked 100% certainty, were acceptable but PGD, which guaranteed that certainty, was not. Focusing only on the sexism and gender discrimination issue, the chair of the ethics committee, in a widely publicised letter, found that PGD for gender balancing would be acceptable.[21] When the full committee reconsidered the matter, it concluded that it had not yet received enough evidence that the need for gender variety was so important in families that it justified creating and discarding embryos for that purpose.[19] In the future if such evidence was forthcoming then PGD for gender variety might also be acceptable.

What might constitute such evidence? One source would be families with two or more children of one gender who very much would like to have another child but only if they could be sure that it would be a child of the gender opposite of existing children. Given the legitimacy of wanting to raise children of both genders, reasonable persons might find that this need outweighs the symbolic costs of creating and discarding embryos for that purpose.

Another instance would be a case in which a couple has had a girl, but now wants a boy in order to meet cultural norms of having a male heir or a male to perform funeral rituals or play other cultural roles. An IVF programme in India is now providing PGD to select male offspring as the second child of couples who have already had a daughter.[22] Because of the importance of a male heir in India, those couples might well consider having an abortion if pregnant with a female fetus (even though illegal in India for that purpose). In that setting PGD for gender selection for gender variety appears to be justified.

PGD for Perfect Pitch Perfect or "absolute" pitch is the ability to identify and recall musical notes from memory.[23] Although not all great or successful musicians have perfect pitch, a large number of them do. Experts disagree over whether perfect pitch is solely inborn or may also be developed by early training, though most agree that a person either has it or does not. It also runs in families, apparently in an autosomal dominant pattern.[23] The gene or genes coding for this capacity have not, however, been mapped, much less sequenced. Because genes for perfect pitch may also relate to the genetic basis for language or other cognitive abilities, research to find that gene may be forthcoming.

Once the gene for perfect pitch or its linked markers are identified, it would be feasible to screen embryos for those alleles, and transfer only those embryos that test positive. The prevalence of those genes is quite low (perhaps three in 100) in the population, but high in certain families.[23] Thus only persons from those families who have a strong interest in the musical ability of their children would be potential candidates for PGD for perfect pitch. Many of them are likely to take their chances with coital conception and exposure of the child to music at an early age. Some couples, however, may be willing to undergo IVF and PGD to ensure musical ability in their child. Should their request be accepted or denied?

As noted, the answer to this question depends on the importance of the reproductive choice being asserted, the burdens of the selection procedure, its impact on offspring, and its implications for deselected groups and society generally. The strongest case for the parents is if they persuasively asserted that they would not reproduce unless they could select that trait, and they have a plausible explanation for that position. Although the preference might appear odd to some, it might also be quite understandable in highly musical families, particularly ones in which some members already have perfect pitch. Parents clearly have the right to instill or develop a child's musical ability after birth. They might reasonably argue that they should have that right before birth as well.

If so, then creating and discarding embryos for this purpose should also be acceptable. If embryos are too rudimentary in development to have inherent rights or interests, then no moral duty is violated by creating and destroying them.[24] Some persons might think that doing so for trivial or unimportant reasons debases the inherent dignity of all human life, but having a child with perfect pitch will not seem trivial to parents seeking this technique. Ultimately, the judgment of triviality or importance of the choice within a broad spectrum rests with the couple. If they have a strong enough preference to seek PGD for this purpose and that preference rationally relates to understandable reproductive goals, then they have demonstrated its great importance to them. Only in cases unsupported by a reasonable explanation of the need—for example, perhaps creating embryos to pick eye or hair colour, should a person's individual assessment of the importance of creating embryos be condemned or rejected.

A third relevant factor is whether musical trait selection is consistent with respect for the resulting child. Parents who are willing to undergo the costs and burdens of IVF and PGD to have a child with perfect pitch may be so overly invested in the child having a musical career that they will prevent it from developing its own personality and identity. Parents, however, are free to instill and develop musical ability once the child is born, just as they are entitled to instill particular religious views. It is difficult to say that they cross an impermissible moral line of risk to the welfare of their prospective child in screening embryos for this purpose. Parents are still obligated to provide their child with the basic education and care necessary for any life plan. Wanting a child to have perfect pitch is not inconsistent with parents also wanting their child to be well rounded and equipped for life in other contexts.

A fourth factor, impact on deselected groups, is much less likely to be an issue in the case of perfect pitch because there is no stigma or negative association tied to persons without that trait. Persons without perfect pitch suffer no stigma or opprobrium by the couple's choice or public acceptance of it, as is arguably the case with embryo selection on grounds of gender, sexual orientation, intelligence, strength, size, or other traits. Nor is PGD for perfect pitch likely to perpetuate unfair class advantages, as selection for intelligence, strength, size, or beauty might.

A final factor is the larger societal impact of permitting embryo screening for a non-medical condition such as perfect pitch. A valid concern is that such a practice might then legitimise embryo screening for other traits as well, thus moving us toward a future in which children are primarily valued according to the attractiveness of their expected characteristics. But that threat is too hypothetical to justify limiting what are otherwise valid exercises of parental choice. It is highly unlikely that many traits would be controlled by genes that could be easily tested in embryos. Gender is determined by the chromosome, and the gene for perfect pitch, if ever found, would be a rare exception to the multifactorial complexity of such traits. Screening embryos for

perfect pitch, if otherwise acceptable, should not be stopped simply because of speculation about what might be possible several decades from now.

PGD for Other Non-Medical Traits The discussion of PGD for perfect pitch illustrates the issues that would arise if single gene analysis became possible for other traits, such as sexual orientation, hair or eye colour, or height, intelligence, size, strength, and memory. In each case the ethical assessment depends on an evaluation of the importance of the choice to the parents and whether that choice plausibly falls within societal understandings of parental needs and choice in reproducing and raising children. If so, it should usually be a sufficient reason to create and screen embryos. The effect on resulting offspring would also be of key moral importance. Whether selection carries a public or social message about the worth of existing groups should also be addressed.

Applying this methodology might show that some instances of non-medical selection are justified, as we have seen with embryo selection for gender variety and perhaps for having a child with perfect pitch. The acceptability of PGD to select other non-medical traits will depend on a careful analysis of the relevant ethical factors, and social acceptance of much greater parental rights to control the genes of offspring than now exists.

CONCLUSION

Although new indications are emerging for PGD, it is likely to remain a small part of reproductive practice for some time to come. Most new indications serve legitimate medical purposes, such as screening for single gene mutations for late onset disorders or susceptibility to cancer. There is also ethical support for using PGD to assure that a child is an HLA match with an existing child.

More controversial is the use of PGD to select gender or other non-medical traits. As with medical uses, the acceptability of non-medical screening will depend upon the interests served and the effects of using PGD for those purposes. Speculations about potential future non-medical uses should not restrict new uses of PGD which are otherwise ethically acceptable.

ACKNOWLEDGMENT

Professor Robertson was supported by the Ethical, Legal, and Social Issues Program of the National Institute of Human Genome Research, US National Institutes of Health (USA).

REFERENCES

 1 International Working Group on Preimplantation Genetics. Preimplantation genetic diagnosis: Experience of 3000 clinical cycles. Report of the 11th annual meeting, May 15, 2001. *Reprod Biomedicine Online* 2001; 3:49–53.

 2 Verlinsky Y. Rechitsky S, Verlinsky O., *et al.* Preimplantation diagnosis of P53 tumor suppressor gene mutations. *Reprod Biomedicine Online* 2001; 2:102–5.

 3 Verlinsky Y. Rechitsky S, Schoolcraft W, *et al.* Preimplantation diagnosis for fanconi anemia combined with HLA matching. *JAMA* 2001; 285:3130–3.

 4 Verlinsky Y. Rechitsky S., Verlinsky O., *et al.* Preimplantation diagnosis for early-onset alzheimer's disease caused by V717L mutation. *JAMA* 2002; 283:1018–21.

 5 Fukuyama F. *Our postmodern future: consequences of the biotechnology revolution.* New York: Farrar, Strauss, & Giroux, 2002.

 6 Stock G. *Redesigning humans: our inevitable genetic future.* New York: Houghton Mifflin, 2002.

 7 Simpson J. L. Celebrating preimplantation genetic diagnosis of p53 mutations in Li-Fraumeni syndrome. *Reprod Biomedicine Online* 2001; 3: 2–3.

 8 Towner D., Loewy R. S., Ethics of preimplantation diagnosis for a woman destined to develop early-onset alzheimer disease. *JAMA* 2002; 283:1038–40.

 9 Human Fertilisation and Embryology Authority. *Opinion of the ethics committee. Ethical issues in the creation and selection of preimplantation embryos to produce tissue donors.* London: HFEA, 2001 Nov 22.

10 Pennings G., Schots S., Liebaers I. Ethical considerations on preimplantation genetic diagnosis for HLA typing to match a future child as a donor of haematopoietic stem cells to a sibling. *Hum Reprod* 2002; 17:534–8.

11 Robertson J. A., Kahn J., Wagner J. Conception to obtain hematopoietic stem cells. *Hastings Cent Rep* 2002; 32:34–40.

12 Sen A. More than 100 million women are missing. *New York Review of Books* 1990; 37:61–8.

13 Eckholm E. Desire for sons drives use of prenatal scans in China. *The New York Times* 2002 Jun 21:A3.

14 Jaccoby E. E., Jacklin C. N., *The psychology of sex differences.* Palo Alto: Stanford University Press, 1974.

15 Robertson J. A., Preconception gender selection. *Am J Bioeth* 2001; 1:2–9.

16 Grubb A., Walsh P., Gender-vending II. *Dispatches* 1994; 1:1–3.

17 Mahowald M. B., *Genes, women, equality.* New York: Oxford University Press, 2000: 121.

18 American Society of Reproductive Medicine, Ethics Committee. Preconception gender selection for nonmedical reasons. *Fertil Steril* 2001; 75:861–4.

19 Robertson J. A., Sex selection for gender variety by preimplantation genetic diagnosis. *Fert Steril* 2002; 78:463.

20 American Society of Reproductive Medicine, Ethics Committee. Sex selection and preimplantation genetic diagnosis. *Fertil Steril* 1999; 72:595–8.

21 Kolata G. Society approves embryo selection. *The New York Times* 2001 Sept 26:A14.

22 Malpani A., Malpani A., Modi D., Preimplantation sex selection for family balancing in India. *Hum Reprod* 2002; 17:11–12.

23 Blakeslee S. Perfect pitch: the key may lie in the genes. *The New York Times* 1990 Nov 30:1.

24 American Society of Reproductive Medicine, Ethics Committee. Ethical considerations of assisted reproductive technologies. *Fertil Steril* 1994; 62(suppl):32–7S.

SELECTING EMBRYOS FOR DESIRED TRAITS
President's Council on Bioethics

In this brief passage, the President's Council on Bioethics considers whether it is likely that significant demand will emerge for preimplantation genetic diagnosis (PGD) to select embryos *for* desired traits, in contrast to the established practice of using PGD to select *against* embryos with genetic or chromosomal disorders. In the council's view, several practical problems confront this possible extension of PGD use, making it unlikely that the use of PGD to select embryos for desired traits will "become widespread in the forseeable future." Still, the council argues, there are reasons to believe that "the use of this approach toward 'better children' might well become the practice of at least a significant minority."

. . . [T]he possibility of genetic enhancement of children through embryo selection cannot be easily dismissed. This approach . . . would not introduce new genes but would merely select positively among those that occur naturally. It depends absolutely on IVF, as augmented by the screening of the early embryos for the presence (or absence) of the desired genetic markers, followed by the selective transfer of those embryos that pass muster. This would amount to an "improvement-seeking" extension of the recently developed practice of preimplantation genetic diagnosis (PGD), now in growing use as a way to detect the presence or absence of genetic or chromosomal abnormalities *before* the start of a pregnancy.

As currently practiced, PGD works as follows: Couples at risk for having a child with a chromosomal or genetic disease undertake IVF to permit embryo screening before transfer, obviating the need for later prenatal diagnosis and possible abortion. A dozen or more eggs are fertilized and the embryos are grown to the four-cell or the eight-to-ten-cell stage. One or two of the embryonic cells (blastomeres) are removed for chromosomal analysis and genetic testing. Using a technique called polymerase chain reaction to amplify the tiny amount of DNA in the blastomere, researchers are able to detect the presence of genes responsible for one or more genetic disorders.[1] Only the embryos free of the genetic or chromosomal determinants for the disorders under scrutiny are made eligible for transfer to the woman to initiate a pregnancy.

The use of IVF and PGD to move from disease avoidance to baby improvement is conceptually simple, at least in terms of the techniques of screening, and would require no change in the procedure. Indeed, PGD has already been used to serve two goals unrelated to the health of the child-to-be: to pre-select the sex of a child, and to produce a child who could serve as a compatible bone-marrow or umbilical-cord-blood donor for a desperately ill sibling. (In the former case, chromosomal analysis of the blastomere identifies the embryo's sex; in the latter case, genetic analysis identifies which embryos are immunocompatible with the needy recipient.) It

is certainly likely that blastomere testing can be adapted to look for specific genetic variants at *any* locus of the human genome. And even without knowing the precise function of specific genes, statistical correlation of the presence of certain genetic variants with certain phenotypic traits (say, with an increase in IQ points or with perfect pitch) could lead to testing for these genetic variants, with selection following on this basis. As Dr. Francis Collins, director of the National Human Genome Research Institute, noted in his presentation to the Council, the time may soon arrive in which PGD is practiced for the purpose of selecting embryos with desired genotypes, even in the absence of elevated risk of particular genetic disorders.[2] Dr. Yury Verlinsky, director of the Reproductive Genetics Institute in Chicago, has recently predicted that soon "there will be no IVF without PGD."[3] Over the years, more and more traits will presumably become identifiable with the aid of PGD, including desirable genetic markers for intelligence, musicality, and so on, as well as undesirable markers for obesity, nearsightedness, color-blindness,[4] etc.

Yet, as Dr. Collins also pointed out to the Council, there are numerous practical difficulties with this scenario. For one thing, neither of the parents may carry the genetic variant they are most interested in selecting for. Also, selecting for highly polygenic traits would require screening a large number of embryos in order to find one that had the desirable complement. With only a dozen or so embryos to choose from, it will not be possible to optimize for the many necessary variants.[5]

The practice of PGD and selective transfer is still quite new, and fewer than 10,000 children have been born with its aid. How likely or widespread such a practice might become is difficult to predict. As we have already indicated, a number of practical issues would need to be addressed before PGD could be extended to permit selection of desirable traits beyond the absence of genetic disorders. First are questions of possible harm caused by removing blastomeres for testing (up to a sixth or even a quarter of the embryo's cells are taken). Although current evidence (from limited practice) suggests that the procedure inflicts neither any immediately visible harm on the early embryos, nor any obvious harm on the child that results, more attention to long-term

Reprinted from President's Council on Bioethics, *Beyond Therapy: Biotechnology and the Pursuit of Happiness* (2003), pp. 40–44.

risks to the child born following PGD is needed before many people would consider using it for "improvement" purposes only. Because many of the desirable human phenotypic traits are very likely polygenic, the contribution of any single gene identifiable by blastomere testing is likely to be small, and the likelihood of finding all the "desired" genetic variants in a single embryo is exponentially smaller still. Testing for multiple genetic variants using the DNA from a single blastomere is likely to be limited—for a time—by the quantities of DNA available, the sensitivity of the genetic tests, and the ability to perform multiple tests on the same sample. But it seems only a matter of time before techniques are perfected that will permit simultaneous screening of IVF embryos for multiple genetic variants. And should some of the "desirable" genes come grouped in clusters, selection for at least some desired traits might well be possible.

Finally, even if PGD could be used successfully to select an embryo with a number of desirable genetic variants, there is simply no guarantee that the child born after this procedure would grow up with the desired traits. The interplay of nature and nurture (genes and environment) in human development is too complex and too little understood to make such results predictable. Given that IVF combined with PGD is an inconvenient and expensive alternative to normal procreation, and given that success is doubtful at best, the purely elective use of this procedure seems unlikely to become widespread in the foreseeable future. . . .

Nevertheless, we think it would be imprudent to ignore completely this approach to "better children." More and more people are turning to assisted reproduction technologies (ART): in parts of western Europe, roughly five percent of all births involve ART; in the United States, it is roughly one percent and climbing, as the average maternal age of childbirth keeps rising and family size keeps declining. More and more people are using IVF not merely to overcome infertility but to screen and select embryos free of certain genetic defects. Women who plan to delay childbearing are being encouraged to consider early removal and cryopreservation of their own youthful ovarian tissue, to be reintroduced into their bodies at sites easily accessible for egg harvesting when they decide to have children. Other novel methods of obtaining supplies of eggs for IVF—possibly including deriving them in bulk from stem cells[6]—would make the procedure less burdensome, and would, in theory, permit the creation of a large enough population of embryos to make screening for polygenic traits feasible.

The anticipated vast extension of genetic screening will make many more couples aware of the risks they run in natural reproduction, and they may choose to turn to IVF to reduce them—especially if obtaining eggs became easy. Once more and more couples start screening embryos for disease-related concerns, and once scientists have identified those genes that correlate with various admirable traits, the anticipated expansion of improved and more precise screening techniques might enable users of IVF to screen for "desirable genes" as well. People already using PGD to screen for disease markers might seek information also about other traits, as they have with sex or histocompatibility. And if, once screening becomes automated, its cost comes down, or if society decides to reimburse for PGD (regarding it as less expensive than the care of genetically diseased children), the use of this approach toward "better children" might well become the practice of at least a significant minority. Under these circumstances, should genuine and significant improvements be achieved for a few highly desired attributes (say, in maximum lifespan . . .), one can easily imagine that there would be an increased demand for the practice, inconvenient or not. In the meantime, we would do well to consider the ethical implications not only of such future prospects but also of our current practices that make use of genetic knowledge.

NOTES

1 Although scientists are able to identify thousands of human genes and their variants, the fact that at present blastomere testing is done on the minute quantity of DNA present in one or two cells limits the reach of PGD in any given embryo to a handful of genetic variants. However, ongoing research on techniques for whole genome amplification will likely permit PGD in the future to test simultaneously for hundreds or even thousands of genetic variants in the same embryo. Of course, because of the complex relationship between genes and traits, the mere ability to screen for multiple genetic variants in no way guarantees that numerous phenotypic traits will soon be detectable.

2 Collins, F., "Genetic Enhancements: Current and Future Prospects," Presentation at the December 2002 meeting of the President's Council on Bioethics, Washington, D.C. Transcript available on the Council's website at www.bioethics.gov.

3 Mandavilli, A., "Fertility's new frontier takes shape in the test tube," *Nature Medicine* 9(8): 1095, 2003.

4 Color-blindness, a single-gene defect, can already be screened for.

5 If, for example, a desired trait required the concurrence of only seven specific genetic alleles and (to take the simplest case) there were only two alternate variants of each gene,

one would need (on the average) 128 embryos (and even more eggs) to get the full complement (2 to the seventh power). . . . Today, in the average IVF cycle, twelve to fifteen eggs are obtained by superovulation, and roughly only half make it to the stage where screening could occur. Of course, if the oocyte supply could be increased, say by deriving oocytes from embryonic stem cells, this problem might be soluble.

6 Hübner, K., et al., "Derivation of oocytes from mouse embryonic stem cells," *Science* 300(5620): 1251–1256, 2003.

GENE THERAPY

THE DANGEROUS PROMISE OF GENE THERAPY
Sophia Kolehmainen

Kolehmainen discusses the tragic case of Jesse Gelsinger, a young man who volunteered for a 1999 gene therapy protocol and died as a result of his participation. In Kolehmainen's view, the Gelsinger case pointedly illustrates the need for more effective regulation and oversight of gene therapy research. In this regard, she considers problems associated with (1) the safety of gene therapy protocols, (2) commercial interests in gene therapy, and (3) the recruitment of research subjects for gene therapy protocols.

In the mid-1980s scientists began to extol the promises of gene therapy. Conceptually (and if you consider the world only at the sub-microscopic level), gene therapy is a logical, straightforward solution to genetic disease: if a gene seems to be causing a disease, then to cure the disease scientists must remove the "bad" gene, and substitute or add a "good" gene. The reality is much more complex. Scientists have faced hurdles at every step of the gene therapy process as the multiple relationships among genes and between genes, disease, proteins, and the immune system (to name just a few of the relevant factors) have undermined the simplicity of the theory and added to the already difficult technicalities of inserting new genes into humans. Though more than

three hundred gene therapy protocols, involving more than four thousand patients, have been approved for human trials in the United States, gene therapy has yet to fulfil its promise of curing any genetic disease.

On September 17th, 1999, 18-year-old Jesse Gelsinger died as a result of his voluntary participation in a gene-therapy experiment, becoming the first known human victim of this technology. Jesse's experience illuminates important elements in gene therapy that should make government agencies, scientists, and the public take the need to regulate and oversee this technology very seriously.

Jesse had a rare genetic disease, known as ornithine transcarbamylase (OTC) deficiency, which affected his ability to rid his body of ammonia, a usual, but toxic, breakdown product of protein. In healthy individuals, as proteins are broken down,

Reprinted with permission from *GeneWatch*, vol. 13, no. 1 (February 2000).

enzymes in the liver rid the body of the ammonia. People who have OTC (usually males, as the associated gene appears to be located on the X chromosome, making it much rarer for women, who have two X chromosomes, to have the condition) lack the enzymes needed to rid the body of ammonia, and so the ammonia builds up in the blood, can travel to the brain, and, in extreme cases, lead to coma, brain damage and death.

In its severest form, OTC induces coma and usually brain damage just seventy-two hours after birth. One half of children with OTC die in their first month of life, and half of the rest die before their fifth birthday. Jesse had a mild form of the disease because some of his enzymes were functioning normally. He was therefore able to control the disease with diet and drugs, though he needed to take 32 pills a day. However, as long as he stuck to the restrictive diet and drug regimen, Jesse was not sick.

The experimental protocol for which Jesse volunteered had no chance of providing him, or any of the other volunteers, with any benefit. It was designed only to test the safety of a treatment that would be used on babies with the fatal form of OTC. The scientists who designed the protocol at the University of Pennsylvania's Institute for Gene Therapy, Dr. James Wilson and Dr. Mark Batshaw, believed that OTC could be surmounted with gene therapy. They hoped to infuse babies who had OTC with genes that would help them produce the missing enzymes. In order to get these genes into the patient's cells, Dr. Wilson developed a weakened cold virus (known as adenovirus) which was designed to enter the cells as any virus would, but, instead of delivering disease, it was supposed to deliver the corrective OTC gene. Wilson and Batshaw hoped that the infusion of adenovirus and corrective genes could be used to reduce infant fatalities by controling the high levels of ammonia in babies with OTC immediately after birth.

Wilson and Batshaw worked together to develop the protocol and, in 1995, they submitted their OTC protocol to the National Institute of Health's (NIH) Recombinant DNA Advisory Committee (RAC) and the Food and Drug Administration (FDA) for review and approval, as is required for all human experiments involving gene therapy. Their human gene therapy trial called for 18 patients with OTC in six groups of three, to receive increasing doses of the genetically altered adenovirus carrying the corrective OTC gene. The adenovirus-OTC infusion was to be delivered to the patients through a catheter into an artery that leads directly to the liver. The goal of the trial was to find the maximum tolerated dose of adenovirus and OTC: high enough to work, and low enough to avoid serious side effects.

Jesse found out about the trial from his pediatric geneticist when he was seventeen and, though he wanted to sign up right away, regulations required him to wait until his eighteenth birthday. Four days after his eighteenth birthday, Jesse was at the University of Pennsylvania meeting with Dr. Raper, the surgeon in charge of patient and medical care for the gene therapy trial. Jesse was deemed eligible for the study and assigned to the final test subject group— the group that would receive the highest dose of adenovirus. At the time, the researchers believed that in the worst case, the trial might result in an inflamed liver. When Jesse was to begin the experiment on September 13, 1999, he traveled to Pennsylvania from Arizona by himself; his father had made plans to fly out later for the liver biopsy— the procedure that was considered to carry the most serious risk.

On September 13, 1999 Dr. Raper injected 30 milliliters of the adenovirus with the corrective OTC gene into Jesse's bloodstream. That evening Jesse was sick with a fever of 104.5 degrees. Dr. Raper was not particularly concerned because other patients in the study had had a similar reaction. By the morning of September 14, however, Jesse seemed disoriented and exhibited signs of jaundice—a condition which usually results from either liver failure or blood clotting, both of which would be serious for an individual with a liver already weakened by OTC. That evening, Jesse had dangerously high ammonia levels in his blood and was in a coma. Jesse's father arrived on the morning of September 15th. Later that day Jesse's lungs began to fail and he went into kidney failure the next day. According to the physicians, Jesse's severe immune system reaction led to multiple-organ-system failure and he died on September 17th, 1999, four days after the gene-therapy injection.

THE SAFETY OF GENE THERAPY

Human gene therapy trials raise the question of how safe an experiment must be before it is ethical to try it on humans. Prior to the human protocol, Batshaw and Wilson had done animal studies to help prove that OTC gene therapy was ready for human trial. They cited more than twenty experiments on mice to prove the efficacy of the treatment, and twelve safety studies in mice, Rhesus monkeys and baboons.

In Wilson and Batshaw's early animal experiments with adenovirus, several Rhesus monkeys died after intense immune system reactions like Jesse's to high doses of adenovirus. Wilson then experimented with the adenovirus itself, removing different combinations of its DNA to make it safer. Wilson believed that the adenovirus variation he used in the human protocol was significantly less toxic than the one which caused the death of the monkeys. The U. Penn researchers also decided to reduce the highest dose to be used in the human trial two-hundredfold from that used in the animal experiments.

In addition to safety measures suggested by the animal experiments, the mandatory review of human gene therapy experiments by the FDA and RAC is supposed to add another level of precaution. However, critics of this process have often stated that the current regulatory framework—review by the NIH's RAC and approval by the FDA—creates an ineffectual review process. When Wilson and Batshaw first presented their protocol for review by the RAC, both of the RAC scientists reviewing the protocol had reservations about approving it. They felt that the protocol was too dangerous to test on asymptomatic individuals as it was the first time heavy doses of adenovirus would be injected directly into the bloodstream and the experiment had no chance of lasting benefit to the human subjects. However, continued negotiations between the federal reviewers (including RAC and FDA officials) and the University of Pennsylvania scientists resulted in approval of the protocol.

Following the report of Jesse Gelsinger's death, and subsequent revelations of six other deaths in gene therapy experiments in New York and Massachusetts, the National Institute of Health (NIH) RAC convened a three-day public inquiry into Jesse's death, the conduct of gene therapy research, and the

safety of using adenovirus. The inquiry was covered in the media, and attended by officials of the FDA, the University of Pennsylvania scientists, other gene therapy researchers, and family and friends of Jesse Gelsinger.

In what was described as a tumultuous exchange on the first day of the inquiry, the FDA argued that Jesse's liver was not functioning well enough at the time of the infusion of adenovirus, and he should not have been eligible for the study; that the Pennsylvania scientists had violated FDA regulations by failing to report information about patients who had experienced serious side effects that could have ended the trial; and that the informed consent document that Jesse signed deviated from the one approved by the agency when it reviewed the protocol. The new consent form had made no mention of the severe immune system responses to adenovirus that led to the deaths of the monkeys.

Dr. Wilson and the scientists from the University of Pennsylvania countered that they had no evidence from human or animal testing that could have foretold Jesse's death; and that at the time Jesse enrolled in the study he was eligible. On the second day of the inquiry, the University of Pennsylvania stated that they still could not explain Jesse's death, though they had found some evidence in his bone marrow of another virus which might have increased his susceptibility to the effects of the adenovirus.

On January 21, 2000, the FDA indefinitely shut down human gene therapy experiments at the University of Pennsylvania, citing "numerous serious deficiencies" in ensuring patient safety, and issued a report detailing 18 specific violations. This action by the FDA halted eight experiments at Dr. Wilson's Institute for Gene Therapy at the University of Pennsylvania, including five active clinical trials. The trials will remain "on-hold" until the Institute responds formally to the FDA's report, and convinces the FDA that it can properly follow the federal rules designed to ensure the safety of study volunteers.

The human gene therapy trials at the University of Pennsylvania were not the only trials affected by the inquiry into Jesse's death. The FDA also suspended enrollment in gene therapy trials for advanced liver cancer patients being run by the Schering-Plough Corporation of Madison, NJ and the University of California San Francisco. The Schering-Plough trials were using high doses of adenovirus in the liver and researchers there had also found evidence of serious side effects from the use of adenovirus in gene therapy.

Since the news of Jesse's death was first brought to the attention of government regulators and the public in September 1999, further evidence of serious risks to patient safety in other gene therapy experiments has come to light. In response to reminders sent out by regulators, the NIH received 691 reports of "serious adverse events" in gene therapy experiments, and although the current regulatory structure requires researchers to promptly notify the NIH as problems arise, 652 of the reports had never been presented to the NIH. Reports from at least two gene therapy trials revealed that volunteers had died during the course of the experiments. The scientists in both cases decided that the deaths were not related to the gene therapy treatment. However, their reports indicate that, in fact, they cannot conclusively say what caused the deaths of some of the volunteers.

CORPORATE INTERESTS IN GENE THERAPY

In addition to questions of safety, the massive amount of corporate interest in the development of gene therapy technology raises questions that can only be addressed with diligent oversight. Intense commercial interest in gene therapy may create conflicts between business decisions and medical decisions.

In the case of the gene therapy trial that led to Jesse's death, Dr. James Wilson, the head of the Institute for Gene Therapy at the University of Pennsylvania, also owns a private company called Genovo Inc, which he founded in 1992. Genovo has the rights to any discoveries made by Wilson at his University of Pennsylvania lab. Through this arrangement, Genovo has access to Wilson's discoveries, at the same time minimizing its business risks as the company can let the lab run the clinical trials prior to deciding to invest. The NIH, further reduced Genovo's risk and maximized the company's benefits by funding the OTC trial in which Jesse took part. Genovo also has a financial stake in the adenovirus variation Wilson developed and tested on

Jesse in the human gene therapy trial, which would have been very marketable if it had been successful.

In addition, BIOGEN, a Cambridge-based biotechnology company, has paid Genovo thirty-seven million dollars since 1995 for the right to eventually market any liver and lung related therapies developed by Genovo. Genovo shares the money from BIOGEN with Dr. Wilson's Institute at U.Penn, and in fact the Biogen money accounts for twenty percent of the Institute's budget. The Genovo-Biogen deal (which is up for renewal this year) calls for Genovo to make progress in moving gene therapy towards a marketable product.

In August, 1999, Genovo entered into an agreement with GENZYME (another Cambridge-based biotech company), to develop liver-directed gene therapy for metabolic disorders.

Wilson has stated many times that his business interests do not influence his judgment during trials and, also, that his involvement in gene therapy is not about money, but about "leadership, notoriety, and accomplishment." Even so, the existence of the financial stakes and relationships described above, which seem to be typical in the gene therapy research industry, require vigilant oversight to ensure that the medical decisions, as much as possible, are based on considerations of health and not money.

WILLING AND ABLE VOLUNTEERS

The intense corporate interest in human gene therapy becomes even more disturbing when considered in conjunction with the fact that people are literally lining up to be test subjects for clinical trials. Gene therapy gives promise to people who are desperately searching for hope. It is a technology marketed as a cure for genetic disease—diseases which often lead to suffering which is entirely unjustifiable. If a friend or a family member had a genetic disease, and you watched him or her suffer without respite or chance of cure, wouldn't you jump at any opportunity to end that? This scenario raises serious concerns since it puts a most vulnerable and well-meaning group of people at serious risk without adequate protections.

One of the most important questions Wilson and Batshaw faced in designing their human trial of OTC gene therapy was determining who were the appropriate test subjects for their research. Initially, they believed that the protocol should be tried on infants with severe OTC, as the therapy was designed specifically for these babies. But Arthur Caplan, the resident bioethics expert at the University of Pennsylvania, disagreed. He stated that it would be unethical to experiment with sick babies because the parents of dying infants are too stressed to be able to give informed consent.

Consequently, Wilson and Batshaw decided to use stable adults for the protocol—men like Jesse who had the disease but were surviving with drugs and diet, and women who carry the gene linked to OTC. This shift from dying infants to stable adults meant that people who were living with their disease and benefiting from conventional treatments were put at risk in situations which would not produce any benefit for them.

The NIH/RAC hearings after Jesse's death also made public the fact that some of the volunteers for this study were recruited in a coercive manner—using Internet sites and newsletters which detailed the promise of the therapy if it worked and which stressed the need for human subjects. This type of information, placed where it would be seen by a population sensitive to the problems of living with a genetic disease raises further issues about getting truly informed and voluntary subjects for human experimentation.

Human gene therapy experimentation raises many issues. The promise of the technology is represented as very great and the reality of it is very dangerous, that human gene therapy must be seriously and cautiously evaluated. Without increased and more effective oversight, Jesse's death could be the first of many in gene therapy. Though Jesse's participation in the human trial did not provide him or the infants with OTC with any benefit, it did perhaps lead to something even more important in this field. Jesse's death has forced researchers and government officials to reappraise the current framework and structure of gene therapy research, to reexamine informed consent procedures, and to take public responsibility for their actions.

THE FUTURE OF GENE THERAPY: BALANCING THE RISKS AND THE BENEFITS OF CLINICAL TRIALS

Marina Cavazzana-Calvo, Adrian Thrasher, and Fulvio Mavilio

In this brief selection, three European researchers involved in clinical trials of gene therapy for the treatment of children suffering from severe combined immunodeficiencies (SCIDs) discuss these trials and some of the ethical and policy issues associated with them. Maintaining that the risk/benefit ratio is the only relevant standard for the ethical assessment of gene therapy, the authors argue that clinical trials of gene therapy should not be unnecessarily delayed. They also argue that harmonization of regulatory control is of crucial importance, especially among various European states and between Europe and the United States.

Gene therapy has the potential to treat devastating inherited diseases for which there is little hope of finding a conventional cure. In the late 1990s, our groups in Paris, London and Milan began treating children suffering from rare immune disorders (severe combined immunodeficiencies, or SCIDs). The successful treatment of the first patients was greeted with excitement when it was first reported in 2000 and 2002 (refs[1, 2]). Sadly, this euphoria turned to alarm at the end of 2002, when two of the ten children treated in France developed leukaemia-like conditions.[3]

Reprinted with permission of the publisher from *Nature*, vol. 427, February 2004, pp. 779–781.

In all of these patients, the genetic defect was corrected by inserting a therapeutic gene into a 'disabled' retrovirus, known as a vector. This vector was then used to 'infect' bone-marrow stem cells taken from each patient before being injected back into their bloodstream, where it was hoped they would multiply into normal immune cells. As it turned out, the ability of these viruses to insert themselves into DNA was also responsible for activating a cancer-promoting gene. News of the leukaemia immediately raised concerns about using a therapeutic approach that may cause cancer at such an alarming frequency. Patient safety is, of course, the first and foremost concern of anybody trying to develop a new medical treatment. But it would be unfortunate if the future of gene therapy was decided by emotive issues rather than careful analysis of its risks and benefits.

The leukaemia cases generated enormous interest among scientists, regulators and the general public. Reactions from regulatory authorities in the United States and Europe varied widely. . . . Some asked clinicians to revise the eligibility criteria for future trials and to update procedures for obtaining informed consent from patients, whereas others imposed a general moratorium on trials involving the use of retroviruses. In the United Kingdom, clinical studies were never put on hold, whereas in Italy treatment for individuals was approved during 2003 only when there was an imminent threat to life. The combination of bad press, scepticism from colleagues, and mixed reactions from regulators has effectively thrown the field into recession.

The current 'gene-therapy-causes-cancer' mood and uncertainty about the effects of tighter regulations is discouraging scientists from starting new clinical trials, and scaring investors and the biotechnology industry away from the field. In 2003 leading industrial players either closed their operations (Gene Therapy, Maryland) or redirected their efforts away from retroviral vectors (Cell Genesys, California). This is unfortunate, because in the absence of industrial investment it is unlikely that gene therapy will eventually deliver on its promises.

What can or should be done? As scientists, we are used to learning from crises and developing solutions to emerging problems. But restoring confidence in the future of gene therapy is going to be a tough sell—much of the debate is no longer about scientific concerns. We would like gene therapy to be seen, and treated, as any other experimental therapy, and that means recognizing the successes as well as the failures.

THE SUCCESSES

SCIDs are rare genetic failures in the development of the immune system that are fatal in the first years of life.[4] The patients treated in Italy suffered from adenosine deaminase-deficient (ADA⁻) SCID, which means that they lacked an essential enzyme involved in DNA metabolism. The patients treated in France and Britain suffered from X-SCID, caused by a defect in a gene on the X chromosome. For both diseases, transplantation of bone marrow from perfectly matched donors is the treatment of choice, although it is available to less than one in three patients. For the others, transplantation from mismatched donors carries a 75% overall chance of survival, with a 15–20% risk of developing severe immunological complications and a 20–30% risk of early mortality.[5]

In the early 1990s, attempts to treat ADA-SCID with gene therapy achieved only partial success, owing to problem in transferring genes into the patients' stem cells. But recent developments in both vector and cell transplantation technology led to the successful treatment of both forms of SCID.[1,2] Of the 18 SCID patients treated so far in Paris, Milan and London, 17 benefited from life-saving reconstitution of their immune functions for up to five years. All these patients are currently alive.

THE FAILURES

The optimism generated by what was considered to be the first true success of gene therapy turned into disappointment at the news of the two leukaemia cases. Genetic analysis of the malignant cells showed that in both cases the retroviral vector had inserted into, and activated, an oncogene called *LMO2* that is associated with childhood leukaemia. The activated oncogene was not the only cause of the malignancy, but was most likely the event that triggered it.[3]

The leukaemias came as a surprise, partly because none of the preclinical studies had shown any evidence of cancer in animals treated with the same approach. Moreover, although scientists had always considered the possibility that gene insertion would activate oncogenes, no such event had been observed in more than a decade of clinical trials in humans involving large numbers of genetically modified blood cells.[6] The apparently high (15%) risk to X-SCID patients of developing malignant cells suggests that there are specific risk factors for this disease—one possibility being an association between the therapeutic gene and the activated oncogene.[3,7] More research is needed into this question.

THE TRADE-OFF

The patients who developed the leukaemias received a particularly high number of genetically modified stem cells. The issue of dose is an important one. By considering what we know about the likelihood of retroviruses inserting into active genes and the number of potential oncogenes in the human genome, a recent analysis estimates that up to one in every 10,000 modified cells might harbour a dangerous insertion.[8] Although these predictions need to be checked against actual clinical data, it is likely that the higher the number of cells given to a patient, the higher the probability of receiving one that is potentially malignant. This possibility poses a real ethical dilemma. The effectiveness of gene therapy has been limited for years by inefficient technology. The SCID trials changed that by increasing both gene transfer and cell transplantation efficiency. Scaling back this efficiency might reduce the risk of side effects, but will almost certainly lower the chances of success. Is there a sensible risk/benefit balance in such situations?

After the leukaemia cases occurred, scientists and regulatory authorities called for a halt to clinical experiments. In most countries, trials were allowed to resume after a temporary hold, on the basis that the potential benefits to patients outweighed the risks. Many argued that there is a need to develop new, safer vectors that avoid the problem of oncogene activation, and for more preclinical studies to enable better assessment of the risks. It is hard to disagree with these positions. Research must go on, particularly on vector design. Nevertheless, this

work may take many years, and even the best animal model is far from being able to predict all of the possible risk factors when treating patients. This was certainly true in the X-SCID case.

In the meantime, we are left with a lifesaving treatment that works for most patients, and several patients with no alternative treatments or with alternatives that carry even higher risks. Gene therapy, just like any other treatment, has side effects, and we have to deal with them—as we would do for any other treatment. Even with the risk of leukaemia, gene therapy is still a much better therapy than mismatched bone-marrow transplantation for SCID patients, and a fair assessment of the risk/benefit ratio should really be the only ethical criterion underlying the decision to use it. Ultimately, when assessing actual risk, there is no substitute for clinical trials on many patients. Delaying these trials would prevent researchers from assessing its full therapeutic potential, postpone its development into an effective therapy, and ultimately affect the right of patients to have access to a better treatment.

PREDICTION AND MONITORING OF RISKS

Decisions on how to carry out further trials are complicated by the availability of technology to analyse genetically modified stem cells before and after they are given to patients. It has been proposed that using such analysis would prevent patients being given potentially malignant cells. Although regulatory authorities in Europe and the United States have not yet demanded this type of monitoring, the jury is still out on the issue. Could such 'molecular monitoring' provide useful information to clinical investigators and reduce the risks to patients?

As discussed above, there could be potentially dangerous gene insertions in all samples of genetically modified cells. Unfortunately, the molecular analysis destroys the cells. So screening all samples before transplantation, as argued by some,[9] is technically impossible—each modified stem cell is unique, and taking 10% of the cells for analysis will tell you nothing about the other 90%. In addition, until we know more about what causes cells to become malignant, there is no evidence that detecting certain insertions would inevitably lead to leukaemia, for example. There are many factors that prevent cells with potentially dangerous insertions from developing into a malignant cell,[8] and the risk could vary greatly in different patients and for different diseases.

More realistically, molecular monitoring could be carried out during the follow-up phase of clinical trials. Such analysis could help to estimate the frequency of potentially harmful events, and provide a better risk assessment for future clinical trials. In the case of the French X-SCID patients, retrospective analysis of blood samples taken at regular intervals revealed how clones of the malignant cells grew and proliferated in the patients' blood.[3] This provided a wealth of information on the causes and development of the leukaemia. However, monitoring gene insertions has less value than we would like for predicting and diagnosing cancer in individual patients. For diagnostic purposes, proliferating cell clones cannot indicate cancer alone, which requires other clinical information. We therefore argue that mandatory molecular monitoring would put an unnecessary burden on clinical centres running gene-therapy trials, without significantly reducing the risk of leukaemia. Instead, we recommend systematic archiving of bone marrow and blood samples from all patients undergoing stem-cell gene therapy, to allow retrospective analysis at any time.

REGULATORY HARMONY

The varied responses from regulatory authorities add greatly to the uncertainty surrounding gene therapy. By creating a complex web of different rules in different countries, multicentre clinical trials become harder to plan and execute. Harmonization of legislation among European states, and between Europe and the United States, is urgently needed. Although talks are ongoing between the US Food and Drug Administration (FDA) and the European Medical Evaluation Agency (EMEA) on this point, the picture remains bleak.

The EMEA has no formal jurisdiction over early clinical trials, and individual European countries resist the idea of giving up national authority on this matter. The Gene Therapy Expert Group within the EMEA has done an outstanding job in providing accurate information on the cancer-related risks, and sensible suggestions about the regulatory options.[10] However, unless measures are rapidly taken to harmonize the decision-making process of European states on gene-therapy regulation, it is unlikely that any agreement between the FDA and the EMEA will have the beneficial impact that investigators and industry—and ultimately patients—are waiting for.

Retroviruses are the only clinical tool currently available to introduce a permanent genetic modification into stem cells and to treat life-threatening conditions such as SCIDs. We believe it is essential to find a rational balance between feasibility, safety and efficacy when deciding on the clinical uses of these vectors, as well as when devising suitable regulations and guidelines.

ACKNOWLEDGMENTS

The authors report the shared opinion of the scientists and clinicians who developed and performed gene therapy of SCIDs in France, Italy and the United Kingdom, and in particular of Alessandro Aiuti, Claudio Bordignon, Alain Fischer, Salima Hacein-Bey-Abina and Maria Grazia Roncarolo.

REFERENCES

1 Cavazzana-Calvo, M. *et al. Science* **288,** 669–672 (2000).
2 Ajuti, A. *et al. Science* **296,** 2410–2413 (2002).
3 Hacein-Bey-Abina, S. *et al. Science* **302,** 415–419 (2003).
4 Fischer, A. *Lancet* **357,** 1863–1869 (2001).
5 Antoine, C. *et al. Lancet* **361,** 553–560 (2003).
6 Bonini, C. *et al. Nature Med* **9,** 367–369 (2003).
7 Dave, U. P., Jenkins, N. A. & Copeland, N. G. *Science* **303,** 333 (2004).
8 Baum, C. *et al. Blood* **101,** 2099–2114 (2003).
9 Williams, D. A. & Baum, C. *Science* **302,** 400–401 (2003).
10 http://www.emea.eu.int/index/indexh1.htm

GERM-LINE GENE THERAPY
LeRoy Walters and Julie Gage Palmer

Walters and Palmer begin by presenting four scenarios in which germ-line gene therapy, if it were available, would be very useful. Their subsequent analysis of the ethics of germ-line gene therapy is based on the assumption that effective (and safe) germ-line intervention methods will eventually be developed. Surveying the major ethical arguments for and against germ-line gene therapy, the authors identify and articulate five arguments in support of germ-line gene therapy and eight arguments against it. Ultimately supportive of germ-line gene therapy, Walters and Palmer explicitly endorse three of the five pro arguments and offer replies to the eight con arguments.

. . . It should be recognized that the various alternatives for approaching genetic disease have differing effects on the germ line of the treated patient. Standard medical therapies, like somatic cell gene therapy, are somatic treatments and do not correct genetic defects in a patient's germ line. They may allow patients to live and to reproduce, passing on genetic mistakes which, without treatment, would not be perpetuated. Preimplantation and prenatal selection, like somatic medicine, may also result in a higher incidence of germ-line genetic defects because, unless they employ selective discard and selective abortion of unaffected carriers, both strategies increase the number of carriers of genetic defects that are born.

Successful germ-line gene replacement, on the other hand, will not perpetuate genetic mistakes. It will not only cure the patient at hand; it will also prevent the disease in question from arising in that patient's descendants. Applied to heterozygous carriers on a large scale, it could theoretically eliminate chosen disease-causing genes from the human gene pool.

As long as germ-line gene therapy must be performed on human zygotes or embryos one at a time after in vitro fertilization, it is likely to remain an expensive technology with limited use. Only if a technique is developed for performing gene replacement or gene repair within the reproductive cells of hu-

man adults—perhaps through the injection of highly refined vectors that "home in" only on those cells (or their precursors in males)—are we likely to see the widespread diffusion of germ line genetic intervention for disease prevention. . . .

FOR WHAT CLINICAL SITUATIONS WILL GERM-LINE GENE THERAPY BE PROPOSED?

It is difficult to predict the precise context in which germ-line gene therapy will first be considered. Tables 1 through 4 show four scenarios where the issue of germ-line intervention may at least be discussed at some point in the future.

TABLE 1   Mode of Inheritance 1

Both the wife and the husband are afflicted with a recessive genetic disorder. That is, both have two copies of the same malfunctioning gene at a particular site in their chromosomes. Therefore, all of their offspring are likely to be affected with the same genetic disorder.

TABLE 2   Mode of Inheritance 2

Both the wife and the husband are carriers of a recessive genetic disorder. That is, each has one copy of a properly functioning and one copy of a malfunctioning gene at a particular site in their chromosomes. Following Mendel's laws, 25% of the couple's offspring are likely to be "normal," 50% are likely to be carriers like their parents, and 25% are likely to be afflicted with the genetic disorder.

TABLE 3 Disease Condition 1

A diagnosable genetic disorder results in major, irreversible damage to the brains of affected fetuses during the first trimester of pregnancy. There is no known method for making genetic repairs in the uterus during pregnancy. If any genetic repair is to be made, it must be completed before the embryo begins its intrauterine development.

TABLE 4 Disease Condition 2

A diagnosable genetic disorder affects many different cell types in many different parts of the bodies of patients affected by the disorder. Somatic cell gene therapy that targets a particular cell type is therefore unlikely to be successful in combating the disorder. Therefore, germ-line gene therapy delivered early enough to affect *all* cell types may be the only feasible way to prevent disease in a particular future person.

The kind of situation described in Table 1 is likely to arise as medical care succeeds in prolonging the lives of people with genetic disorders such as sickle cell disease or cystic fibrosis. If somatic cell gene therapy is employed in significant numbers of people afflicted with recessive genetic diseases, some of those people's somatic cells will be able to function normally, but their reproductive cells will remain unchanged, thus assuring that they will be carriers of genetic disease to the next generation. If two such phenotypically cured people marry and have children, all or almost all of their children will be afflicted with the disease which their parents had. Each succeeding generation of these children will need somatic cell gene therapy for the treatment of their disease.

Table 2 sketches a scenario frequently encountered by genetic counselors. In this case, germ-line genetic intervention could be viewed as an alternative to prenatal diagnosis and selective abortion of affected fetuses or to preimplantation diagnosis and the selective discard of affected early embryos. A couple might also elect germ-line genetic intervention in order to avoid producing children who are *carriers* of genetic defects, even if the children

are not themselves afflicted with genetic disease. The parents would know that children who are carriers may one day face precisely the kind of difficult reproductive decisions that they as parents are facing.

In the type of case outlined in Table 3, somatic cell gene therapy might be effective if one could deliver it to the developing embryo and fetus during the earliest stages of pregnancy, that is, shortly after the embryo has implanted in the uterus. However, there is no known method of administering intrauterine therapy to an early first-trimester embryo, and a deferral of treatment until the second or third trimester would probably allow irreversible damage to occur. Preimplantation treatment, which would almost certainly affect the future germ-line cells as well as the future somatic cells, could be the only feasible approach to producing children who are not brain damaged, especially for couples who reject the alternative of selectively discarding early embryos.[1]

The scenario presented in Table 4 may be especially relevant to the development of particular kinds of cancers as a result of inborn genetic factors and subsequent mutations. For example, about 40% of people with a cancer of the retina called *retinoblastoma* transmit a dominant gene for this disorder to their children. In patients with this germ-line type of retinoblastoma, somatic mutational events that occur after birth seem to activate the cancer-causing gene and can result in multiple types of cancer developing in different cell types within the patient's body. For example, a kind of cancer called *osteogenic sarcoma* frequently develops later in life in patients who have been successfully treated for retinoblastoma.[2] With germ-line retinoblastoma, the only effective antidote to the development of multiple types of cancers may be early germ-line gene therapy that effectively repairs *all* of the cells in a developing embryo.[3]

THE NEEDED TECHNOLOGICAL BREAKTHROUGH: GENE REPLACEMENT OR GENE REPAIR

As we noted earlier in this chapter [of *The Ethics of Human Gene Therapy*], the current technique for somatic-cell gene therapy relies on rather imprecise methods of gene addition. For safe and effective germ-line gene therapy, it seems likely that a more precisely targeted method of gene replacement or gene repair will be necessary. The most obvious reason for preferring gene replacement is that gene addition in embryos would result in their (later-developing) sperm or egg cells containing *both* the malfunctioning and the properly functioning genes. Thus, one undesirable effect of researchers' treating present or future reproductive cells by gene addition is that the researchers would be directly contributing to an increase in the number of malfunctioning genes in future generations. In addition, if any of the germ-line disorders are dominant, as retinoblastoma seems to be, then only gene replacement is likely to eradicate the deleterious effects of the malfunctioning gene.

MAJOR ETHICAL ARGUMENTS IN FAVOR OF GERM-LINE GENE THERAPY

In this and the following section we will analyze the major ethical arguments[4] for and against germ-line gene therapy.[5] For this analysis we will make the optimistic assumption that germ-line intervention methods will gradually be refined until they reach the point where gene replacement or gene repair is technically feasible and able to be accomplished in more than 95% of attempted gene transfer procedures. Thus, the following analysis presents the arguments for and against germ-line intervention under the most favorable conditions for such intervention.

A first argument in favor of germ-line intervention is that it may be the only way to prevent damage to particular biological individuals when that damage is caused by certain kinds of genetic defects. This argument is most closely related to the last two scenarios presented above. That is, only genetic modifications introduced into preimplantation embryos are likely to be early enough to affect all of the important cell types (as in retinoblastoma), or to reach a large enough fraction of brain cells, or to be in time to prevent irreversible damage to the developing embryo. In these circumstances the primary intent of gene therapy would, or at least could, be to provide gene therapy for the early embryo. A

side effect of the intervention would be that all of the embryonic cells, including the reproductive cells that would later develop, would be genetically modified.[6]

A second moral argument for germ-line genetic intervention might be advanced by parents. It is that they wish to spare their children and grandchildren from either (1) having to undergo somatic cell gene therapy if they are born affected with a genetic defect or (2) having to face difficult decisions regarding possibly transmitting a disease-related gene to their own children and grandchildren. In our first scenario, admittedly a rare case, two homozygous parents who have a genetic disease know in advance that all of their offspring are likely to be affected with the same genetic disease. In the second scenario, there is a certain probability that the parents' offspring will be affected or carriers. An assumption lying behind this second argument is that parents should enjoy a realm of moral and legal protection when they are making good-faith decisions about the health of their children. Only if their decisions are clearly adverse to the health interests of the children should moral criticism or legal intervention be considered.

A third moral argument for germ-line intervention is more likely to be made by health professionals, public-health officials, and legislators casting a wary eye toward the expenditures for health care. This argument is that, from a social and economic point of view, germ-line intervention is more efficient than repeating somatic cell gene therapy generation after generation. From a medical and public health point of view, germ-line intervention fits better with the increasingly preferred model of disease prevention and health promotion. In the very long run, germ-line intervention, if applied to both affected individuals and asymptomatic carriers of serious genetic defects, could have a beneficial effect on the human gene pool and the frequency of genetic disease.[7]

A fourth argument refers to the roles of researchers and health professionals. As a general rule, researchers deserve to have the freedom to explore new modes of treating and/or preventing human disease.[8] To be sure, moral rules set limits on how this research is conducted. For example, animals involved in the preclinical stages of the research should be treated humanely. In addition, the human subjects involved in the clinical trials should be treated with respect. When and if germ-line gene therapy is some day validated as a safe and effective intervention, health care providers should be free to, and may have a moral obligation to, offer it to their patients as a possible treatment. This freedom is based on the professional's general obligation to seek out and offer the best possible therapeutic alternatives to patients and society's recognition of a sphere in which health professionals are at liberty to exercise their best judgment on behalf of their patients.

A fifth and final argument in favor of germ-line gene therapy is that this kind of intervention best accords with the health professions' healing role and with the concern to protect rather than penalize individuals who have disabilities. This argument is not simply a plea for protecting all embryos and fetuses from the time of fertilization forward. Both authors of this book [*The Ethics of Human Gene Therapy*] think that abortion is morally justifiable in certain circumstances. However, prenatal diagnosis followed by selective abortion and preimplantation diagnosis followed by selective discard seem to us to be uncomfortable and probably discriminatory halfway technologies that should eventually be replaced by effective modes of treatment. The options of selective abortion and selective discard essentially say to prospective parents, "There is nothing effective that the health care system has to offer. You may want to give up on this fetus or embryo and try again." To people with disabilities that are diagnosable at the prenatal or preimplantation stages of development the message of selective abortion and selective discard may seem more threatening. That message may be read as, "If we health professionals and prospective parents had known you were coming, we would have terminated your development and attempted to find or create a nondisabled replacement."

This argument is not intended to limit the legal access of couples to selective abortion in the case of serious health problems for the fetus. We support such access. Rather, it is an argument about what the long-term goal of medicine and society should be. In our view, that long-term goal should be to prevent disability and disease wherever possible. Where prevention is not possible, the second-best alternative is a cure or other definitive remedy. In cases where neither prevention nor cure is possible, our goal should be to help people cope with disability and disease while simultaneously seeking to find a cure.

MAJOR ARGUMENTS AGAINST GERM-LINE GENE THERAPY

First, if the technique has unanticipated negative effects, those effects will be visited not only on the recipient of the intervention himself or herself but also on all of the descendants of that recipient. This argument seems to assume that a mistake, once made, could not be corrected, or at least that the mistake might not become apparent until the recipient became the biological parent of at least one child. For that first child, at least, the negative effects could be serious, as well as uncorrectable.

Second, some critics of germ-line genetic intervention argue that this technique will never be necessary because of available alternative strategies for preventing the transmission of diagnosable genetic diseases. Specifically, critics of germ-line gene therapy have sometimes suggested that preimplantation diagnosis and the selective discard of affected embryos might be a reasonable alternative to the high-technology, potentially risky attempt to repair genetic defects in early human embryos. Even without in vitro fertilization and preimplantation diagnosis, the option of prenatal diagnosis and selective abortion is available for many disorders. According to this view, these two types of selection, before embryos or fetuses have reached the stage of viability, are effective means for achieving the same goal.

The third argument is closely related to the second: this technique will always be an expensive option that cannot be made available to most couples, certainly not by any publicly funded health care system. Therefore, like in vitro fertilization for couples attempting to overcome the problem of infertility, germ-line gene therapy will be available only to wealthy people who can afford to pay its considerable expense on their own.

The fourth argument builds on the preceding two: precisely because germ-line intervention will be of such limited utility in preventing disease, there will be strong pressures to use this technique for genetic enhancement at the embryonic stage, when it could reasonably be expected to make a difference in the future life prospects of the embryo. Again in this case, only the affluent would be able to afford the intervention. However, if enhancement interventions were safe and efficacious, the long-term effect of such germ-line intervention would probably be to exacerbate existing differences between the most-well-off and the least-well-off segments of society.

Fifth, even though germ-line genetic intervention aims in the long run to treat rather than to abort or discard, the issue of appropriate respect for preimplantation embryos and implanted fetuses will nonetheless arise in several ways. After thorough-going studies of germ-line intervention have been conducted in nonhuman embryos, there will undoubtedly be a stage at which parallel studies in human embryos will be proposed. The question of human embryo research was recently studied by a committee appointed by the director of the National Institutes of Health.[9] Although the committee specifically avoided commenting on germ-line intervention, its recommendation that certain kinds of human embryo research should be continued and that such research should be funded by NIH provoked considerable controversy. Critics of the committee's position would presumably also oppose the embryo research that would be proposed to prepare the way for germ-line gene therapy in humans.[10] Their principal argument would be that the destruction or other harming of preimplantation embryos in research is incompatible with the kind of respect that should be shown to human embryos.

Even after the research phase of germ-line genetic intervention is concluded, difficult questions about the treatment of embryos will remain. For example, preimplantation diagnosis may continue to involve the removal of one or two totipotential cells from a four- to eight-cell embryo. While the moral status of totipotential human embryonic cells has received scant attention in bioethical debates, there is at least a plausible argument that a totipotential cell, once separated from the remainder of a preimplantation embryo, is virtually equivalent to a zygote; that is, under favorable conditions it could develop into an embryo, a fetus, a newborn, and an adult. This ob-

jection to the destruction of totipotential embryonic cells will only be overcome if a noninvasive genetic diagnostic test for early embryos (like an x-ray or a CT scan) can be developed. Further, even if a noninvasive diagnostic test is available, as we have noted above, a postintervention diagnostic test will probably be undertaken with each embryo to verify that the intervention has been successful. Health professionals and prospective parents will probably be at least open to the possibility of selective discard or selective abortion if something has gone radically wrong in the intervention procedure. Thus, germ-line genetic intervention may remain foreclosed as a moral option to those who are conscientiously opposed to any action that would directly terminate the life of a preimplantation embryo or a fetus.

The sixth argument points to potential perils of concentrating great power in the hands of human beings. According to this view, the technique of germ-line intervention would give human beings, or a small group of human beings, too much control over the future evolution of the human race. This argument does not necessarily attribute malevolent intentions to those who have the training that would allow them to employ the technique. It implies that there are built-in limits that humans ought not to exceed, perhaps for theological or metaphysical reasons, and at least hints that corruptibility is an ever-present possibility for the very powerful.

The seventh argument explicitly raises the issue of malevolent use. If one extrapolates from Nazi racial hygiene programs, this argument asserts, it is likely the germ-line intervention will be used by unscrupulous dictators to produce a class of superior human beings. The same techniques could be also used in precisely the opposite way, to produce human-like creatures who would willingly perform the least-attractive and the most-dangerous work for a society. According to this view, Aldous Huxley's *Brave New World* should be updated, for modern molecular biology provides tyrants with tools for modifying human beings that Huxley could not have imagined in 1932.

The eighth and final argument against germ-line genetic intervention is raised chiefly by several European authors who place this argument in the context of human rights.[11] According to these commentators, human beings have a moral right to receive from their parents a genetic patrimony that has not been subjected to artificial tampering. Although the term "tampering" is not usually defined, it seems to mean any intentional effort to introduce genetic changes into the germ line, even if the goal is to reduce the likelihood that a genetic disease will be passed on to the children and grandchildren of a particular couple. The asserted right to be protected against such tampering may be a slightly different formulation of the sixth argument noted above—namely, that there are built-in limits, embedded in the nature of things, beyond which not even the most benevolent human beings should attempt to go.

A BRIEF EVALUATION OF THE ARGUMENTS

In our view, the effort to cure and prevent serious disease and premature death is one of the noblest of all human undertakings. For this reason the first pro argument—that germ-line intervention may be the only way to treat or prevent certain diseases—seems to us to be of overriding importance. We also find the third pro argument to be quite strong, that a germ-line correction, if demonstrated to be safe and effective, would be more efficient than repeated applications of somatic cell gene therapy. In addition, the final pro argument about the overall mission of the health professions and about society's approach to disabilities seems to us to provide a convincing justification for the germ-line approach, when gene replacement is available.

Our replies to the objections raised by critics of germ-line intervention are as follows:

1. *Irreversible mistakes.* While we acknowledge that mistakes may be made in germ-line gene therapy, we think that the same sophisticated techniques that were employed to introduce the new genes will be able to be used to remove those genes or to compensate for their presence in some other way. Further, in any sphere of innovative therapy, a first step into human beings must be taken at some point.

2. *Alternative strategies.* Some couples, perhaps even most couples, will choose the alternative strategies of selective abortion or selective discard. In our view, a strategy of attempting to prevent or treat potential disease or disability in the particular biological individual accords more closely with the mission of the health sciences and shows greater respect for children and adults who are afflicted with disease or disability.

3. *High cost, limited availability.* It is too early to know what the relative cost of germ-line intervention will be when the technique is fully developed. In addition, the financial costs and other personal and social harms of preventable diseases will need to be compared with the financial costs of germ-line gene therapy. It is at least possible that this new technology could become widely diffused and available to many members of society.

4. *Use for enhancement.* Prudent social policy should be able to set limits on the use of germ-line genetic intervention. Further, some enhancements of human capabilities may be morally justifiable, especially when those enhancements are health related. We acknowledge that the distribution of genetic enhancement is an important question for policy makers. (The issue of enhancement is discussed in greater detail in [Chapter 4 of *The Ethics of Human Gene Therapy*].)

5. *Human embryos.* In our view, research with early human embryos that is directed toward the development of germ-line gene therapy is morally justifiable in principle. Further, we acknowledge the potential of a totipotential cell but think that the value of a genetic diagnosis outweighs the value of such a cell. We also accept that, if a serious error is made in germ-line gene therapy, terminating the life of the resulting embryo or fetus may be morally justifiable. In short, there is a presumption in favor of fostering the continued development of human embryos and fetuses, but that presumption can in our view be overridden by other considerations like serious harm to the developing individual or others and the needs of preclinical research.

6. *Concentration of power.* We acknowledge that those who are able to use germ-line

intervention will have unprecedented ability to introduce precise changes into the germ lines of particular individuals and families. However, in our view, it is better for human beings to possess this ability and to use it for constructive purposes like preventing disease in families than not to possess the ability. The central ethical question is public accountability by the scientists, health providers, and companies that will be involved with germ-line intervention. Such accountability presupposes transparency about the use of the technology and an ongoing monitoring process aimed at preventing its misuse.

7. *Misuse by dictators.* This objection focuses too much attention on technology and too little on politics. There is no doubt that bona fide tyrants have existed in the 20th century and that they have made use of all manner of technologies—whether the low-tech methods of surgical sterilization or the annihilation of concentration camp inmates with poison gas or high-tech weapons like nuclear warheads and long-range missiles—to terrify and to dominate. However, the best approach to preventing the misuse of genetic technologies may not be to discourage the development of the technologies but rather to preserve and encourage democratic institutions that can serve as an antidote to tyranny. A second possible reply to the tyrannical misuse objection is that germ-line intervention requires a long lead time, in order to allow the offspring produced to grow to adulthood. Tyrants are often impatient people and are likely to prefer the more instantaneous methods of propaganda, intimidation, and annihilation of enemies to the relatively slow pace of germ-line modification.

8. *Human rights and tampering.* It is a daunting task to imagine what the unborn and as-yet-unconceived generations of people coming after us will want.[12] Even more dif-

ficult is the effort to ascribe rights to [future] human beings. Insofar as we can anticipate the needs and wants of future generations, we think that any reasonable future person would prefer health to serious disease and would therefore welcome a germ-line intervention in his or her family line that effectively prevented cystic fibrosis from being transmitted to him or her. In our view, such a person would not regard this intervention as tampering and would regard as odd the claim that his or her genetic patrimony has been artificially tampered with. Cystic fibrosis was not a part of his or her family's heritage that the future person was eager to receive or to claim. . . .

NOTES

1 It is perhaps worth noting that researchers performing somatic-cell gene therapy have carefully avoided diseases and subtypes of diseases that affect mental functioning. One thinks, for example, of Lesch-Nyhan syndrome, of certain subtypes of Gaucher disease and Hunter syndrome, of Tay-Sachs disease, and of metachromatic leukodystrophy.

2 We owe the suggestion of retinoblastoma as a candidate disorder to Kevin FitzGerald, S.J. We are also indebted to Nelson A. Wivel for information on the genetics of retinoblastoma. See Nelson A. Wivel and LeRoy Walters, "Germ-Line Gene Modification and Disease Prevention: Some Medical and Ethical Perspectives," *Science* 262(5133): 533–538; 22 October 1993. See also Stephen H. Friend et al., "A Human DNA Segment with Properties of the Gene That Predisposes to Retinoblastoma and Osteosarcoma," *Nature* 323(6089): 643–646; 16 October 1986; and Ei Matsunaga, "Hereditary Retinoblastoma: Host Resistance and Second Primary Tumors," *Journal of the National Cancer Institute* 65(1): 47–51; July 1980.

3 Although the genetics of the germ-line p53 gene mutation are more complex than the genetics of the germ-line mutation that causes retinoblastoma, p53 may turn out to be another important tumor suppressor gene to which the same comments apply. On the germ-line p53 mutation, see Frederick P. Li et al., "Recommendations on Predictive Testing for Germ Line p53 Mutations Among Cancer-Prone Individuals," *Journal of the National Cancer Institute* 84(15): 1156–1160; 5 August 1992; and Curtis C. Harris and Monica Hollstein, "Clinical Implications of the *p53* Tumor-Suppressor Gene," *New England Journal of Medicine* 329(18): 1318–1327; 28 October 1993.

4 Eric T. Juengst, "Germ-Line Gene Therapy: Back to Basics," *Journal of Medicine and Philosophy* 16(6): 589–590; December 1991.

5 Burke K. Zimmerman, "Human Germ-Line Therapy: The Case for Its Development and Use," *Journal of Medicine and Philosophy* 16(6): 596–598; December 1991.

6 For a detailed discussion of and justification for germ-line intervention in this setting, see Marc Lappé, "Ethical Issues in Manipulating the Human Germ Line," *Journal of Medicine and Philosophy* 16(6): 621–639; December 1991.

7 As noted above, already in 1962 Joshua Lederberg was arguing against H. J. Muller's proposals for improving the human gene pool through programs of "voluntary germinal choice" by appealing to the prospect of rapid, global genetic intervention by means of germ-line gene therapy. See Joshua Lederberg, "Biological Future of Man," in Gordon Wolstenholme, ed., *Man and His Future* (London: J. & A. Churchill, 1963), pp. 265 and 269.

8 On the general issue of the freedom of scientific inquiry, see Loren R. Graham, "Concerns About Science and Attempts to Regulate Inquiry," *Daedalus* 107(2): 1–21; Spring 1978.

9 National Institutes of Health, Human Embryo Research Panel, *Report* (Bethesda, MD: NIH, 27 September 1994).

10 See, for example, the following critiques of human embryo research: "The Inhuman Use of Human Beings," *First Things* 49: 17–21; January 1995; Dianne N. Irving, "Testimony Before the NIH Human Embryo Research Panel," *Linacre Quarterly* 61(4): 82–89; November 1994; and Kevin O'Rourke, "Embryo Research: Ethical Issues," *Health Care Ethics USA* 2(4): 2–3; Fall 1994.

11 Alex Mauron and Jean-Marie Thévoz, "Germ-Line Engineering: A Few European Voices," *Journal of Medicine and Philosophy* 16(6): 654–655; December 1991.

12 There is a rather substantial literature on this topic. See, for example, Ruth Faden, Gail Geller, and Madison Powers, eds., *AIDS, Women and the Next Generation* (New York: Oxford University Press, 1991); LeRoy Walters, "Ethical Issues in Maternal Serum Alpha-Fetoprotein Testing and Screening: A Reappraisal," in Mark I. Evans et al., eds., *Fetal Diagnosis and Therapy: Science, Ethics and the Law* (Philadelphia: J.B. Lippincott, 1989), pp. 54–60; and Lori B. Andrews et al., eds., *Assessing Genetic Risks: Implications for Health and Social Policy: Report* (Washington, DC: National Academy Press, 1994).

GENETIC ENHANCEMENT

GENETIC ENHANCEMENT
Walter Glannon

Glannon distinguishes between gene therapy and genetic enhancement, and he defends the treatment-enhancement distinction, most directly against the objection that a clear line cannot be drawn between treatment and enhancement. He is committed to the view that genetic interventions are morally legitimate only when the underlying intention is therapeutic in nature—that is, when the interventions are directed at treating disease and restoring function to a normal or adequate level; genetic interventions intended to enhance functions that are already normal are morally objectionable. Glannon advances four arguments against genetic enhancement. (1) Some people would have an unfair advantage over others based on their ability to pay for access to enhancement procedures. (2) Universal access to genetic enhancement would not provide an adequate remedy for the first problem because this approach would be "collectively self-defeating." (3) Inequality resulting from enhancements could threaten our "conviction in the fundamental importance of equality," with resulting damage to self-respect, social harmony, and stability. (4) Enhancement of noncompetitive, virtuous dispositions would threaten to undermine our autonomy and moral agency.

Gene therapy must be distinguished from genetic enhancement. The first is an intervention aimed at treating disease and restoring physical and mental functions and capacities to an adequate baseline. The second is an intervention aimed at improving functions and capacities that already are adequate. Genetic enhancement augments functions and capacities "that without intervention would be considered entirely normal."[1] Its goal is to "amplify 'normal' genes in order to make them better."[2] In chapter 1 [of *Genes and Future People*], I cited Norman Daniels's definitions of health and disease as well as what the notion of just health care entailed. This involved maintaining or restoring mental and physical functions at or to normal levels, which was necessary to ensure fair equality of opportunity for all citizens. Insofar as this aim defines the goal of medicine, genetic enhancement falls outside this goal. Furthermore, insofar as this type of intervention is not part of the goal of medicine and has no place in a just health care system, there are no medical or moral reasons for genetically enhancing normal human functions and capacities.

Some have argued that it is mistaken to think that a clear line of demarcation can be drawn between treatment and enhancement, since certain forms of enhancement are employed to prevent disease. LeRoy Walters and Julie Gage Palmer refer to the immune system as an example to make this point:

> In current medical practice, the best example of a widely accepted health-related physical enhancement is immunization against infectious disease.
>
> With immunizations against diseases like polio and hepatitis B, what we are saying is in effect, "The immune system that we inherited from our parents may not be adequate to ward off certain viruses if we are exposed to them." Therefore, we will enhance the capabilities of our immune system by priming it to fight against these viruses.
>
> From the current practice of immunizations against particular diseases, it would seem to be only a small step to try to enhance the general function of the immune system by genetic means. . . . In our

view, the genetic enhancement of the immune system would be morally justifiable if this kind of enhancement assisted in preventing disease and did not cause offsetting harms to the people treated by the technique.[3]

Nevertheless, because the goal of the technique would be to prevent disease, it would not, strictly speaking, be enhancement, at least not in terms of the definitions given at the outset of this section. Genetically intervening in the immune system as described by Walters and Palmer is a means of maintaining it in proper working order so that it will be better able to ward off pathogens posing a threat to the organism as a whole. Thus, it is misleading to call this intervention "enhancement." When we consider what is normal human functioning, we refer to the whole human organism consisting of immune, endocrine, nervous, cardiovascular, and other systems, not to these systems understood as isolated parts. The normal functioning in question here pertains to the ability of the immune system to protect the organism from infectious agents and thus ensure its survival. Any preventive genetic intervention in this system would be designed to maintain the normal functions of the organism, not to restore them or raise them above the norm. It would be neither therapy nor enhancement but instead a form of maintenance. Therefore, the alleged ambiguity surrounding what Walters and Palmer call "enhancing" the immune system does not impugn the distinction between treatment and enhancement.

If enhancement could make adequately functioning bodily systems function even better, then presumably there would be no limit to the extent to which bodily functions can be enhanced. Yet, beyond a certain point, heightened immune sensitivity to infectious agents can lead to an overly aggressive response, resulting in autoimmune disease that can damage healthy cells, tissues, and organs. In fact, there would be a limit to the beneficial effects of genetic intervention in the immune system, a limit beyond which the equilibrium between humoral and cellular response mechanisms would be disturbed.[4] If any intervention ensured that the equilibrium of the immune system was maintained in proper working order, then it would be inappropriate to consider it as a form of enhancement.

To further support the treatment-enhancement distinction, consider a nongenetic intervention, the use of a bisphosphonate such as alendronate sodium. Its purpose is to prevent postmenopausal women from developing osteoporosis, or to rebuild bone in women or men who already have osteoporosis. Some might claim that, because it can increase bone density, it is a form of enhancement. But its more general purpose is to prevent bone fractures and thus maintain proper bone function so that one can have normal mobility and avoid the morbidity resulting from fractures. In terms of the functioning of the entire organism, therefore, it would be more accurate to consider the use of bisphosphonates as prevention, treatment, or maintenance rather than enhancement.

Some might raise a different question. Suppose that the parents of a child much shorter than the norm for his age persuaded a physician to give him growth hormone injections in order to increase his height. Suppose further that the child's shortness was not due to an iatrogenic cause, such as radiation to treat a brain tumor. Would this be treatment or enhancement? The question that should be asked regarding this issue is not whether the child's height is normal for his age group. Rather, the question should be whether his condition implies something less than normal physical functioning, such that he would have fewer opportunities for achievement and a decent minimum level of well-being over his lifetime. Diminutive stature alone does not necessarily imply that one's functioning is or will be so limited as to restrict one's opportunities for achievement. Of course, being short might limit one's opportunities if one wanted to become a professional basketball player. But most of us are quite flexible when it comes to formulating and carrying out life plans. Robert Reich, the treasury secretary in President Clinton's first administration, is just one example of how one can achieve very much in life despite diminutive stature. If a child's stature significantly limited his functioning and opportunities, then growth-hormone injections should be considered therapeutic treatment. If his stature were not so limiting, then the injections should be considered enhancement.

Admittedly, there is gray area near the baseline of adequate functioning where it may be difficult to distinguish between treatment and enhancement.

Accordingly, we should construe the baseline loosely or thickly enough to allow for some minor deviation above or below what would be considered normal functioning. An intervention for a condition near the baseline that would raise one's functioning clearly above the critical level should be considered an enhancement. An intervention for a condition making one's functioning fall clearly below the baseline, with the aim of raising one's functioning to the critical level, should be considered a treatment. For example, an athlete with a hemoglobin level slightly below the norm for people his age and mildly anemic may want to raise that level significantly in order to be more competitive in his sport. To the extent that his actual hemoglobin level does not interfere with his ordinary physical functioning, an intervention to significantly raise that level would be an instance of enhancement. In contrast, for a child who has severe thalassemia and severe anemia, with the risk of bone abnormalities and heart failure, an intervention to correct the disorder would be an instance of treatment.

The main moral concern about genetic enhancement of physical and mental traits is that it would give some people an unfair advantage over others with respect to competitive goods like beauty, sociability, and intelligence. . . . Enhancement would be unfair because only those who could afford the technology would have access to it, and many people are financially worse off than others through no fault of their own. Insofar as the possession of these goods gives some people an advantage over others in careers, income, and social status, the competitive nature of these goods suggests that there would be no limit to the benefits that improvements to physical and mental capacities would yield to those fortunate enough to avail themselves of the technology. This is altogether different from the example of immune-system enhancement. There would be no diminishing marginal value in the degree of competitive advantage that one could have over others for the social goods in question and presumably no limit to the value of enhancing the physical and mental capacities that would give one this advantage. Not having access to the technology that could manipulate genetic traits in such a way as to enhance these capacities would put one at a competitive disadvantage relative to others who would have access to it.

Advancing an argument similar to the one used by those who reject the treatment-enhancement distinction, one might hold that competitive goods collapse the categorical distinction between correcting deficient capacities and improving normal ones. This is because competitive goods are continuous, coming in degrees, and therefore the capacities that enable one to achieve these goods cannot be thought of as either normal or deficient.[5] Nevertheless, to the extent that any form of genetic intervention is motivated by the medical and moral aim to enable people to have adequate mental and physical functioning and fair equality of opportunity for a decent minimum level of well-being, the goods in question are not *competitive* but *basic*. In other words, the aim of any medical intervention by genetic means is to make people better off than they were before by raising or restoring them to an absolute baseline of normal physical and mental functioning, not to make them comparatively better off than others. Competitive goods above the baseline may be continuous; but the basic goods that enable someone to reach or remain at the baseline are not. Given that these two types of goods are distinct, and that they result from the distinct aims and practices of enhancement and treatment, we can affirm that enhancement and treatment can and should be treated separately. We can uphold the claim that the purpose of any genetic intervention should be to treat people's abnormal functions and restore them to a normal level, not to enhance those functions that already are normal.

As I have mentioned, genetic enhancement that gave some people an advantage over others in possessing competitive goods would entail considerable unfairness. A likely scenario would be one in which parents paid to use expensive genetic technology to raise the cognitive ability or improve the physical beauty of their children. This would give them an advantage over other children with whom they would compete for education, careers, and income. Children of parents who could not afford to pay for the technology would be at a comparative disadvantage. Even if the goods in question fell above the normal functional baseline, one still could maintain that such an advantage would be unfair. It would depend on people's ability to pay, and inequalities in income are unfair to the extent that they result from some factors beyond people's control.

We could not appeal to the notion of a genetic lottery to resolve the problem of fairness regarding genetic enhancement. For, as I argued in the last section [of *Genes and Future People*], such a lottery is better suited to meeting people's needs than their preferences, and enhancements correspond to people's preferences. Moreover, a lottery might only exacerbate the problem by reinforcing the perception of unfairness, depending on how losers in the lottery interpreted the fact that others won merely as a result of a random selection. One suggestion for resolving the fairness problem (short of banning the use of the technology altogether) would be to make genetic enhancement available to all. Of course, how this system could be financed is a question that admits of no easy answer. But the more important substantive point is that universal access to genetic enhancement would not be a solution. Indeed, the upshot of such access would provide a reason for prohibiting it.

Universal availability of genetic enhancement would mean that many competitive goods some people had over others would be canceled out collectively. The idea of a competitive advantage gradually would erode, and there would be more equality among people in their possession of goods. There would not be complete equality, however. Differing parental attitudes toward such goods as education could mean differences in the extent to which cognitive enhancement was utilized. Some parents would be more selective than others in sending their children to better schools or arranging for private tutors. So, there still would be some inequality in the general outcome of the enhancement. But quite apart from this, the process of neutralizing competitive goods could end up being self-defeating on a collective level.[6] More specifically, one probable side-effect of boosting children's mental capacity on a broad scale would be some brain damage resulting in cognitive and affective impairment in some of the children who received the genetic enhancement. The net social cost of using the technology would outweigh any social advantage of everyone using it. If no one is made better off than others in their possession of social goods, but some people are made worse off than they were before in terms of their mental functioning, then the net social disadvantage would provide a reason for prohibiting collective genetic enhancement.

There is another moral aspect of enhancement that should be considered. I have maintained that inequalities above the baseline of normal physical and mental functioning are of no great moral importance and may be neutral on the question of fairness. Although equality and fairness are closely related, one does not necessarily imply the other. Again, fairness pertains to meeting people's needs. Once these needs have been met, inequalities in the possession of goods relating to preferences are not so morally significant. Thus, if the idea of an absolute baseline implies that people's basic physical and mental needs have been met, and if people who are comparatively better or worse off than others all have functioning at or above the baseline, then any inequalities in functioning above this level should not matter very much morally. If this is plausible, then it seems to follow that there would be nothing unfair and hence nothing morally objectionable about enhancements that made some people better off than others above the baseline. Nevertheless, this could undermine our belief in the importance of the fundamental equality of all people, regardless of how well off they are in absolute terms. Equality is one of the social bases of self-respect, which is essential for social harmony and stability.[7] Allowing inequalities in access to and possession of competitive goods at any level of functioning or welfare might erode this basis and the ideas of harmony and stability that rest on it. Although it would be difficult to measure, this type of social cost resulting from genetic enhancement could constitute another reason for prohibiting it.

Yet, suppose that we could manipulate certain genes to enhance our noncompetitive virtuous traits, such as altruism, generosity, and compassion.[8] Surely, these would contribute to a stable, well-ordered society and preserve the principle of fair equality of opportunity. Nothing in this program would be incompatible with the goal of medicine as the prevention and treatment of disease. But it would threaten the individual autonomy essential to us as moral agents who can be candidates for praise and blame, punishment and reward. What confers moral worth on our actions, and indeed on ourselves as agents, is our capacity to cultivate certain dispositions leading to actions. This cultivation involves the exercise of practical reason and a process of critical self-reflection, whereby we modify, eliminate, or reinforce

dispositions and thereby come to identify with them as our own. Autonomy consists precisely in this process of reflection and identification. It is the capacity for reflective self-control that enables us to take responsibility for our mental states and the actions that issue from them. Given the importance of autonomy, it would be preferable to have fewer virtuous dispositions that we can identify with as our own than to have more virtuous dispositions implanted in us through genetic enhancement. These would threaten to undermine our moral agency because they would derive from an external source.[9] Even if our genes could be manipulated in such a way that our behavior always conformed to an algorithm for the morally correct course of action in every situation, it is unlikely that we would want it. Most of us would rather make autonomous choices that turned out not to lead to the best courses of action. This is because of the intrinsic importance of autonomy and the moral growth and maturity that come with making our own choices under uncertainty. The dispositions with which we come to identify, imperfect as they may be, are what make us autonomous and responsible moral agents. Enhancing these mental states through artificial means external to our own exercise of practical reason and our own process of identification would undermine our autonomy by making them alien to us.

In sum, there are four reasons why genetic enhancement would be morally objectionable. First, it would give an unfair advantage to some people over others because some would be able to pay for expensive enhancement procedures while others would not. Second, if we tried to remedy the first problem by making genetic enhancement universally accessible, then it would be collectively self-defeating. Although much competitive unfairness at the individual level would be canceled out at the collective level, there would be the unacceptable social cost of some people suffering from adverse cognitive or emotional effects of the enhancement. Third, inequalities resulting from enhancements above the baseline of normal physical and mental functioning could threaten to undermine the conviction in the fundamental importance of equality as one of the bases of self-respect, and in turn social solidarity and stability. Fourth, enhancement of noncompetitive dispositions would threaten to undermine the autonomy and moral agency essential to us as persons.

NOTES

1 Jon Gordon, "Genetic Enhancement in Humans," *Science* 283 (March 26, 1999): 2023–2024.

2 Eric Juengst, "Can Enhancement Be Distinguished from Prevention in Genetic Medicine?" *Journal of Medicine and Philosophy* 22 (1997): 125–142, and "What Does Enhancement Mean?" in Erik Parens, ed., *Enhancing Human Traits: Ethical and Social Implications* (Washington, DC: Georgetown University Press, 1998): 27–47, at 27. Also, Dan Brock, "Enhancements of Human Function: Some Distinctions for Policymakers," Ibid., 48–69.

3 *The Ethics of Human Gene Therapy* (New York: Oxford University Press, 1997), 110. Instead of distinguishing between treatments and enhancements, Walters and Palmer distinguish between health-related and non-health-related enhancements. But I do not find this distinction to be very helpful.

4 Brock points this out in "Enhancements of Human Function," 59. Marc Lappe makes a more compelling case for the same point in *The Tao of Immunology* (New York: Plenum Press, 1997).

5 Kavka develops and defends the idea that competitive goods are continuous in "Upside Risks: Social Consequences of Beneficial Biotechnology," in Carl Cranor, ed., *Are Genes Us? The Social Consequences of the New Genetics* (New Brunswick, NJ: Rutgers University Press, 1994): 155–179, at 164–165.

6 Kavka, "Upside Risks," 167. Also, Brock, "Enhancements of Human Function," 60; and Buchanan et al., *From Chance to Choice* (New York: Cambridge University Press, 2000), chap. 8.

7 Rawls makes this point in *A Theory of Justice* (Cambridge, MA: Harvard Belknap Press, 1971), 7–11, and in "Social Unity and Primary Goods," in A. Sen and B. Williams, eds., *Utilitarianism and Beyond* (Cambridge: Cambridge University Press, 1982), 162. See also Daniels, *Just Health Care* (New York: Cambridge University Press, 1985).

8 Walters and Palmer present this thought-experiment in *The Ethics of Human Gene Therapy*, 123–128. As they note, Jonathan Glover introduced this idea in *What Sort of People Should There Be?* (Harmondsworth: Penguin, 1984).

9 Drawing on the work of Lionel Trilling and Charles Taylor, Carl Elliott discusses cognitive and affective enhancements that undermine what he calls the "ethics of authenticity" in "The Tyranny of Happiness: Ethics and Cosmetic Psychopharmacology," in Parens, *Enhancing Human Traits*, 177–188. Also relevant to this issue is Harry Frankfurt, "Identification and Externality," in Frankfurt, *The Importance of What We Care About* (New York: Cambridge University Press, 1989): 58–68.

GENETIC ENGINEERING

Dan W. Brock

Brock defends the prospective use of genetic engineering to enhance human traits and functions against various moral objections. He rejects the idea that genetic engineering (of an embryo) would change the fundamental identity of an individual in a way that the efforts of parents to develop the capacities of their children by manipulating environmental factors do not. He also rejects the idea that the treatment of disease is objectively beneficial for an individual in a way that enhancement of normal function would not be. Brock acknowledges that some enhancements of normal human traits and functions would be beneficial only within a limited range. He also briefly considers whether there is any justified basis to the moral concern that the use of genetic engineering to enhance particular human capacities would transform and devalue the associated human activities. Next, he argues that any moral assessment of genetic engineering for purposes of enhancement must take account of *who* is employing the relevant genetic technology (e.g., whether it is government or parents), and he concludes his analysis by acknowledging that the use of genetic engineering to enhance capacities that would confer competitive advantages on recipients raises serious issues about fairness and equality of opportunity.

In June 2000 government and industry groups jointly announced that the goal of the worldwide Human Genome Project (HGP) to map and sequence the entire human genome had essentially been completed. Of course, enormous work still lay ahead to understand the specific genes that contribute to human disease and disability, much less to the multitude of complex physical, cognitive, emotional, and behavioral traits of normal humans. No one can confidently predict the rate at which that understanding will be achieved in the future nor the ultimate limits on it. The way in which genes interact with other genes and with different environments only multiplies what we still for the most part do not yet understand. But, despite how much remains to be learned, we have already made great strides in beginning to understand the genetic bases of human nature. Much of the initial work in the HGP has focused on a search for the specific genetic contributions to human disease and disability. The gene has been identified, and tests for it developed, that allow prediction with a very high degree of certainty of whether an individual will develop Huntington's chorea, an adult-onset, single gene disease that leads to devastating neurological deterioration and death over a period of years. In other cases, genes have been identified, and tests for them developed, that only increase individuals' risks of developing diseases like breast cancer.

At present, this new information still allows only limited and relatively crude control over the genetic inheritance of our progeny. A couple who know from family history or other means that one or both are at risk of passing on a particular genetic disease to their children can test for their risk of doing so before conception. If a risk is found to be present, various means, such as sperm or egg donation, *in vitro* fertilization (IVF), pre-implantation embryo testing, or forgoing conception, are now available to avoid transmission of the genetic disease to future children. After conception, testing of the fetus is sometimes possible to determine whether it carries the gene or genes for the disease, and the parents can

then decide whether to abort an affected fetus. While such testing is now possible for only a quite limited number of diseases or disabilities for which there is a significant genetic component, we can expect these capacities to continue to expand rapidly in the future. Moreover, the capacity to detect deleterious genes is likely to be combined with new abilities for *in utero* therapeutic interventions or genetic manipulations to correct for the deleterious gene(s). Thus, we can expect that advances in genetic knowledge and technology will increase our ability to prevent or to reduce the prevalence of disease caused in significant part by deleterious genes.

It is not just much disease, however, but virtually all normal human traits that have some significant genetic basis. The same advances in genetic knowledge and technology that will enable us to prevent disease will ultimately enable us to undertake interventions to manipulate the genes underlying normal traits and functions and to enhance those traits and functions in the absence of any disease or disability; it may become possible to manipulate genes to enhance normal intelligence or memory, immune responses to many human diseases, physical strength or dexterity, and life expectancy, to take only a few examples. Thus, we face the prospect of being able to take control over and to design human nature and the nature of our progeny. What was once in the hands of God or the natural lottery will come increasingly within deliberate human choice and control. This [essay] is about some of the ethical issues we can expect to face when we gain that control.

In the limited space available here, I will not pursue the technical means by which these genetic interventions will likely occur. While some bases for them are already in place, how they will develop is speculative and uncertain at this time and while some of the ethical concerns will be specific to particular technical means as they develop over time, most of the deepest ethical concerns do not turn on the specific technical details of genetic interventions. I will understand "genetic engineering" here to mean the deliberate alteration or addition of genes in a human embryo; this includes somatic cell genetic interventions that affect only the subject of the intervention as well as germ cell interventions where

Reprinted with permission of the publisher from *A Companion to Applied Ethics* (2003), edited by R. G. Frey and Christopher Heath Wellman, pp. 356–357, 361–367. © 2003 by Blackwell Publishing Ltd.

the changes will be passed on to the progeny of the subject of the intervention. This means that our current means noted above of preventing the passing on of genetic disease are not instances of genetic engineering as I will understand it here. . . .

USE OF GENETIC ENGINEERING TO ENHANCE NORMAL FUNCTION

To use genetic engineering . . . to seek to prevent genetic diseases and the suffering and disabilities that they cause does not seem morally wrong and may sometimes be morally required. This is in keeping with efforts in medicine more generally to prevent or treat disease and the suffering and disability it causes. However, many people worry that the use of genetic engineering to enhance normal function in persons who are without disease raises fundamentally different and deeper moral concerns than the medical use of genetic engineering. Yet what could be wrong with parents using the technology of genetic engineering if it becomes available to improve their children's lives and opportunities? Parents are generally regarded as having permission, and in some cases an obligation, to produce the best children they can. They are expected, for example, to keep their children as healthy as possible. If genetic techniques gave parents a way to enhance their children's immune systems, and the intervention posed only risks comparable to vaccination, should parents not be free, or even required in some cases, to use them? Parents invest time, efforts, and resources in developing athletic talents, intellectual abilities, and prudential or moral virtues in their children. If parents have great leeway in attempting to produce the best children they can, according to their own view of what is best, why not extend this liberty to genetic means?

ENVIRONMENTAL VERSUS GENETIC CHANGES

Some opponents of genetic engineering mistakenly see it as changing the fundamental identity of a person in a way that parents' environmental efforts do not. They see parental efforts as environmental in helping to develop the capacities their children already have, as bringing out the potential that is already there. In contrast, genetic interventions are seen as changing children in some more fundamental way,

making them different from who they otherwise would have been. But this contrast is problematic. When parents use their control over environmental factors to "bring out the best" in their children, they modify phenotype. Given their children's genotypes, the range of traits and capabilities—both physical and behavioral—that constitute the phenotype of the child we see and interact with is very much a result of the environment that parents and others create. There is no pre-existing and fixed best in the child that is brought out by parental manipulation of environmental causes; such manipulation has enormous effects in shaping and determining phenotype. Why not then add to parents' arsenal of methods whatever genetic interventions make it easier to accomplish their goals for their children?

Part of what disturbs many people is the mistaken belief that genetic interventions modify the essence or identity of the individual, whereas environmental interventions only modify accidental features and leave identity unchanged. The idea seems to be that genetic interventions result in a new individual, whereas environmental interventions merely modify the same individual. But our genes do not constitute our identity in any deep sense. Suppose the operation of our immune system could be enhanced or our eye color changed by a genetic intervention. We would not be inclined to muse: "I wonder who I would have been if my parents had not altered my immune system or eye color in this way?" We might have very different responses if they altered genes that produced major changes in aspects of the self that we consider central to our sense of self or personal identity. For each of us, it is particular elements of our phenotype, such as being intelligent, compassionate, or witty, not every aspect of our genotype, that we take to be central to our conceptions of self and to our essence as a particular individual. These traits are produced by interactions between our genotype and our environment and neither means of altering them is more fundamental.

WHEN ARE ENHANCEMENTS BENEFITS?

Treatment of disease that restores normal human function is typically and uncontroversially assumed to benefit persons. One source of moral concern and unease about genetic engineering is whether enhancing individuals' normal human traits would in fact be beneficial for them. In *Brave New World,* Aldous Huxley (1946) imagined engineering some persons to have limited abilities and aspirations, and to be happy doing menial jobs in society. While this might be beneficial for the society, it was morally objectionable in exploiting those individuals for the benefit of the rest of society. Morally acceptable genetic engineering of individuals should, certainly in the great majority of cases, plausibly be of benefit to those individuals from their own perspective.

Are treatments of disease objectively good for a person in respects in which enhancements are not? For example, treatment that prevents paraplegia seems uncontroversially and objectively beneficial to anyone whereas enhancement of a capacity to excel in athletics or play a musical instrument may only be beneficial for a person with interests in these activities. However, this is not a contrast between genetic engineering used for treatment versus enhancement, but rather a contrast between abilities that are all-purpose means, useful in virtually any plan of life, and abilities useful in some plans of life but not in many others. Some enhancements of capacities like memory or the ability to focus attention on tasks for extended periods of time would likewise be useful in nearly any plan of life, whereas treatment, for example, of a disease that impairs fine motor skills might be very important to a pianist but of little importance to a person who did not make significant use of those skills. There is no systematic contrast between treatment of disease and enhancement of normal function that makes the former objectively beneficial in a way the latter is not.

THE MAGNITUDE OF ENHANCEMENT

If disease is understood roughly as a condition causing an adverse deviation in normal species function, however, treatment that prevents or treats disease and so maintains or restores normal function will be at least prima facie beneficial for a person. Moreover, the attaining of normal function provides a rough stopping point for successful treatment. On the other hand, in the use of genetic engineering for enhancement the limits of possible changes in people's genetic inheritance are more open ended both in the capacities that might be enhanced and in the degree to which the capacities might be improved; there is no obvious end-point to potential enhancements comparable to the role normal function plays with treatment. How much stronger or smarter or more memory should we aim at?

It might seem that the more a desirable trait is enhanced by genetic engineering the better, but that would be a mistake for at least two reasons. First, some enhancements would only be beneficial within a limited range because of how the enhanced capacity or trait would interact with the individual's other capacities or traits. For example, enhancing some forms of memory beyond a limited range might so interfere with other forms of memory or other cognitive processes as to be, overall, undesirable instead of a benefit. The second reason why some enhancements would only be beneficial within a limited range is that beyond that range individuals would become unsuited for human social life. For example, there are well-known social benefits to being tall. That is why growth hormone—a pharmacological intervention—that raised a normal individual's height to several inches above the norm might be a beneficial enhancement. But there are limits to how much of an increase in height would be beneficial. To grow to be 9 ft tall, certainly not now possible with growth hormone, would be on balance harmful in nearly any human society because our social world is constructed for persons whose height rarely reaches beyond 7 ft at most. One would literally become, in a physical respect, unfit for human company. And if the change were still more dramatic, as in the case of Gulliver in Lilliput, it could become hard to see the individual still as a member of the same species. Many changes in human features and capacities by genetic engineering would only be beneficial within some range, and public policy could quite appropriately regulate its use to ensure that it stays within the beneficial range.

THE MEANS USED FOR ENHANCEMENT

Is it morally important that genetic engineering is the means used to enhance human capacities? Of course, means may vary in various morally important ways, such as the risks they carry, but is there something about genetic manipulation itself that raises moral worries? Many people admire others who have developed skills and abilities through long hard effort that they would not admire when the means used was genetic engineering. Moreover, sometimes a valued activity is defined in part by the means it employs, not just by the end at which it aims. It was a great achievement several years ago when IBM's computer "Big Blue" beat the then world chess champion Gary Kasparov. But it surely was a very different achievement from the one in which a human challenger recently beat Kasparov. And suppose an IBM engineer who designed Big Blue's program and implemented the moves it chose claimed that he was the new world chess champion. Here, means make all the difference in the chess skills and successes with which the engineer should be credited. In many valued human activities, the means of acquiring the capacities are as much valued and admired as the performance itself. Opponents of genetic engineering on these grounds will need to show that enhancing particular human capacities by genetic engineering as opposed to other means transforms and devalues important activities that employ those capacities.

WHO IS USING GENETIC ENGINEERING?

It will often be morally important who is using genetic engineering technologies to enhance a particular capacity. I believe the most important differences are between three cases: first, when government employs or strongly encourages their use; second, when individuals use them on others, most importantly parents on their children; third, when individuals use them to enhance their own capacities (strictly, this last would not be genetic engineering as defined above, but genetic interventions may become possible later than the embryo stage of development). The most obvious difference is between the first two cases and the third, since the first two raise the issue of the justification of some persons acting to affect someone else; for example, it is widely held that individuals are justified in taking risks for themselves that they would not be justified in imposing on others. Less obvious, but at least as important, are the

different degrees and forms of neutrality about what is a good life that are properly expected from the state, from parents toward their children, and from individuals in their own lives.

In liberal democracies, it is widely held that the state should seek to be neutral between different comprehensive conceptions of a good life that its citizens may hold. This liberal neutrality places substantial limits on governmental action to employ, encourage, or require the use of genetic engineering that would only be beneficial in some specific conceptions of a good life. The genetic engineering compatible with this liberal state neutrality is roughly that which enhances what John Rawls (1971) called primary goods, that is, general purpose means useful in a wide variety of, if not virtually all, plans of life. Placing fluoride in the water supply is justified on these grounds: enhancing resistance to tooth decay is beneficial no matter what one's particular plan of life. Enhancing memory by genetic engineering might be as well.

Consider now parents' use of genetic engineering for their children. Whoever has primary responsibility for raising children—in most societies, parents—must have substantial discretion in the values they impart and the particular capacities they seek to develop and enhance in their children. There are moral limits, however, on parents' authority to enhance their children's capacities, whether by genetic engineering or other means, as the following case illustrates. Suppose parents put their 7-year-old daughter into an intensive tennis training program to develop her potential to become a professional tennis player; whether wise or not, parents are generally accepted to have the right to do this. But suppose the parents also proposed to withdraw her from school because they believed her education was interfering with her tennis training. Public policy, quite properly, would not permit them to do so because, although it might enhance her tennis skills, it would be at the cost of severely limiting or neglecting many other capacities and opportunities she would otherwise have later to choose and pursue other, different, life plans. Parents do not have an unlimited moral right to shape their children and their children's capacities at the cost of denying them a reasonable array of opportunities to select and pursue their own conception of a good life as they mature and develop the capacities to make those choices. Children have what Joel Feinberg (1980) has called a right to an "open future," which is derivative from the more fundamental right of adults to self-determination in making significant choices about their lives for themselves and according to their own values or conception of a good life. Disagreements will arise, of course, about the extent or scope of a child's right to an open future and what would violate that right, but the right places significant limits on the use of genetic engineering by parents for their children.

If individuals could use genetic engineering for themselves, neither of these forms of neutrality would be required because their doing so would be an exercise, not an infringement, of self-determination or autonomy. Public policy might legitimately seek to ensure that such choices are well informed, particularly when there are significant and irreversible risks, but it should not substitute its own judgments about when genetic engineering would be desirable for the voluntary, informed judgments of competent adults. As a general matter, we have seen that who would be using genetic engineering could be important for the moral justification of that use.

IMPACT OF GENETIC ENGINEERING ON FAIRNESS AND INEQUALITY

I want finally to provide what I believe is the most important example of the moral issues public policy will face in responding to widespread new capacities for genetic engineering that enhances normal capacities. The problem arises when an enhancement by genetic engineering would confer a substantial competitive or positional advantage on its recipient, thereby strengthening an individual's position relative to others in competitions for scarce roles or benefits. If the genetic engineering is expensive and distributed on the basis of an ability to pay for it, then only the economically well off will get it. This will raise concerns about fairness and equality of opportunity, specifically whether those who cannot afford genetic engineering have a fair opportunity to compete for the benefit against those whose capacities to compete have been enhanced by genetic en-

gineering. Imagine that the children of the higher socioeconomic classes not only have the social advantages they now typically have, but that they also have certification that their intelligence, memory, immune system, and capacity to concentrate attention on tasks for extended periods of time have all been enhanced by genetic engineering. This would be a very significant advantage in work and other contexts; it would likely significantly increase inequality and would raise serious issues of fairness and equality of opportunity for public policy. Public policy could reasonably regulate the use of genetic engineering that would unfairly increase inequality, but there would be an important moral complication in doing so, quite apart from generating the necessary political will to do so.

Many real enhancements that may become possible through genetic engineering will in part confer positional or competitive advantages, but will in part confer non-competitive or intrinsic benefits as well. Take the example of enhancing individuals' capacities to focus their attention more intensely for significant periods of time on a particular task or activity. Many adults with no disease or deficit now use the drug Ritalin for this purpose. This would confer a significant advantage in work contexts. But it would also increase individuals' intrinsic satisfactions from activities like listening to music, watching films or sunsets, and so forth, none of which are competitive benefits that make anyone else worse off. The quandary for public policy is that concerns about fairness and equality of opportunity would support limits on this use of genetic engineering, but these limits would at the same time deny individuals the opportunity of gaining significant, non-competitive benefits in their lives.

Public policy will face other difficult issues in responding to new capacities for genetic engineering, including regulation of competitive enhancements that would be self-defeating if widely used and regulation of the risks that will be inherent in their use. Whether used for treatment of disease or for enhancement, genetic engineering in humans should take place only after careful evaluation to ensure that its risks are justified by its potential benefits—this will be especially important for any germ-line interventions. But the potential long-term adverse impact on inequality and fairness may well prove to be the greatest challenge.

The moral and policy issues that will likely be raised in the future by new capacities to employ genetic engineering to prevent disease and disability and to enhance normal human capacities will ultimately concern how we are to shape our nature as humans. Some people will condemn any such interventions as "playing God," but I believe the potential for human benefit makes any general moral bar to their use unjustified. What I have tried to do in this [essay] is to articulate some of the moral and policy issues that we must confront if we are to use genetic engineering wisely, safely, and ethically.

ACKNOWLEDGMENTS

This [essay] draws heavily on Brock (1998) and Buchanan et al. (2000).

REFERENCES

Brock, D. W. (1998) Enhancement of human function: Some distinctions for policy makers. In E. Parens (ed.), *Technologies for the Enhancement of Human Capacities.* Washington, DC: Georgetown University Press.

Buchanan, A. E., Brock, D. W., Daniels, N., and Wikler, D. (2000) *From Chance to Choice: Genetics and Justice.* Cambridge: Cambridge University Press.

Feinberg, J. (1980) The child's right to an open future. In W. Aiken and H. LaFollette (eds.), *Whose Child? Children's Rights, Parental Authority, and State Power.* Totowa, NJ: Rowman and Littlefield.

Rawls, J. (1971) *A Theory of Justice.* Cambridge, MA: Harvard University Press.

ANNOTATED BIBLIOGRAPHY

Adams, Harry: "A Human Germ-line Modification Scale," *Journal of Law, Medicine & Ethics* 32 (Spring 2004), pp. 164–173. Adams suggests the following categories as a framework for the assessment of possible germ-line modifications, whether therapeutic in nature or enhancements: (1) those that should be prohibited, (2) those that should be available to everyone, (3) those that may be available to anyone with adequate resources, and (4) those that should be mandatory for everyone.

Alpern, Kenneth D., ed.: *The Ethics of Reproductive Technology* (New York: Oxford University Press, 1992). This anthology is designed to address both normative and conceptual questions associated with innovations in human reproduction—both technological innovations (e.g., IVF) and social innovations (e.g., surrogate motherhood).

Boone, C. Keith: "Bad Axioms in Genetic Engineering," *Hastings Center Report* 18 (August/September 1988), pp. 9–13. Boone warns against reliance on simplistic axioms (e.g., we must not "play God" or "interfere with nature") in making ethical judgments in the area of genetic engineering. He emphasizes the need for balanced judgment and attempts to identify in the case of each simplistic axiom a partial truth wrongly represented as the whole truth.

Boss, Judith A.: *The Birth Lottery: Prenatal Diagnosis and Selective Abortion* (Chicago: Loyola University Press, 1993). The first two chapters of this book provide useful factual information on genetic disorders and prenatal diagnostic procedures. In later chapters, Boss examines various proposed justifications for selective abortion and ultimately concludes that the practice cannot be justified.

Botkin, Jeffrey R.: "Ethical Issues and Practical Problems in Preimplantation Genetic Diagnosis," *Journal of Law, Medicine & Ethics* 26 (Spring 1998), pp. 17–28. Botkin discusses the risks, limitations, and costs of PGD, clarifies the purposes that the procedure might serve, and provides an analysis of the ethical issues raised by the procedure.

Brock, Dan W.: "An Assessment of the Ethical Issues Pro and Con," in *Cloning Human Beings: Report and Recommendations of the National Bioethics Advisory Commission* (Rockville, MD: NBAC, June 1997), Volume II, Section E, pp. 1–23. This valuable paper provides an overall survey of the moral arguments for and against human cloning.

Buchanan, Allen, Dan W. Brock, Norman Daniels, and Daniel Wikler: *From Chance to Choice: Genetics and Justice* (Cambridge: Cambridge University Press, 2000). The authors examine a wide range of ethical issues associated with the use of genetic technologies.

Cameron, C., and R. Williamson: "Is There an Ethical Difference Between Preimplantation Genetic Diagnosis and Abortion?" *Journal of Medical Ethics* 29 (2003), pp. 90–92. The authors argue that PGD and implantation of an unaffected embryo, while allowing affected embryos to die, is ethically preferable to prenatal diagnosis and selective abortion.

Cohen, Cynthia B., ed.: *New Ways of Making Babies: The Case of Egg Donation* (Bloomington: Indiana University Press, 1996). This collection includes a set of articles addressing the ethical and policy issues associated with egg donation.

Klotzko, Arlene Judith, ed.: *The Cloning Sourcebook* (New York: Oxford University Press, 2001). Part I of this anthology deals with the science of cloning, Part II considers the context of cloning, Part III is dedicated to the ethics of cloning, and Part IV addresses policy issues.

Journal of Medicine and Philosophy 16 (December 1991). This issue features a series of articles under the general title of "Human Germ-Line Engineering." A wide range of arguments for and against germ-line gene therapy can be found in the various articles.

Lauritzen, Paul: *Pursuing Parenthood: Ethical Issues in Assisted Reproduction* (Bloomington: Indiana University Press, 1993). Lauritzen considers the ethics of AIH, IVF, donor insemination (AID), and surrogate motherhood. His final chapter is entitled "The Myth and Reality of Current Adoption Practice."

Law, Medicine & Health Care 16 (Spring/Summer 1988). This special issue is entirely dedicated to surrogate motherhood. Articles are organized under the headings of (1) civil liberties, (2) ethics, and (3) women's autonomy. Material is also provided on the case of Baby M.

New York State Task Force on Life and the Law: *Assisted Reproductive Technologies: Analysis and Recommendations for Public Policy* (April 1998). This report provides a wealth of information about the various reproductive technologies used in clinical practice. Clinical, legal, and policy issues are identified, and analysis of these issues culminates in an extensive set of conclusions and recommendations.

Overall, Christine: *Ethics and Human Reproduction: A Feminist Analysis* (Boston: Allen & Unwin, 1987). Overall embraces a feminist perspective on reproductive ethics and contrasts a feminist approach with nonfeminist and antifeminist approaches. She discusses sex preselection in Chapter 2, surrogate motherhood in Chapter 6, and artificial reproduction in Chapter 7.

Parens, Erik, and Adrienne Asch, eds.: *Prenatal Testing and Disability Rights* (Washington, DC: Georgetown University Press, 2000). This valuable collection of articles provides divergent viewpoints on the various claims associated with the disability rights critique of prenatal diagnosis and selective abortion.

Pence, Gregory E.: *Who's Afraid of Human Cloning?* (Lanham, MD: Rowman & Littlefield, 1998). Pence constructs an overall case for the moral acceptability of human cloning.

Purdy, Laura M.: "Surrogate Mothering: Exploitation or Empowerment?" *Bioethics* 3 (January 1989), pp. 18–34. Purdy argues against the view that surrogate mothering is necessarily immoral. She acknowledges the danger that surrogate mothering could deepen the exploitation of women but also insists that surrogacy has the potential to empower women.

Robertson, John A.: *Children of Choice: Freedom and the New Reproductive Technologies* (Princeton, NJ: Princeton University Press, 1994). Emphasizing the importance of procreative freedom, Robertson provides an analysis of the ethical, legal, and social issues associated with various reproductive technologies. He considers IVF in Chapter 5; sperm donation, egg donation, and gestational surrogacy in Chapter 6; and the selection and shaping of offspring characteristics in Chapter 7.

Rothman, Barbara Katz: *The Tentative Pregnancy: Prenatal Diagnosis and the Future of Motherhood* (New York: Viking Penguin, 1986). Rothman raises a host of concerns about the social impact of prenatal diagnosis.

Tong, Rosemarie: *Feminist Approaches to Bioethics: Theoretical Reflections and Practical Applications* (Boulder, CO: Westview Press, 1997). Chapter 7 of this book provides discussions of artificial insemination and IVF. Chapter 8 provides a discussion of surrogacy. Chapter 9 includes discussions of prenatal diagnosis and gene therapy.

Walters, LeRoy, and Julie Gage Palmer: *The Ethics of Human Gene Therapy* (New York: Oxford University Press, 1997). This useful book provides chapters on somatic-cell gene therapy, germ-line gene therapy, and enhancement engineering.

SOCIAL JUSTICE AND HEALTH-CARE POLICY

INTRODUCTION

No honest and well-informed discussion of health care in the United States can deny that our system is in crisis and that American-style managed care has failed to achieve several commonly accepted goals of health care. In the first comprehensive study of the medical impact of not having health insurance, the Institute of Medicine states that "lack of health insurance for tens of millions of Americans has serious negative consequences and economic costs not only for the uninsured but also for their families, the communities they live in, and the whole country. The situation is dire and expected to worsen."[1] Lack of insurance, the 2004 study indicates, leads to delayed diagnoses, life-threatening complications, and 18,000 premature deaths in the United States every year. For present purposes, the assertion that the American health-care system is in a deepening crisis can be supported by considering the system's performance in terms of certain goals.

Perhaps the most commonly accepted goals of a health-care system and, therefore, of health-care reform are the following: universal access, cost controls, comprehensiveness of benefits, freedom of choice and freedom from hassle for patients, and quality of care. How well does American health care perform by reference to these benchmarks?

First, the United States does not come close to achieving universal access. In 1986, 37 million Americans lacked health insurance. In 2004 (the time of this writing) the number hovers between 44 million and 45 million. By contrast, most industrial countries provide universal access to health care.

Second, despite not covering one sixth of its population, the American system has controlled costs poorly. In 1986 the United States spent almost 11 percent of its gross domestic product (GDP) on health care, a figure that rose to about 14 percent by 1994. For several years in the mid-1990s, health-care inflation slowed significantly (due in part to some of the techniques of managed care), but at the end of the decade overall spending was again rising quickly. From 2000 to 2004 costs rose steeply—four times as fast as wages—with health insurance premiums rising at double-digit rates each year. Moreover, Americans spend far more *per person* (including the uninsured) on their health care than citizens of any other country spend. In 1998 U.S. per capita spending on health care was $4,270 (compared with a median of $2,000 among twenty-three industrial countries); in 2004, according to one estimate, the figure is $5,540 per capita.

Third, coverage provided by both private plans and public insurance programs in this country is typically not comprehensive. Even the best plans and programs provide only limited coverage for psychiatric care and limited or no coverage for dental care; many provide limited coverage for long-term and chronic care and commonly force patients to leave hospitals before they feel well, leading to such piecemeal legislation as laws prohibiting health plans from denying new mothers a second day in the hospital. Despite one trend in the opposite direction—increasing coverage for prescription drugs—the benefit packages for the citizens of Canada, Germany, Great Britain, France, Sweden, and many other countries are more complete.

Fourth, while (insured) Americans long enjoyed considerable freedom in choosing doctors, hospitals, and the like, managed care has imposed severe restrictions on patient choice. Moreover, while for many years the administrative complexity of American health care has been criticized for greatly inconveniencing patients, managed care has exacerbated this problem with additional layers of restrictions. By comparison, the systems of countries that provide universal access commonly extend much more freedom of choice to patients while imposing less inconvenience.

Finally, quality of care is commonly regarded as the pride of the American system. The best American health care is as good as care anywhere else in the world, and America's prowess in high-technology medicine is reputedly second to none. At the same time, one could argue that most people need good basic care more than they need high-technology virtuosity, and persons lacking insurance or covered by relatively weak private plans or public programs tend to receive substandard care. Also sobering is the estimated 98,000 American deaths per year due to medical error.[2]

Some of the difficulties of the American approach to financing and delivering health care can be understood in terms of its experience with managed care. The nonprofit group health plans of a generation ago—the earliest health maintenance organizations (HMOs)—rightly claimed to provide high-quality care while reducing costs by emphasizing prevention and health maintenance within a coordinated system of care. But today the for-profit managed care organizations (MCOs) that dominate health care are mainly responsive to the bottom line, or maximizing profits. Having much higher turnover of patients than old-fashioned HMOs, they do not find it so economically sensible to invest in patients' lifetime wellness. Meanwhile, although the basic purpose of health insurance is to spread risk among a population, thereby protecting the less fortunate, today's dominant MCOs try to avoid covering people who are sick or likely to get sick and try to minimize the costs of treating individuals they do cover. One wonders whether the logic of insurance is compatible with the logic of Wall Street.

Consequently, the American experiment of allowing the free market to determine the shape of health-care finance and delivery has failed to yield progress in connection with the basic goals of health care. Current reluctance to involve the government in significant overhaul of our system has entailed piecemeal initiatives that increase expenditures without improving the efficiency of our overall system. Examples include the Health Insurance Portability and Accountability Act of 1996, which makes it easier for those who change jobs or become unemployed to retain coverage, and the 1997 State Children's Health Insurance Program, which has reduced the number of uninsured children.

Because most Americans are disadvantaged by the health-care status quo, it is not surprising that, as reflected in polls, the American public has favored significant health-care reform for many years. Political interest in reform was clearly dampened after President Clinton's reform proposal, associated with the term "managed competition," was soundly defeated in 1994. Nevertheless, the public's interest in reform remains high, as suggested by a 2003 *Washington Post* poll that found that 80 percent of Americans consider it more important to achieve universal coverage than to hold down taxes.[3] But, to understate the point, the public's preferences are not the only ones that carry weight. Powerful special-interest groups with a financial stake in the shape of health-care finance and delivery—such as the private insurance industry, drug companies, and to some extent even the American Medical Association (which resisted major reform several times in the twentieth century)—have collectively invested many millions of dollars in an effort to preserve the status quo or something relatively close to it. Thus, while the experience of industrial countries around the world strongly suggests that the major goals of health care are achievable only if the government plays a significant organizing role—at least in the financing of health care—there are few indications that the United States will soon take such a step.

Whatever the current trends may be, what does justice require in the way of health-care reform? Is rationing morally defensible and, if so, what kinds of rationing? How should the methods of managed care be morally evaluated? And what sorts of systems would satisfy the demands of justice while meeting other appropriate objectives of health care? This chapter explores these and related questions.

JUSTICE, RIGHTS, AND SOCIETAL OBLIGATIONS

Does society have a moral obligation to ensure that everyone has access to at least some level of health care? In other words, is the popular goal of universal access morally sound? If so, what level of care is the appropriate standard? For example, should society ensure access to all needed services, or should only basic care be guaranteed? Answering such questions requires an understanding of various conceptions of justice as well as other possible bases of societal obligations regarding health care.

Justice, Liberty, Equality, and the Right to Health Care Three broad *conceptions* or *visions* of justice dominate social-political theory: libertarian, socialist, and liberal. These conceptions or visions are sometimes sharpened into specific *theories* of justice. Two moral values, liberty and equality, are of key importance. (Utility also plays a role insofar as everyone agrees that efficiency and practicality are important values. But utility does not unambiguously favor one of the three basic conceptions.) The *libertarian* conception of justice holds liberty to be the ultimate moral ideal; the *socialist* conception of justice takes social equality to be the ultimate moral ideal; and the *liberal* conception tries to combine equality and liberty into one moral ideal.

The Libertarian Conception of Justice On a libertarian view, individuals have moral rights to life, liberty, and property, which any just society must recognize and respect. These are conceived as negative rights or rights of noninterference: If A has a right to X, no one should prevent A from pursuing X or deprive A of X. According to libertarians, the sole function of government is to protect the individual's life, liberty, and property against force, theft, and fraud. Providing for the welfare of those who cannot or will not provide for themselves is not a morally justifiable function of government. To make such provisions, the government would have to take from some against their will in order to give to others. This is perceived as an unjustifiable limitation on individual liberty. Individuals own their own bodies and, therefore, the labor they exert. It follows, for the libertarian, that individuals have the right to whatever income or wealth their labor can earn in a free marketplace, and no one has the right to take part of that income to provide health care or other goods for other persons.

The Socialist Conception of Justice A direct challenge to libertarians comes from those who defend the socialist conception of justice. Although socialist views differ in many respects, one common element is a commitment to social equality, however specified, and to government or collective measures furthering that equality. Since social equality is the ultimate value, limitations on individual liberty that are necessary to promote equality are seen as justified. Socialists challenge libertarian views on the primacy of liberty in at least two ways. First, they defend their ideal of social equality. (Their arguments take various forms and need not concern us here.) Second, they assert the meaninglessness of rights of noninterference to those who lack adequate food, health care, and so forth. For those who lack the money needed to buy food and health care needed to sustain life, the libertarian right to life is an empty sham. Liberty rights, such as the right to exchange goods freely, are meaningless to those who cannot exercise such rights because of economic limitations. Where libertarians stress freedom from government interference, socialists stress the government's obligation to promote the welfare of its citizens by ensuring that their most important needs are met. Where libertarians stress *negative rights,* socialists stress *positive rights*—that is, rights to be provided with certain things. Where libertarians criticize socialism for the limitations it imposes on liberty, socialists criticize libertarianism for allowing gross inequalities among those who are "equally human."

The Liberal Conception of Justice Liberals reject the libertarian conception of justice for failing to include what liberals perceive as a fundamental moral concern: the requirement that those who have more than enough must help those in need. Like the socialist, the liberal recognizes the extent to which economic constraints can limit the exercise of negative rights by those lacking economic means. The liberal, however, is likely to perceive more of the negative rights claimed by the libertarian as extremely important; while some socialists agree with liberals that civil liberties (e.g., freedom of speech) are very important, liberals generally place greater importance than socialists do on, for instance, the value of economic liberty or noninterference. At the same time, liberals defend institutions that provide for the basic needs of disadvantaged members of society. Not opposing all social and economic inequalities, they differ among each other concerning both the morally acceptable extent of those inequalities and their justification. A utilitarian liberal, for example, might hold that inequalities are justified to the extent that they increase the total amount of good in society. A different approach is taken by liberal contemporary philosopher John Rawls, who maintains that inequalities in the distribution of primary social goods (e.g., income, opportunities) are justified only if they benefit everyone in society, especially the least advantaged.[4] The primary concern here is not with the total amount of good in a society but with the good of the least advantaged.

Theories of Justice and a Right to Health Care What, if anything, can be inferred from theories of justice regarding the existence of a moral right to health care? Allen Buchanan in this chapter asks this question in regard to both a libertarian and a liberal theory of justice. After discussing the libertarian approach as exemplified in the work of Robert Nozick, Buchanan points out that for the libertarian, there is no moral right to health care and no societal obligation to provide it. (Note that a right to health care, as an entitlement to be provided some good, would be a *positive* right.) Citing Rawls's view as an example of a liberal position, Buchanan explains Rawls's central principles of justice before speculating about their implications regarding what constitutes justice in health care. According to Buchanan, the implications of Rawls's theory for a right to health care are far from clear.[5]

Buchanan also discusses the stance a utilitarian might take regarding a right to health care. He has in mind rule-utilitarianism, which (as explained in Chapter 1) can support the assertion of certain rights. In rule-utilitarianism, the correct conception of justice and of related moral rights is the one whose application maximizes the net amount of good in society. Buchanan examines some of the implications of a utilitarian approach for a right to health care and the scope of any such right. In another reading in this chapter, Kai Nielsen argues from a socialist position in defending a right to health care based on a view of justice whose fundamental principle is that of moral equality—a principle he interprets to mean that everyone's life matters equally. On his account, any society committed to moral equality must make publicly funded medical treatment of the same quality and extent available to all.

Societal Obligations or Commitments to Provide Health Care Some arguments supporting a societal obligation to provide health care do not involve the claim that individuals have a *right* to health care. These arguments often appeal to considerations of beneficence as well as considerations of the special nature of health-care needs, a strategy adopted by the President's Commission for the Study of Ethical Problems in Medicine and Biomedical and Behavioral Research.[6] In its influential report, the Commission asserts that society has an obligation to ensure that every citizen has access to adequate care without being subject to excessive burdens. This assertion is grounded in (1) the special moral significance of health care, (2) the fact that many health-care needs are undeserved, and (3) the implausibility of expecting everyone to be able to meet their needs using their own resources when these needs are so unpredictable, costly, and unevenly distributed among people. Because the Commission contends only that society has an obligation to ensure universal access to an *adequate* level of care, its view is consistent with a two-tier medical system in which the well-to-do can purchase additional services beyond what is available to everyone.

Other arguments support a societal obligation to provide health care without assuming a right to health care. One approach focuses on what universal access to health care (or lack thereof) expresses about a society's character. No decent and compassionate society, according to this line of thinking, could fail to provide health care to its members when it has the financial resources to do so. This argument amounts to an appeal to *virtue;* someone advancing such an argument might not even use the term *societal obligation* (since virtue ethics downplays the concept of obligation), preferring instead to speak of *appropriate societal commitments.* A similar argument could be developed from the perspective of *the ethics of care*: A caring society would commit itself to guaranteeing adequate health care to its people, thereby strengthening the social bonds among them. (See Chapter 1 for discussions of virtue ethics and the ethics of care.)

RATIONING, MANAGED CARE, AND HEALTH-CARE REFORM IN THE UNITED STATES

In the United States, policy decisions about the allocation of health-care resources are regularly made by Congress, state legislatures, managed care organizations, and other health insurance companies, plans, and programs. These allocation decisions about health-care expenditures and the distribution of health-care resources are sometimes called *macroallocation* decisions. They are contrasted with *microallocation* decisions, those made by particular hospital staffs, individual professionals, or even plan administrators about the allocation of scarce health-care resources (e.g., transplantable organs) to particular patients.

Macroallocation may be thought of as beginning with two especially fundamental questions. First, how much of our total economic resources should be devoted to health care and biomedical research? This question requires that we ask about the importance of these goods vis-à-vis other goods. For example, current biomedical technology is making it possible to save and prolong lives that could not have been saved before. Should other social goods, such as education, receive less funding in order to prolong individual lives as long as possible? A second fundamental macroallocation question concerns how the slice of the economic pie devoted to biomedicine should be further divided. How large a piece should be devoted to preventive measures, to curative measures, to the production of new equipment used in treatment and diagnosis, and to research? Then, of course, more specific questions present themselves, such as "Out of the slice going to biomedical research, how much should be devoted to AIDS research, to various sorts of cancer research, and so on?" Further questions concern both the best procedures or processes for making macroallocation decisions and the values that should guide those decisions.

The concept of rationing is often invoked in the context of macroallocation. Though the term *rationing* is used in several ways, it may be broadly understood for our purposes as relating to the second question in the previous paragraph and involving choices within a particular area of biomedicine concerning the relative weight to be given to competing needs. For example, concerning the allocation of public funds, should the funding of prenatal care take precedence over the funding of heart transplants? One sense of rationing is that of *denying* individuals services they need or want because of limited resources. It is in this sense of the term that some commentators assert that the American system rations by the ability to pay; persons lacking adequate health insurance or sufficient funds are often denied health care they need or want. Especially when health-care costs are rising quickly, a commonly asked question is whether more explicit forms of rationing should be accepted.

Whether or not such explicit rationing should be accepted, it occurs regularly in the context of managed care. Indeed, the topics of rationing and managed care are inextricably connected in American health care today. As Allen Buchanan explains in an article reprinted in this chapter, *managed care* combines health insurance and the delivery of a broad range of integrated health-care services for some population of enrollees, paying for those services prospectively from an estimated, limited budget. Thus, within a managed care plan, money devoted to costly, marginally effective treatments is simply unavailable for other purposes. Because not every possible treatment that might benefit enrollees (patients) can be funded within the limited budget, managed care plans need to make decisions about what sorts of health-care services to cover, whether to cover a particular treatment in a particular case, or both. (Whereas policy decisions in managed care regarding what sorts of services to cover involve macroallocation, case-by-case decisions that are not determined by general policies involve microallocation.) American managed care is currently dominated by *for-profit* MCOs, creating further pressure to ration: Money that is taken for profits cannot be devoted to services for patients, effectively shrinking the economic pie from which all patients must eat. More will be said about managed care later in this section.

If it is necessary or desirable to ration health care explicitly, what are the morally appropriate criteria to use? The state of Oregon has directly confronted the problems of access to health care and rising costs by developing an explicit rationing plan, whose purpose is to ensure that all Oregonians have access to basic health care. The Health Services Commission, appointed in 1989, had the task of ranking, for Medicaid, medical conditions and associated treatments in terms of their overall importance. Rankings were to take into account both the costs of services and their likely effects on patients' quality of life. The plan called for funding as many of the services as possible within the limits of the state budget, provided that all Oregonians at or below the federal poverty line would be covered. The state commission's long list of ranked condition-treatment pairs, presented in 1990, stirred ethical and political debate about particular rankings, criteria used for ranking, and the list's consequences for particular groups of patients.

Norman Daniels explores in this chapter the question of whether the Oregon rationing plan is fair or just. His analysis considers such aspects of the plan as (1) extending health-care coverage to those who had lacked it, (2) removing coverage of some (relatively low-ranked) services for persons who had already been covered by Medicaid, and (3) attempting to base health-care priorities on values expressed in public meetings. Readers should note that while Daniels's discussion is exceptionally in-depth with regard to fundamental ethical issues, chapters have been added to the Oregon rationing story since the time of his article.

In 1992 the (first) Bush administration rejected the Oregon plan, claiming that its list discriminated against disabled persons, since the ranking of condition-treatment pairs was partly based on an assessment of the possibility of restoring a full quality of life (one lacking infirmity or disability), an outcome precluded for the disabled. In response, the Health Services Commission produced a substantially revised list in which each condition-treatment pair was analyzed in terms of the probability of death with and without treatment. (For example, pancreatic cancer will cause death with or without treatment, whereas bacterial meningitis is very likely to cause death without treatment but less likely to do so with treatment.) In 1993 the Clinton administration approved the plan, which went into effect the next year.

One interesting development in the Oregon experiment is that a public list of prioritized condition-treatment pairs has led to an overall expansion of services covered—no doubt because rationing of valuable services is more difficult to sustain in the bright light of public scrutiny. Today, for example, all enrollees are eligible for dental care and organ transplants, as well as mental health and chemical dependency services; indeed, most of the listed services that are not covered are only marginally effective. Moreover, services "below the line" are often provided even though the state does not reimburse them. Thus, it is not clear that the Oregon rationing plan has significantly restricted access to needed services despite the negative publicity the plan received prior to its implementation. In any event, having encountered difficulties in financing its plan and various other challenges, Oregon continues to experiment with ways of controlling costs, producing useful practice guidelines for doctors, and encouraging Medicaid enrollees to sign up with managed care plans connected with the program.

Debates over appropriate criteria for rationing (e.g., effects on quality of life, likelihood of forestalling death) and how to implement a rationing plan are fueled by the assumption that rationing is inevitable or necessary. When the term *rationing* is used to refer to the withholding of care that certain patients need, or strongly believe they need, such rationing may be difficult to justify in the absence of a persuasive case for its necessity. Disagreement about whether a particular medical service ought to be withheld, or its supply significantly limited, may trace to disagreement about whether this service provides any significant benefit. Yet, even if two people agree on the matter of benefit, they may disagree on whether the medical service in question should be rationed due to differing views on another matter: whether changes in the relevant insurance program or in the health-care system as a whole might make that service affordable. Perhaps cost savings through a more efficient health-care program or system would permit the provision of services that now appear unaffordable due to inefficiency. Therefore, just as the topics of rationing and managed care are inextricably linked in the present context of American health care, both topics are closely tied to the issue of health-care reform in the United States.

In an article reprinted in this chapter, Leonard M. Fleck argues that rationing is unavoidable—the demand for services always exceeding an affordable supply—but that fairness in health-care reform will require rationing *for everyone.* "Last chance" therapies, he contends, demonstrate the unavoidability of rationing decisions. These therapies represent the last chance at prolonging the lives of certain patients, who often want them desperately, yet they also tend to be very expensive and only marginally beneficial. Fleck argues that public insurance programs and MCOs should not have to cover them, because doing so would drive up health-care costs, in turn making it harder to expand access to health care, which ought to be the foremost priority of health-care reform. As our society confronts the issues connected with systemic reform, he continues, philosophers can play several important roles in facilitating the needed discussion.

In considering what sort of health-care reform we should seek, we need to revisit the status quo. The American health-care system features a mix of private and public elements. A large percentage of the United States population has some form of private health insurance, often largely paid for by employers—although presently there is a trend of employers dropping health–care benefits for employees. Federal funds provide insurance for people over 65 (Medicare) and, in combination with state funds, for those below a certain income level (Medicaid), though income thresholds vary greatly from state to state. In addition, special groups, such as veterans and military personnel, are directly cared for in hospitals operated by the government. As noted previously, nearly 45 million Americans today have neither private nor public insurance. As also noted, MCOs have become a primary force in health insurance. Not only do they currently dominate the private insurance market; many enrollees in public programs such as Medicare and Medicaid are strongly encouraged to sign up with MCOs. On the whole, the American health-care system has fared rather poorly in terms of the basic goals of a health-care system. Hence the calls for reform.

Assuming some type of health-care reform in the United States is morally imperative, for what system of health-care delivery and finance should we aim? What models are available? According to one influential school of thought, represented by Ezekiel Emanuel in an article reprinted in this chapter, any realistic answer must assume that managed care will play a major role. For unless—as seems extremely unlikely in the near future—the federal government *radically* overhauls our health-care system through legislation, we will have to work within a system in which managed care dominates.

Comparing the current crisis in American health care with that of the early 1990s, Emanuel draws several lessons from the Clinton administration's politically unsuccessful reform effort. According to Emanuel, these lessons indicate that any viable approach to health-care reform will retain private managed care delivery, break the link between employment and insurance, include realistic mechanisms for controlling costs, and assume a form that is palatable across the American political spectrum. A system of universal health-care vouchers, he contends, holds the greatest promise for meeting these criteria. In this approach, every individual or family would receive a voucher from the government or from employers who opt to retain this responsibility. Vouchers would be used to purchase health insurance from a private MCO or insurance system. A quasi-public body would have responsibility for monitoring and certifying the adequacy of the insurance companies.

Whatever merits this or other proposals may have, it may be a long time before American health care undergoes significant change. In the meantime, there are important moral concerns about the way in which particular MCOs currently deliver care. On what basis—or by what standards—can the performance of MCOs be morally evaluated? In one of this chapter's readings, Norman Daniels and James Sabin focus on decisions by MCOs to ration or set limits on desired, potentially beneficial care. Citing data from a study of how MCOs actually make decisions about coverage for new technologies, the authors argue that fairness in setting limits and making other allocation decisions is more important than closure, the making of these decisions within a fixed budget. Fairness, they elaborate, requires decision making based on acceptable reasons, openness about the reasons underlying particular decisions, and opportunities for revisiting disputed decisions.

While Daniels and Sabin address the question of appropriate standards for evaluating particular MCOs—with special reference to their rationing decisions—a broader sort of evaluation examines the moral adequacy of American managed care as a whole. Widespread unhappiness with this system motivates major reform, as noted earlier in this Introduction and by several of our authors. But unhappiness is one thing, appropriate moral criticism another. How *should* we evaluate American managed care? One approach would be to compare its overall performance with either (1) some view of what justice (and perhaps other moral values) demand or (2) the performance of health-care models represented by other nations or by a state like Oregon, which makes use of managed care yet finances and organizes health-care delivery in a unique way.

In connection with the first approach, as Buchanan points out, some critics have faulted American managed care for the following: (a) not contributing to the expansion of access to health care; (b) rationing, thereby depriving patients of care to which they have a right; and (c) pressuring doctors to ration, thereby encouraging them to fail in their duty to serve patients' best interests. But are these criticisms compelling? According to Buchanan, criticism (a) is based on the false premise that our society has divided up the moral burden of expanding access to health care and assigned a portion of that burden to MCOs. Criticisms (b) and (c), he argues, incorrectly suppose that our society has articulated an "adequate level of care" to which everyone is supposedly entitled. In response to Buchanan, one might note that a theory of justice in health care can offer at least a sketch of such an adequate level. But the authority of any such theory might be questioned if it is not widely embraced within our society. Since American society seems significantly pluralistic with respect to theories of social justice, is there a reasonable standpoint from which to evaluate our current experiment with managed care?

It would certainly seem so. While Americans differ significantly with respect to theories of justice, they agree much more on the appropriate goals of health care. Accordingly, as in the second approach suggested previously, American health care can be compared with other real-world models in terms of success in achieving such widely accepted goals.

SYSTEMS OF HEALTH-CARE DELIVERY AND FINANCE: FOUR INTERNATIONAL PERSPECTIVES

The Canadian System As noted by Pat Armstrong in this chapter, the Canadian single-payer approach is a form of managed care. It combines insurance and the delivery of integrated health-care services for a population of enrollees (the citizens of a particular province), paying for those services prospectively from a limited budget (in the form of medical expenditure caps). But in Canadian-style managed care—known as medicare—universal coverage is achieved while costs are successfully controlled by a greatly streamlined form of administration and a lack of profiteering.

Canada is just one of numerous industrial nations with single-payer systems affording universal access to health care. While spending considerably less per capita on health care than the United States does ($2,250 versus $4,270 in 1998), Canada provides high-quality care and achieves health indices that are comparable to those of its southern neighbor. Significantly, Canada provides a comprehensive package of health-care services for its citizens, covering inpatient and ambulatory care, long-term care for the chronically disabled elderly, and psychiatric services. Only some provinces cover dental services, chiropractic care, optometric care, and prescription drugs. The administrative simplicity of the Canadian system allows it to spend only about one-eighth of every health-care dollar on administration, while the United States spends about one-quarter of each dollar for this purpose. The United States has more than 1,000 different payers. Most of them, as part of the private sector, must advertise, determine patient eligibility, elaborate restrictions on coverage, conduct patient-by-patient utilization reviews, try to collect on bad debts, and pay huge executive salaries, while seeking a profit. In contrast, Canada funds almost all of its care through the federal and provincial governments. Patients are rarely billed. Providers are either paid a fixed sum for each patient enrolled in their practices or they submit simple, standardized forms and get paid on a fee-for-service basis. While some private insurance companies offer elective services not covered by the universal Medicare plan (e.g., cosmetic surgery), the role of private insurance is marginal, due in part to the illegality of private companies' providing the same services that are offered in the universal Medicare package.

Canadians and others familiar with this single-payer system generally agree that it provides universal access to a comprehensive array of high-quality health services in a cost-effective manner that affords considerable patient freedom. Pressures to reduce costs, however, are a reality that actually led to *decreased* public expenditures for several years in the 1990s, generating concerns about not meeting some health needs. There have also been, over the years, complaints about lengthy waits in line for elective services. While the vast majority of Canadians would not trade their health-care system for the American system, according to polls, some wealthy Canadians have sought high-technology services in the United States rather than wait for them in Canada. (Meanwhile, several American states have found it cost-effective to import medications from Canada rather than purchase them domestically, where the absence of price controls makes them much more expensive.)

In one of this chapter's selections, John Iglehart's interview of Allan Rock, Canada's Minister of Health, identifies some of the current challenges that confront the Canadian system. According to Rock, the system's basic structure remains sound, continuing to afford both social equity and economic efficiency. But its difficulties include an inadequate range of community-based services and long-term care; insufficient federal funding for health care, leaving too great a burden on provincial governments' finances; overreliance on fee-for-service practice, which fails to ensure twenty-four-hour accessibility; and a failure to ensure that rural care is sufficiently accessible and of adequate quality. Rock offers several suggestions for how the Canadian health-care system can meet these and other challenges.

The German Model A different model for financing and delivering health care is offered by Germany. As explained by Gerd Richter in this chapter, the most distinctive feature of this system is its "sickness funds." These nonprofit, semi-private organizations, of which there were (at the time of his writing) more than 1,000, together offer coverage to all citizens. Sickness funds set premiums based on one's ability to pay and not on risk factors such as occupational risks or one's health history. One tenth of the population either opts for alternative coverage from for-profit private insurance—which offers more amenities but not additional medical services—or, in the case of civil servants, enjoys governmental insurance. Members of sickness funds choose their own physicians. The medical coverage includes inpatient and ambulatory care, prescription drugs, dental services, psychiatric care, and chiropractic and optometric care; coverage also includes cash benefits in special circumstances (e.g., maternity, necessary travel, burials). At the same time, long-term care for chronically disabled elderly persons is means-tested and some dental and medical services require modest copayments by patients.

In order to keep costs reasonably under control, the system's financing has always featured global budgeting, including controls on the prices and volume of services, equipment, and products. Additionally, hospital doctors and nurses are salaried. Such cost control measures have been reasonably successful: At the time of Richter's writing, roughly 10 percent of the German GDP was devoted to health care and only 3 percent of the population reported serious problems in being able to pay medical bills.

According to Richter, defects of the German system include a glut of doctors, increasing costs, and weak integration between primary care and hospital care. Despite these difficulties, he notes, most Germans are satisfied with the quality of care and freedom of choice within a system that ensures equal access for all citizens while costing much less than the American health-care system. Providing some support for Richter's optimistic conclusion are surveys finding that German patients and physicians express more overall satisfaction with their health-care system than American patients and physicians express with their system.[7]

One important transformation in the system is a result of 1993 legislation that gave Germans the right to choose among a range of sickness funds, rather than being assigned to one, resulting in a sort of managed competition: Funds compete with each other, but do so within national restrictions such as fee schedules for paying health-care professionals and specific salary agreements. Perhaps the most conspicuous consequence of the 1993 legislation is that the number of sickness funds decreased from about 1,000 in 1993 to 477 in 1998 as less competitive funds sought safety in mergers.[8]

The British Approach A distinct model of health-care delivery and finance is found in Great Britain. In one of this chapter's readings, Nicholas Mays and Justin Keen offer a descriptive overview of the British health-care system along the following lines. Founded in the middle of the twentieth century, the National Health Service (NHS) immediately provided all British citizens equitable access to health care. Importantly, private care and insurance were not abolished. British citizens may choose to pay for private insurance, while their tax contributions fund the NHS. Unlike their Canadian counterparts, British physicians may provide a particular type of medical service both within the public system and outside of it, and private insurance companies may cover services that are provided in the NHS. For several decades, as overall health-care spending has greatly increased, so has the demand for services. Can the NHS keep pace with current demand for expensive treatments and prescription drugs? According to Mays and Keen, the most likely scenarios include expanding the private sector. But any radical changes in this direction, in their view, would seriously threaten the goals of equity, efficiency, patient satisfaction, and access—as suggested by the record of the American system dominated by the private sector. In view of the high level of public satisfaction with the present health-care system, the authors conclude, Great Britain should exercise caution in pursuing structural changes in the face of increasing demand for services.

Whatever the future may hold in store for British health care, further details about how the system currently operates may be helpful. First, the benefits offered by the NHS are even more comprehensive than those offered in Canada and Germany. In addition to inpatient, ambulatory, and long-term care, the NHS covers dental services, prescription drugs (with a copay), psychiatric care, chiropractic care, and optometric services. At the same time, this system controls costs in part by more aggressively limiting the supply of medical services and equipment (e.g., limiting the supply of dialysis machines). As a single-payer system, the NHS also saves a great deal through simplified administration. NHS physicians are either salaried or receive a fixed sum for assuming the care of particular patients. In the public system, however, patients have limited choice of their primary care physicians, whose referrals they need to see specialists. On the whole, British patients' freedom of choice may be comparable to that of many American patients insured by MCOs (though it is clearly greater than that of uninsured Americans) while British patients on average seem to encounter less bureaucratic inconvenience.

British health-care expenditures are a double-edged sword.[9] On the one hand, cost controls have been remarkably successful. Providing one indication, 2000 per capita health spending in Great Britain totaled only $1,813 as compared with $2,580 in Canada, $2,780 in Germany, and $4,540 in the United States. On the other hand, the system has arguably undersupplied health care, causing long waits for routine surgeries and failing to update infrastructure sufficiently as buildings and equipment become outdated. The Labor administration headed by Tony Blair decided to invest more heavily in health care. Thus, taxes have increased in recent years, projecting a rise in health spending from 6.8 percent of the GDP in 2003 to an estimated 9.4 percent in 2007–08 (high by European standards but much lower than the American level of 14–15 percent).

Italian Health Care In the final reading of this chapter, Giovanna Ruberto provides an overview of the Italian National Health Service (NHS). As she explains, Italy's Constitution guarantees free comprehensive health care to all citizens; a 1998 law guarantees the same coverage to all foreign visitors, including illegal immigrants. Funded by tax revenues and budgeted yearly by Parliament, the Italian NHS consumes approximately 7 percent of the country's GDP. Health care is delivered through a network of territorial agencies, each funded by a state budget. Agencies, in turn, purchase health-care services from public health facilities and, occasionally, from private hospitals. Private health insurance is nonexistent while supplementary insurance, which no one really needs, is rare. In 2000 the World Health Organization ranked the Italian health-care system second in the world (to France), evaluating systems by the criteria of "(1) attainment of health for the population, (2) responsiveness, and (3) fair financing."

Despite these indications of success, the Italian NHS faces challenges. For example, there are regional differences in the quality of health care, the north enjoying an advantage over the south. Other problems include rising costs, a population whose average age is increasing, and unrealistic expectations for certain interventions such as gene therapy. One necessary response to some of these difficulties, Ruberto submits, will be establishing criteria for withholding certain types of care.

Broadening the American Perspective Early in the twenty-first century, the variety of health-care systems around the world all face significant financial and other challenges. As Americans reflect on the shape of our own health-care system, and how it might be changed, reflections will improve by being well-informed. Surprisingly, many discussions in the United States assume that the major goals of health care, such as the five discussed in this Introduction, cannot be achieved in a harmonious way. Indeed, Americans often assume that the two major goals of universal access and reasonable cost controls are incompatible. These common assumptions are false, as evidence from around the world amply demonstrates. While no system is free of significant difficulties, widely accepted goals of health care are achievable. The question for Americans, then, is how much longer we will tolerate a system that often seems to favor the interests of big business and other special-interest groups more than the interests of patients and society as a whole. If the answer is "not much longer," then the really difficult—and largely political—challenge is to identify and start moving down the path to meaningful reform.

D.D.

NOTES

1 Institute of Medicine, *Insuring America's Health: Principles and Recommendations* (Washington, DC: National Academies Press, 2004), p. 1.

2 Information presented in these five paragraphs was gathered from the following sources: George J. Schieber, Jean-Pierre Poullier, and Leslie M. Greenwald, "Health System Performance in OECD Countries, 1980–1992," *Health Affairs* 13 (4) (1994), pp. 100–112; Colleen Grogan, "Deciding on Access and Levels of Care: A Comparison of Canada, Britain, Germany, and the United States," *Journal of Health Politics, Policy, and Law* 17 (Summer 1992), pp. 213–232; Karen Donelan et al., "All Payer, Single Payer, Managed Care, No Payer: Patients' Perspectives in Three Nations," *Health Affairs* 15 (2) (1996), pp. 254–265; Richard B. Saltman and Josep Figueras, "Analyzing the Evidence on European Health-Care Reforms," *Health Affairs* 17 (2) (1998), pp. 85–98; Gerard F. Anderson, Jeremy Hurst, Peter Sori Hussey, and Melissa Jee-Hughes, "Health Spending and Outcomes: Trends in OECD Countries, 1960–1998," *Health Affairs* 19 (3) (2000), pp. 150–157; and David S. Broder, "Our Broken Health Care System," *The Washington Post* (July 15, 2004), p. A23.

3 Washington Post-ABC News Poll, *The Washington Post* (October 20, 2003), p. A17.

4 John Rawls, *A Theory of Justice* (Cambridge, MA: Harvard University Press, 1971).

5 Philosophers have, in fact, emphasized different elements in Rawls's theory of justice in spelling out consequences for health-care allocation. See, e.g., Ronald M. Green, "Health Care and Justice in Contract Theory Perspective," in Robert M. Veatch and Roy Branson, eds., *Ethics and Health Policy* (Cambridge, MA: Ballinger, 1976), pp. 111–126; Norman Daniels, "Health Care Needs and Distributive Justice," *Philosophy and Public Affairs* 10 (Spring 1981), pp. 146–179; and David DeGrazia, "Grounding a Right to Health Care in Self-Respect and Self-Esteem," *Public Affairs Quarterly* 5 (October 1991), pp. 301–318.

6 President's Commission for the Study of Ethical Problems in Medicine and Biomedical and Behavioral Research, *Securing Access to Health Care* (Washington, DC: Government Printing Office, 1983).

7 See Robert Blendon et al., "Satisfaction with Health Systems in Ten Nations," *Health Affairs* 9 (3) (1990), pp. 185–192; and Robert Blendon et al., "Physicians' Perspectives on Caring for Patients in the United States, Canada, and West Germany," *New England Journal of Medicine* 328 (April 8, 1993), pp. 1011–1016.

8 Lawrence D. Brown and Volker E. Amelung, "'Manacled Competition': Market Reforms in German Health Care," *Health Affairs* 18 (2) (1999), pp. 76–91.

9 The information in this paragraph comes from Simon Stevens, "Reform Strategies for the English NHS," *Health Affairs* 23 (May/June 2004), pp. 37–38.

JUSTICE, RIGHTS, AND SOCIETAL OBLIGATIONS

JUSTICE: A PHILOSOPHICAL REVIEW
Allen Buchanan

Buchanan begins by setting out three theoretical approaches to justice: (1) a utilitarian approach, (2) Rawls's theory of justice as fairness, and (3) Nozick's libertarian theory. He confronts each position with several questions about health care. These questions deal with a right to health care, the relative importance of health care or health-care needs vis-à-vis other goods or needs, the relative importance of various forms of health care, and the compatibility of our current health-care system with the demands of justice. Buchanan concludes that none of the three theoretical approaches provides clear answers to all the questions raised and that the application of each depends upon numerous unavailable empirical premises. This leaves a great deal of work to be done in developing an account of justice in health care.

INTRODUCTION

The past decade has seen the burgeoning of bioethics and the resurgence of theorizing about justice. Yet until now these two developments have not been as mutually enriching as one might have hoped. Bioethicists have tended to concentrate on micro issues (moral problems of individual or small group decisionmaking), ignoring fundamental moral questions about the macro structure within which the micro issues arise. Theorists of justice have advanced very general principles but have typically neglected to show how they can illuminate the particular problems we face in health care and other urgent areas.

Micro problems do not exist in an institutional vacuum. The parents of a severely impaired newborn and the attending neonatologist are faced with the decision of whether to treat the infant aggressively or to allow it to die because neonatal intensive care units now exist which make it possible to preserve the lives of infants who previously would have

died. Neonatal intensive care units exist because certain policy decisions have been made which allocated certain social resources to the development of technology for sustaining defective newborns rather than for preventing birth defects. Limiting moral inquiry to the micro issues supports an unreasoned conservatism by failing to examine the health care institutions within which micro problems arise and by not investigating the larger array of institutions of which the health care sector is only one part. Since not only particular actions but also policies and institutions may be just or unjust, serious theorizing about justice forces us to expand the narrow focus of the micro approach by raising fundamental queries about the background social, economic, and political institutions from which micro problems emerge.

On the other hand, the attention to individual cases which dominates contemporary bioethics can provide a much needed concrete focus for refining and assessing competing theories of justice. The adequacy or inadequacy of a moral theory cannot be determined by inspecting the principles which constitute it. Instead, rational assessment requires an ongoing process in which general principles are revised and refined through confrontation with the rich complexity of our considered judgments about particular cases, while our judgments about particular cases are gradually structured and modified by our provisional acceptance of general principles. Since our considered judgments about particular cases may often be more sensitive and sure than our assessments of abstract principles, careful attention to accurately described, concrete moral situations is essential for theorizing about justice.

Further, it is not just that the problems of bioethics provide one class of test cases for theories of justice among others: the problems of bioethics are among the most difficult and pressing issues with which a theory of justice must cope. It appears, then, that the continued development of both bioethics and of theorizing about justice in general requires us to explore the problems of justice in health care. In this essay I hope to contribute to that enterprise by first providing a sketch of three major theories of justice and by then attempting to ascertain some of their implications for moral problems in health care.

THEORIES OF JUSTICE

Utilitarianism Utilitarianism purports to be a comprehensive moral theory, of which a utilitarian theory of justice is only one part. There are two main types of comprehensive utilitarian theory: Act and Rule Utilitarianism. Act Utilitarianism defines rightness with respect to particular acts: an act is right if and only if it maximizes utility. Rule Utilitarianism defines rights with respect to rules of action and makes the rightness of particular acts depend upon the rules under which those acts fall. A rule is right if and only if general compliance with that rule (or with a set of rules of which it is an element) maximizes utility, and a particular action is right if and only if it falls under such a rule.

Both Act and Rule Utilitarianism may be versions of either Classic or Average Utilitarianism. Classic Utilitarianism defines the rightness of acts or rules as maximization of *aggregate* utility; Average Utilitarianism defines rightness as maximization of utility *per capita*. The aggregate utility produced by an act or by general compliance with a rule is the sum of the utility produced for each individual affected. Average utility is the aggregate utility divided by the number of individuals affected. 'Utility' is defined as pleasure, satisfaction, happiness, or as the realization of preferences, as the latter are revealed through individuals' choices.

The distinction between Act and Rule Utilitarianism is important for a utilitarian theory of justice, since the latter must include an account of when *institutions* are just. Thus, institutional rules may maximize utility even though those rules do not direct individuals as individuals or as occupants of institutional positions to maximize utility in a case by case fashion. For example, it may be that a judicial system which maximizes utility will do so by including rules which prohibit judges from deciding a case according to their estimates of what would maximize utility in that particular case. Thus the utilitarian justification of a particular action or decision may not be that it maximizes utility, but rather that it falls under some rule of an institution or set of institutions which maximizes utility.[1]

Some utilitarians, such as John Stuart Mill, hold that principles of justice are the most basic moral principles because the utility of adherence to them is especially great. According to this view, utilitarian principles of justice are those utilitarian moral principles which are of such importance that they may be *enforced,* if necessary. Some utilitarians, including Mill perhaps, also hold that among the utilitarian principles of justice are principles specifying individual rights, whether the latter are thought of as enforceable claims which take precedence over appeals to what would maximize utility in the particular case. Indeed, some contemporary rights theorists such as Ronald Dworkin define a (justified) right claim as one which takes precedence over mere appeals to what would maximize utility.

A utilitarian moral theory, then, can include rights principles which themselves prohibit appeals to utility maximization, so long as the justification of those principles is that they are part of an institutional system which maximizes utility. In cases where two or more rights principles conflict, considerations of utility may be invoked to determine which rights principles are to be given priority. Utilitarianism is incompatible with rights only if rights exclude appeals to utility maximization at all levels of justification, including the most basic institutional level. Rights founded ultimately on considerations of utility may be called *derivative,* to distinguish them from rights in the *strict* sense.

Utilitarianism is the most influential version of teleological moral theory. A moral theory is teleological if and only if it defines the good independently of the right and defines the right as that which maximizes the good. Utilitarianism defines the good as happiness (satisfaction, etc.), independently of any account of what is morally right, and then defines the right as that which maximizes the good (either in the particular case or at the institutional level). A moral theory is *deontological* if and only if it is not a teleological theory, i.e., if and only if it either does not define the good independently of the right or does not define the right as that which maximizes the good. Both the second and third theories of justice we shall consider are deontological theories.

John Rawls's Theory: Justice as Fairness In *A Theory of Justice* Rawls pursues two main goals. The first is to set out a small but powerful set of principles of justice which underlie and explain the considered moral judgments we make about particular actions, policies, laws, and institutions. The second is to offer a theory of justice superior to Utilitarianism. These two goals are intimately related for Rawls because he believes that the theory which does a better job of supporting and accounting for our considered judgments is the better theory, other things being equal. The principles of justice Rawls offers are as follows:

1. The principle of greatest equal liberty: Each person is to have an equal right to the most extensive system of equal basic liberties compatible with a similar system of liberty for all ([6], pp. 60, 201–205).

2. The principle of equality of fair opportunity: Offices and positions are to be open to all under conditions of equality of fair opportunity—persons with similar abilities and skills are to have equal access to offices and positions. ([6], pp. 60, 73, 83–89).[2]

3. The difference principle: Social and economic institutions are to be arranged so as to benefit maximally the worst off ([6], pp. 60, 75–83).[3]

The basic liberties referred to in (1) include freedom of speech, freedom of conscience, freedom from arbitrary arrest, the right to hold personal property, and freedom of political participation (the right to vote, to run for office, etc.).

Since the demands of these principles may conflict, some way of ordering them is needed. According to Rawls, (1) is *lexically prior* to (2) and (2) is *lexically prior* to (3). A principle 'P' is lexically prior to a principle 'Q' if and only if we are first to satisfy all the requirements of 'P' before going on to satisfy the requirements of 'Q.' Lexical priority allows no trade-offs between the demands of conflicting principles: the lexically prior principle takes absolute priority.

Rawls notes that "many kinds of things are said to be just or unjust: not only laws, institutions, and social systems, but also particular actions . . . decisions, judgments and imputations. . . ." ([6], p. 7). But he insists that the primary subject of justice is the *basic structure* of society because it exerts a pervasive and profound influence on individuals' life prospects. The basic structure is the entire set of major political, legal, economic, and social institutions. In our society the basic structure includes the Constitution, private ownership of the means of production, competitive markets, and the monogamous family. The basic structure plays a large role in distributing the burdens and benefits of cooperation among members of society.

If the primary subject of justice is the basic structure, then the primary problem of justice is to formulate and justify a set of principles which a just basic structure must satisfy. These principles will specify how the basic structure is to distribute prospects of what Rawls calls *primary goods.* They include the basic liberties (listed above under (2)), as well as powers, authority, opportunities, income, and wealth. Rawls says that primary goods are things that every rational person is presumed to want, because they normally have a use, whatever a person's rational plan of life ([6], p. 62). Principle (1) regulates the distribution of prospects of basic liberties; (2) regulates the distribution of prospects of powers and authority, so far as these are attached to institutional offices and positions, and (3) regulates the distribution of prospects of the other primary goods, including wealth and income. Though the first and second principles require equality, the difference principle allows inequalities so long as the total system of institutions of which they are a part maximizes the prospects of the worst off to the primary goods in question.

Rawls advances three distinct types of justification for his principles of justice. Two appeal to our considered judgments, while the third is based on what he calls the Kantian interpretation of his theory.

The first type of justification rests on the idea, mentioned earlier, that if a set of principles provides the best account of our considered judgments about what is just or unjust, then that is a reason for accepting those principles. A set of principles accounts for our judgments only if those judgments can be derived from the principles, granted the relevant facts for their application.

Rawls's second type of justification maintains that if a set of principles would be chosen under conditions which, according to our considered judgments, are appropriate conditions for choosing principles of justice, then this is a reason for accepting those principles. The second type of justification includes three parts: (1) A set of conditions for choosing principles of justice must be specified. Rawls labels the complete set of conditions the 'original position.' (2) It must be shown that the conditions specified are (according to our considered judgments) the appropriate conditions of choice. (3) It must be shown that Rawls's principles are indeed the principles which would be chosen under those conditions.

Rawls construes the choice of principles of justice as an ideal social contract. "The principles of justice for the basic structure of society are the principles that free and rational persons . . . would accept in an initial situation of equality as defining the fundamental terms of their association" ([6], p. 11). The idea of a social contract has several advantages. First, it allows us to view principles of justice as the object of a *rational collective choice.* Second, the idea of *contractual obligation* is used to emphasize that the choice expresses a basic commitment and that the principles agreed on may be rightly enforced. Third, the idea of a contract as a *voluntary agreement* which set terms for mutual advantage

suggests that the principles of justice should be "such as to draw forth the willing cooperation" ([6], p. 15) of all members of society, including those who are worse off.

The most important elements of the original position for our purposes are a) the characterization of the parties to the contract as individuals who desire to pursue their own life plans effectively and who "have a highest-order interest in how . . . their interests . . . are shaped and regulated by social institutions" ([8], p. 64); b) the 'veil of ignorance,' which is a constraint on the information the parties are able to utilize in choosing principles of justice; and c) the requirement that the principles are to be chosen on the assumption that they will be complied with by all (the universaliz ability condition) ([6], p. 132).

The parties are characterized as desiring to maximize their shares of primary goods, because these goods enable one to implement effectively the widest range of life plans and because at least some of them, such as freedom of speech and of conscience, facilitate one's freedom to choose and revise one's life plan or conception of the good. The parties are to choose "from behind a veil of ignorance" so that information about their own particular characteristics or social positions will not lead to bias in the choice of principles. Thus they are described as not knowing their race, sex, socioeconomic, or political status, or even the nature of their particular conceptions of the good. The informational restriction also helps to insure that the principles chosen will not place avoidable restrictions on the individual's freedom to choose and revise his or her life plan.[4]

Though Rawls offers several arguments to show that his principles would be chosen in the original position, the most striking is the maximin argument. According to this argument, the rational strategy in the original position is to choose that set of principles whose implementation will maximize the minimum share of primary goods which one can receive as a member of society, and principles (1), (2), and (3) will insure the greatest minimal share. Rawls's claim is that because these principles protect one's basic liberties and opportunities and insure an adequate minimum of goods such as wealth and income (even if one should turn out to be among the worst

nal thing is to choose them, rather than ⌐ith one's life prospects by opting for alⸯative principles. In particular, Rawls contends that it would be irrational to reject his principles and allow one's life prospect to be determined by what would maximize utility, since utility maximization might allow severe deprivation or even slavery for some, so long as this contributed sufficiently to the welfare of others.

Rawls raises an important question about this second mode of justification when he notes that this original position is purely hypothetical. Granted that the agreement is never actually entered into, why should we regard the principles as binding? The answer, according to Rawls, is that we do in fact accept the conditions embodied in the original position ([6], p. 21). The following qualification, which Rawls adds immediately after claiming that the conditions which constitute the original position are appropriate for the choice of principles of justice according to our considered judgments, introduces his third type of justification: "Or if we do not [accept the conditions of the original position as appropriate for choosing principles of justice] *then perhaps we can be persuaded to do so by the philosophical reflections*" (emphasis added [6], p. 21). In the Kantian interpretation section of *A Theory of Justice,* Rawls sketches a certain kind of philosophical justification for the conditions which make up the original position (based on Kant's conception of the 'noumenal self' or autonomous agent).

For Kant an autonomous agent's will is determined by rational principles and rational principles are those which can serve as principles for all rational beings, not just for this or that agent, depending upon whether or not he has some particular desire which other rational beings may not have. Rawls invites us to think of the original position as the perspective from which autonomous agents see the world. The original position provides a "procedural interpretation" of Kant's idea of a Realm of Ends or community of "free and equal rational beings." We express our nature as autonomous agents when we act from principles that would be chosen in conditions which reflect that nature ([6], p. 252).

Rawls concludes that, when persons such as you and I accept those principles that would be cho-

sen in the original position, we express our nature as autonomous agents, i.e., we act autonomously. There are three main grounds for this thesis, corresponding to the three features of the original position cited earlier. First, since the veil of ignorance excludes information about any particular desires which a rational agent may or may not have, the choice of principles is not determined by any particular desire. Second, since the parties strive to maximize their share of primary goods, and since primary goods are attractive to them because they facilitate freedom in choosing and revising life plans and because they are flexible means not tied to any particular ends, this is another respect in which their choice is not determined by particular desires. Third, the original position includes the requirement that they will be principles of rational agents in general and not just for agents who happen to have this or that particular desire.

In the *Foundation of the Metaphysics of Morals* Kant advances a moral philosophy which identifies autonomy with rationality [4]. Hence for Kant the question "Why should one express our nature as autonomous agents?" is answered by the thesis that rationality requires it. Thus *if* Rawls's third type of justification succeeds in showing that we best express our autonomy when we accept those principles in the belief that they would be chosen from the original position, and *if* Kant's identification of autonomy with rationality is successful, the result will be a justification of Rawls's principles which is distinct from both the first and second modes of justification. So far as this third type of justification does not make the acceptance of Rawls's principles hinge on whether the principles themselves or the conditions from which they would be chosen match our considered judgments, it is not directly vulnerable either to the charge that Rawls has misconstrued our considered judgments or that congruence with considered judgments, like the appeal to mere consensus, has no justificatory force.

It is important to see that Rawls understands his principles of justice as principles which generate *rights* in what I have called the strict sense. Claims based upon the three principles are to take precedence over considerations of utility and the principles themselves are not justified on the grounds that a basic structure which satisfies them will maximize utility. Moreover, Rawls's theory is not a teleological theory of any kind because it does not define the right as that which maximizes the good, where the good is defined independently of the right. Instead it is perhaps the most influential current instance of a deontological theory.

Nozick's Libertarian Theory There are many versions of libertarian theory, but their characteristic doctrine is that coercion may only be used to prevent or punish physical harm, theft, and fraud, and to enforce contracts. Perhaps the most influential and systematic recent instance of Libertarianism is the theory presented by Robert Nozick in *Anarchy, State, and Utopia* [5]. In Nozick's theory of justice, as in libertarian theories generally, the right to private property is fundamental and determines both the legitimate role of the state and the most basic principles of individual conduct.

Nozick contends that individuals have a property right in their persons and in whatever 'holdings' they come to have through actions which conform to (1) "the principle of justice in [initial] acquisition" and (2) "the principle of justice in transfer" ([5], p. 151). The first principle specifies the ways in which an individual may come to own hitherto unowned things without violating anyone else's rights. Here Nozick largely follows John Locke's famous account of how one makes natural objects one's own by "mixing one's labor" with them or improving them through one's labor. Though Nozick does not actually formulate a principle of justice in (initial) acquisition, he does argue that whatever the appropriate formulation is it must include a 'Lockean Proviso,' which places a constraint on the holdings which one may acquire through one's labor. Nozick maintains that one may appropriate as much of an unowned item as one desires so long as (a) one's appropriation does not worsen the conditions of others in a special way, namely, by creating a situation in which others are "no longer . . . able to use freely [without exclusively appropriating] what [they] . . . previously could" or (b) one properly compensates those whose condition is worsened by one's appropriation in the way specified in (a) ([5], pp. 178–179). Nozick emphasizes that the Proviso

only picks out one way in which one's appropriation may worsen the condition of others; it does not forbid appropriation or require compensation in cases in which one's appropriation of an unowned thing worsens another's condition merely by limiting his opportunities to appropriate (rather than merely use) that thing, i.e., to make it his property.

The second principle states that one may justly transfer one's legitimate holdings to another through sale, trade, gift or bequest and that one is entitled to whatever one receives in any of these ways, so long as the person from whom one receives it was entitled to that which he transferred to you. The right to property which Nozick advances is the right to exclusive control over anything one can get through initial appropriation (subject to the Lockean Proviso) or through voluntary exchanges with others entitled to what they transfer. Nozick concludes that a distribution is just if and only if it arose from another just distribution by legitimate means. The principle of justice in initial acquisition specifies the legitimate 'first moves,' while the principle of justice in transfers specifies the legitimate ways of moving from one distribution to another: "Whatever arises from a just situation by just steps is itself just" ([5], p. 151).

Since not all existing holdings arose through the 'just steps' specified by the principles of justice in acquisition and transfer, there will be a need for a *principle of rectification* of past injustices. Though Nozick does not attempt to formulate such a principle he thinks that it might well require significant redistribution of holdings.

Apart from the case of rectifying past violations of the principles of acquisition and transfer, however, Nozick's theory is strikingly anti-redistributive. Nozick contends that attempts to force anyone to contribute any part of his legitimate holdings to the welfare of others is a violation of that person's property rights, whether it is undertaken by private individuals or the state. On this view, coercively backed taxation to raise funds for welfare programs of any kind is literally theft. Thus, a large proportion of the activities now engaged in by the government involve gross injustices.

After stating his theory of rights, Nozick tries to show that the state is legitimate so long as it limits

its activities to the enforcement of these rights and eschews redistributive functions. To do this he employs an 'invisible hand explanation,' which purports to show how the minimal state could arise as an unintended consequence of a series of voluntary transactions which violate no one's rights. The phrase 'invisible hand explanation' is chosen to stress that the process by which the minimal state could emerge fits Adam Smith's famous account of how individuals freely pursuing their own private ends in the market collectively produce benefits which are not the aim of anyone.

The process by which the minimal state could arise without violating anyone's rights is said to include four main steps ([5], pp. 10–25).[5] First, individuals in a 'state of nature' in which (Libertarian) moral principles are generally respected would form a plurality of 'protective agencies' to enforce their libertarian rights, since individual efforts at enforcement would be inefficient and liable to abuse. Second, through competition for clients, a 'dominant protective agency' would eventually emerge in given geographical area. Third, such an agency would eventually become a 'minimal state' by asserting a claim of monopoly over protective services in order to prevent less reliable efforts at enforcement which might endanger its clients: it would forbid 'independents' (those who refused to purchase its services) from seeking other forms of enforcement. Fourth, again assuming that correct moral principles are generally followed, those belonging to the dominant protective agency would compensate the 'independents,' presumably by providing them with free or partially subsidized protection services. With the exception of taxing its clients to provide compensation for the independents, the minimal state would act only to protect persons against physical injury, theft, fraud, and violations of contracts.

It is striking that Nozick does not attempt to provide any systematic *justification* for the Lockean rights principles he advocates. In this respect he departs radically from Rawls. Instead, Nozick assumes the correctness of the Lockean principles and then, on the basis of that assumption, argues that the minimal state and only the minimal state is compatible with the rights those principles specify.

He does, however, offer some arguments against the more-than-minimal state which purport to be independent of that particular theory of property rights which he assumes. These arguments may provide indirect support for his principles insofar as they are designed to make alternative principles, such as Rawls's, unattractive. Perhaps most important of these is an argument designed to show that any principle of justice which demands a certain distributive end state or pattern of holdings will require frequent and gross disruptions of individuals' holdings for the sake of maintaining that end state or pattern. Nozick supports this general conclusion by a vivid example. He asks us to suppose that there is some distribution of holdings 'D_1' which is required by some end-state or patterned theory of justice and that 'D_1'is achieved at time 'T.' Now suppose that Wilt Chamberlain, the renowned basketball player, signs a contract stipulating that he is to receive twenty-five cents from the price of each ticket to the home games in which he performs, and suppose that he nets $250,000, from this arrangement. We now have a new distribution 'D_2.' Is 'D_2' unjust? Notice that by hypothesis those who paid the price of admission were entitled to control over the resources they held in 'D_1' (as were Chamberlain and the team's owners). The new distribution arose through *voluntary exchanges of legitimate holdings,* so it is difficult to see how it could be unjust, even if it does diverge from 'D_1.' From this and like examples, Nozick concludes that attempts to maintain any end-state or patterned distributive principle would require continuous interference in peoples' lives ([5], pp. 161–163).

As in the cases of Utilitarianism and Rawls's theory, Nozick and libertarians generally do not limit morality to justice. Thus, Nozick and others emphasize that a libertarian theory of individual rights is to be supplemented by a libertarian theory of virtues which recognizes that not all moral principles are suitable objects of enforcement and that moral life includes more than the nonviolation of rights. Libertarians invoke the distinction between justice and charity to reply to those who complain that a Lockean theory of property rights legitimizes crushing poverty for millions. They stress that while justice demands that we not be *forced* to contribute to the well-being of others, charity requires that we help even those who have no *right* to our aid.[6]

IMPLICATIONS FOR HEALTH CARE

Now that we have a grasp of the main ideas of three major theories of justice, we can explore briefly some of their implications for health care. To do this we may confront the theories with four questions:

1. Is there a right to health care? (If so, what is its basis and what is its content?)

2. How, in order of priority, is health care related to other goods, or how are health care needs related to other needs? (If there is a right to health care, how is it related to other rights?)

3. How, in order of priority, are various forms of health care related to one another?

4. What can we conclude about the justice or injustice of the current health care system?

In some cases, as we shall see, the theories will provide opposing answers to the same question; in others, the theories may be unhelpfully silent.

We have already seen that the Utilitarian position on rights in general is complex. If by a right we mean a right in the strict sense, i.e., a claim which takes precedence over mere appeals to utility at all levels, including the most basic institutional level, then Utilitarianism denies the existence of rights in general, including the right to health care. If, on the other hand, we mean by right a claim that takes precedence over mere appeals to utility at the level of particular actions or at some institutional level short of the most basic, but which is justified ultimately by appeal to the utility of the total set of institutions, then Utilitarianism does not exclude, and indeed may even require rights, including a right to health care. Whether or not the total institutional array which maximizes utility will include a right to health care will depend upon a wealth of *empirical facts* not deducible from the principle of utility itself. The nature and complexity of the relevant facts can best be appreciated by considering briefly the bearing of Utilitarianism on questions (2) and (3). A utilitarian system of (derivative) rights will pick out certain goods as those which make an especially

large contribution to the maximization of utility. It is reasonable to assume, on the basis of empirical data, that health care, or at least certain forms of health care, is among them. Consider, for example, prenatal care, broadly conceived as including genetic screening and counseling (at least for special risk groups), prenatal nutritional care and medical examinations for expectant mothers, medical care during delivery, and basic pediatric services in the crucial months after birth. If empirical research indicates (1) that a system of institutional arrangements which maximizes utility would include such services and (2) that such services can best be assured if they are accorded the status of a right, with all that this implies, including the use of coercive sanctions where necessary, then according to Utilitarianism there is such a (derivative) right. The strength and content of this right relative to other (derivative) rights will be determined by the utility of health care as compared with other kinds of goods.

It is crucial to note that, for the utilitarian, empirical research must determine not only whether certain health care services are to be provided as a matter of right, but also whether the right in question is to be an equal right enjoyed by all persons. No commitment to equality of rights is included in the utilitarian principle itself, nor is there any commitment to equal distribution of any kind. Utilitarianism is egalitarian only in the sense that in calculating what will maximize utility each person's welfare is to be included.

Utilitarian arguments, sometimes based on empirical data, have been advanced to show that providing health care free of charge as a matter of right would encourage wasteful use of scarce and costly resources because the individual would have no incentive to restrain his 'consumption' of health care. The cumulative result, it is said, would be quite disutilitarian: a breakdown of the health care system or a disastrous curtailment of other basic services to cover the spiraling costs of health care. In contrast (proponents of this argument continue) a *market* in health care encourages 'consumers' to use resources wisely because the costs of the services an individual receives are borne by that individual.

On the other side of the utilitarian ledger, empirical evidence may be marshalled to show that the benefits of a right to health care outweigh the costs, including the costs of possible over-use, and that a market in health care would not maximize utility because those who need health care the most may not be able to afford it.

Similarly, even if there is a utilitarian justification for a right to health care, empirical evidence must again be presented to show that it should be an equal right. For it is certainly conceivable that, under certain circumstances at least, utility could be maximized by providing extensive health care only for some groups, perhaps even a minority, rather than for all persons.

Utilitarians who advocate a right to health care often argue that this right, like other basic rights, should be equal, on the basis of the assumption of diminishing marginal utility. The idea, roughly, is that with respect to many goods, including health care, there is a finite upper bound to the satisfaction a person can gain from being provided with additional amounts of the goods in question. Hence, if in general we are all subject to the phenomenon of diminishing marginal utility in the case of health care and if the threshold of diminishing marginal utility is in general sufficiently low, then there are sound utilitarian reasons for distributing health care equally.

Finally, it should be clear that for the utilitarian the issue of priorities within health care, as well as that of priorities between health care and other goods, must again be settled by empirical research. If, as seems likely, utility maximization requires more resources for prevention and health maintenance rather than for curative intervention after pathology has already developed, then this will be reflected in the content of the utilitarian right to health care. If, as many writers have contended, the current emphasis in the U.S. on high technology intervention produces less utility than would a system which stresses prevention and health maintenance (for example through stricter control of pollution and other environmental determinants of disease), then the utilitarian may conclude that the current system is unjust in this respect. Empirical data would also be needed to ascertain whether more social resources should be devoted to high- or low-technology intervention: for example, neonatal intensive care units versus 'well-baby clinics.' These

examples are intended merely to illustrate the breadth and complexity of the empirical research needed to apply Utilitarianism to crucial issues in health care.

Libertarian theories such as Nozick's rely much less heavily upon empirical premises for answers to questions (1)–(4). Since the libertarian is interested only in preventing violations of libertarian rights, and since the latter are rights against certain sorts of interferences rather than rights to be provided with anything, the question of what will maximize utility is irrelevant. Further, any effort to implement any right to health care whatsoever is an injustice, according to the libertarian.

There are only two points at which empirical data are relevant for Nozick. First, whether or not any current case of appropriation of hitherto unheld things satisfies the Lockean Proviso is a matter of fact to be ascertained by empirical methods. Second, empirical historical research is needed to determine what sort of redistribution for the sake of rectifying past injustices is necessary. If, for example, physicians' higher incomes are due in part to government policies which violate libertarian rights, then rectificatory redistribution may be required. And indeed libertarians have argued that two basic features of the current health care system do involve gross violations of libertarian rights. First, compulsory taxation to provide equipment, hospital facilities, research funds, and educational subsidies for medical personnel is literally theft. Second, some argue that government enforced occupational licensing laws which prohibit all but the established forms of medical practice violate the right to freedom of contract [3]. Those who raise this second objection also usually argue that the function of such laws is to secure a monopoly for the medical establishment while sharply limiting the supply of doctors so as to keep medical fees artificially high. Whether or not such arguments are sound it is important to note that Libertarianism is not to be confused with Conservatism. A theory which would institute a free market in medical services, abolish government subsidies, and reduce government regulation of medical practice to the prevention of injury and fraud and the enforcement of contracts has radical implications for changing the current system.

Libertarianism offers straightforward answers to questions (2) and (3). Even if it can be shown that health care in general, and certain forms of health care more than others, are especially important for the happiness or even the freedom of most persons, this fact is quite irrelevant from the perspective of a libertarian theory of justice, though it is no doubt significant for the libertarian concerned with charity or other virtues which exceed the requirements of justice. Nozick and other libertarians recognize that a free market in medical services may in fact produce severe inequalities and that there is no assurance that all or even most will be able to afford adequate medical care. Though the humane libertarian will find this condition unfortunate and will aid those in need and encourage others to do likewise voluntarily, he remains adamant that no one has a right to health care and that hence none may rightly be forced to aid another.

According to Rawls, the most basic questions about health care are not to be decided either by consideration of utility or by market processes. Instead they are to be settled ultimately by appeal to those principles of justice which would be chosen in the original position. As we shall see, however, the implications of Rawls's principles for health care are far from clear.[7]

No principle explicitly specifying a right to health care is included among Rawls's principles of justice. Further, since those principles are intended to regulate the basic structure of society as a whole, they are not themselves intended to guide the decisions individuals make in particular health care situations, nor are they themselves to be applied directly to health care institutions. We are not to assume that either individual physicians or administrators of particular policies or programs are to attempt to allocate health care so as to maximize the prospects of the worst off. In Rawls's theory, as in Utilitarianism, the rightness or wrongness of particular actions or policies depends ultimately upon the nature of the entire institutional structure within which they exist. Hence, Rawls's theory can provide us with fruitful answers at the micro level only if its implications at the macro level are adequately developed.

If Rawls's theory includes a right to health care, it must be a right which is in some way derivative upon the basic rights laid down by the Principle of Greatest Equal Liberty, the Principle of Equality of Fair Opportunity, and the Difference Principle. And if there is to be such a derivative right to health care, then health care must either be among the primary goods covered by the three principles or it must be importantly connected with some of those goods. Now at least some forms of health care (such as broad services for prevention and health maintenance, including mental health) seem to share the earmarks of Rawlsian primary goods: they facilitate the effective pursuit of ends in general and may also enhance our ability to criticize and revise our conceptions of the good. Nonetheless, Rawls does not explicitly list health care among the social primary goods included under the three principles. However, he does include wealth under the Difference Principle and defines it so broadly that it might be thought to include access to health care services. In "Fairness to Goodness" Rawls defines wealth as virtually any legally exchangeable social asset; this would cover health care 'vouchers' if they could be cashed or exchanged for other goods ([7], p. 540).

Let us suppose that health care is either itself a primary good covered by the Difference Principle or that health care may be purchased with income or some other form of wealth which is included under the Difference Principle. In the former case, depending upon various empirical conditions, it might turn out that the best way to insure that the basic structure satisfies the Difference Principle is to establish a state-enforced right to health care. But whether maximizing the prospects of the worst off will require such a right and what the content of the right will be will depend upon what weight is to be assigned to health care relative to other primary goods included under the Difference Principle. Similarly, a weighting must also be assigned if we are to determine whether the share of wealth one receives under the Difference Principle would be sufficient both for health care needs and for other ends. Unfortunately, though Rawls acknowledges that a weighted index of primary goods is needed if we are to be able to determine what would maximize the prospects of the worst off, he offers no account of how the weighting is to be achieved.

The problem is especially acute in the case of health care, because some forms of health care are so costly that an unrestrained commitment to them would undercut any serious commitment to providing other important goods. Thus, it appears that until we have some solution to the weighting problem Rawls's theory can shed only a limited light upon the question of priority relations between health care and other goods and among various forms of health care. Rawls's conception of primary goods may explain what distinguishes health care from those things that are not primary goods, but this is clearly not sufficient.

Perhaps because he is aware of the exorbitant demands which certain health care needs may place upon social resources, Rawls stipulates that the parties in the original position are to choose principles of justice on the assumption that their needs fall within the 'normal range' ([9], pp. 9–10). His ideal may be that the satisfaction of extremely costly special needs for health care may not be a matter of justice but rather of *charity*. If some reasonable way of drawing the line between 'normal' needs which fall within the gambit of principles of justice and 'special' needs which are the proper object of the virtue of charity could be developed, then this would be a step towards solving the priority problems mentioned above.

It has been suggested that the Principle of Equality of Fair Opportunity, rather than the Difference Principle, might provide the basis for a Rawlsian right to health care ([2], pp. 16–18). While I cannot accord this proposal the consideration it deserves here, I wish to point out that there are four difficulties which make it problematic. First, priority problems still remain. For now we are faced with the task of assigning a weight to health care relative to those other factors (such as education) which are also determinants of opportunity. Further, since the Principle of Equality of Fair Opportunity is lexically prior to the Difference Principle, we must again face the prospect that commitment to the former principle might swallow up social resources needed for providing important goods included under the latter.

Second, because it refers only to opportunities for occupying social *positions* and *offices,* rather than to opportunities in general, the Principle of Equality of Fair Opportunity might be thought too narrow to provide an adequate foundation for a right to health care. Rawls might respond either by defining 'position' rather broadly or by arguing that opportunities for attaining positions and offices are related to opportunities in general in such a way that equality in the former insures equality in the latter.

Third, and more importantly, Rawls's Principle of Equality of Fair Opportunity takes 'abilities' and 'skills' as given, requiring only that persons with equal or similar abilities and skills are to have equal prospects of attaining social positions and offices. Yet clearly inequalities in health care can produce severe inequalities in abilities and skills. For example, poor nutrition and medical care during gestation can result in mental retardation, and many health problems hinder the development of skills and abilities. Hence it might be argued that if the Principle of Opportunity is to provide an adequate basis for a right to health care it must be reformulated to capture the crucial influence of health care or the lack of it upon individual development.

Each of the theories of justice under consideration offers a theoretical basis for answering some basic questions concerning justice in health care. We have seen, however, that none of them provides unambiguous answers to all of the questions and that each depends for its application upon a wealth of empirical premises, many of which may not now be available. Each theory does at least rule out some answers and each supplies us with a perspective from which to pursue issues which we cannot ignore. Nonetheless, almost all of the work in developing an account of justice in health care remains to be done.[8]

NOTES

1 In this essay I shall be concerned for the most part with utilitarianism at the institutional level, and I shall proceed on the assumption that a set of institutions which maximizes utility will include rules which bar other direct applications of the principle of utility itself. Consequently, I will mainly be concerned with Rule Utilitarianism, rather than Act Utilitarianism (the latter being the view that the rightness or wrongness of a given act depends solely upon whether it maximizes utility). For an original and interesting attempt to show that Act Utilitarianism is compatible with social norms that bar direct appeals to utility, see [10].

2 Rawls sometimes refers to the "Principle of Equality of Fair Opportunity" and sometimes to the "Principle of Fair Equality of Opportunity." For convenience I will stay with the former label.

3 The phrase "worst off" refers to those who are worst off with respect to prospects of the social primary goods regulated by the Difference Principle.

4 For a detailed elaboration of this point, see [1].

5 For a fundamental objection to Nozick's invisible hand explanation, see [11].

6 P. Singer [12], expanding an argument developed earlier by R. Titmuss, argues that the existence of markets for certain goods may in fact undermine the motivation for charity.

7 See [2].

8 I would like to thank Earl Shelp and William Hanson for their very helpful comments on an earlier draft of this paper.

REFERENCES

1 Buchanan, A. "Revisability and Rational Choice." *Canadian Journal of Philosophy* 5:395–408, 1975.

2 Daniels, N. "Rights to Health Care and Distributive Justice: Programmatic Worries." *Journal of Medicine and Philosophy* 4:174–191, 1979.

3 Friedman, M. *Capitalism and Freedom.* Chicago: University of Chicago Press, 1962, pp. 137–160.

4 Kant, I *Foundations of the Metaphysics of Morals* (transl. by L. W. Beck), New York: Bobbs-Merrill, 1959, Part III.

5 Nozick, R. *Anarchy, State and Utopia.* New York: Basic Books, 1974.

6 Rawls, J. *A Theory of Justice.* Cambridge, Mass.: Harvard University Press, 1971.

7 Rawls, J. "Fairness to Goodness." *Philosophical Review* 84:536–554, 1975.

8 Rawls, J. "Reply to Alexander and Musgrave." *Quarterly Journal of Economics* 88:633–655, November 1974.

9 Rawls, J. "Responsibility for Ends." Stanford University, Unpublished Lecture, 1979.

10 Sartorius, R. *Individual Conduct and Social Norms.* Encino, Calif.: Dickenson Publishing, 1975.

11 Sartorius, R. "The Limits of Libertarianism." In *Liberty and the Rule of Law,* edited by R. L. Cunningham, 87–131. College Station, Texas: Texas A and M University Press, 1979.

12 Singer, P. "Rights and the Market." In *Justice and Economic Distribution,* edited by J. Arthur and W. Shaw, pp. 207–221. Englewood Cliffs, N.J.: Prentice-Hall, 1978.

AUTONOMY, EQUALITY AND A JUST HEALTH CARE SYSTEM
Kai Nielsen

According to Nielsen, justice requires social institutions that work on the premise of moral equality—the life of everyone matters and matters equally. Beginning with this premise and an analysis of basic needs, Nielsen argues that individuals have a moral right to have their health-care needs met. Furthermore, on his account, a commitment to egalitarianism is incompatible with a two- or three-tier system of medical care. Moral equality requires the open and free provision of medical treatment of the same extent and quality to everyone in society. In his view, a system intended to achieve this end would have to take medicine out of the private sector altogether and place both the ownership and control of medicine in the public sector.

I

Autonomy and equality are both fundamental values in our firmament of values, and they are frequently thought to be in conflict. Indeed the standard liberal view is that we must make difficult and often morally ambiguous trade-offs between them.[1] I shall argue that this common view is mistaken and that

Reprinted with permission of the publisher from *The International Journal of Applied Philosophy,* vol. 4 (Spring 1989), pp. 39–44.

autonomy cannot be widespread or secure in a society which is not egalitarian: where, that is, equality is not also a very fundamental value which has an operative role within the society.[2] I shall further argue that, given human needs and a commitment to an autonomy respecting egalitarianism, a very different health care system would come into being than that which exists at present in the United States.

I shall first turn to a discussion of autonomy and equality and then, in terms of those conceptions, to a conception of justice. In modernizing societies of Western Europe, a perfectly just society will be a society of equals and in such societies there will be a belief held across the political spectrum in what has been called *moral* equality. That is to say, when viewed with the impartiality required by morality, the life of everyone matters and matters equally.[3] Individuals will, of course, and rightly so, have their local attachments but they will acknowledge that justice requires that the social institutions of the society should be such that they work on the premise that the life of everyone matters and matters equally. Some privileged elite or other group cannot be given special treatment simply because they are that group. Moreover, for there to be a society of equals there must be a rough equality of condition in the society. Power must be sufficiently equally shared for it to be securely the case that no group or class or gender can dominate others through the social structures either by means of their frequently thoroughly unacknowledged latent functions or more explicitly and manifestly by institutional arrangements sanctioned by law or custom. Roughly equal material resources or power are not things which are desirable in themselves, but they are essential instrumentalities for the very possibility of equal well-being and for as many people as possible having as thorough and as complete a control over their own lives as is compatible with this being true for everyone alike. Liberty cannot flourish without something approaching this equality of condition, and people without autonomous lives will surely live impoverished lives. These are mere commonplaces. In fine, a commitment to achieving equality of condition, far from undermining liberty and autonomy, is essential for their extensive flourishing.

If we genuinely believe in moral equality, we will want to see come into existence a world in which all people capable of self-direction have, and have as nearly as is feasible equally, control over their own lives and can, as far as the institutional arrangements for it obtaining are concerned, all live flourishing lives where their needs and desires as individuals are met as fully as possible and as fully and extensively as is compatible with that possibility being open to everyone alike. The thing is to provide institutional arrangements that are conducive to that.

People, we need to remind ourselves, plainly have different capacities and sensibilities. However, even in the extreme case of people for whom little in the way of human flourishing is possible, their needs and desires, as far as possible, should still also be satisfied in the way I have just described. Everyone in this respect at least has equal moral standing. No preference or pride of place should be given to those capable, in varying degrees, of rational self-direction. The more rational, or, for that matter, the more loveable, among us should not be given preference. No one should. Our needs should determine what is to be done.

People committed to achieving and sustaining a society of equals will seek to bring into stable existence conditions such that it would be possible for everyone, if they were personally capable of it, to enjoy an equally worthwhile and satisfying life or at least a life in which, for all of them, their needs, starting with and giving priority to their more urgent needs, were met and met as equally and as fully as possible, even where their needs are not entirely the same needs. This, at least, is the heuristic, though we might, to gain something more nearly feasible, have to scale down talk of meeting needs to providing conditions propitious for the equal satisfaction for everyone of their *basic* needs. Believers in equality want to see a world in which everyone, as far as this is possible, have equal whole life prospects. This requires an equal consideration of their needs and interests and a refusal to just override anyone's interests: to just regard anyone's interests as something which comes to naught, which can simply be set aside as expendable. Minimally, an egalitarian must believe that taking the moral point of view requires that each person's good is afforded equal consideration. Moreover, this is not just a bit of egalitarian ideology but is a deeply embedded considered judgment in modern Western culture capable of being put into wide reflective equilibrium.[4]

II

What is a need, how do we identify needs and what are our really basic needs, needs that are presumptively universal? Do these basic needs in most circumstances at least trump our other needs and our reflective considered preferences?

Let us start this examination by asking if we can come up with a list of universal needs correctly ascribable to all human beings in all cultures. In doing this we should, as David Braybrooke has, distinguish *adventitious* and *course-of-life* needs.[5] Moreover, it is the latter that it is essential to focus on. Adventitious needs, like the need for a really good fly rod or computer, come and go with particular projects. Course-of-life needs, such as the need for exercise, sleep or food, are such that every human being may be expected to have them all at least at some stage of life.

Still, we need to step back a bit and ask: how do we determine what is a need, course-of-life need or otherwise? We need a relational formula to spot needs. We say, where we are speaking of needs, B needs x in order to y, as in Janet needs milk or some other form of calcium in order to protect her bone structure. With course-of-life needs the relation comes our platitudinously as in 'People need food and water in order to live' or 'People need exercise in order to function normally or well.' This, in the very identification of the need, refers to human flourishing or to human well-being, thereby giving to understand that they are basic needs. Perhaps it is better to say instead that this is to specify in part what it is for something to be a basic need. Be that as it may, there are these basic needs we *must* have to live well. If this is really so, then, where they are things we as individuals can have without jeopardy to others, no further question arises, or can arise, about the desirability of satisfying them. They are just things that in such circumstances ought to be met in our lives if they can. The satisfying of such needs is an unequivocally good thing. The questions 'Does Janet need to live?' and 'Does Sven need to function well?' are at best otiose.

In this context David Braybrooke has quite properly remarked that being "essential to living or to functioning normally may be taken as a criterion for being a basic need. Questions about whether needs are genuine, or well-founded, come to an end of the line when the needs have been connected with life or health."[6] Certainly to flourish we must have these things and in some instances they must be met at least to a certain extent even to survive. This being so, we can quite properly call them basic needs.

Where these needs do not clash or the satisfying of them by one person does not conflict with the satisfying of the equally basic needs of another no question about justifying the meeting of them arises.

By linking the identification of needs with what we must have to function well and linking course-of-life and basic needs with what all people, or at least almost all people, must have to function well, a list of basic needs can readily be set out. I shall give such a list, though surely the list is incomplete. However, what will be added is the same sort of thing similarly identified. First there are needs connected closely to our physical functioning, namely the need for food and water, the need for excretion, for exercise, for rest (including sleep), for a life supporting relation to the environment, and the need for whatever is indispensable to preserve the body intact. Similarly there are basic needs connected with our function as social beings. We have needs for companionship, education, social acceptance and recognition, for sexual activity, freedom from harassment, freedom from domination, for some meaningful work, for recreation and relaxation and the like.[7]

The list, as I remarked initially, is surely incomplete. But it does catch many of the basic things which are in fact necessary for us to live or to function well. Now an autonomy respecting egalitarian society with an interest in the well-being of its citizens—something moral beings could hardly be without—would (trivially) be a society of equals, and as a society of equals it would be committed to (a) *moral* equality and (b) an equality of *condition* which would, under conditions of moderate abundance, in turn expect the equality of condition to be rough and to be principally understood (cashed in) in terms of providing the conditions (as far as that is possible) for meeting the needs (including most centrally the basic needs) of everyone and meeting them equally, as far as either of these things is feasible.

III

What kind of health care system would such an autonomy respecting egalitarian society have under conditions of moderate abundance such as we find in Canada and the United States?

The following are health care needs which are also basic needs: being healthy and having conditions treated which impede one's functioning well or which adversely affect one's well-being or cause suffering. These are plainly things we need. Where societies have the economic and technical capacity to do so, as these societies plainly do, without undermining other equally urgent or more urgent needs, these health needs, as basic needs, must be met, and the right to have such medical care is a right for everyone in the society regardless of her capacity to pay. This just follows from a commitment to *moral* equality and to an equality of condition. Where we have the belief, a belief which is very basic in non-fascistic modernizing societies, that each person's good is to be given equal consideration, it is hard not to go in that way, given a plausible conception of needs and reasonable list of needs based on that conception.[8] If there is the need for some particular regime of care and the society has the resources to meet that need, without undermining structures protecting other at least equally urgent needs, then, *ceteris paribus,* the society, if it is a decent society, must do so. The commitment to more equality—the commitment to the belief that the life of each person matters and matters equally—entails, given a few plausible empirical premises, that each person's health needs will be the object of an equal regard. Each has an equal claim *prima facie,* to have her needs satisfied where this is possible. That does not, of course, mean that people should all be treated alike in the sense of their all getting the same thing. Not everyone needs flu shots, braces, a dialysis machine, a psychiatrist, or a triple bypass. What should be equal is that each person's health needs should be the object of equal societal concern since each person's good should be given equal consideration.[9] This does not mean that equal energy should be directed to Hans's rash as to Frank's cancer. Here one person's need for a cure is much greater than the other, and the greater need clearly takes precedence. Both should be met where possible, but where they both cannot then the greater need has pride of place. But what should not count in the treatment of Hans and Frank is that Hans is wealthy or prestigious or creative and Frank is not. Everyone should have their health needs met where possible. Moreover, where the need is the same, they should have (where possible), and where other at least equally urgent

needs are not thereby undermined, the same quality treatment. No differentiation should be made between them on the basis of their ability to pay or on the basis of their being (one more so than the other) important people. There should, in short, where this is possible, be open and free medical treatment of the same quality and extent available to everyone in the society. And no two- or three-tier system should be allowed to obtain, and treatment should only vary (subject to the above qualification) on the basis of variable needs and unavoidable differences in different places in supply and personnel, e.g., differences between town and country. Furthermore, these latter differences should be remedied where technically and economically feasible. The underlying aim should be to meet the health care needs of everyone and meet them, in the sense explicated, equally: everybody's needs here should be met as fully as possible; different treatment is only justified where the need is different or where both needs cannot be met. Special treatment for one person rather than another is only justified where, as I remarked, both needs cannot be met or cannot as adequately be met. Constrained by ought implies can, where these circumstances obtain, priority should be given to the greater need that can feasibly be met. A moral system or a social policy, plainly, cannot be reasonably asked to do the impossible. But my account does not ask that.

To have such a health care system would, I think, involve taking medicine out of the private sector altogether including, of course, out of private entrepreneurship where the governing rationale has to be profit and where supply and demand rules the roost. Instead there must be a health care system firmly in the public sector (publicly owned and controlled) where the rationale of the system is to meet as efficiently and as fully as possible the health care needs of everyone in the society in question. The health care system should not be viewed as a business anymore than a university should be viewed as a business—compare a university and a large hospital—but as a set of institutions and practices designed to meet urgent human needs.

I do not mean that we should ignore costs or efficiency. The state-run railroad system in Switzerland, to argue by analogy, is very efficient. The state cannot, of course, ignore costs in running it. But the aim is not to make a profit. The aim is to produce the most rapid, safe, efficient and comfortable service meeting travellers' needs within the parameters of the overall socioeconomic priorities of the state and the society. Moreover, since the state in question is a democracy, if its citizens do not like the policies of the government here (or elsewhere) they can replace it with a government with different priorities and policies. Indeed the option is there (probably never to be exercised) to shift the railroad into the private sector.

Governments, understandably, worry with aging populations about mounting health care costs. This is slightly ludicrous in the United States, given its military and space exploration budgets, but is also a reality in Canada and even in Iceland where there is no military or space budget at all. There should, of course, be concern about containing health costs, but this can be done effectively with a state-run system. Modern societies need systems of socialized medicine, something that obtains in almost all civilized modernizing societies. The United States and South Africa are, I believe, the only exceptions. But, as is evident from my own country (Canada), socialized health care systems often need altering, and their costs need monitoring. As a cost-cutting and as an efficiency measure that would at the same time improve health care, doctors, like university professors and government bureaucrats, should be put on salaries and they should work in medical units. They should, I hasten to add, have good salaries but salaries all the same; the last vestiges of petty entrepreneurship should be taken from the medical profession. This measure would save the state-run health care system a considerable amount of money, would improve the quality of medical care with greater cooperation and consultation resulting from economies of scale and a more extensive division of labor with larger and better equipped medical units. (There would also be less duplication of equipment.) The overall quality of care would also improve with a better balance between health care in the country and in the large cities, with doctors being systematically and rationally deployed throughout the society. In such a system doctors, no more than university professors or state bureaucrats, could

not just set up a practice anywhere. They would no more be free to do this than university professors or state bureaucrats. In the altered system there would be no cultural space for it. Placing doctors on salary, though not at a piece work rate, would also result in its being the case that the financial need to see as many patients as possible as quickly as possible would be removed. This would plainly enhance the quality of medical care. It would also be the case that a different sort of person would go into the medical profession. People would go into it more frequently because they were actually interested in medicine and less frequently because this is a rather good way (though hardly the best way) of building a stock portfolio.

There should also be a rethinking of the respective roles of nurses (in all their variety), paramedics and doctors. Much more of the routine work done in medicine—taking the trout fly out of my ear for example—can be done by nurses or paramedics. Doctors, with their more extensive training, could be freed up for other more demanding tasks worthy of their expertise. This would require somewhat different training for all of these different medical personnel and a rethinking of the authority structure in the health care system. But doing this in a reasonable way would improve the teamwork in hospitals, make morale all around a lot better, improve medical treatment and save a very considerable amount of money. (It is no secret that the relations between doctors and nurses are not good.) Finally, a far greater emphasis should be placed on preventive medicine than is done now. This, if really extensively done, utilizing the considerable educational and fiscal powers of the state, would result in very considerable health care savings and a very much healthier and perhaps even happier population. (Whether with the states we actually have we are likely to get anything like that is— to understate it—questionable. I wouldn't hold my breath in the United States. Still, Finland and Sweden are very different places from the United States and South Africa.)

IV

It is moves of this *general* sort that an egalitarian and autonomy loving society under conditions of moderate scarcity should implement. (I say 'general sort' for I am more likely to be wrong about some of the specifics than about the general thrust of my argument.) It would, if in place, limit the freedom of some people, including some doctors and some patients, to do what they want to do. That is obvious enough. But any society, and society at all, as long as it had norms (legal and otherwise) will limit freedom in some way.[10] There is no living in society without some limitation on the freedom to do some things. Indeed a society without norms and thus without any limitation on freedom is a contradiction in terms. Such a mass of people wouldn't be a society. They, without norms, would just be a mass of people. (If these are 'grammatical remarks,' make the most of them.) In our societies I am not free to go for a spin in your car without your permission, to practice law or medicine without a license, to marry your wife while she is still your wife and the like. Many restrictions on our liberties, because they are so common, so widely accepted and thought by most of us to be so reasonable, hardly *seem* like restrictions on our liberty. But they are all the same. No doubt some members of the medical profession would feel quite reined in if the measures I propose were adopted. (These measures are not part of conventional wisdom.) But the restrictions on the freedom of the medical profession and on patients I am proposing would make for both a greater liberty all around, everything considered, and, as well, for greater well-being in the society. Sometimes we have to restrict certain liberties in order to enhance the overall system of liberty. Not speaking out of turn in parliamentary debate is a familiar example. Many people who now have a rather limited access to medical treatment would come to have it and have it in a more adequate way with such a socialized system in place. Often we have to choose between a greater or lesser liberty in a society, and, at least under conditions of abundance, the answer almost always should be 'Choose the greater liberty.' If we really prize human autonomy, if, that is, we want a world in which as many people as possible have as full as is possible control over their own lives, then we will be egalitarians. Our very egalitarianism will commit us to something like the health care system I described, but so will the realization that, without reasonable health on the part of the population, au-

tonomy can hardly flourish or be very extensive. Without the kind of equitability and increased coverage in health care that goes with a properly administered socialized medicine, the number of healthy people will be far less than could otherwise feasibly be the case. With that being the case, autonomy and well-being as well will be neither as extensive nor so thorough as it could otherwise be. Autonomy, like everything else, has its material conditions. And to will the end is to will the necessary means to the end.

To take—to sum up—what since the Enlightenment has come to be seen as the moral point of view, and to take morality seriously, is to take it as axiomatic that each person's good be given equal consideration.[11] I have argued that (a) where that is accepted, and (b) where we are tolerably clear about the facts (including facts about human needs), and (c) where we live under conditions of moderate abundance, a health care system bearing at least a family resemblance to the one I have gestured at will be put in place. It is a health care system befitting an autonomy respecting democracy committed to the democratic and egalitarian belief that the life of everyone matters and matters equally.

NOTES

1 Isaiah Berlin, "On the Pursuit of the Ideal," *The New York Review of Books* XXXV (March 1987), pp. 11–18. See also his "Equality" in his *Concepts and Categories* (Oxford, England: Oxford University Press, 1980), pp. 81–102. I have criticized that latter paper in my "Formulating Egalitarianism: Animadversions on Berlin," *Philosophia* 13:3–4 (October 1983), pp. 299–315.

2 For three defenses of such a view see Kai Nielsen, *Equality and Liberty* (Totowa, New Jersey: Rowman and Allanheld, 1985), Richard Norman, *Free and Equal* (Oxford, England: Oxford University Press, 1987), and John Baker, *Arguing for Equality* (London: Verso Press, 1987).

3 Will Kymlicka, "Rawls on Teleology and Deontology," *Philosophy and Public Affairs* 17:3 (Summer 1988), pp. 173–190 and John Rawls, "The Priority of Right and Ideas of the Good," *Philosophy and Public Affairs* 17:4 (Fall 1988), pp. 251–276.

4 Kai Nielsen, "Searching for an Emancipatory Perspective: Wide Reflective Equilibrium and the Hermeneutical Circle" in Evan Simpson (ed.), *Anti-Foundationalism and Practical Reasoning* (Edmonton, Alberta: Academic Printing and Publishing, 1987), pp. 143–164 and Kai Nielsen, "In Defense of Wide Reflective Equilibrium" in Douglas

Odegard (ed.) *Ethics and Justification* (Edmonton, Alberta: Academic Printing and Publishing, 1988), pp. 19–37.

5 David Braybrooke, *Meeting Needs* (Princeton, New Jersey: Princeton University Press, 1987), p. 29.

6 *Ibid.*, p. 31.

7 *Ibid.*, p. 37.

8 Will Kymlicka, *op cit.*, p. 190.

9 *Ibid.*

10 Ralf Dahrendorf, *Essays in the Theory of Society* (Stanford, California: Stanford University Press, 1968), pp. 151–78 and G. A. Cohen, "The Structure of Proletarian Unfreedom," *Philosophy and Public Affairs* 12 (1983), pp. 2–33.

11 Will Kymlicka, *op cit.*, p. 190.

RATIONING, MANAGED CARE, AND HEALTH-CARE REFORM IN THE UNITED STATES

IS THE OREGON RATIONING PLAN FAIR?

Norman Daniels

Daniels takes up the question of whether the Oregon rationing plan (which is discussed in the Introduction to this chapter) is fair or just. In exploring this complex question, he notes ways in which particular features can be seen as fair or unfair, depending upon background assumptions about justice. For example, the plan may make those already eligible for Medicaid (the very poor) worse off by not funding some of the services to which they had previously been eligible; this feature counts as unjust, Daniels argues, if justice requires maximally benefiting those who are the worst off. On the other hand, the plan extends coverage to many poor persons previously uncovered by Medicaid—a feature reducing inequity between the poor and others in society. Daniels also examines the way in which (1) political judgments (e.g., regarding the feasibility of alternative strategies for implementing more egalitarian reforms) and (2) judgments about the adequacy of the public process (e.g., regarding which groups were represented at public meetings) affect our moral evaluations of the Oregon plan.

The Oregon Basic Health Services Act mandates universal access to basic care, but includes rationing services to those individuals who are Medicaid recipients. If no new resources are added, the plan may make current Medicaid recipients worse off, but still reduce inequality between the poor and the rest of society. If resources are expanded and benefits given appropriate rankings, no one may be worse off; though inequality will be reduced, alternative reforms might reduce it even further. Whether the outcome seems fair then depends on how much priority to the well-being of the poor we believe justice re-

quires; it also depends on political judgments about the feasibility of alternative strategies for achieving more egalitarian reforms. Oregon makes rationing public and explicit, as justice requires, but it is not clear how community values influence the ranking of services; ultimately, the rationing process is fair only if we may rely on the voting power of the poor.

EXCLUDING PEOPLE VS EXCLUDING SERVICES

In 1987, Oregon drew national attention when it stopped Medicaid funding of soft-tissue transplants. Officials justified the action by claiming that there are more effective ways to spend scarce public dollars than to provide high-cost benefits to relatively

Reprinted with permission of the publisher from *JAMA*, vol. 265 (May 1, 1991), pp. 2232–2235. Copyright © 1991, American Medical Association.

few people. They insisted that the estimated $1.1 million that would have been spent on such transplants in 1987 would save many more lives per dollar spent if invested in prenatal maternal care.[1] Rather than heartlessly turning its back on children in need of transplants, the state was making a "tragic choice" between two instances of rationing by ability to pay. The consequences of ignoring "invisible" pregnant women who cannot afford prenatal maternal care are much worse than are those of refusing to fund highly visible children in need of transplants.

The Oregon Basic Health Services Act boldly couples the rationing of health care with a plan to improve access.[2] It expands Medicaid eligibility to 100% for those individuals who are at the federal poverty level, creates an Oregon Health Services Commission (OHSC) to establish priorities among health services, requires cutting low-priority services rather than excluding people from coverage when reducing expenditures is necessary, mandates a high-risk insurance pool, and requires employers to provide health insurance or to contribute to a state insurance pool. Oregon must obtain a federal waiver to implement the changes in Medicaid.

Oregon explicitly rejects the rationing strategy that predominates in the United States: our rationing system excludes whole categories of the poor and near-poor from access to public insurance, denying coverage to *people,* rather than to low-priority *services.* In contrast, the Oregon plan embodies the following principles: (1) there is a social obligation to guarantee universal access to a *basic level* of health care, (2) reasonable or necessary limits on resources mean that not every beneficial service can be included in the basic level of health care, and (3) a public process, involving consideration of social values, is required to determine what services will be included in the basic level of health care.[1,3]

Though these principles are not a complete account of justice for health care, they have considerable plausibility, derive support from theoretical work on justice and health care, and are, to varying degrees, widely believed in by the US population.[4] Nevertheless, these principles permit rationing care to the poor alone, with serious implications for equality. Thus, critics attack the Oregon plan

for making the poor, specifically poor women and children, "bear the burden" of providing universal access.[5]

To evaluate this criticism, we must ask three questions: (1) Does the plan make the indigent groups better off or worse off? (2) Are the inequalities the plan accepts justifiable? (3) Is the procedure for determining the basic level of health care a just or fair one? These questions raise issues of distributive justice that go beyond the principles underlying the Oregon legislation.

WHAT DOES THE OREGON PLAN DO TO THE WORSE-OFF GROUPS?

Critics of Oregon's plan appeal to widely held egalitarian concerns when they argue that it makes the poor bear the burden of this effort to close the insurance gap. The strongest sense of "bear the burden" is, "being made worse off." Does the plan, as the critics charge, make the poor worse off instead of giving priority to improving their well-being?[6,7]

Consider the simplest case first, a zero sum game with resources. For example, if extrarenal transplants are removed from coverage and no higher-priority services, unavailable before the plan, are added, then current Medicaid recipients will lose some services and the health benefits they produce. They will no doubt then make this complaint: "We bear the burden of the plan. Since we are already the most indigent group, or close to it, we should not have to give up life-saving or other important medical services so that the currently uninsured can get basic level health care."

It is important to grasp the moral force of this complaint. Notice that *aggregate* health status for *all* the poor, including current Medicaid recipients and the uninsured, can be improved by the plan, even though current Medicaid recipients are made worse off. The loss of less important services by current recipients is more than counterbalanced by the gains of the uninsured. As a result, the plan reduces overall inequality between the poor and the rest of society, albeit at the expense of current Medicaid recipients. Therefore, the complaint cannot be that the plan makes society less equal; instead, it is that even greater reductions in inequality are possible if other groups sacrifice instead of Medicaid recipients. It is unfair for current Medicaid recipients to bear a burden that others could bear much better, especially since inequality would then be even further reduced.

How stringent is the priority owed the poorest groups when we seek to improve aggregate well-being? Three positions are possible: (1) help the poor as much as possible *(strict priority);* (2) make sure the poor get some benefit *(modified priority);* or (3) allow only modest harms to the poor in return for significant gains to others who are not well-off *(weak priority).* Critics of the Oregon plan insist that we should not settle for weak priority, especially since feasible alternatives help the poor more. The Oregon plan leaves the bulk of the health care system intact. By eliminating the inefficiencies it contains, eg, by establishing a low-overhead public insurance scheme (as in Canada), or by developing treatment protocols that eliminate unnecessary services, we might be able to avoid making current Medicaid recipients any worse off. Alternatively, by broadening rationing to cover most of society, as in Canada or Great Britain, we could avoid the criticism that only the poor are being made to bear the burden of improving access.

Proponents of the Oregon plan aim for a more complex case than a zero sum game with services, however, hoping to add either new services or new revenue sources.[1,3,8] Suppose, for example, the plan makes available "high-priority" services that are currently not adequately provided, such as prenatal maternal care, mental health, and chemical dependency services, while "low-priority" services, e.g., soft-tissue transplants, are not funded. Then current Medicaid recipients will have a *higher* expected payoff from the revised benefits. Since the currently uninsured are also made better off, and no one is made worse off (except that taxes may be increased), we have what economists call a *pareto superior* outcome. Of course, those particular Medicaid recipients who need the newly rationed services will be worse off, but it is reasonable to judge the effects of the system *ex ante,* and the poor as a whole are better off despite the loss to some individuals who would require soft-tissue transplants.

Thus, with appropriate revisions of Medicaid benefits, the poor will be better off than they are now. Nevertheless, current Medicaid recipients can object, "We achieve our gain in health status by giving up beneficial services that better-off groups receive; in that sense we 'bear the burden' of the Oregon plan. The poor would improve even more if better-off groups contributed more." The complaint is that social inequality could be reduced in a way that benefits the poor even more.

One version of this complaint appeals to long-term considerations: the Oregon plan makes the poor better off in the short run but worse off than they would be in the longer run if a national health insurance scheme were introduced. This claim depends on particular political assumptions about the likelihood of alternative scenarios for reform. In reply, some proponents see the current legislation in Oregon as but the first step in a comprehensive, incremental reform; ultimately, the state would become the major insurer and most powerful purchaser by substituting its basic insurance plan for many private insurance plans as well as for Medicare and long-term care under Medicaid (Sen John Kitzhaber, verbal communication, January 1991). The debate then focuses on the means to health reform, not its ends; disagreement results from complex political, not moral, judgments.

A second complaint about reducible inequality derives from the Children's Defense Fund's charge that the Oregon plan "exempts" the elderly who are Medicaid recipients from the ranking of services.[5] Poor women and children, who constitute 75% of the Medicaid recipients, receive only 30% of the benefits in dollars. Much of the rest goes to the elderly who have "spent down" their resources in order to be eligible for long-term care, but these services—as well as all acute care for the elderly who are covered under Medicare—are not included in the prioritization or rationing process. By not establishing priorities among health care services for the elderly, and by financing expansion of Medicaid coverage, primarily by rationing to women and children, the plan seems to suggest that any use of long-term medical services by the elderly is more important than short-term medical services for the young. This would be an irrational ranking on the face of it. If we did not know how old we were and had to allocate resources over our life span, taking our needs at each stage of life into account, we would not consider this ranking a prudent one.[9] A reasonable rationing plan would consider the importance of all health care services, short-term medical as well as long-term care, over an individual's life span, at each stage of life. To avoid what seems to be discrimination by age, rationing should include all age groups. In reply and as noted, some Oregon proponents intend to expand the plan to cover Medicare and long-term Medicaid care.

Advocates for the Oregon plan argue that additional revenue, which would further reduce inequality, will be easier to obtain when the legislature must visibly cut beneficial services and cannot disguise rationing by raising eligibility requirements for Medicaid. This political judgment ignores evidence from the 1980s, when various states, as well as the federal government, cut important services to the poor, including prenatal maternal care and the Women, Infants, and Children's Program's distribution of food supplements to pregnant women and neighborhood mental health care services. Explicit rationing to the poor made neither politicians nor their constituents so uncomfortable that the cuts were stopped.

In short, we cannot answer the basic question about how the worse off will fare under the current legislation until we are told what they will get, that is, until the Medicaid benefit package is ranked by OHSC, is funded by the legislature, and is approved for a Medicaid waiver by the Department of Health and Human Services, sometime later in 1991. If the current Medicaid recipients are made worse off, there is a serious, though not necessarily fatal, objection to the Oregon plan. If we hold only a weak version of the requirement that we give priority to the worse off, we might still think the plan acceptable even though some of the poor bear the burden of reducing overall inequality. In any case, the Oregon planners hope that rationing will yield a result in which all the poor are better off than now. Political judgments differ about the likelihood of this preferred outcome.

ARE THE INEQUALITIES THE OREGON PLAN ACCEPTS JUSTIFIABLE?

By rationing lower-priority services to the poor, rather than excluding whole groups of the poor and near-poor from insurance, the Oregon plan reduces inequality in our society, even if current Medicaid recipients are, to some extent, worse off than they are now. Somewhat paradoxically, even under the scenario in which no one is worse off, there is still a sense in which the poor bear the burden of the plan, since the plan accepts as official policy an unjustifiable inequality in the health care system.

To see this point, contrast the kind of inequality the Oregon plan accepts with the inequality that arises in the heavily rationed British system.[10] Although about 10% of the British public buys private insurance coverage in order to procure various rationed services, the overwhelming majority abides by the consequences of rationing. This produces a more acceptable structure of inequality than would result if the bottom 20% of the Oregon population has no access to some services that are available to the great majority.[11]

To see why one structure of inequality seems worse than the other, consider how the poor would feel under both. Under the Oregon plan, the poor can complain that society as a whole is content not only to leave them economically badly off, but also to deny them medical services that would protect the range of opportunities that are open to them.[6] There is a basis here for reasonable regrets or resentment, for society as a whole seems content to shut the poor out of mainstream opportunities. They may reasonably feel that the majority is too willing to leave them behind under terms in which the benefits of social cooperation do not reflect their moral status as free and equal agents.[12,13] Alternatively, if health care protects opportunity in a way that is roughly equal for all, except that the most advantaged group has some extra advantages, then this may seem somewhat unfair, but no one group is then singled out for special disadvantages that are viewed as "acceptable" by the economically and medically advantaged majority. Consequently, no group would have a basis for the strong and reasonable regrets that the poor have under the Oregon plan, despite their improvement relative to the current situation.

Thus, even if the poor are better off under the Oregon plan than now, the plan still accepts an inequality that is not ideally just. It is more just—perhaps much more just—than what we now have, but still not what justice requires. Does this mean we should not implement it? The answer seems to depend on political judgments about the feasibility of alternatives. If one thinks that a uniform, universal plan, like Canada's, is a political impossibility in the United States, or if one thinks that introducing the Oregon plan makes further reform in the direction of a uniform plan more likely, then the Oregon plan, even if it is not ideally just, seems reasonable. But if one thinks that introducing the Oregon reform makes more radical reform of the system less likely, then one might well prefer not to make a modest improvement in the justice of the system in order to facilitate a more significant improvement later.

IS THE PUBLIC PROCESS FOR DECIDING WHAT IS 'BASIC CARE' FAIR?

The Oregon plan involves public, explicit rationing; it disavows rationing hidden by the covert workings of a market, or buried in the quiet, professional decisions of providers. Its rationing decisions are the result of a two-step process involving separate, publicly accountable bodies. First (step 1), OHSC, which is charged with taking "community values" into consideration, determines priorities among services in a possible benefit package. Second (step 2), the legislature decides how much to spend on Medicaid, given competing demands on state funds. Some lower-priority services may thus not be covered, but the resulting Medicaid benefit package must still be approved by the Department of Health and Human Services. Assessing the fairness of the rationing process requires examining both steps.

Oregon's insistence on publicity is controversial. Calabresi and Bobbit[14] argue that "tragic choices" are best made out of the public view in order to preserve important symbolic values, such as the sanctity of life. Despite the importance of such symbols, however, justice requires publicity. People

who view themselves as free and equal moral agents must have available to them the grounds for all decisions that affect their lives in fundamental ways, as rationing decisions do. Only with publicity can they resolve disputes about whether the decisions conform to the more basic principles of justice that are the accepted basis of their social cooperation.[15]

Actually, going beyond a concern for publicity, Oregon calls for broad public participation in the development of priorities. Public participation is desirable because it may yield agreement about how to resolve disputes among winners and losers in a fair way. It also makes it more likely that outcomes reflect the consent of those individuals who are affected and, since there may not be one uniquely fair or just way to ration services, participation allows the shared values of a community to shape the result. Is the public participation process itself fair, and does it have a real effect on outcomes?

OHSC held public hearings on health services and asked Oregon Health Decisions to hold community meetings throughout the state "to build consensus on the values to be used to guide health resource allocation decisions."[16] At 47 meetings that were held during the early part of 1990, citizens were asked to rank the importance of various categories of treatment and were asked, "Why is this health care service *important to us?*" From these discussions, an unranked list of 13 "values" was distilled. A tally was kept of how often each value was discussed, but we cannot rank the importance of the values on that basis.

One frequent criticism of the community meeting procedure is that it did not involve a representative cross section of Oregonians. Some 50% were health professionals; too many were college educated, white, and relatively well-off. Moreover, whereas 16% of Oregonians are uninsured, only 9.4% of community meeting participants were uninsured, and Medicaid recipients, the only direct representatives of poor children, were underrepresented by half.[5,16] Even if there was no evidence of bias in the meetings, the process is still open to the charge that it consisted of the "haves" deciding what is "important" to give the "have-nots." The charge is twofold. Not only is the composition of the meetings unrepresentative of the interests of those who will be affected, but the task set for the meetings presupposes that rationing will primarily have an impact on an underrepresented minority.

It is difficult to assess the importance of either charge of bias, for we have no way to compare the outcome with an unbiased alternative. Suspicions about the effects of compositional bias would be reduced, however, if there were no bias in the task, that is, if the Oregon plan called for rationing services to the great majority rather than to the poor. We worry less about who is making a decision if it has an equal impact on everyone, including the decision makers.

The charge of bias is important only if the meetings actually influence the ranking of services (otherwise they are just window dressing). Contrary to public and media understanding, however, the community meetings do not yield a ranking of services, only a general list of community values. Moreover, the list of values cannot be used in any direct way in determining priorities among health services. Some of the "values" are really only categories of services, eg, mental health and chemical dependency, or prevention. Other values, such as equity (guaranteeing access to all) or respecting personal choice, are things we desire of the system as a whole, not of individual services. And the values relevant to ranking services, such as quality of life or cost-effectiveness or ability to function, are not themselves ranked.

OHSC is well aware of this limitation and views the list of values only as a "qualitative check" on the process of ranking services (Paige Sipes-Metzler, personal communication, June and July 1990). Thus, it believes the community concern for equity is met because the system guarantees universal access to basic care. Community concerns about mental health and chemical dependency, or prevention, are met by making sure that these services are included in the ranking process. Although no weights were assigned to values such as quality of life or cost-effectiveness, they are included as factors in the formal ranking process. The only direct community input into the first attempt at ranking services, however, came from a telephone survey aimed at finding how Oregonians ranked particular health outcomes that affect their quality of life. By combining this in-

formation with expert judgments about the likely outcomes of using particular procedures to treat certain conditions, as well as with information about the costs of treating a population with those procedures, OHSC generated a preliminary cost-benefit ranking of services. Because this ranking drew extensive criticism (*New York Times,* July 9, 1990; sect A:17) and failed to match its own expectations about priorities, OHSC modified its procedure for ranking services. As a result, the OHSC commissioners themselves ranked general categories of services according to their importance to the individual, to society, and to the health plan and "adjusted" other items.[17] It remains unclear how this process reflects community values, and until we know just how the final rankings were "adjusted," we cannot know what influence public participation has had.

The rationing process involves two decisions, not one. Suppose that we have a fair procedure and a perfect outcome at step 1: the ranking of services captures relevant facts about costs and benefits and represents community values fairly. Unfortunately, fairness at step 1 does not assure it at step 2, because the voting power of the poor is negated in a political process that generally underrepresents them, judging from past voting patterns and outcomes. Therefore, even if there is a consensus at step 1 about what the basic, minimum package should be, there may be well-founded worries that the legislature will not fund it. Indeed, the situation is somewhat worse because OHSC only ranks services, it does not decide what is basic. The funding decision of the legislature determines what basic care is provided.

Clearly, political judgments diverge on how much we can trust the legislature. The crucial issue from the point of view of process, however, is this: because the Oregon plan explicitly involves rationing primarily for the poor and near-poor, funding decisions face constant political pressure from more powerful groups who want to put public resources to other uses. In contrast, if the legislature were deciding how to fund a rationing plan that applied to themselves and to all their constituents, then we might expect a careful and honest weighing of the importance of health care against other goods. The legislature would then have stronger reasons not to concede to political pressures to divert resources, and other groups would be less likely to apply such pressure. If the plan is expanded to include other groups, then the poor may find important allies.

Worries about fairness in the Oregon rationing process thus come from the plan's being aimed at the poor rather than at the population as a whole. Concerns about fairness in the process thus converge with concerns about the kinds of inequality the system tolerates. This does not mean that the Oregon experiment should not be tried; it may produce less overall inequality in health status than we now have. But we should recognize from the start that a system that rations only to the poor is less equitable and less fair than alternative systems that ration for the great majority of people. To the extent that the inequality ends up troubling many participants in the system, including physicians who will be able to do only certain things for some children and more for others, the strains of commitment to abiding by the rationing will be greater, and rationing may get a worse name than it deserves.

Oregon's plan retains the structure of inequality that it does because states must respond to the problems imposed by a highly inequitable and inefficient national health care system. The plan contains a bizarre irony: the state's Medicaid budget is in crisis because of rapidly increasing costs, largely the result of the burden of long-term care imposed by the elderly, yet the rationing plan focuses on poor children. Oregon did not design a Medicaid system that forces the most vulnerable children and the most vulnerable elderly to compete for scarce public resources. As long as states must respond to problems created by the national system, however, their solutions will inherit its major flaws. Uncoordinated responses by states cannot solve the problems caused by the continuing rapid dissemination of technology, inefficiencies in administering a mixed system, and a growing demand for services in our aging and acquired immunodeficiency syndrome–threatened society.

Oregon offers important lessons for any national effort to address these problems. Nationally, we should embrace Oregon's commitment to provide universal access to basic care and to make rationing a subject of open, political debate, but we should not simply expand the current legislation into a national plan. That would not only reproduce on a larger scale the unjustifiable inequality that the Oregon plan permits. It would also retain at the state level competition for funds between poor children and poor elderly, and it would leave unaddressed the basic problems of inefficiency and rapidly rising costs. In contrast, rationing within a single-payer, public insurance scheme that covered all age groups would more easily address these problems. Whether such a comprehensive scheme is best introduced all at once (on the model of the Canadian system), or is phased in (building on an Oregon-style starting point), is a complex issue. In any case, we have yet to see whether the Oregon plan gives us a clear model for how community values or public participation should influence the design of a national benefit package.

ACKNOWLEDGMENTS

This work was generously supported by grant RH-20917 from the National Endowment for the Humanities and grant 1RO1LM05005 from the National Library of Medicine, Washington, DC.

Helpful information, materials, or comments were provided by Dan Brock, PhD, Arthur Caplan, PhD, Michael Garland, PhD, John Golenski, SJ, Bruce Jennings, PhD, Sen John Kitzhaber, and Paige Sipes-Metzler, DPA.

REFERENCES

1 Golenski J. *A Report on the Oregon Medicaid Priority Setting Project.* Berkeley, Calif: Bioethics Consultation Group; 1990.
2 Senate Bills 27, 534, 935. 65th Oregon Legislative Assembly; 1989 regular sess.
3 Kitzhaber J. *The Oregon Basic Health Services Act.* Salem, Ore: Office of the Senate President; 1990.
4 Blendon R. J., Leitman R., Morrison I, Donelan K. Satisfaction with health systems in ten nations. *Health Aff.* Summer 1990:185–192.
5 *An Analysis of the Impact of the Oregon Medicaid Reduction Waiver Proposal on Women and Children.* Washington, DC: Children's Defense Fund; 1990:1–7.
6 Daniels N. *Just Health Care.* New York, NY: Cambridge University Press; 1985.

7 Rawls J. *A Theory of Justice.* Cambridge, Mass: Harvard University Press; 1971.

8 *Preliminary Report.* Salem: Oregon Health Services Commission; 1990.

9 Daniels N. *Am I My Parents' Keeper? An Essay on Justice Between the Young and the Old.* New York, NY: Oxford University Press Inc; 1988.

10 Aaron H. J., Schwartz W. B. *The Painful Prescription: Rationing Health Care.* Washington, DC: The Brookings Institution; 1984.

11 Temkin L. Inequality. *Philosophy Public Aff.* 1986; 15:99–121.

12 Cohen J. Democratic equality. *Ethics.* 1989; 99:727–751.

13 Scanlon T. M. Contractualism and utilitarianism. In: Sen A. K., Williams B, eds. *Utilitarianism and Beyond.* New York, NY: Cambridge University Press; 1982:103–128.

14 Calabresi G, Bobbit P. *Tragic Choices.* New York, NY: WW Norton & Co Inc; 1978.

15 Rawls J. Kantian constructivism in moral theory: The Dewey Lectures. *J Phil.* 1980; 77:515–572.

16 Hasnain R., Garland M. *Health Care in Common: Report of the Oregon Health Decisions Community Meetings Process.* Portland: Oregon Health Decisions; 1990.

17 Kitzhaber J. *Summary: The Health Services Prioritization Process.* Salem: Oregon State Senate; 1990.

MANAGED CARE: RATIONING WITHOUT JUSTICE, BUT NOT UNJUSTLY

Allen Buchanan

Buchanan argues that three common criticisms of managed care in the United States are misguided and obscure its most central ethical problem. First, the claim that managed care organizations (MCOs) fail in their obligation to improve—or at least not worsen—access because they seek healthier, wealthier patients rests on a false assumption: that the American health-care system has a feasible division of responsibility that assigns obligations regarding access to MCOs. Two other common criticisms, Buchanan continues, are that MCOs, by employing rationing, deprive patients of care to which they are entitled, and that MCOs, by pressuring physicians to ration, threaten physicians' commitment to serve patients' best interests. Both criticisms, he argues, are vitiated by their false assumption that the United States has articulated what should count as an adequate level of care to which everyone is entitled. According to the author, the central flaw of American managed care is that "it operates in an institutional setting within which no connection can be made between the activities of rationing and the basic requirements of justice."

ETHICAL CRITICISMS OF MANAGED CARE

Managed care, the latest manifestation of efforts to privatize health care, is often passionately criticized on *ethical* grounds.[1] The ethical criticisms most frequently voiced are these: (1) by "skimming the cream" of the patient population, managed care organizations fail to discharge their obligations to improve (or at least to not worsen) the access problem; (2) in order to contain costs, managed care organizations engage in rationing techniques that withhold some types of beneficial care and that reduce the quality of care, depriving patients of care to which they are entitled; and (3) by pressuring physicians to ration care, managed care organizations interfere with physicians fulfilling their professional fiduciary obligation to provide the best care for each patient (Council 1995; Emanuel and Dubler 1995; Rodwin 1993: 135–153; Spece, Shimm, and Buchanan 1996: 1–11).

From *Journal of Health Politics, Policy and Law,* vol. 23, no. 4 (August 1998), pp. 617–634. Copyright 1998, Duke University Press. All rights reserved. Reprinted with permission.

I shall argue that each of these allegations is radically misconceived. . . .

WHAT MANAGED CARE IS

For our purposes a simple characterization of managed care will suffice. A managed care organization *combines* health care *insurance* and the *delivery* of a broad range of integrated health care services for *populations* of plan enrollees, financing the services *prospectively* from a predicted, limited budget. At present the following cost-containment techniques are often identified with managed care: (1) payment limits (e.g., diagnosis-related groupings [DRGs] for Medicare hospital fees); (2) requirement of preauthorization for certain services (e.g., surgeries); (3) the use of primary care physicians as "gatekeepers" to control referral to specialists; (4) so-called "de-skilling" (using less highly trained providers for certain services than was customary during the pre–managed care, third-party fee-for-service era); and (5) financial incentives for physicians to limit utilization of care (e.g., year-end bonuses or holdbacks of payments that physicians receive only if they do not exceed specified utilization limits). In addition, managed care increasingly employs data from outcome (efficacy) studies to develop practice guidelines and for the ongoing assessment and refinement of diagnostic services and treatment services.

THE HISTORICAL RATIONALE FOR MANAGED CARE

Managed care is the result of a "payers' revolt" against the alarming escalation in the cost of health care in the United States under the third-party, fee-for-service system. The payers include employers in the private sector who provide health care benefits for their employees, the federal government in the Medicare program, and federal and state governments in Medicaid. The initial stages of the managed care revolution occurred in the private sector, but government has begun to try to curb the increases in its health care costs by utilizing the cost-containment measures developed in the private sector. For example, there are efforts to encourage Medicare and Medicaid patients to join health maintenance organizations (HMOs). Some analysts predict that the

only solution to the projected severe underfunding of Medicare, as the population ages and the workforce shrinks, is to enroll all or most Medicare patients in managed care organizations.

It is extremely important to emphasize that the transition to managed care was primarily an effort at cost containment by the corporate purchasers of health care. Employers reached a point at which they were no longer willing to keep paying for services for their employees while the percentage of the gross domestic product (GDP) devoted to health care climbed toward 15 percent and the proportion of the cost of producing their goods and services devoted to paying premiums for their employees steadily rose.

In other words, the motivation for moving to managed care on the part of those whose efforts actually brought it about had nothing to do with addressing what might be called *the primary access problem*. By the primary access problem, I mean the fact that over 40 million people in the United States lack secure access to anything other than emergency care because they have no private health care insurance and are not covered by any government program.

The only plausible—though somewhat tenuous and uncertain—connection between the payers' revolt that produced managed care and the primary access problem is this: By reducing the rate at which the cost of health care was rising, managed care may be preventing the access problem from worsening, by making insurance continue to be affordable for most of those who are now lucky enough to be insured. Even the most ardent defenders of managed care have not been able to make an empirical case for the claim that managed care will have any significant impact on, much less solve, the primary access problem.

Indeed, what is most remarkable about the vociferous popular debate about managed care— from an ethical point of view—is that the issue of access for the uninsured seems to have dropped off the public's radar screen entirely. If the primary access problem is mentioned at all, what is said is this: Unless the cost escalation is curbed, there is no hope of extending access to the uninsured; and managed care is the only realistic means of curbing the cost spiral.

This latter claim is astonishing, if it is understood as contributing in any way to the *justification* for the transition to managed care, in that it overlooks a simple but enormously important fact: There is simply no reason to expect that whatever cost savings do result from managed care will be used to make a significant contribution at all to ameliorating the primary access problem. As will become clearer as the analysis proceeds, we should not expect managed care cost savings to contribute to ameliorating the primary access problem because managed care has developed in a system in which there is (1) no social consensus on, or authoritative political determination of, what health care services every citizen is entitled to (the "decent minimum" or "adequate level" of care) and (2) there are no institutional mechanisms capable of ensuring that resources saved through the cost-containment measures of managed care are utilized to ensure that all citizens have access to such an entitlement (Daniels 1986).

The chief reason why such institutional mechanisms are lacking is that the United States lacks something even more basic, something that virtually every other developed country has: a central government that takes ultimate responsibility for ensuring that every citizen has access to a decent minimum or adequate level of health care. Instead of this fundamental commitment, we in the United States have only an ideology: the naive belief (or cynical pretense) that everyone will have adequate access through a division of labor between government programs and private insurance, if both private and public entities fulfill their obligations. I argue, however, that without a politically effective societal consensus on what the right to health care includes, and without concrete institutional arrangements that embody a commitment to ensure that every citizen has access to the level of care included in the right, there is no reason to believe that the uncoordinated action of the private and public sectors will achieve a reasonable approximation of universal access.

WHY MANAGED CARE ORGANIZATIONS HAVE NO OBLIGATIONS OF JUSTICE TO ENSURE ACCESS

Although they seem oblivious to the fact, those who currently criticize managed care organizations for marketing strategies and benefit designs that "skim the cream" of the patient population and exclude those with costly health conditions are simply repeating a fundamental mistake that the opponents of the first wave of privatization made a decade ago. In the mid-1980s, privatization of health care in the United States took the form of the rapid growth of for-profit hospitals. Critics complained that for-profit hospitals were shunning uninsured or underinsured patients and that this had the effect of dumping such patients on already financially precarious public hospitals, thereby worsening the access problem.

That such behavior on the part of for-profits has made it harder for public hospitals to serve the medically indigent is probably true. But it does not follow that in behaving in this way, for-profit hospitals are violating their obligations to help ensure access to care. They would only be guilty of violating obligations to help ensure access if they had such obligations, but they do not.

To understand why they do not, it is important to draw a distinction between two models for how access to a decent minimum or adequate level of health care for all might be achieved through the combined operation of the private sector and government entities (Buchanan 1992: 235–250).[2] According to the first model, a private health care insurance market is expected to provide adequate care at affordable prices for a substantial portion (perhaps even a majority) of the total population, and government recognizes and acts on a commitment to fill whatever gaps in access remain. Private commercial entities, whether they are for-profit hospitals or managed care organizations, have no obligations to help ensure access. They are under no obligation to provide care that is not profitable for them to provide.

According to the second model, there is an institutionally prescribed *division of obligations to secure access* between the private and public sectors. Political processes at the highest level assign private-sector entities determinate obligations regarding access. In the first model, the role of government is to fill whatever gaps in access remain after the market has done its job, but commercial entities in the private sector have no obligations regarding access.[3] In the second model, private-sector entities are not simply agents in the market; they have special obligations to act in ways they would not act if they simply acted as agents in the market.

Those who charge that managed care organizations are violating ethical obligations when they engage in practices that exclude especially costly patients from coverage altogether (and thereby increase the financial strain on public providers) are implicitly assuming that in doing so, these organizations are not bearing their fair share of the burden of securing access for all. But this last assumption would only be true if the United States had adopted the second model, that is, if it actually had an institutional division of labor that assigned obligations concerning access to private commercial entities. It does not. Nor does it have a government that is willing to play the gap-filling role required by the first model (nor, apparently, is there a majority of citizens that is willing and able to demand that their representatives act so as to make government play that role).

In the absence of a political assignment of obligations to private-sector entities such as for-profit hospitals or managed care organizations, there is no more reason to assume that such entities have obligations regarding access than there is to assume that grocers have obligations to supply the poor with food or that home builders are obligated to furnish free housing (Brock and Buchanan 1986: 224–249). It will not do to say that health care is unique. Food and shelter are also essential for life.

Of course, for-profit entities, like grocers, home builders, and anyone who has the resources to help the needy without excessive cost to themselves, may have what moral theorists traditionally have called "imperfect" obligations of charity (Buchanan 1987). Such obligations, unlike obligations of justice, are said to be indeterminate, with a large area of discretion for the benefactor to choose whom he will benefit and in what manner, and always within the limits of the provision that doing so is not "excessively costly." Under conditions of increasingly vigorous competition, private-sector commercial entities can plausibly argue that engaging in charity toward those who lack access may be an excessive cost. In other words, in a competitive environment, there is a predictable tendency for private agents to construe their imperfect obligations less and less generously.

The simple but important point is that without an authoritative political assignment of determinate obligations of access to private-sector commercial entities, and without some effective system of sanctions to ensure each entity that its competitors are fulfilling their prescribed duties, we cannot say that the activities of managed organizations deprive anyone of what they are entitled to as a matter of the right to health care.

Moreover, unless a mixed private-public health care system is an instance of one of the two models sketched above, there is no realistic hope that the combined operation of the public and private sectors will result in access to an "adequate level" or "decent minimum" of health care for all. The natural operation of a competitive market in health care insurance (especially if, as in the United States, insurance is largely employment-based) will result in some of those who most need health care not being able to get it in the market. And if government fails to fulfill the gap-filling role, as it has in the United States, then some, perhaps many, will be without access to even a decent minimum of care.

It should be clear at this point that the chief *conceptual* mistake that prevents the U.S. public and policy makers from dealing with the primary access problem (and from even framing the ethical issues of managed care in a coherent and fruitful way) is that we overlook the unpleasant fact that our system is neither an instance of model one nor of model two. My point is not that we have an access problem due to a purely conceptual mistake. Rather, what I am suggesting is that this conceptual mistake aids and abets both our unwillingness to confront the primary access problem and our confusion about what the real ethical problems of current arrangements are. This is nowhere clearer than in the muddled terms with which the debate over rationing in managed care is framed. The lack of (1) a societal agreement on what the entitlement to health care includes and of (2) concrete institutional arrangements for seeing that all have access to a decent minimum of care through the combined operations of the private and public sectors (the implementation of either model one or model two of a mixed private-public system) undercuts the very assumptions under which the current ethical debate about rationing in managed care is conducted. This fundamental point will become clearer as we examine the controversy over rationing in managed care.

RATIONING IN MANAGED CARE: RATIONING FOR COST CONTAINMENT, NOT FOR JUSTICE

We have just seen that by acting competitively, managed care organizations do not violate obligations of justice, even if their behavior worsens the access problem by shifting costs to public sector providers or by refusing to enroll individuals who would be very costly to treat. Frequently, however, a different allegation concerning rationing is leveled at managed care organizations: They are accused of acting unethically in their rationing practices toward those whom they *do* serve.

WHY THE DENIAL OF CARE IN MANAGED CARE IS NOT SUBSTANTIVELY UNJUST

There are three chief ways in which rationing practices may be unethical. Rationing practices are (1) *contractually unjust* if they violate the special rights of enrollees that are generated through the contract offering the plan. Rationing practices are (2) *procedurally unjust* if there is discrimination (say, on the basis of sex or race), if the rules for limiting care are applied inconsistently, or if there are no reasonable institutional mechanisms for informing patients that rationing choices are being made and giving them opportunities to appeal decisions they believe to be unfair. Rationing practices are (3) *substantively unjust* if the principles of rationing upon which they rely are themselves unjust, even when applied consistently, without discrimination, and under conditions of adequate disclosure and due process.

Sometimes the complaint about managed care rationing practices is that they are contractually or procedurally unjust, but often it is stated or implied that they are substantively unjust. For example, there has been considerable public outrage (and several lawsuits) in response to the fact that some patients who might have benefited from autologous bone marrow transplant have been denied this treatment for breast cancer by their HMOs. In some cases, the complaint has been that denial of such

care violates contractually generated rights. However, even here there is often the suggestion that contractual language concerning the provision of "comprehensive care" is to be interpreted ultimately by reference to the notion of an adequate level or decent minimum of care to which the individual is supposed to be entitled. The complaint about denial of care is then based on the assumption that the care denied falls within the adequate level or decent minimum to which each individual is entitled and that ultimately defines the "comprehensive care" that HMOs promise to deliver.

If such complaints about denial of care are understood as charges of substantive injustice, as opposed to procedural or contractual injustice, then they must rest upon an assumption that the form of treatment being denied is included in the array of services to which the individual is entitled, independently of the particular nature of the plan contract. But we have already seen that at present in the United States there is no authoritative standard for defining the scope of this entitlement. For this reason an individual who is denied some service cannot plausibly argue that the rationing practice of the organization commits an injustice by excluding a service that ought to be immune from exclusion. In the absence of an authoritative determination of what is included in the adequate level or decent minimum, virtually *no* service is in principle immune from exclusion.

It would be quite different if there were an authoritative political determination or even a rough but deep societal consensus on what the adequate level or decent minimum includes. Then disputes about whether a particular service may be denied would in principle be resolvable. But in the United States we have not settled on a standard because we have not been forced to do so as a prerequisite of trying to implement a commitment to provide universal access. Yet in the absence of a societal agreement about what services the individual is entitled to, we cannot say that a managed care organization rations unfairly when it refuses to pay for a particular form of care (unless doing so is contractually or procedurally unjust). So, unless they are construed narrowly as disagreements about contractual rights or procedural injustice, charges that managed care wrongs patients by denying certain services are simply muddled.

This is not to say that procedural injustices and contractual injustices do not occur, or that when they do they are not serious ethical problems. Marketing schemes can oversell a plan, misleading potential enrollees about what they can reasonably expect by way of coverage. And both the contract between the payer and the managed care organization and the policy upon which the individual relies may be ambiguous or even intentionally misleading. Moreover, a fair interpretation of a contract or a policy must take into account the historical cultural context in which it exists, and it can be argued that until very recently, the U.S. context encouraged insured individuals to believe that they were entitled to "everything." Nevertheless, the further we proceed into the "managed care revolution," the less convincing it is to claim that enrollees have a reasonable expectation that there will be no limits on care. If contracts and policies are reasonably clear, if rationing policies are applied in a nondiscriminatory way, if marketing does not misrepresent coverage, and if a reasonable person should know that managed care means limits, there is no basis for inferring that injustice has occurred simply because a patient does not get some beneficial care or receives care of less than the highest quality. Efforts at ethical reform within the managed care system should focus on procedural and contractual injustices and on educating patients so that their expectations are realistic, not based on imagined substantive injustices.

WHY THE REDUCTION OF QUALITY OF CARE IN MANAGED CARE IS NOT IN ITSELF UNETHICAL

The situation is similar in the case of allegations that managed care is undermining the *quality* of care. The lack of an institutional commitment to securing access to an adequate level of care for all deprives us of any rational basis for saying that anyone is *wronged* by reductions in quality for the sake of cost containment, so long as contractual rights are respected and procedural justice is observed. For example, frequently there are complaints that managed care organizations are reducing the quality of care by so-called de-skilling—using less highly trained

individuals to perform certain services (e.g., having nurses do some tasks physicians have customarily performed or using social workers to do what psychiatrists used to do). Or, to take another common example, there are complaints that some HMOs are using cheaper medications that have more side effects or that are less efficacious than the best drugs available for the condition in question (e.g., using older generation tricyclic anti-depressants rather than the newer serotonin-uptake inhibitors).

Using a drug that is less efficacious or that has more side effects or using a provider with lesser skills may indeed reduce the quality of care. But it does not follow that there is anything unjust or in any way unethical about doing so. Rationing practices that reduce quality of care are only unethical if they are contractually unjust, procedurally unjust, or substantively unjust. Suppose for a moment that neither of our two examples of rationing-produced reductions in care quality involve violations of contractual obligations or of the requirements of procedural justice. Is there anything unethical per se about reducing quality to reduce costs?

The answer must be no, unless one of two assumptions is granted: (1) that every patient is entitled to the highest quality care that is technically feasible, regardless of cost; or (2) that these particular reductions in quality result in the care provided falling below the level of quality that is included in the adequate level or decent minimum of care to which every individual is entitled.

At this stage of the debate over health care costs, the falsity of the first assumption should be obvious to everyone. Providing the highest quality of care for everyone all the time is neither politically feasible nor required by any reasonable theory of just health care. Only if one denies that resources are scarce (or fails to understand that there are other goods in life besides health care) would one assume that everyone is entitled to the highest quality of care that is technically feasible, without regard to cost.

So if lower quality care is substantively unjust, it must be because it falls below the adequate level or decent minimum of care to which all are entitled. But as we have already seen, there is no societal consensus on what this is and political processes have yielded no authoritative determination of it. Of course, there may be some services that are so inexpensive and so efficacious in preventing or curing serious diseases that we can assume that they would be included in any reasonable societal consensus. But many reductions in quality wrought by managed care organizations will not fall within this uncontroversial core. For these latter quality reductions, there is no basis for saying that the organizations that effect them are acting wrongly, or that their enrollees are being deprived of something to which they are entitled.

WHY THE DENIAL OF CARE AND LOWER QUALITY ARE NOT INCOMPATIBLE WITH ETHICAL BEHAVIOR ON THE PART OF PROVIDERS

It is often said that participation in the rationing practices of managed care is incompatible with ethical behavior on the part of physicians (and nurses, etc.). The most vigorous critics seem to assume that it is unethical for physicians to provide anything other than all services that are expected to be of any benefit for the patient at the highest level of quality that is technically feasible.

This assumption, however, is indefensible. In any system, but especially in a system in which coverage is primarily financed by private employers, there must be limits on which services are provided and on the quality with which they are delivered. It is simply wishful thinking to assume that cost containment in managed care can succeed in controlling health care costs without having a negative impact on coverage and quality. (It is worth noting that some managed care organizations have explicitly acknowledged that reductions in quality are sometimes justified by emphasizing that they seek to maximize *value,* where value is understood as a function of quality and cost.)

So, in itself the fact that managed care rationing denies services and lowers quality provides no basis for saying that these organizations are requiring physicians to act unethically. In the absence of an authoritative standard for what counts as adequate care, such behavior on the part of physicians would only be unethical if physicians were obligated to provide all beneficial care and to provide only care

of the highest quality. Of course, some assume that physicians have this obligation simply by virtue of being medical professionals. But if a realistic appreciation of the need to control costs in health care is to count for anything, such an understanding of the role of physicians must be rejected. There is every reason to believe that effective cost containment can only be achieved if physicians refrain from insisting on the highest quality care that is expected to be of any benefit, regardless of costs and regardless of the ratio of costs to benefits.

If this is so, then the alternatives are stark but simple: Either we hold fast to the assumption that medical professionalism is incompatible with physicians providing anything less than the highest quality care in every case, but must conclude that a system that effectively controls costs has no place for medical professionals; or we rethink our conception of medical professionalism to make room for the idea that providing less than the highest quality of care is sometimes acceptable.

The former alternative is unacceptable. There is no reason why cost control in our health care system should be held hostage to an indefensible "essentialist" conception of medical professionalism that, in effect, says that a physician cannot be a true physician or an ethical physician unless he ignores the fact that resources are scarce.[4] None of this is to deny that physicians face serious ethical challenges in managed care. It is only to reject the groundless claim that whenever physicians do not provide all beneficial care or provide less than the highest quality care, they act wrongly. Once this point is appreciated, it becomes clear just how debilitating the absence of a standard for adequate care is. In the absence of such a standard for what patients are entitled to there is no answer to the question, "Which denials of care and how much reduction in quality is acceptable?" And there is no answer to the question: "When does the physician's participation in efforts at cost containment violate his or her fiduciary obligation to the patient?"

A disclaimer is in order at this point. My contention is not that no standards of ethical behavior apply to the actions of physicians in managed care, nor that everything physicians are asked to do by managed care organizations is ethically permissible.

I have only argued that the fact that physicians do not provide potentially beneficial care, or that they provide care that is not of the highest quality, does not in itself constitute a breach of their obligations. There are other ways that physicians can go wrong ethically in the managed care environment, however. For example, if physicians encourage their patients to believe that they are acting solely as advocates for the patient's best interests, but in fact make decisions that do not maximize the patient's interests, then they act wrongly. Similarly, given the pervasive and long-standing cultural expectation that physicians are to give their patients all reasonable information about alternatives for treatment, "gag clauses" that prohibit physicians from informing their patients of potentially beneficial treatments available elsewhere that are not provided by the patient's managed care organization are unethical. . . .

CONCLUSION

I began this essay by noting that the problems of managed care seem to have eclipsed the primary access problem in the United States—the fact that over 40 million people lack health insurance (along with at least another 20 million who are radically underinsured). Before we become excessively preoccupied with the ethical dilemmas of managed care, we should pause to note that all the parties to the controversy over managed care are the "haves"—the insured population that worries about denial of beneficial care, the payers who want to control costs, and the providers who fear losing their professional autonomy and forfeiting patient trust. Conspicuously absent from this triad are the millions of uninsured. If my analysis is correct, the "haves" cannot so easily escape the "have nots"—that is, the ethics of managed care will remain a confused muddle of blame-shifting until the primary access problem is addressed. For until a societal consensus emerges on what forms of health care at what level of quality all are entitled to, and until an authoritative and realistic division of responsibilities for access is institutionalized in our mixed private-public system, the ethical debate about rationing and quality of care *in* managed care will continue to be confused and sterile.

The ethical indignation over managed care, though sometimes conceptually confused, is both un-

derstandable, and—if properly redirected—potentially a force for progress. Given the expectations that the third-party fee-for-service system engendered, it is not surprising that people should tend to assume that if they have health care insurance, they are entitled to "the best care," and that they should be deeply troubled by some of the reductions in coverage that are now occurring. If these negative sentiments can be informed by a recognition that the problem, ultimately, lies with the system, rather than with particular organizations or agents within it, they may eventually motivate systemic reform.

Instead of blaming managed care organizations for failing to fulfill obligations concerning access and quality that they do not have, excoriating them for giving patients less care than they are entitled to when what they are entitled to is wholly unclear, and accusing them of causing physicians to fail to discharge alleged fiduciary obligations that are incompatible with any reasonable hope of cost control, perhaps we should focus our energies on the primary access problem. What is most ethically problematic about managed care is not that it denies beneficial care, reduces quality, and pressures physicians to act as rationers. What is most ethically problematic about managed care is the system of which it is a part, for whose most basic ethical flaw it provides, and can provide, no remedy.

NOTES

1 Privatization is used to refer to a broad range of initiatives, including the following: (1) selling public health care facilities and delivery organizations to private enterprises; (2) contracting out publicly provided services to private enterprises through competitive bidding; (3) using government policies to encourage the growth of for-profit health care entities (hospitals, nursing homes, and outpatient facilities); (4) using government policies to encourage greater reliance on private health insurance (including combination insurer-provider organizations such as HMOs); and (5) implementing de-insurance practices, such as the introduction or escalation of out-of-pocket payment for health care services (copayments, deductibles, and charges for prescription drugs)

2 Of course, a mixed system is only one way to achieve access to an adequate level or decent minimum of care for all. A purely public system could also achieve this. The topic of the present article, however, is the ethical status of rationing in managed care, which exists in a mixed system.

3 Of course, some contend that there would be no access gap in an unencumbered, competitive market for health care insurance—all would receive what they are entitled to, according to their preferences and ability to pay, if they were free to purchase from among the full range of leaner to more generous benefit packages which such a market would offer. This free-market view of just health care rests on either of two assumptions: (1) that there is no market-independent health care entitlement—just health care is whatever the free market delivers; or (2) that there is an independent entitlement, but as a matter of fact an unencumbered, competitive market for health care insurance would ensure that this entitlement was available to all. The former assumption weds the free-market theory of just health care to a larger free-market theory of justice, according to which the outcomes of competitive markets, whatever they turn out to be, are just. Virtually no one has actually espoused this view, since it is very implausible to argue that market outcomes are just regardless of the initial distribution of assets people bring to the market. Once it is admitted that the justice or injustice of the initial distribution of assets is relevant to the justice of the outcomes of market processes, the first assumption must be abandoned. The second assumption is equally implausible, in my view, because there are some individuals, including those unable to work (such as children and the severely disabled) who would not be able to get the "decent minimum" of services (under any reasonable description of the latter) at affordable prices in a competitive insurance market. However, for my purposes, it is not necessary to show that this is so; all that is necessary is to point out that in order to know whether or not the second assumption is true, we need first to settle the issue of what counts as a "decent minimum" (or "adequate level") of care. Until we know what this is, we cannot establish that a competitive market does (as assumption 2 contends) deliver it to all (Brock and Buchanan 1986: 224–249; Buchanan 1987).

4 For a prominent instance of the "essentialist" view that rationing care is incompatible with being an ethical physician, see Pellegrino and Thomasma 1988: 172–173.

REFERENCES

Brock, Dan W., and Allen Buchanan. 1986. Ethical Issues in For-Profit Health Care. In *For-Profit Enterprise in Health Care,* ed. Bradford H. Gray. Washington, DC: National Academy.

Buchanan, Allen. 1987. Justice and Charity. *Ethics* 97(3):558–575.

—. 1992. Private and Public Responsibilities in the U.S. Health Care System. In *Changing to National Health Care,* ed. Robert P. Huefner and Margaret P. Battin. Salt Lake City: University of Utah Press.

Council on Ethical and Judicial Affairs, American Medical Association. 1995. Ethical Issues in Managed Care. *Journal of the American Medical Association* 273(4): 330–335.

Daniels, Norman. 1986. Why Saying No to Patients in the United States Is So Hard. *New England Journal of Medicine* 314(21):1380–1383.

Emanuel, Ezekiel J., and Nancy Neveloff Dubler. 1995. Preserving the Physician-Patient Relationship in the Era of Managed Care. *Journal of the American Medical Association* 273(4):323–329.

Pellegrino, Edmund, and David Thomasma. 1988. *For the Patient's Good: The Restoration of Beneficence in Health Care.* New York: Oxford University Press.

Rodwin, Marc. 1993. *Medicine, Money, and Morals: Physicians' Conflicts of Interest.* New York: Oxford University Press.

Spece, Roy G., Jr., David S. Shimm, and Allen Buchanan, eds. 1996. *Conflicts of Interest in Clinical Practice and Research.* New York: Oxford University Press.

RATIONING: DON'T GIVE UP
Leonard M. Fleck

Asserting that fairness in health-care reform in the United States will require rationing for all, Fleck argues that philosophers can play an important role in a necessary public conversation. "Last chance" therapies, he contends, demonstrate the indispensability of rationing decisions in that they represent a final opportunity at prolonging the lives of certain patients, but are extremely expensive while providing only marginal benefits. Fleck argues that managed care organizations and public insurance programs should not be required to cover these therapies because doing so would drive up health-care costs, thereby making it harder to insure the currently uninsured— which should be the highest priority of health-care reform. The contribution that philosophers can make to reform efforts, according to Fleck, includes (1) educating the public about the need for their input regarding these moral issues, (2) motivating the public to take part in rational democratic deliberations, and (3) facilitating these deliberations about rationing and health-care reform.

There can be no health reform without health care rationing. There can be no *fair* health reform without health care rationing *for all*. This is my first large point. Second, philosophers can have, and ought to have, a substantial role in achieving health reform, but it will not be as academic scholars or as political shills or as masters of the media sound bite. Rather, it will be as facilitators (honest brokers) of a certain sort of public conversation.

The problem of health care rationing will become more painfully acute during this decade, especially because we are likely to see the rapid proliferation of costly "last chance" therapies. I have in mind three examples that have achieved some media prominence in the past year. They are the totally implantable artificial heart (TIAH), the left ventricular assist device (LVAD), and Herceptin, a drug now available to women with metastasized breast cancer, specifically, the 30 percent of such women with HER-2 receptors that have the unfortunate effect of speeding up the metastatic process. For our purposes, the defining features of these therapies are that they represent the last chance at prolonging life for individuals who otherwise face death in the near future; they are very expensive at the individual level and in the aggregate; and they typically yield what from some social point of view would be judged marginal benefits relative to costs. All the same, they are interventions that patients are very likely to want. Is a just and caring society, or employer, or managed care plan morally obligated to provide them?

To concretize the issue a bit, there is a potential annual need of 350,000 TIAHs at an aggregate cost of $52 billion. If this number seems high, the reader should know that we currently perform about 650,000-bypass surgeries in the United States each

year and another 600,000 coronary angioplasties. Projections are that the TIAH will provide an average of five extra years of life expectancy, although the range around that average could be quite large. If we provide the device to anyone at social expense (through Medicare, for example), would justice require that we provide it to someone whose predicted life expectancy with the device might be only one year? This is the "ragged edge" problem that Daniel Callahan has insightfully identified.

There will be a potential need of 200,000 LVADs each year for patients with end-stage congestive heart failure, although predicted survival on average for that device might be only one to two years. Herceptin therapy might be needed by 12,000 women each year at a likely cost of $70,000 per case. As reported in the *New England Journal of Medicine* (15 March 2001), the average gain in life expectancy for this therapy is five months, with some women gaining significantly more than that. This translates to a cost per life-year saved of about $160,000. But there is nothing else that can be offered these women, who are doubly unfortunate because they have both a terminal illness and a genetic predisposition to faster progression of the disease. Is a just and caring society morally obligated to provide them with access to this therapy at social expense?

We can imagine "compassionate" legislative mandates that would require Medicare and private insurance companies to cover these "last chance" therapies. But would that be a good thing to do? Should we applaud such efforts as another incremental step on the road to health reform?

My response to both questions would be negative, mainly for two reasons. First, these are the "early" last chance therapies. There will be many more, and there will be no morally or rationally obvious place to draw a line. Second, these therapies will dramatically increase health costs for the already insured, thereby making it all the more unlikely that we will have the political and economic resources to address the health needs of the uninsured, which is where the health reform effort really needs to begin.

What should be the role of the philosopher in addressing the issues of health reform and health care rationing? There are three critical roles. One is to educate the public, especially community and professional leaders, about the urgency and importance of these questions, and to explain that they are *moral issues requiring their engagement.* They are not discussions best shunted to experts of one sort or another. It must be emphasized that this is not a "pure" philosophic role; philosophers, to be credible, must be willing to educate themselves about the relevant empirical and policy literature so that the moral issues are realistically contextualized.

Second, philosophers must be able to effectively motivate the public to engage in rational democratic deliberation about these issues over a sustained period of time. I have found an essay by Allen Buchanan to be a nearly perfect example of the sort of argument that is needed to motivate the public. [See "Managed Care: Rationing Without Justice, But Not Unjustly," *Journal of Health Politics, Policy, and Law* 23 (1998).] He calls attention to the unceasing cries of unjust treatment by members of managed care plans who have had one or another rationing decision imposed upon them. But he points out that there is no shared conception of justice for determining what health care resources a person has a just claim to; their complaints are just rhetorical fulminations. If they are unhappy with that state of affairs, then they need to engage in the public deliberations that can create and legitimate a shared conception of health care justice. For such legitimation to occur, the safe and indifferent middle class ensconced in managed care plans will have to address the problem of the uninsured; their conception of health care justice cannot (logically) be their private creation.

Third, philosophers ought to serve as facilitators of these rational democratic deliberations about health reform and health care rationing. That means philosophers cannot pose as prophets or experts. Rather, they need to facilitate these conversations in the Deweyan problem-solving mode of honest public inquiry, as opposed to lecturing from some point of view.

The basic message that frames these discussions would be this: We cannot escape the need to make these rationing decisions, especially the very painful decisions associated with last chance therapies. Someday, virtually all of us will likely be affected by this problem. We can make these rationing decisions collectively in ways that we judge to be "just enough" and "caring enough," given that there are no perfectly just options available to us. Or we can allow bureaucrats and administrators and employers and stockholders to make these decisions *for* us on whatever grounds they choose, moral or non-moral. There is nothing wise or virtuous in the healthy segregating themselves from the ill.

There are many reasonable and just rationing choices that we might make with respect to TIAHs and LVADs and therapy for metastasized breast cancer. But we must in fact *make* those decisions, and make them on rationally explicit grounds, if we want to avoid arbitrary and discriminatory access and limitation decisions. And we must make those decisions in the context of a socially endorsed universal package of health benefits.

There are many ways in which these public deliberations might be subverted or perverted. The critical role of the philosopher is to use her skills to protect them from subversive social currents and to help the conversation move toward a mutually respectful overlapping consensus. Socrates, Dewey, and Rawls would all be proud.

CLOSURE, FAIR PROCEDURES, AND SETTING LIMITS WITHIN MANAGED CARE ORGANIZATIONS

Norman Daniels and James Sabin

Daniels and Sabin address the question of what conditions are necessary for the moral legitimacy of decisions made by managed care organizations (MCOs) to ration or set limits on desired, potentially beneficial care. Drawing on preliminary data from a study of how MCOs make decisions about coverage for new technologies, the authors argue that closure—the making of allocation decisions for an insured population within the constraints of a fixed budget—is not strictly necessary for legitimacy even if it is preferable. More important, they maintain, is fairness in the process involved in setting limits and making other allocation decisions. Fairness, according to Daniels and Sabin, requires decision making based on reasons that reasonable people will accept, openness about the reasons underlying decision making, and the opportunity for revisiting disputed decisions.

Managed care organizations (MCOs) and other insurers sometimes deny access to new technologies that patients and clinicians think medically appropriate or believe are a medical last chance. In the climate of considerable public distrust that exists in the United States, these denials are sometimes met with litigation or even legislative mandates requiring coverage for the treatment, even though a solid case can be made that these technologies are still experimental and that contractual language excludes their coverage. For example, attempts by MCOs to restrict access to unproven uses of high-dose chemotherapy with bone marrow transplants were greeted by both responses. Distinct from the problem of distrust, however, is another problem, which we will refer to here as the legitimacy problem. It is posed by the question: Under what conditions would patients, members of health plans, and clinicians come to accept limit-setting decisions by MCOs as fair or legitimate? We will discuss this question drawing on preliminary observations from a study of how MCOs make decisions about coverage for new technologies (see Acknowledgment section). First, however, we will revisit briefly the concept of closure—roughly the idea that resource allocation decisions for a covered population are made within a budget—in order to modify the importance that one of us attributed to it earlier, in light of the discussion of the legitimacy problem.

Reprinted with permission of Blackwell Publishing Ltd. from *Journal of the American Geriatrics Society,* vol. 46, no. 3 (March 1998), pp. 351–354.

CLOSURE: BRIEF HISTORY OF AN IDEA

After the introduction of diagnosis-related groups (DRGs) in 1983, when caps on hospital reimbursements began to affect physician decisions about hospital stays for Medicare patients, many people complained that physicians were being pressured to make medical decisions that were not in the best interests of their patients. Early discharge for a frail older patient, for example, might not be in her best interest. Physicians complying with pressures from DRGs would thus be denying medically beneficial services and would fail to act as the fiduciary agents of their patients. Why did it seem so hard to say no? Would such denials ever be fair?

Daniels suggested at the time that "saying no" to beneficial treatments was particularly difficult in the US, compared with Canada or Great Britain, for example, because denials in the US are not made in a closed system.[1] A closed system is one in which (1) a determinate quantity of resources is devoted to health care, presumably as the result of a democratic decision to devote just so much of the social budget to health care rather than to other things, and (2) there is a process for allocating those resources to meet the needs of the covered population. In a closed system, what is spent on one thing is not available for something else, and what is saved by avoiding one use can then be allocated to something else. Specific decisions about which needs to meet must consider the "opportunity cost" of using resources for one need rather than another. Such decisions can be made in various ways. For example, a Canadian primary care physician once explained why he would not game the queuing system for CT scans by rating a patient as more urgent than the patient was. Doing so, he said, would reduce his credibility with the gatekeepers for that resource and would work to the disadvantage of all of his patients. Under closure, with reliable procedures in place, it would be possible to say to patients who were denied treatment that the resources saved by not meeting their needs were in fact being used to meet more important needs of others. Not only would it be possible to say that, but it would be possible to document whether it was true.

Patients (or clinicians) might still disagree with the specific judgments about which needs were more important to meet, but they would presumably accept the overarching principle that limited resources should be allocated to meet more important needs before meeting less important ones. If a reasonable set of judgments were made about how to allocate limited resources fairly, and if the limit on resources were itself reasonable and fair, then we could say to losers, "Every system will have some people who lose out to others, but you are not worse off than anyone need be under feasible alternative arrangements." This principle governing fair treatment would seem to be widely accepted and derivable within various accounts of justice and health care, including the one we endorse.[2]

Cost-containment measures in the US, however, operated outside of a closed system at that time. There was—and still is—no assurance that expenditures not made for one patient will be used for others for whom treatment is more important. We cannot say to the Medicare patient experiencing a premature discharge that the savings will be used to meet more urgent needs elsewhere in the system, for the savings might actually be returned to investors in a for-profit hospital or they might be used to invest in services that meet less important needs. A physician might then plausibly think, "I should aim for the good I can definitely control, my patient's extra days, not the questionable good from savings, for those may disappear into black holes in the system." This rationale for noncompliance expresses the deep strain of commitment that results when the open system prevents any assurance that the sacrifice is fair. The rationale justifies gaming the system in various ways.

CLOSURE AND MANAGED CARE: THE LEGITIMACY PROBLEM

Do managed care organizations (MCOs) offer a way around this problem by providing appropriate closure? After all, they cover a defined population with a specific set of resources derived from members' premiums. For that population, don't they form a closed system that would permit the appropriate reassurances to patients and clinicians about fairness in reallocating savings?

We answer this question with three points. First, it is not clear that all MCOs form closed systems in the relevant sense. Second, at least with regard to decisions about coverage for new technologies, MCOs do not make decisions about opportunity costs under closure. Third, MCOs face a legitimacy problem in their decision-making about setting limits, including their decision-making about coverage for new technologies. Consequently, the nature of the process for making those decisions is crucial to providing reassurances about fairness and legitimacy.

The first point, that not all MCOs are perceived to be closed systems in the relevant sense, becomes apparent when we consider the problem of medical loss ratios (the percent of expenditures not actually spent on medical services) and what might be meant by saying that resources available to meet health-care needs for a defined population are limited in a closed system. In the Canadian or British systems, resources are limited by a democratic decision about global budgets for health care that are applied to provinces or regions. The budget allows a specific amount for administrative costs, in effect specifying a medical loss ratio. In these systems, administrative costs tend to be extremely low by American standards.

In MCOs, medical loss ratios—the portion of a health-care dollar not spent on medical services—vary widely, from nearly 10% for some nonprofit organizations to nearly 30% for some for-profit companies,[3] although there is controversy about whether some variation is caused by variations in accounting methods, e.g., across the boundary between non-profits and for-profits.[4] In our competitive system, some of the nonmedical expenditures will go to marketing costs, some to high upper-level management salaries, and, in for-profit MCOs, to returns to investors. If a patient (or practitioner) encounters a limit on services that are arguably beneficial, he would be persuaded that savings from the limit worked to meet the greater needs of other patients only if he believed that the competitive system were so efficient that patients as a whole did better under it than under alternative arrangements. For example, he would have to believe that an adequate return to investors was part of the mechanism that made the system more efficient than any noncompetitive system and that, despite the high medical loss ratio, more resources were available for meeting patient needs than would be available under alternative systems. Absent such a conviction in the competitive system, or in for-profits organizations within it, health-care dollars that flow into the pockets of investors or advertisers in charge of marketing will be perceived as "leaks" from the system, violating closure.

The second point came as a surprise. When we began studying how leading managed care organizations made decisions about coverage for new technologies, we expected to find some form of comparative decision-making. That is, we expected MCOs to have a relatively fixed budget for coverage of new technologies, especially in the current climate in which employers and the government were shopping for lowest premiums that MCOs could offer, and we expected to find some consideration of which among the new technologies it would be most important to offer under those budget constraints. We did not find what we expected.

So far, we have found only noncomparative decision-making at the organizations we have studied. This finding is true whether assessments of technologies for safety and efficacy are done internally, by committees that do their own literature review and assemble their own expert panels, or partly externally, using assessments made by commercial vendors. We see no evidence that coverage decisions reflect a prior budgeting decision. Each technology seems to be on the table by itself. There is no comparison with competing technologies except with alternative treatments for the same condition. When a decision to cover a new technology is made, however, it is usually not a simple yes or no. Rather, a much more detailed decision is generally made, specifying approval for aspects of the technique (if there are important variants), selection criteria for patients, and even selection criteria for providers, e.g., centers of excellence for doing certain surgeries or cancer treatments.

We have interviewed key figures in the technology assessment process at six collaborating sites. Among them, there is almost universal rejection of the idea that MCOs are in a position to make comparative decisions about new technologies. They tend to see the task of technology assessment as limited: it is primarily intended to prevent the dissemination of technologies that provide no net benefit compared with alternatives for that condition. The criteria used by the national Blue Cross/Blue Shield Medical Advisory Panel of the Technology Evaluation Center are limited to that purpose. Cost-effectiveness may be considered among alternative strategies for treating the same condition. (Because comparative decisions are not in evidence, more controversial uses of cost-effectiveness to compare technologies for treating different conditions are also not in evidence.) Through interviews with participants in coverage decisions and observations of meetings at which such decisions are made, we find a great reluctance to be put in the situation of making choices about relative importance among new treatments that show reasonable net benefit. No one seems willing to be put in the position of having to say to patients or clinicians demanding such technologies that the coverage committee thought one set of needs was more important to meet than another. The dominant sentiment was that such decisions should be societal, not the prerogative of medical directors and other specialists in a committee appointed by a private organization. Some have said explicitly that they would not be able to defend such decisions in court. Others raise explicit concerns that when further sources of waste are squeezed out of the healthcare, system, e.g., when we have shortened hospital stays as much as it is reasonable to do so, then consideration of "opportunity cost" will become more pressing (that is, we will have to compare the value of investment in this technology with the value of alternatives to see if we are getting the highest value use of our resources).

There is an important irony here. The American public was scared away from national health-care reform, including talk about nationally mandated benefit packages, in part because it feared big government making health-care decisions. When members of the Ethics Working Group of the Clinton Health Care Task Force argued that there should be some discussion of the mechanism for making decisions about coverage under budget constraints, they were told that rationing (the R word) could not be used in any documents the task force produced.[5] The fear was that openness would backfire and that the Clinton plan would seem to be admitting it would ration health care and would be attacked (it was attacked anyway). The effect of the failure of comprehensive reform is to leave many decisions about coverage in private hands, specifically in the hands of managers of MCOs (and other insurers). But these organizations fear being accused of rationing as much as did advocates of specific comprehensive legislative reforms. The result is that new technologies are disseminated only through the filter of judgments about safety and net benefit. Because many view new technologies as a primary driving force for health-care costs across all variations in health-care systems,[6] these organizations ultimately will increase the pressures they face to reduce costs. When the main sources of savings are exhausted—e.g., reducing hospital stays or extracting higher discounts from various providers—there will be less room to escape from the need for comparative decision-making.

BEYOND CLOSURE: TOWARD SOLVING THE LEGITIMACY PROBLEM

The climate of distrust that surrounds large insurers and managed care organizations in the US makes solving the legitimacy problem more urgent, but it does not constitute that problem. Rather, the legitimacy problem derives from the fundamental fact that decisions to limit use of (arguably) beneficial services, including new technologies, are moral and not simply technical decisions. Indeed, they are morally controversial. The issue, then, is why we should view MCOs as a legitimate authority for making moral decisions about the well-being of members.

Even noncomparative decisions about new technologies raise morally difficult and controversial questions. For example, an MCO may believe that it has an obligation to all covered members to conserve resources and adhere to a principle, often reflected in contractual language, that says investigational or unproven treatments are not covered benefits. This principle might be defended further on the grounds that, over time, knowledge of efficacy derived from controlled clinical trials is the proper basis for making further decisions about how to meet healthcare needs of a covered population. In addition, the MCO may feel that it cannot take the chance of imposing unacceptable risk/benefit ratios on patients by covering unproven therapies. Whereas these are powerful reasons for restraint, there are also opposing considerations. If a patient faces a life-threatening illness, for example, a respect for shared decision-making about risk taking might argue for not putting so much weight on the MCO's judgment about uncertainty and unacceptable risk/benefit ratios. The medical urgency of the condition might also be viewed as a reason to relax the concern about conserving resources or for modifying the standard of what counts as investigational. It is possible for reasonable people to disagree about these matters.

When we face comparative decisions about new technologies, because, for example, budget constraints begin to apply to coverage decisions for them, as they currently do in some globally budgeted systems, we face even more difficult moral problems. For example, Daniels has argued that a principle assuring equality of opportunity, like other general principles of distributive justice, is too indeterminate to solve some of the key rationing problems we face.[7,8] The concern for equal opportunity tells us, for example, that we must give some priority to those with the most restricted opportunities, but it cannot give a principled account of how much priority to give. Similarly, we know that to protect opportunity in a whole population, we must sometimes aggregate modest benefits to larger numbers in favor of significant benefits to very few. Here, too, we have no principled account of how to aggregate (although Kamm explores this issue in pathbreaking ways[9]). Similarly, we do not know how to weight, in a principled way, promoting best outcomes against giving people fair chances at getting some benefit.

When general principles of distributive justice fail to give principled solutions, we must either look for more fine-grained principles or we must turn to fair procedures and treat their outcomes as fair. Just as general principles of justice prove too indeterminate to solve crucial rationing problems, so, too, do general specifications of the goals of medicine. Agreeing, for example, that reducing premature death is a reasonable goal of medicine whereas eliminating all fatal disease is not[10] does not provide us with solutions to the kinds of rationing problems noted here.

We are pushed to emphasize fair publicly accountable procedures by another line of reasoning. Only such procedures can establish legitimacy for the setting of limits on beneficial medical services. This point is true in universal public systems, in which rationing is often carried out covertly and hidden in budget-setting practices, and it is particularly pressing in our mixed system, in which the grounds for decision-making may even be viewed as trade secrets. Why should a patient or a clinician who takes her agency role seriously accept limits set by managed care organizations? For those limits to seem fair and reasonable, they would have to reflect concerns about how to meet the more important needs of other patients under resource constraints. Because most or all managed care organizations do not provide any reasons at all for their coverage decisions, even where some good reasons may under-

lie the actual decision, they feed the suspicion of many people that decisions are largely motivated by efforts to reduce costs and improve the bottom line, whether the organization is for-profit or not.

What would a fair decision-making procedure involve, given that these decisions have a moral content, that people may disagree about what outcomes count as fair, and that the stakes are high? If we were talking about decisions in a public agency (like the Oregon Health Resources or Health Services Commissions), we might be tempted to emphasize public participation, and we might be lulled into thinking that the key element was a democratic procedure, such as a majority vote among appropriate officials, including patient representatives and representatives of other interest groups. The problem with this procedural view, even in public agencies, is that voting among such representatives may seem to be simply a way of aggregating preferences. Nevertheless, moral decisions about public policy, we are inclined to think, should not simply be the result of maximizing the satisfaction of preferences.[11-13] Good reasons matter, and deliberation about them is key. Given pluralism about values, we cannot expect that all moral reasons and reasoning will be persuasive to everyone, but if fundamental interests are at stake, we at least should seek to base our decisions on reasons that all free and equal citizens can accept.

We need to adapt this insight from the theory of deliberative democracy to the context of managed care organizations, where institutional structures may not permit us to insist on direct public participation in public deliberation about limit setting.[14] The key element in adaptation, we suggest, is the focus on reasons that all can accept as a reasonable basis for deliberation about how to protect normal functioning for a defined population under budget constraints. If the reasons for decisions about coverage for new technologies are made explicit and are available to clinicians, patients, and would-be members, then there is the basis for a wider social conversation and deliberation about the goals of medicine. The fair procedure would also involve grievance or dispute-resolution mechanisms and opportunity for revisiting decisions.

An example will help. Suppose a MCO decides to cover growth hormone treatment but only for children who are growth hormone deficient or who have Turner's syndrome. It should state the reason for its limitations on coverage. This statement might appear, for example, in its medical director's letter to clinicians, where such policies are often published (generally without reasons or rationale). Reasons should also be provided in support materials used in informing would-be patients or families in an attempt to secure informed consent or, better, to engage in "shared decision-making" about the procedure.

Good reasons for limiting coverage to these categories of patients might be that there is inadequate evidence of efficacy, or inadequate evidence of good risk/benefit ratios, for other children. Such reasons are clearly aimed at a public good that all can understand, the provision of effective and safe treatment to a defined population under resource constraints. Of course, if new evidence of broader efficacy or safety emerges, then the decision may have to be revisited if that is the only reason for the limits.

Another defensible but more controversial reason for the limited coverage might be that coverage should be restricted to treatment of disease or disability (departures from normal functioning), whereas being very short, with no other diagnosable condition, is not a disease or disability. This reason requires a moral argument. Not all will accept it; they may have a more expansive view of the tasks of medicine.[15, 16]

Over time, through this reason-giving process, MCOs would articulate a fine-grained conception of how to provide high-quality care to a defined population under resource constraints. The decisions and the accompanying reasons would constitute a form of case law. Through interaction, challenge, and deliberation among all those affected by these decisions, the decisions can be modified. Over time, if these organizations are responsive to some combination of market forces and public regulation, the social deliberation that the reason-giving enables becomes the basis for our articulating acceptable goals of medicine. Through this process, we can flesh out in practical decision-making acceptable reasons for setting limits. To the extent that the kinds of reasons that then play a visible role in articulating the goals of the organization are reasons that all must view as

appropriate and reasonable, the organization appealing to them will be perceived to have a legitimate decision-making procedure.

Notice that addressing the legitimacy problem in these ways does not require that an organization actually satisfy the condition of closure discussed earlier. Even without true closure, progress could be made on the legitimacy problem, and some assurance could be given about fairness. We believe, however, that closure reduces uncertainty about the fairness of some reallocation decisions, uncertainty that would be hard to remove when we consider the nature of some kinds of leakage from MCOs. Conversely, if there is closure, there may still be a problem of legitimacy. Closed European systems that have denied some last-chance treatments have sometimes been challenged by patients, clinicians, the media, and politicians who are not persuaded that the denial is based on sound reasons, often because these public systems are as secretive about their deliberations as are our private health plans. Although closure helps, my main point is that the nature of the process involved in limit-setting and other allocation decisions is more important in establishing legitimacy than is the mere fact of closure itself.

ACKNOWLEDGMENTS

The research on which this paper draws is part of a project titled "Decisions to Limit the Use of New Technologies at HMOs and Other Insurers: Principles, Process, and Guidelines." The project involves five major nonprofit managed care organizations, the Oregon Health Resources Commission, and two for-profit managed care organizations. We are indebted for discussion of these ideas to Susann Wilkinson, a collaborator on this research.

REFERENCES

1 Daniels N. Why saying no to patients in the United States is so hard: Cost containment, justice, and provider autonomy. N Engl J Med 1986; 314:1381–1383.

2 Daniels N. Just Health Care. Cambridge: Cambridge University Press, 1985.

3 Nudelman P. M., Andrews L. M. The 'value added' of not-for-profit health plans. N Engl J Med 1996; 334:1057–1059.

4 Hasan M. Let's end the nonprofit charade. N Engl J Med 1996; 334:1055–1057.

5 Daniels N., Light D. W., Caplan R. L. Benchmarks of fairness for health care reform. New York: Oxford University Press, 1996.

6 Newhouse J. P. An iconoclastic view of health cost containment. Health Aff 12(suppl):152–171.

7 Daniels N. Rationing fairly: Programmatic considerations. Bioethics 1993; 7:724–733.

8 Daniels N. Four unsolved rationing problems. Hastings Cent Rep 1994; 24:27–29.

9 Kamm F. M. Morality and mortality: Death and whom to save from it, Vol 1. Oxford: Oxford University Press, 1993.

10 Callahan D. The goals of medicine: Setting new priorities. Hastings Cent Rep 1996; 6(suppl):S1–28.

11 Rawls J. Political liberalism. New York: Columbia University Press, 1993.

12 Cohen J. Deliberation and democratic legitimacy. In: Hamlin A, Petit P, eds. The Good Polity. Oxford: Blackwells, 1989, p. 17–34.

13 Sunstein C. The partial constitution. Cambridge, MA: Harvard University Press, 1993.

14 Daniels N., Sabin J. E. Limits to health care: Fair procedures, democratic deliberation, and the legitimacy problem for insurers. Philos Public Aff 1997; 26:303–350.

15 Daniels N. Growth hormone therapy for short stature: Can we support the treatment/enhancement distinction? Growth Gener Horm 1992; 8(suppl 1):46–48.

16 Sabin JE, Daniels N. Determining 'medical necessity' in mental health practice. Hasting Cent Rep 1994; 24:5–13.

HEALTH CARE REFORM: STILL POSSIBLE

Ezekiel Emanuel

Citing widespread unhappiness with the American health-care system, relentlessly rising costs, increasing numbers of uninsured Americans, and less comprehensive coverage for those who are insured, Emanuel argues that the United States is entering a major health-care crisis and needs a plan for reform. Comparing the impending crisis with that of the early 1990s—which created a social mandate, ultimately squandered, for systematic health-care reform—he draws several lessons from that experience. Together these lessons suggest, he continues, that any viable approach to health-care reform would retain private managed care delivery, separate insurance from employment, include realistic cost-control mechanisms, and prove palatable to both liberals and conservatives. According to Emanuel, a system of universal health-care vouchers stands the best chance of meeting these criteria.

Without much public notice, health care is entering a crisis. The events of 11 September and the Enron collapse have made that crisis more imminent, serious, and even more likely to come on the American public and politicians unnoticed. September 11 gave the economy another major hit, led to a military build up that will consume whatever budget surplus there might have been, and drew whatever political and public attention exists away from domestic issues. Nevertheless, we should attend to health care

reform. There will soon be a major crisis, and we need to be ready with a reasonable policy for politicians who will suddenly find themselves in need of answers.

Consider four descriptive and five prescriptive propositions that lead to the outlines of a politically palatable and ethically justifiable strategy.

(1) *No one is happy with the current health care system.* Doctors and patients hate the encroachment on their choice, feel they have no control over their health plan, and trust no one. Managed care organizations and employers feel that doctors and patients have unrealistic demands, are unwilling to confront the need to cut costs, and are unwilling to be held

Reprinted with permission of the publisher from *Hastings Center Report,* vol. 32 (March-April 2002), pp. 32–34. Copyright © 2002 by The Hastings Center.

accountable; managed care is asked to do the impossible to simultaneously improve quality and keep costs down.

(2) *Health care costs are going up and will continue to go up in the foreseeable future.* Whatever savings there were in the 1990s from managed care, they are gone, and they will not return. With pharmaceuticals rising at 20 to 30 percent per year, and hospitals and doctors demanding more money, premiums are heading up at double digit rates with no end in sight.

(3) *The number of uninsured Americans is going up and the range of health benefits for those who are insured is going down.* Increases in unemployment and increases in health care premiums mean more people will lose their health insurance. Decreases in corporate profits mean that those still insured will have skimpier benefit packages and bear more of the premium price with higher copayments.

(4) *Pressure on state budgets will also mean close looks at Medicaid budgets.* As the economy declines, state coffers shrink. Coincidentally, rises in unemployment and health care costs will increase Medicaid expenditures, further squeezing state budgets and crowding out other vital state programs, including education and infrastructure improvements.

This is the crisis. But we have been here before. This was almost exactly the situation in the early 1990s, except that then managed care had the potential to constrain costs. And yet, as we all know, health care reform failed. In part, it failed because Clinton spectacularly misplayed the politics of health care reform, and in part because employers embraced managed care—and abandoned Clinton's plan—on the premise that managed care was a more certain path to controlling costs.

What better proof is there that everyone makes big—multibillion dollar—mistakes? But we can learn five key lessons from that stunning and tragic failure that might help develop universal health care coverage.

(5) *The big hurdle for health care reform is not ethics or economics but politics.* Ethics supports universal coverage. Both ethics and economics urge the need for cost constraint. But even when everyone agrees that there is a problem, that is no guarantee they all—or even a majority of them—will support the same solution. The key is to provide a solution that

both liberals and conservatives can endorse, making it harder for any single interest group to kill it.

(6) *Retain a private health care delivery system.* "Harry and Louise" ads proved that the health care insurance industry is strong and can torpedo almost any reform package that tries to eliminate it. After all, its survival is at stake, and the industry has nothing to lose in such a life-and-death struggle. More importantly, no delivery system that is dominantly public will have any chance of widespread public support in the United States. It is important to emphasize ad nauseam that there is a difference between finance and delivery and that predominantly public finance can happily coexist with private delivery. This occurs in lots of spheres—defense procurement, biomedical research, highway construction. But recall Lyndon Johnson's problem with selling Medicare to the American medical establishment and don't underestimate the difficulty of communicating this basic distinction between finance and delivery.

(7) *Break the employer-health insurance link.* This is purely a quirk of history and it persists because of inertia. No reasonable person defends it. With the end of lifetime employment, with American residential and employment mobility, with small businesses as the driving force behind job creation, it makes no sense to have health coverage provided by employers. More importantly, employers no longer want this responsibility. Health care costs are unpredictable and rising; employers need predictability. They would rather compete for employees on salary than on health benefits. For employees, having the employer control which insurance company they get and which doctor they see is odious and constraining.

(8) *Some kind of managed delivery system is here to stay.* While everyone has the managed care blues and many people are writing its obituary, some form of managed health care seems here to stay. Leaving health care decisions to each doctor's discretion has been undermined by quality and cost data. When everyone is talking about the importance of systems for delivering safe, high quality, and cost effective care it is hard to imagine that we will dismantle the very delivery system capable of doing this. It is much more likely that a new form of management will arise.

(9) *Permit a multitiered delivery system as long as the bottom rung is reasonable.* Ethicists often worry about tiered systems in which the the rich have access to better medical care. This worry is mistaken. Justice does not require that every person receive the same health care services. The only key ethical questions are whether the range of medical services guaranteed to all as the minimum is just, and whether allowing the rich to buy more undermines what the less well-off get. We should expect the rich to spend their money to get more of everything, but this should not disturb us if the poor are guaranteed a sufficient package.

So the question is: Is there a health care system that retains private, managed care delivery, breaks the employer link, will not break the bank, and can be politically palatable to both liberals and conservatives? After a century of repeated failures to enact a national health care system, the most hopeful answer that can be given is *maybe.*

The only thing I can imagine that fulfills these requirements is a universal health care voucher system. Vouchers would be provided to individuals and families by the government or by private employers who prefer—or are forced by union contracts—to retain this responsibility. Individuals and families would use vouchers to purchase health insurance from a private managed care or insurance system. A quasi-public body would certify managed care or health insurance companies based on their ability to provide the minimum services, fiscal health, and adequate delivery capacity. This body would also have responsibility for monitoring quality of these delivery systems.

Could this work? This is the barest of outlines and there are a huge number of details to be worked out. I can only sketch some answers to the most critical questions. Politically it has certain attractive qualities. "Universal health care voucher" is a simple sound-bite slogan. The public will like the control it provides over choice of insurance company, as well as the prospect of secure coverage that does not change with every change in employer. For liberals it provides for universality in health insurance—a long-sought goal. Liberals have opposed vouchers in education and for Medicare. But these are existing universal, public provision programs in which a

voucher system seems to take something away. There is no universal entitlement in health care; a voucher may well be the only way to achieve that cherished goal. For conservatives it is a voucher that gives individuals choice over their own health coverage. Conservatives have never met a voucher system they did not like. This would be especially popular with conservatives if Medicare and Medicaid were included either immediately or phased in with new beneficiaries, thereby getting the government completely out of health care.

To ensure fiscal responsibility the value of the voucher would have to be established. The infusion of money required to establish its value would be a net redistribution from the rich to the poor, politically the most problematic of its characteristics. But then the value of the voucher would increase with overall inflation, plus a bit for the aging of the population. This would provide a perfect fiscal rheostat. People who want more services would pay higher premiums and co-payments. As prices increase, people would opt for fewer added services and use their services more prudently and cost consciously. When the gap between the value of the voucher and the premiums increased too much, requiring more out-of-pocket payments, there would be political pressure by the public to significantly increase the value of the voucher. But that would require raising taxes to pay for a higher voucher value. Thus the system would provide perfect individual and social incentive to control costs.

To minimize cherry picking by the managed care and insurance companies, the value of the voucher payment to the companies would be "risk adjusted" or based on partial capitation. This would mean that incentives to exclude the sickest members of society would be minimized or eliminated. Simultaneously, to the public the voucher would appear the same, ensuring universality and popular support.

If we are to have any chance of reforming the health care system to ensure universal health care coverage while controlling costs in a politically palatable form, I think the universal health care voucher is the only way forward. Will it solve all problems? Clearly not. Is a universal health care voucher better than what we have? Definitely.

MANAGING CARE THE CANADIAN WAY

Pat Armstrong

Armstrong argues that Canada's publicly administered, mainly nonprofit health-care system represents an approach to managed care that is superior to the largely privately administered and for-profit American approach. Canada's days of rapid cost escalation, Armstrong points out, ended more than three decades ago when it adopted its current system—medicare—which provides universal access to care; indeed, in recent years per capita spending has actually declined. By contrast, in the United States managed care services are increasingly withheld to lower costs, and overall costs in the system are rapidly rising with greater restrictions on patient choice and no improvement on access to care. Two major factors contributing to this inefficiency, she argues, are enormous administrative expenditures and profiteering by private insurance companies. Armstrong notes that, despite the comparative strengths of the Canadian approach to managing care, there are indications that Canada may experiment with certain features of American-style managed care—an unfortunate development, in her view, considering all the evidence suggesting that the Canadian approach better achieves the goals of health care.

For over 30 years, Canada has had a system for managing care that usually is called "medicare." When the federal government introduced first hospital insurance and then medical insurance, it began one of the world's largest natural experiments in managing care. This experiment has demonstrated that the Canadian publicly administered, mainly nonprofit care is superior to the largely for-profit and privately administered services in the United States. Despite this, Canada is now importing American managed care, in the form of managed care corporations and managed care practices.

The appeal of the U.S. models may be found in their public promises. The *Managed Health Care Dictionary*[1] defines managed care as "any method of health care designed to reduce unnecessary utilization of services, contain costs, and measure performance, while providing accessible, quality, effective health care." Competition, financial incentives and new managerial strategies are the primary methods used to cut costs; service integration, infor-

mation technology and utilization review are the main means of improving quality and access. But the evidence contradicts the claims made about these methods, and about managed care itself. U.S. managed care has not controlled costs, reduced the volume and intensity of service utilization, nor increased access and quality.[2]

Compared to Canada, or any other country with publicly administered care, costs have not been controlled in the United States. Indeed, health economist Robert Evans demonstrates that Canada's period of rapid cost escalation ended with medicare.[3] Our per capita spending has declined in recent years while it has been rising in the United States. The main cost savings with managed care have come through reducing hospital expenditures, primarily through shortening patient stays, a strategy that already has reached its limit here and in the United States. Meanwhile, U.S. outpatient costs have continued to rise parallel with the profits taken from care.

One managed care strategy that is gaining popularity among Canadian health-care planners is capitation, or rostering as it is sometimes called. In this

Reprinted with permission of the publisher from *Humane Health Care International,* vol. 13, no. 1 (Spring 1997), pp. 13–14.

approach, a fixed payment is made to the provider for the patients enrolled in his/her practice, regardless of the number of services supplied. In theory, this gives the providers an incentive to make the most effective use of their time and to keep their patients healthy. At the same time, this arrangement prevents patients from doctor shopping and from abusing the system in other ways. Increasingly, the way into any part of the system is through a single provider, theoretically offering integrated care through "one-stop shopping."

In the United States, this strategy has produced "skimming"—the selection by the plan of healthy patients and the rejection of those who are ill or likely to become so. Also, the plans have introduced incentives to withhold services, in that the more services a physician provides, the lower his/her income. Thus the insurance companies exert enormous pressure on the gatekeepers—an increasing number of whom are employees of the companies. Under the managed care plan, with only one way in, a patient refused enrollment has no alternative service available. Moreover, with this integration of services, large profitable corporations, which own the entire range of services, have been able to reduce the competition that was central to the managed care concept: as competition declines so too do people's choices. In some states one company may provide the only hospital, laboratory and doctors services in town. They may also become the only employer of health-care providers in the area.

Canada already has a capitation system—it is called medicare. People sign up with their provincial or territorial government through a single, administratively efficient entry point in each region. Nevertheless, governments now propose to sign individuals up with a particular provider rather than with the system itself. Recognizing the dangers of "skimming," its proponents suggests legal restrictions on the providers to prevent them from rejecting patients. Also, they propose to restrict a patient's ability to change providers, although there is little evidence that many Canadians "doctor shop" without reason. In any event, second opinions often are warranted, because medicine is an art as well as a science and also because doctors are subject to error or to limited knowledge. Moreover, as people travel to

work or seek employment, it is increasingly difficult for them to ensure that they will have their accidents or fall ill within range of their designated provider.

The U.S. plans run up tremendous administrative costs through their efforts to enroll and control patients, and to manage the perverse underutilization incentives in each of their panels. The plans now employ more administrators than care providers. This practice also shifts the risks of patient illness onto the provider and American practitioners have responded to this risk by joining together into larger and larger provider pools.[4] However, Canadians developed medicare to share these risks and developed a national plan to ensure equitable access to quality care. Services in Canada have become increasingly integrated, while still allowing for variety, choice, and small, community-based services. However, it appears that greater integration patterned on the American system will increase costs and, at the same time, will reduce access and patient choice.

Utilization review, another important strategy in managed care, is also coming to Canada. Based on patterns of practice, in theory utilization review is an assessment that determines whether a practice is medically necessary and efficient. Organizations such as Ontario's Institute for Clinical and Evaluative Sciences (ICES) have developed data on incidence of treatment and use that can be applied to utilization review. ICES cautions that factors other than particular physician practices may influence the data and asserts that the data should provide guidelines rather than formulas for care. Nevertheless, these data often are transformed into formulas in managed care, and commonly utilization data may be used to assess a diagnosis before proceeding to treatment. Usually the assessment is made by someone sitting at a computer examining the data, rather than by a provider examining a patient. Too often, refusal of service may be based on economic considerations; not even on practice patterns. In this way, managed care "increasingly strips physician and hospitals of critical decision-making authority,"[5] although the provider remains responsible for the patient and liable for malpractice action. Meanwhile, the formulas based on patterns may prescribe care. In health care, although there may be only a 10% chance that the symptoms are due to cancer, it is essential that the necessary tests not be denied even though the probabilities are low. Yet such denial would be routine under managed care, if acceptable utilization is based on probability formulas. In the United States, formulas for care have become so restrictive that increasingly patients have sought redress from the courts. New Jersey, for example, has enacted legislation to give women the option of staying in the hospital 48 hours after the birth of a baby, when insurers began to demand that such women leave a day after delivery.[6]

These, and other managed care practices, combined with hospital closures, delisting and other service reductions, set the stage for the takeover of health care by corporations from the United States. Already some managed care firms have moved into the vacuum created by downsizing; indeed the provisions of the North American Free Trade Agreement will make it difficult to reclaim this territory for public care once it is lost. As the President and CEO of Aetna Health Management Canada Inc., a subsidiary of an American insurance company, explained, "Growing government cutbacks in health care such as hospital closures, have created business opportunities."[7] Equally important, the deterioration of services has reduced Canadians' vested interest in our publicly administered system and has increased demands for alternatives. Managed care seems to promise everything we used to have, but at lower cost and delivering better quality.

The plans that began in the United States as health maintenance organizations (HMOs) similar to the Community Clinic in Sault St. Marie, have become giant corporations that amass huge profits from limiting access to care. A large part of the money that could go to human care now goes to profit and increasingly to administrative measures that prevent people from receiving care. As noted earlier, this monitoring that reduces choices for both patients and providers requires an expensive and extensive bureaucracy. In response, American citizens have appealed to the courts and to the legislators, thus producing more regulations and more bureaucracy. Canada's system has not been perfect. However, we have developed a system that provides equitable access for many more people to far better care than managed care has provided in the United States. We have done this with less bureaucracy, more choice and at a lower cost. Why would we look to the U.S. and managed care for models to emulate?

REFERENCES

1 Rognehaugh R. Gaitherburg, Maryland: Aspen, 1996; 109.

2 Finkel, M. L. Managed Care Is Not the Answer. *J Health Politics Policy Law* 1993; 18(1).

3 Health Care Reform: The Issue from Hell. *Policy Options* 1993; 37.

4 Robinson J. C, Casalino L. P. Vertical Integration and Organizational Networks in Health Care. *Health Affairs* 1996.

5 Sederer L. I., Mirin S. M. The Impact of Managed Care on Clinical Practice. *Psychiatric Quarterly* 1994; 65 (3):179.

6 Sullivan J. F. Officials Scrutinizing Doctor Bonuses in Managed Care Plans. *New York Times* 1995; B6.

7 Quoted in Slocum D. Aetna Health Makes First Acquisition. *The Globe and Mail* 1996; B3.

RESTORING THE STATUS OF AN ICON: A TALK WITH CANADA'S MINISTER OF HEALTH

John K. Iglehart

This excerpt from a longer article records most of the author's interview of Allan Rock, Canada's Minister of Health. Whereas Armstrong describes the basic structure of the Canadian health-care system, this interview reveals several of the key challenges facing the system as well as changes designed to help meet these challenges. The picture emerging from the interview includes the following important points. Reduced governmental spending and a gradual transition from hospital-based to community-based services have generated concerns about the accessibility and quality of needed health care. Canadians place a high priority on "restoring our iconic health-care system to the condition it must be in if it's to provide timely access to high-quality care." The basic structure of the system—including the illegality of private companies' providing the same services as are available in the public system—is sound, in terms of both social equity and economic efficiency, according to Rock. But the current range of community-based services and long-term care is inadequate, requiring an integration of such services into the standard benefit package to which all Canadians are entitled. Moreover, the federal government must assume responsibility for fully half of health-care expenditures, up from the current level of about one quarter. Meanwhile, provincial health plans should move away from fee-for-service practice to a rostered approach to primary care in order to ensure twenty-four-hour accessibility and greater efficiency. Finally, ways must be found to ensure that health care delivered in rural areas is of adequate quality and accessibility.

Iglehart: The dean of the University of Toronto's medical school recently characterized Canada's publicly funded health care system as "more than a social program, it is a unifying force and national obsession." Yet in the 1990s public confidence in the system has fallen precipitously. To what do you attribute this erosion of faith?

Rock: The health care system is iconic in Canada because Canadians overwhelmingly believe that it reflects their values and that making medical care available as needed, without barriers with respect to income, is tied into our sense of sharing and caring as a nation. But two activities over the past decade have led to an increasing gulf between the ideal and the principles of the Canada Health Act and the reality on the ground. The first has been a reduction in funding, as federal and provincial governments cut back to overcome the deficit spending of the 1980s and early 1990s and to balance their books. Health care spending accelerated in the 1970s and 1980s almost without restriction, and these expenditures were gobbling up provincial budgets to the tune of almost 40 percent. The federal government ran a huge, crippling deficit, so all governments had to reduce spending. And when you constrain the public portion of health spending, consumers feel it acutely.

Reprinted with permission from *Health Affairs,* vol. 19, no. 3 (May/June 2000), pp. 132–140.

The other development that has roiled the system is its partial restructuring—which would (and should) have happened regardless of the budgetary restraints—from the hospital-based services of the past toward the more community-based services of the future. When both of these things happened together, there were consequences for accessibility, quality, and responsiveness in the system. When you combine that with some problems with long-term planning on human resources in health care, you're going to have challenges with the delivery of services. That undermines the confidence of the public.

Iglehart: One of the consequences of the budget cutbacks was that the national government, which in the early years of the system contributed about half of the resources, now provides provinces less than 25 percent of the funds to operate their health insurance plans. How does Ottawa reconcile its strong determination to remain a full partner with the provinces in the system, when it is providing so little of the funding to operate it?

Rock: If we're going to keep a national health care system, the federal government in Ottawa has to have moral authority and leverage to encourage respect for the national principles and to monitor compliance with national standards. As you point out, when this system started, the federal government picked up about half of the overall cost. The federal government currently covers about 23 percent of overall costs and about 33 percent of the publicly funded costs.

In February 1999 we had what we called the health budget, in which we undertook over five years to greatly increase transfers to the provinces. When those increases are fully felt, our total contribution to health care costs rises to the level of 23 percent. I don't think that's enough. For the Canadian government to continue to have the moral authority to influence reform in the system, to encourage change, and to enforce the principles and standards of the national system, we have to be a more robust contributor.

Let me just give you a brief overview. Of every dollar spent on health care in Canada (out of about $90 billion spent a year), the federal government contributes about twenty-three cents. The consumer, the public—out of their own pockets—contributes about thirty-one cents; the balance, about forty-five cents, is contributed by the provinces. So the government now contributes less to health care costs than the public, whether through private insurance or out-of-pocket spending. We have to increase that, and we should increase it, so that we maintain a place of influence in the discussion of changes in health care and in respect of national principles.

Iglehart: Is this a tough argument to win with the prime minister and his other ministers?

Rock: We're coming out of a period of enormous public restraint. Not only did we not spend additional money in the period 1993–1998, but we actually cut back, shrinking the role of the federal government and reducing program spending by a significant amount. Now that we've balanced the books, although we still have a significant national debt, we at least don't have to worry about an annual deficit in spending, and, in fact, we have a surplus that is growing year by year.

But you can just imagine the pent-up demands, first of all, to restore basic government services to their previous level, whether in national defense or in fisheries; second, to provide additional spending, whether for the needs of children through early intervention programs, in justice by increasing crime prevention, or in immigration by providing for more officers at the border. And quite apart from increased spending demands by Cabinet colleagues, you also have pressure for tax cuts, because the tax burden in Canada is unacceptably high. Personal and corpo-

rate income taxes must come down. Some argue that the consumer tax (the goods and services tax) should be reduced. All of these pressures converge at the same time.

My case, John, is that when you ask Canadians, and we have, they answer in remarkable unanimity (we believe nine out of ten) that the first priority of their government when there's a dollar available should be restoring our iconic health care system to the condition it must be in if it's to provide timely access to high-quality care. Last year we had a health budget that reflected that priority, and I'll continue to argue for health as a top priority every year until we get the numbers right.

MOVING TOWARD PRIVATE COVERAGE?

Iglehart: The squeeze on public expenditures in Canada has rekindled the long-standing debate about the ban on private insurance for publicly insured services. Canada is, after all, the only Organization for Economic Cooperation and Development (OECD) country that does not allow private companies to sell products that offer the same benefits that the provincial health insurance plans provide. Do you think that the growing public pressure for more access to specialists and other services is going to force a change in national policy?

Rock: I believe that we can meet the needs of Canadians within the principles of the Canada Health Act without resorting to private parallel services—because, in my view, the principles of the act allow for all the flexibility that's needed to overcome our problems. But let me say at the outset that I'm firmly convinced that the Canadian system makes sense not only from a social equity point of view, but also from an economic point of view. It makes economic sense because it has been proved again and again that the single-payer, publicly financed, universal system is more cost-effective and constitutes a competitive advantage for Canadian businesses, compared with their U.S. counterparts.

Let me just give you a couple of examples. As a percentage of GDP (gross domestic product) in the United States, health care is almost 14 percent. Canada's figure is 9.5 percent. The public component of spending is about 6 percent in both countries.

The difference is primarily accounted for by overhead and administrative costs. An American professor pointed out last year in Toronto that if you look at a Toronto hospital and a hospital of equal size in Boston, I believe, the Boston hospital had 317 people in the billing and collections department and the Toronto hospital had 17. We don't have to worry about the cost of rating the population or assessing risk, because everybody's in. We don't have to worry about the multipayers, because there's only one. And that administrative difference makes it possible for us to have a much leaner and more efficient health care system. The competitive advantage for employers is that it's much less of a burden for Canadian employers to provide health coverage for their employees; they do so at a fraction of what U.S. employers spend, which is one of the reasons why we have by far the lowest payroll costs of any country in the OECD.

So I'm determined to maintain the current public system, not out of stale dogma or rigid catechism, but because I believe profoundly that it is the best from the social perspective and also makes the most economic sense. And for those who want to have efficiency and effectiveness in government, I say to you that the Canadian system has no peer.

Iglehart: Within the context of the issues over whether or not private resources should be infused into the system, the most recent threat to current national policy seems to be the call of Alberta's premier for the introduction of private hospitals. Would this be a legal action under the Canada Health Act?

Rock: We haven't seen the legislation, so it's impossible to assess whether it's lawful or consistent with the federal act. But from what I know of the proposal, from reading the policy paper, it looks as though it's the wrong thing to do, the wrong solution to the problem that it's intended to address. The problem is, according to the premier, waiting lists of people who cannot get ready access to surgical services. At the same time, public hospitals in Alberta have operating rooms whose lights have been turned off and whose surgeons are idle, because they don't have the funds to go back into the operating room, turn on the lights, and proceed with the surgery.

I fail to understand how the appropriate response to the unmet need is to contract with private facilities when the public facility is already there, idle, waiting for funding. And the orthopedic surgeons themselves in Alberta have called for the money to be put, instead of in the hands of private contractors, into the public hospital, which has already proved to be a more effective and efficient way of meeting the population's surgical needs.

Also, Calgary, Alberta, has already had some experience with contracting out private services for surgical care, including cataract surgery. And the comparative data that we now have on the relative performance of the private facility contracting to provide cataract procedures versus those available in public facilities show that the waiting lists are shorter, the patient outcomes are better, and the costs are less in the public than in the private facility. I don't understand why the premier proposes this course, and I don't think that the last chapter in this saga has yet been written.

LONG-TERM CARE IN CANADA

Iglehart: Long-term care in Canada seems to be a system of services controlled by the provinces, patchwork in their adequacy and the amount of money invested. In your mind, as the population ages, how adequate is the current range of community-based services and long-term care?

Rock: It's not adequate. The transition that I spoke of earlier, which occurred in the 1990s when the hospital sector was downsized, has not been accompanied by a corresponding increase in investment in home and community care. We all know that differences in technology, innovations in pharmaceuticals, new techniques, and greater efficiencies have allowed us to shorten hospital stays. In Canada, twenty-five years ago, hospitals accounted for almost half of health spending; today they're less than a third. I visited a major hospital in one of our big cities recently, where I was told that 72 percent of their surgery is now done on an outpatient basis. Each month our medical journals report breathtaking changes in the kinds of surgical procedures that can be done on an out-patient basis—it's remarkable.

But at the same time, in Canada we have not recognized the corresponding need to increase home and community care supports if we're expecting patients to spend less time in the acute care setting.

What's more, our system has not, in my view, devoted sufficient resources to the whole spectrum of community care, from preacute to postacute care, to supportive housing for the frail elderly, to long-term care, to palliative care for those who want to die at home. My own parents died at home, one after the other in 1994 and 1995, each from cancer, and I had firsthand exposure to the difficulties in getting access to home-care services, the variability in quality, and the lack of connectiveness of home-care services to the rest of the system. It was disturbing.

We're at a point where we need two things: first, a greater recognition of the importance of home and community care as an integrated part of our health care in Canada, and second, a nationwide approach that will ensure that a Canadian, no matter where she or he lives, will have access as part of publicly insured health care services to certain home and community care support. I am working now with my provincial counterparts, negotiating toward a national approach that will weave home and community care into public health care as an integral part of services to which all Canadians are entitled.

Iglehart: Will this proposal eventually become part of the standard provincial benefit package?

Rock: Yes, that's the objective. Just as surgery is covered without cost at the time of service, so would home and community care be made available through the provincial plans. The difficult issues that we're now examining are the scope of coverage, how do we price that coverage, how is it most effectively delivered, what are the standards that we should anticipate, what training is required, and what staffing resources must be put in place. The approach toward which we're tending is to look at national objectives expressed broadly, allowing each province to fulfill those objectives in ways it finds most appropriate, so that there's a maximum degree of flexibility in the hands of provincial ministers of health to meet the national objectives. The government of Canada would pay its share.

Iglehart: Do you see that as a fifty-fifty sharing of costs, or is that still on the table?

Rock: I see it as fifty-fifty. But negotiations with provinces will determine the exact mechanisms for funding, and the amounts.

THE FEDERAL/PROVINCIAL SPLIT

Iglehart: I have the sense that for services that are not covered in the basic package, whether it's home care or pharmacare, there's something of a dilemma involving both the provinces and the federal government, in that the provinces are reluctant to move forward to expand services, say, in pharmacare, because they're uncertain of Ottawa's willingness to sustain a flow of funds, once it has been initiated. How do you work through that? Am I characterizing that right, Allan, as something of a dilemma between the central government and provinces? I cite, for instance, the recommendation of the National Health Care Forum for new benefits in home care and pharmacare, Ottawa apparently agreeing on supporting this or that recommendation, but then a reluctance or even opposition occurs at the provincial level.

Rock: I don't think that's the main issue in pharmacare, because if provincial concern about a consistent federal commitment were the root of the problem, we wouldn't be talking about home care, either.

In pharmacare, I think it's more complicated than that. We had a national conference on pharmacare in 1998, at which the provinces and all of the stakeholders were present, and all of us were impressed with the complexity of the challenge. What we're trying to work toward in this federal mandate, in the period from now until 2001, is agreement on an overall approach to how a national pharmacare plan might work, and then a realistic timetable for its achievement. About 85 percent of the population is already covered in certain circumstances, whether through private plans or public plans because of age or income status. There are many forces to reconcile: the complexity of the infrastructure already in place for approving drugs, which is done federally; decisions about which drugs are included in insurance plans, which is done provincially; the interests of the pharmaceutical companies, both brand-name and generic; and various interest groups representing senior citizens and others. We also have to worry about the sustainability of such a plan going forward, in terms of the increased costs of many prescription drugs.

Clearly this is not something that can be done overnight. We're now trying to put together a plan that will accommodate those interests and achieve a simple national objective: to make sure that price doesn't become a barrier to needed medication for any Canadian. How we achieve that is complex. By the end of this government's term of office in 2001, we hope to have general agreement on a broad plan and a timetable toward its implementation, but I do not believe that the implementation will occur in this term of office.

MARKETING DRUGS TO CONSUMERS

Iglehart: As you know, direct-to-consumer pharmaceutical advertising is running rampant in the United States, in terms of expenditures. Canada does not allow direct-to-consumer advertising—is that correct?

Rock: That's right.

Iglehart: Will that change? Is that a steadfast law that Ottawa believes deeply in?

Rock: I believe that direct-to-consumer drug advertising runs the risk of encouraging demand, which ought to be a clinical, not a consumer-driven, decision. The information should be available to consumers, so that they know the range of services available. That's done, for example, by the Canadian Health Network that we have just launched on the Internet. But allowing direct-to-consumer advertising by the drug companies, I think, is inappropriate. I think clinical decisions about whether a drug should be prescribed should be left in the hands of the clinician.

CHANGING HEALTH CARE DELIVERY MODELS

Iglehart: Over the past decade the managed care model has become dominant in the United States. In Canada provincial health insurance plans have enshrined the small-business model of fee-for-service practice. Do you see any indication that Canada will move away from this mode of physician payment and its emphasis on solo practice?

Rock: Yes, and in my view, it has to happen. If we're going to keep Canada's public health care system, primary health care reform—moving away from fee-for-service as the standard form of remuneration—has to occur. I'm encouraged by movement in that direction.

Even as we speak (in January 2000), our annual emergency room crunch is going on in Canada.

Every January, it's the same. It's perhaps worse this year than others, because of a combination of the flu and other seasonal problems overwhelming the hospital emergency departments and causing difficulties in providing access to genuine emergency cases.

There are two main reasons this happens. The first is that when their primary care physician is unavailable, patients are advised to go to the emergency room, regardless of the urgency of their need. The second is that often persons with genuine emergencies are waiting to be admitted to the hospital but can't be because all of the beds are occupied by people who are ready to be moved to community-based care, which doesn't exist, or moved home, but home care isn't available.

The two greatest challenges are to change the way primary health care is delivered, so that people have access to something other than the emergency room, and to beef up home and community care, so that acute care hospital beds can be freed up for people who really need them.

Coming back to your question, there is now growing support for a rostered approach to primary care, delivered to a defined population by a team of family doctors working in partnership not only with each other but also with nurse practitioners, nurses, midwives, nutritionists, physiotherapists, and perhaps others. This would ensure a much more responsive mechanism for primary health care needs, so that people are not forced to go to the emergency room after five P.M. This includes twenty-four-hour accessibility and a method of payment for a physician that is other than fee-for-service. It has to be fair compensation, worked out with the involvement of the doctors to respect their professionalism. It has to provide for holidays, continuing medical education, and a fair pension. And it could involve negotiations between a given hospital and a team, depending whether or not physicians wanted to work full time or be on call. More and more of the provinces seem to be moving toward negotiating for this type of care approach as they sit down with their medical associations to work out compensation arrangements for the coming years.

Iglehart: I have a strong sense sense that there's support within the Conservative political party, as well as your own Liberal party to move in this direction.

Rock: I'm very encouraged by this. In fact, just this morning I said publicly how much I welcome the Ontario premier's comments (from the Conservative opposition party), and I'm prepared to support him in every way in working toward that goal.

Iglehart: What is the attitude of organized medicine—is that a major obstacle to primary care reform? Not only would such a change entail a new way of paying physicians, but government also would be changing the configuration of the delivery system, something that Canada has not done in the past.

Rock: I believe that views are changing within medical associations, particularly among young physicians, who are more open to alternative compensation approaches than their older peers. Some of the provincial medical associations have helped to mount pilot projects to test different approaches. Also, as more women enter medicine, the flexibility this would provide will be seen as a welcome innovation. In the medical profession generally there is a greater openness, because some doctors find that the current scheme forces on them a lifestyle that is not always fulfilling and rewarding. The nursing profession is also open to these changes.

HEALTH PROFESSIONALS SUPPLY

Iglehart: Canada's medical association believe that the country faces a shortage of physicians, particularly in certain specialties, and Canada's nursing associations believe that the same is true for nurses. Both are calling for an increase in the number of new trainees and perhaps the need to infuse the system, at least temporarily, with more foreign-trained physicians and nurses. What is the national government's view on these questions of supply?

Rock: We met with provincial ministers in September 1999 to talk about this issue. Provincial ministers are responsible for the funding of medical schools. So while I'm not anxious to spend their money for them, I am entitled to a view. That view, which I think is shared by most of my provincial counterparts, is that before we determine whether we have enough doctors, we have to determine how health services are going to be provided. There's a real connection between the last subject we discussed and this one: How are you delivering primary care? If you determine that, it'll help you understand how many family doctors you need in practice, because allocating health staffing resources depends upon the way in which they're deployed.

Most of the provincial ministers, I believe, want to determine, with their medical associations, how to structure the delivery of health services to the community over the coming three or four years, before they come to a final conclusion about enrollment in medical schools. On nursing, I think there's broad agreement that we do have a shortage of nurses now and will in the future, so efforts are being made to recruit and retain nurses.

One last point: The medical associations in the provinces also understand that we have to accelerate the process for accrediting foreign-trained doctors so that in the short term we can meet whatever needs are not being met by taking advantage of foreign-trained doctors who are already in this country.

Iglehart: Canada has the same problem that virtually every industrialized country has: Everybody wants to practice in the attractive cities—San Francisco, Boston, Toronto, Vancouver—and nobody wants to go up north or to the rural areas.

Rock: Quite right. When I first became minister of health and began looking more closely at the situation here, I concluded that the real threat of two-tier medicine in Canada is not rich and poor or haves and have-nots; it's urban and rural. The rural population is demographically older, enjoys less good health than the urban population, and is more prone to accidents, and yet it has less access than the urban population does to everything from ambulances to emergency rooms to doctors and specialists.

And while the delivery of health services is a provincial responsibility, this problem has a national dimension because it happens all across Canada. For that reason, I've opened up a new office of Health Canada devoted to rural health. We're creating a network of rural health researchers across the country. We've set aside a substantial sum of money for pilot projects, exploring better ways of meeting rural health needs through delivering services in different ways. . . .

THE GERMAN HEALTH CARE SYSTEM
Gerd Richter

Richter provides a descriptive overview of the German health-care system. As he explains, the most distinctive feature of this system is the more than 1,000 "sickness funds," nonprofit organizations that provide insurance to about 90 percent of the population, setting premiums based on ability to pay and not on risk factors. About 8 percent of the population is covered by for-profit private insurance companies, while the remaining 2 percent—civil servants—are covered by the government. Members of sickness funds choose their own physicians, and coverage includes a comprehensive set of medical and dental benefits as well as cash benefits in special circumstances (e.g., maternity, necessary travel, burials). Richter also explains other major components of the German health-care system: the differing roles and prerogatives of office-based and hospital-based physicians; the financing of hospitals, whose physicians and nurses are salaried; and the pharmaceutical sector, in which all drug prescriptions are covered by sickness funds and most private insurers. Defects of the German system, he suggests, include a glut of doctors, increasing costs, and weak integration between primary care and hospital care. Despite these difficulties, Richter notes, most Germans are satisfied with the quality of care and freedom of choice within a system that ensures equal access for all citizens; moreover, the total costs of health care in Germany are much lower than they are in the United States.

The German insurance system has its roots in a communitarian/solidarity principle that states that all citizens should receive health care benefits according to their needs and should pay according to their ability. This system is founded on the three principles of self-governance, social partnership, and social security. First, self-governance refers to the fact that the insured and the providers operate as self-managing private organizations under public law, with as little interference from the government as possible. Second, social partnership indicates that both employees and employers share the financial burdens of health care. Third, the principle of social security reflects the attitude that the economically stronger members of a society should support the weaker members to ensure equality of access to health care. The German health care system can be summarized as follows:[1]

Reprinted with permission of the publisher from Gerd Richter, "Customers or Members: An Important Distinction Between the U.S. and German Health Care Systems," *BioLaw,* vol. II, August–September 1995, Special Section, pp. 74–77.

- the younger and healthier members subsidize the older and less healthy members of society;
- those with higher incomes subsidize those with lower incomes;
- the single and childless subsidize families and those with children; and
- the employed subsidize those who are unemployed.

The system is financed by employees and employers in a government-mandated way, and care is provided by four main players: the so-called sickness funds *(Krankenkassen),* associations of office-based ambulatory care physicians, hospitals, and the pharmaceutical sector.

SICKNESS FUNDS

The statutory sickness funds are the most characteristic component of the German health care system. They came into effect as the Health Insurance Act of 1883 under the centralizing force of Otto von Bismarck, driven by the poor conditions of the industrial working class, which posed a risk to family structure and therefore to society in general. These consequences of industrialization and urbanization challenged the economic, political, and social structures of Germany, challenges that health care in Germany was designed to meet, within the context of the solidarity principle and the general rights of a citizen to participate in and benefit from the goods of the state. Along with statutory health care insurance came work-related accident insurance (in 1884), retirement funds (in 1889), and unemployment insurance (in 1927). These four pillars remain the basis of the German system.

These health care provisions became German political traditions, connecting the concept of community with forms of social insurance. Sickness, accident, and aging were circumstances that could be managed more fairly within the conceptual framework of community than within the framework of individual freedom and self-determination. The health insurance system represented a political commitment to structure medical care not on the basis of an individual's ability to pay for a commodity but on the communitarian basis of providing for a general need. Today, Germany's comprehensive health care system is based on a compulsory insurance scheme in which approximately 90 percent of the population participate. The remaining 10 percent includes 8 percent who are fully covered by for-profit private insurance companies and 2 percent, mostly civil servants, for whom the government provides health care.[1,2]

The insurance scheme is highly decentralized and consists of more than one thousand insurance or sickness funds of different types. These are non-profit organizations and membership is compulsory. They are required to accept all persons who qualify. Their premium rates are not permitted to reflect differences on the basis of age, gender, or risk factors. This mandatory acceptance of diversity efficiently distributes the risk.

Premiums are set in such a way as to prevent the accumulation of either excessive reserves or deficits. Individual contributions are linked to income, and the one-to-one contribution of employer and employee, which amounts, on average, to 12.8

percent of one's gross salary.[1] Spouses below a minimum income are covered, as are dependents. In addition to a comprehensive set of medical and dental benefits, fund members are also entitled to cash benefits in special circumstances: sickness, maternity, necessary travel costs, burial allowances, and so forth. If one is above a certain income level (approximately $47,000 in 1992) one may opt for private insurance, a decision generally irreversible unless one's income drops permanently below the established threshold.

PHYSICIANS

In Germany there is a sharp line between office-based physicians and hospital-based clinicians. Primary care and hospital care are almost completely separated. Office-based physicians play the dominant role in the health care sector as a whole: they provide ambulatory care, prescribe drugs and medical appliances, and decide who is to be hospitalized. All members of sickness funds may choose their own physician; at each visit they present an insurance card that identifies the patient for the invoice to the sickness fund.

Office-based physicians are organized into regional associations, and those associations negotiate the annual budget with the sickness funds. Primary care physicians are usually paid on a fee-for-service basis, the schedule for which is established through negotiation on a state level. Primary care physicians receive payment from their regional association, which is compensated by the sickness funds.

In 1977 the Health Care Cost Containment Act was passed into law, which created the Uniform Evaluation Standard (Einheitlicher Bewertungsmabstab) so that the schedule of charges for medical services and their relative point value to one another was defined. This is similar to the resource-based relative value scale (RBRVS) used by Medicare.[3] The point values are translated in a monetary valued schedule of charges by the conversion factor so that physicians can be paid fee-for-service. Since 1987 the growth in physicians' overall expenditures has been tied to the growth in income per sickness fund member, and because of this the conversion factor was and is dependent on the overall expenditure level and the number of sevices provided. If the physicians provide more services than expected the point value will decrease, if they provide less than expected they will receive more money for each point. This way of remunerating physicians should help to control costs, so that expenditure does not increase faster than wages. But at the same time it embodied the positive incentives of a fee-for-service scheme, encouraging physicians to overdiagnose and overtreat patients, and encouraged the growth of the number of specialists at the expense of primary care physicians.

To avoid the latter, in 1987 the Uniform Evaluation Standard was reformed to increase the point values of consultations, physical examinations, and preventive care relative to technical services. This modification could be seen as an attempt to increase the level of personal medicine provided by general practitioners in relation to the level of technical services provided by specialists, but had only a small effect on the relative income of general practitioners versus specialists.[3] As in the United States, general practitioners are at the bottom end of the income scale; despite various initiatives, the overall ranking of physicians' incomes has not changed dramatically.

HOSPITALS

German hospitals operate within three related sectors: public, private, and church affiliated. But investment and capital expenditures for all three sectors come primarily from the state, with some local government budget funds. The establishment of hospitals is regulated through government planning. A hospital's costs are financed primarily by per diem payments, which are fixed in such a way as to cover all administrative costs and are negotiated annually with sickness funds on a regional level. There are also special per diem rates for such services as hemodialysis, intensive care, and pediatric oncology, and cost-per-case rates for transplants or cardiothoracic surgery.

Hospital budgets are linked to the growth of the incomes of sickness fund members and are in this way relatively fixed and controlled. New regulation, however, aims to increase efficiency and reduce the length of hospital stays by moving toward cost-per-case reimbursement.

Hospital-based physicians and nurses are paid by salary at levels negotiated between unions (representing clinicians) and the German Hospital Association (representing hospitals). These representational bodies serve essential and efficient roles outside of the strictly political role of government. The strict division, however, between inpatient care and primary care creates costly inefficiencies due to the number of diagnostic and therapeutic procedures that are done twice, once in each setting. The 1993 German Health Care Act attempts to improve integration and increases the essentially symbolic copayment rates for inpatients to approximately $9 per day for the first fourteen days. Although primarily symbolic, these payments are still payments one wishes to avoid and which thus create some incentive toward efficiency.

PHARMACEUTICAL SECTOR

Drug expenditures in Germany are high, due to excessive consumption and artificially high prices. Surveys indicate that German physicians prescribe on average about eleven medicines per person per year, almost three times more than their American colleagues.[4] This is probably because all prescriptions are covered by all sickness funds and by most private insurers. The German legislature has set reference prices for prescriptions, requiring patients to pay the difference between the reference price and higher priced brands. One must co-pay for all medicine whether or not there is an established reference price. To protect the chronically ill and the poor, however, there is an annually determined copayment cap that is essentially income dependent.

The deficiencies in the German system are the high number of doctors (in 1990 the unified Germany had 3.11 physicians per thousand residents compared with 2.32 in the United States),[3] the increasing costs of technical specialization, the lack of integration between primary care and hospital care, and the length of time patients remain in the hospital. These have resulted in increasingly high costs to the whole system. Despite these expenses, the total cost of the system amounts to about 9 percent of the gross domestic product, which is a comparatively moderate rate by international measures.

most people are satisfied with their
...d with the system's ability to meet the
...of equal access for all, freedom of
choi..., ...igh quality of care. Costs of the system will continue to rise in the future, due primarily to the aging of the population and the
increasing ability of the system to sustain the
chronically ill.

The total costs of health care in Germany remain much lower than they are in the United States.
German society as a whole is, however, no more
willing than American society to bear the increasing
burden promised in the future. . . .

NOTES

[1] U. Hoffmeyer, "The Health Care System in Germany" in
Financing Health Care, Vol. 1, U. Hoffmeyer and T. R.
McCarthy, eds. (Kluwer: Dordrecht/Boston/London, 1994).

[2] M. Arnold, *Solidarit't 2000: Die medizinische Versorgung
und ihre Finanzierung nach der Jahrtausendwende* (Enke:
Stuttgart, 1993).

[3] K. D. Henke, M. A. Murray, and C. Ade, *Global Budgeting
in Germany: Lessons for the United States,* Health Affairs
(Fall 1994), pp. 7–21.

[4] J. M. Graf von der Schulenburg, "The German Health Care
System: Concurrent Solidarity, Freedom of Choice, and Cost
Control" in *Health Care Systems and Their Patients. An
International Perspective,* M. M. Rosenthal and M. Frenkel,
eds. (Westview Press: Boulder/San Francisco/Oxford, 1992),
pp. 83–104.

WILL THE FUDGE ON EQUITY SUSTAIN THE NHS INTO THE NEXT MILLENNIUM?

Nicholas Mays and Justin Keen

Mays and Keen offer a descriptive overview of the British health-care system that is
both historical and forward-looking. As they explain, when the National Health Service (NHS) was founded in 1946, it provided equitable access to health care for all
citizens without abolishing private care; in Britain, citizens may choose to pay for private insurance while physicians may provide services outside of the NHS (even if they
also provide services within the public system). Since the late 1960s, overall spending on health care has greatly increased, along with the demand for services, leading
to the question of whether the NHS can keep up with current demand for expensive
drugs and treatments. The most likely scenarios, the authors continue, include an increased proportion of private finance and delivery of services, yet any radical movement in this direction seriously threatens the goals of equity, efficiency, patient
satisfaction, and access—as suggested by the poor performance, by these criteria, of
the largely privatized American system. Mays and Keen conclude that, considering the
high level of British satisfaction with the NHS, Great Britain should exercise caution
in pursuing changes in both the public and private health-care sectors.

The NHS [National Health Service] was established
as a compromise between key parties; it allowed
those patients who could afford it to have access to

This article was first published in the *British Medical Journal,* vol. 317
(1998), pp. 66–69, and is reproduced by permission of the BMJ
Publishing Group.

both private health care and the NHS and it permitted consultants to have access to income from private practice while working in the NHS. This safety
valve for excess demand was developed contrary to
the founding principles of equity, but it has been a
feature of health care in the United Kingdom ever

since; it allows more affluent patients to circumvent the periodic funding crises in the NHS while maintaining their support for health care funded by taxes. However, the share of total health-care spending contributed by the private sector has risen steadily. This trend has led some commentators to argue that the NHS is not sustainable, primarily because funding through taxation will lead to an increasing gap between the demand for and supply of health care. Alternatives to the NHS would involve requiring a larger private contribution to the costs of health care but such systems require complex regulation and seem to produce inequities that reveal the specific interests of their proponents. In contrast, expanding the funding of the NHS in line with increases in the gross national product is affordable and broadly equitable.

Whether the UK compromise between public and private interests will be sustained cannot be predicted. Recent developments suggest that major change may occur unintentionally through the cumulative effects of small or unplanned changes, or both, or result from applying policy thinking from other fields of welfare, such as social security reform.

HEALTH CARE WAS RATIONALISED, NOT NATIONALISED

There is a tendency in commentary on the NHS to discuss it as though it is the only healthcare system in the United Kingdom but this has never been an accurate reflection of the situation. The early history of the NHS shows clearly that the newly nationalised service did not represent a clean break with the past even though it rapidly consigned private health care to a residual role that served a small minority of the population.[1] Rather, it was a partial rationalisation of what existed, conditioned by a need to reassure and encourage, rather than coerce, a number of conservative professional interest groups to participate. Thus from the outset the NHS was entangled in a wide range of relationships (with both private finance and those who supplied health care and related goods and services privately) which compromised its goal of ensuring that health services were available exclusively on the basis of need.

Over the 50 years some of the large scale features of this compromise have remained remarkably stable, both within the NHS and in its relationships with the private sector [(see the accompanying box)]. Thus the 1946 act which founded the NHS represents a long-term compromise between the interests of the state and the interests of professional, commercial, middle income, and upper income groups. This compromised fudged the equity principle in the 1946 act by permitting, and at times encouraging, private health care to develop alongside the NHS as a safety valve for people with the resources to make additional provision for themselves. The question now is whether the compromise will continue to protect the NHS into the 21st century.

CONTINUITY AND CHANGE

Despite successive funding crises threatening the comprehensiveness and sustainability of the NHS, an increasing level of criticism of its apparently poor performance, and the tolerance of private health care by successive governments the main developments in NHS policy since 1948 have done little directly to undermine the fundamental principles of the NHS as being predominantly funded by taxes and providing universal access to services. Instead, changes in policy have attempted, as in the case of the internal market,[2] to improve efficiency and responsiveness to patients' needs within a publicly funded system.

Over time there have been shifts in the perception of what is possible and desirable in the future. Perhaps the biggest change has been in the perception that there is a widening gap between what the NHS might be able to provide with more resources and what it can provide at current levels of funding. For example, the increasing numbers of high cost drugs that the NHS is required to purchase lead to contentious priority decisions and fuel the demand for more spending. One result of this perceived gap is that successive government changes to the NHS have not reduced the attraction of private health care. Far from private practice diminishing as the NHS has grown, the private sector has become steadily more important both in financing and supplying health care, but this has not threatened the founding principles of the NHS.[3] The [accompanying box] summarises some of the main trends in the balance between private and public finance and the provision of health services.

Public-private ties established with the founding of the NHS

· General practitioners work as independent contractors, not salaried employees

· Specialist doctors and other professionals can maintain both NHS and private practices

· NHS pay beds (essentially private beds in NHS hospitals which allow the trust to charge for the bed and consultants to charge separately for services)

· Prescription and other charges to users for NHS services

· Patient access to both NHS and private treatment, sometimes for the same condition; access to private treatment on the basis of ability to pay rather than need

· Reliance of the NHS on pharmaceutical and other industries to develop new products with the NHS contributing resources to development and testing

---

ARGUMENTS FOR CHANGES IN THE NHS

The NHS continues to have high levels of public support. Seventy seven per cent of the population support the principle of a health service available to all, although this does not necessarily mean that they oppose people having the choice of paying for private health care.[8] Although it is difficult to believe when you are on an NHS waiting list, people are more satisfied with arrangements in the United Kingdom than are people in either Canada or the United States.[9] The United Kingdom also compares favourably internationally in terms of fairness of funding, equality of access, and efficiency.[10]

Nevertheless, arguments persist that a higher share of private funding in a mixed economy of public and private care is inevitable and desirable. Crit-

ics tend to argue that a publicly funded system, particularly one funded through general taxation, cannot provide the volume and standard of health care that an increasingly affluent, aged, and sophisticated population wants (despite the fact that we cannot determine objectively what level of spending is correct). The main difference between the United Kingdom and other comparable countries lies not in the amount of public funding for health care but in the lower level of private funding. There is a clear gap between NHS resources and demand, shown particularly clearly in the provision of expensive new drugs such as interferon beta. Yet more public spending is not an option if the United Kingdom is to remain internationally competitive in increasingly global markets, and additional spending is political suicide for any government. If more affluent people are only able to spend more of their money on health care provided outside the NHS then, inevitably, the private sector will and should grow to meet the unmet demand in the public sector.

Governments, including the current one, have responded to this argument by vowing to keep taxes and public spending down which further encourages the suspicion that institutions like the NHS are unsustainable and that more private finance is the only alternative. A range of solutions to the perceived financial unsustainability of the NHS has been proposed. For example, Hoffmeyer and McCarthy[11] propose a model to replace the NHS and meet increasing demand with a guaranteed package of health care for all; their model comprises competing health insurance agencies, compulsory insurance, premiums based on income and (health) risk, a central fund designed to share the costs of high risk groups, safety nets for individuals unable to afford or find insurance, providers competing for the business of insurance agency purchasers, and a prohibition against insurers excluding whole groups of patients or insisting on unreasonable terms to avoid risk.

This model has something in common with the different forms of insurance that were available in the United Kingdom before the formation of the NHS. The central ideas are that patients can choose between different packages and insurers, and more affluent patients can insure themselves for higher levels of care, which would increase the level of funding for health care beyond that permitted by successive parsimonious governments. Behind the scenes the government would attempt to ensure that each insurer had roughly equal funds in relation to the requirements of those enrolled in their plan.

But is it the case that we cannot afford the NHS, and would it be a good thing to abandon the basic architecture of health care in the United Kingdom for something new? Analysis indicates that given even conservative estimates of economic growth the United Kingdom can continue to pay for the welfare state and the NHS through taxation, if it chooses.[12] Whether we should spend more is a separate question to which there is no objective answer.

As to whether the United Kingdom should opt for a more explicitly mixed system with much more private finance and a basic publicly subsidised sector for the less well off, 40 years' experience from all over the world cautions against it.[13] Such systems, like that in the United States, tend to perform poorly in terms of public satisfaction, health outcomes, efficiency, access, and equity of finance, and are difficult to manage and regulate. They do, however, tend to increase expenditure, jobs, and incomes in the health sector. For this reason, they are supported by providers and private insurers. They are also attractive to upper income taxpayers since they enable such people to benefit at the expense of poorer people, because user charges and the cost of private insurance impose more of a burden on those who are poor and who are more likely to make higher use of services. The greater the reliance on private finance and the less the reliance on taxation or social insurance, the greater the opportunity for people to purchase more services for themselves without having to pay to support a similar standard of care for everyone else. Since those in need in any one year will be a small proportion of the population—and they will be disproportionately elderly people and those with chronic illnesses, who are least able to pay—private finance tends to improve access to care for those who are least likely to need it. Healthcare financing changes in the United Kingdom would thus have profound consequences for the equitable distribution of resources.

Trends in the mix of public and private financing

· Total spending in the NHS and in the private health-care sector rose from 3.9% of gross domestic product in 1960 to 7.1% of gross domestic product in 1992[4]

· The private sector's share of total spending on health care rose from around 3% in the 1960s to 14% in 1985 and to 16% in 1992[3]

· Public and private expenditure on private hospital care and private nursing home care increased from 9.9% of total health-care expenditure in 1986 to 19.9% in 1996[5]

· The number of subscribers to private heath insurance policies increased from 2.45 million in 1986 to 3.17 million in 1996[6]

· Payments by patients for NHS services rose from £35m in 1960 to £919m in 1996

· Investment in new hospitals under the private finance initiative announced since 1 May 1997 was £660m (Department of Health press release 98/123)[7]

THE SHAPE OF THINGS TO COME

Irrespective of the merits of these arguments—and they have made little headway in most countries that have systems providing universal access to care—there is little doubt that a more mixed economy is emerging in the United Kingdom (box [above]), albeit not always as a direct result of explicit reform of health policy. Further changes could occur simply through the accumulation of seemingly separate smaller scale changes which would further reduce the contribution of publicly funded health services; the box [across] summarises a few of these changes.

Change may also come about unintentionally if the proposals contained in the government white paper *The New NHS*,[14] which sets out Labour's plans for the abolition of the internal market, are acted on. One theory is that the unwitting combination of the new primary care groups (groups of practices responsible both for commissioning hospital and community health services and developing general practitioner services) in England and the use of the private finance initiative (a scheme under which private finance is used to build hospitals which are then leased back to the NHS) will lead to something akin to an American style system developing in the United Kingdom; general practitioners might in effect function outside the NHS and this could possibly trigger an unplanned shift to a system in which patients choose to enrol with a range of competing primary care based total healthcare plans using vouchers from the NHS together with private insurance to cover additional services.[15]

Developments that are altering the mix of financing for health care

- Charging for eye tests on the NHS
- Moving NHS dental care into the private sector
- Commercial funding for all major NHS capital schemes
- Changes in social security leading to a requirement for personal insurance against accident and sickness
- Plans for compulsory private insurance for long term care
- Proposals from some NHS health-care trusts for additional contributions from local people
- Government plans to charge insurers for the full cost of NHS treatment of motorists and passengers involved in road accidents.

Some of the changes would emphasise more strongly the difference between the privately insured haves and the publicly subsidised have nots, along the lines of the American model,[16] which could undermine the current majority support for the NHS. However, this does not seem to be the intention of the government, which has signalled that its priority is to support the NHS and to reduce the likelihood that people will use the private sector by making the reduction of NHS waiting lists a priority.[17] Like its predecessor, this government's aim seems to be to improve efficiency within the publicly funded system using management techniques borrowed from the private sector.

CONCLUSION

The overall position at the moment is one where most of the main elements of the 1946 compromise settlement remain in place—for better or for worse. The fact that the compromise was not simply between public and private interests but was more complex has made it difficult to change. Gazing into a crystal ball is rarely rewarding but it seems that the NHS may move in one of at least three different directions. In the first scenario key elements of the 1946 settlement, including the privileged position of consultants, will be renegotiated, with sources of finance staying broadly the same. The rapid evolution of the debate on clinical self regulation, particularly following the case in Bristol in which three surgeons were accused of continuing to operate despite high mortality,[18] suggests that this may already be happening. The second scenario is of more radical change, whether planned or unplanned, with a far larger role for private finance. Some of the signs suggest that this is not out of the question. The third scenario, which tends already to be the outcome of the periodic crises in the NHS, is that it will continue to muddle through, with its current least worst settlement largely in place. As time goes on and if the private sector continues to grow this third path may become less likely, since an increasing proportion of the population will come to rely on the private sector for more of its health care.

Maybe the most important development will be in our sensibilities. Having been told for so long that change is inevitable, the prospect of change does not seem quite so alarming, even though the evidence that it will solve the enduring problems of health care in the United Kingdom is lacking.

REFERENCES

1 Rivett G. *From cradle to grave: Fifty years of the NHS.* London: King's Fund, 1998.

2 Secretaries of State. *Working for patients.* London: HMSO, 1989. (Cm 555.)

3 Propper C. *Who pays for and who gets health care?* London: Nuffield Trust, 1998. (Health economics series, no. 5.)

4 Organisation for Economic Cooperation and Development. *Health care reform: The will to change.* Paris: OECD, 1996.

Thanks for helpful comments, but no responsibility for the contents of this paper, are due to Tony Harrison and Sean Boyle.

5 Laing W. *Laing's review of private healthcare*. London: Laing and Buisson, 1997.

6 Association of British Insurers. *The private medical insurance market*. London: ABI, 1997.

7 McGuigan S. *Office of Health Economics compendium of health statistics 1997*. London: OHE, 1997

8 Judge K., Mulligan J. A, New B. The NHS: new prescriptions needed? In: Jowell R., Curtice J., Park A., Brook L., Thomson K., Bryson C., eds. *British social attitudes, the 14th report: the end of Conservative values?* Aldershot: Ashgate/Social and Community Planning Research, 1997:49–72.

9 Blendon R. J, Leitman R., Morrison I., Donelan K. Satisfaction with health systems in ten nations. *Health Aff (Millwood)* 1990: 9; 185–92.

10 Wagstaff A., van Doorslaer E. Equity in the finance of health care: some international comparisons. *J Health Economics* 1992; 11:361–87.

11 Hoffmeyer U. K., McCarthy T. R. *Financing health care*. Amsterdam: Kluwer Academic, 1995.

12 Hills J. *The future of welfare: a guide to the debate*. Rev ed. York: Joseph Rowntree Foundation, 1997.

13 Evans R. G. Health care reform: who's selling the market and why? *J Public Health Med* 1997; 19:45–9.

14 Secretary of State for Health. *The new NHS*. London: Stationery Office, 1997. (Cm 3807.)

15 Pollock A. The American way. *Health Serv J* 1998; 108:28–9.

16 Reinhardt U. A social contract for 21st century health care: Three-tier health care with bounty hunting. *Health Economics* 1996; 5:479–99.

17 Milburn A. The chance we've been waiting for. *Health Serv J* 1998; 108:20.

18 Treasure T. Lessons from the British case. *BMJ* 1998; 316:1685–6.

ETHICS, POLITICS, AND PRIORITIES IN THE ITALIAN HEALTH-CARE SYSTEM
Giovanna Ruberto

Ruberto provides an overview of the Italian National Health Service (NHS). As she explains, Italy's Constitution guarantees free health care to all citizens; a recent law has guaranteed that same coverage to foreign visitors, even illegal immigrants, in the country. The Italian NHS, which is funded by tax revenues and budgeted yearly by Parliament, consumes approximately 7 percent of the Italian gross domestic product (in comparison with 14 to 15 percent of the GDP in the United States). Health care is delivered through a network of territorial agencies, each funded by a state budget. Each agency purchases health-care services from public health facilities and, occasionally, from private hospitals. Private health insurance is nonexistent. Like the British NHS, the Italian NHS provides universal coverage to a wide array of health-care services. In 2000 the World Health Organization ranked the Italian health-care system second in the world (to France). Despite these indications of success, the Italian NHS has problems, including regional differences in the quality of health care, rising costs, unrealistic expectations on the part of the public, and a population whose average age is increasing. One necessary response to some of these difficulties, according to Ruberto, will be establishing criteria for the withholding of care.

The constitutions of all Western countries revised after World War II incorporated a new focus on citizens' rights: the right to personal liberty, to health, to well-being, and so forth. In fact, equal and free access to health care and to education are now seen as fundamental rights throughout Western Europe. They are considered to be as basic as the right to freedom of speech, and they are seen as necessary constituents of and means to freedom.

From *Medicine and Social Justice: Essays on the Distribution of Healthcare*, edited by Rosamond Rhodes et al., pp. 191–196. Copyright © 2002 by Oxford University Press, Inc. Reprinted by permission of Oxford University Press, Inc.

In the Constitution of Italy, individuals' right to health care is specifically decreed in Article 32 where the government pledges free health care to all, including the indigent. Legislation related to the health-care system was revised in 1978 by Law 883 and also by subsequent legislative decrees. As recently as 1998, Law 40 was passed, which clearly asserts that all foreign citizens, even illegal immigrants, have an equal right of access to health care. The sum total of this legislation makes health care a fundamental right for everyone in Italy. Access to the health-care system is free for everyone living in or simply visiting the nation.

The Italian National Health System (NHS) is financed by the general tax revenue and an additional health-care tax. Expenditures of the NHS are based on a budget that is voted every year by Parliament. The annual appropriation for the NHS is approximately 7% of the Italian gross domestic product (GDP). Wealthy people pay more taxes, but all people receive the same comprehensive health-care assistance without regard to income or tax contribution. Health care is provided through a structured network of territorial agencies, each financed by a state budget. These agencies purchase treatments or social services from public health facilities and occasionally from private hospitals when a specific treatment is needed and the patient cannot wait for it from the usual public sources. The National Health Care Plan, which sets the standards for medical care and social services, is formulated by the Ministry of Health in collaboration with regional health councillors. In sum, the state takes responsibility for the health care of all people through a regionally organized system that is completely patient-oriented. In Italy, there is no private health insurance system, and even supplemental health insurance is very uncommon because, in effect, no one needs it. Private donations are only used in a supplementary way to support research and sometimes to purchase new equipment.

Traditionally in Italy, public services are better than private services. Medicine is no exception. The Italian public health hospital system offers more comprehensive treatment options than do private hospitals, and the quality of the services is also better than what is available through the private sector.

Like the British National Health Service, the Italian National Health System provides uniform and universal coverage. This means that everyone has free access to hospital care (e.g., medical, surgical), to sophisticated therapies (e.g., transplantation, genetic counseling), to preventive medicine (e.g., vaccination), and to continuing care from family physicians.

In 2000 the World Health Organization (WHO) published *World Health Report 2000,* its evaluation of the performance of health-care systems in 190 countries around the globe according to how well they met three goals: *(1)* attainment of health for the population, *(2)* responsiveness, and *(3)* fair financing. Western European countries achieved the highest rankings on the list. Italy was ranked second only to France as having the best health-care system in the world.

Despite our extraordinarily high ranking on performance in health-care delivery, some of the problems inherent in our system were not reflected in the WHO assessment. The level of our assistance has grown nationally, but allocation and development is organized regionally. The consequence of this regional design is that there are some regional differences in health care. Most of the hospitals, and specifically most of the excellent hospitals, are located in the northern part of the Italy (Lombardia, Emilia-Romagna, Toscana). Nevertheless, because we have the freedom to travel and receive health care anywhere in the country, a kind of health migration has developed to allow people to utilize the highest quality of medical care and the most effective diagnosis and treatment. For example, the hospital where I work is in Pavia. More than 40% of its patients come from outside the city and the region.

While Italy has thus far been able to offer its people exemplary health care, the rising costs are putting the system in jeopardy. To continue to provide its excellent level of comprehensive health-care assistance, the nation will have to adopt a number of measures to contain costs. We have heard the call for moving away from the traditional public management of the system and for the introduction of strong professional private sector management styles. We have also heard the demand for a clear definition of explicit objectives for our National Health System as a prelude to rationing. And we have heard the demand for family doctors to take on a crucial role in filtering access to care and controlling the use of expensive prescription drugs. Setting priorities for a health-care system encompasses three main issues:

- the allocation of resources (the portion of resources to be spent on health care and how these resources should be divided among the various types of services)
- optimal production (how health care can be efficiently put together in both ethical and economic terms)
- distribution (how health care should be distributed among the people).

Yet, in our recent efforts in allocating health-care resources we encounter a number of problems (*Hastings Center Report,* 1996).

Recent goals and reforms in the health-care system are economically unsustainable. They tend to generate unaffordable medicine, which in itself is going to be the most unacceptable problem in the future. Bloated expectations tend to widen the inequitable gap between the rich and the poor in the same country and between developed and developing countries.

The situation is also clinically confusing. It is hard to find a good balance between care and cure, between conquering disease and improving the quality of life, between reducing mortality and morbidity, and between investing social resources in health care and the actual improvement in the health of the population. In reality, the enormous investment of resources directed toward achieving good health has undeniably increased the average life span and improved the quality of life in general. Nevertheless, we must acknowledge that people die from medical conditions associated with their way of life or social status even in countries that spend more than others on their health-care system. This should make us seriously ponder how we spend the resources we have before deciding how much of them to spend.

Recent efforts to resolve the problem have been socially frustrating, fostering false and unrealistic hopes in the public and creating expectations of wonders from modern medical technology that cannot be met or that can only be met at an unaffordable

and exorbitant cost. It is worth noting, for example, that great hopes have been invested in gene therapies that are still ineffective. Consider also how we fool ourselves into believing that we have found the cure for cancer every time new and more costly drugs are developed. In reality, our form of medicine is still essentially diagnostic, it primarily treats symptoms and is less than modestly curative. Many previously acute diseases can now be maintained in the chronic phase. We can cure only very few. This situation raises another problem, namely the cost of chronic treatment for an increased number of people who live with disease for a significant number of years.

Regional reforms lack coherent direction and purpose. They respond to pressures from special-interest groups (multinational pharmaceutical companies, the academic world, etc.) with unrelated objectives or in the name of market freedom. These piece-meal changes accept no direction, no vision of worthy goals oriented toward the needs and desires of people, and no meaningful picture of medicine's contribution to the individual's well-being.

The aging population is yet another complicating factor. It is a real problem now and it is expected to become an even greater problem in the future. The number of people over the age of 65 is constantly increasing. It is obvious that this is an important achievement, but it is equally obvious that we must begin to consider the age factor as an increasingly important variable in the public health-care system.

Many factors are responsible for increasing the average life span: greater attention is given to prevention, improved living conditions (e.g., hygiene, nutrition) and increased ability to maintain people with diseases in the chronic phase when only a few years ago these same diseases ended with death in the acute phase (e.g., renal failure, cardiovascular diseases, neurodegenerative diseases, cancer). As a consequence, we find ourselves confronting patients who cannot be considered healthy and who need costly medications and/or surgical procedures for many years. Many new medical technologies now in the research and development phase will further extend the lives of the elderly and, at the same time, raise the cost of caring for them. Every developed nation is going to face a significant increase in the number of people over the age of 85. This problem will be intensified by further technological developments, which will not only allow us to treat the elderly more effectively, but also increase the cost of their care, both in long-term care facilities and in the home-care setting.

We are also going to face a greater public demand for good medical care. Publicized research results create expectations that are typically followed by people clamoring for the newest technology. Researchers and the media have fed the hunger for results and nourished the belief that medicine can cure every illness, or at least provide treatment. We have also communicated the idea that money can allow you to avoid disease and its fatality.

All these factors together, an increased life span, more "state of the art" medical procedures, and higher expectations have made it necessary for us to reexamine the dimensions our public health-care budget and to scrutinize our values and our conception justice. If, for example, we decided to treat only the sick with acute conditions, neglecting those with chronic conditions, we could be valuing productivity and efficiency because by favoring the patients who can be cured, the cost-benefit ratio becomes more efficient. Doing the contrary, as Callahan (1987, 1998) polemically and paradoxically suggests, treating only chronically ill patients who cannot be successfully cured, results in increased costs for less benefit. The values that support this type of choice are solidarity and the dignity of the person. We need to forge a strong bond among bioethics, health-care economics, and politics so as to decide together what is the common good. To make the choices that cannot be avoided, we must find a consensus on where to start rationing and from which criteria.

The history of the Italian health-care system reveals that Italy chose to let supply direct demand. For example, The National Health Care Plan, which represents the government's health-care objectives at the practical level, has the task of determining "the level of health care services which in any case must be guaranteed to all its citizens." In fact, this strong commitment to universe access to health-care keeps the cost-benefit concept from rendering the aims of the health care system meaningless. The National Health Care Plan is committed to defend and

promote the dignity of the people, especially those who are most fragile. As with most Scandinavian and southern European countries, Italy has also chosen to guarantee access to the health care system to everyone by utilizing tax revenues as the main financing source. Public funding of medicine is widely accepted because it guarantees a fair distribution of resources and allows everyone to utilize the system.

Nevertheless, Italian health professionals are aware that as medical procedures become more complex and costly, we will be obligated to establish criteria for withholding treatment. We will have to develop a system that will not only protect those utilizing the system but that also reflects solidarity by not excluding or selecting individuals based on their social condition, culture, income, physical or psychological weaknesses. The development of health-care policy should be based on the concept of a renewed agreement among citizens, health care workers, and elected officials.

All questions do not have an immediate or a single answer. Starting with the premise that the present standard of universal access to health-care services must continue, we can imagine the first step in limiting health care. For example, we can start from an issue that is rarely mentioned in resource-allocation discussions, which is serious consideration of the role of medical education. We teach our students to be hi-tech doctors, forgetting about the primacy of the doctor—patient relationship. Today, the ability to take a patient's medical history, to examine the patient, and to listen to the patient are replaced by an emphasis on hi-tech diagnostic tests and analyses. In a certain sense, we teach as if making a diagnosis based on the results of hi-tech equipment (CT scan, MRI, etc.) is more objective than basing diagnosis on the signs and symptoms of an illness. Most freshly trained doctors do not know how to interpret the sounds they hear with their stethoscope, yet they know details about every single laboratory test that has just been discovered. This excessive reliance on technology also reflects deterioration of the doctor-patient relationship. Today the doctor's fear of legal action is constantly present and prompts the call for tests and analyses just to avoid being accused of malpractice. Recuperating trust in the doctor–patient relationship can help family practitioners to treat their patients better without wasting resources. The problem of allocating scarce medical resources makes rethinking and reviewing the framework that sustains the doctor–patient relationship crucially important. The context of rationing provides pressing reasons for restoring dignity to the doctor who must cease to be a mere provider of medical services and must reclaim responsibility to the patient who must not regard medicine as a store where one gets whatever health care one desires.

Another aspect of the current view that we can correct is tied to the idea that medicine should only treat or cure. We invest enormous resources to study new diagnostic procedures, to provide more sophisticated transplants, to develop more costly drug ther-

apies, and to perform extravagant procedures for assisted reproduction, yet little is spent on prevention. Patients, doctors, and elected officials must unite around the concept of "shared responsibility." The government has to guarantee fair and equal access to medical treatment. The doctor has to utilize the knowledge and skills of medicine to treat and cure patients without wasting resources. The citizen has to learn and practice a way of life that keeps diseases at bay or that limits their impact and progress. Diet, lifestyle, and physical exercise are fundamental components in maintaining well-being. Smoking is unhealthy, and so is being overweight and leading a sedentary lifestyle. In fact, the government is now focused on these strategies to contain the cost of the medication expenses. (See Table 1) We also need to

TABLE 1   Alternative Strategies for Cost-Containment in the Pharmaceutical Sector in the EU Member States

Strategies Regarding the Supply

Fixed estimated budgets for doctors	Family practitioners in the UK
Estimated cost guidelines for doctors	Germany
Fixed estimated budgets for medications	Germany, Italy
Training	France
Evaluating economic feasibility	UK
Checking prescriptions	Almost every country except the UK
Disease management	France, UK
Positive and/or negative lists	Every country
Limit the number of products	Denmark, The Netherlands, Norway
Create a market for generic drugs	Almost every country except France

Strategies Regarding the Demand

Sharing the costs	Almost every country except the Netherlands
Health-education programs	The Netherlands, UK, Italy

Strategies Aimed at the Market as a Whole

Keeping prices low	France, Italy, Sweden, Norway
Regulating profits	UK
Referencing prices	Denmark, Germany, The Netherlands
Expected earnings or fixed estimated budgets for industry	France, Spain
Taxes on promotional expenses	France, Spain, Sweden
Creating a market for generic drugs	Almost every country

Source: E. Mossialos and B. Abel-Smith, Cost-containment in the pharmaceutical sector in the EU Member States. London: London School of Economics, 1996.

take care of the environment in which we live. Consider the cost of diseases related to environmental pollution (e.g., the treatment of asthma or allergies).

Furthermore, we need a strong cultural effort to encourage people to accept the idea of limits and the inevitability of suffering and sickness as they once did. If a child is hyperactive today, he is quickly medicated. If one feels unhappy or depressed for a very serious personal problem, she takes a pill.

Health-care workers, patients, and citizens are aware that we are at a medical frontier. We are about to reach goals in understanding biological processes and curing diseases that were, until recently, unimaginable. This knowledge should not become the privilege of a few at the expense of the health of the majority. Fair allocation of these resources is what we should all want. We therefore need to consider seriously about quickly building a value system for just allocation before economic needs dictate the allocation policies and before we lose the heritage that the European health-care systems have constructed and strengthened over the last 20 years.

ACKNOWLEDGMENT

I want to thank Caterina Campani, who helped with the final version of the chapter.

NOTE

1 The *Hastings Center Report* provides a systematic overview of the health-care problem. The expert panel classified the reasons for reestablishing the priorities of health care into four categories.

REFERENCES

Callahan, D. (1987). *Setting Limits: Medical Goals in an Aging Society.*

Callahan, D. (1998). *False Hopes.* New York: N.Y. Simon & Schuster.

Hastings Center Report (1996). The goals of medicine: Setting new priorities. Special Supplement, November, pp. S1–S27.

ANNOTATED BIBLIOGRAPHY

Bodenheimer, Thomas: "The Oregon Health Plan—Lessons for the Nation (First of Two Parts)," *New England Journal of Medicine* 337 (August 28, 1997), pp. 651–655. Bodenheimer provides a helpful description of the Oregon rationing plan, including changes in the system since its federal approval in 1994.

Childress, James F.: "Ensuring Care, Respect, and Fairness for the Elderly," *Hastings Center Report* 14 (October 1984), pp. 27–31. While granting that, under ideal conditions, some age-based rationing would be ethically defensible in principle, Childress contends that such rationing in our less-than-ideal world would be morally problematic. For the purposes of thinking creatively about allocation alternatives, he suggests replacing the military metaphor that dominates our thinking about medicine with the metaphor of nursing.

Daniels, Norman: *Justice and Justification: Reflective Equilibrium in Theory and Practice* (Cambridge: Cambridge University Press, 1996). In this collection of essays, Daniels explores the idea that ethical justification involves the achievement of coherence or "reflective equilibrium" in a system of beliefs. Among the practical topics explored are the design of health-care systems as well as age-based and other forms of rationing.

———: *Am I My Parent's Keeper?* (New York: Oxford University Press, 1988). Daniels seeks a principled approach to allocating health care, income support, and other types of resources to members of different age groups in society. Because we all age, he argues, each of us passes through different life stages. Thus, if we can determine how we would prudently allocate our fair share of social goods to ourselves over different life stages, we can discover what justice demands in the way of allocation between age groups.

DeGrazia, David: "Why the United States Should Adopt a Single-Payer System of Health Care Finance," *Kennedy Institute of Ethics Journal* 6 (June 1996), pp. 145–160. Drawing on evidence from other countries, especially Canada, DeGrazia argues that the most likely path to successful health-care reform in the United States involves adopting the single-payer model. Additionally, the author identifies several political and cultural factors that make it difficult for Americans to view this option clearly, and he argues that rationing cannot be profitably discussed while questions about the broader health-care system are bracketed.

Dougherty, Charles J.: *American Health Care: Realities, Rights, and Reform* (New York: Oxford University Press, 1988). Dougherty provides a moral evaluation of American health care. The book divides into (1) a review of access to health care ("realities"), (2) a pluralistic philosophical defense of a moral right to health care ("rights"), and (3) an assertion of what reforms are needed to achieve justice ("reforms").

Fleck, Leonard M.: "Just Caring: Oregon, Health Care Rationing, and Informed Democratic Deliberation," *Journal of Medicine and Philosophy* 19 (August 1994), pp. 367–388. Fleck argues that American efforts at health-care reform should be informed by lessons that can be extracted from Oregon's experiment with rationing. Most generally, we must learn that the need for rationing is inescapable, that any rationing process must be public, and that fair rationing plans must be developed through rational democratic deliberation.

Grogan, Colleen M.: "Deciding on Access and Levels of Care: A Comparison of Canada, Britain, Germany, and the United States," *Journal of Health Politics, Policy, and Law* 17 (1992), pp. 213–232. Noting that Americans tend to believe universal coverage is feasible only if a minimal benefit package is guaranteed, Grogan provides data demonstrating that Canada, Great Britain, and Germany all achieve universal access to very comprehensive benefit packages while largely succeeding in controlling costs. She argues that in Canada, Great Britain, and Germany difficult rationing decisions are obviated by confronting difficult political decisions about the structure of the health-care system, while in the United States, the avoidance of such difficult political decisions makes rationing problems seem intractable.

Jarvis, Rupert: "Join the Club: A Modest Proposal to Increase Availability of Donor Organs," *Journal of Medical Ethics* 21 (1995), pp. 199–204. After reviewing and rejecting several possible approaches to meeting the demand for transplantable organs, Jarvis defends a scheme whereby only those who agree to be donors may be recipients of organs.

Journal of Medicine and Philosophy 26 (April 2001). This special issue is entitled "Do Children Get Their Fair Share of Health and Dental Care?" Several leading contributors to bioethics literature address the question contained in the title of this special issue.

Moreno, Jonathan D.: "Recapturing Justice in the Managed Care Era," *Cambridge Quarterly of Healthcare Ethics* 5 (1996), pp. 493–499. Moreno examines and critically evaluates the recent managed care movement in the United States, noting with concern the near disappearance of discussions of social justice in the bioethics community. Because managed care is headed in a direction that is ethically unsound and politically unsustainable, he maintains, bioethics needs to ensure that justice recaptures its place in the public mind.

Nelson, James Lindemann: "Measured Fairness, Situated Justice: Feminist Reflections on Health Care Rationing," *Kennedy Institute of Ethics Journal* 6 (March 1996), pp. 53–68. In this article, Nelson attempts to demonstrate the fruitfulness of an interchange between mainstream discussions of justice in health care and feminist reflections on power, privilege, and justice.

Nord, Erik: *Cost-Value Analysis in Health Care: Making Sense Out of QALYs* (New York: Cambridge University Press, 1999). This book provides an in-depth exploration of quality-adjusted life years, a type of outcomes measure frequently used in discussions of health care.

Powers, Madison: "Managed Care: How Economic Incentive Reform Went Wrong," *Kennedy Institute of Ethics Journal* 7 (4) (1997), pp. 353–360. Giving special attention to economic incentives, Powers argues that, following the Clinton administration's failed health-care reform effort, managed care has demonstrated its inability to meet the goals of reasonable cost controls and universal access.

President's Commission for the Study of Ethical Problems in Medicine and Biomedical and Behavioral Research: *Securing Access to Health Care,* Vol. 1: *Report* (Washington, DC: U.S. Government Printing Office, 1983). This influential report presents the commission's conclusions about (1) an ethical framework grounding a societal obligation to provide an adequate level of health care to all citizens, (2) the state of health care in America, and (3) changes in health-care delivery that can move the United States in the direction of meeting its societal obligation.

———: *Securing Access to Health Care,* Vol. 2: *Appendices: Sociocultural and Philosophical Studies.* This volume contains sociological, philosophical, and ethical studies pertaining to the issue of health-care access.

———: *Securing Access to Health Care,* Vol. 3: *Appendices: Empirical, Legal, and Conceptual Studies.* The three parts of this volume are entitled "Ethical Implications of Health Care Distribution," "Allocation in Varied Medical Settings," and "Legal Implications of Allocation Policies."

Veatch, Robert M.: *The Foundations of Justice: Why the Retarded and the Rest of Us Have Claims to Equality* (New York: Oxford University Press, 1986). Veatch examines current conceptions of justice, equality, and social responsibility as he grapples with the question of how to allocate limited resources fairly, especially to people with inexhaustible needs and little capacity for improvement.

Wellstone, Paul D., and Ellen R. Shaffer: "The American Health Security Act: A Single-Payer Proposal," *New England Journal of Medicine* 328 (May 20, 1993), pp. 1489–1493. The authors argue for the adoption of a single-payer system of health-care financing and delivery, citing its likely success in controlling costs while providing universal access. Their proposal permits insurance companies to offer services not covered by the public system, such as elective cosmetic surgery.

CASE STUDIES

This appendix contains a set of case studies for analysis and discussion. Some of the cases are essentially records of actual situations. Others, however, are only loosely based on actual happenings, and a few have been constructed simply for their perceived pedagogical value. Most of the cases have been developed only up to a crucial "decision point." Although retrospective case review—concerned with the appropriateness of decisions actually made in any given case—is called for in a few of the cases presented here, most of the cases ask for a prospective rather than a retrospective analysis. Thus, the more common task is to provide an analysis of what should be done within the context of a developing case rather than an analysis of what has actually been done in a case that has already run its course.

When case descriptions feature a richness of factual detail and nuance, they are sometimes characterized as "thick." By way of contrast, case studies of the type presented here may be characterized as relatively "thin," and their somewhat schematic character may cause discomfort. Individuals involved in analyzing such cases often feel that it would be desirable to have more factual details, especially clinical ones. This recurrent desire reflects the well-based axiom that good decision making must be based on "good facts." However, a perceived lack of factual detail should not be allowed to paralyze analysis and discussion. If the proper decision in a certain case is thought to be dependent upon information not provided in the case description, and if it is reasonable to believe that the desired information would or could be available to those confronted with the decision, a discussion of the case can include an examination of the precise way in which the desired information is relevant to the decision.

Two final points are worth noting. First, the last paragraph of each case study identifies some questions raised by the case. These questions are not the only ones worthy of consideration, but they can be used to facilitate analysis and discussion. Second, the title of each case study is followed by a number or numbers within brackets. These numbers refer to the various chapters in this book. Thus, the chapter or chapters most directly relevant to each case are identified.

CASE 1
WITHHOLDING INFORMATION ABOUT RISKS [2]

Marcia W is a 40-year-old female with multiple myeloma, who upon diagnosis shows great interest in having all the information that is necessary to make a decision about further treatment. Dr. C tells her that the response rates to chemotherapy with this disease are very good and that recent research has shown that 50 percent of patients can hope for long-term survival rates, which are tantamount to cure. The other 50 percent of patients die within a year or two. What Dr. C neglects to tell her is that preliminary studies are showing that, over a twenty-year period subsequent to chemotherapy, 10 percent of those who survive the myeloma will contract a form of leukemia that is highly resistant to treatment. When her treatment is discussed in a staff meeting, Dr. C says that he does not want to tell Marcia W about the 10 percent because he is afraid that it might unduly alarm her and cause her not to take treatment, thereby spoiling her chances for long-term survival. Moreover, he states (1) that the research is not conclusive enough to suit him and (2) that 10 percent is such a low figure that he is not morally required to communicate the risk. After all, he suggests, one cannot inform a patient of *every* risk.

(1) Does Marcia W have a right to the information about the possible risk of leukemia? (2) Is this 10 percent chance of contracting leukemia significant for her decision making? (3) Will this information harm her by making it impossible for her to make an autonomous decision? (4) Is the refusal to disclose justified by the low 10 percent figure and the serious consequences of refusing treatment?

CASE 2
A PATIENT'S REQUEST FOR A POSSIBLY USELESS TREATMENT [2]

After arriving at his doctor's office, Jeff R complains of the flu and requests an antibiotic. His description of symptoms convinces Dr. T that he has the flu. Dr. T explains to Jeff R that antibiotics are physiologically useless against the flu and other conditions caused by viruses (as opposed to bacteria). In dealing with patients who have the flu, she ordinarily recommends rest and fluids and sometimes recommends over-the-counter drugs. But Jeff R insists on an antibiotic, so she considers writing a prescription. On the one hand, she figures that an antibiotic will cause Jeff R no harm and might even help psychologically by making him feel that something is being done for his condition. On the other hand, she is aware that overuse of antibiotics makes it more likely that bacteria in the environment will become resistant to available antibiotics.

(1) Should Dr. T honor Jeff R's request for antibiotics? (2) Is it appropriate for physicians to offer treatments whose sole purpose is to provide psychological comfort when that comfort is based on a false belief or misunderstanding?

CASE 3
PATIENT RESPONSIBILITY [2]

For years Brian B has visited a public clinic that provides health care to uninsured persons. He has established a relationship with Dr. L, who always inquires about Brian's smoking habits and advises him to quit or at least curtail his smoking. Despite repeated warnings, Brian B has continued to smoke heavily, even after developing signs of emphysema in his early fifties. Now, at age 57, Brian B has a severe case of emphysema and goes frequently to the clinic—sometimes clearly for medical purposes, but sometimes apparently just to talk. The clinic, meanwhile, has been hit with budget cuts that have resulted in fewer staff to see patients. Dr. L is irritated with Brian B for ignoring all warnings and worsening his own medical condition. Dr. L tells him that, in the future, he must call before coming to the clinic and that there might not always be a staff member available to see him. Dr. L adds, "These days I am very busy with patients—patients who, by the way, follow doctor's orders—and I will be unable to see you."

(1) To what extent is Brian B responsible for his severe case of emphysema? (2) Does Dr. L have an obligation to continue to be available to Brian B? Does virtue require his continued availability?

CASE 4
VOLUNTARY STERILIZATION AND A YOUNG, UNMARRIED MAN [2]

Gregory X, who is 25 years old, unmarried, and childless, wants a vasectomy. (Vasectomy is a sterilization procedure that, until recently, had been considered irreversible but at present can sometimes be surgically reversed.) He goes to Dr. H, a urologist in a clinic in a large city hospital, because he cannot afford the surgery elsewhere. He tells Dr. H that he has decided, after several years of thought, never to be a parent. The vasectomy will now ensure that and make it unnecessary for any woman he loves to run the various risks associated with the available means of contraception. Dr. H has doubts about performing the surgery on a young, unmarried man. He asks Gregory X to consider the feelings of a possible future wife who will not have any say about the sterilization decision. Gregory X insists on the surgery.

(1) Should Dr. H accede to Gregory X's request despite his reservations, since Gregory X cannot afford the vasectomy elsewhere? (2) Is there anything morally problematic about Gregory X's request?

CASE 5
THE DENTIST AND PATIENT AUTONOMY [2]

A 36-year-old man, Patrick M, contacts the office of an endodontist. (Endodontics is a specialized field of dentistry.) Patrick M wants to arrange for a procedure commonly called a "root canal" to be performed on each of his teeth. A root canal is a common (somewhat involved) procedure used as an alternative to extracting a diseased tooth. It consists of removing the damaged or diseased blood vessels and nerves contained within the tooth. The tooth is thus "devital" but functions normally. If this procedure is not done on a diseased tooth or if the tooth is not extracted, infection will very likely develop in the necrotic tissue and spread into the jaw bone and surrounding tissues.

The endodontist is startled by the idea of performing a root canal on all of Patrick M's teeth. Further discussion makes Patrick M's motivation clear. He is a fervent survivalist, dedicated to planning for every contingency in the expectation that some conflagration is about to destroy society. Patrick M is attempting to ensure—by having all of his teeth desensitized—that he will never suffer a toothache. Although the endodontist cannot escape a sense of amusement over what he considers a bizarre situation, Patrick M seems fully prepared both to undergo a difficult set of procedures and to pay what will be a huge overall bill. Still, the endodontist feels that it would be unethical to remove healthy tissue. He feels that he is being asked to perform a procedure that is not indicated by the existing conditions and may never be indicated, judging by the excellent overall health of the teeth.

(1) Is there any significant difference between the dentist-patient relationship and the physician-patient relationship? (2) Should the endodontist accede to Patrick M's desires?

CASE 6
LIBERTY AND THE ELDERLY PATIENT [2]

Ronald X is 71 years old. A widower, he lives alone in an apartment, but he receives some assistance from a cleaning woman and a friendly neighbor. Ronald X is presently in a hospital because of a broken leg, but he is ready to be discharged. Ronald X also suffers from arteriosclerosis, a condition that results in his experiencing periods of confusion during which he sometimes wanders purposelessly around the city, running some risks to himself. Ronald X's children do not want him to return to his home. They believe that he needs the supervised care provided in a nursing home. Ronald X, when not in a confused state, repeatedly expresses his awareness of the problems he faces stemming from his arteriosclerosis and of the resultant risks he runs. Nonetheless, he would rather run those risks than be confined to institutional care. The health-care professionals and Ronald X's children decide that he will not be discharged from the hospital until an appropriate nursing home is found. At that time, he will be sent to the nursing home. When Ronald X insists on being discharged from the hospital, the medical professionals sedate him to a level sufficient to gain his compliance.

(1) Are the health-care professionals and Ronald X's children making an unjustified leap from his occasional risk-running behavior to the conclusion that he lacks sufficient competence to determine the shape of his own life? (2) Is this paternalistic limitation on Ronald X's liberty morally obligatory? morally permissible? morally reprehensible?

CASE 7
RITALIN FOR A NORMAL BOY [2]

Teresa T and George L, two highly educated and successful professionals, bring their son, Mike, into the office of his pediatrician, Dr. S, with some concerns about Mike's behavior. In school the boy has had difficulties sitting still and following directions, and sometimes has trouble concentrating on his studies both in school and at home. After an extensive discussion with Mike and his parents, Dr. S is convinced that the boy does not have Attention Deficit/Hyperactivity Disorder or any other condition meriting a diagnosis. Mike appears to be a normal, energetic boy who faces many of the behavioral challenges that normal, energetic boys commonly face in school and other highly structured environments.

Despite this reassurance, Teresa T and George L ask Dr. S to write a prescription for Ritalin for Mike. As they explain, they have read that Ritalin can help children (and adults) to improve their concentration regardless of whether they have a medical diagnosis. "Besides," Teresa T asks, "who can draw a bright line between illness and normalcy these days?" Although Dr. S is aware that Ritalin and other stimulants are sometimes prescribed to children like Mike, he expresses reservations about prescribing cognition-affecting medications for children who are basically well. His reservations persist when further discussion reveals that Teresa T and George L are thinking of administering Ritalin to Mike only occasionally, when he needs to prepare for and take a test or complete a difficult assignment.

(1) Do physicians have a responsibility to restrict prescriptions to those patients who have a diagnosable illness or disorder? Does it matter whether the medication in question affects cognition? Does it matter whether the patient is a child? (2) Is there a meaningful boundary between illness, dysfunction, and other medical conditions on the one hand and medical normalcy on the other? If so, does this boundary determine the limits of appropriate medical practice? (3) Does the provision of medications to children who lack a diagnosable condition—in order to enhance their performance in competitive contexts—pose a social threat that merits our serious attention? If so, what is the nature of this threat and how might the medical profession or society address it?

CASE 8
AGGRESSIVE ADVERTISING FOR COSMETIC SURGERY [2]

"Shape Up for Summer!" the advertisement advises. "Don't Be Ashamed to Hit the Beach." Appearing in a variety of magazines for teenage girls and women, the ad offers several types of cosmetic surgery, including breast augmentation and liposuction. Although the five versions of the ad feature different models, each model is a Caucasian woman of college age who is slim, large breasted, and dressed in a bikini. The ad provides contact information for a team of physicians who specialize in cosmetic surgery.

(1) Is it ethically acceptable for physicians to provide services that employ their medical skills for ends other than treating a medical illness, dysfunction, or other diagnosable condition? (2) Is it ethically acceptable for physicians to stimulate demand for such services with attention-grabbing advertisements that may take advantage of some people's insecurities (e.g., about their physical attractiveness)? (3) Is medicine best understood as a business or as a profession with stricter moral norms than those governing business?

CASE 9
MANAGED CARE AND THE TEMPTATION TO SKIMP ON SERVICES [2]

Dr. W, a primary care physician, works for a managed care organization that provides her a monthly capitated sum for each patient in her care. All money spent on providing tests or services for one of her patients comes out of her own pocket; at the end of the month, she keeps whatever money is saved. Recently, many of Dr. W's patients have been sick, requiring considerable medical attention, resulting in a significant drop in her income. Tom D arrives in her office, complaining of irregularities in his heartbeat; sometimes, he reports, it seems that his heart either has a double beat or misses a beat. Using a stethoscope, Dr. W is unable to detect any cardiac abnormalities. At this point, Dr. W is unsure how to proceed. She considers that many people experience slightly irregular heartbeats with no negative consequences for their health. Moreover, Tom D has often struck her as an anxious person who sometimes worries excessively about insignificant symptoms (although he does not seem to need psychiatric care). If she orders a cardiology consult, the cardiologist is likely to order at least one sensitive test, costing Dr. W hundreds of dollars. "He's probably worried about nothing," she thinks. "But can I accept a slight risk that he has a significant heart condition?"

(1) Is it unethical for doctors to consider their own financial interests when they conflict with a patient's best interests? (2) Is it unethical for managed care organizations to create such strong financial incentives for physicians to withhold medical services? (3) What should Dr. W do in this situation?

CASE 10
HOSPITALS, SURGEONS, AND ECONOMIC INCENTIVES [2, 3]

A large, for-profit hospital chain (RASA) offers to share the profits generated by the use of its operating rooms with the staff surgeons who use them. Dr. G is one of these surgeons. Thus, she benefits financially in two ways when she operates on a patient in a RASA hospital—she is paid for the operation and she receives a share of the hospital's profits. There are other, equally equipped hospitals in the community whose facilities Dr. G could use.

(1) Is Dr. G acting in a morally acceptable way by referring her patients to a RASA hospital? (2) Is RASA's profit-sharing policy morally acceptable? (3) Does RASA's policy work to the detriment of the patient?

CASE 11
THE NURSE AND INFORMED CONSENT [2, 3]

Michael G, who is dying of leukemia, is in a hospital, where he is receiving chemotherapy. A registered nurse involved in his care, Nurse L, learns that he has never received information about alternative natural therapies. She gives Michael G the information and discusses the advantages and disadvantages of the various alternatives. After extensive reflection and consultation with his family, Michael G decides to leave the hospital and to make arrangements to try one of the alternative therapies. He informs the attending oncologist of his decision. When the oncologist learns about the source of Michael G's information, he charges Nurse L with unprofessional conduct and asks that her nursing license be revoked. Nurse L argues that the patient has the right to know about the alternatives and that a failure to inform him vitiates his "informed consent" to the chemotherapy.

(1) Was Nurse L acting in a morally correct way when she gave Michael G the information? (2) Should the physician in charge have the final word about the information a patient receives? (3) If Michael G did not know about the alternative therapies, was his agreement to the chemotherapy *informed* consent?

CASE 12
THE OFFICE NURSE AND INFORMED CONSENT [2, 3]

Joan R is going through menopause. Her physician, Dr. W, wants her to begin estrogen therapy. After talking with the physician, Joan R agrees to the therapy. She stops at the nurse's desk in Dr. W's office to pick up her prescription. In the course of the conversation, Nurse M realizes that Dr. W has not informed Joan R that other options are available to her and that there is wide disagreement about which option is preferable. Instead of taking only estrogen, Nurse M reasons, Joan R could choose to take estrogen together with a progestin, or she could choose to take no hormones at all. Each of these options is thought to carry different potential benefits and risks.

(1) Should Nurse M provide Joan R with that information? (2) Should Nurse M suggest to Joan R that she initiate an additional discussion with Dr. W in order to obtain more information? (3) Should Nurse M express her concern in this matter to Dr. W? If so, how should she approach him?

CASE 13
PAIN RELIEF, CULTURAL BELIEFS, AND THE ROLE OF A FAMILY MEMBER [2, 3]

Marie F, a 40-year-old Haitian immigrant, is hospitalized with terminal lung cancer. Initially, the nurse responsible for Marie's care complied with her (competent) request for pain medication. Then Marie's brother, Jean, arrived from another city and found his sister delirious and mumbling incomprehensibly (as patients often do under a heavy dose of pain medication). In accordance with the voodoo religion of his family's culture, Jean took Marie's behavior to suggest the presence of evil spirits in her body; if not exorcised, he thought, the spirits would bring harm to their entire family. Upon learning that Marie's delirious mumbling occurred after she was given pain medication, Jean demanded that the medication be discontinued, explaining, "The medicine brought the spirits into her, so we need to stop the medicine to get the spirits out!" At this point, the nurse feels conflicted between honoring Marie's request for pain control measures and respecting her family's religion. (She also wonders whether this religion assumes that an adult male should make medical decisions on behalf of female family members—as some traditional belief systems assume—but she is reluctant to broach this issue with Jean.)

(1) How should the nurse responsible for Marie's care handle this predicament? (2) Does the principle of self-determination apply to competent adults regardless of cultural

context? (3) Would continuing to administer pain medication to Marie entail a failure to respect the religious beliefs expressed by Jean?

CASE 14
CONFLICT BETWEEN THE INTERESTS OF A PATIENT AND HIS WIFE [2, 3]

An elderly man, Bill S, has been paralyzed by a stroke but apparently retains decision-making capacity. There is no significant chance that the paralysis can be reversed. The patient's physician, Dr. Z, believes the patient should enter a nursing home when he is ready to be discharged from the hospital. Bill S, however, insists on returning home, although the only available caretaker is his rather frail, elderly wife, Amy S, who has a heart ailment. Amy S knows that she is incapable of the physical demands required to care for her husband, and she knows that he will refuse nursing care at home. She explains to her husband that, if her health fails, he will have to enter a nursing home anyway and she may become bedridden or die. Amy S pleads with Dr. Z to intercede when her husband remains adamant. Because Bill S is very attached to his physician, Dr. Z believes that by threatening to withdraw from the case he might be able to get Bill S to change his mind.

(1) How should Dr. Z deal with this situation? (2) Should the interests of family members, when they conflict with a patient's interests, have any bearing on medical decision making? (3) Is it ever appropriate for a physician to pressure a patient to do what is morally right?

CASE 15
AN HIV-INFECTED SURGEON AND A DUTY TO DISCLOSE [2, 3]

Dr. M, a surgeon, has learned that he has been infected with the human immunodeficiency virus (HIV). A prominent study estimates that surgeons cut themselves, on average, 2.5 times for every 100 surgical procedures and that, in approximately one-third of those cases, the patient is touched with the instrument carrying the surgeon's blood. According to the study, for every 1,000 cases in which an HIV-infected surgeon's blood mixes with that of a patient, a patient will become infected in at most 3 cases. Thus, there is *some* risk that a patient operated on by Dr. M will be infected.

(1) Does Dr. M have an obligation to refrain from performing surgery? (2) If not, does Dr. M have an obligation to inform those on whom he plans to operate that he is infected with the virus? (3) Suppose the positions were reversed and a patient, Dorothea L, is the one infected. Is Dorothea L obligated to inform Dr. M of her infection?

CASE 16
"WOULD A COCHLEAR IMPLANT BE BEST FOR OUR CHILD?" [3]

Having become parents one year ago, Sean and Mary McG are considering cochlear implant surgery for their infant child, Gregory, who, like his parents, was born deaf. Cochlear implants are surgically implanted devices that often, but not always, enable partial hearing and speech comprehension in deaf individuals. Neither Sean nor Mary McG has had cochlear implant surgery, which was unavailable when they were young; both speak and read English, their first language, but now rely mostly on American Sign Language (ASL) in each other's company. When they first heard about cochlear implant surgery, the parents were enthusiastic about the possibility of reducing the effects of deafness, which they consider a serious disability, in their child. But some deaf friends of theirs have expressed strong opposition to cochlear implants, stressing their limited efficacy and criticizing efforts to assimilate deaf people into mainstream hearing culture. "Take more pride in being deaf," they say to Sean and Mary McG. "Take pride in our shared language, ASL, and Deaf culture. The whole attitude that says deafness is a disability reflects the majority's prejudice against deafness and the preference that everyone adjust to hearing culture and lifestyle." The McGs feel conflicted. Although they might allow their son to decide for himself when he is older—say, ten or even fifteen—they understand that success rates for cochlear implants are much higher when the surgery is performed in the first few years of life.

(1) Is being deaf objectively disadvantageous, notwithstanding the many achievements of deaf individuals and the deaf community? Or does the classification of deafness as a disability largely reflect the hearing majority's prejudices? (2) What decision regarding cochlear implant surgery would best promote Gregory's long-term interests?

CASE 17
AN INTERSEX INFANT AND DECISIONS ABOUT "NORMALIZATION" [3]

Accompanied by her husband, Fred, Jenny D has just given birth to a boy. The infant's penis is extremely small, creating an appearance of sexual ambiguity ("Is that a boy or a girl?"). In confronting cases involving "intersex" or ambiguous genitalia, many physicians have assumed that healthy psychosexual development requires early social assignment to one gender and a corresponding genital appearance. Accordingly, the attending physician—in consultation with colleagues including a sexologist—ask Jenny and Fred D to consider surgical removal of their infant's testicles, additional surgery, and hormonal treatment to make the child more female in appearance, and a plan to raise their infant as a girl. The parents consider this option along with an alternative approach: avoiding surgery and hormone treatment, raising their child as a boy, providing any psychological counseling he may need, and allowing him to make any major decisions about his sexuality when he is older.

(1) What decision for the present would seem most conducive to the child's long-term interests? (2) What should the medical team do to facilitate the parents' decision making?

CASE 18
UNPROTECTED SEX AND PATIENT CONFIDENTIALITY [3]

For two months, Brian P, who suffers from depression, has been seeing Dr. A in weekly psychotherapy sessions. Brian P, who is gay, has long struggled with feelings of social rejection and with insecurity about his attractiveness; in the past year, he has also experienced the trauma of learning that he is HIV-positive. Shortly after Dr. A feels that he and Brian P have established a strong rapport, Brian P explains that he and a man he has been dating, George S, have begun to have unprotected sex. Even more startling to Dr. A is Brian P's stated intention not to tell George S that he (Brian) is HIV-positive. Careful to avoid a judgmental tone, Dr. A presents the advantages of safe sex and recommends that Brian P inform George S. But Brian P fears that either of those options would lead to his being rejected. While he does not want to harm his partner, Brian P—apparently in denial—claims that unsafe sex is not very likely to transmit HIV (despite Dr. A's assertions to the contrary). Moreover, Brian P reasons, HIV infection is not as bad as it used to be, since a combination of drug therapies now makes long-term survival possible for many HIV-infected individuals.

Dr. A is deeply disturbed by Brian P's intention to continue to have unsafe sex with George S without disclosing his HIV-positive status to him. While Dr. A is sure he would breach confidentiality (as a last resort) if a patient intended to kill an identified third party, Brian P does not intend to kill his partner. Moreover, Dr. A and Brian P have achieved a trust that makes psychotherapy more likely to succeed, a trust that would be put at risk if Brian P's confidentiality were breached. Still, Dr. A feels some obligation to protect George S by warning him if Brian P continues on the present course.

(1) Do health professionals have a "duty to warn" that can override their obligation to maintain patient confidentiality? (2) If so, does this duty extend to cases like the present one? (3) What should Dr. A do?

CASE 19
PRIVACY AND MONITORING SYSTEMS IN A PSYCHIATRIC HOSPITAL [3]

The new superintendent of the Meller Valley Psychiatric Hospital, Dr. R, has decided to install television monitoring devices in all the patients' rooms, as well as in the hallways and visiting rooms of the hospital. His primary purposes are to make it easier to locate personnel when they are needed in a hurry and to help the staff, which is shorthanded, keep an eye on the doings of patients, a small number of whom are prone to violence. Patients know about the surveillance, but visitors are not informed. Some of the members of Dr. R's staff object, arguing that the system is a gross violation of the privacy of both patients and visitors.

(1) Is Dr. R morally justified in establishing the monitoring system? (2) Are patients' and visitors' rights being violated?

CASE 20
A RANDOMIZED CLINICAL TRIAL AND A PHYSICIAN'S RESPONSIBILITY TO A PATIENT [2, 4]

Dr. L has agreed to request the participation of his patients in an RCT designed to test a new drug whose purpose is to treat and cure a disease that is about 70 percent fatal. One of the participants in the trial, Bruce W, has been a patient of Dr. L's for eleven years. There are 90 participants in the RCT. Placebos have been given to 36. The other 54 have been given the new drug. None of the patients is told which treatment he or she is receiving, although all know they are taking part in an RCT. After 24 of the 36 patients on placebos and 15 of those receiving the new drug die, Bruce W asks Dr. L whether he is a placebo recipient and whether there is any good reason to think the new drug is effective. Dr. L knows that Bruce W is a placebo recipient and that the data so far tend to support the view that the experimental drug is effective and prevents death. Dr. L and other physicians involved in the trial prefer not to end it at this time because of concerns about the validity of the study if it is terminated prematurely.

(1) Should the experiment be ended and the remaining patients put on the new therapy immediately? (2) Should Dr. L decline at this point to provide Bruce W with the requested information? (3) Does Dr. L have an obligation to his patient, Bruce W, which should take precedence over concerns about establishing the validity of the RCT's results?

CASE 21
ENROLLING INELIGIBLE PATIENTS IN A CLINICAL TRIAL [2, 4]

Participation in the clinical trial of a drug intended to benefit cancer patients is contingent upon the fulfillment of certain requirements. These include having only a certain type of cancer; having at least an eight-week life expectancy; having normal kidney, liver, and heart functioning; and having the ability to perform everyday functions. The validity of the trial depends upon the enforcement of these requirements. The trial is being conducted by colleagues of Dr. T who have asked him to enroll eligible patients in the trial, with the latter's consent, of course. Dr. Y, who is Dr. T's patient, has exhausted the therapies available for his form of cancer. Dr. Y hears about the clinical trial. Although he knows that he cannot meet all the requirements for participation, he tells Dr. T that he wants to be enrolled and asks that Dr. T fudge the data, if necessary, since otherwise he has no chance for survival.

(1) Should Dr. T fudge the data to give Dr. Y one last chance? (2) Since Dr. Y is also a physician and understands that his participation will compromise the validity of the trial, is his insistence on participation incompatible with his professional commitment?

CASE 22
A TEENAGER'S CONSENT TO PARTICIPATE IN RESEARCH [4]

One hundred high school sophomores are asked to participate in an experimental trial of a new soap intended to prevent acne or at least to mitigate its severity. In the planned randomized clinical trial, half the students will receive the new soap, while the other half will be given a facsimile without the ingredients thought to be effective against acne. No risks to the students are anticipated. The students are given consent forms to take home for their parents' signature. Because they are fearful of the possibility of unknown risks, Lisa H's parents refuse to consent on Lisa's behalf, although Lisa wants to participate in the project.

(1) Should Lisa's consent override her parents' refusal? (2) Would the answer be different if a similar situation occurred involving children whose ages ranged from seven to nine?

CASE 23
BRAIN-DAMAGED GIBBONS AND THE MARCH OF SCIENCE [4]

In 2017, the United States Air Force commences a study to learn about "the basic mechanisms responsible for brain damage in head-injured fighter pilots." In this study, which involves the use of gibbons (one of the "lesser ape" species), a subject's head is cemented tightly in a helmet and subjected to a sudden jerking movement, generating an extremely strong impact. While the gibbon's skull is not fractured, neurological damage is caused by the impact of the brain against the hard skull. Anesthesia is carefully used so that the gibbons are completely unconscious during the procedure. The head trauma causes some subjects to become permanently comatose; others become conscious after anesthesia wears off (and are then given standard pain medications as needed). All become irreversibly brain-damaged and too disabled to feed themselves. Each lives alone in a small cage for approximately one month—during which time various tests are conducted—before they are killed and their brains analyzed.

(1) Can nonhuman animals be harmed by loss of freedom, disability, or death (as distinct from pain, distress, and suffering)? Does social isolation constitute a harm for highly sociable animals, such as primates? (2) Are some harms so great that no animal subjects should ever be forced to incur them? (3) Does the species of animal subjects matter in con-

sidering whether a study is justified? If so, how? (4) Does the importance of the research objective justify the study? Thousands of head-injured humans are hospitalized every year. Should they be considered as possible subjects for studies that cause no additional harm to them? Could more use be made of autopsy studies?

CASE 24
PHYSICIAN DISAGREEMENT REGARDING A PATIENT'S WISHES [2, 5]

John H, a 59-year-old male, has been diagnosed as having cancer, the primary site of which is the pancreas. His condition is rapidly deteriorating. John H has requested that he not be resuscitated if he should go into cardiac arrest. He has also stated that he wishes no further treatment. Dr. W, who is John H's personal physician, and Dr. R, the oncologist in the case, agree that he should not be resuscitated, and "Do not resuscitate" is written on his chart. However, when John H begins to experience severe internal bleeding, he asks his physicians if they can do something. Whether John H is competent at this point is unclear. Dr. W does not want to take measures to stop the bleeding, in keeping with John H's original request for no further treatment. Dr. R sees the request "to do something" as taking precedence over the earlier request for no additional treatment. If they do not act quickly to stop the internal bleeding, John H will die as a result of blood loss.

(1) What is the most appropriate response in this situation? (2) When a patient who is in a great deal of pain, weak, and close to death makes a request that seems at odds with a decision he made when he may have been more fully autonomous, which request should guide those caring for him?

CASE 25
HONORING A LIVING WILL [2, 5]

Esther K, a 65-year-old woman with a long history of diabetes, has been diagnosed as having pancreatic cancer. At the time of diagnosis, she refused all aggressive therapies and later wrote a living will, in which she stated clearly that she did not want any "extraordinary means" used to prolong her life. She specified the "extraordinary means" as chemotherapy, respirators, or resuscitation efforts. Three months after diagnosis, Esther K was admitted to the hospital in a confused state with discoloration on her foot and some evidence of necrotic tissue on the top of her foot. Observation over the next couple of days revealed that the necrosis had spread, and the surgeon, Dr. P, diagnosed gangrene. Dr. P wanted to remove the foot before the gangrene spread. Esther K was somewhat confused but nonetheless agreed to the surgery. The family was very upset with Dr. P for suggesting the surgery and for considering her competent to give consent. The family thinks that in the spirit of the living will she would not want the surgery, which would fall into the class of "extraordinary means." Furthermore, the family thinks that Esther K is too confused to give reflective consent, and this may be borne out by the fact that the patient whispered to the nurse that she consented only because she was afraid Dr. P would no longer take care of her and might order her out of the hospital.

(1) How specific must a living will be in order for it to be morally decisive? (2) Is there a danger of assuming that a consent is valid merely because it coincides with what the physician wishes to do? (3) What weight should be given to the family's judgment in this case?

CASE 26
REFUSAL OF LIFE-SUSTAINING TREATMENT BY A MINOR [2, 3, 5]

Jimmy T is an 11-year-old boy who suffers from lymphoma. The oncologist has indicated that without chemotherapy Jimmy is likely to die within six months. She has also indicated that chemotherapy provides an effective cure in only 20 percent of cases like Jimmy's; in most of the cases, chemotherapy produces at best an additional three-month to six-month extension of life. Jimmy is also compromised by an incurable neurological disease. This disease will eventually make it impossible for him to walk, talk, use his hands effectively, or control his excretory functions. Already his speech is slurred, and he cannot hold a pencil. Even without the lymphoma, the prognosis for him because of the neurological disease is death by the age of 18. Jimmy has been raised in a strong religious environment, and his belief in God has been an important comforting factor for him. After having the facts fully explained to him, he has accepted his situation and the inevitability of his death at a young age. He says that he does not want the chemotherapy and that he is ready to "go to God." His parents, however, cannot reconcile themselves to losing Jimmy. They override Jimmy's decision and tell the oncologist to proceed with the chemotherapy.

(1) Should minors of Jimmy's age be permitted to participate in decisions of this magnitude? (2) Whose decision, the parents' or the child's, should be decisive? (3) How should the oncologist deal with this situation?

CASE 27
A POSSIBLE CONFLICT OF INTEREST FOR A PROXY DECISION MAKER [3, 5]

Joe and Liz C married fifteen years ago. (Before that, he was a widower and she was divorced.) For the past seven years the marriage has been relatively unhappy, due to the revelation of Liz C's affair with one of her husband's colleagues. Two weeks ago Liz C had a stroke. It is clear that some of her capacities will be damaged by the stroke, but the extent of incapacitation is currently unknown. Right now she cannot speak and has incurred respiratory difficulties and an acute infection. Joe C has requested that her conditions not be treated. "Make her as comfortable as possible and let her die in peace," he urged the medical team. "After all, she always said she didn't want to be an invalid. I'm sure she wouldn't want to live." But the attending physician, Dr. H, remembers Joe C's remarking a couple of times that he could not imagine taking care of an invalid wife. Moreover, Dr. H, who has known the couple for years, is aware of the affair that took place long ago, and he has often sensed a deep bitterness on the part of Joe C toward his wife. Dr. H therefore wonders about Joe C's motives and about whose interests would be served if Liz C were allowed to die. Without being quite sure how to proceed, he decides he cannot simply take for granted Joe C's testimony about his wife's preferences.

(1) If the medical team is unable to uncover more information regarding Liz C's wishes regarding treatment in her present circumstances, how should her best interests be determined? (2) If her best interests favor treatment of her infection and breathing difficulties as well as rehabilitative therapy—in apparent conflict with Joe C's wishes—should these interventions be initiated? Should Joe C's interests be given any significant consideration?

CASE 28
ANENCEPHALIC NEWBORNS, ORGAN DONATION, AND SOCIAL POLICY [5]

It is estimated that 1,000 to 2,000 babies are born in the United States each year with anencephaly, the total or almost total absence of the cerebral hemispheres. Many of these infants are stillborn; the prognosis for those born alive is that they will live for only a few hours, days, or weeks. Although the organ systems of some anencephalic infants are under-developed, there are many cases in which organs (e.g., a heart or kidneys) could be transplanted to other infants whose lives might thereby be saved. Some parents of anencephalic infants would undoubtedly consent to organ donation as a way of creating some redeeming value out of a tragic situation. Still, numerous reservations have been expressed about the idea of transplanting the organs of anencephalic infants. In particular, for transplants to have a reasonable prospect of success, the vital organs must be taken from an anencephalic infant before it meets the criteria of (whole) brain death; thus, harvesting its vital organs is tantamount to killing the infant. At present, there is no legal mechanism through which this sort of organ donation can be accomplished.

(1) Is it disrespectful, unfair, or otherwise immoral to transplant the organs of an anencephalic infant? (2) Should we adopt a social policy that would permit (with parental consent) harvesting the organs of an anencephalic infant? (3) If an anencephalic infant is stillborn, would it be justifiable to attempt resuscitation purely for the purpose of keeping organs intact until they can be harvested? (4) If it is justifiable to harvest the organs of an anencephalic infant, would it be justifiable to harvest the organs of someone in a permanent vegetative state?

CASE 29
NEONATAL CARE AND THE PROBLEM OF UNCERTAINTY [5]

Bobbie C is now 6 months old. He was born prematurely with a birth weight of 800 grams and had multiple problems from the beginning. Bobbie developed hyaline membrane disease due to his undeveloped lungs and the need for a respirator. He also developed rickets. A CAT scan revealed some calcium deposits in the brain, which might or might not compromise his mental functions. Within the first month, Bobbie developed thrombocytopenia (low platelet count), for which he was given transfusions. He now suffers from a depression of his immunological system, perhaps related to the transfusions. He shows little interest in eating, and all attempts to bottle-feed him have failed after a couple of days. His health-care costs are being supported by Medicaid, and they are estimated to be in the neighborhood of $550,000 for his six months of hospitalization. Now the health-care staff and the attending physician are considering the possibility of a bone marrow transplant to deal with the thrombocytopenia and the immunosuppression. The chances of success in an infant this small are minimal, and the procedure is largely experimental in infants having this condition. If the transplant is successful, it will alleviate only one of his many problems.

(1) In view of the many uncertainties in this case, what is the proper treatment decision? (2) Should society be expected to shoulder such an expense for an infant who is so physiologically and, perhaps, mentally compromised? (3) Do the parents have a right to reject further aggressive therapies? to insist on them?

CASE 30
IS NUTRITION EXPENDABLE? [5, 6]

Mildred D, a 78-year-old woman, suffers from diabetes, which has been controlled largely by diet. She has a history of heart disease and has suffered two heart attacks. She has now had a stroke, which has rendered her semicomatose and paralyzed. She must be fed through an NG (nasogastric) tube, and the sustenance that she receives in this way is the only thing that keeps her going. Mildred D has previously indicated to her family that in such a circumstance she would not want to be resuscitated. Her condition is slowly deteriorating, but it looks as though the dying process will be a long one. It seems that she will never return from the twilight zone in which she now resides. Angiography indicates that a substantial portion of the brain has been destroyed by the stroke. Her three children want to stop the tube feedings, but the physician objects that it is unethical to "starve" a patient so that she will die sooner.

(1) Is it morally legitimate to withhold nutrition in this case? (2) Does the family have the right to make such a decision for the patient? (3) Should the refusal of resuscitation be considered an indicator that the patient would also refuse nutrition?

CASE 31
DEATH BY DEHYDRATION [5, 6]

Roberta W is a 67-year-old unmarried female. A retired teacher, she is cared for by her brother and his wife in their home. Roberta W suffers from severe emphysema and related heart problems. She also suffers from a collection of nagging medical problems, including bloatedness, hemorrhoids, and a hernia. She is largely confined to her bed. Occasionally she feels well enough to sit up for an hour or so, but eating, going to the bathroom, and personal grooming are experienced as exhausting and burdensome. Roberta W is weary of the circumstances of her life, and she regrets being a burden to her brother and his wife, although they do not seem to resent the demands placed upon them by her care. Roberta W's prognosis is somewhat unclear, and she may well live for several years in her present state, but she continually says that she would rather be dead. At one point, when her hernia was especially bothersome to her, she had a conversation with her physician, Dr. R. He said that the hernia could easily be corrected by surgery but that it was very unlikely that she would survive the surgery because of her emphysema and heart problems. She said that she wanted the surgery anyway. "If I die, fine; if I survive, at least I have one less problem." Dr. R responded that no responsible surgeon would perform an operation in such circumstances.

Roberta W now asks Dr. R to admit her to the hospital. Her plan is to stop drinking and to refuse any form of medical hydration, but she wants to be in the hospital so that any discomfort can be controlled through medication. She has read that patients who refuse all hydration will usually die within a week or so.

(1) If Roberta W refuses all hydration, is she committing suicide? (2) Should Dr. R accept Roberta W's plan and cooperate with her in executing it? Should his cooperation be understood as physician assistance in suicide? (3) Would it have been morally justified for a surgeon to have provided the hernia surgery that she had wanted at an earlier time?

CASE 32
ACTIVE EUTHANASIA AND PHYSICIAN-ASSISTED SUICIDE IN THE NETHERLANDS [6]

Both voluntary active euthanasia (VAE) and physician-assisted suicide (PAS) have been openly available to patients in The Netherlands for many years. For example, a government-sponsored study reported that in 1990 there were 2,300 cases of VAE and 400 cases of PAS, accounting for about 3 percent of overall mortality that year. And yet, until more recently, these practices were not strictly legal. Rather, the operational understanding was that physicians would be immune from prosecution as long as they adhered to a set of guidelines worked out by agreement of the medical and legal communities. In 2002, however, the year in which the Termination of Life on Request and Assisted Suicide Act (TLRASA) went into effect, VAE and PAS were formally legalized in The Netherlands.

The TLRASA stipulates that any physician who properly conforms to "due care criteria" in the provision of VAE/PAS and promptly reports to a Regional Review Committee any case in which VAE or PAS has been provided will be immune from prosecution. Further, in order to comply with the due care criteria, the physician must: "(a) be satisfied that the patient has made a voluntary and carefully considered request; (b) be satisfied that the patient's suffering was unbearable, and that there was no prospect of improvement; (c) have informed the patient about his situation and his prospects; (d) have come to the conclusion, together with the patient, that there is no reasonable alternative in the light of the patient's situation; (e) have consulted at least one other, independent physician, who must have seen the patient and given a written opinion on the due care criteria referred to in (a) to (d) above; and (f) have terminated the patient's life or provided assistance with suicide with due medical care and attention." A Regional Review Committee is charged with the responsibility of reviewing each reported case of VAE/PAS in order to determine if physician actions have properly conformed to the due care criteria.

The TLRASA explicitly allows for the possibility of active euthanasia in accordance with an advance-directive principle. That is, in essence, active euthanasia may be provided for a presently incompetent patient who, while competent, made a written declaration requesting that his or her life be terminated under specified circumstances. The TLRASA further allows for the possibility of VAE/PAS in the case of a minor who is at least 12 years old and "is deemed to be capable of making a reasonable appraisal of his own interests." Requests from 16- and 17-year-olds can be complied with but only on the condition of *consultation* with parents (or guardian), although parental/guardian approval is not required. Requests from 12- to 15-year-olds can also be complied with but only on the condition of parental/guardian *consent.*

(1) Is the Dutch system for the practice of active euthanasia and physician-assisted suicide morally sound? (2) Does the Dutch model incorporate adequate safeguards against abuse? (3) Are the TLRASA provisions related to minors morally sound? (4) Should active euthanasia be legalized in the United States along the lines of the Dutch model?

CASE 33
A BRAIN-DEAD MOTHER GIVES BIRTH [5, 7]

Rosa J suffered a fatal seizure while she was 23 weeks pregnant. Although Rosa J was declared brain-dead the day after the seizure, cardiopulmonary function was maintained by means of a respirator and allied technology for nine weeks, until she gave birth to a healthy baby girl by cesarean section. During this time, the physicians used steroids to help the lungs of the fetus mature and monitored fetal growth with ultrasound examinations. Rosa J was fed intravenously and given antibiotics for infections when necessary. After the birth, the respirator was disconnected. The baby was given an excellent chance to survive, although she weighed only three pounds. From the time of the seizure, all decisions about Rosa J and the fetus she was carrying were made by physicians in consultation with Rosa J's family.

(1) Should Rosa J have been maintained on a respirator for nine weeks after being declared brain-dead simply in order to give the child she was carrying a better chance to survive? (2) Was Rosa J being used merely as a means to others' ends? (3) Is someone who is brain-dead a "person" and, therefore, on a Kantian account an individual who cannot be used merely as a means to others' ends?

CASE 34
EMBRYONIC STEM CELLS AND A PRESIDENTIAL DECISION [7, 8]

In a short speech delivered to the nation August 9, 2001, President George W. Bush offered some general reflections on the ethics of research on embryonic stem cells and also announced a decision he had made about the use of federal funding to support such research.

"As a result of private research, more than sixty genetically diverse stem cell lines already exist. They were created from embryos that have already been destroyed, and they have the ability to regenerate themselves indefinitely, creating ongoing opportunities for research. I have concluded that we should allow federal funds to be used for research on these existing stem cell lines, where the life and death decision has already been made.

"Leading scientists tell me research on these sixty lines has great promise that could lead to breakthrough therapies and cures. This allows us to explore the promise and potential of stem cell research without crossing a fundamental moral line, by providing taxpayer funding that would sanction or encourage further destruction of human embryos that have at least the potential for life."

The President's decision was widely viewed as an effort to craft a political compromise on a volatile policy issue. The essence of the decision was this: Research on preexisting stem cell lines—that is, those already in existence as a result of the prior destruction of embryos—would be eligible for federal funding, but research on stem cell lines derived from embryos destroyed after August 9, 2001, would not be eligible for federal funding.

(1) Is the Bush federal funding policy morally defensible? (2) Is the Bush federal funding policy too restrictive? Is it too permissive?

CASE 35
MATERNAL PKU AND FETAL WELFARE [7]

Martha J, a 23-year-old female, was born with PKU (phenylketonuria), an enzyme deficiency that prevents the metabolization of phenylalanine. Children born with PKU are ordinarily placed on a special low-phenylalanine diet for at least the first five years of their life. Although the diet is necessary to prevent severe retardation, it is very burdensome, not only because normal foods are very limited but also because the main source of protein is a bad-tasting "medical food." Because Martha J was placed on this special diet in her childhood, she does not suffer from retardation.

Martha J is four months pregnant. Although her inability to metabolize phenylalanine is no longer a problem for her own well-being, there is a problem for the fetus she is carrying. Unless Martha J maintains the same low-phenylalanine diet throughout the course of her pregnancy, her fetus is at grave risk for severe retardation, microcephaly, congenital heart disease, and other disorders. Martha J's religious beliefs have motivated her to decide against abortion. Nevertheless, she is ambivalent about her pregnancy, because she is unmarried and depressed by the breakdown of her relationship with the child's father. She is also finding it very difficult to adhere to the same dietary restrictions that she found so oppressive in her childhood. Dr. R, the obstetrician who is caring for Martha J, has repeatedly emphasized the importance of adhering to the prescribed diet, but Martha J acknowledges that she has been inconstant in doing so.

(1) Should Dr. R encourage Martha J to reconsider the possibility of abortion? (2) If Martha J is resolved to carry her fetus to term, how should Dr. R deal with the fact that she is not maintaining the prescribed diet? (3) If all else fails, should Dr. R seek a court order that would place Martha J in a supervised setting where dietary restrictions could be enforced?

CASE 36
A FETUS WITH TURNER'S SYNDROME [7, 8]

Barbara J is a 37-year-old woman who is pregnant and in her 20th week. She is married and has one child, a 4-year-old girl. At the advice of her obstetrician, Barbara J has undergone amniocentesis, so that tests could be performed for chromosomal abnormalities and neural-tube defects. The tests have just come in, and Barbara J is told that the fetus has been diagnosed with a chromosomal abnormality known as Turner's syndrome.

A normal female has two X chromosomes. In Turner's syndrome, one of the two X chromosomes is missing; there is a total of only 45 chromosomes. Females who have Turner's syndrome have a characteristic appearance: short stature, webbing of the neck, sagging eyelids, low hairline on the back of the neck, and multiple moles. The syndrome is also characterized by narrowing of the aorta, the failure of menstruation and breast development, and infertility. Although many patients with Turner's syndrome have difficulty performing tasks that require spatial orientation, they can otherwise function normally in society.

(1) How serious are the appearance and developmental problems associated with Turner's syndrome? (2) Would abortion be morally justified in this case? Does it make a difference that the fetus is already at 20 weeks?

CASE 37
PRENATAL DIAGNOSIS AND SEX SELECTION [7, 8]

A 32-year-old woman, Lisa B, goes to the prenatal diagnostic center of a major hospital. She is intent on arranging for chorionic villi sampling (CVS) in order to determine the sex of the fetus she is carrying. A genetic counselor explains to her that the center has an established policy against making prenatal diagnosis (whether CVS or amniocentesis) available for purposes of sex selection. The genetic counselor, in defending the policy, tells her that there is a collective sense at the center that abortion purely on grounds of sex selection is both morally and socially problematic.

Lisa B proceeds to explain her situation. She and her husband already have three children, all of whom are girls. They want very much to have a male child but, for economic reasons, are determined to have no more than one more child. Indeed, if they had a boy among their three children, they would not even consider having a fourth. They feel so strongly about this fourth child's being a boy that, if they cannot gain assurance that it is a male, they will elect abortion. Lisa B insists that it is unfair for the center to deny her access to prenatal diagnosis.

(1) Should the center consider this case an exceptional one and make CVS available? (2) Would the center be well advised to develop a different policy regarding the availability of prenatal diagnosis for purposes of sex selection?

CASE 38
PREIMPLANTATION GENETIC DIAGNOSIS AND HUNTINGTON'S DISEASE [7, 8]

Heather D is a 24-year-old female whose father suffers from Huntington's disease, an autosomal dominant genetic disease whose symptoms first emerge (ordinarily) between the ages of 30 and 50. Huntington's disease is characterized by a progressive physical and mental deterioration leading to death in ten to fifteen years. Heather D knows that there is a 50 percent chance that she has inherited the defective gene from her father, but she has decided not to undergo testing to determine whether she has inherited the gene, because she would rather not know. Heather D and her husband want to have a child, but both of them have a strong desire that their child not be at risk for Huntington's disease. They have rejected the possibility of prenatal diagnosis and selective abortion, in part because Heather D realizes that diagnosis of her fetus as carrying the defective gene would entail the knowledge that she also carries the gene, and because Heather D's husband is morally opposed to abortion. A genetic counselor has suggested an alternative involving preimplantation genetic diagnosis. Several embryos could be formed in vitro using Heather D's eggs and her husband's sperm. These embryos could be tested for the presence of the Hungtington's gene, with only embryos free of the gene being transferred to Heather's uterus. If any embryos were found to carry the defective gene, they would be quietly discarded.

(1) Is Heather D's decision not to be tested for the Huntington's gene a wise one? (2) Does the genetic counselor's suggestion provide a satisfactory solution to the problem? (3) Is preimplantation genetic diagnosis and the discarding of affected embryos morally equivalent to prenatal diagnosis and selective abortion?

CASE 39
CYSTIC FIBROSIS AND A FINDING OF NONPATERNITY [8]

At the age of 19 months, Jennifer C was diagnosed with cystic fibrosis (CF), an autosomal recessive genetic disease. The characteristic pattern is that a child inherits the CF gene from both parents, each of whom is a carrier. Jennifer C's parents, who have been married about three years, are anxious to clarify their risk for having another child with this disorder. They are referred to a genetic counselor, who arranges for DNA testing to confirm their carrier status. The results from the laboratory indicate that Jennifer's mother is a carrier but her husband is not. In fact, DNA analysis shows clearly that he is not the biological father of the child. The genetic counselor is unsure how to proceed.

(1) Should the genetic counselor communicate the finding of nonpaternity to the couple, perhaps jeopardizing their young marriage? Should the genetic counselor first speak privately with the woman? (2) If the woman is willing to identify the biological father, should the genetic counselor notify him that he is almost certainly a carrier of the CF gene?

CASE 40
IVF AND A POSTMENOPAUSAL WOMAN [8]

Emily L is a 59-year-old woman who plans to retire at the age of 60 from her job as a financial executive. She has been married for ten years to a man who also plans to retire within the next year. He is presently 64 years of age. Both Emily L and her husband are in good health and look forward to carving out a new life in retirement. In fact, they have decided that this would be a good time for them to raise a child, so they want to arrange for Emily L to become pregnant. They are aware that it is now possible for postmenopausal women to bear children by employing egg donation, in vitro fertilization (IVF), and embryo transfer to the womb of the postmenopausal woman, who would receive hormonal treatments. The idea is that Emily L's husband would provide the sperm for IVF, making him the biological father of the child. When Emily L and her husband explain their plan to Dr. T at the Metropolitan Fertility Clinic, Dr. T is uncertain whether the clinic should support Emily's attempt to become pregnant. Dr. T has successfully produced pregnancies in women who have experienced early menopause, but she is not comfortable with the age of the prospective parents in this particular case.

(1) Is the plan formulated by Emily L and her husband morally sound? If not, what is problematic about it? (2) Should Dr. T and the clinic support Emily L's attempt to become pregnant?

CASE 41
BABY M [8]

In February 1985, Mary Beth Whitehead entered into a commercial surrogacy agreement with a married couple, Elizabeth and William Stern. Mary Beth Whitehead agreed, for a fee of $10,000, to be artificially inseminated with William Stern's semen and to bear a child that upon birth would be given over to the couple and adopted by Elizabeth Stern. Elizabeth Stern was living under a possible diagnosis of multiple sclerosis and was reluctant to bear the risks associated with pregnancy. Mary Beth Whitehead was married and had two children at the time she entered into the surrogacy contract.

Mary Beth Whitehead eventually became pregnant and Baby M was born March 27, 1986. (The baby was named Sara by Mary Beth Whitehead and Melissa by the Sterns.) Upon giving birth, Mary Beth Whitehead realized that she did not want to part with the child, but she did give the child over to the Sterns on March 30. The next day, clearly in emotional turmoil, she implored the Sterns to let her keep the baby for another week. The Sterns reluctantly agreed. When Mary Beth Whitehead subsequently refused to return Baby M to the Sterns, William Stern filed a complaint seeking legal enforcement of the surrogacy contract. In response, Mary Beth Whitehead and her husband fled with Baby M from New Jersey to Florida. The Whiteheads continually changed their location in Florida in an effort to escape detection, but Florida authorities eventually located Baby M when she was about four months old. The child was returned to New Jersey and placed in the temporary custody of the Sterns while the trial court considered how the matter was to be resolved.

Eight months later, when Baby M was about one year old, the trial court announced its judgment. The trial court (a) found the surrogacy contract to be valid, (b) ordered the termination of Mary Beth Whitehead's parental rights, (c) awarded sole custody of Baby M to William Stern, and (d) authorized adoption by Elizabeth Stern.

The New Jersey Supreme Court ultimately took a very different position. The court concluded that commercial surrogacy contracts are invalid and unenforceable in New Jersey.

Four principal concerns were expressed. First, a surrogate mother cannot be forced by a pre-birth contract to surrender her child because she is in no position to make an *informed* choice prior to birth. Second, commercial surrogacy contracts are tantamount to baby selling. Third, commercial surrogacy contracts would allow the rich to exploit the poor. Fourth, there is a risk of psychosocial harm to the resultant child. Although consideration of Baby M's best interests led the court to award primary custody to the Sterns, the court found no basis for the termination of Mary Beth Whitehead's parental rights and therefore concluded that she (as the child's legal mother) was entitled to visitation.

(1) Is it the trial court or the New Jersey Supreme Court that provided the best overall resolution of the issues involved in this case? (2) Should commercial surrogacy contracts be recognized as valid and legally enforceable? (3) Who should be recognized as the legal mother of Baby M? Would it make a difference if Mary Beth Whitehead, instead of being both the genetic and gestational mother of Baby M, had been only the gestational mother of Baby M, that is, if an egg provided by Elizabeth Stern had been fertilized with her husband's sperm and then transferred to the uterus of Mary Beth Whitehead?

CASE 42
IVF, EMBRYO SPLITTING, AND DELAYED TWINNING [8]

Karen T and Roger T, a married couple in their late 30s, have been trying for several years to start a family. After consulting with Dr. M at the University Reproductive Center, the couple decided to try IVF, even though their expenses for this procedure would amount to at least $8,000. Karen T expressed worries about the possible hazards of the fertility drugs commonly used to enhance the production of mature eggs, but she ultimately agreed to undergo drug treatment, and several eggs were recovered via a minor but uncomfortable surgical procedure. The eggs were subsequently fertilized with Roger T's sperm. Of the seven embryos ultimately produced by this process, four were frozen at the four-cell stage, and the other three were transferred to Karen T's uterus, but without success. Later, three of the remaining embryos were thawed and transferred to Karen T's uterus, again without success.

Concerned about the risks of fertility drugs, the risks and discomfort of the egg-recovery process, and the overall expense of the procedure, the couple is now reluctant to start another course of IVF. They propose the following plan to Dr. M. The one remaining embryo should be thawed and split into four cells, so that each can begin the process of division and growth. Implantation should be attempted with two of the newly formed embryos; the other two should be frozen. Further, they suggest, if Karen T becomes pregnant and gives birth to a healthy child, the couple can wait two or three years and then attempt to achieve pregnancy with the remaining embryos. This plan could result in genetically identical children of different ages.

(1) Should Dr. T act in accordance with the wishes of the couple? (2) Is embryo splitting morally defensible as an adjunct to IVF and embryo transfer? (3) Is embryo splitting and delayed twinning less morally problematic than cloning via somatic cell nuclear transfer?

CASE 43
JUSTICE AND ABORTION FUNDING [7, 9]

Sara G is a 35-year-old mother of four children whose husband deserted her about a month after she became pregnant with her fifth child. The ages of her four children range from 1 to 6 years. She knows nothing about her husband's whereabouts and is currently being supported by public assistance. Sara G is less than three months pregnant and wants an abortion. Her reasons are as follows: (1) She does not have the skills to get a job whose earnings will even come close to the public assistance she receives. If she has to pay for child care from whatever meager wages she could earn, the money left could not support her family at even the subsistence level, so, at least until the children are older, she will be dependent upon public assistance. The sums she receives are barely adequate to take care of her present family. Adding another member would mean even further deprivation for her present family. (2) Her caseworker has agreed that, when the four children are a bit older, Sara G will go into a job-training program that will enable her to get a job paying enough to get the family off public assistance and to give her children a better start in life. Sara G has undergone a battery of psychological tests to help determine what kind of work she should be capable of doing with the right education and training. The social worker and psychological counselor are both confident that Sara G can do the work necessary to make a good living for herself and her family. Having another child would only postpone the time when Sara G will be self-supporting, and in the meantime her family would be living at a very inadequate level.

Because Sara G is on public assistance, she must get an authorization from the social work agency to secure funding for any medical procedure that is not necessitated by an emergency. In cases involving abortion, the final decision is made by a social worker.

(1) Should the social worker authorize funding for the abortion? (2) What moral justification could be advanced to support an authorization? a refusal to authorize? (3) What restrictions, if any, should there be on the Medicaid funding of abortion?

CASE 44
JUSTICE, MENTAL DISABILITY, AND PUBLIC POLICY [9]

State representative Jeremy H has introduced a state bill that would establish homes for the care and education of children with major learning disabilities, such as severe retardation and autism. The bill would provide one home for every twelve children presently institutionalized in five state institutions for children with such disabilities. The present annual cost of maintaining the five institutions is $100 million. Providing the new form of care for the present institutionalized population of 8,000 is expected to cost about $130 million annually.

Jeremy H argues that the currently institutionalized children live in antiquated buildings lacking basic human necessities and amenities. The children frequently spend whole days in their cheerless rooms; many are not even properly clothed. Supervised by an overworked, largely untrained staff, they receive almost nothing in the way of education, entertainment, or structured activities. Jeremy H argues that justice requires removing these individuals from such subhuman conditions and offering them an opportunity for a more "normal" life.

A physician, Dr. M, is opposed to the bill and testifies at a legislative hearing. He argues that the money required to make the change could be used more efficiently to provide health care for three groups: normal children, women lacking access to gynecological and prenatal services, and working adults whose employers do not provide health insurance. He also argues that the occurrence of retardation and other mental disabilities can be greatly reduced through prenatal diagnosis.

(1) Should the proposed bill be enacted into law? (2) Do the mentally retarded have a right to lead a life as "normal" as possible, given their limitations?

CASE 45
JUSTICE, AGE, AND PERSONAL RESPONSIBILITY [9]

The intensive care unit (ICU) at a local hospital has one available bed. Two patients are in immediate and desperate need of ICU care. The first is Jeffrey O, who is 71 years old and has been severely injured in an automobile accident. Jeffrey O was in good physical shape prior to the accident and does not suffer from any debilitating condition. However, his present condition is extremely critical due to the accident. The second patient is Donald R, a 22-year-old drug addict whose present condition, equally critical, is the result of drug use.

(1) Which of the two should receive the ICU bed? (2) Would the answer be different if Donald R were 71 years old and Jeffrey O were 22? (3) Suppose Donald R was not a drug addict but a previously healthy 22-year-old severely injured in an automobile accident. Furthermore, suppose that Jeffrey O had been admitted to the hospital about an hour before Donald R, but the decision about putting each of them in the ICU is being made at the same time. Who should get the bed?

CASE 46
JUSTICE, HEALTH CARE, AND POVERTY [9]

Amanda R is 25 years old. Although she holds both a full-time and a part-time job, she has a very low income and does not have any health-care insurance. At the same time, Amanda R's income is just high enough to prevent her from qualifying for any government-funded health care such as that provided by Medicaid. While experiencing severe chest pain and difficulty in breathing, Amanda R goes to the emergency room of a local for-profit hospital. Before she receives any care, clerical personnel in the hospital determine her financial status and the fact that she is uninsured. By the time she is examined, Amanda R's chest pains stop, and her breathing difficulties disappear. A medical staff member gives her a cursory examination, which does not include an electrocardiogram, and sends her home, suggesting that she go to her own physician the next day for a more thorough examination.

(1) If the medical staff member's decision not to give Amanda R a more thorough examination and not to admit her for further observation was based on her lack of health-care insurance, can that decision be morally justified? (2) Suppose that Amanda R's symptoms had not eased while she was in the emergency room and that the medical staff member had decided that Amanda R did need hospital admittance, observation, and testing. However, suppose that, instead of admitting her to the for-profit hospital, Amanda R had been sent by ambulance to a community (not-for-profit) hospital. Would that behavior have been morally acceptable?

ABOUT THE CONTRIBUTORS

TERRENCE F. ACKERMAN is Professor and Chair of the Department of Human Values and Ethics at the College of Medicine, University of Tennessee, Memphis.

MARCIA ANGELL is Senior Lecturer, Department of Social Medicine, Harvard University.

GEORGE J. ANNAS is Edward R. Utley Professor at the Boston University School of Public Health, where he is also Chair of the Department of Health Law, Bioethics, and Human Rights.

PAT ARMSTRONG is Professor of Sociology, York University (Toronto, Ontario).

JOHN D. ARRAS is Porterfield Professor of Biomedical Ethics and Professor of Philosophy at the University of Virginia.

MARTIN BENJAMIN is Professor Emeritus of Philosophy at Michigan State University.

JAMES L. BERNAT is Professor in the Department of Medicine, Section of Neurology, Dartmouth Medical School.

R. B. BRANDT was Professor of Philosophy at the University of Michigan.

DAN W. BROCK is Professor of Medical Ethics and Director, Division of Medical Ethics and University Program in Ethics and Health, Department of Social Medicine, Harvard University.

BARUCH BRODY is Leon Jaworski Professor of Biomedical Ethics and Director of the Center for Medical Ethics and Health Policy, Baylor College of Medicine, and is also Professor of Philosophy at Rice University.

HOWARD BRODY is Professor of Family Practice and Philosophy at Michigan State University.

BARRY F. BROWN is Emeritus Professor of Philosophy at the University of Toronto.

ALLEN E. BUCHANAN is Professor of Philosophy at the University of Arizona.

DANIEL CALLAHAN is a cofounder of The Hastings Center (Garrison, New York), where he is presently Director of International Programs.

NORMAN L. CANTOR is Professor of Law and is Justice Nathan L. Jacobs Scholar, Rutgers University School of Law at Newark (New Jersey).

ALEXANDER MORGAN CAPRON is Henry W. Bruce University Professor of Law and Medicine, University of Southern California.

CHRISTINE K. CASSEL is President and Chief Executive Officer of the American Board of Internal Medicine and the ABIM Foundation.

MARINA CAVAZZANA-CALVO is a physician and researcher at the Immunology and Pediatric Haematology Unit, Hospital Necker (Paris, France).

JAMES F. CHILDRESS is Edwin B. Kyle Professor of Religious Studies and Professor of Medical Education at the University of Virginia.

KEVIN C. CHUNG is Associate Professor of Plastic Surgery and Director, University of Michigan Hand Center, University of Michigan.

CARL COHEN is Professor of Philosophy at the University of Michigan.

CHARLES M. CULVER is Professor of Medical Education, School of Graduate Medical Science, Barry University (Miami Shores, Florida).

NORMAN DANIELS is Professor of Ethics and Population Health, Department of Population and International Health, Harvard University.

REBECCA DRESSER is Professor of Law and Professor of Ethics in Medicine at Washington University School of Law.

EZEKIEL EMANUEL is Chair of the Department of Clinical Bioethics, National Institutes of Health.

LEONARD M. FLECK is Professor of Philosophy and Medical Ethics at Michigan State University.

JOHN C. FLETCHER was Emily Davie and Joseph S. Kornfield Professor of Biomedical Ethics in the School of Medicine, University of Virginia.

BENJAMIN FREEDMAN was Professor at the McGill Center for Medicine, Ethics, and Law and Clinical Ethicist at the Sir Mortimer B. Davis Jewish General Hospital in Montreal, Canada.

BERNARD GERT is Stone Professor of Intellectual and Moral Philosophy at Dartmouth College and Adjunct Professor of Psychiatry at Dartmouth Medical School.

WALTER GLANNON is Assistant Professor, Centre for Applied Ethics, University of British Columbia, and Clinical Ethicist at the Children's and Women's Health Centre of British Columbia.

LEONARD H. GLANTZ is Associate Dean for Academic Affairs, School of Public Health, Boston University.

LAWRENCE O. GOSTIN is Professor of Law at the Georgetown University Law Center, Professor of Public Health at the Johns Hopkins University, and Director of the Center for Law and the Public's Health.

MICHAEL A. GRODIN is Professor of Health Law, Pediatrics, Psychiatry, and Socio-Medical Sciences and Community Medicine at Boston University, where he is also Director of the Law, Medicine, and Ethics Program.

SHERRI A. GROVEMAN is an attorney who serves on the Board of Directors of both the Androgen Insensitivity Support Group and the Intersex Society of North America.

AMY M. HADDAD is Professor at the School of Pharmacy and Health Professions and Associate Director, Creighton Center for Health Policy and Ethics, Creighton University (Omaha, Nebraska).

DEBORAH S. HELLMAN is Associate Professor of Law at the University of Maryland.

SAMUEL HELLMAN is A. N. Pritzker Distinguished Service Professor in the Department of Radiation and Cellular Oncology, University of Chicago.

EDWIN CONVERSE HETTINGER is Professor of Philosophy at the College of Charleston (South Carolina).

ROGER HIGGS is Professor of General Practice and Primary Care at the School of Medicine and Dentistry, King's College, London.

JOHN K. IGLEHART is Editor-in-Chief of *Health Affairs* and a national correspondent for *The New England Journal of Medicine.*

LEON R. KASS is Addie Clark Harding Professor, the Committee on Social Thought and the College, University of Chicago, and Chair of the President's Council on Bioethics.

JUSTIN KEEN is Professor of Health Politics and Information Management at the Nuffield Institute, University of Leeds (Leeds, England).

PATRICIA A. KING is Carmack Waterhouse Professor of Law, Medicine, Ethics, and Public Policy, Georgetown University.

KENNETH KIPNIS is Professor of Philosophy at the University of Hawaii at Manoa.

SOPHIA KOLEHMAINEN is Deputy Director of the Cedar Tree Foundation (Boston).

HELGA KUHSE is Honorary Senior Research Fellow at the Centre for Human Bioethics, Monash University (Melbourne, Australia).

MARGARET OLIVIA LITTLE is Associate Professor of Philosophy and Senior Research Scholar, Kennedy Institute of Ethics, Georgetown University.

BRUCE LOWENSTEIN has a private practice in psychotherapy and provides outpatient services for Helen Hayes Hospital (West Haverstraw, New York).

RUTH MACKLIN is Professor of Bioethics at the Albert Einstein College of Medicine (New York).

WENDY K. MARINER is Professor of Law and Professor of Socio-Medical Sciences and Community Medicine at Boston University, where she is also Director of the Patient Rights Program.

DON MARQUIS is Professor of Philosophy at the University of Kansas.

FULVIO MAVILIO is a researcher at the Instituto Scientifico H. San Raffaele (Milan, Italy) and in the Department of Biomedical Sciences, University of Modena (Modena, Italy).

NICHOLAS MAYS is Professor of Health Policy at the School of Hygiene and Tropical Medicine, University of London.

DIANE E. MEIER is Professor in the Department of Geriatrics and Adult Development and also Catherine Gaisman Professor of Medical Ethics, Mount Sinai School of Medicine (New York).

VICKI MICHEL is a bioethics and law consultant who also serves as Adjunct Professor at Loyola Law School, Los Angeles.

FRANKLIN G. MILLER is Special Expert, Intramural Research Program, National Institute of Mental Health, and Bioethicist, Department of Clinical Bioethics, National Institutes of Health.

CLAUDIA MILLS is Associate Professor of Philosophy at the University of Colorado, Boulder.

R. PETER MOGIELNICKI is Professor of Medicine (General Internal Medicine) at Dartmouth Medical School.

THOMAS H. MURRAY is President and Chief Executive Officer of The Hastings Center (Garrison, New York).

LISA H. NEWTON is Professor of Philosophy and Director of the Program in Applied Ethics at Fairfield University (Connecticut).

KAI NIELSEN is Professor Emeritus of Philosophy at the University of Calgary (Alberta, Canada) and Adjunct Professor of Philosophy at Concordia University (Montreal, Quebec).

DAVID ORENTLICHER is Samuel R. Rosen Professor of Law and Codirector of the Center for Law and Health at Indiana University School of Law–Indianapolis.

JULIE GAGE PALMER is Lecturer in Law, University of Chicago Law School.

EDMUND D. PELLEGRINO is John Carroll Professor Emeritus of Medicine at Georgetown University Medical Center and Senior Research Scholar at the Kennedy Institute of Ethics, Georgetown University.

TIA POWELL is Executive Director of the New York State Task Force on Life and the Law.

LAURA M. PURDY is Professor of Philosophy at Wells College (Aurora, New York).

TIMOTHY E. QUILL is Professor of Medicine, Psychiatry, and Medical Humanities at the University of Rochester School of Medicine and Dentistry, and Director of the Palliative Care Program at Strong Health, University of Rochester Medical Center.

JAMES RACHELS was Professor of Philosophy at the University of Alabama at Birmingham.

GERD RICHTER is Professor of Internal Medicine and of Biomedical Ethics at Philipps University (Marburg, Germany).

JOHN A. ROBERTSON holds the Vinson & Elkins Chair of Law at the University of Texas Law School.

GIOVANNA RUBERTO is Professor of Immunology at the University of Pavia (Italy).

JAMES SABIN is Associate Clinical Professor of Psychiatry, Harvard Medical School.

SUSAN SHERWIN is University Research Professor of Philosophy and Women's Studies at Dalhousie University (Fairfax, Nova Scotia).

MARK SIEGLER is Professor of Medicine, the Lindy Bergman Distinguished Service Professor, and Director of the Maclean Center for Clinical Medical Ethics at the University of Chicago.

PETER SINGER is Ira W. DeCamp Professor of Bioethics, Center for Human Values, Princeton University.

BONNIE STEINBOCK is Professor of Philosophy at the University at Albany, State University of New York.

JUDITH JARVIS THOMSON is Professor of Philosophy at the Massachusetts Institute of Technology.

ADRIAN THRASHER is Reader, Molecular Immunology Unit, Institute of Child Health (London, England).

TOM TOMLINSON is Professor in the Department of Philosophy and Director of the Center for Ethics and Humanities in the Life Sciences at Michigan State University.

BONNIE POITRAS TUCKER is Professor Emerita of Law at Arizona State University.

ROBERT WACHBROIT is Research Scholar at the Institute for Philosophy and Public Policy, University of Maryland.

LEROY WALTERS is Joseph P. Kennedy Professor of Christian Ethics, Kennedy Institute of Ethics, and Professor of Philosophy at Georgetown University.

MARY ANNE WARREN is Professor of Philosophy at San Francisco State University.

MARK R. WICCLAIR is Professor of Philosophy and Adjunct Professor of Community Medicine at West Virginia University and is Adjunct Professor of Medicine and Center for Bioethics and Health Law faculty, University of Pittsburgh.

JANE S. ZEMBATY is Professor Emerita of Philosophy at the University of Dayton.